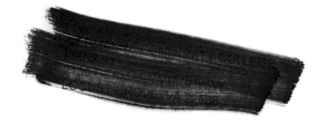

FIFTH EDITION

Counseling *the* Nursing Mother

A Lactation Consultant's Guide

Judith Lauwers, BA, IBCLC, FILCA
Anna Swisher, MBA, IBCLC

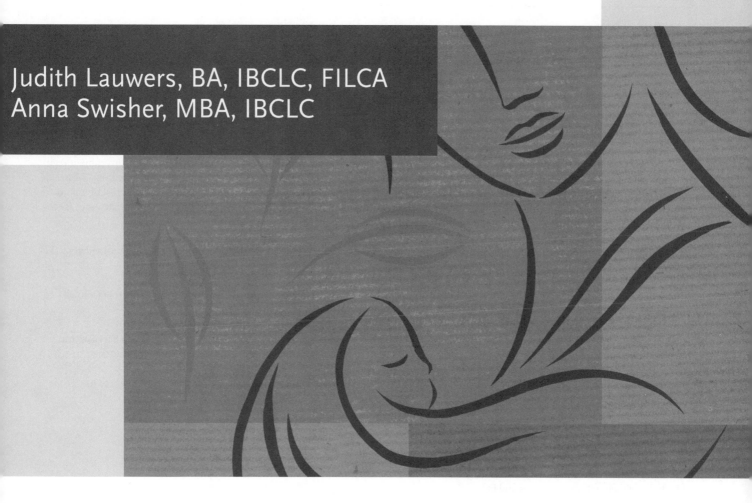

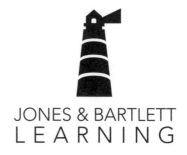

JONES & BARTLETT
LEARNING

World Headquarters
Jones & Bartlett Learning
40 Tall Pine Drive
Sudbury, MA 01776
978-443-5000
info@jblearning.com
www.jblearning.com

Jones & Bartlett Learning Canada
6339 Ormindale Way
Mississauga, Ontario L5V 1J2
Canada

Jones & Bartlett Learning International
Barb House, Barb Mews
London W6 7PA
United Kingdom

Jones & Bartlett Learning books and products are available through most bookstores and online booksellers. To contact Jones & Bartlett Learning directly, call 800-832-0034, fax 978-443-8000, or visit our website, www.jblearning.com.

Substantial discounts on bulk quantities of Jones & Bartlett Learning publications are available to corporations, professional associations, and other qualified organizations. For details and specific discount information, contact the special sales department at Jones & Bartlett Learning via the above contact information or send an email to specialsales@jblearning.com.

Production Credits
Publisher: Kevin Sullivan
Acquisitions Editor: Amy Sibley
Associate Editor: Patricia Donnelly
Editorial Assistant: Rachel Shuster
Senior Production Editor: Carolyn F. Rogers
Production Assistant: Sara Fowles
Marketing Manager: Rebecca Wasley

V.P., Manufacturing and Inventory Control: Therese Connell
Cover Design: Kristin E. Parker
Associate Photo Researcher: Sarah Cebulski
Composition: Publishers' Design and Production Services, Inc.
Cover Image: © Claire Fraser/Imagezoo/age fotostock
Printing and Binding: Courier Westford
Cover Printing: Courier Westford

Library of Congress Cataloging-in-Publication Data
Lauwers, Judith, 1949–
    Counseling the nursing mother : a lactation consultant's guide / Judith Lauwers, Anna Swisher. — 5th ed.
        p. ; cm.
    Includes bibliographical references and index.
    ISBN 978-0-7637-8052-4 (casebound)
    1. Lactation consultants. 2. Breastfeeding. 3. Lactation. 4. Breastfeeding promotion. 5. Mothers—Counseling of.
I. Swisher, Anna. II. Title.
    [DNLM: 1. Breast Feeding. 2. Counseling—methods. 3. Infant Nutritional Physiological Phenomena. 4. Lactation—
physiology. WS 125 L391c 2011]
    RJ216.L354 2011
    649′.33—dc22
                                                                                            2010016445

6048

Printed in the United States of America
15 14 13 12 11   10 9 8 7 6 5 4 3 2

Dedication

We dedicate this edition to two friends and colleagues who were pioneers in the lactation consultant profession and who left us too early.

JoAnne Scott was a La Leche League leader for 31 years before becoming the founding Executive Director of the International Board of Lactation Consultant Examiners in 1985, a position she held until her illness forced her to step down in 2005. When *Counseling the Nursing Mother* was first published, Joanne commented that it was a book she had in her head and planned to write until she found that someone beat her to it! Her vision and persistence steered our profession through a period of exceptional growth from 1985 to 2005. JoAnne Scott passed away in 2006, 1 year after our profession celebrated its 20th anniversary.

Mary Rose Tully took the first IBLCE exam in 1985 and was instrumental in the acceptance of the lactation consultant as a member of the healthcare team. She served in leadership roles in the Human Milk Banking Association of North America, the American Public Health Association, the International Lactation Consultant Association, the U.S. Breastfeeding Committee, and other organizations. In 2006, Mary Rose co-founded the Carolina Global Breastfeeding Institute at the University of North Carolina, where she was also Director of Lactation Services at UNC's hospital and a faculty member in the schools of medicine and nursing. She passed away in 2009 afer a brief illness.

JoAnne and Mary Rose were valued friends and visionary colleagues who are missed by all who were privileged to cross their paths. Both women are remembered for their ready smiles and their passionate commitment to providing excellent care to breastfeeding mothers, infants, and families. It is with immeasurable respect and poignant remembrance that we dedicate this fifth edition of *Counseling the Nursing Mother* to JoAnne Scott and Mary Rose Tully.

Contents

PART **4**
SPECIAL CARE

PART **5**
ROLE OF THE IBCLC

Preface

I can't hear a word you're saying.
Who you are speaks too loudly.

—Ralph Waldo Emerson

We release this fifth edition of *Counseling the Nursing Mother* in the 25th year of the lactation consulting profession, a celebration of all that has been achieved and the promise of the years to come. *Counseling the Nursing Mother* is unique among all other lactation texts in its focus on counseling and communication skills. We hope you will gain an appreciation for the significance of counseling techniques and how your style and approach can enhance your interactions with mothers and thus your effectiveness. Topics are presented within a counseling framework, and practical suggestions are interwoven with evidence-based information throughout the text. We hope the insights shared within these pages will assist you in applying knowledge and research into day-to-day clinical practice with an appreciation for counseling challenges and how to meet them.

The text also serves as a significant tool for teaching interns and others in the healthcare profession. It is ideal as the first text in the journey to becoming an IBCLC, enabling the learner to understand lactation in easy-to-read terminology before advancing to more scientific texts. The extensive glossary and index and the *Key Terms* and *At a Glance* features in each chapter make the text a valuable study guide for the certification exam as well as a quick reference when working with mothers.

The strong features from the fourth edition continue, with the timeless chapter on critical reading of research that explains the process in easy-to-understand descriptions. The text is written from a teaching perspective to help the reader grow professionally in the lactation field, with a focus on reaching out to the current generation of mothers. The comprehensive glossary has been expanded to over 600 terms used in lactation practice—a great study tool for the certification exam!

New features in the fifth edition include:

- mPINC survey and breastfeeding rates
- Joint Commission initiative
- AAP endorsement of the Ten Steps
- Lactation staffing levels
- Knowledge gaps on the healthcare team
- Feminism and breastfeeding
- Electronic breastfeeding support
- Obesity research
- Warnings about induction and elective cesareans
- WHO growth charts
- Biological nurturing and baby-led breastfeeding
- Subclinical mastitis
- Paternal postpartum depression
- Breastfeeding in emergencies
- Same sex partners
- H1N1 influenza
- Insulin resistance and metabloic syndrome
- Bariatric (weight loss) surgery
- Hepatitis B
- HTLV-1
- IBCLC Scope of Practice

Several topics have been expanded, including:

- History of wet nursing and formula manufacturing
- Baby-Friendly Hospital Initiative
- Infant assessment
- Gastroesophageal Reflux (GER)

- Teen mothers
- Cultural competence
- NICU, including needs of fathers
- Late preterm infant
- Autoimmune disorders
- HIV and breastfeeding
- Human milk banking
- Breastfeeding promotion

Part 1 (Chapters 1–6) focuses on the IBCLC in action, beginning in Chapter 1 with a historical perspective of infant feeding and the growth of the lactation profession. Various work settings for IBCLCs are explored in Chapter 2. Chapter 3 presents new material on the sociological perspective of breastfeeding assistance and support. Chapters 4 and 5 focus on empowering mothers and using effective counseling strategies and techniques, elements which set this text apart from others in the lactation field. Chapter 6 addresses practical elements in consultations with mothers and babies, including anticipatory guidance, problem solving, and documentation.

Part 2 (Chapters 7–10) covers the science of lactation. Chapter 7 describes the newest understanding of breast anatomy, growth and development, and variations in structure and function. Chapter 8 provides a basic understanding of nutrients, nutrition in pregnancy and lactation, and how to teach nutrition to mothers. Properties of human milk are studied in Chapter 9, with attention to its lifelong health benefits and a comparison to artificial feeding. Chapter 10 studies safety issues of medications, social toxicants, and environmental contaminants in the mother's milk.

Part 3 (Chapters 11–18) spans across the prenatal to postpartum phase, from the woman's decision to breastfeed through to weaning. Chapter 11 discusses issues involved with decision making, preparing for breastfeeding, and selecting a physician. Hospital practices are explored in Chapter 12, with an emphasis on early breastfeeding, a supportive climate, and comprehensive care plans. Chapter 13 examines newborn assessment, infant behavior and growth, and strategies for infant crying. Practical aspects of breastfeeding are presented in Chapter 14, including positioning, multiples, tandem nursing, and assisting with a feeding. Factors related to the baby's attachment and suckling are discussed in Chapter 15, with practical suggestions for assisting with problems. Chapter 16 presents common occurrences during the early weeks, including the establishment of lactation, leaking, nipple soreness, engorgement, plugged ducts, and mastitis. Chapter 17 relates factors inherent in breastfeeding

beyond the first month, from patterns of growth, infant development, breastfeeding an older baby, and supplementary and complementary feedings, to weaning. Finally, Chapter 18 addresses the consequences of compromised milk production and transfer on the health outcome and growth of the infant.

Part 4 (Chapters 19–25) addresses special care situations and counseling challenges, beginning in Chapter 19 with changes that occur within the family in terms of parenting, sexual adjustments, fertility, and sibling reactions. Lifestyle variations such as low income, single parenting, adolescent mothers, and cultural differences are explored in Chapter 20, as well as dealing with opposition to breastfeeding. Chapter 21 discusses various breastfeeding techniques and devices and their appropriate use. Temporary breastfeeding situations such as jaundice, relactation, induced lactation, and delayed breastfeeding are presented in Chapter 22. Chapter 23 describes the special needs of high-risk infants, with a sensitive approach to counseling a mother whose baby has died. Interruptions in breastfeeding are explored in Chapter 24, with practical suggestions for managing feedings and combining working and breastfeeding. A wide variety of long-term special needs for mothers and babies are presented in Chapter 25, with advice on how to counsel mothers in these situations.

Part 5 (Chapters 26–28) examines the important role of the IBCLC as professional and advocate. Educational preparation and certification are emphasized in Chapter 26, along with standards of practice, promoting your services, educating other healthcare providers, and maturing in the role of IBCLC. Chapter 27 provides a clear and easy-to-understand review of how to read and review research critically, with illustrations provided through mock articles. The text ends with Chapter 28 and the important role of the IBCLC in promoting breastfeeding, policy changes, and creating baby-friendly healthcare.

Lactation consultants, like other professionals, need to embrace change as the amount of new information accelerates. We must be lifelong learners! In *Counseling the Nursing Mother*, we have helped accommodate that need by providing resources for your ongoing learning and research. We recognize the need to teach and mentor a new generation of lactation consultants and other healthcare providers. We urge our readers to accept that challenge and responsibility. This text provides a starting point for that journey.

Judith Lauwers
Anna Swisher

Acknowledgments

A text of this scope is the result of collaboration with scores of colleagues throughout the history of the lactation consultant profession. Our thanks and appreciation go to all who have enriched our understanding of the art and science of breastfeeding and of the lactation consulting profession. Their generosity and selfless sharing of resources and insights for this and previous editions of *Counseling the Nursing Mother* help promote lactation consulting to new generations of professionals. There is always the inadvertent possibility of omitting the name of an important contributor. If any contribution has been omitted, we apologize.

Special thanks for assistance with this fifth edition to Stacie Aguilar, Kathy Amell, Sarah Burton, Janis Cook, Leila Farber, Amy Hanson, Leslie Jackson, Mary Knudson, Phyllis Kombol, Hollye Long, Kori Martin, Amy Noack, Cathy Thomsen, Kat Shealy, and Kim Updegrove. For previous editions, thanks to James Akré, Pam Allyn, Tammy Arbeter, Helen Armstrong, Lois Arnold, Jan Barger, Genevieve Becker, Cheston Berlin, Debi Bocar, Priscilla Bornmann, Sarah Emery Bradley, Sandra Breck, Cathy Carothers, K. Jean Cotterman, Sarah Coulter Danner, Deanna Diodato, Lee Anne Dobos, Patricia Donohue-Carey, Dianne Flury, Karen Foard, Scott Franklin, Teresa Gonzalez, Cynthia Good Mojab, Anh Gordon, Linda Gort-Walton, Thomas Hale, Peter Hartmann, Kay Hoover, Pat Houck, Kathleen Huggins, Sharon Kelly, Connie Kishbaugh, Kyle Knisely, Linda Kutner, Miriam Labbok, Mary Grace Lanese, Cathy Liles, Deanna Lockett, Margot Mann, John Mann, Becky Mannel, Lisa Marasco, Chele Marmet, Patricia Martens, Debbie Matisse, Carol Mavity, Valerie McClain, James McKenna, Valerie Mick, Maureen Minchin, Nancy Mohrbacher, Chris Mulford, Jack Newman, Jeanette Panchula, Denise Parker, Molly Pessl, Carole Peterson, Ellen Petok, Maureen Polivka, Donna Ramsay Geddes, Steve Rein, Jan Riordan, Kathy Romberger, JoAnne Scott, Debbie Shinskie, Barbara Shocker, Gina Solomon, Ruth Solomon, Amy Spangler, Marian Tompson, Mary Toporcer, Mary Rose Tully, Beverly Vaugh, Marsha Walker, Catherine Watson-Genna, Nancy Williams, Karen Wilson, Barbara Wilson-Clay, Michael Woolridge, and Lisa Wyatt.

We owe tremendous thanks to the wonderful team at Jones & Bartlett Learning, including Kevin Sullivan, Tricia Donnelly, and the amazing Carolyn Rogers, Sarah Cebulski, and Rachel Shuster for shepherding us through a very tight production schedule with cheerfulness and grace.

Also, for the first and second editions published by Avery Publishing, we profoundly thank Candace Woessner, coauthor, mentor, and friend. We also acknowledge and thank M. Elaine Adams, Barbara Bernard, Celeste Marx, Gerry McKeegan, and Mary Jo Stine. Other individuals who were key in developing information that provided the basis of the first edition are Ditta and Frank Hoeber, Joanne Hill, Louise Stevens, and numerous volunteers with the Childbirth Education Association of Greater Philadelphia. We also thank the many mothers and babies from whom we have learned so much about the miraculous bonds of breastfeeding and parenting.

Finally, we wish to acknowledge our families for their patience and support throughout the writing and editing process. We thank Judi's husband Dave; sons Mike and Chris; and grandchildren Molly, Juliette, Matthew, and Samantha. We thank Anna's children Travis, Faith, and Kristin; and nieces Lee Anne, Misty, Shannon, and Leila, who have reclaimed breastfeeding as the norm. You ignited and nurtured our passion for babies, mothers, and families.

1

PROMOTION AND SUPPORT

1

Breastfeeding Promotion in the Modern World

The promotion of breastfeeding among caregivers and parents is much more complex than it might seem on the surface. The superiority of human milk over substitutes is well documented and widely acknowledged by the scientific and medical communities and the general population. It is, therefore, not easy to explain why parents choose artificial milk in spite of that knowledge. Many caregivers fail to recommend breastfeeding to their clients or provide questionable advice when complications arise. The factors driving these behaviors are complex. To understand such contradictions requires examining the many issues involved with infant feeding practices. These practices have evolved and will continue to evolve, along with other changes in society. Understanding the dynamics of this evolution, as well as the political and sociological factors involved, is essential to effecting tangible and enduring change that will enhance maternal and infant health.

∼ Key Terms

Baby-Friendly Hospital
   Initiative (BFHI)
Complementary feeding
Exclusive breastfeeding
Global Data Bank on
   Breastfeeding
*Global Strategy for Infant
   and Young Child
   Feeding*
Healthy People 2010
Healthy People 2020
Innocenti Declaration
International Code of
   Marketing of
   Breastmilk Substitutes
Lactation consultant
Malnutrition

Morbidity
Mortality
Osteoporosis
Paradigm shift
*Protecting, Promoting, and
   Supporting Breastfeeding*
Ten Steps to Successful
   Breastfeeding
United Nations Children's
   Fund (UNICEF)
U.S. Department of
   Agriculture
U.S. Surgeon General
Wet nurse
World Health Assembly
World Health
   Organization (WHO)

∼ Infant Feeding Practices Throughout History

Breastfeeding our young is so intrinsic to our existence that it defines humans as a class: mammals. The human infant is one of more than 4200 types of mammals, all of which feed their young with the mother's milk. Human milk historically has been the predominant means of nourishing infants—either the milk of the baby's mother or the milk of another woman (Figure 1.1). Nevertheless, throughout history, some women have made a conscious choice not to breastfeed their children. Women of wealth often chose the use of wet nurses or hand feeding in an effort to stay beautiful, to get pregnant again, or as a status marker. As a result, human milk substitutes have been available for centuries. It has been only in recent history, however, that more infants in the United States and other developed countries have received artificial baby milk

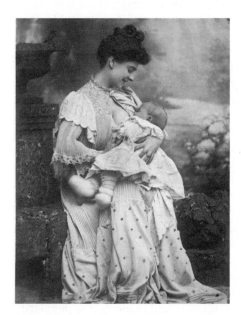

FIGURE 1.1 A mother breastfeeding her baby in the early 1900s.

Source: Printed with permission of breastfeedingart.net.

than have been breastfed. Globally, breastfeeding still predominates as the method for feeding infants.

Wet Nursing

Wet nursing—the act of a woman nursing a baby other than her own—dates back to at least 2500 BC in ancient Egypt. Prior to the advent of mass manufacturing, women who could not produce enough milk or who did not nurse their babies used wet nurses (i.e., other lactating women) to nurse their babies. Obstetrician Pierre Budin, the founder of neonatalogy, kept meticulous records on the wet nurses whom an orphanage used. The wet nurses produced an average of 2230 mL of milk per day, and one even produced 2840 mL (96 oz) (Budin, 1907)! Historically, casual cross-nursing of infants has been practiced in many cultures.

Advent of Infant Formula

During the 18th and 19th centuries, the advent of modern medicine, science, and technology generated great changes in infant feeding. Budin recognized in the late 19th century the link between increased infant mortality and gastroenteritis resulting from contaminated cow's milk. He introduced the concept of well-baby check-ups and educating mothers on maintaining breastfeeding and substituting with sterilized milk if natural nutrition failed (Toubas, 2007). Artificial formula became available in the mid-19th century, primarily to provide nutrition for infants in institutions. By the late 1890s, milk factories provided pasteurized milk and home sterilizers to the public (Wolf, 2001), making it easier for infants to be raised on human milk substitutes. As formula became available in increasing supply, parents turned to it as an acceptable substitute for human milk (Wolf, 2003). When the increase in artificial feeding led to greater numbers of infant deaths, efforts regrettably focused on improving artificial baby milk rather than increasing breastfeeding rates.

A new profession of pediatricians emerged as infant feeding experts to guide mothers in selecting the appropriate food for their babies. As the baby grew, the pediatrician gave the mother a prescription for a formula appropriate to her baby's age. It was soon determined that babies could receive a standard formula irrespective of age. Pediatricians, by then a firmly established profession, then evolved into specialists in well-baby care and preventive medicine. Pediatrics—a profession that sprang from the manufacturing of artificial baby milk—continues to be influenced by the infant formula industry.

Formula feeding continued to increase in popularity in the 20th century, with cow's milk products being promoted as the "modern and civilized" way to nourish infants. As the popularity of formula feeding grew, the attractiveness and accessibility of artificial feeding became associated with higher-class, more highly educated women. Breastfeeding, in turn, became associated with lower social status, and women who chose to breastfeed were given little support or encouragement. The popularity of artificial baby milk eventually trickled down through all social strata until babies throughout the industrialized world were predominantly fed artificial baby milk from a bottle rather than being nurtured at their mothers' breast. Furthermore, Western society began to regard the breast in a sexual context in the 1950s when pornography entered "men's" magazines and infiltrated the media at large (Palmer, 2009). This sexual objectification subverted breasts' biological function to nourish and nurture babies.

Separation of Mothers and Babies

With the Industrial Revolution came greater accessibility of artificial baby milk, providing women of all social strata with new options for feeding their infants. As a consequence, when women gave birth to babies, they were no longer required to invest themselves totally in feeding and raising their babies throughout infancy.

By the time men began returning home at the end of World War II, they found a new landscape in family life. Women, who had entered the workforce in large numbers while men served in the military, found that they enjoyed the freedom and challenge of working outside the home. When men returned from the war, some of these women did not want to return to a life confined to child care at home. Artificial baby milk made it possible for mothers to work or pursue other activities outside the home while still raising a family. Although their female ancestors had been bound by biology to nurture their young, modern women now had a choice and the ability to determine their future. The feeding practices that liberated mothers from their babies were attractive to some women. Thus the prevailing cultural belief in many industrialized societies evolved to one in which the feeding of artificial baby milk became the norm, and breastfeeding the exception.

At the same time, dramatic changes took place in birth practices throughout the industrialized world. By the early part of the 20th century, industrialized medicine had removed much of the danger from the birth process. Prior to that time, women traditionally had given birth at home with female family members and a midwife in attendance, thus enjoying a strong and continuous support system throughout labor and delivery. Breastfeeding was regarded as part of the birth process, with the baby being put to breast as the end stage of labor and birth.

As medical technology advanced, however, childbirth moved from the home to the hospital, compromising both mother's and baby's personal needs and moving control of the birth from the mother to medical staff. Women now gave birth primarily in a sterile hospital setting surrounded by technology, without the support of female relatives that had been standard in the past. Birthing practices separated mothers from their babies, regimented infant care, and interfered with the initiation of breastfeeding (Davis-Floyd & St. John, 1998; Leavitt, 1986). Mothers had limited access to their babies during their critical first week of life, with babies brought out for brief feeding periods on a strict schedule.

Breastfeeding Revisited

Early in the 20th century, some members of the medical community began to question the wisdom of the prevalence of feeding babies artificial baby milk. In 1921, Julius P. Sedgwick advocated for students to spend more time in medical school observing and studying breastfeeding and less time studying artificial feeding and formula making (Sedgwick, 1921). The Brooklyn Pediatric Society, in 1924, addressed inclusion of breastfeeding instruction in postgraduate medical education. Its members concluded that breastfeeding was a matter of medical education and lay instruction (McKay, 1924). The scarcity of lactation education in medical and nursing schools continues to be a challenge in the 21st century (Brodribb et al., 2009; Grossman et al., 2009; Szucs et al., 2009; Philipp et al., 2007).

In 1929, studies identified a correlation between a child's cognitive development and the method of infant feeding. They noted that all of the babies studied with IQs exceeding 130 were breastfed (Hoefer & Hardy, 1929). Around the same time, however, many parents began to rely on childcare books to help them rear their children. These books promoted regimented feeding schedules, stressed the need to trust scientific development in infant feeding, gave poor breastfeeding advice, and robbed women of trusting their own instincts.

By the early 1950s, recognition of the importance of breastfeeding to infant health led to the publication of books for parents. Professional articles on breastfeeding and infant feeding began to appear in medical literature. Mother-to-mother support groups also emerged in the early 1950s. Grassroots efforts by La Leche League and other breastfeeding support organizations actively promoted breastfeeding as the preferred method of infant feeding—messages that continue to resonate today (Figure 1.2).

The 1960s ushered in a feminist movement, in which women sought a lifestyle liberated from male control. Some committed to healthful living. Breastfeeding held little appeal for some of these women, whose lives focused on personal achievement and freedom (Thulier, 2009). Others regarded breastfeeding as the natural and culturally appropriate method of infant feeding. The two opposing viewpoints created a dilemma for women and

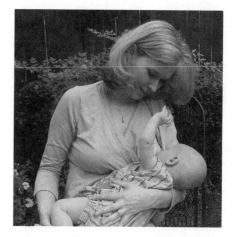

FIGURE 1.2   A modern day mother breastfeeding her baby.
Source: Printed with permission of Anna Swisher.

generated debate about feminist ideals, which continues to this day.

Just as the move to artificial feeding had begun among more educated women and those belonging to higher social classes, so, too, did the movement back to breastfeeding. Enlightened women of the 18th and 19th century had led society to infant feeding practices that would liberate them and enable them to pursue personal challenges. Enlightened women of the 20th century refocused society on reasserting the needs of the family, reestablishing women's autonomy, and protecting the health of infants and children.

Breastfeeding, and in particular exclusive breastfeeding for the first six months of a child's life, ranks among the most effective interventions for improving child survival and health (Chan, 2008). As a society, we have an obligation to establish conditions that facilitate sound child feeding practices. This mandate requires that parents receive objective, consistent, evidence-based information that supports informed, sound feeding choices for their infants. Breastfeeding is the right of both the mother and her child (Kent, 2006).

Breastfeeding Rates

Breastfeeding rates vary significantly throughout the world, and the quality of the data about breastfeeding also varies. Definitions of exclusive breastfeeding vary from one country to another, presenting a challenge when attempting to compile meaningful statistics. Exclusive breastfeeding, as defined by the World Health Organization (WHO), means that breastfeeding babies receive no food or drink other than their mother's milk.

WHO established a Global Data Bank on Breastfeeding in 1982 in an effort to disseminate identical indicators and definitions worldwide that will ensure consistent and comparable results in breastfeeding studies. Now known as the Global Data Bank on Infant and Young Child Feeding (WHO, 2010), the bank pools information mainly from national and regional surveys, and studies dealing specifically with the prevalence and duration of breastfeeding and complementary feeding. The data bank is continually updated as new studies and surveys become available.

Fueled almost entirely by the efforts of the grassroots movement that began in the 1950s, breastfeeding rates reached a peak of 61.9 percent of U.S. mothers by the early 1980s. Rates then began to decline, inspiring the U.S. Surgeon General to convene a work group to study breastfeeding and human lactation in 1984. U.S. breastfeeding rates continued to drop, reaching 51.5 percent in 1990, before rising again to initiation rates of between 65.1 percent (Li et al., 2003) and 69.5 percent in 2001 (Ryan et al., 2002).

Some groups where the prevalence of breastfeeding was lowest have shown the greatest increase in breastfeeding rates since 1989. For example, between 1988 and 1997, rates of breastfeeding among African American women during the postpartum period increased 65 percent. During the same period, rates of African American women breastfeeding at 6 months postpartum grew 81 percent. Breastfeeding rates among women aged 20 years and younger at both periods also increased substantially, as did the rates among women with a grade-school education (*Healthy People 2010*, 2003).

The United States' *Healthy People 2010* target rates were 75 percent initiation, 50 percent at 6 months, and 25 percent at 12 months. Nearly half of U.S. states achieved the national objectives for breastfeeding initiation, although fewer have achieved the objectives for breastfeeding duration and exclusive breastfeeding (Centers for Disease Control and Prevention [CDC], 2008b). A U.S. study found that breastfeeding rates in this country increased from 60 percent in 1994 to 77 percent in 2006. Rates among non-Hispanic black women rose from 36 percent to 65 percent during the same period (McDowell et al., 2008).

The CDC published the Breastfeeding Report Card 2008 to report the extent to which infants are breastfed in each U.S. state. The report indicators, which were derived from the breastfeeding goals outlined in *Healthy People 2010*, show where a state has been successful and where more work is needed (CDC, 2008c). While encouraging trends in breastfeeding rates have emerged in a few countries, global data show that only 38 percent of infants worldwide are exclusively breastfed for 6 months, 56 percent are breastfed with complementary food at 6 to 9 months, and 39 percent continue to breastfeed with complementary foods at 20–23 months. (UNICEF, 2007). *Healthy People 2020*, released in midyear 2010, includes goals for exclusive breastfeeding as well as increases in worksite lactation programs and live births in facilities that provide recommended breastfeeding care (*Healthy People 2020*, 2009).

This underachievement in breastfeeding rates contributes to the unnecessary deaths of more than 1 million children each year—lives that could be saved if mothers and families were adequately encouraged and supported to breastfeed (Chan, 2008). Interventions to promote exclusive breastfeeding are estimated to have the potential to prevent 13 percent of all deaths involving children younger than age 5 years in developing countries and are the single most important preventive intervention against child mortality (Bhandari et al., 2008). When translated into healthcare dollars, cost savings in the United States alone could amount to $13 billion per year, according to a 2010 study (Bartick & Reinold, 2010). The study reported that 911 preventable deaths occur annually in the United States because breastfeeding rates fail to reach global recommendations. Sudden infant death syndrome, necrotizing enterocolitis, and lower respiratory infections in preterm infants accounted for 95 percent of the deaths. Breastfeeding is protective against all three of these illnesses. The researchers assert that most of the annual costs could be saved if breastfeeding initiation and duration rates increase to recommended levels.

Factors That Affect Breastfeeding Rates

Rates of breastfeeding continue to be highest among college-educated women and women aged 35 years and older. In one study, 95.5 percent of the highest-educated mothers initiated breastfeeding, compared to 73.1 percent of the lowest-educated mothers. At 6 months following childbirth, 39.3 percent of highest-educated mothers and 15.2 percent of lowest-educated mothers were still breastfeeding (van Rossem et al., 2009). The lowest rates of breastfeeding occur among women whose infants are at highest risk of poor health and development (those aged 21 years and younger and those with low educational levels). Analysis of data from U.S. National Immunization Surveys shows that children of college graduates are more likely to meet the target breastfeeding rates. By comparison, rates are lowest among children of single mothers, less educated mothers, and participants in the federally funded WIC (Women, Infants, and Child) nutritional program. No groups met the target for exclusive breastfeeding (Forste & Hoffmann, 2008).

In a Canadian study, women who attended or completed college were more likely to breastfeed. A higher level of education was also associated with longer duration of breastfeeding (Simard et al., 2005). A Taipei study revealed significant regional variations in the rate of breastfeeding within different parts of the country (Chien et al., 2005). Another study reported significant improvements in breastfeeding initiation and exclusivity following efforts to change behavior on a large-scale community level in Africa and Latin America (Quinn et al., 2005). It is suggested that interventions in hospitals and the community are needed to increase exclusivity (Haiek et al., 2007).

~ Breastfeeding as an Infant Health Issue

Numerous studies illustrate global recognition of the impact of breastfeeding on infant morbidity and mortality. The medical community acknowledges that breastfeeding is healthiest for infants. Human milk is, in fact, regarded as a baby's first immunization, as babies are born "autoimmune deficient" (Labbok et al., 2004). Human milk's unique constitution fosters the infant's health and growth and makes it easily digested and efficiently used by the body.

The multitude of health benefits for the baby, discussed in depth in Chapter 9, is a clear testimony to the significance of human milk in infant feeding. The longer an infant breastfeeds, the greater protection he or she receives (Chen, 2004; Habicht, 1986). Antibodies in the mother's milk are highly targeted against infectious agents in the mother's environment, those to which the infant is likely to be exposed shortly after birth (Brandtzaeg, 2007). As the baby grows, this child develops his or her own active immunity as the child's own body begins to produce antibodies. Human milk contains a variety of anti-

bodies capable of enhancing infant antibody response (Van de Perre, 2003).

Human milk protects the infant from infectious diseases and reduces the chance of infections. Therefore, infants who are not breastfed are at increased risk of many diseases and infections (see Table 1.1). In fact, having been breastfed continues to protect the child long into adulthood. Not having been breastfed, therefore, places a person at increased risk for an array of childhood and adult anomalies (see Table 1.2). These protections are discussed in detail in various chapters throughout this book.

The mechanics involved in breastfeeding promote optimal development of the oral cavity, thus lowering the incidence of malocclusion (Labbok & Hendershot, 1987). A breastfed child also develops a proper swallowing pattern that extends into adulthood. Both of these outcomes may reduce the risk of obstructive sleep apnea in adulthood (Palmer, 2004). With the greatest increment of craniofacial development occurring within the first four years of life (Shepard et al., 1991), the avoidance of bottles and artificial nipples during infancy can have far-reaching health consequences.

Breastfed children may have different early relationships with their mothers as well. Breastfeeding is a physical embodiment of the mother–baby relationship that continues long after birth. The bonding that accompa-

TABLE 1.1 Infant Health Risks from Not Being Breastfed

Health Risk	References
Necrotizing enterocolitis	Henderson et al., 2009; Chauhan et al., 2008; Ip et al., 2007; Buescher, 2004, 1994; McGuire, 2003; Caplan, 1993; Dugdale, 1991; Lucas, 1990
Nosocomial (hospital-acquired) sepsis	Meinzen-Derr et al., 2004; Schanler et al., 1999; El-Mohandes et al., 1997
Otitis media (or middle ear infection)	Ip et al., 2007; Turck & Comité de Nutrition de la Société Française de Pédiatrie, 2005; Hanson et al., 2002; Scariati et al., 1997; Dewey et al., 1995; Aniansson et al., 1994; Duncan et al., 1993
Respiratory infections and asthma	Ogbuanu et al., 2009; Mihrshani et al., 2008; Ip et al., 2007; Brandtzaeg, 2007; Turck & Comité de Nutrition de la Société Française de Pédiatrie, 2005; Oddy & Glenn, 2003b; Bulkow et al., 2002; Levine et al., 1999
Digestive infections, including diarrhea	Newburg et al., 2004; Mihrshahi et al., 2008; Newburg, 2009; Ip et al., 2007; Coppa, 2006; Turck & Comité de Nutrition de la Société Française de Pédiatrie, 2005; Van Veen et al., 2004; Vieira et al., 2003; Tellez et al., 2003; Escuder et al., 2003; Mahmud et al., 2001; Kelly & Coutts, 2000; Orrhage & Nord, 1999; Clemens et al., 1997
Bacterial infections	Kohler et al., 2002; Fernandes et al., 2001; Wold & Adlerhath et al., 2000
Allergies	Mihrshahi et al., 2008; Bener et al., 2007; Monterrosa et al., 2008; Turck & Comité de Nutrition de la Société Française de Pédiatrie, 2005; Newburg et al., 2004; Bachrach et al., 2003; Tellez et al., 2003; Van Odijk et al., 2003; Silfverdal et al., 2002
Urinary tract infections	Hanson, 2004; Marild et al., 2004
Rotavirus	Gianino, 2002; Mastretta et al., 2002
Protracted oxidative stress in preterm infants	Ledo et al., 2009
Sudden infant death syndrome	Ip et al., 2007

TABLE 1.2   Childhood and Adult Health Risks from Not Being Breastfed

Health Risk	References
Lower cognitive abilities	Rees & Sabia, 2009; Kramer et al., 2008; Horta et al., 2007; Elwood et al., 2005; Gomez-Sanchiz et al., 2004; Smith et al., 2003; Rao et al., 2002; Anderson et al., 1999; Horwood & Fergusson, 1998; Lucas et al., 1992
Meningitis	Hylander et al., 1998
Juvenile arthritis	Mason et al., 1995
Childhood cancers	Smulevich et al., 1999
Leukemia and lymphoma	Perrilat, 2002; Bener et al., 2001; Shu et al., 1999
Hodgkin's disease	Davis, 1998
Neuroblastoma	Daniels, 2002
Type 1 diabetes	Ip et al., 2007; Young et al., 2002; Monetini, 2001; Kimpimaki et al., 2001
Type 2 diabetes	Ip et al., 2007; Horta et al., 2007; Owen et al., 2006
Inflammatory bowel disease such as Crohn's disease and ulcerative colitis	Thompson et al., 2000; Corrao, 1998
Multiple sclerosis	Tarrats et al., 2002; Pisacane et al., 1994
Celiac disease	Ivarsson et al., 2002
Hypertension	Singhal et al., 2001
High cholesterol and heart disease	Owen et al., 2002, 2008; Singhal et al., 2004; Ravelli et al., 2000; Fall et al., 1992
Obesity	Butte, 2009; Aydin et al., 2006, 2008; Griffiths et al., 2008; Rudnicka et al., 2007; Turck & Comité de Nutrition de la Société Française de Pédiatrie, 2005; Owen et al., 2005; Martin, 2004; Grummer-Strawn et al., 2004; Toschke et al., 2002; Binns et al., 2003
Bed-wetting during childhood	Barone et al., 2006

nies breastfeeding fosters a special closeness and forms a deep and lasting attachment between mother and child. The early sensory stimulation from skin-to-skin contact that takes place during breastfeeding helps develop the baby's perceptual and response mechanisms. It also aids respiration by stimulating blood flow, which may partly explain the reduced incidence of respiratory ailments in breastfed babies.

A breastfeeding mother is able to respond quickly to her baby's hunger cries without the delay imposed by the need to prepare and heat a bottle. This immediate response to the baby's needs instills a sense of security and trust that may help the child accept the demands of socialization later in life.

In the United States, one-fourth of all child abuse and neglect victims are younger than one year of age (CDC, "Child Maltreatment," n.d.). Most infant deaths involve very young infants, and most occur in ethnic groups with the lowest breastfeeding rates (CDC & Bernard, n.d.). With more than 60 percent of substantial maltreatment perpetrated by the mother, it is significant that breastfeeding may help to protect against child maltreatment, particularly child neglect. In a 15-year cohort Australian study, nonbreastfed infants had a 2.6 greater risk of neglect than infants breastfed for 4 months or more (Strat-

hearn et al., 2009). The researchers concluded that "the most basic etiologic factor underlying child neglect may be an impaired ability to form interpersonal relationships" and that breastfeeding "may be an important means of 'training' a new mother in how to form a secure interpersonal relationship with her new infant."

~ Breastfeeding as a Women's Health Issue

In many ways, breastfeeding is as much a women's health issue as it is an infant feeding issue. A study conducted in Taiwan reported that mothers who breastfed for 6 months or longer demonstrated a better health-related quality of life. In addition, their physical functioning, general health perception, and mental health scores were higher than those of mothers who did not breastfeed. Family income, the mother's parity, and the child's health status were also associated with the mother's quality of life (Chen et al., 2007).

Women's health traditionally has received little attention in the U.S. healthcare agenda. Part of the challenge in promoting breastfeeding in today's climate stems from this persistent failure in the healthcare system. The healthcare arena needs to view breastfeeding as part of women's health and treat it as such. Whatever healthcare providers can do to help empower the women in their care will benefit women and their families for years to come.

Both giving birth and breastfeeding are empowerment issues for women (Davis-Floyd & St. John, 1998; Van Esterik, 1994). Women who gain more control over their birth and breastfeeding experiences achieve a greater sense of power, self-esteem, and ego (Locklin & Naber, 1993). Medical technology often strips a woman of this power by placing external controls on pregnancy, birth, and breastfeeding—the three life functions that belong solely to women.

Breastfeeding is a part of the entire childbearing cycle. The female body is designed to progress from pregnancy to birth and then on to breastfeeding. Interrupting this cycle by not breastfeeding interrupts the normal continuum. Put simply, breastfeeding is the normal transition from intrauterine maternal-based nutrition to extrauterine maternal-based nutrition. For this reason, anthropologist Ashley Montagu suggested that gestation is actually an 18-month process, with a baby spending 9 months in utero and 9 months nurtured at the breast (Montagu, 1986).

For breastfeeding to be a real choice for all women, society needs to become more woman- and child-friendly (Hausman, 2008; Smith, 2008; Heller, 1997). Breastfeeding and mothering are only two strands in the weaving of women's lives. To ignore the rest of the fabric is to fail to see how all the strands are connected. Lactation consultants and other caregivers help breastfeeding women by considering the total fabric. As Van Esterik (1994) states, "breastfeeding is a holistic act and is intimately connected to all domains of life: sexuality, eating, emotion, appearance, sleeping, and parental relationships." It is an integral part of the whole fabric of women's lives.

Physical and Emotional Effects of Breastfeeding on Women

Breastfeeding has a significant impact on women's health. For example, oxytocin released during breastfeeding contracts the uterus and helps stop bleeding after delivery. It is, therefore, important that breastfeeding begin immediately after birth and that it continue frequently. Oxytocin, known as the "mothering" hormone, may also pass to the infant through breastmilk (Lawrence & Lawrence, 2005). Prolactin and oxytocin play a role in maternal feelings of well-being, relaxation, and mothering. A positive breastfeeding experience can contribute to a woman feeling good about herself, which raises her self-esteem and empowers her as a woman.

Breastfeeding may also have a significant positive impact on both systolic and diastolic blood pressures of mothers. One study measured maternal blood pressure before, during, and after a breastfeed, initially at 2 days

postpartum and then during the following 25-week breastfeeding period. Blood pressure fell significantly in response to breastfeeding in both time periods (Jonas et al., 2008).

Breastfeeding women are energy efficient (Illingworth et al., 1986) and can produce milk even when they are subjected to limited caloric intake. The increased caloric demand that accompanies breastfeeding allows the mother to supplement her usual eating pattern—provided that it is nutritionally sound—and still control her weight and return to her prepregnancy size more quickly. As discussed in Chapter 19, exclusive breastfeeding is 98 percent effective in delaying pregnancy naturally without the use of artificial contraceptives for the first 4 to 6 months postpartum.

The risk of premenopausal breast cancer is reduced with breastfeeding, and the longer a woman breastfeeds, the greater the protection (Ip et al., 2007; Turck & Comité de Nutrition de la Société Française de Pédiatrie, 2005; Becher et al., 2003; Beral et al., 2002; Zheng et al., 2000). The risk of ovarian cancer is also decreased with breastfeeding (Ip et al., 2007; Turck & Comité de Nutrition de la Société Française de Pédiatrie, 2005; Tung et al., 2003; Yen et al., 2003; Rosenblatt & Thomas, 1993).

Continued research into the correlation between lactation and osteoporosis has provided reassurance to breastfeeding women that the bone loss experienced as a result of breastfeeding is regenerated after weaning and that lactation provides protection against osteoporosis (Turck & Comité de Nutrition de la Société Française de Pédiatrie, 2005; Paton et al., 2003; Carranza-Lira & Mera Paz, 2002). Exclusive breastfeeding for 6 months could also eliminate weight retention by 6 months postpartum in many women (Baker et al., 2008). The researchers who drew this conclusion cited problems with previous research that failed to limit the studies to the recommended exclusive breastfeeding for 6 months, which produced inconsistent findings and called into question the correlation between breastfeeding and weight loss.

Women in developed countries continue to get fatter; obesity, in turn, increases the risk of diabetes. Women who have gestational diabetes are at higher risk of converting to type 2 diabetes (Bentley-Lewis et al., 2008). Women who develop gestational diabetes and who do not subsequently breastfeed their babies are at a higher risk for this conversion. Research has also found that the risks for hypertension (and strokes), hyperlipidemia (high cholesterol), and cardiovascular disease are higher among women who do not breastfeed (Stuebe & Schwarz, 2010).

∿ Cultural Influences on Infant Feeding

People generally acknowledge that breastfeeding is best for babies. Even the infant formula industry makes that declaration sometimes in its advertising. However, the messages that permeate the media in the United States and other developed countries do little to support breastfeeding. Despite a renewed interest in breastfeeding, bottle feeding is still recognized as the cultural norm. Adolescent girls and boys, as well as many adults, are generally uncomfortable with the topic or embarrassed at seeing a baby breastfed. At the same time, it is common to see babies and toddlers of all ages in public with feeding bottles or pacifiers. Shelves in grocery stores, toy stores, and discount stores abound with bottle feeding devices and infant formula. News media, Internet sites, children's books, parenting magazines, and medical journals carry scores of bottle feeding messages. Many U.S. states have found it necessary to pass legislation safeguarding the right of women to breastfeed in public or making it illegal to interfere with them when they do so.

A paradigm shift in the way society views infant feeding must accompany breastfeeding promotion efforts. For several decades, promotion efforts have focused defensively on the benefits of breastfeeding, enumerating all the reasons why mothers should breastfeed their babies. Nevertheless, for healthful practices such as breastfeeding to be promoted more effectively, public awareness must shift to the hazards of *not* breastfeeding and the reasons mothers should not feed their babies artificial baby milk. The U.S. Ad Council adopted this approach in a 2004 breastfeeding awareness campaign (Merewood & Heinig, 2004).

Efforts to educate the American public about the benefits of breastfeeding date back to the late 19th century. Physicians "constantly decried the 'children with weak and diseased constitutions belonging to that generally wretched class called bottle fed. . . .' Today's medical community recognizes what their predecessors knew a century ago—that the American propensity to shun human milk is a public health problem and should be exposed as such" (Wolf, 2003).

This shift in approach is illustrated with results of a classic study by Lucas et al. (1992), who found that preterm infants receiving human milk have higher IQ levels than those receiving infant formula. These study results need to be considered within the context that the biological norm is for infants to receive human milk. Therefore, it is not the case that breastfed infants have higher IQs. Rather, they have normal IQs, and artificially fed infants have lower than normal IQs because they failed to receive their mothers' milk. Likewise, all the health outcomes for breastfed infants and mothers enumerated in this chapter are not simply benefits of breastfeeding: They are indisputable evidence of the risk of not breastfeeding. When the public makes this subtle shift in attitude, perceiving the negative consequences of feeding their babies artificial baby milk, parents will be more likely to make informed and healthy choices.

⌇ Breastfeeding as an Economic Issue

The economic costs of not breastfeeding are staggering. A March 2001 analysis from the U.S. Department of Agriculture (USDA) stated that a minimum of $3.6 billion would be saved if breastfeeding were increased from the 2001 levels of 64 percent while mother and child are in the hospital following childbirth and 29 percent until the child reaches 6 months of age to 75 percent and 50 percent, respectively, the levels recommended by the U.S. Surgeon General and *Healthy People 2010*. The analysis calculated cost savings from treating only three childhood illnesses: otitis media, gastroenteritis, and necrotizing enterocolitis (Weimer, 2001). U.S. taxpayers would save $112 million in Medicaid costs and $478 million in government subsidy costs if WIC infants were breastfed for as little as 3 months. (WIC is a supplemental food program for low-income women, infants, and children.) A 50 percent reduction in pharmacy costs was also projected from increasing the breastfeeding rate (Montgomery & Splett, 1997).

⌇ International Breastfeeding Promotion Initiatives

Worldwide, the practice of substituting artificial baby milk for human milk, either partially or fully, has resulted in greater incidents of malnutrition, infections, diarrheal diseases, impaired growth, and even infant deaths. By the mid-1970s, health experts realized a need for a global effort to stem the tide of these negative outcomes for children. Beginning in 1981, several major global initiatives began to promote breastfeeding. They are introduced here and discussed further in Chapter 28.

International Code of Marketing of Breastmilk Substitutes

A 1978 U.S. Senate hearing led by Senator Edward Kennedy provided the impetus for global action to monitor corporate practices in the marketing of infant formula. In 1981, the World Health Assembly created the International Code of Marketing of Breastmilk Substitutes, which was subsequently affirmed by all member states of the World Health Organization. The International Code still awaits enactment into legislation or enforceable regulations at the national level in many countries. The United States delayed signing onto the International Code for many years because of aggressive lobbying by the infant formula industry; indeed, this country was the last nation to sign the agreement.

Table 1.3 highlights the main points of the International Code, which calls for regulating the marketing and distribution of products represented to be suitable as a partial or total replacement for human milk. Any product that is promoted for use during the exclusive breastfeeding period for children younger than age 6 months will have the effect of replacing human milk in the child's intake. The intent of the International Code is to regulate the advertising and promotional techniques used to sell infant formula and other human milk substitutes. It covers all foods marketed or otherwise represented to replace human milk, as well as feeding bottles and artificial nipples (WHO, 2008).

Because of delays in national implementation of the International Code, and continued disregard of its provisions by manufacturers and distributors, artificial feeding continued to increase and breastfeeding rates continued to decline throughout the 1980s. In an effort to improve breastfeeding rates throughout the world, UNICEF and WHO issued a 1989 joint statement entitled *Protecting, Promoting, and Supporting Breastfeeding*. The statement led to the formation of the Ten Steps to Successful Breastfeeding (Figure 1.3) as a guide to promote sound breastfeeding practices and policies worldwide (WHO, 1989). In 1990, WHO and UNICEF reaffirmed their commitment to breastfeeding with the *Innocenti Declaration on the Protection, Promotion and Support of Breastfeeding*. This declaration called for the establishment of national breastfeeding coordinators in all countries, universal use of the Ten Steps to Successful Breastfeeding by maternity services, implementation of the International Code, and legal protections for employed breastfeeding women.

TABLE 1.3   The International Code of Marketing of Breastmilk Substitutes

Code Provision	Implications to Consider
Under the scope of the Code, items marketed or otherwise represented to be suitable as human milk substitutes can include foods and beverages such as: • Infant formula • Other milk products • Cereals • Vegetable, fruit, and other puréed preparations • Juices and baby teas • Follow-on milks • Bottled water	Whether or not a product is considered to be within this definition will depend on how it is promoted for infants. Any products that are marketed or represented as suitable substitutes to human milk will fall into this category. Since babies should receive *only* human milk for the first six months, any other food or drink promoted for use during this time will be a human milk substitute.
Regarding advertising and information, the Code recommends that: • Advertising of human milk substitutes, bottles, and teats to the public not be permitted • Educational materials explain the benefits of breastfeeding, the health hazards associated with bottle feeding, the costs of using infant formula, and the difficulty of reversing the decision not to breastfeed • Product labels clearly state the superiority of breastfeeding, the need for the advice of a healthcare worker, and a warning about health hazards; and they show no pictures of babies, or other pictures or text idealizing the use of infant formula	Health workers such as lactation consultants and breastfeeding counselors need to press their legislators for measures that will implement the Code in full. This would protect mothers from advertising in parent magazines and on television. It would also prevent direct company contact with mothers through hotlines, Internet sites, mailings, home-delivered supplies of formula, and baby clubs.
Regarding samples and supplies, the Code recommends that: • No free samples be given to pregnant women, mothers, or their families • No free or low-cost supplies of human milk substitutes be given to maternity wards, hospitals, or any other part of the healthcare system	Under the Code, free or low-cost supplies can be distributed only outside of the healthcare system and must be continued for as long as the infant needs them. In the United States, this is usually for one year. Elsewhere, it is for at least six months. The healthcare system encompasses healthcare workers, including lactation consultants *and* breastfeeding counselors.
Regarding healthcare facilities and healthcare workers, the Code recommends that: • There be no product displays, posters, or distribution of promotional materials • No gifts or samples be given to healthcare workers • Product information for health professionals be limited to what is factual and scientific	This provision also covers bottles that are provided and shown in advertisements by breast pump companies that are clearly feeding bottles, even when no teats are shown. Pens and pads of paper with the name of a formula company are examples of gifts.

Every facility providing maternity services and care for newborn infants should:

1. Have a written breastfeeding policy that is routinely communicated to all healthcare staff.
2. Train all healthcare staff in skills necessary to implement this policy.
3. Inform all pregnant women about the benefits and management of breastfeeding.
4. Help mothers initiate breastfeeding within a half hour of birth.
5. Show mothers how to breastfeed and how to maintain lactation even if they should be separated from their infants.
6. Give newborn infants no food or drink other than breastmilk unless medically indicated.
7. Practice rooming in—allow mothers and infants to remain together 24 hours a day.
8. Encourage breastfeeding in response to feeding cues.
9. Give no artificial teats or pacifiers (also called dummies or soothers) to breastfeeding infants.
10. Foster the establishment of breastfeeding support groups and refer mothers to them on discharge from the hospital or clinic.

FIGURE 1.3   Ten Steps to Successful Breastfeeding.

Source: World Health Organization (WHO). *Protecting, Promoting, and Supporting Breastfeeding: A Joint WHO/UNICEF Statement.* Geneva: WHO; 1989.

Baby-Friendly Hospital Initiative

The Baby-Friendly Hospital Initiative (BFHI) was launched in 1991 by UNICEF and WHO as an effort to ensure that all maternity services, whether free-standing or residing in a hospital, become centers of breastfeeding support. A maternity facility can be designated "Baby-Friendly" when it does not accept free or low-cost breastmilk substitutes, feeding bottles, or teats, and has implemented the Ten Steps to Successful Breastfeeding. The process is controlled by national breastfeeding authorities, using global criteria that can be applied to maternity care in every country. The internationally defined term "Baby-Friendly" may be used only by maternity services that satisfy the global criteria for the BFHI.

A Baby-Friendly designation means that a facility meets high global standards and has at least 75 percent of mothers exclusively breastfeeding at discharge. The global process for receiving Baby-Friendly recognition involves an internal self-assessment, an external assessment by outside evaluators, and a presentation of the findings by UNICEF. The process may vary from one country to another, as government officials make adaptations that will complement their country's standards. See Chapter 28 for further discussion of the implementation of the BFHI program.

Health facilities worldwide are being designated as "Baby-Friendly," with the initiative being adopted more slowly in some countries than in others. Since the BFHI began, more than 15,000 facilities in 156 countries have been officially designated as Baby-Friendly (UNICEF, 2009). In 2005, 10,441 hospitals and maternities were designated as Baby-Friendly hospitals in the WHO Western Region alone, with the charge being led by the Philippines, Myanmar, China, and Mongolia (WHO, 2007). Globally, fewer than 2 percent of Baby-Friendly facilities are located in developed countries such as the United States, Canada, and Australia. By 2009, there were only 79 Baby-Friendly facilities in the United States (BFHIUSA, 2009).

Research overwhelmingly points to the Baby-Friendly initiative as increasing breastfeeding rates, reducing complications, and improving mothers' healthcare experiences, as presented in Chapter 28. In addition to increasing the rate of in-hospital exclusive breastfeeding, BFHI-advocated practices have a positive effect on mothers' planned duration of breastfeeding, mothers' and babies' health, and mothers' breastfeeding knowledge (Abolyan, 2006; Gau, 2004). The impact of several risk factors on exclusive breastfeeding was significantly reduced after adapting the BFHI approach to the neonatal intensive care unit (NICU) setting (Dall'Oglio et al., 2007).

After 49 of Cuba's 56 hospitals and maternity facilities became Baby-Friendly, exclusive breastfeeding rates at 4 months rose from 25 percent in 1990 to 72 percent in 1996. Likewise, thanks to the more than 6000 Baby-Friendly hospitals in China, exclusive breastfeeding rose from 29 percent in 1992 to 68 percent in 1994 in rural areas of that country and from 10 percent to 48 percent in urban areas (UNICEF, 2009).

Several countries have reported increased breastfeeding rates when any of the Ten Steps were used. They include Australia (Oddy, 2003b), Brazil (de Oliveira et al., 2003; Bicalho-Mancini & Velasquez-Melendez, 2004), Germany (Dulon, 2003), Italy (Banderali, 2003; Cattaneo, 2001), Saudi Arabia (Fida, 2003), Switzerland (Merten, 2004), Taiwan (Gau, 2004), and the United States (Merewood, 2003; Philipp, 2003, 2001).

The Promotion of Breastfeeding Intervention Trial (PROBIT) studied more than 17,000 births in 31 maternity facilities in the Republic of Belarus that employed a breastfeeding promotion intervention based on the Baby-Friendly Hospital Initiative. Infants from the intervention sites were significantly more likely than control infants to be breastfed to any degree at 12 months, and were more likely to be exclusively breastfed at 3 and 6 months. They also had a significant reduction in the risk of gastrointestinal tract infections and atopic eczema in the first year of life (Kramer et al., 2009).

One study conducted in the United Kingdom suggests that practices in Baby-Friendly maternity units are likely to increase breastfeeding initiation but not duration (Bartington et al., 2006). Another study found that babies born in Baby-Friendly facilities are more likely to be breastfed for a longer time, particularly if the hospital shows high compliance with UNICEF guidelines. The researchers acknowledge that breastfeeding rates have improved in non-Baby-Friendly facilities as well, perhaps due to increased public awareness of the benefits of breastfeeding. Mothers who intended to breastfeed longer may have chosen to give birth in a Baby-Friendly hospital, which would have an indirect influence on duration rates (Merten et al., 2005)

A general increase in breastfeeding initiation in Switzerland since 1994 may be a consequence of the increasing number of Baby-Friendly health facilities there. In that country, Baby-Friendly hospitals actively use their certification by UNICEF as a promotional asset. As a result, the differences in breastfeeding duration might be attributable to the fact that mothers who intend to breastfeed longer deliberately choose to give birth in a Baby-Friendly hospital and would be more willing to comply with the recommendations. The fact that breastfeeding rates have generally improved even in non-Baby-Friendly health facilities may be indirectly influenced by the BFHI; its publicity and training programs for health professionals have raised public awareness of the benefits of breastfeeding, and the number of professional lactation counselors has increased continuously (Merten et al., 2005).

Global Strategy for Infant and Young Child Feeding

In 2003, in a bid to further strengthen world attention on infant feeding practices, WHO and UNICEF collaborated to create the *Global Strategy for Infant and Young Child Feeding* (WHO, 2003). This document builds on the 1981 International Code of Marketing of Breastmilk Substitutes; the 1990 *Innocenti Declaration on the Protection, Promotion and Support of Breastfeeding;* and the 1991 Baby-Friendly Hospital Initiative. It places those initiatives in the overall context of national policies, programs on nutrition and child health, and a number of other declarations and conventions. The *Global Strategy* addresses appropriate, evidence-based feeding practices for infants and young children that are essential for attaining and maintaining proper nutrition and health.

The *Global Strategy* identifies essential interventions to ensure that children develop to their full potential, free from the adverse consequences of compromised nutritional status and preventable illness. The initiative charges governments, international organizations, and other concerned parties with ensuring that their collective action contributes to the attainment of these goals. Major components of the *Global Strategy* include the following measures:

- Development of comprehensive national policies on infant and young child feeding
- Use of an evidence-based, integrated, comprehensive approach
- Consideration of the physical, social, economic, and cultural environment
- Healthcare support of exclusive breastfeeding for 6 months
- Supportive work environments to increase exclusive breastfeeding rates
- Support of breastfeeding with complementary foods for up to 2 years and beyond
- Provision of adequate, timely, safe complementary foods
- Guidance to families in exceptionally difficult circumstances
- Legislation and regulations to ensure adherence to the International Code of Marketing of Breastmilk Substitutes and subsequent World Health Assembly resolutions

Country-Specific Breastfeeding Initiatives

Several country-specific initiatives are also in place to promote and protect breastfeeding. In the United States, the CDC collects data through the National Immunization Registry, provides significant funding for breastfeeding projects, and has published the *CDC Guide to Breastfeeding Interventions* with evidence-based strategies for supporting mothers (CDC, 2009). The U.S. Department of Health and Human Services' Maternal and Child Health Bureau published *The Business Case for Breastfeeding*, a national breastfeeding resource kit and training initiative to improve worksite support for breastfeeding (Health Resources and Services Administration [HRSA], 2008). The *Health and Human Services Blueprint for Action on Breastfeeding*, published by the Office of the Surgeon General, provides evidence-based strategies for workplaces, families, and healthcare providers to support new mothers (USDHHS, 2000). A European blueprint followed in 2004 (European Commission, 2004). Similar initiatives are taking place in other countries throughout the world.

U.S. mPINC Survey

In 2007, the CDC collaborated with Battelle Centers for Public Health Research and Evaluation to conduct the Maternity Practices in Infant Nutrition and Care (mPINC) survey. The survey measured breastfeeding-related maternity care practices at all intrapartum care facilities across the United States and compared the extent to which such practices vary by state. Thus the state mPINC score represented the extent to which each state's birth facilities provided maternity care that supports breastfeeding. The survey, which was sent to all U.S. hospitals and birth centers with registered maternity beds, obtained data from 82 percent of these facilities. Results from the survey indicate that birth facilities in most states are not providing maternity care that is fully supportive of breastfeeding. The CDC plans to repeat the survey to assess changes over time (CDC, 2008a).

The Joint Commission Initiative

In 2009, a U.S. initiative occurred that shows promise for improving services to breastfeeding mothers and babies. The Joint Commission (2009) launched a new perinatal care measure set, including a requirement for hospitals to report the rate of exclusive breastfeeding among mothers who intend to breastfeed. The Joint Commission accredits U.S. hospitals and, therefore, is very instrumental in improving the quality of care patients receive. Requiring the reporting of breastfeeding rates will encourage maternity hospitals to institute policies that improve rates, and hence the hospital's support of breastfeeding families.

American Academy of Pediatrics' Endorsement of the Ten Steps

Another landmark event was the American Academy of Pediatrics' endorsement of the Ten Steps to Successful Breastfeeding (Tayloe, 2009). Because of their stance on pacifier use relative to reducing the incidence of Sudden Infant Death Syndrome, the AAP did not support a categorical ban on pacifiers. Nevertheless, the AAP voiced strong support for the remaining tenets of the Ten Steps, thus strengthening efforts within the U.S. healthcare system to institute practices that support breastfeeding.

U.S. Government Initiatives

The Patient Protection and Affordable Care Act of 2010 requires employers to provide a reasonable break time and a place for breastfeeding mothers to express milk for one year after their child's birth (U.S. Congress, 2010). In addition, the White House Task Force on Childhood Obesity, with input from 12 federal agencies and thousands of parents, included support for breastfeeding in their action plan to solve the problem of childhood obesity in the United States (Barnes, 2010). Championed by First Lady Michelle Obama, the task force agenda included working in strong partnership with states, local communities, and the private sector to accomplish their goals. Four recommendations were made regarding breastfeeding:

- Hospitals and healthcare providers should use maternity care practices that empower new mothers to breastfeed, such as the Baby-Friendly hospital standards.

- Healthcare providers and insurance companies should provide information to pregnant women and new mothers on breastfeeding, including the availability of educational classes, and connect pregnant women and new mothers to breastfeeding support programs to help them make an informed infant feeding decision.

- Local health departments and community-based organizations, working with healthcare providers, insurance companies, and others should develop peer support programs that empower pregnant women and mothers to get the help and support they need from other mothers who have breastfed.

- Early childhood settings should support breastfeeding.

∼ Current Breastfeeding Recommendations

The ultimate goal of global promotion, protection, and support of breastfeeding is breastfeeding-friendly health care. Such a climate will empower and enable women to breastfeed exclusively for the first six months following childbirth and will create circumstances that enable mothers to continue to breastfeed for two years or longer with complementary foods. Exclusive breastfeeding means that breastfeeding babies receive no drinks or foods other than their mothers' milk, with the exception of vitamin and mineral drops or medicines. For exclusive breastfeeding to go easily, infants should receive no pacifiers or artificial teats (nipples). The mother (or caregiver providing expressed milk) feeds the baby in response to hunger cues, and no limits are placed on frequency or length of feedings. When they are exclusively breastfed, most infants receive at least 8 to 12 breastfeeds in 24 hours, including night feedings.

In light of what is known about the numerous health benefits of human milk and lactation, the American Academy of Pediatrics (2005) recommends that all mothers breastfeed exclusively for 6 months and continue breastfeeding with appropriate complementary food through 12 months and beyond. Further, it asserts that "there is no upper limit to the duration of breastfeeding and no evidence of psychological or developmental harm from breastfeeding into the third year of life or longer." In support of this recommendation, the AAP cites both the psychological value afforded the breastfeeding mother and infant and the protection against disease received by the maturing infant.

The World Health Organization recommends that all babies around the world be breastfed exclusively for 6 months and continue to breastfeed with appropriate complementary food for up to two years and beyond (WHO, 2003). The American Academy of Family Physicians supports breastfeeding past infancy, including tandem nursing (AAFP, 2007). Optimal health of the mother and baby forms the basis of these recommendations, as well as minimal cost to the family, community, and environment.

∼ Summary

The infant feeding climate today is one in which many parents embrace the idea of breastfeeding. For the most part, healthcare providers share a conviction that breastfeeding is the optimal method for infant nutrition. Despite this intellectual agreement, breastfeeding women need support and advice in societies dominated by bottle feeding messages, sometimes hostile societal attitudes, and aggressive formula industry marketing. Caregivers, agencies, lactation consultants, and breastfeeding counselors can provide this support. They can educate parents about breastfeeding management and empower them to reach their breastfeeding goals. Breastfeeding is a basic human right of all mothers and babies. The WHO and UNICEF initiatives will help ensure these rights, when enforced. They provide a framework for true progress in breastfeeding promotion and the establishment of breastfeeding-friendly healthcare.

∼ Chapter 1—At a Glance

Facts you learned—

The breastfeeding context:

- There is a cultural belief in many countries that bottle feeding is the norm.
- There is a scarcity of lactation education in medical and nursing schools.
- Women with the lowest breastfeeding rates are 21 years old and younger, with low education.
- Breastfeeding rates among African American women are increasing.
- Media in the United States do little to support breastfeeding.
- An increase in breastfeeding rates could save billions of healthcare dollars.
- Babies should be breastfed exclusively for the first 6 months after their birth.
- Mothers should be empowered to breastfeed for 2 years or longer.

International promotion and support efforts:

- Baby-Friendly Hospital Initiative
- *Global Strategy for Infant and Young Child Feeding*
- *Innocenti Declaration*
- International Code of Marketing of Breastmilk Substitutes

- *Protecting, Promoting and Supporting Breastfeeding*
- Ten Steps to Successful Breastfeeding
- UNICEF
- *Healthy People 2010 and 2020* (United States)
- U.S. Surgeon General
- Global Data Bank on Breastfeeding
- World Health Organization

Risks of artificial feeding for babies:

- Lowers cognitive development
- Increases the incidence of malocclusion
- May increase the risk of obstructive sleep apnea in adulthood
- May reduce attachment between mother and child
- Hampers development of the baby's perceptual and response mechanisms
- Hinders respiration by decreasing blood flow
- Many other risks, described in Chapter 9

Risks of not breastfeeding for mothers:

- Lack of empowerment
- Increased risk of hemorrhage after delivery
- No protection from lactation hormones against stress
- Slower return to prepregnancy weight
- No natural delay in ovulation
- Increased risks of breast and ovarian cancer
- Increased risk of osteoporosis
- Increased risk of converting from gestational diabetes to type 2 diabetes
- Increased risks of hypertension, stroke, hyperlipidemia, and cardiovascular disease

∼ References

Abolyan LV. The breastfeeding support and promotion in Baby-Friendly maternity hospitals and not as yet Baby-Friendly Hospitals in Russia. *Breastfeed Med.* 2006;1(2):71-78.

American Academy of Family Physicians (AAFP). AAFP policy statement on breastfeeding. 2007. http://www.aafp.org/online/en/home/policy/policies/b/breastfeedingposition-paper.html. Accessed February 16, 2009.

American Academy of Pediatrics (AAP), Work Group on Breastfeeding. Breastfeeding and the use of human milk. *Pediatrics.* 2005;115(2):496-506.

Anderson J, et al. Breastfeeding and cognitive development: a meta-analysis. *Am J Clin Nutr.* 1999;70:525-535.

Aniansson G, et al. A prospective cohort study on breastfeeding and otitis media in Swedish infants. *Pediatr Infect Dis J.* 1994;13:183-188.

Aydin S, et al. Ghrelin is present in human colostrum, transitional and mature milk. *Peptides.* 2006;27(4):878-882.

Aydin S, et al. Presence of obestatin in breast milk: relationship among obestatin, ghrelin, and leptin in lactating women. *Nutrition.* 2008;24(7-8):689-693.

Bachrach VR, et al. Breastfeeding and the risk of hospitalization for respiratory disease in infancy: a meta-analysis. *Arch Pediatr Adolesc Med.* 2003;157(3):237-243.

Baker JL, et al. Breastfeeding reduces postpartum weight retention. *Am J Clin Nutr.* 2008;88:1543-1551.

Barnes M. White House Task Force on Childhood Obesity, Report to the President. Solving the problem of childhood obesity within a generation. May 2010. www.letsmove.gov/tfco_fullreport_may2010.pdf. Accessed May 11, 2010.

Banderali G, et al. Monitoring breastfeeding rates in Italy. *Acta Paediatr.* 2003; Suppl 91(441):6-8.

Barone JG, et al. Breastfeeding during infancy may protect against bed-wetting during childhood. *Pediatrics.* 2006; 118(1):254-259.

Bartick M, Reinhold A. The burden of suboptimal breastfeeding in the United States: a pediatric cost analysis. *Pediatrics.* Apr 5, 2010; DOI: 10.1542/peds.2009-1616. http://pediatrics.aappublications.org/cgi/reprint/peds.2009-1616v1. Accessed May 5, 2010.

Bartington S, et al. Are breastfeeding rates higher among mothers delivering in Baby Friendly accredited maternity units in the UK? *Int J Epidemiol.* 2006;35(5):1178-1186.

Becher H, et al. Reproductive factors and familial predisposition for breast cancer by age 50 years: a case-control-family study for assessing main effects and possible gene-environment interaction. *Int J Epidemiol.* 2003;32(1):38-48.

Bener, A, et al. Longer breast-feeding and protection against childhood leukaemia and lymphomas. *Eur J Cancer.* 2001; 37(2):234-238.

Bener, A, et al. Role of breast feeding in primary prevention of asthma and allergic diseases in a traditional society. *Eur Ann Allergy Clin Immunol.* 2007;39(10):337-343.

Bentley-Lewis R, et al. Gestational diabetes mellitus: postpartum opportunities for the diagnosis and prevention of type 2 diabetes mellitus. *Nat Clin Pract Endocrinol Metab.* 2008; 4(10):552-558.

Beral V, et al. (Collaborative Group on Hormonal Factors in Breast Cancer). Breast cancer and breastfeeding: collaborative reanalysis of individual data from 47 epidemiological studies in 30 countries, including 50,302 women with breast cancer and 96,973 women without the disease. *Lancet.* 2002;360(9328):187-195.

BFHIUSA. Baby-Friendly Hospitals and Birth Centers. 2009. http://www.babyfriendlyusa.org/eng/03.html. Accessed May 12, 2009.

Bhandari N, et al. Mainstreaming nutrition into maternal and child health programmes: scaling up of exclusive breastfeeding. *Matern Child Nutr.* 2008; 4(suppl 1):5-23.

Bicalho-Mancini P, Velasquez-Melendez G. Exclusive breastfeeding at the point of discharge of high-risk newborns at a neonatal intensive care unit and the factors associated with this practice. *J Pediatr (Rio J).* 2004;80(3):241-248.

Binns C, et al. Breastfeeding and the prevention of obesity. *Asia Pac J Public Health.* 2003;15:S22-S26.

Brandtzaeg P. Why we develop food allergies. *Am Sci.* 2007; 95:28-35.

Brodribb W, et al. Breastfeeding knowledge: the experiences of Australian general practice registrars. *Aust Fam Physician.* 2009;38(1-2):26-29.

Budin P. Neonatology on the web. The nursling: lecture 3. 1907. http://www.neonatology.org/classics/nursling/nursling.3.html, Accessed July 20, 2009.

Buescher S. Anti-infective Properties of Human Milk with Special Reference to the Pre-term Baby. Presentation, Human Lactation: Current Research and Clinical Implications; October 21, 2004; Amarillo, TX.

Buescher S. Host defense mechanisms of human milk and their relations to enteric infections and necrotizing enterocolitis. *Clin Perinatol.* 1994;21:247-226.

Bulkow, L, et al. Risk factors for severe respiratory syncytial virus infection among Alaska native children. *Pediatrics.* 2002;109(2):210-216.

Butte NF. Impact of infant feeding practices on childhood obesity. *J Nutr.* 2009;139(2):412S-416S.

Caplan MS, MacKendrick W. Necrotizing enterocolitis: a review of pathogenetic mechanisms and implications for prevention (review). *Pediatr Pathol.* 1993;13(3):357-369.

Carranza-Lira S, Mera Paz J. Influence of number of pregnancies and total breastfeeding time on bone mineral density. *Int J Fertil.* 2002;47(4):169-171.

Cattaneo A, Buzzetti R. Effect on rates of breast feeding of training for the baby-friendly hospital initiative. *BMJ.* 2001; 323(7325):1358-1362.

Centers for Disease Control and Prevention (CDC). *2007 CDC National Survey of Maternity Practices in Infant Nutrition and Care (mPINC).* 2008a. http://www.cdc.gov/breastfeeding/data/mpinc. Accessed November 16, 2009.

Centers for Disease Control and Prevention (CDC). *Breastfeeding Among U.S. Children Born 1999–2005: CDC National Immunization Survey.* 2008b. http://www.cdc.gov/breastfeeding/data/NIS_data/index.htm. Accessed February 8, 2009.

Centers for Disease Control and Prevention (CDC). *Breastfeeding Report Card.* 2008c. http://www.cdc.gov/breastfeeding/data/report_card.htm. Accessed February 8, 2009.

Centers for Disease Control and Prevention (CDC). *Child Maltreatment: Facts at a Glance.* http://www.cdc.gov/ncipc/dvp/CM_Data_Sheet.pdf. Accessed November 12, 2009.

Centers for Disease Control and Prevention (CDC), Bernard SJ. *Fatal Injuries Among Children by Race and Ethnicity—United States, 1999–2002.* http://www.cdc.gov/mmwr/preview/mmwrhtml/ss5605a1.htm. Accessed November 12, 2009.

Centers for Disease Control and Prevention (CDC). *The CDC Guide to Breastfeeding Interventions.* 2009. http://www.cdc.gov/breastfeeding/resources/guide.htm. Accessed February 22, 2009.

Chan M. Going for the gold by supporting mothers to breastfeed: statement by WHO Director-General Dr Margaret Chan on the occasion of World Breastfeeding Week 2008. http://www.who.int/mediacentre/news/statements/2008/s08/en. Accessed February 8, 2009.

Chauhan M, et al. Enteral feeding for very low birth weight infants: reducing the risk of necrotising enterocolitis. *Arch Dis Child Fetal Neonatal Ed.* 2008;93(2):F162-F166.

Chen YC, et al. The association between infant feeding pattern and mother's quality of life in Taiwan. *Qual Life Res.* 2007;16(8):1281-1288.

Chen A, Rogan W. Breastfeeding and the risk of postneonatal death in the United States. *Pediatrics.* 2004;113(5):e435-e439. http://pediatrics.aappublications.org/cgi/content/abstract/113/5/e435.

Chien L, et al. National prevalence of breastfeeding in Taiwan. *J Hum Lact.* 2005;21(3):338-344.

Clemens J, et al. Breastfeeding and the risk of life-threatening enterotoxigenic *Escherichia coli* diarrhea in Bangladeshi infants and children. *Pediatrics.* 1997;100(6):E2. http://pediatrics.aappublications.org/cgi/content/abstract/100/6/e2.

Coppa G, et al. Human milk oligosaccharides inhibit the adhesion to Caco-2 cells of diarrheal pathogens: *Escherichia coli, Vibrio cholerae, and Salmonella fyris.* Pediatr Res. 2006;59(3):377-382.

Corrao G, et al. Risk of inflammatory bowel disease attributable to smoking, oral contraception and breastfeeding in Italy: a nationwide case-control study. *Int J Epidemiol.* 1998; 27(3):307-404.

Dall'Oglio I, et al. Breastfeeding promotion in neonatal intensive care unit: impact of a new program toward a BFHI for high-risk infants. *Acta Paediatr.* 2007;96(11):1626-1631.

Daniels J, et al. Breast-feeding and neuroblastoma, USA and Canada. *Cancer Causes and Control.* 2002;13(5):401-440.

Davis M. Review of the evidence for an association between infant feeding and childhood cancer. *Int J Cancer.* 1998; (Suppl 11):29-33.

Davis-Floyd R, St. John G. *From Doctor to Healer: The Transformative Journey.* New Brunswick, NJ: Rutgers University Press; 1998.

de Oliveira M, et al. A method for the evaluation of primary health care units' practice in the promotion, protection, and support of breastfeeding: results from the state of Rio de Janeiro, Brazil. *J Hum Lact.* 2003;19(4):365-373.

Dewey K, et al. Differences in morbidity between breast-fed and formula-fed infants. *J Pediatr.* 1995;126(5 Pt 1):696-702.

Dugdale A. Breast milk and necrotising enterocolitis. *Lancet.* 1991;337(8738):435-436.

Dulon M, et al. Breastfeeding promotion in non-UNICEF-certified hospitals and long-term breastfeeding success in Germany. *Acta Paediatr.* 2003;92(6):653-658.

Duncan B, et al. Exclusive breastfeeding for at least 4 months protects against otitis media. *Pediatrics.* 1993;91:867-872.

El-Mohandes A, et al. Use of human milk in the intensive care nursery decreases the incidence of nosocomial sepsis. *J Perinatol.* 1997;17:130-134.

Elwood PC, et al. Long-term effect of breast feeding: cognitive function in the Caerphilly cohort. *J Epidemiol Community Health.* 2005;59(2):130-133.

Escuder M, et al. Impact estimates of breastfeeding over infant mortality. *Rev Saude Publica.* 2003;37(3):319-325.

European Commission, Directorate Public Health and Risk Assessment. *EU Project on Promotion of Breastfeeding in Europe. Protection, Promotion and Support of Breastfeeding in Europe: A Blueprint for Action.* Luxembourg; 2004. http://europa.eu.int/comm/health/ph_projects/2002/promotion/promotion_2002_18_en.htm. Accessed October 12, 2009.

Fernandes R, et al. Inhibition of enteroaggregative Escherichia coli adhesion to HEp-2 cells by secretory immunoglobulin A from human colostrum. *Pediatr Infect Dis J.* 2001;20(7): 672-678.

Fall CH, et al. Relation of infant feeding to adult serum cholesterol concentration and death from ischaemic heart disease. *BMJ.* 1992;304(6830):801-805.

Fida N, Al-Aama J. Pattern of infant feeding at a university hospital in Western Saudi Arabia. *Saudi Med J.* 2003; 24(7): 725-729.

Forste R, Hoffmann JP. Are US mothers meeting the *Healthy People 2010* breastfeeding targets for initiation, duration, and exclusivity? The 2003 and 2004 National Immunization Surveys. *J Hum Lact.* 2008;24(3):278-288.

Gau M. Evaluation of a lactation intervention program to encourage breastfeeding: a longitudinal study. *Int J Nurs Stud.* 2004;41(4):425-435.

Gianino P. Incidence of nosocomial rotavirus infections, symptomatic and asymptomatic, in breast-fed and non-breast-fed infants. *J Hosp Infect.* 2002;50(1):13-17.

Gomez-Sanchiz M, et al. Influence of breast-feeding and parental intelligence on cognitive development in the 24-month-old child. *Clin Pediatr (Phila).* 2004;43(8):753-761.

Griffiths LJ, et al. Effects of infant feeding practice on weight gain from birth to 3 years. *Arch Dis Child.* 2008;94:577-582.

Grossman X, et al. Hospital Education in Lactation Practices (Project HELP): does clinician education affect breastfeeding initiation and exclusivity in the hospital? *Birth.* 2009; 36(1):54-59.

Grummer-Strawn L, et al. Does breastfeeding protect against pediatric overweight? Analysis of longitudinal data from the Centers for Disease Control and Prevention Pediatric Nutrition Surveillance System. *Pediatrics.* 2004;113(2):e81-e86. http://pediatrics.aappublications.org/cgi/content/full/113/2/e81.

Habicht J, et al. Does breastfeeding really save lives, or are apparent benefits due to biases? *Am J Epidemiol.* 1986; 123(2):279-290.

Haiek LN, et al. Understanding breastfeeding behavior: rates and shifts in patterns in Québec. *J Hum Lact.* 2007;23(1):24-31.

Hanson L, et al. Breast-feeding, a complex support system for the offspring. *Pediatr Int.* 2002;44(4):347-352.

Hanson L. Protective effects of breastfeeding against urinary tract infection. *Acta Paediatr.* 2004;93(2):154-156.

Hausman B. Women's liberation and the rhetoric of "choice" in infant feeding debates. *Intl Breastfeed J.* 2008;3:10.

Health Resources and Services Administration (HRSA). The business case for breastfeeding/steps for creating a breastfeeding friendly worksite: bottom line benefits [kit]. 2008. http://ask.hrsa.gov/detail.cfm?PubID=MCH00254. Accessed February 22, 2009.

Healthy People 2010. 2003. http://www.healthypeople.gov/document/html/objectives/16-19.htm. Accessed February 3, 2010.

Healthy People 2020 Public Meetings: 2009 draft objectives. 2009. www.healthypeople.gov/HP2020. Accessed May 5, 2010.

Heller S. *The Vital Touch*. New York: Henry Holt; 1997.

Henderson G, et al. Enteral feeding regimens and necrotising enterocolitis in preterm infants: a multicentre case-control study. *Arch Dis Child Fetal Neonatal Ed.* 2009;94(2): F120-F123.

Hoefer C, Hardy MC. Later development of breastfed and artificially fed infants. *JAMA.* 1929;92:615.

Horta BL, et al. *Evidence on the Long-Term Effects of Breastfeeding: Systematic Reviews and Meta-analyses.* World Health Organization; 2007.

Horwood L, Fergusson D. Breastfeeding and later cognitive and academic outcomes. *Pediatrics.* 1998;101:1.

Hylander M, et al. Human milk feedings and infection among very low birth weight infants. *Pediatrics.* 1998;102(3):E38. http://pediatrics.aappublications.org/cgi/content/full/102/3/e38.

Illingworth PJ, et al. Diminution in energy expenditure during lactation. *Br Med J.* 1986;292:437.

Ip S, et al. *Breastfeeding and Maternal and Infant Health Outcomes in Developed Countries* (Report 153). Rockville, MD: Agency for Healthcare Research and Quality; 2007.

Ivarsson A, et al. Breast-feeding protects against celiac disease. *Am J Clin Nutr.* 2002;75(5):914-921.

The Joint Commission. National Hospital Inpatient Quality Measures: Perinatal Care Core Measure Set. September 2009. http://www.jointcommission.org/PerformanceMeasurement/PerformanceMeasurement/Perinatal+Care+Core+Measure+Set.html. Accessed November 16, 2009.

Jonas W, et al. Short- and long-term decrease of blood pressure in women during breastfeeding. *Breastfeed Med.* 2008;3: 103-109.

Kelly D, Coutts A. Early nutrition and the development of immune function in the neonate. *Proceedings of the Nutrition Society.* 2000;59(2):177-185.

Kent G. Child feeding and human rights. *Int Breastfeed J.* 2006; 18(1):27.

Kimpimaki T, et al. Short-term exclusive breastfeeding predisposes young children with increased genetic risk of Type 1 diabetes to progressive beta-cell autoimmunity. *Diabetologia.* 2001;44(1):63-69.

Kohler H, et al. Antibacterial characteristics in the feces of breast-fed and formula-fed infants during the first year of life. *J Pediatr Gastroenterol Nutr.* 2002;34(2):188-193.

Kramer MS, et al. A randomized breast-feeding promotion intervention did not reduce child obesity in Belarus. *J Nutr.* 2009;139(2):417S-421S.

Kramer S, et al. Breastfeeding and child cognitive development: New evidence from a large randomized trial. *Arch Gen Psychiatry.* 2008;65(5):577-584.

Labbok MH, et al. Breastfeeding: maintaining an irreplaceable immunological resource. *Nat Rev Immunol.* 2004;4(7):565-572.

Labbok M, Hendershot G. Does breastfeeding protect against malocclusion? *Am J Prev Med.* 1987;3:227-232.

Lawrence R, Lawrence R. *Breastfeeding: A Guide for the Medical Profession.* 6th ed. St. Louis, MO: Elsevier-Mosby; 2005.

Leavitt J. *Brought to Bed: Childbearing in America, 1750–1950.* New York: Oxford University Press; 1986.

Ledo A, et al. Human milk enhances antioxidant defenses against hydroxyl radical aggression in preterm infants. *Am J Clin Nutr.* 2009;89:210-215.

Levine O, et al. Risk factors for invasive pneumococcal disease in children: a population-based case-control study in North America. *Pediatrics.* 1999;103(3):E28. http://pediatrics.aappublications.org/cgi/content/extract/105/5/1172. Accessed May 26, 2010.

Li R, et al. Prevalence of breastfeeding in the United States: the 2001 National Immunization Survey. *Pediatrics.* 2003; 111(5 part 2):1198-1201.

Locklin M, Naber S. Does breastfeeding empower women? Insights from a select group of educated, low-income minority women. *Birth.* 1993;20:30-35.

Lucas A. Breastmilk and neonatal NEC. *Lancet.* 1990;336:1519-1523.

Lucas A, et al. Breast milk and subsequent intelligence quotient in children born preterm. *Lancet.* 1992;339:261-264.

Mahmud M, et al. Impact of breast feeding on *Giardia lamblia* infections in Bilbeis, Egypt. *Am J Trop Med Hyg.* 2001; 65(3):257-260.

Marild S, et al. Protective effect of breastfeeding against urinary tract infection. *Acta Paediatr.* 2004;93(2):164-168.

Martin L, et al. Presence of adiponectin and leptin in human milk. 2004 Pediatric Academic Societies' Annual Meeting,, May 2, 2004; San Francisco.

Mason T, et al. Breast feeding and the development of juvenile rheumatoid arthritis. *J Rheumatol.* 1995;22(6):1166-1170.

Mastretta, E, et al. Effect of *Lactobacillus* GG and breast-feeding in the prevention of rotavirus nosocomial infection. *J Pediatr Gastroenterol Nutr.* 2002;35(4):527-531.

Meinzen-Derr J, et al. The role of human milk feedings in risk of late-onset sepsis. 2004 Pediatric Academic Societies' Annual Meeting, May 1, 2004; San Francisco, CA.

McDowell MM, et al. Breastfeeding in the United States: findings from the National Health and Nutrition Examination Surveys, 1999–2006. *NCHS Data Brief.* 2008;(5):1-8.

McGuire W, Anthony M. Donor human milk versus formula for preventing necrotising enterocolitis in preterm infants: systematic review. *Arch Dis Child.* 2003;88(1)SI:11-14.

McKay F. Infant mortality in relation to breastfeeding. *NY State J Med.* 1924;24:433-438.

Merewood A, Heinig J. Efforts to promote breastfeeding in the United States: development of a national breastfeeding awareness campaign. *J Hum Lact.* 2004;20(2):140-145.

Merewood A, et al. The baby-friendly hospital initiative increases breastfeeding rates in a US neonatal intensive care unit. *J Hum Lact.* 2003; 19(2):166-171.

Merten S, Ackermann-Liebrich U. Exclusive breastfeeding rates and associated factors in Swiss baby-friendly hospitals. *J Hum Lact.* 2004; 20(1):9-17.

Merten S, et al. Do Baby-Friendly hospitals influence breastfeeding duration on a national level? *Pediatrics.* 2005; 116(5) e702-e708. http://pediatrics.aappublications.org/cgi/content/abstract/116/5/e702. Accessed May 26, 2010.

Mihrshahi S, et al. Association between breastfeeding patterns and diarrhoeal and respiratory illness: a cohort study in Chittagong, Bangladesh. *Int Breastfeed J.* 2008;3(1):24-28.

Monetini L. Bovine beta-casein antibodies in breast- and bottle-fed infants: their relevance in Type 1 diabetes. *Diabetes Metab Res Rev.* 2001;17(1):51-54.

Montagu A. *Touching: The Human Significance of the Skin.* New York: Harper & Row; 1986.

Monterrosa EC, et al. Predominant breast-feeding from birth to six months is associated with fewer gastrointestinal infections and increased risk for iron deficiency among infants. *J Nutr.* 2008;138(8):1499-1504.

Montgomery D, Splett P. The economic benefit of breastfed infants enrolled in WIC. *Am J Diet Assoc.* 1997;97:379-385.

Newburg D. Neonatal protection by an innate immune system of human milk consisting of oligosaccharides and glycans. *J Anim Sci.* 2009;87(13 suppl):26-34.

Newburg D, et al. Innate protection conferred by fucosylated oligosaccharides of human milk against diarrhea in breast-fed infants. *Glycobiology.* 2004;14(3):253-263.

Oddy W, Glenn K. Implementing the baby-friendly hospital initiative: the role of finger feeding. *Breastfeed Rev.* 2003b; 11(1):5-10.

Ogbuanu IU, et al. The effect of breastfeeding duration on lung function at age 10 years: a prospective birth cohort study. *Thorax.* 2009;64:62-66.

Orrhage K, Nord C. Factors controlling the bacterial colonization of the intestine in breastfed infants. *Acta Paediatr.* 1999;88(430):47-57.

Owen CG, et al. Infant feeding and blood cholesterol: a study in adolescents and a systematic review. *Pediatrics.* 2002; 110(3):597-608.

Owen CG, et al. Effect of infant feeding on the risk of obesity across the life course: a quantitative review of published evidence. *Pediatrics.* 2005;15(5):1367-1377.

Owen CG, et al. Does breastfeeding influence risk of type 2 diabetes in later life? A quantitative analysis of published evidence. *Am J Clin Nutr.* 2006;84(5):1043-1054.

Owen CG, et al. Does initial breastfeeding lead to lower blood cholesterol in adult life? A quantitative review of the evidence. *Am J Clin Nutr.* 2008;88(2):305-314.

Palmer B. Sleep Apnea from an Anatomical, Anthropologic and Developmental Perspective. Paper presented at the Academy of Dental Sleep Medicine; Philadelphia, PA. June 4, 2004; www.brianpalmerdds.com. Accessed July 20, 2009.

Palmer G. *The Politics of Breastfeeding: When Breasts Are Bad for Business.* 3rd ed. London: Pinter & Martin; 2009.

Paton L, et al. Pregnancy and lactation have no long-term deleterious effect on measures of bone mineral in healthy women: A twin study. *Am J Clin Nutr.* 2003;77(3):707-714.

Perrilat F. Day-care, early common infections and childhood acute leukaemia: a multicentre French case-control study. *Br J Cancer.* 2002;86(7):1064-1069.

Philipp B, et al. Baby-Friendly Hospital Initiative improves breastfeeding initiation rates in a US hospital setting. *Pediatrics.* 2001;108(3):677-681.

Philipp B, et al. Breastfeeding information in nursing textbooks needs improvement. *J Hum Lact.* 2007;23(4):345-349.

Philipp B, et al. Sustained breastfeeding rates at a US baby-friendly hospital. *Pediatrics.* 2003;112(3 Pt 1):e234-e236.

http://pediatrics.aappublications.org/cgi/content/full/112/3/e234.

Pisacane A, et al. Breastfeeding and multiple sclerosis. *Br J Med.* 1994;308:1411-1412.

Quinn VJ, et al. Improving breastfeeding practices on a broad scale at the community level: success stories from Africa and Latin America. *J Hum Lact.* 2005;21(3):345-354.

Rao M, et al. Effect of breastfeeding on cognitive development of infants born small for gestational age. *Acta Paediatrica.* 2002;(91)3:267-274.

Ravelli A, et al. Infant feeding and adult glucose tolerance, lipid profile, blood pressure, and obesity. *Arch Dis Child.* 2000; 82(3):248-252.

Rees D, Sabia J. The effect of breast feeding on educational attainment: evidence from sibling data. *J Human Capital.* 2009;3:43-72.

Rosenblatt KA, Thomas DB. Lactation and the risk of epithelial ovarian cancer: the WHO collaborative study of neoplasia and steroid contraceptives. *Int J Epidemiol.* 1993;22(2):192-197.

Rudnicka AR, et al. The effect of breastfeeding on cardiorespiratory risk factors in adult life. *Pediatrics.* 2007;119(5) e1107-e1115. http://pediatrics.aappublications.org/cgi/content/abstract/119/5/e1107.

Ryan A, et al. Breastfeeding continues to increase into the new millennium. *Pediatrics.* 2002;110(6):1103-1109.

Scariati P, et al. A longitudinal analysis of infant morbidity and the extent of breastfeeding in the US. *Pediatrics.* 1997;99(6): E5-E7. http://pediatrics.aappublications.org/cgi/content/abstract/99/6/e5?maxtoshow=&HITS=10&hits=10&RESULTFORMAT=&titleabstract=breastfeeding&searchid=1056999920090_4568&stored_search=&FIRSTINDEX=30&journalcode=pediatrics.

Schanler R, et al. Feeding strategies for premature infants: Beneficial outcomes of feeding fortified human milk versus preterm formula. *Pediatrics.* 1999;104(6 Pt 1):1150-1157.

Sedgwick JP, Fleishner EC. Breastfeeding in the reduction of infant mortality. *Am J Public Health.* 1921;11:153-157.

Shepard JWJ, et al. Evaluation of the upper airway in patients with OSA/SDB. *Sleep.* 1991;14:361-371.

Shu X, et al. Breast-feeding and risk of childhood acute leukemia. *J Natl Cancer Inst.* 1999;91(20):1765-1772.

Silfverdal S, et al. Long term enhancement of the IgG2 antibody response to *Haemophilus influenzae* type B by breast-feeding. *Pediatr Infect Dis J.* 2002;21(9):816-821.

Simard I, et al. Factors influencing the initiation and duration of breastfeeding among low-income women followed by the Canada Prenatal Nutrition Program in 4 regions of Quebec. *J Hum Lact.* 2005;21(3):327-337.

Singhal A, et al. Breastmilk feeding and lipoprotein profile in adolescents born preterm: follow-up of a prospective randomised study. *Lancet.* 2004;363(9421):1571-1578.

Singhal A, et al. Early nutrition in preterm infants and later blood pressure: two cohorts after randomised trials. *Lancet.* 2001;357(9254):413-419.

Smith MM, et al. Influence of breastfeeding on cognitive outcomes at age 6–8 years: Follow-up of very low birth weight infants. *Am J Epidemiol.* 2003;158(11):1075-1078.

Smith P. "Is it just so my right?" Women repossessing breastfeeding. *Intl Breastfeed J.* 2008;3:12.

Smulevich V, et al. Parental occupation and other factors and cancer risk in children: 1. Study methodology and non-occupational factors. *Int J Cancer.* 1999;83(6):712-717.

Strathearn L, et al. Does breastfeeding protect against substantiated child abuse and neglect? A 15-year cohort study. *Pediatrics.* 2009;123:483-493.

Stuebe A, Schwarz E. The risks and benefits of infant feeding practices for women and their children. *J Perinatol.* 2010;30(3):155-162.

Szucs K, et al. Breastfeeding knowledge, attitudes, and practices among providers in a medical home. *Breastfeed Med.* 2009;4(1):31-42.

Tarrats R, et al. Varicella, ephemeral breastfeeding and eczema as risk factors for multiple sclerosis in Mexicans. *Acta Neurol Scand.* 2002;105(2)88-89.

Tellez A, et al. Antibodies in mother's milk protect children against giardiasis. *Scand J Infect Dis.* 2003;35(5):322-325.

Tayloe D. Letter of endorsement to WHO and UNICEF on behalf of Executive Committee of the Board of Directors of the American Academy of Pediatrics (AAP). August 25, 2009. http://www.aap.org/breastfeeding/files/pdf/TenStepswosig.pdf. Accessed May 13, 2010.

Thompson N, et al. Early determinants of inflammatory bowel disease: Use of two national longitudinal birth cohorts. *Eur J Gastroenterol Hepatol.* 2000;12(1):25-30.

Thulier D. Breastfeeding in America: A history of influencing factors. *J Hum Lact.* 2009;25(1):85-94.

Toschke A, et al. Overweight and obesity in 6- to 14-year-old Czech children in 1991: protective effect of breast-feeding. *J Pediatr.* 2002;141(6):764-769.

Toubas PL. Dr. Pierre Budin: promoter of breastfeeding in 19th century France. *Breastfeed Med.* 2007;2(1):45-49.

Tung K, et al. Reproductive factors and epithelial ovarian cancer risk by histologic type: a multiethnic case-control study. *Am J Epidemiol.* 2003;148:629-638.

Turck D, Comité de Nutrition de la Société Française de Pédiatrie. Breast feeding: health benefits for child and mother [in French]. *Arch Pediatr.* 2005;12S3:S145-S165.

United Nations Children's Fund (UNICEF). The Baby-Friendly Hospital Initiative. 2009. http://www.unicef.org/programme/breastfeeding/baby.htm. Accessed May 12, 2009.

United Nations Children's Fund (UNICEF). The state of the world's children 2008. December, 2007: p 221. http://www.unicef.org/sowc08/docs/sowc08.pdf. Accessed February 4, 2010.

U.S. Congress. Section 4207 ("Reasonable Break Time for Nursing Mothers") of the Patient Protection and Affordable Care Act of 2010, Pub.L.No 111-148. January 5, 2010. http://democrats.senate.gov/reform/patient-protection-affordable-care-act-as-passed.pdf. Accessed May 11, 2010.

U.S. Department of Health and Human Services (USDHHS), Department of Health and Human Services for Action on Breastfeeding Office on Women's Health. *Health and Human Services Blueprint for Action on Breastfeeding.* 2000. http://www.womenshealth.gov/archive/breastfeeding/programs/blueprints/bluprntbk2.pdf. Accessed February 22, 2009.

Van Odijk J, et al. Breastfeeding and allergic disease: a multidisciplinary review of the literature (1966–2001) on the mode of early feeding in infancy and its impact on later atopic manifestations. *Allergy.* 2003;58(9):833-843.

Van de Perre P. Transfer of antibody via mother's milk. *Vaccine.* 2003;21(24):3374-3376.

Van Esterik P. Guest editorial. *J Hum Lact.* 1994;10(2):71.

van Rossem L, et al. Are starting and continuing breastfeeding related to educational background? The Generation R study. *Pediatrics.* 2009;123(6):e1017-e1027.

Van Veen H, et al. The role of N-linked glycosylation in the protection of human and bovine lactoferrin against tryptic proteolysis. *Eur J Biochem.* 2004;271(4):678-684.

Vieira G, et al. Child feeding and diarrhea morbidity. *J Pediatr (Rio J).* 2003;79(5):449-454.

Weimer J. *Economic Benefits: A Review and Analysis.* Economic Research Service, U.S. Department of Agriculture, Food Assistance and Nutrition Research Report 13. March 2001.

Wold AE, Adlerbeth I. Breast feeding and the intestinal microflora of the infant: implications for protection against infectious diseases. *Adv Exp Med Biol.* 2000;478:77-93.

Wolf J. Don't kill your baby: Public health and the decline of breastfeeding in the nineteenth and twentieth centuries. The Ohio State University; 2001.

Wolf J. Low breastfeeding rates and public health in the US. *Am J Pub Health.* 2003;93(12):2001–2010.

World Health Organization (WHO). *Protecting, Promoting, and Supporting Breastfeeding: A Joint WHO/UNICEF Statement.* Geneva: WHO; 1989.

World Health Organization (WHO). *Global Strategy for Infant and Young Child Feeding.* Geneva: WHO; 2003.

World Health Organization (WHO). Global data bank on infant and young child feeding; 2010. http://www.who.int/nutrition/databases/infantfeeding/en/index.html. Accessed February 3, 2010.

World Health Organization (WHO). *Key Strategies for Promotion of Breastfeeding.* World Health Organization Regional Office for the Western Pacific; 2007.

World Health Organization (WHO). The International code of marketing of breastmilk substitutes: frequently asked questions. 2008. http://whqlibdoc.who.int/publications/2008/9789241594295_eng.pdf. Accessed February 8, 2009.

Yen ML, et al. Risk factors for ovarian cancer in Taiwan: a case-control study in a low-incidence population. *Gynecol Oncol.* 2003;89(2):318-324.

Young T, et al. Type 2 diabetes mellitus in children–prenatal and early infancy risk factors among native Canadians. *Arch Ped Adol Med.* 2002;146(7):651-655.

Zheng T, et al. Lactation reduces breast cancer risk in Shandong Province, China. *Am J Epidemiol.* 2000;152:1129-1135.

2

Lactation Consultants as Part of the Healthcare Team

Until breastfeeding becomes the societal norm and several generations of women are comfortable with breastfeeding self-care and management, breastfeeding care will be an integral part of maternal and infant health care. The mother and the baby form a nursing dyad—one unit, each dependent on the other. The goal of breastfeeding is for mother and baby to function smoothly as a team. Breastfeeding assistance is most effective when caregivers work collaboratively, both with one another and with parents. All members of the healthcare team must support the nursing dyad and provide consistent care for mothers to achieve their breastfeeding goals. The role of lactation consultant emerged in the mid-1980s; the healthcare team member who fills this role has breastfeeding as a primary focus. Volunteer lay counselors remain important members of the healthcare team as well. They provide peer support and guidance as a complement to the assistance provided by health professionals.

∾ Key Terms

Accreditation and
    Approval Review
    Committee on
    Education in Human
    Lactation and
    Breastfeeding (AARC)
Certification
Clinical competencies for
    IBCLC practice
Community outreach
Discharge planner
Health consumer
ICD-9 code
International Board
    Certified Lactation
    Consultant (IBCLC)
International Board of
    Lactation Consultant
    Examiners (IBLCE)

International Lactation
    Consultant Association
    (ILCA)
Lactation consultant
Lay counselor
Mother-to-mother
    support group
Networking
Outreach counseling
Private practice
Standards of practice
Superbill
Third-party
    reimbursement
Warmline
WIC (Special
    Supplemental Food
    Program for Women,
    Infants and Children)

∾ The Healthcare Team Approach

Because the profession is so young, lactation consultants sometimes find it challenging to establish themselves as integral members of the mother's and baby's healthcare team. Your role as a lactation consultant may be new to many medical professionals. Demonstrating the need for a certified lactation consultant, developing credibility, overcoming medical elitism, and addressing practical employment issues are some of the challenges you may face while establishing yourself in this profession. The services you offer and the manner in which you work with other healthcare providers will influence both your reputation and the cooperation you receive. Communicating with primary care practitioners is the key means of becoming a part of the healthcare team. Inform caregivers of your services, and help them understand your role on the team. Mothers are more likely to continue breastfeeding when they receive encouragement from their clinician to breastfeed (Kutlu et al., 2007; Nakar et al., 2007; Labarere et al., 2005; Taveras et al., 2003).

A team approach to the mother's and baby's care correlates to a "medical home," a term originally used to describe care of special-needs children (American Academy of Pediatrics [AAP], 2009). A medical home is an approach to comprehensive primary care that is accessible, continuous, comprehensive, family-centered, coordinated, compassionate, and culturally effective. Providers' attitudes and cultures within the medical home affect the level of breastfeeding promotion and support (Szucs et al., 2009). Closing any gaps in communication, knowledge, and counseling skills is integral to meeting the needs of mothers and babies.

∾ The Lactation Consulting Profession

With the increase in artificial infant feeding and the accompanying decrease in breastfeeding, some women who breastfeed find they need professional help. Whereas women in earlier generations could turn to their elders for advice and support, women initiating breastfeeding in a bottle feeding culture often have no experienced women in their families to help them. Pregnant women and new mothers ideally would receive appropriate breastfeeding advice and support from their healthcare providers. That is, all caregivers—physicians, nurses, midwives, physician assistants, dieticians, physical therapists, occupational theraists, and childbirth educators—would incorporate breastfeeding teaching and support into their existing practices. In an age of specialization, however, it is no surprise that a healthcare professional has emerged who specializes in human lactation and breastfeeding support.

The professional lactation consultant is a member of the mother's healthcare team who serves as an advocate for the breastfeeding mother and her baby. This advocacy extends beyond the nursing couple to advocate separately for the infant as well, with the lactation consultant using specialized knowledge and skills in conjunction with a willingness to work at the baby's pace. As the only member of the healthcare team whose primary focus is breastfeeding, the lactation consultant may need to suggest alternative plans of breastfeeding care if recommendations by other members of the healthcare team could potentially jeopardize breastfeeding. Lactation consultants offer an adjunct service that builds on the physician–patient relationship. The best way to change physicians' practices is through the sharing of clinical data and positive feedback from families. Lactation consultants can help facilitate communication between mothers and their physicians to improve the support mothers receive.

Growth of the Profession

Individuals enter the lactation consultant profession from a variety of backgrounds, with some possessing advanced degrees in the healthcare field. Because of their professional education and experience, it is a natural progression for those working in maternal/child health to expand their services and specialize in lactation consulting (Figure 2.1). Many nutritionists and dieticians move into lactation support because of their understanding of the importance of human milk to lifelong health. Others begin their careers as lay counselors and then acquire the advanced education and skills that enable them to work professionally as part of the healthcare team. Still others enter lactation consulting from unrelated fields after breastfeeding their own children and developing a desire to help other mothers achieve their breastfeeding goals.

Interest in a specialized field began in the early 1980s, with the advent of professional education for lactation management through various private programs. Several professional texts on lactation management emerged— some directed to the medical profession and others directed to practical aspects of counseling. In 1984, U.S. Surgeon General C. Everett Koop convened a Workshop

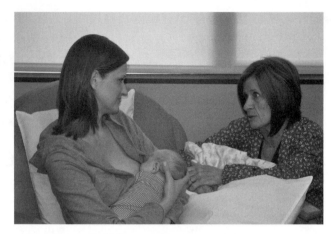

FIGURE 2.1   IBCLC on staff in the hospital.
Source: Printed with permission of Anna Swisher.

on Breastfeeding and Human Lactation, which identified professional education as one of six core areas to be addressed in the lactation field. In 1985, a pioneering group of leaders solidified the new lactation consulting profession with the creation of a certification board and a professional association.

The International Board of Lactation Consultant Examiners (IBLCE) was established in 1985 to develop and administer a certification examination to measure the knowledge and skills necessary for safe and effective practice as a lactation consultant. In 2009, the IBLCE examination was administered in 14 languages in more than 40 countries across all major continents (Gross, 2009). Candidates for the exam must meet minimal requirements regarding education in lactation management and clinical experience. Upon successful completion of the exam, IBLCE grants the designation "International Board Certified Lactation Consultant" (IBCLC). IBLCE later added "Registered Lactation Consultant" (RLC) in the United States as an additional trademark designation. Only an IBCLC may use this trademark. Recertification is required every 5 years, with retesting every 10 years. See Appendix H for IBLCE's contact information to get current requirements.

The International Lactation Consultant Association (ILCA), formed in 1985 as an association for professional lactation consultants, has as its mission to "advance the profession of lactation consulting worldwide through leadership, advocacy, professional development, and research" (ILCA, 2009). ILCA publishes the *Journal of Human Lactation*, a peer-reviewed scientific quarterly journal, and offers an extensive website with a variety of professional resources. An annual conference, with information on cutting-edge lactation practices and research, offers continuing education opportunities to those who assist mothers and babies with breastfeeding. National affiliates are available in most parts of the world.

Several documents have been developed to guide the lactation consulting profession, including a Code of Ethics (Appendix A), a Scope of Practice (Appendix B), Standards of Practice (Appendix C), and Clinical Competencies (Appendix D). A Core Curriculum for IBCLC Practice was published in 2002 as a first step in establishing educational standards for the lactation profession (Mannel et al., 2007). Clinical internships soon began to emerge for aspiring lactation consultants, providing supervised clinical practice with experienced IBCLCs.

In 2003, IBLCE launched a pilot clinical pathway for qualifying to take the certification exam. This pathway, which utilizes the Clinical Competencies, soon became a permanent pathway toward certification. The number of educational offerings increased and by 2008, the Accreditation and Approval Review Committee (AARC) on Education in Human Lactation and Breastfeeding formalized an accreditation process through the Commission on Accreditation of Allied Health Education Programs (ILCA, 2009). This move coincided with the development of a model academic curriculum framework to guide post-secondary institutions in launching programs for lactation consultants.

Practicing as a Lactation Consultant

Healthcare practitioners care for breastfeeding mothers and babies in a variety of settings. For example, lactation consultants may work in hospitals, physicians' offices, public health clinics, home health care, and private practice. The experience you bring to the job may dictate the practice setting you choose. In many cases, hospitals, physicians' offices, and home healthcare agencies prefer that the lactation consultant possess additional training in health care, such as nursing. Health clinics may employ a lactation consultant who is also a registered dietician or nutritionist. A lactation consultant in private practice requires extensive experience with a great variety of babies and breastfeeding situations. The discussion in this chapter explores each of these practice settings. Some provisions are relevant to all practice settings, including appropriate space that provides privacy for consultations or calls, an area for office work, and breastfeeding equipment and supplies.

Equipment and Furniture for an Office-Based Practice

Having appropriate equipment will increase your efficiency in processing the necessary paperwork in a busy practice. You will need a desk, chair, filing cabinet, and any other furnishings that will provide for efficiency and comfort. A computer, fax machine, and printer will enable you to maintain accurate client records and produce professional reports and correspondence. There are now many Internet faxing services available that enable you to send and receive fax reports electronically; this saves both paper and time. A dedicated cell phone or land telephone line with your business voice mail greeting will ensure that you receive all calls and can answer them professionally. You may also consider offering e-mail access to mothers and setting up a business website or blog to provide educational information to a new generation of mothers who turn first to the Internet for information and for seeking help. You will also need a reference library accessible to you both during the consultation and when writing reports directed to physicians.

Mothers will need a comfortable chair or couch with arms where they can sit and nurse, preferably one you can wipe clean. A footstool placed in front of the chair will help you teach mothers good body positioning. Pillows of various shapes and sizes will enable mothers to get comfortable for feedings and to position their babies at the breast. Using pillows with removable pillowcases will assure mothers of safe hygiene practices. A baby sling will allow you to hold the baby while the mother is pumping and to complete your paperwork for the visit at the same time.

In addition, you will need a place where you can lay the baby for examining him or her and where you can secure the baby while you are assessing and working with the mother. A highly sensitive, calibrated digital scale is standard equipment in clinic and private practice settings, as well as in hospital nurseries. You will need either paper products or linens for use on your changing table and scale. Many lactation consultants in clinic and private practice settings provide toys for toddlers to keep them busy while they work with the mother and baby. If you do so, make sure you select toys you can clean adequately.

Breastfeeding Supplies and Inventory

Mothers appreciate having easy access to various breastfeeding devices for rental or purchase. Some lactation consultants provide pump rentals and purchases; many do not. If you do not rent or sell pumps, then you should be ready to provide your clients with a list of places and bona fide websites that do. Appendix H contains the names of some breast pump companies.

Rental programs for breast pumps usually allow clients to lease a pump at a daily, weekly, or monthly rate. In many cases, special rates for long-term use (i.e., 5 or 6 months) are available as well.

In the beginning, you may wish to serve as a rental station on consignment with a breast pump company. Later, after you have firmly established a rental station, changing to a flat rate may be a better option financially. In addition to large rental electric breast pumps, you can provide smaller electric pumps for purchase, motor adapters, power packs, feeding cups, and bottles. Providing replacement parts for breast pumps and breast pump kits is a convenience that mothers greatly appreciate. You can also provide instructions that address common questions regarding refunds for early returns, special rental rates, care of the pump, and arranging for its return.

Identify a place where disposable supplies can be stored and that is easily accessible during consultations. These items may include medicine droppers, small cups, nipple shields, and nursing supplementers. You may also need small amounts of formula to feed babies who need calories when the mother's expressed milk is not available. If you use olive oil to improve the vacuum of the breast pump flange, make sure you have small medicine cups to provide individual amounts to mothers. Keep track of items you do not have that would either make a consultation go more smoothly or make it more comfortable for the mother. Weigh the cost of such items against the time frame during which you will use or sell them. Ordering a small number of new items will allow you to test the market before making a large investment. If an item has a high turnover rate, you might consider purchasing it in quantity and prepaying to save money on shipping and handling.

Lactation consultants in high-volume practices may decide to accept Web-generated orders for equipment. Unless you are comfortable with the process of building and maintaining your own website, you may find that hiring a third party to build and maintain your site is more appropriate. Be sure to keep links up-to-date. If you offer online services, you will need to provide credit card and electronic payment options (such as PayPal). Word-of-mouth recommendations from colleagues may save you both time and money when it comes time to set up your own website.

As part of your practice, you must observe any applicable privacy regulations, such as the Health Portability and Accountability Act (HIPAA) privacy guidelines in the United States. Forms should include a privacy statement and the patient will need to sign a release form for you to share information with her other healthcare providers (Bornmann, 2008).

∾ *Practicing in a Hospital*

A large percentage of lactation consultants work in hospitals. Providing support and guidance to mothers as they welcome their new baby into their family can be very rewarding. Hospital-based lactation consultants have the potential to greatly influence a mother's self-confidence and competence as she begins breastfeeding. One of the most important jobs of a hospital-based lactation consultant is ensuring that someone who is skilled in breastfeeding assessment observes every mother breastfeed her baby before discharge. While the lactation consultant attempts to see all mothers, it is often a staff nurse who spends the most time teaching and supporting mothers as they learn how to breastfeed their babies. Although you may not be able to see every breastfeeding mother, you will most likely see any who are having problems.

An essential role of the hospital-based lactation consultant, therefore, is providing breastfeeding instruction and guidance for maternity staff to achieve consistency and continuity of care. Training hospital nursery staff is a potential, cost-effective intervention even in settings with relatively high rates of breastfeeding (Shinwell, 2006). Having maternity staff trained in basic breastfeeding care and prepared to handle some of the more common challenges encountered in the immediate postpartum period permits the lactation consultant to respond to referrals for situations that are more complex. Chapter 12 further discusses the lactation consultant's role in postpartum breastfeeding care.

Work hours in a hospital will depend on the amount of time allocated for lactation coverage. Being a member of a hospital staff has some notable advantages—namely, a steady income and work, as well as employment benefits. Lactation consultants working in a hospital generally receive an hourly wage (non-exempt), although some may be salaried (exempt). The salary range is comparable to that of a nurse clinician or a registered nurse certified in a specialty. Hospital employment offers the flexibility of working on a full-time or part-time basis, or *pro re nata* ("PRN"), meaning, as needed.

Challenges of Hospital Practice

As a member of the hospital staff, you will be part of a team that includes the maternity and nursery staff as well as the mothers' and babies' physicians. Having such a wide-ranging group of colleagues can provide a source of reference and moral support. At the same time, unsupportive staff or administrators may create obstacles or frustrations for you, especially when a conflict in philosophy or priorities arises. Because the rest of the staff will view you as an expert, they may tend to rely on you to handle aspects of mothers' breastfeeding teaching and care that could actually be managed by the mother's or baby's nurse.

Lactation consultants often work longer hours than personnel in other staff positions as they make an effort to see every breastfeeding mother and baby. This is especially the case for those who are the sole lactation consultant at a hospital. Being on staff makes providing inpatient and staff education convenient. Ensuring that the nursing staff knows how to provide basic breastfeeding care can lighten your load, although you may then primarily see mothers and babies with complicated problems, which increases the potential for professional burnout.

As a hospital employee, because you are accountable to the administration, hospital policies and limitations may restrict your role as a breastfeeding advocate. There may be some battles you cannot win, requiring you to make compromises that conflict with your personal code of breastfeeding support. When hospitals experience downsizing, administrators may regard the lactation consultant's position as less critical than other positions. Consequently, you may lose your job or assume duties unrelated to breastfeeding, especially if you have other clinical skills such as nursing, dietetics, or occupational therapy. This outcome can be very frustrating to someone whose primary interest is breastfeeding support.

On the bright side, many hospitals are willing to fund their lactation consultants' attendance at conferences and memberships to professional organizations. You may also have an opportunity to develop a strong lactation program and to be instrumental in designing and improving the care that breastfeeding mothers and babies in your community receive.

Hospital Lactation Program

The hospital setting enables you to influence large numbers of people. How hospital-based lactation consultants function varies, based on the setting. You may provide services to both inpatients and outpatients and serve as a resource for hospital staff in the care of normal breastfeeding couples. This includes assisting with the care of couples who are having difficulty, as well as providing in-service education and training for staff. You may make rounds on some or all breastfeeding mothers and babies, including those who are patients elsewhere in the hospital, such as surgery or the emergency room. Alternatively, depending on the size and staffing of the facility, you may see only mothers and babies whom other medical or nursing staff refer to you. Administratively, you may develop breastfeeding policies and procedures, competency guidelines, performance evaluations, and patient documentation forms. You may also develop information for the hospital's website, as well as handouts and reading materials for breastfeeding parents.

Follow-up is an essential element of breastfeeding care. Engaging in routine contact with mothers after discharge will increase their competence and self-confidence. Some hospitals provide outpatient visits on a fee-for-service basis or as a billable service; others provide it at no additional cost to the patient. Some hospitals make follow-up telephone calls after discharge. Still others provide no outpatient or telephone lactation services, instead referring mothers to outside resources such as community support groups.

Referral of mothers to peer support groups, community-based lactation consultants, and other health professionals is an essential part of hospital follow-up. You can also assist the mother in obtaining breastfeeding devices, when appropriate, and teach her how to use them. Another outpatient service provided by many lactation consultants is conducting classes about infant feeding, incorporating practical information about breastfeeding and the realities and risks of artificial infant feeding.

Lactation Staffing Levels

Ideally, every hospital would provide 24-hour assistance for breastfeeding mothers and babies. When the number of lactation consultants on staff is limited, however, lactation coverage may occur only during the daily work week or for only one shift. From a staffing perspective, it is important to recognize that lactation programs often provide much more than clinical coverage. Caring for high-acuity breastfeeding patients, educating large numbers of staff and physicians, and administering a busy, complex lactation service all require significantly more staffing than is commonly believed. Almost one-third of a lactation consultant's time can be spent in indirect clinical activities such as education, research, program development, and administration (Mannel & Mannel, 2006). Administration tasks encompass issues such as policies, procedures, documentation, staffing, personnel management, patient information, statistics, quality assurance, and hospital leadership. All of these nonclinical responsibilities need to be accounted for when calculating staffing needs that are realistic and that provide optimal care for mothers and infants.

Based on data collected in the Mannel and Mannel study, a community hospital with 1,500 deliveries and an 85 percent breastfeeding rate would require about 2.5 full-time employees (FTEs) for the care of healthy, full-term newborns. This coverage provides for 3 inpatient clinical consults of approximately 30 minutes each for every mother/baby dyad, as well as a follow-up phone call (see Table 2.1). The recommended number of FTEs would increase if the practice involves caring for special care infants and engaging in post-discharge visits of mothers and babies. Clinical time spent with each mother/baby dyad in the NICU would be about 5.5 hours compared to 2.2 hours for healthy, full-term infants.

～ Practicing in a Health Clinic

Public health clinics offer many avenues of employment for lactation consultants. Research suggests that IBCLCs working in these kinds of outpatient primary care settings may promote a longer duration of breastfeeding (Thurman & Allen, 2008). Many health clinics offer one-on-one breastfeeding counseling, classes, and postpartum support groups. In this setting, you may counsel mothers or supervise and train peer counselors. You may also provide information and education to agencies that deliver prenatal, labor and delivery, postpartum, pediatric, or daycare services. In addition, many lactation consultants

TABLE 2.1 IBCLC Staffing in a Community Hospital

1,500 Deliveries with 85% Breastfeeding Rate	FTE Ratio	Calculation	FTEs
Mother/baby care with three 30-minute consults	1:783	1,275/783	1.6
Telephone follow-up clinical consult	1:3,915	2,500/3,915	.6
Education	0.1:1,000	1.5 × .01	.1
Program development and administration	0.1:1,000	1.5 × .01	.1
Research	0.1–0.2		.1
Total FTEs (1 FTE = 1,900 work hours)			2.5

FTE = full-time employee.

Source: Adapted from Mannel R, Mannel RS. Staffing for hospital lactation programs: Recommendations from a tertiary care teaching hospital. *J Hum Lact.* 2006;22:(4)409.

in public health participate in state breastfeeding workshops, consortiums, and committees.

You will encounter many diverse lifestyles when working in a public health clinic. Consequently, it is important to be sensitive to families' cultural and socioeconomic values. Many clients move frequently, making ongoing contact challenging. Because lifestyles and priorities among clinic clients may be quite different from your personal experience, you need to remain flexible and adaptable. You can find common ground with mothers by focusing on their love and concern for their children.

Nutrition Assistance Programs

In the United States, the Special Supplemental Food Program for Women, Infants, and Children (WIC) is geared toward helping pregnant women choose nutritious foods and providing services to breastfeeding mothers, infants, and children up to 5 years of age. To qualify for WIC assistance, family income must be 185 percent of the poverty level. In other words, if the poverty level is $10,000 in annual income, a person would need to make $18,500 per year or less to receive WIC benefits (U.S. Department of Agriculture [USDA], 2009). Breastfeeding rates among WIC participants are increasing, at a time when rates in the overall population remain unchanged. The WIC program saves tax dollars by encouraging healthy eating, which in turn lowers healthcare costs.

The Canada Prenatal Nutrition Program (CPNP) provides many of the same services as the U.S.-based WIC program. A distinguishing feature of the Canadian program is that it provides no free formula except as a compassionate response to a woman who has run out of formula and cannot afford to buy more. CPNP believes that free supplies of formula affect women's choice of feeding method. For this reason, the program places heavy emphasis on promotion and support of breastfeeding. By comparison, one cross-generational study found that free

formula from WIC affected breastfeeding rates (Fooladi, 2001).

Breastfeeding Promotion in WIC

With a long history of promoting and supporting breastfeeding, WIC's focus on breastfeeding is intended to help mothers make an informed choice about infant feeding through evidence-based information. WIC encourages mothers to breastfeed exclusively, provides anticipatory guidance, and helps create and advocate for a supportive environment that will help mothers carry out their breastfeeding intentions. Its philosophy is to help participants become healthier and more self-sufficient through education and application of sound nutritional principles.

At no cost to participants, the program provides nutritious foods to supplement the diet, information on healthy eating, and referrals for health care. As part of its scope, the WIC program engages in extensive breastfeeding promotion efforts at the local, state, and national levels. The USDA encourages breastfeeding among WIC participants through regulatory provisions, publications, cooperative efforts with other federal agencies and private organizations, and funding of breastfeeding grants and studies.

The variety of approaches employed contributes to increasing the rates of breastfeeding among WIC participants. Breastfeeding mothers in WIC receive follow-up support through peer counselors and are eligible to participate in WIC longer than non-breastfeeding mothers. Those who exclusively breastfeed their infants receive an enhanced food package. Breastfeeding mothers can also receive breast pumps, breast shells, or nursing supplementers to help support the initiation and continuation of breastfeeding. In addition, WIC provides prenatal classes, toll-free telephone lines that supply information about and assistance with breastfeeding, and health professional training.

As part of its wide-ranging coverage, WIC promotes the use of peer counselors to provide ongoing support to breastfeeding clients who are participating in the program. Peer counselors reach mothers on their level, dispel cultural myths, and offer advice on other lifestyle issues based on personal experience. For that reason, WIC peer counselors must be representative of the community they serve (see Chapter 20 for a discussion of cultural issues). A lactation consultant working under WIC's aegis may train and supervise peer counselors or initiate a peer counselor program if none exists.

WIC has access to a significant segment of low-income, at-risk mothers and infants in the United States. In fact, nearly half of all mothers and babies in this country qualify for participation in WIC. Nutritional information and healthy foods were first provided to disadvantaged American families through a pilot WIC program in 1972. The program grew rapidly, until today it serves 8 million people, including 2 million infants and nearly 2 million mothers. The program is administered through 90 state agencies. Given this high degree of expo-

sure, the USDA has ample opportunities to contribute to achieving the Department of Health and Human Services' *Healthy People 2010* goals for breastfeeding as well as the program's own nutritional goals. The USDA's national breastfeeding promotion campaign augments breastfeeding efforts already under way in communities throughout the United States. The campaign promotes breastfeeding awareness and support among women of childbearing age, their families, and others who influence their infant feeding decisions.

The Pediatric Nutrition Surveillance 2007 Report conducted by the Centers for Disease Control and Prevention (CDC) found that among WIC participants in 2007, 59.8 percent of infants were ever breastfed, 25.4 percent were breastfed for at least 6 months, and 17.5 percent were breastfed for at least 12 months (USDHHS, 2009a). Table 2.2 summarizes the breastfeeding trends among WIC participants. By way of comparison, the 2006 National Immunization Survey (NIS) indicates that

TABLE 2.2   Breastfeeding Trends Among WIC Participants*

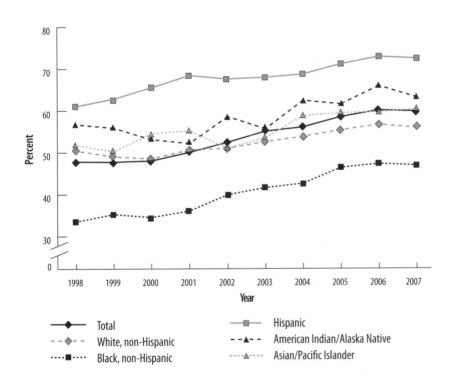

*Among infants born during the reporting period. Year 2010 target: increase the proportion of mothers who breastfeed their babies in the early postpartum period to 75 percent.

Data from: 2007 National PedNSS Data Table 19D. Available at http://www.cdc.gov/pednss/pednss_tables/tables_numeric.htm.

Source: Polhamus B, et al. *Pediatric Nutrition Surveillance 2007 Report*. Atlanta, GA: U.S. Department of Health and Human Services, Centers for Disease Control and Prevention; 2009. Centers for Disease Control and Prevention, 1600 Clifton Rd, Atlanta, GA 30333. (800-232-4636). cdcinfo@cdc.gov.

among all children born in the United States in 2006, 74 percent initiated breastfeeding, 43 percent were breastfeeding at 6 months, and 23 percent were breastfeeding at 12 months. Approximately 33 percent of infants born in 2006 were exclusively breastfed through 3 months of age, and 14 percent were exclusively breastfed for 6 months (USDHHS, 2009b).

Many socioeconomic characteristics common among the WIC population are associated with lower rates of breastfeeding and may contribute to this discrepancy—notably, race, age (younger than 20 years), and education (less than high school graduate).Within each income group, the breastfeeding rates for non-Hispanic black infants were significantly lower compared with the breastfeeding rates among non-Hispanic white and Mexican American infants (McDowell et al., 2008).

A portion of WIC funding for breastfeeding goes toward paying the salaries of healthcare professionals and peer counselors. This funding offers an ideal opportunity for the establishment of a lactation consultant position. Some states or agencies have breastfeeding promotion positions funded on a percentage basis. For example, the time allocated to a registered dietician job position may be divided as follows: 80 percent for regular WIC job functions and 20 percent for breastfeeding promotion and support.

Most states designate a WIC breastfeeding coordinator for each agency. The responsibilities shouldered by these individuals are diverse, and the backgrounds of potential coordinators vary as well. For example, one position may require a lactation consultant to be certified through the IBLCE; another may include non-breastfeeding functions that require a nursing or dietetic degree; and still another may require someone with experience in marketing, fundraising, or promotional activities to provide expertise in community outreach.

∾ Working in a Physician Group

Working with an obstetrician, pediatrician, or family practice group offers an opportunity to care for mothers and babies through many stages of breastfeeding. In this type of setting, most of the practice is preventive and you will see healthy, normal babies as well as those who experience difficulties. Working with only a few physicians will make it easier for you to come to agreement on breastfeeding issues.

You may work specific hours in the physician's office or work via an on-call system from home. Your client load, and therefore the hours you work, will be dependent on the physician's patient load. Breastfeeding complications are not limited to specific hours, of course, so you will need to be available around the clock. In addition, mothers will need a way to contact you directly. A cell phone, beeper, or voice mail system will enable you to contact clients at your convenience. It will also be important to ensure that coverage is available from another lactation consultant or other caregiver for times when you are unavailable.

Having a lactation consultant on staff attracts mothers to the practice. There is great marketing potential if yours is the first physician practice in the community to employ a certified lactation consultant. If you wish to develop a lactation program for a physician or group practice, prepare a brief proposal outlining specific services you could provide for their patients. Chapter 26 contains further suggestions for developing a job proposal or job description.

Working with a physician group sometimes means that downsizing could eliminate your position. To address this possibility, you should prepare and keep up-to-date documentation that illustrates your importance to the practice. Recording breastfeeding statistics within the practice will help you to document your effectiveness. For example, you can record the number of mothers who initiate breastfeeding and those who continue to breastfeed for 6 weeks, 3 months, 6 months, and 1 year after their babies are born. You can also document the frequency and nature of problems and the assistance you provided.

Lactation Services Geared Toward a Physician Practice

Having a lactation consultant in the practice frees up time for physicians and office personnel who would otherwise spend helping patients with breastfeeding, both prenatally and postpartum. Of course, the preventive education, hospital counseling, and telephone follow-up that the lactation consultant provides are far more effective than the crisis management that becomes necessary when problems surface suddenly. Being able to turn the care of a slow-gaining infant over to a lactation consultant relieves the physician's patient load and ensures that the cause of the problem is identified and that breastfeeding is preserved.

As a lactation consultant, you will be a valuable resource to the practice in updating physicians and staff on new research in your field. Your expertise will prove valuable to others in the practice who have limited time to research breastfeeding literature to stay current with practice guidelines. To help them keep abreast of new developments, you can make sure that your colleagues have the latest information on breastfeeding management, treatment of problems, and compatibility of medications with breastfeeding. You can also provide in-service programs for the nursing staff to help them in their discussions with breastfeeding patients.

If you make rounds in the hospital for the patients in your practice, you may need to be creative with your schedule. You will want to see every mother at least once before discharge and observe her breastfeeding technique. You may be there at a time when the baby is not ready for a feeding, or early discharge could make it difficult for you to see every breastfeeding mother in a timely manner. To ensure that you work efficiently, you can contact the hospital in the morning to determine which mothers need a visit and plan your rounds to make sure you see all who need a visit.

Postpartum breastfeeding classes and a breastfeeding support group are natural extensions of your services to mothers in a pediatric practice. You may also promote prenatal breastfeeding classes to obstetricians who generally refer their patients to your pediatric practice. Having contact with women on a prenatal basis provides an opportunity to help them in their decision to breastfeed and to dispel any misconceptions. You also can explore a woman's breastfeeding goals, evaluate her previous history, and assess her breasts and nipples in preparation for breastfeeding.

As part of the physician practice's services, you can provide follow-up after hospital discharge to guide mothers through the early weeks of breastfeeding. Ideally, follow-up calls will occur at 2 to 3 days after discharge, 3 to 4 days after that, and again at 2 weeks. Providing anticipatory guidance through follow-up telephone calls helps the mother avoid complications; additional follow-up can then take place more frequently as warranted. If specific problems or concerns arise, an office visit or home visit may be necessary to evaluate the situation. To prepare for offering telephone support, you might consider using a separate cell phone or installing a separate telephone line in your home. You can establish a 24-hour telephone "warmline," where the caller leaves a message on an answering machine or voice mail system and you respond to the call later (as opposed to a "hotline" where incoming calls are answered). Depending on your service, you may also choose to carry a pager or to be available by cell phone.

When working as part of a physician group, you will need to have available a private room with a comfortable chair, a variety of pillows, charting forms, a breast pump and other breastfeeding devices, literature, diapers, and other items discussed under private practice. You may incorporate breast pump rentals and other breastfeeding devices into the physician's practice or provide them as a service separate from your arrangement with the physician. You may also write your own breastfeeding handouts to provide up-to-date, evidence-based information that reflects the philosophy of your practice.

You might consider dividing your time between an outpatient pediatric clinic and an obstetrical clinic. Challenges with this arrangement include timing of the consultations, educating staff and patients on preparation for consultations to make sure the baby will be ready for a

feed, increasing awareness of service availability among mothers and healthcare staff, and collaborating with various clinic personnel (Lukac et al., 2006).

Financial Considerations

You can negotiate billing for your services with the physician at the time of your interview. Once an agreement is reached, a specific contract should be drawn up specifying your services and salary. You may want to renegotiate the arrangement at the end of the first year to reflect any changes in your services. Wages in a physician's practice may range between those of an office staff nurse and a hospital-based lactation consultant. Compensation may be on a per-client basis to cover such services as hospital rounds, follow-up telephone calls, establishment of a basic chart, and a warmline. The practice can bill breastfeeding classes and office or home visits separately or include it in the physician's fee. In some cases, the practice may prefer to compensate for the lactation consultant's services with an hourly salary. If the position is part-time, employment benefits such as health insurance or vacation time may not be included as part of the compensation package.

If clients pay you directly on a fee-for-service basis, they can submit the bill to their insurance company for reimbursement, or the physician can include your services on the bill submitted to the insurance company. Individual insurance companies will determine whether to reimburse for your services. This may be the least desirable arrangement, as many mothers will not use your services until they are in full-blown crisis, in an effort to avoid paying the upfront cost. Information on third-party reimbursement is available from United States Lactation Consultant Association (USLCA, 2009).

Practicing in Home Health Care

The home care lactation consultant provides follow-up to mothers and babies after hospital discharge. Home health services begin with discharge planning and continue through home visits and community referrals. It is essential that home care nurses be well educated in breastfeeding management so that they can give effective care and advice. Ideally, every home care agency that provides maternity services will have a lactation consultant on staff. Hospitals customarily contract with managed care companies to provide home care service. Home care staff see only mothers with insurance coverage.

In today's environment, which is characterized by short hospital stays, home care services are essential to mothers and babies. If the mother does not stay in the hospital at least 48 hours after delivery, the hospital staff may not be able to observe a breastfeeding for every mother and baby. Many families elect to stay only 24 hours, especially when it is not their first birth. Knowing that a home care lactation consultant will visit the mother shortly after discharge provides greater assurance that these mothers will receive the breastfeeding advice and care they need.

Breastfeeding advocates have had varying degrees of success in obtaining health maintenance organization (HMO) coverage for home care services. Some HMOs may be more likely to provide coverage for lactation services if the lactation consultant is also a registered nurse. In some places, home health staff see mothers only if they have a health problem. The American Alliance of Health Plans lists health plans that offer lactation coverage (www.aahp.org).

Home Health Lactation Program

Home health agency lactation services will vary, but the program described here may serve as a model for a continuum of breastfeeding support. The home healthcare staff in this program received comprehensive instruction through the WHO/UNICEF "18-Hour Course for Breastfeeding Management and Promotion in a Baby-Friendly Hospital," tailored to fit the needs of home care staff. Agencies differ in their policies for determining which mothers are eligible for home visits, as well as the duration of the visits. The average length of a lactation visit made by employees of this home health agency is 90 minutes; other agencies require that visits be no longer than 45 minutes. Some limit visits to mothers who are at risk, have given birth by cesarean section, or have preterm babies.

A maternity discharge planner visits every mother/baby dyad on the day of discharge to evaluate the mother and baby and review their charts. She discusses breastfeeding progress and concerns, gives the mother instructions until her first home visit, and documents her visit for the lactation consultant. Breastfeeding mothers receive a home visit by a lactation consultant who is also a nurse. The mother receives information to help her detect potential breastfeeding problems and a breastfeeding diary in which she can track feedings, voids, and stools. Mothers eligible for home health services receive information about the home care nursing and lactation consultant services. After hospital discharge, the lactation consultant contacts the home care department to arrange for follow-up.

The Lactation Consultant's Role

In preparation for the visit, the mother is encouraged to think of herself still as a patient and to not worry about showering, dressing, or preparing for a visitor. Helping the mother lower her expectations encourages her to continue getting the rest she needs. A home environment is less controlled than a hospital room, requiring you to be flexible in your expectations and the manner in which you provide care.

On the first visit, you may open the door to an excited sibling or a frantic mother who needs reassurance. The visit may begin with social amenities and emotional support substantially different from that provided in a hospital setting. Likewise, family dynamics may be quite different from those observed in the hospital environment, with the baby's father, siblings, and grandparents often present. As a result, you may able to assess the mother's support system and capitalize on teaching opportunities with other family members in the comfort of their own environment. Often, speaking loudly enough for a family member in another room to hear what the mother is being told goes a long way in enlisting support from a skeptical relative. However, you need to be careful to protect your client's privacy. Do not ask her personal medical questions in the presence of others without verifying that it is acceptable to her to speak freely in front of other family members or friends.

On the first visit, the lactation consultant will focus on observing and assessing a breastfeeding and building the mother's self-confidence. This activity includes learning how breastfeeding is going, checking the breastfeeding diary, and discussing the mother's labor and delivery to identify potential problems with breastfeeding such as the possibility of a sleepy baby because of birth interventions. It also gives the mother an opportunity to talk about her birth and any disappointments, thereby helping her gain perspective and move on to other parenting issues such as breastfeeding. Anticipatory guidance will help the mother avoid potential complications such as low milk production, nipple soreness, or engorgement.

The mother may seem more relaxed and reassured on the second home visit, as she is likely feeling more rested and confident. She is now more prepared to "take in and take hold," as described by Reba Rubin (1957). Guiding her in long-term issues such as managing feedings after returning to work and accessing community support provides a vital link for the mother in reaching her breastfeeding goals. This visit will include another complete assessment of mother and baby, including a breast exam. By this second visit, which occurs around day 5 or 6 after childbirth, the mother should report at least six to eight wet diapers and three to five stools in 24 hours. Infant weight loss should be stabilized or less than 7 percent of birth weight.

～ Working in Private Practice

Private practice is a reasonable option for a seasoned lactation consultant who has many years of experience working with a wide variety of breastfeeding mothers and infants. Some private practice lactation consultants have another medical credential beyond their IBCLC designation (e.g., RN, MD, or RD). These credentials can be important when working on a referral basis. Also, licensed credentials make it more likely that insurance companies will provide reimbursement. The impetus for licensing board-certified lactation consultants is increasing, with the ultimate goal being that more states will cover lactation services for Medicaid patients. Because "registered" is a more familiar term to many U.S. insurers than "certified," IBLCE designated its lists of certificants in every country as a registry in 1999. As a consequence, IBCLCs can state that they are registered with the IBLCE and list "Registered Lactation Consultant" (RLC) after their IBCLC credential.

Challenges of Private Practice

Private practice lactation consultants are dependent on referrals to maintain and expand their client base. Establishing a large referral base from contacts with other lactation consultants, hospitals, caregivers, and previous clients can take several years. However, because your referral base does not rely on a single source, you will be able to advocate for breastfeeding more assertively. It is easier to speak your mind when you are autonomous!

Many private practice lactation consultants enjoy the autonomy of being their own boss. On the upside, they can set their own work hours and arrange their schedules around family functions and other responsibilities. On the downside, working in private practice usually results in minimal contact with staff at the hospitals and thus provides limited opportunities to forge peer relationships. Working on community coalitions can provide effective networking with other professionals. They will learn more about you and your practice, and you will become acquainted with new colleagues. Some of the tips in Chapter 28 may help guide the manner in which you relate to other professionals.

Subscribing to relevant journals will help you stay current on medical and practice issues; membership in ILCA will entitle you to receive its publication, *Journal of Human Lactation*. Journal articles are also available in medical libraries and on the Internet, often at little or no cost. Most medical disciplines have large numbers of websites that send out e-mail news updates.

You can overcome the challenges associated with private practice, especially if you are a self-starter who enjoys autonomy. Ultimately, the key to your success will be engaging in sound business practices, making the time commitment necessary to see clients, following through with necessary paperwork, and marketing your services.

Business Structure

Establishing a private practice is a serious business decision that will require work to succeed. You may want to take a small-business course from your local community college if you do not have a business background. In addition, many books and seminars are available that explain how to start a small business and run a home office. The U.S. Internal Revenue Service offers free business seminars to educate entrepreneurs about federal tax requirements and provides extensive information on this topic on its website (www.irs.gov). Although you will not have employee benefits, being self-employed may provide you with some tax benefits, which an accountant can help you identify.

Most private practice IBCLCs operate as sole proprietors. If you possess other professional credentials, establishing a professional association or S corporation may confer certain tax advantages. For instance, an IBCLC may also be a marriage and family therapist or an occupational therapist.

Limited liability corporations (LLCs) are also popular choices as business structures for entrepreneurs. They combine the personal liability protection of a corporation with the tax benefits and simplicity of a partnership. In addition, they are more flexible and require less paperwork than corporations require.

Consulting with an accountant or tax attorney prior to beginning your practice can help you avoid potential tax and business pitfalls associated with running your own business.

Office Location

The first decision regarding your office location is whether you will work from home or will locate your office elsewhere in the community. If you base your practice in your home, check with your local zoning board to determine whether there are any restrictions on signs, parking, or storage of supplies. If you plan for clients to enter and leave your home, you may need additional coverage on your homeowner's insurance. Be aware that some insurance companies charge higher rates when pregnant women will be entering and leaving the home.

If you decide to establish a home office, it is important that the consultation take place where the client cannot see or hear family members and where others cannot hear what you and the client discuss. Conversations between you and your clients are confidential, and you do not want to risk others overhearing anything said as part of those dialogues. You may discuss delicate issues such as abuse, rape, and sexually transmitted diseases. For this reason, you will need to establish an environment that is conducive to a mother who chooses to confide such sensitive issues. You will also need bathroom facilities, safe and easy access into and out of your home, and convenient parking. Given these demands, some lactation consultants use their home offices only to conduct business aspects of their practice and see mothers only through home visits.

To create a professional appearance, remove all family items from the area you use for your practice. A few attractively framed pictures of your family may be appropriate on your desk and confer credibility as an experienced mother. Invest in quality framing for your educational credentials, including your IBCLC certification. Framing local awards and certificates of appreciation reflects that you are a committed member of your community. Signs of academic and community achievement will help mothers feel secure in choosing you as a member of their healthcare team.

If you have a busy practice, paperwork and other items can clutter your office. Clear away any clutter before the client arrives so that you present an organized appearance. You can store items in a drawer or closet until after the consultation. You can save time by preparing several client charts ahead of time and giving the client a clipboard containing the consent form and intake form at the beginning of the consultation.

For an off-site setting, a carefully selected location can be your key to a successful practice. You need to be sure that clients will feel comfortable visiting you at this location. You will want good outdoor lighting for evening appointments, security, snow removal, and adequate parking. An office in a commercial building will require rent, insurance, utilities, a business sign, and maintenance. Many commercial offices offer secretarial services for small businesses, including copiers, fax machines, telephones, and voice mail systems. A commercial leasing service can help you determine if this setup is a viable option for your practice. See the earlier discussion of equipment and supplies you will need for consultations.

Marketing Your Practice

After you establish your business structure and location, you need to consider a marketing strategy that will ensure the success of your practice. Decide before you open your practice how busy you want to be. Your life stage may determine the number of clients you want to see on a daily, weekly, or monthly basis. If you have small children or a nursling, you may want to limit your advertising to word-of-mouth to limit your practice to fewer clients. If your children are in school or no longer at home, you might market your services more assertively to attract more clients. Planning for the anticipated response of your target market will help you attract the number of clients you wish for your practice. Talk with other lactation consultants who work in private practice to find out which marketing strategies work best for them. What mistakes did they make that you can avoid? Most lactation consultants will be happy to share their experience in setting up a private practice. Learn from the successes and mistakes of others. You do not have to reinvent the wheel!

Your clients will come primarily from medical referrals, referrals from past clients, and your listing in the telephone directory. Placing an ad in the yellow pages section of your local directory is a good use of your marketing dollars. You may automatically get a listing in the white pages (business pages) and the yellow pages when you install a business telephone line. If so, check with your telephone company to ensure that your listing and category also appear online in the Internet yellow pages. In addition, many IBCLCs establish websites that offer basic breastfeeding information and links to other breastfeeding and parenting sites. IBCLCs who are ILCA members are listed in the association's "Find a Lactation Consultant" database at www.ilca.org.

Contact local practitioners, hospitals clinics, birthing centers, and childbirth educators to acquaint them with the services you provide. Sending letters to such groups and individuals will introduce your services to the community, and making a follow-up visit will allow them the opportunity to ask questions and get to know you. Be sure to keep a file of business cards, noting on the back of the card the date you received it and the circumstances of the contact. Ask for an e-mail address if one does not appear on the business card. Such contacts will prove helpful to you and your clients at various times in your practice.

A press release in your local paper can garner you free publicity. Check with the program director of radio stations in your area as well. Often call-in radio shows (especially healthcare shows) will conduct on-air interviews about breastfeeding and lactation services.

Many aspects of your daily routine as a private practice lactation consultant will provide marketing opportunities. For example, you can meet with physicians and their staff at their offices to confer about clients and to discuss breastfeeding care. Offer to present a free in-service session on breastfeeding to the staff. After you have seen a client, send a report to the physicians involved (usually the pediatrician and the obstetrician). Some circumstances may warrant enclosing a copy of relevant research articles. Such actions will reinforce your credibility as a member of the mother's and infant's healthcare team and increase the likelihood that the physician will refer other mothers to you.

Of course, satisfied clients are the best sources of referrals. Your attention to meeting the needs of mothers in your care will reap marketing benefits as those satisfied clients recommend your services to friends and family and return for help with future babies.

Financial Issues

Private practice will require you to process billing and collect fees. Few private practice lactation consultants have the luxury of relegating this task to another person. Plan a regular time monthly to update your records and mail bills for any outstanding accounts. If you do not have provider status with the mother's insurance carrier, you will want to collect the fee directly from the client rather than from the insurance company. The client can then send your receipt to her insurance company for reimbursement.

You will need to keep a monthly record of all business expenses and income. An inexpensive accounting software program (such as QuickBooks or Quicken) can simplify this process for you, as these programs provide for easy record retention and quick reference. In addition, you may want to use spreadsheets to identify your profits and losses and assist you in business planning. Income records may include items such as consultations and services, rental and sale of breast pumps and other devices, breastfeeding classes, and speaking engagements. It is important to keep track of all expenses related to the business, such as office supplies and equipment, utilities, insurance, educational materials and programs, professional memberships, advertising, donations, and taxes. Software designed specifically for lactation practices is available for this purpose.

Clients need to know what your charges will be before any consultation takes place. When the nature of a telephone call requires a consultation, you can say to the mother, "I will be happy to see you. I have an opening at the following times . . . You will need to be here for about 2 hours and my fee is. . . ." If a mother says she cannot afford your services, it may help her to realize that she is paying the same fee for 1 hour of your time as she does for a 10-minute appointment with her primary caregiver. At that rate, your services are quite a bargain! You can help mothers be comfortable paying for your services by approaching the topic in a self-assured and practical manner.

Third-Party Reimbursement

Be sure to provide clients with appropriate forms with which they can seek reimbursement from their insurance companies. Third-party reimbursement is a legislative and policy issue related to healthcare insurance in the United States. A reimbursement tool kit is available from USLCA, with information about coding, coverage of lactation care and services, filing of claims, and a list of insurance commissioners in each U.S. state (USLCA, 2009).

A three-part carbonless superbill, available from the UCLA Lactation Alumni Association, is designed specifically for reimbursement of lactation consulting services (see Appendix H for contact information). The copy the client submits to her insurance company must include your name and federal tax identification number. The second copy becomes part of the client's records; she can use it as documentation for a tax deduction at the end of the year as a childcare expense if she works outside the home. The third copy is for y~~ou~~

companies require submission of their own insurance forms for reimbursement rather than accepting the superbill. Encourage the client to contact her insurance carrier to learn its requirements.

Figure 2.2 illustrates a sample referral letter from a physician that may be helpful in seeking reimbursement for a breast pump rental. The mother can attach it as a cover letter to her insurer. To facilitate reimbursement, you may choose to attach a physician's prescription requesting your services, dated and made out in the client's name. You may create a form for the physician with information that needs to be reflected on the prescription, including specific ICD-9 (International Classification of Diseases) codes relevant to breastfeeding.

[Date]

To insurance carrier for: [client's name]

Name of policyholder:

Policy number: _____

The following explanation of medical need is provided in order to expedite insurance coverage for the rental of an electric breast pump.

[Name of mother] delivered the high-risk infant [name of baby] on [date]. The child is too immature or ill to nurse directly at the breast. However, it is well established that human milk provides optimal infant nutrition for the first 6 months of life. Thus, the mother of a premature or high-risk newborn is encouraged to pump her breasts in order to supply milk for her hospitalized baby and to maintain lactation until the baby can nurse at the breast.

The intermittent electric breast pump is by far the most efficient, effective, and physiologic means of simulating the sucking action of a normal infant. Inexpensive manual, battery-operated, or small electric breast pumps are an adjunct to milk expression for occasional use when a large intermittent suction pump is unavailable. A piston-type electric breast pump is essential for the maintenance of an adequate milk supply whenever a child is unable to breastfeed normally. Such pumps cost approximately $1,400 and thus are far more economical to rent.

The electric pump will be necessary until the baby is able to take all required nutrition by feeding at the breast. An electric breast pump is not a convenience for the mother; rather it is a medical necessity in the best interest of the child's health.

Sincerely,

[Pediatrician]

FIGURE 2.2   Physician letter for insurance coverage for ~~a~~ breast pump.

Be aware that some codes may apply only if the physician is present for the consultation. Information to include on a prescription includes the following items:

- For a consultation: Consult [your name] for evaluation, assessment, and treatment of [diagnosis and ICD-9 code].
- For breast pump rental: Feed baby mother's milk. Obtain the mother's milk by use of a hospital-grade electric breast pump. Classified as durable medical equipment.
- For breast pump rental: Electric breast pump for treatment of [diagnosis and ICD-9 code].
- For infant feeding supplies: To ensure adequate caloric intake, use a [name of device].

Availability to Clients

As a private practice lactation consultant, you will need to be available to clients at established times. In addition, you will need to arrange coverage for times you are away from your practice. Carefully select the person who will cover for you in your absence. Agree ahead of time how she will respond to clients. You will want to know that she approaches breastfeeding with a philosophy that is compatible with yours. Also, learn whether she has an answering machine and determine any times when the practice may not be covered.

Telephone calls must be able to get through to your office at all times. For this reason, you will need a cell phone, an answering machine, or voice mail. Be aware that you are legally required to respond if a client leaves a message for you.

Maintain a professional demeanor during all telephone contacts with clients, including when you answer the telephone and in the greeting you leave on your answering machine or voice mail. It is helpful in your recorded greeting to ask callers to say their telephone number twice, very clearly, or to ask for two separate telephone numbers. You may receive calls from distraught mothers whose telephone numbers are unintelligible, or not even given. To help with this issue, you may want to add caller ID to your phone service.

If you are unable to see a client because of a personal commitment, simply say that you are unavailable at that time and suggest the next available time. It is unnecessary and unprofessional to explain the reason you are not available. Make sure that family members know not to answer the business telephone.

If your private practice includes visits to mothers' homes, you should equip your car with the necessary supplies and equipment, because you will not be able to run back to your office easily for something you forgot. Be aware that all mothers may not have items you need for teaching positioning, such as footstools or comfortable pillows. Take a cell phone in case you become lost or if you expect to drive to an unsafe neighborhood. Always obtain clear directions to your client's home, including cross streets and landmarks. If your vehicle has a GPS unit, so much the better. If not, use a new map or print a copy of the location from www.mapquest.com or another Internet map service. Verify with your client that it is correct before you leave for your appointment.

Documentation

A signed consent form is important to obtain with every new client. You may wish to include in the consent form a statement granting permission for photographs you might take for teaching purposes. As a courtesy, ask permission again before taking any pictures. You will also want to develop standard assessment forms that elicit the information you need from each client. If you make it a practice to use these forms with all clients, you will avoid forgetting to ask an important question.

At the end of the consultation, you will need to complete a report to the client's physicians, usually the pediatrician and the obstetrician. Schedule time to write the physician's report immediately after the client leaves. Do not consider your consultation completed until you have written and sent this important report. See Chapter 6 for discussion of documenting breastfeeding assessments and writing physician reports.

Lactation consultants in private practice advise keeping records for at least 7 years. This information includes appointment books, client folders, telephone logs, financial records, and receipts. You can place everything for each calendar year in a separate box and label it clearly. If you maintain client files on your computer, be sure to back up these files on another storage medium frequently. Online backup services are available, in which your private data resides on another secure server. At some time in the future, you may need a duplicate of a client's records, financial information for tax reporting, or other such paperwork. Your diligence in retaining files will facilitate locating material when you need it. See Chapter 26 for further discussion of documentation as it relates to legal liability.

∽ Other Members of the Healthcare Team

It is helpful to recognize that parents, nurses, physicians, midwives, and educators all share your goal of ensuring good health for mothers and babies. By keeping current with research and literature from all disciplines that affect lactation and breastfeeding management, you can exchange relevant information with medical professionals and work with them to provide parents with optimal breastfeeding care. Sharing appropriate information among the various disciplines will help broaden your sphere of influence and will be a welcome contribution to your community.

Encourage mothers to participate actively in their care, as their buy-in is integral to the functioning of the healthcare team. Multiple institutional and personal factors lead to inconsistent professional breastfeeding support, an inconsistency intensified by the fact that multiple practitioners assist each mother (Nelson, 2007). These barriers underscore the importance of forming a strong healthcare team and delivering a coordinated effort.

Knowledge Gaps on the Healthcare Team

Research has revealed significant gaps in knowledge among members of the healthcare team. For example, a survey of pediatricians, obstetricians, pediatric nurses, obstetric nurses, breastfeeding triage nurses, public health nurses, WIC personnel, lactation consultants, and peer counselors in the United States revealed gaps in breastfeeding knowledge, counseling skills, and professional education and training (Szucs et al., 2009). A study in Greece revealed that trends in developed countries influenced many health professionals to advocate feeding practices that failed to promote exclusive breastfeeding (Pechlivani et al., 2008).

Nursing education does not adequately prepare its students for helping mothers with breastfeeding (Register et al., 2000; Freed et al., 1996; Anderson, 1991). Pediatric nurse practitioners and nurse midwives, although very supportive of breastfeeding, receive little experience in breastfeeding support and management as part of their educational programs (Hellings & Howe, 2004). For example, a study in Australia demonstrated that although midwives recognized the importance of immediate skin-to-skin contact for newborn infants, few understood its significance for facilitating correct attachment and effective suckling (Cantrill et al., 2004).

When giving information to patients, physicians rely on their background and training in a particular field. Unfortunately, most medical schools devote little, if any, time to the practical management of breastfeeding. Biochemistry or breastfeeding problems of a medical nature are often the focus, rather than practical breastfeeding management and support. An Australian study rated attitudes and knowledge of medical students in their final year of schooling. Those who had more than 26 weeks of personal experience with breastfeeding (self or partner) had higher levels of breastfeeding knowledge, attitudes, confidence, and perceived effectiveness in helping mothers. Notably, those who had negative breastfeeding experiences were more likely to have less positive breastfeeding attitudes than those who had positive experiences. In addition, many lacked sufficient breastfeeding knowledge

for their clinical role and had significant knowledge deficits in all subject areas (Brodribb et al., 2008).

Keeping up with the latest information in journal articles can be difficult in a busy practice. As a result, many physicians rely primarily on conferences, seminars, and the breastfeeding experiences of their families and patients to inform their practice. If these experiences were negative or problematic, it may bias the information and advice they give to patients. In addition, physicians' gender and personal experience with breastfeeding often influence their attitudes and confidence with breastfeeding issues. Brodribb and colleagues (2007) stress that physicians need to learn practical breastfeeding information and skills to assist breastfeeding women, rather than relying on personal or spousal breastfeeding experience.

While physicians generally are aware of the benefits of human milk, their practices often do not reflect an understanding of the day-to-day management of breastfeeding. An Israeli study reported a low level of breastfeeding knowledge among physicians despite a positive disposition toward breastfeeding (Nakar et al., 2007). In a Turkish study, the knowledge level of health professionals did not translate into their own or their spouses' breastfeeding practices (Yaman & Akçam, 2004). An Iraqi study found that primary healthcare physicians had good basic knowledge about the process of breastfeeding but were deficient in problem solving (Al-Zwaini et al., 2008). In addition, research shows that obstetricians tend to be least confident in their ability to resolve problems involving low milk production whereas pediatricians are least confident in their ability to resolve problems involving breast pain or tenderness or cracked or painful nipples (Taveras et al., 2004).

Many physicians welcome research-based information and materials on lactation management. Unfortunately, much of the infant feeding literature that physicians currently receive pertains to the use of artificial formula. Often, the literature they receive about breastfeeding is provided "free" of charge and written by infant formula companies. Physicians need sound, unbiased, evidence-based breastfeeding information from a source that does not have a vested interest in women not breastfeeding. The lactation consultant is an important resource for providing this information to physician practices. The solid knowledge base that lactation consultants provide will benefit a busy physician practice. Chapter 26 provides further discussion of the need for improving breastfeeding education among the members of the mother's healthcare team.

Physicians on the Team

New mothers flourish in their breastfeeding and parenting when they are supported and validated in their decisions. Mothers need to be empowered as parents and welcomed as equal members of their baby's and their own healthcare teams. Physicians are customarily considered the primary member of a mother's healthcare team and, therefore, exert tremendous influence over her practices. Thus supportive physicians with a solid knowledgeable base in breastfeeding can positively influence breastfeeding initiation and continuation.

Some physicians, despite having received training in breastfeeding benefits, fail to support women with practices that promote exclusive breastfeeding (Leavitt et al., 2009). One 2004 survey showed that compared with their peers of 10 years earlier, pediatricians were more likely to consider difficulties or inconvenience associated with breastfeeding to outweigh its benefits, and more failed to believe that almost all mothers are able to breastfeed. Despite these beliefs, more physicians were likely to recommend exclusive breastfeeding and to follow supportive hospital policies than was the case for their predecessors (Barclay, 2008).

Another reason for physician nonsupport is a reluctance to advocate breastfeeding because it may pressure mothers or make them feel guilty about their choice to bottle feed. Adopting a middle-of-the-road stance regarding breastfeeding transmits a message to parents that artificial formula is equally healthy for their infant. Such an ambivalent approach fails to safeguard optimal nutrition and preserve infant health. Parents would not expect their infant's physician to be noncommittal about the importance of immunizations, car seat use, dental checkups, or avoidance of cigarette smoking and other social toxicants—and breastfeeding is no different. The issue of guilt is explored further in Chapter 4.

Physicians need to adopt an approach that protects the continuation of breastfeeding for mothers and babies in their care. Indeed, results of a study in China indicate that healthcare providers need to be more actively involved in educating and motivating mothers and their family members to adopt optimal breastfeeding practices (Shi et al., 2008). When they encounter a problem requiring specialized care, they can be encouraged to refer mothers to an IBCLC. They can also refer mothers to a community group that will provide mother-to-mother support.

Research suggests that support through an early, routine, preventive visit by a trained primary care physician increases breastfeeding efficacy (Labarere et al., 2005). General practitioners are an important resource for breastfeeding women, particularly those who live in rural and remote areas (Brodribb et al., 2007). Some physicians now specialize in breastfeeding support, with several physician-led clinics in the United States specializing in providing outpatient clinical support for breastfeeding-related issues. Physicians in most of these "breastfeeding medicine clinics" also provide primary care services within the same clinical setting (Shaikh, 2008).

Peer Counselors

A reciprocal and cooperative working relationship with breastfeeding counselors and other support people will enhance the effectiveness of any lactation consultant. In addition to WIC peer counselors, who are usually of the same ethnic origin as the other women in the community, lay counselors are available in most communities through mother-to-mother support groups such as La Leche League and Nursing Mothers. Whether the counselor works for an agency or as part of a mother-to-mother support group, you can all cooperate to support women in your community. Peer supporters combined with a breastfeeding support group are an effective way of increasing breastfeeding prevalence in areas characterized by low continuation rates (Ingram et al., 2005).

Several studies have suggested that support groups do not increase breastfeeding significantly (Hoddinott, 2009; MacArthur, 2009; Muirhead et al., 2006). Other studies have reported on the benefits of peer support groups among low-income women in the United States (Ahluwalia et al., 2000; Shaw & Kaczorowski, 1999; Grummer-Strawn et al., 1997). In another study, peer counseling programs were found to help increase breastfeeding among preterm infants (Merewood et al., 2007).

The findings that suggest support groups have no effect on continuation of breastfeeding suggest that a support group, when it operates in isolation, is not effective and demonstrate the multifaceted influences on mothers' decisions to initiate and continue breastfeeding. For example, the median time for mothers to begin participation in the support groups in the Hoddinott study was 5 weeks postpartum, long after the sensitive period in the weeks immediately after the baby's birth, when premature supplementation and weaning take place. Additionally, the support groups were not studied in correlation to the quality of assistance and support at the time of breastfeeding initiation.

The greater effectiveness of support groups reported by other studies was observed when the support groups were combined with practical hands-off teaching and home visits (Hannula et al., 2008), WHO/UNICEF professional training (Britton et al., 2007), and needs-based, one-to-one, informal education before and after the birth by a trained breastfeeding professional or peer counselor (Dyson et al., 2005). Support groups alone do not provide all that mothers need. In establishing a support group intervention, one must study what has worked in the past and design the intervention as part of evidence-based practices.

Mother-to-Mother Support Groups

Mother-to-mother support groups provide a much needed service to women in the community and further the pro-

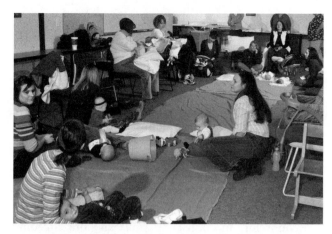

FIGURE 2.3 Mothers and their babies in a support group.
Source: Courtesy of St. John's Hospital, Springfield Illinois.

motion of breastfeeding. Thanks to increasing breastfeeding rates, a majority of babies now leave the hospital being breastfed, either partially or exclusively. Unfortunately, many of these mothers fail to continue breastfeeding because they lack the necessary support and information to do so. Those who have no female relatives or friends to guide their breastfeeding will benefit from the services of a mother-to-mother support group. These groups provide support through written materials, counseling services, regular discussion groups, and special programs (Figure 2.3). They reinforce women's traditional patterns of seeking and receiving advice from relatives and friends. As Wiessinger (2002) notes, mother-to-mother support groups function as "breastfeeding support in its oldest, most enduring form—women learning without pressure, over time, from women they want to emulate."

Research suggests that women find group-based peer coaching to be more empowering than one-to-one coaching. One study concluded, "Groups provided flexibility, a sense of control, and a diversity of visual images and experiences, which assisted women to make feeding-related decisions for themselves, and they offered a safe place to rehearse and perform breastfeeding in front of others, in a culture where breastfeeding is seldom seen in public" (Hoddinott, 2006). Additionally, peer support respects diversity, ensures inclusivity, and stimulates community empowerment (Dykes, 2005).

The goal of a mother-to-mother support group is to educate women about options and to help them make informed choices. Step 10 of the Ten Steps to Successful Breastfeeding guideline created by WHO and UNICEF calls for the establishment of breastfeeding support groups and the referral of mothers to them when they are discharged from the hospital or clinic (WHO, 1989). If a mother-to-mother support group does not exist in your community, you might consider beginning one among the women in your care.

Participating in a support group's activities increases mothers' satisfaction and self-confidence. A support group should accommodate the style and needs of the women and the community it serves. In many communities, breastfeeding support groups need to be more accessible to breastfeeding women (Clifford & McIntyre, 2008). Research continues to document increases in breastfeeding initiation and duration rates as a result of peer counselor support. In addition, researchers have identified increased levels of self-esteem, empowerment, and satisfaction among mothers who receive support from peer counselors (Rossman, 2007). Mutual sharing and observing mothers breastfeed their babies greatly enhance the participants' own breastfeeding and parenting experiences. In one study, mothers who attended a breastfeeding support group more often continued breastfeeding for at least 6 months if they decided to breastfeed after birth, intended to breastfeed for longer than 6 months, had higher monthly household income, and did not smoke during pregnancy (Bosnjak et al., 2008).

Role of the Peer Counselor

Today, many mothers live in a culture where they do not have access to older, experienced family members and friends to support and teach them how to breastfeed. Peer counselors can fill this gap and help to build a culture of breastfeeding (Rossman, 2007). Peer counselors find their role in helping mothers very rewarding (Meier et al., 2007). One of their most valuable services to mothers is the validation and support they provide. Studies show that women tend to deal with their personal stresses by talking about them with others who share or understand their situation. Oxytocin is released when women are affirmed and feel validated, relaxing women and helping to build trust (Brizendine, 2006).

To serve as peer counselors, individuals must acquire training in counseling and breastfeeding care. They can then provide an invaluable service to mothers by offering anticipatory guidance to help mothers learn what to expect, avoid potential problems, and resolve issues before they become unmanageable. Peer counselors are capable of dealing with many types of breastfeeding situations without a background of extensive lactation education. They educate mothers about their options and encourage them to participate actively in decisions about their babies' care. They typically emphasize exclusive breastfeeding for at least 6 months, baby-led weaning, and limited separation of mother and baby. Helping mothers manage breastfeeding and working, supporting early weaning, and other variations in breastfeeding styles that require compromises will reflect counselors' flexibility and acceptance.

Inviting women to mother-to-mother group meetings is an effective form of outreach for advocates of breastfeeding. At group meetings, counselors lead discussion groups and offer support to new mothers, helping them gain a feeling of self-reliance and reassurance. Regular meetings for breastfeeding mothers in the community provide a valuable counseling opportunity. Meeting formats should encourage friendly and informal discussion and provide a supportive environment. Networking and visiting with other mothers are especially effective for mothers who lack contact with other breastfeeding women. The primary factors influencing meetings should be the needs of the women who will be attending. The goal should be to involve mothers as much as possible and help them feel comfortable in taking part, through questions, demonstrations, small-group discussions, and book reviews.

The Lactation Consultant's Role

For the lactation consultant, forging a positive working relationship with peer counselors, the mothers they counsel, and their caregivers contributes to meeting the needs of breastfeeding women in the community. Be careful not to place yourself, counselors, or mothers in opposition to other members of the medical community, as this "us versus them" mentality could discourage healthcare providers from referring mothers to you and diminishes your credibility within the community. Maintaining open communication and cooperation with and between the medical community and breastfeeding counselors is essential, enabling the mother to make decisions based on consistent information from all sources.

Being aware of and involved in the lactation services and support available within your community will help you ensure that mothers receive continuing care and consistent information. In the absence of a community support group, it is especially important that you provide support, follow-up, and appropriate written materials after hospital discharge and whenever new mothers experience difficulty. You might also help develop a mother-to-mother support group, train group leaders, and make yourself available as a resource to the group. Other ways to actively reach out to women include speaking at childbirth classes and clinics, sharing information with professionals, and visiting high school health classes.

The services you offer to mother-to-mother support groups generally will be voluntary, but the value of the ensuing good public relations often outweighs the drawbacks of foregoing monetary gain. Judge each service according to its impact and the scope of your commitment when deciding whether to charge a fee. By working with other members of the community as a team, you can present a unified program of support to breastfeeding mothers.

The following suggestions may increase your effectiveness as well as that of the mother-to-mother support group:

- Maintain a reciprocal referral system whereby you refer mothers to the support group for continuing outreach support and the support group, in return, refers mothers to you and other IBCLCs when a special situation requires a higher level of expertise. This system ensures that a greater number of mothers receive necessary support and information.

- Ensure that the support group provides quality counseling and accurate information by training its peer counselors in counseling skills and breastfeeding information. It is important that the support and education they offer to mothers is consistent with your philosophy and approach. You can offer continuing education in the form of study nights, seminars, and workshops; be available as an advisor and stand ready to answer questions from counselors; and review written materials for counselors and parents.

- Assist with support group activities, offer to speak at parent or counselor meetings, and help organize outreach programs run by the group. Encourage community programs that address both parents and the medical community.

- Assist as a liaison between the support group and the medical community. Maintain two-way communication when mothers have problems, and keep both physicians and the support group informed.

∼ The Mother's Role on the Healthcare Team

As a lactation consultant, you should encourage mothers to share the positive features of breastfeeding with their physicians. When mothers share what works well for them, they can help modify or change physician attitudes, opinions, and practices. Remind mothers that physicians are usually very busy and may not recall all the details of a situation. As issues arise, a mother can convey her desire to breastfeed and summarize plans previously discussed with caregivers. She and her physician then can decide how to adapt the plans to her present situation.

Mothers need to be assertive and clear when communicating with both their physicians and lactation consultants. Most tend to focus their comments on problems, which could cause physicians to prescribe unnecessary practices for what they perceive to be a mother's concern. If a mother mentions that her baby is fussy, her physician may respond by prescribing a formula supplement, thinking that the mother is worried that she doesn't have enough milk. In reality, she may simply have general questions about caring for a fussy baby and had not considered a correlation between breastfeeding and her baby's fussiness. Mothers need to be clear with the messages they send, and they need to be assertive regarding their wishes.

The Mother's Education

Mothers can learn about breastfeeding through reading, classes, and personal assistance. Your role in the mother's education is to serve as a facilitator who gently guides her, acting as a consultant and using your scientific knowledge and practical experience to nurture and protect the relationship between the mother and her infant.

Several basic elements are important in a comprehensive program of breastfeeding education and support for parents. Ideally, the mother's education begins before or during her pregnancy and continues through the postpartum period. Prenatal and postnatal breastfeeding education and support have been shown to improve breastfeeding initiation and continuation rates (Kutlu et al., 2007). Mothers benefit most from a program that provides the following range of services:

- Prenatal and postpartum classes
- Daily rounds in the hospital
- Assistance with breastfeeding problems before and after hospital discharge
- Routine long-term follow-up
- Telephone warmline for advice and support
- Breastfeeding literature
- Referral to a mother-to-mother support group

Approach to Educating Mothers

Your primary role with mothers is to teach practical information about breastfeeding, point out options, and offer useful suggestions. Explaining why a certain technique works the way it does and giving the mother the reasons behind your suggestions will help her understand them, relate to them, and adapt them to her situation. Educating her in this manner will give her the tools to handle future similar circumstances and to grow in self-confidence. (See the discussion of adult learning in Chapter 4.)

When you share information with mothers, be sure to communicate clearly and simply. Offer the least complicated explanation in lay terms. Relate the information in a friendly and low-key manner, neither overwhelming a mother nor making her appear uninformed. Relate only information that you are certain is up-to-date, correct, and evidence based—not opinion or one person's experience. If your information conflicts with information the mother obtained from another source, check your sources for accuracy and try to help the mother resolve the conflict. Always check your sources if you are uncertain. If

you cannot answer a question, tell the mother you will research it and follow up with her later.

For you to share information effectively, you must thoroughly understand the process of milk production, typical breastfeeding patterns, and factors that may affect them. If you are incorporating lactation consulting into a wider medical role, such as a hospital-based nurse or midwife, you may focus primarily on basic breastfeeding management. You will then need to be aware of potential complications and unusual circumstances, as well as resources for making appropriate referrals. If you are specializing in the lactation field as a board-certified lactation consultant, you will need expertise in more complicated and unusual breastfeeding circumstances.

Whatever the level of breastfeeding care that you deliver, it is important to remain current with relevant literature and practices. Lactation research is dynamic and extensive, and continuing your lactation education will enable you to give appropriate advice to mothers. It is imperative in lactation—as in most fields today—that you become a lifelong learner and embrace change when warranted.

Sharing Medical Information

It is especially important that the information and advice you give to mothers is obtained from a reliable source. Anything beyond the scope of the lactation consultant must be presented in a manner of educating the mother, not prescribing treatment. (This is not the case for those who have prescriptive authority, such as a medical doctor, nurse practitioner, or physician's assistant.) Information on prescription drugs changes frequently based on current research, and you must be sure to have the most up-to-date information when you relate it to mothers. One authoritative source on medications and lactation is *Hale's Medications and Mothers' Milk* (Hale, 2010). When discussing drugs with a mother, always recommend that she consult her baby's physician concerning their advisability. The baby's physician ultimately should have the final decision.

Conflicting Advice and Informed Choice

You can be instrumental in promoting health consumerism and encouraging parents to assume an active role in their family's health care. Of course, some parents may need more guidance than others in assuming this new role. You can assist them by providing options and advice and by suggesting ways in which they can interact with their physicians. Your primary function in this regard is to coordinate the mother's breastfeeding care and empower her to breastfeed with minimal intervention or complications.

In recent years, great strides have been made in family-centered maternity care and breastfeeding. Nevertheless, the breastfeeding advice you give in some situations may conflict with the advice given by other healthcare providers. This disagreement is not necessarily a sign that one side is incorrect, but rather reflects the fact that there are a variety of medical opinions concerning obstetrics and pediatrics. You can present information to the mother and urge her to make her own choices and to work toward suitable solutions with her physicians. When your guidance contradicts that of the physician, it can cause confusion and concern for the mother. Acknowledge this conflict and help the mother to develop a plan.

When a conflict exists, parents must resolve it with their other caregivers. Take care to avoid alienating people in your medical community. In some cases, you may communicate directly with the mother's or baby's physician. At other times, you may share information with the mother that she, in turn, will discuss with her physician. Polite assertiveness, a positive attitude, and a willingness to work with the physician to resolve the conflict to everyone's mutual satisfaction will strengthen the parents' position. Informing and educating parents places this responsibility on them. If parents fail to accept this active role, recognize that you have fulfilled your responsibility of informing them of their options, whether or not you agree with their decisions. See Chapter 4 for further discussion of health consumerism and informed consent.

∽ Summary

The professional lactation consultant has a variety of employment options. Each particular work setting differs from others in many ways. A constant thread among all settings is the role of the lactation consultant as part of a strong healthcare team that provides consistent care to mothers as they establish breastfeeding. Mothers who receive support from a strong healthcare team will be empowered to participate in decision making as informed health consumers. Whether you work in a hospital, clinic, physician group, home health care, or private practice, a commitment to breastfeeding mothers and babies is the driving force behind all lactation consultations. Volunteer counselors continue to play a valuable role in the mother's support. You can help coordinate this care by maintaining a reciprocal relationship with community support groups.

∽ Chapter 2—At a Glance

Facts you learned—

Members of the healthcare team:

- Mothers share positive aspects of breastfeeding with physicians.
- Physicians empower parents as equal members of the healthcare team.

- IBCLCs provide lactation expertise:
  - Read research and literature, and use evidence-based materials.
  - Refer mothers to support groups.
  - Teach prenatal and postpartum classes.
  - Share medical information appropriately.
  - Help mothers sort through conflicting advice.
  - Teach and advise peer counselors.

IBCLCs in hospital practice:

- Make rounds with mothers.
- Provide inpatient and staff education.
- Provide equipment and supplies for mothers.
- Establish a hospital-based lactation program.

IBCLCs in WIC programs:

- Serve low-income mothers and infants.
- Counsel mothers with cultural, socioeconomic, and lifestyle differences.
- Teach classes and facilitate support groups.
- Teach and supervise peer counselors.

IBCLCs in a physician practice:

- See both healthy mothers and babies and those experiencing difficulties with breastfeeding.
- Have patient loads that depend on the physician's patient load.
- Teach classes and facilitate support group.
- Meet pregnant women.
- Make rounds in hospital.
- Provide follow-up calls and a warmline.

IBCLCs in home health care:

- Follow up with mothers after discharge.
- Assess the mother, baby, and breastfeeding.
- Provide anticipatory guidance on long-term issues.

IBCLCs in private practice:

- Are typically seasoned IBCLCs with extensive experience.
- Establish a small business and obtain office and lactation equipment.
- Market the practice and establish a referral base.
- Bill for services and facilitate third-party reimbursement.
- Provide office and home visits and telephone follow-up.
- Document consultations, send physician reports, and retain records.

～ References

Ahluwalia IB, et al. Georgia's breastfeeding promotion program for low-income women. *Pediatrics*. 2000;105:E85l.

Al-Zwaini EJ, et al. Knowledge of Iraqi primary healthcare physicians about breastfeeding. *East Mediterr Health J*. 2008; 14(2):381-388.

American Academy of Pediatrics (AAP). *Children's health topics*. 2009. www.medicalhomeinfo.org. Accessed April 28, 2009.

Anderson E, Geden E. Nurses' knowledge of breastfeeding. *JOGNN*. 1991;20(1):58-63.

Barclay L. Pediatrician promotion of breast-feeding among their patients has declined. *Arch Pediatr Adolesc Med*. 2008;162: 1142-1149.

Bornmann PG. A legal primer for lactation consultants. In: International Lactation Consultant Association; Mannel R, Martens PJ, Walker M, eds. *Core Curriculum for Lactation Consultant Practice*. 2nd ed. Sudbury, MA: Jones and Bartlett; 2008:159-190.

Bosnjak AP, et al. Influence of sociodemographic and psychosocial characteristics on breastfeeding duration of mothers attending breastfeeding support groups. *J Perinat Med*. 2008;37(2):185-192.

Britton C, et al. Support for breastfeeding mothers. *Cochrane Database System Rev*. 2007;1:CD001141.

Brizendine L. *The Female Brain*. New York: Morgan Road Books/ Random House; 2006.

Brodribb WE, et al. Gender and personal breastfeeding experience of rural GP registrars in Australia: a qualitative study of their effect on breastfeeding attitudes and knowledge. *Rural Remote Health*. 2007;7(3):737.

Brodribb W, et al. Breastfeeding and Australian GP registrars: their knowledge and attitudes. *J Hum Lact*. 2008;24(4):422-430.

Cantrill R, et al. Midwives' knowledge of newborn feeding ability and reported practice managing the first breastfeed. *Breastfeed Rev*. 2004;12(1):25-33.

Clifford J, McIntyre E. Who supports breastfeeding? *Breastfeed Rev*. 2008;16(2):9-19.

Dykes F. Government funded breastfeeding peer support projects: implications for practice. *Matern Child Nutr*. 2005; 1(1):21-31.

Dyson L, et al. Interventions for promoting the initiation of breastfeeding. *Cochrane Database System Rev*. 2005;2: CD001688.

Fooladi M. A comparison of perspectives on breastfeeding between two generations of black American women. *J Am Acad Nurse Pract*. 2001;13(1):34-38.

Freed G, et al. Methods and outcomes of breastfeeding instruction for nursing students. *J Hum Lact*. 1996;12:105-110.

Gross LJ. *Statistical Report of the 2009 IBLCE Examination*. International Board of Lactation Consultant Examiners; 2009. www.iblce.org. Accessed May 6, 2010.

Grummer-Strawn LM, et al. An evaluation of breastfeeding promotion through peer counseling in Mississippi WIC clinics. *Matern Child Health J*. 1997;1:35-42.

Hale T. *Medications and Mothers' Milk*. Amarillo, TX: Hale Publishing; 2010.

Hannula L, et al. A systematic review of professional support interventions for breastfeeding. *J Clin Nurs*. 2008;17:1132-1143.

Hellings P, Howe C. Breastfeeding knowledge and practice of pediatric nurse practitioners. *J Pediatr Healthcare*. 2004;18: 8-14.

Hoddinott P, et al. Effectiveness of policy to provide breastfeeding groups (BIG) for pregnant and breastfeeding mothers in primary care: cluster randomised controlled trial. *BMJ*. 2009;30:338.

Hoddinott P, et al. One-to-one or group-based peer support for breastfeeding? Women's perceptions of a breastfeeding peer coaching intervention. *Birth*. 2006;33(2):139-146.

Ingram J, et al. Breastfeeding peer supporters and a community support group: evaluating their effectiveness. *Matern Child Nutr*. 2005;1(2):111-118.

International Lactation Consultant Association (ILCA). 2009. www.ilca.org. Accessed February 15, 2009.

Kutlu R, et al. Assessment of effects of pre- and post-training programme for healthcare professionals about breastfeeding. *J Health Popul Nutr*. 2007;25(3):382-386.

Labarere J, et al. Efficacy of breastfeeding support provided by trained clinicians during an early, routine, preventive visit: a prospective, randomized, open trial of 226 mother–infant pairs. *Pediatrics*. 2005;115(2):e139-e146. http://pediatrics .aappublications.org/cgi/content/abstract/115/2/e139.

Leavitt G, et al. Knowledge about breastfeeding among a group of primary care physicians and residents in Puerto Rico. *J Community Health*. 2009;34(1):1-5.

Lukac M, et al. How to integrate a lactation consultant in an outpatient clinic environment. *J Hum Lact*. 2006;22(1):99-103.

MacArthur C, et al. Antenatal peer support workers and breastfeeding initiation: cluster randomised controlled trial. *BMJ*. 2009;338:b131.

Mannel R, et al. (eds.). *Core Curriculum for Lactation Consultant Practice*. 2nd ed. Sudbury, MA: Jones and Bartlett; 2008.

Mannel R, Mannel R. Staffing for hospital lactation programs: recommendations from a tertiary care teaching hospital. *J Hum Lact*. 2006;22(4):409-417.

McDowell M, et al. *NCHS Data Brief Number 5: Breastfeeding in the United States: Findings from the National Health and Nutrition Examination Survey, 1999–2006*. U.S. Department of Health and Human Services (USDHHS), Centers for Disease Control and Prevention (CDC), National Center for Health Statistics (NCHS); April 2008. www.cdc.gov/nchs/data/databriefs/db05.htm. Accessed July 21, 2009.

Meier E, et al. A qualitative evaluation of a breastfeeding peer counselor program. *J Hum Lact*. 2007;23(3):262-268.

Merewood A, et al. The effect of peer counselors on breastfeeding rates in the neonatal intensive care unit: results of a randomized controlled trial. *J Pediatr*. 2007;150(3):318.

Muirhead PE, et al. The effect of a programme of organised and supervised peer support on the initiation and duration of breastfeeding: A randomised trial. *Br J Gen Pract*. 2006;56 (524):191-197.

Nakar S, et al. Attitudes and knowledge on breastfeeding among paediatricians, family physicians, and gynaecologists in Israel. *Acta Paediatr*. 2007;96(11):1712-1713.

Nelson AM. Maternal–newborn nurses' experiences of inconsistent professional breastfeeding support. *J Adv*. 2007;60 (1):29-38.

Pechlivani F, et al. Infant feeding and professional advice in the first half of the 20th century in Greece. *Breastfeed Rev.* 2008;16(3):23-28.

Register N, et al. Knowledge and attitudes of pediatric office nursing staff about breastfeeding. *J Hum Lact.* 2000;16:210-215.

Rossman B. Breastfeeding peer counselors in the United States: helping to build a culture and tradition of breastfeeding. *J Midwifery Women's Health.* 2007;52(6):631-637.

Rubin R. Attainment of the maternal role. *Nurs Res.* 1957;16(3): 237-245.

Shaikh U, Smillie CM. Physician-led outpatient breastfeeding medicine clinics in the United States. *Breastfeed Med.* 2008; 3(1):28-33.

Shaw E, Kaczorowski J. The effect of a peer counseling program on breastfeeding initiation and longevity in a low-income rural population. *J Hum Lact.* 1999;15(1)19-25.

Shi L, et al. Breastfeeding in rural China: association between knowledge, attitudes, and practices. *J Hum Lact.* 2008;24 (4):377-385.

Shinwell ES, et al.The effect of training nursery staff in breast-feeding guidance on the duration of breastfeeding in healthy term infants. *Breastfeed Med.* 2006;1(4):247-252.

Szucs KA, et al. Breastfeeding knowledge, attitudes, and prac-tices among providers in a medical home. *Breastfeed Med.* 2009;4(1):31-42.

Taveras EM, et al. Clinician support and psychosocial risk fac-tors associated with breastfeeding discontinuation. *Pedi-atrics.* 2003;112(1 Pt 1):108-115.

Taveras EM, et al. Opinions and practices of clinicians associated with continuation of exclusive breastfeeding. *Pediatrics.* 2004;113(4): e283-e290. http://pediatrics.aappublications .org/cgi/content/abstract/113/4/e283?maxtoshow=&HITS= 10&hits=10&RESULTFORMAT=&fulltext=breastfeeding +lactatiom&searchid=1&FIRSTINDEX=0&sortspec= relevance&resourcetype=HWCIT.

Thurman SE, Allen PJ. Integrating lactation consultants into primary healthcare services: are lactation consultants affecting breastfeeding success? *Pediatr Nurs.* 2008;34(5): 419-425.

United States Department of Agriculture (USDA), Food and Nutrition Services. Women, Infants and Children: Fre-quently asked questions. 2009. www.fns.usda.gov/wic. Ac-cessed February 17, 2009.

United States Department of Health and Human Services (USD-HHS), Centers for Disease Control and Prevention (CDC). *Pediatric Nutrition Surveillance 2007 Report.* January 2009a. www.cdc.gov/pednss/pdfs/PedNSS_2007.pdf. Ac-cessed July 23, 2009.

United States Department of Health and Human Services (USD-HHS), Centers for Disease Control and Prevention (CDC). *Breastfeeding Among U.S. Children Born 1999–2006, CDC National Immunization Survey.* July 28, 2009b. www.cdc .gov/breastfeeding/data/NIS_data. Accessed July 23, 2009.

United States Lactation Consultant Association (USLCA). 2009. www.uslca.org. Accessed February 15, 2009.

Wiessinger D. On behalf of breastfeeding: last step first. *Cur Iss Clin Lact.* 2002:69-73.

World Health Organization (WHO). *Protecting, prompting, and supporting breastfeeding: A joint WHO/UNICEF statement.* Geneva: WHO; 1989.

Yaman H, Akçam M. Breastfeeding practices of health profes-sionals and care workers in Turkey. *Collegium Antropo-logicum.* 2004;28(2):877-844.

A Sociological Perspective on Breastfeeding Support

The norms and perceptions of society determine much of what transpires in the context of breastfeeding promotion and support. This chapter explores breastfeeding support from a sociological perspective, including insights into the needs of breastfeeding women and the most effective strategies to help them meet those needs. Awareness of social thinking and social behavior will help you, as a lactation consultant, understand women's perceptions and processing of breastfeeding information and media messages. These insights will, in turn, enhance your interactions with mothers and the assistance you provide.

Auguste Comte conceived the new academic discipline of "sociology" in 1838 as a formal study of society. The term comes from two Latin words, *socius* and *-logia*, reflecting the scientific study of human society and social interactions (Tischler, 2006). Sociology examines the history, development, organization, and problems of people living together as social groups. It is a scientific study of social behavior, thought, and the manner in which we depend upon, interact with, influence, and are influenced by others.

∼ Key Terms

Attachment
Attitude
Attribution
Behavior
Bonding
Cognitive learning
Compliance
Conformity
Culture
Decision making
Demographics
Empowerment
Ethics
Evidence-based practice
Group behavior

Intention
Involvement theory
Motivation
Perception
Primary groups
Retention and recall
Role
Secondary groups
Self-efficacy
Self-image
Sensory input
Social marketing
Social thinking
Split-brain theory
Status

∼ Organization of a Society

A society is defined as a collection of people who share a common culture, territory, and identity. This commonality binds people together through relationships and interactions. The pattern of these relationships forms the social structure of a society. Culture, status, roles, groups, organizations, social institutions, and community are all elements of this social structure.

Culture

Culture involves all that we learn in the course of social life and transmit across generations. It is the "learned, socially transmitted heritage of artifacts, knowledge, beliefs, values, and normative expectations that provides the members of a particular society with the tools for coping with recurrent problems" (Goodman, 1992). Culture shapes and structures social life by defining the foods we eat, the clothes we wear, the language we speak, the values and beliefs we hold, and the practices we follow. Societies differ in their values and in the norms that define appropriate behavior. Such cultural diversity demonstrates the flexibility and variability of human conditions.

Subcultures are individual groups within a culture that vary by social class, ethnicity, race, religion, lifestyle, goals, and interests. The identity of a subculture may revolve around its ethnic heritage, economic circumstance, or geographic region. A subculture often has a distinctive language and form of communication. We tend to evaluate others' customs, practices, and behaviors in light of our own culture and experience. At the same time, we need to understand each cultural practice in terms of its place in the larger cultural context. Social values correspond to each individual subculture that exists within society. We cannot easily dismiss the worth of practices within a subculture merely based on what we consider to be "right" and "wrong." Rather, we need to approach and assess each culture individually and with an open mind.

When working with people from cultures different from your own, it can be easy to dismiss certain dietary or infant care practices as unimportant or senseless. For the mother in that culture, however, these practices may carry deep meaning or reflect familial tradition, and thus may contribute positively to her breastfeeding and overall mothering identity. Some cultures promote beneficial practices such as carrying a baby close, breastfeeding on demand, and long-term breastfeeding. Some believe that pinning a band around the baby's abdomen will prevent an umbilical hernia; such a practice is not harmful to the baby and does not need to change. The custom of restricting the mother's consumption of fresh fruit for several weeks postpartum may have some effect on her nutritional status. The belief that colostrum is harmful to the baby leads to delaying breastfeeding in some cultures until the mother's milk changes to mature milk—a practice that can affect the baby's health and the establishment of breastfeeding.

The degree to which a mother merges into a new culture depends on how firmly she clings to traditional values. Mothers who wish to integrate their families into Western culture may perceive artificial infant milk to be the desired method of infant feeding. Despite the fact that breastfeeding is the norm in their native culture, they may choose to formula feed in an attempt to fit into their new surroundings. Chapter 20 explores cultural issues related to breastfeeding.

Status

We tend to think of status in terms of prestige, wealth, or power. In a sociological context, status refers to a person's position within a network of social relationships. Status may denote a place in the family, such as mother, father, daughter, or son. It can also refer to a position in the workplace, religious community, or other segment of society. The social statuses people occupy strongly influence the aspects of a culture they will experience. Although everyone occupies a variety of statuses within their social structure, people tend to identify themselves through one "master" status. Men traditionally define themselves in terms of their occupation. Women traditionally have defined themselves as mothers.

Definitions of self tend to evolve in response to societal changes. Over the past several decades, women in Western culture increasingly define themselves through their professional role in society rather than their personal role within the family. It is important to consider this trend in your interactions with working mothers. When working with a professional woman who plans to return to work, it will help to recognize that she has invested heavily in her career. She may have conflicting feelings about leaving her baby versus losing her career "momentum." Acknowledging these conflicts and helping the mother explore her reservations will empower her both as a mother and in her career.

Our motivations and goals change from childhood to old age as each season of our lives unfolds. The encouragement you can offer mothers to sequence their seasons of life may be a refreshing "new" thought for women who are merging motherhood with a career. By understanding this cultural dynamic, you will be able to tailor your approach and sensitively help women meet their needs and reach their breastfeeding goals.

The findings of a Swedish study confirm that socioeconomic status influences breastfeeding duration. In this study, maternal educational level, maternal unemployment benefits, social welfare, and equivalent disposable income were strongly associated with breastfeeding when examined individually in mothers of preterm and term infants (Flacking et al., 2007). An Australian study found that, although overall breastfeeding rates during a 10-year period remained unchanged, there was a significant disparity in breastfeeding rates based on socioeconomic level. The study found a wide gap in breastfeeding rates between the most and least disadvantaged families (Amir & Donath, 2008), with the highest rates of breastfeeding being observed among the most advantaged families.

Role

Social status determines our expectations and behavior and the resulting societal roles. Role differs from status in that a person occupies a status and performs a role within that status. Individuals who occupy the status of parent, for instance, hold certain values regarding the importance of children. Parents are subject to specific norms regarding the obligation to provide their children with emotional, physical, and financial support—these are their role expectations. The manner in which they perform their parental role (i.e., their role behavior) reflects on their status as a parent.

Parental norms vary widely between subcultures. Bottle feeding is very much the norm among minority populations within the United States. Some immigrants consider the ability to provide formula as a status symbol, and the breastfeeding they would have done at home is denigrated. Well-educated, upper-middle-class, older parents tend to regard breastfeeding as the biologically superior way to feed infants. The expectation to breastfeed or at least "try" to do so is a part of their parental status.

Groups and Organizations

The set of expectations shared by people with a common status and role forms the basis of their interactions with one another. Most activities take place in the context of groups such as families, teams, peer groups, and work groups. Social life, therefore, is group life. Members of a group have a sense of shared identity. This group membership may be figurative, or it may exist within an organized structure. By definition, an organization is a group created specifically to carry out a particular task. It has a formal structure through which it attempts to accomplish that task.

When a young couple begins a family, they become parents and, therefore, part of the peer group of other parents, whether formally or informally. Many first-time parents bond with other parents in their childbirth education classes. Indeed, they may seek the company of other new parents. They may judge their parenting abilities against those of other parents. They may join a parenting group or a playgroup with their children. They may desire the formal structure of a parenting class, with specific goals for learning parenting skills. All of these group identities are important to the couple's perceptions of themselves as parents and to the manner in which they perform their parental role.

Mothers who join breastfeeding support groups often form long-term intimate friendships with other mothers who are also adapting to the parental role. One study found that mothers tend to rate social support as more important than health service support. Health service support was described unfavorably because of time pressures, lack of availability of healthcare professionals or guidance, promotion of unhelpful practices, and delivery of conflicting advice (McInnes & Chambers, 2008).

Social Institutions

Statuses, roles, and groups combine to form social institutions. Most societies are composed of five major institutions: economy, education, family, politics, and religion. A social institution has relatively stable clusters of values, norms, statuses, roles, social groups, and organizations that relate to a specific area of human activity. The institution of education, for example, satisfies society's need to provide its members with a basic set of knowledge and skills enabling them to function in society.

Major institutions tend to be founded based on similar norms, values, and goals. As a consequence, when a change occurs in one institution, it usually triggers a change in others. Family structure, relationships, and mobility, for example, have all changed tremendously over the past century. This transformation of the family represents a social change that has affected the nature of society as well as each person's childhood and adult experiences (Tischler, 2006). Attitudes, beliefs, and values all play roles in future societal changes.

Recognizing the interdependence among social institutions can provide insights into determining the needs of mothers and their families. For example, when working with a mother who is a member of a religious community, it will help you to understand that the high value placed on the family by the mother's community of faith will support her desire to stay home with her children, and probably to breastfeed.

Community

As a social group, a community shares an identity, a structured pattern of interaction, and a common geographical territory. The geographic proximity of community members enhances the frequency of their interactions as well as the consequences of those interactions. The demographic study of a population takes into account social, cultural, and environmental factors that influence behavior and change. The population within a particular community is a key defining element in its social structure and culture.

Understanding a community's demographics will assist you in framing your interactions with families within that community. Most large population centers contain great diversity in family subcultures. An awareness of your city's characteristics will enhance your sensitivity to your clients' cultural beliefs. For example, a burgeoning East Indian population can be found in many U.S. cities. Educating yourself about Indian beliefs concerning childbirth and breastfeeding will help you establish credibility with the Indian mothers you serve. For example, it is considered polite to remove your shoes when entering an Indian home. Members of this culture prepare special foods for the postpartum mother and keep both mother and baby warm. The paladai—a cup feeding device—has been used to feed babies in India for many years and is sometimes used in the Western world as well (Sideman, 1999).

If you are unsure about a cultural practice, do not hesitate to ask your client. Most families are receptive to explaining cultural practices to people who are sincerely interested.

⌒ The Process of Socialization

Scholars continue to argue over the issue of "nature versus nurture," questioning whether our identity and behavior are determined biologically or by our social experiences. We all enter the world as potentially social beings dependent on others for survival. Both heredity and environment then contribute to the development of the person we become. Society teaches each new member how to think, feel, and live. This is the essence of socialization. Through social interaction, we develop an identity, a set of beliefs, and a range of skills that allow us to participate in society.

The process of socialization maintains social order. Socialization is a lifelong process in which our social development progresses through a series of stages. The quality of intellectual, social, and emotional behavior at one stage of development differs fundamentally from the next stage. Over the life course, families, schools, and other socializing institutions instill socially acceptable values into the members of the society.

Those who go against the majority opinion and challenge the dominant system of ideas are often deemed rebellious and perhaps even radical. Sometimes, however, a challenge to a practice or set of beliefs evolves into a movement that creates real change. Such is the case with promotional efforts to empower women to breastfeed in a climate that embraces bottle feeding. This challenge is also evident in many cultures when women breastfeed their children beyond the first year.

Social Thinking

Social behavior usually begins with social cognition—that is, social thinking. Most behavior results from deliberation, judgment, beliefs, and expectations. Through cognition, we form inferences from social information before we act. The study of cognition involves the manner in which we acquire, organize, and use knowledge and information, or data. It focuses primarily on perception, attention, memory, thought, and language. Within a social context, social thinking is a study of how we perceive, react to, and remember things about ourselves and other people. It encompasses how different social situations influence our thinking process, how we perceive ourselves, and how we form impressions of others.

People rarely collect social data with a truly open mind. Instead, our life experiences invariably lead us to have certain expectations that help us sift through new information. These expectations can bias our interpretations, especially if they are based on few or unique experiences. Additionally, negative expectations can cause us to reject the opportunity to collect new information. To arrive at a meaningful conclusion, we must recognize that prior expectations influence our beliefs and actions. We must select from among the data we collect, and judge whether information is or is not relevant and useful.

The integration of our prior expectations and experiences helps us to interpret our social environment and evaluate new experiences and social encounters. Recognizing the effects of this cognitive process on those whom you counsel will help you to devise effective helping strategies. In a primarily bottle feeding culture such as the United States and other developed countries, a young woman might react with distaste or discomfort when she sees a mother breastfeeding a toddler or older child in public. Her perceptions are based on a cultural belief of breasts as sexual objects, as evidenced by the preponderance of such images transmitted through print media, commercials, television programs, movies,

and the Internet. Consequently, she may view breastfeeding as a sexual act, not a biological act of love and nurturing, and consider it inappropriate in public or with an older child.

Social policies that affect educational attainment may be important factors in breastfeeding. One California study reported that breastfeeding rates may be influenced by health education specifically or by more general levels of schooling among mothers and their partners (Heck et al., 2006). Another study demonstrated a positive association between breastfeeding duration, a mother's level of educational attainment, and her breastfeeding knowledge (Kronborg & Vaeth, 2004). High levels of knowledge were associated with long duration of breastfeeding among primiparous mothers, but this association was not found among multiparous mothers.

Women in a U.S. WIC population (i.e., those receiving benefits from the Women, Infants, and Children nutritional program) who intended to breastfeed had higher levels of breastfeeding knowledge, reported fewer barriers to breastfeeding, and demonstrated greater self-efficacy (Mitra et al., 2004). Given the clear relationship between knowledge and behavior related to breastfeeding, interventions should focus on improving breastfeeding knowledge, enhancing confidence in the ability to breastfeed, and overcoming barriers. Further, targeting breastfeeding initiatives toward low-income, less educated mothers who lack breastfeeding support from their loved ones may improve breastfeeding rates among urban first-time mothers (Persad & Mensinger, 2008).

Cognitive Learning

Learning is the process by which we acquire knowledge and experience that we apply to future related behavior. Newly acquired knowledge combines with experience to serve as feedback and influence future behavior in similar situations. The process of learning ranges from the most simple, almost reflexive responses to abstract concepts and complex problem solving.

When confronted with a problem, we sometimes see the solution instantly. More often, however, we are likely to search for information on which to base a decision and then carefully evaluate what we learn so that we can make the best decision. This is the essence of cognitive learning. The process of problem solving enables us to gain some control over our environment and is pivotal to producing the desired response.

For learning to occur, four basic elements must be present: motivation, cues, response, and reinforcement. The learning process begins with a personal need or goal that is unmet. The motivation to satisfy this need or goal acts as a stimulus to learning. The degree to which we are actively involved in learning will depend on our level of motivation. Cues are the stimuli that give direction to our motives and guide our actions toward the desired outcome. The way we respond to these cues—in other words, how we behave—constitutes our response. The response we choose depends greatly on both previous learning and responses reinforced in the past. Reinforcement increases the likelihood of a specific future response as the result of particular cues or stimuli. Such repetition increases the strength of the association and slows the process of forgetting.

For a new mother, learning how to hold her baby at the breast and practicing that positioning with the assistance of a skilled caregiver enables her to hone her technique. The new mother will become increasingly more confident with each successive feeding as she is able to anticipate and respond to her baby's cues. When a mother responds to her baby's hunger cues by putting him or her to the breast, she teaches her baby to anticipate that she will meet his or her needs for food and comfort. It also reinforces the mother's future nurturing of her child. The repetition of breastfeeding throughout the child's nursing years reinforces the child's learning of parental concern and a mother's learning to put the child's welfare ahead of her own. This helps to set the pattern for lifelong maternal love and selflessness.

Processing Information

The human mind processes information it receives as input in much the same way as a computer processes data. The manner in which the brain processes information depends on two factors: our cognitive ability and the complexity of the information to be processed. For instance, our ability to form mental images influences the degree to which we can recall information. Differences in the way we process images, in turn, reflects our preference for and frequency of both visual and verbal processing. Figure 3.1 illustrates the process of receiving and retrieving sensory input, using an example of showing a mother how to position her baby at the breast.

Receiving and Storing Information

Processing information occurs in stages. To begin, a series of memory "storehouses" in the brain temporarily collect information. The image of a sensory input lasts for only 1 or 2 seconds in the mind's sensory store. It is lost immediately if it is not processed and transferred to the short-term store. The short-term store constitutes the working memory, where information is processed and held for a brief period. The amount of information that can be held in short-term storage is limited to four or five items. At this stage, the information will be lost in approximately 30 seconds unless it is mentally repeated through the process of rehearsal. Information we rehearse is transferred to the long-term store within 2 to 10 seconds. We can retain the information that is placed in long-term storage for days, weeks, or even years.

Retention and Recall of Information

The degree to which we repeat information or relate it to other data greatly affects retention. Rehearsal enables us to hold information in short-term storage long enough for encoding to take place. When we encode information, we select a word or visual image to represent an object we have perceived. Although both verbal and visual images are important in forming an overall mental image, verbal images take less time to learn than visual images (Goodman, 1992). Thus one-on-one assistance with a breastfeeding mother produces better retention than just asking the mother to watch a how-to video.

Information can be lost when the short-term store receives a great deal of input at the same time, which reduces its capacity to only two or three pieces of information. When we receive too much information—a situation referred to as information overload—we find it difficult to encode and store it all. The result of this overload is confusion, less effective choices, and poor decision making. In the vulnerable immediate postpartum period, most parents receive an overwhelming amount of instruction on all aspects of maternal and infant care. This makes it unlikely the mother can even locate the breastfeeding information, much less process any of it!

Information in long-term storage is constantly organized and reorganized as new links are forged between chunks of information. As we gain more knowledge, we expand the network of relationships between data and sometimes are motivated to search for additional information. This process of activation relates new data to old data, thereby making the retained information more meaningful. Along the way, the data that we have already encoded may be re-encoded to include larger amounts of information.

Encounters with chunks of information that do not match our frame of reference and prior knowledge hamper retention and recall. We are more likely to spend time interpreting and elaborating on information we find relevant to our needs, re-encoding this information and thus activating such relevant knowledge from long-term memory. Retrieval is the process by which we recover this information. When the retrieval system fails, forgetting takes place. New mothers often find it difficult to recall specific instructions regarding breastfeeding. Reinforcing verbal instruction with written materials and other visual aids will provide the necessary support at this time of change and confusion.

Involvement and Relevance

The way we process information depends on how relevant it is to us and our level of involvement. High involvement

**Sensory input is received: Mother is shown how to position her baby at the breast.
Input collects in the SENSORY STORE, where it is stored for 1–2 seconds.**

When It Works	Why It Works	When Things Go Wrong	
Input is *processed* within 1–2 seconds. ⇩	Mother is alert. It is a teachable moment. Mother is motivated.	Input is not processed in time. ⇒	Information is lost immediately.
Input transfers to the *short-term store* and is retained for 30 seconds. ⇩	Process is described and demonstrated with a doll while mother brings baby to breast.	**Why It Went Wrong** Mother is tired or in pain. Mother lacks motivation. Mother is distracted.	

When It Works	Why It Works	When Things Go Wrong	
Input is *rehearsed* within 30 seconds. ⇩	Mother practices putting her baby to breast. Mother is given assistance and support in the early days.	Input is not rehearsed in time. ⇒	Information is not retained.
		Why It Went Wrong Mother doesn't do a return demonstration. No one visits to reinforce. Mother forgets important features.	

When It Works	Why It Works	When Things Go Wrong	
Less than 5–6 items of input are received and rehearsed. ⇩	Mother is given printed and verbal instructions about what to expect in the first week: frequency, duration, feeding cues, number of stools and voids.	More than 5–6 items of input are received and rehearsed within 30 seconds. ⇒	Information overload. Information is not retained. Confusion takes place. Less effective choices. Poor decision making.

RESULT FOR MOTHER
⬇
Mother has a solid grasp of basic management.

Mother is ready to focus on additional factors for the next several months.

Why It Went Wrong
Mother is given 2 pages of printed and verbal instructions that include:
  frequency, duration, feeding cues, number of stools and voids, what to eat, various positions for holding the baby at feedings, how to end a feeding, how to soothe a fussy baby, what to do about leaking, how to treat sore nipples and engorgement, when to start supplements, how and when to wean, how to express milk, how to manage breastfeeding and returning to work, how to increase milk production, and how to nurse in public.

Input is *encoded*.
⇩
Input transfers within 10 seconds to *long-term store*, where 2–3 items are retained for days, weeks, or years.
⇩

Activation of input takes place to:
◆ Organize with new links.
◆ Expand network of relationships.
◆ Motivate search for more information.
⇩

Mother applies what she knows to new situations.

| *Recoding* of input takes place to: ◆ Accommodate more information. ◆ Interpret and elaborate. ◆ Match frame of reference. ◆ Match prior knowledge. ◆ Activate long-term memory. ⇩ | Mother continues to learn more about breastfeeding at each stage of her baby's development and responds appropriately. | Does not match frame of reference or prior knowledge.   ⇒ | Retention and recall are hampered. Retrieval system fails. Forgetting takes place. |

Retrieval of information.

Mother feels confident about her breastfeeding knowledge and management techniques.

Mother applies what she knows when she breastfeeds subsequent babies.

RESULT FOR MOTHER
⬇
Mother doesn't know how to feed on cue; starts early supplements and solids.
Mother doesn't get a good latch; gets sore nipples.
Mother weans early.
Mother doesn't breastfeed subsequent babies.

FIGURE 3.1   Pathway for sensory input.

produces more extensive processing of information. Level of involvement is a critical factor in determining which method of persuasion is likely to be effective. As the message becomes more personally relevant and our involvement increases, we become more willing to spend the cognitive effort required to process the message. We seek information, weigh it carefully, and evaluate its merits. When we are highly involved or have a strong opinion about an issue, we may interpret something as being more positive than it actually is if it agrees with our opinion (Schiffman & Kanuk, 2006). Those who are uninvolved will be more receptive to arguments both for and against an issue, or they will take no position at all. For these people, learning is enhanced by visual cues and repetition. Lactation consultants involved in complex cases often find that the healthcare provider (such as an endocrinologist or occupational therapist) least involved with the infant or mother's care may be the most willing to try new approaches.

Involvement theory evolved from a stream of research referred to as split-brain theory, which describes how the right and left hemispheres of the brain specialize in the kinds of information they process (see Figure 3.2). The left brain focuses on cognition; it is considered to be rational, active, and realistic. Cognitive information requires a high degree of active involvement. Conversely, the right brain is considered nonverbal, emotional, symbolic, impulsive, and intuitive—all characteristics that involve affect. Affect refers to the manner in which a person projects his or her emotions. We process and store right-brain information passively—that is, without active involvement.

The right and left hemispheres of the brain work together to process information, and normally both hemispheres are engaged and integrated during the process. Integrated processors show greater overall recall of both verbal and visual input. Both sides of the brain are capable of high or low involvement. For instance, there is some initial engagement of the right brain in a high-involvement cognitive (left-brain) process; similarly, some engagement of the left brain occurs in a high-involvement affective (right-brain) process.

Left Brain: Cognition

rational
active
realistic

Right Brain: Affect

nonverbal
emotional
symbolic
impulsive
intuitive

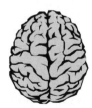

FIGURE 3.2   Split-brain theory.

∼ Social Behavior

Human behavior is more than just the action of isolated individuals—it is social action. Perceptions and social norms govern our social behavior, even though much of the time we are unaware of these influences. The meaning individuals ascribe to their action is what creates society. The foundations of most societies are intrinsically adaptable and durable and can accommodate people consciously making and altering the social order around them.

As a society increases in complexity, the individual parts of society grow increasingly dependent upon one another, becoming interconnected. Society sets boundaries for behavior. Our social surroundings either have helped to create or are affected by whatever we undergo as individuals. As an example, consider a breastfeeding woman who experiences resistance from her employer and fellow workers when she returns to work after having her first baby. She receives support from a breastfeeding counselor and ultimately becomes a counselor herself. She works with her employer to establish a lactation room and a positive work environment for mothers. When she returns to work after giving birth to her second baby, her work environment is dramatically more supportive of her continuing to breastfeed.

Each of us belongs to a social group whose membership to a greater or lesser degree dictates our behavior. Other determinants of our behavior include our personality, ethical values, and attitudes.

Personality

Our inner psychological characteristics both determine and reflect how we respond to our environment. Specific qualities, attributes, traits, and mannerisms distinguish one person from another, creating a unique combination of factors that explains why no two individuals are exactly alike. Although personality is largely consistent and firmly grounded, specific needs, motives, attitudes, or reactions can influence a change in behavior. For example, we may alter our personality as part of a gradual maturing process or in response to major life events, such as childbirth. Becoming a mother enables a woman to embrace unconditional love and learn unselfishness as she tends to her child's needs.

The hormone oxytocin, which is released during breastfeeding, increases women's ability to do repetitive tasks, a vital ability for daily childcare (Taylor et al., 2000). Oxytocin also lowers maternal response to stress, and may reduce the child's stress response later in life (Pedersen & Boccia, 2002). Breastfeeding mothers tend to be more extroverted and are more agreeable and open than those who formula feed (Wagner et al., 2006). In a 2009 study, factors that influenced breastfeeding duration included the mother's parenting and breastfeeding self-efficacy as well as her priorities, adaptability, and stress (O'Brien et al., 2009).

Self-Image

We all have an image of ourselves as having certain traits, habits, possessions, relationships, and ways of behaving. This self-image is likely to influence the manner in which we act with different people and in different situations. Our self-image is unique and is the outgrowth of our background and experience. It is influenced by how we see ourselves, how we would like to see ourselves, how we believe others see us, and how we would like others to see us. How we expect to see ourselves at some specified future time also influences our self-image and provides an opportunity for change. The manner in which these various self-images guide our attitudes and behavior depends on the specific situation.

As a lactation consultant, you may see mothers who feel pressured by their spouse or peer group to breastfeed but who personally do not want to do it. The mother's self-image is in conflict. She sees her role as a mother as including breastfeeding, but internally (perhaps because of physical abuse, sexual abuse, domestic violence, or social conditioning), she recoils from the physicality of feeding her baby at the breast.

Compared with mothers who exclusively formula feed their infants, exclusively breastfeeding mothers have higher levels of self-concept including self-satisfaction, behavior, moral worth, value as a family member, and physical appearance (Britton & Britton, 2008). An Australian study reported on mothers' psychological factors that correlated with breastfeeding duration. Attributes associated with longer duration included optimism, self-efficacy, faith in breastmilk, breastfeeding expectations, anxiety, planned duration of breastfeeding, and the time of the infant feeding decision (O'Brien et al., 2008). The study found that these psychological factors were more predictive of breastfeeding duration than were sociodemographics. Studies also show that the duration of breastfeeding has a positive association with a mother's intention to breastfeed, her previous experience with breastfeeding, and her self-efficacy and self-confidence (Wilhelm et al., 2008; Kronborg & Vaeth, 2004).

Unconscious Needs

Unconscious needs or drives lie at the heart of human motivation and personality. Freud believed that human drives are largely unconscious and that people are primarily unaware of the true reasons for their actions. In the case of the hypothetical mother described previously, she may feel discomfort with breastfeeding but not consciously know why. The unconscious reason could be repressed sexual abuse or a distorted understanding of breastfeeding due to sexual teasing. Perhaps the woman has an ill-defined self-image and believes that breasts are only sexual organs, so that breastfeeding is seen as a sexual act.

Personality Types

There are many theories about personality types; three of the leading theories are discussed here. Carl Jung, a contemporary of Freud, stressed the influence of personality on behavior. His personality types are used in the Myers-Briggs Type Indicators, a personality inventory that measures several psychological characteristics—sensing, intuiting, thinking, feeling, extroversion, introversion, judging, and perceiving. The pairing of these attributes can be used to classify distinctly different personality types. Identifying these proclivities offers a picture of how individuals will respond to their world.

The combinations of some of these indicators are especially useful in determining how people obtain and process information and how they make decisions. Learning how these particular personality types influence information processing and decision making enables us to better satisfy another person's needs. The four Myers-Briggs personality types describe personalities that combine sensing and thinking, sensing and feeling, intuitive and thinking, or intuitive and feeling (see Figure 3.3).

A neo-Freudian approach to understanding personality contends that social relationships are fundamental to the formation and development of personality. Alfred Adler believed that human beings seek to attain various rational goals, which he termed "style of life." In his theory, Adler emphasized an individual's efforts to overcome feelings of inferiority as a key factor in driving that person's behavior. In contrast, Harry Stack Sullivan believed that people continually attempt to establish significant and rewarding relationships with others. He was particularly concerned with an individual's efforts to reduce tension and anxiety.

Another premise, known as trait theory, focuses on the measurement of personality in terms of specific psychological characteristics. A "trait" is defined as any distinguishing, relatively enduring way in which one individual differs from another. Inner-directed people, for example, tend to rely on their own values or standards. They may respond favorably to an approach that stresses personal benefits. Conversely, other-directed individuals tend to look to other people for direction about what is "right" or "wrong." They focus more on social acceptance, in keeping with their tendency to look to others for guidance.

Specific personality traits can identify those persons who are more likely to be responsive to the influence of others. Individuals who are most susceptible to interpersonal influence tend to be less self-confident than those

	Thinking	Feeling
Sensing	*Sensing-Thinking* • Rational in decision making • Driven by logic rather than values • Practical and pragmatic • Expends considerable effort to search for information • Avoids risk • Identifies with material objects • Makes decisions for the short term	*Sensing-Feeling* • Practical and pragmatic • Driven by values rather than logic • Makes decisions based on subjectivity • Likely to consider others when making a decision • Shares risks with others • Aware of how material objects influence others • Makes decisions for the short term
Intuitive	*Intuiting-Thinking* • Takes a broad view of personal situation • Relies on imagination, yet uses logic to approach decisions • Imagines a wider range of options in making a decision • Willing to take a risk • Makes decisions for the long term	*Intuitive-Feeling* • Takes a broad view of personal situation • Imagines a wide range of options in making a decision • Highly people oriented and likely to consider views of others • Makes decisions based on subjectivity • Seeks risk • Makes decisions for an indefinite period of time

FIGURE 3.3 Personality types and behavior.

who are less susceptible to such influence. Lactation consultants, for example, may see both strong self-confidence and lack of confidence when working with teen mothers. On the one hand, the teen mother may be clearly inner directed and strong beyond her years in advocating for her baby. On the other hand, she may sometimes be other directed, looking to her mother, her caseworker, or another adult to make decisions for her.

Ethics

Morals and ethics greatly influence an individual's social behavior. The word "ethics" is derived from the Greek term *ethos*. Every culture develops its own form of ethics. In Western civilization, ethics is synonymous with character or morals. That is, ethics are principles or standards of human conduct. In an attempt to define the highest good, sociologists have identified three principal standards of conduct: happiness or pleasure; duty, virtue, or obligation; and perfection ("Ethics," 2009). Although moral customs change with each new generation, ethical values are enduring. They may or may not coincide with what is currently and locally moral.

Early Theories on Ethics

Philosophers first began to theorize about moral behavior in 6th-century Greece, which led to the development of philosophical ethics. One notable thinker, Pythagoras, suggested that moral philosophy should be based on the beliefs that our intellectual nature is superior to our sensual nature and that the best life is one devoted to mental discipline. A century later, the group of Greek philosophers known as Sophists opposed moral absolutes and taught rhetoric, logic, and civil affairs. The Sophist Protagoras, for example, put forth the theory that human judgment is subjective and that an individual's perception of himself or herself is valid only for that person and cannot be generalized.

Socrates and his student Plato opposed the Sophist philosophy, teaching instead that virtue is knowledge and that people will be virtuous if they know what virtue is. They believed that education has the capacity to make people moral. Later Greek philosophers espoused these same beliefs, maintaining that the essence of virtue is self-control and that self-control can be learned. A sound knowledge base will provide a foundation for lactation consultants to evaluate moral judgments and character and make ethical decisions (Noel-Weiss & Walters, 2006).

Plato taught that good is an essential element of reality and maintained that human virtue lies in the fitness of a person to perform his or her proper function in the world. He described the human soul as having three elements: intellect, will, and emotion. Intellect leads to wisdom, will leads to courage or the capacity to act, and emotion leads to temperance or self-control. Of the three, Plato believed that intellect is the highest virtue and that emotion should be subject to intellect and will.

Plato's student Aristotle believed that happiness is the aim of life and that virtues are essentially good habits. In other words, one must develop two habits to attain happiness. The habit of mental activity consists of knowledge and contemplation. Practical action and emotion form the other habit, courage. Aristotle taught that moral virtues must be flexible to accommodate the differences among people and conditions. He saw intellectual and moral virtues as a means toward the attainment of happiness, which results when a person realizes his or her full human potential.

In 3rd-century Rome, the school of philosophy known as Stoicism held that nature is orderly and rational and that only a life led in harmony with nature can be good. The Stoics believed that material circumstances influence life and that we should strive to be independent of such influences. They concluded that practical wisdom, courage, discretion, and justice could achieve independence. The Epicureans shared this philosophy, advocating that we postpone immediate pleasure to attain more secure and lasting satisfaction in the future. They taught that self-discipline must regulate the good life.

The advent of Christianity revolutionized the concept of ethics. Western thought now had a religious notion of good, one positing that humans are totally dependent on God and can achieve goodness only with the help of God's grace, not by means of will or intelligence. Christianity gave rise to the "golden rule": Treat others as we wish to be treated and love others as we love ourselves.

Deontological ethics or deontology (from the Greek word meaning "obligation or duty") is an approach to ethics that emerged in the 1930s. It focuses on the intentions or motives behind an action, with respect for rights, duties, and principles (Olson, 2003). Because of its emphasis on rights, duties and principles, deontological ethics form a good framework for healthcare providers (Aiken, 2004).

Living an Ethical Life

The works of the early Greek, Roman, and Christian philosophers gave birth to the tenets that form the basis of modern ethics. John Locke, for example, believed in the natural goodness of humanity. He maintained that the pursuit of happiness and pleasure leads to cooperation when conducted rationally. Locke argued that private happiness and general welfare coincide, and that immediate pleasures must give way to a prudent regard for ultimate good.

This perspective reveals the ultimate dilemma of trying to live an ethical life. Ethical living in its fullest sense is an aspiration we can only approach. In reality, none of us practices ethical habits all the time. Everyone has internal personal needs and external social needs—the challenge is to integrate these two selves. Individuals who seek power may not accept customary ethical rules, but may conform to rules that can help them become successful. They will seek to persuade others that they are moral in an attempt to mask their power seeking and to gain social approval of their actions, presenting themselves as morally motivated.

This perspective is evident in the actions by formula manufacturing executives. They pressured the American Academy of Pediatrics in an attempt to prevent a public service ad campaign promoting breastfeeding (Merewood & Heinig, 2004). Although the campaign still aired, the message was weakened by the formula industry's tactics. Members of the formula industry in the past have superficially acknowledged the value of human milk. This acknowledgment has been subverted by "yes, but" tactics in their advertising. Moreover, the industry strenuously lobbied against an advertising campaign designed to dramatically increase breastfeeding rates. Formula makers' moral appeal that they be recognized as supporting optimal health is eclipsed by their self-interests in selling their products.

We steer our lives by trial and error and by intuition and reason. Our assumptions about the world determine our direction, our identity, and ultimately the character of our society. A community is composed of unique and interdependent beings who ideally relate to one another in a way that elicits the best from every person. Our ethical values determine how we behave, how we treat one another, and how we create the social conditions and habits necessary for others to thrive, both individually and collectively.

Elements of an Ethical Culture

An ethical culture is one that creates a humane environment in which we treat others as unique individuals, value their worth, and treat them with respect. In doing so, we elicit the best from each and every person. This effort enhances our own personal growth, because when we see and encourage good in others, we discover it in ourselves. In an ethical culture, therefore, we live by habits that enable everyone to thrive. We reach beyond ourselves to decrease suffering and to increase creativity in the world. We allow others to make choices and to be accountable for their mistakes. For instance, cultures that value mothering and children promote practices that support the worth of mothering and breastfeeding. Sweden, Norway, and several other European nations provide generous maternity leaves for mothers, enabling them to breastfeed without separation from their babies (Honeyball, 2009).

Ethical theory provides a framework for determining right from wrong and guides ethical decision making (Beauchamp & Childress, 2001). An ethical culture advocates a life of integrity in which we keep commitments. We are more open, honest, caring, and responsive to others. We make significant choices in our lives and build ethical relationships. We are committed to educating ourselves so that we can grow, both in wisdom and socially. We remain true to our values and standards. We recognize that words have limited value without actions to support them, and that ultimately we are judged by what we do, not by what we say. Any lapse in ethics, or even the appearance of a lapse, can significantly harm one's reputation.

IBLCE's Code of Ethics guides the behavior of lactation consultants. The IBLCE expects these professionals to support the Code of Ethics and incorporate it into their careers (see Appendix A). Ethical issues relevant to the lactation profession are discussed further in Chapters 26 and 28.

Attribution

Sociology includes a consideration of how people attribute causes to their behavior and to the behavior of others. We want to know why we and others act—or do not act—in certain ways. We seek reasons for behavior, and we expect excuses and apologies when an error occurs or when we are disappointed. This process of explaining behavior is known as attribution.

When we believe we understand the causes of behavior, we react with thoughts, feelings, and responses specific to those causes. A Hong Kong study revealed that mothers attributed their infant feeding decisions to their own decision-making process, followed by advice from their husbands. The mothers' personal feelings of responsibility, self-worth, and closeness to the baby influenced their decision in favor of breastfeeding (Kong & Lee, 2004).

The manner in which we attribute causes and reasons for past events influences our expectations of the future. When we attribute cause, we search for and use information about the person and the social context in which the behavior under consideration took place. We seek to explain other people's behavior in an attempt to reduce uncertainty about what is likely to happen in the future, given similar conditions. This enables us to predict and to feel some measure of control over the world in which we live. A new mother may encounter this line of thought when she is told by her own mother, "I wanted to breastfeed you, but I didn't make enough milk." This information could set the stage for the new mother to expect that she, too, will not "make enough milk."

It is important to recognize that how we perceive the cause of behavior may differ from the actual cause. Such discrepancies in perception are common and explain how individuals can draw such different conclusions about a particular event or behavior. What we expect to see often strongly influences what we do see. Our perception of the cause of a particular behavior depends on our personality, the features of the behavior, and the social context of the behavior. In addition, our perception influences the degree of responsibility we attribute to someone for his or her actions. For example, parents may ascribe conscious motivation to a baby's feeding behaviors with comments such as "He's being lazy; he's just using me as a pacifier; he doesn't want to nurse."

Perception

Perception is the process by which an individual selects, organizes, and interprets stimuli into a meaningful and coherent picture of the world. An almost infinite number of stimuli bombard us during every minute and every hour of every day. A stimulus is any unit of input to any of the five senses of sight, hearing, sound, taste, and touch. We subconsciously add to and subtract from these raw sensory inputs to produce our private picture of the world. This picture is influenced by our own expectations, motives, and learning, which are all based on our previous experiences.

We consciously exercise a great deal of selectivity as to which stimuli—which aspects of the environment—we perceive. The stimuli we select depend on the nature of the stimulus, our previous experience, and our motives at the time. As mentioned previously, we usually see what we expect to see. Familiarity, previous experience, and preconditioned expectations all interact to determine what we expect to see. We also tend to perceive things we need or want: The stronger the need or want, the stronger our awareness is of those stimuli and the greater our tendency to ignore unrelated stimuli. Our process of perception simply attunes itself more closely to elements in the environment that are important to us.

Preconditioned expectations mean that we tend to attribute the qualities we associate with certain people to others who may resemble them. We also tend to carry images in our minds of the meanings of various kinds of stimuli. Recognizing this fact can help us understand the implications of our perceptions and appreciate how they may influence our behavior and our expectations of others. For the lactation consultant, it is important to "know thyself," and to recognize personality types that irritate or disturb you. When you encounter a mother with that personality, recognize your emotional reaction. You can consciously choose to interact with this client in a respectful, healthy way and leave your bias at the door. Awareness strengthens your ability to help this mother and not react solely to her personality or allow her to "push your buttons."

In addition to perceiving overt stimuli, people can be stimulated below their level of conscious awareness. In other words, we can perceive stimuli without being consciously aware that we are doing so. Stimuli that are too weak or too brief to be consciously seen or heard may nevertheless be strong enough to be perceived by one or more receptors. Such subliminal perception can result from a brief visual presentation, from accelerated speech in low-volume auditory messages, or from embedded or hidden imagery or words. Subliminal messages can motivate people to exhibit a certain behavior without being aware of why they are motivated to behave in that manner.

Infant formula manufacturers and other companies well understand this relationship—which explains why they are willing to spend millions of dollars on advertising to ensure that the image of a baby bottle or their particular logo connotes quintessential babyhood. Such advertising typically depicts a mother feeding a bottle to her baby, warmly portraying optimal eye contact and a wide smile. In comparison, the same ad might portray a breastfeeding mother with her eyes averted and minimal facial expression. The subliminal projection casts the bottle feeding mother as being more engaged with her baby and enjoying feeding time more completely. Some media placements are even more overtly anti-breastfeeding, as evidenced by Cow & Gate's 2006 ad: "I'm thinking of getting a t-shirt made—'Danger! Sore boobs!'" (Palmer, 2009).

Attitude

Attitudes are an expression of inner feelings that reflect whether we are favorably or unfavorably predisposed to something. We cannot observe others' attitudes directly; instead, we infer them from what people say or do. Attitudes evaluate a message ("Do I want to do this?") and may either propel us toward or repel us away from a particular behavior. The process of trying and evaluating a behavior is the primary means by which we form attitudes. Among adolescents, knowledge and social influence are important predictors of positive beliefs about breastfeeding and future intention to breastfeed (Swanson et al., 2006). A significant relationship also exists between positive attitudes toward breastfeeding and exposure to breastfeeding among university undergraduate students (Marrone et al., 2008). Clearly, an understanding of attitudes among adolescents and young adults is important to breastfeeding promotion efforts.

Many healthcare professionals were trained in an era of formula feeding and schedules as the norm, and most of them bottle fed their children. They often believe that formula is "just as good" as breastmilk. Formula manufacturers promote this attitude through aggressive marketing targeted specifically to the medical community. As discussed in Chapter 2, physicians' attitudes can have a major influence on the choices their patients make.

In general, the more information we have about something, the more likely we are to form attitudes about it, either positive or negative. Individuals often use only a portion of the total amount of information available to them and are not always ready or willing to process more. For this reason, it is important to narrow your focus to the few key points that are at the heart of your message. When you have the opportunity to interact with another healthcare professional, keep your message simple and succinct. He or she may be more open to one fact about breastfeeding than to a barrage of emotional information. This point is especially salient when you are interacting with people in the medical field who are unfamiliar with the concepts of breastfeeding as the biological norm and artificial feeding as suboptimal and possessing health risks to the infant.

Determining Attitudes Part of the information we use in developing attitudes are the mores and cultural norms of society. The rules of behavior within a peer group contribute to that group's uniformity. In other words, cultural norms regarding personal conduct and ethical standards are responsible for a certain degree of uniformity among individual members of that culture. Attitude formation is linked to personal experience and the influence of family and friends. Our early childhood, family background, educational level, and subculture all contribute to differences among us and, consequently, to differences among our attitudes.

Direct marketing efforts and the mass media constantly expose us to new ideas, products, opinions, and advertisements and attempt to influence our attitudes through their messages. Parents, for example, are besieged with promotional messages about products they "must" have for their baby. Members of the lactation profession must be careful not to send similar messages about the need for breastfeeding devices.

Predicting Behavior Knowledge of people's attitudes provides insight that facilitates understanding and predicting their behavior. Although attitudes are relatively enduring, they are easier to change than beliefs and values. Our central beliefs and values—those that influence and determine how we think and act—are highly resistant to change. By comparison, beliefs and values that are more peripheral have less influence on how we see the world, and are more easily changed.

Attitudes are often influenced by circumstances. Individuals may hold a variety of attitudes toward a particular behavior, each corresponding to a particular situation. Therefore, it is important to consider the situation in which a behavior takes place so as to interpret it correctly. A healthcare provider who espouses support for breastfeeding may be surprisingly quick to recommend supplementing with formula. You may understand this inconsistency better if you learn that the provider has adopted more aggressive protocols for treating hyperbilirubinemia in light

- I definitely will
- I probably will
- I am uncertain whether I will
- I probably will not
- I definitely will not

FIGURE 3.4 Scale of intent.

of revised American Academy of Pediatrics guidelines (AAP, 2004).

Intention The intention to act is the best predictor of behavior. A person's attitude toward something will occur at some point along a scale of intent (see Figure 3.4) that ranges from positive to negative intentions (Schiffman & Kanuk, 2006). To understand intention, we must understand what influences our intent to act. We are primarily influenced by people who are significant and important in our life—family, friends, and coworkers. We consider first how we believe they would respond to the decision and then whether their response will affect our motivation to act.

When it comes to infant feeding, the support of the child's father is one of the main determinants in whether a woman breastfeeds (Chang & Chan, 2003; Chen & Chi, 2003; Scott et al., 2001; Arora et al., 2000; Kessler et al., 1995). His attitude influences the mother's motivation, intention, and, therefore, her behavior. Further, intention to breastfeed is predictive of breastfeeding behavior, and advice received prenatally and postpartum is significantly correlated with hospital feeding method (Mistry et al., 2008).

Attitude Changes Attitudes can change because of personal experience and exposure to new sources of information. Personality plays a pivotal role in the speed with which attitudes are likely to change. Individuals who crave information and enjoy thinking (cognition) are likely to form positive attitudes in response to messages that are rich in information. In contrast, those who rank relatively low in their need for cognition are more likely to respond to messages and impressions that appeal to their emotions.

An effective strategy for changing attitudes is to help the individual recognize how the new behavior serves a positive purpose and is superior to the alternative. An Australian study reported that 87 percent of women who had not intended to breastfeed on a long-term basis changed their opinion as they saw their child enjoy breastfeeding, as their knowledge about breastfeeding increased, and as they were exposed to long-term breastfeeding role models (Gribble, 2008).

Healthcare providers who receive education about the improved health outcomes of breastfed infants may change their early, less favorable attitudes toward this type of infant feeding. If a woman can see that her attitude toward a behavior is in conflict with another attitude, she may change her evaluation of the behavior in question. Another useful strategy is to change the individual's beliefs about the attributes of the alternative. The emphasis on advertising the risks of formula feeding instead of the benefits of breastfeeding exemplifies this approach (Walker, 2007; Merewood & Heinig, 2004).

Motivation

As we have seen, motivation is a driving force behind behavior. Our individual thinking and learning influence the specific goals we select, as well as the manner in which we act to achieve those goals. Experiencing an unfulfilled need, want, or desire creates internal tension. This tension provides the motivation to engage in behavior that will ultimately reduce the tension. To take action and exhibit this new behavior, we engage in a process of thinking, learning new information, and recalling previous learning. The new behavior, in turn, helps us fulfill the goal or need that initially provided the motivation. Finally, reaching the goal reduces tension and enables us to manage the situation that precipitated these actions. Figure 3.5 illustrates this path (Weber, 1992).

Intrinsically motivated women—that is, those who internally desire to breastfeed—may nevertheless need both support and instruction to begin and continue

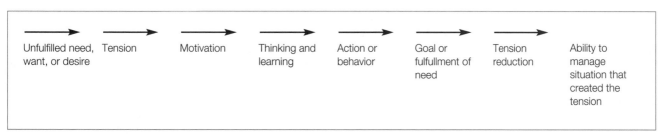

FIGURE 3.5 Path of motivation.

breastfeeding. In contrast, those mothers who are extrinsically motivated—that is, influenced by others—may benefit from motivational interviewing. Successfully experienced women may need only minimal breastfeeding counseling (Racine et al., 2009). Conversely, disincentives are significantly associated with a mother's motivation to stop breastfeeding (Racine et al., 2008).

In one study, researchers studied the use of motivational interviewing to promote sustained breastfeeding. Motivational interviewing is a counseling approach that explores and resolves ambivalence within the client. The goals of the study were to increase breastfeeding to 6 months and to increase breastfeeding self-efficacy. Although results were not statistically significant, the researchers suggested that motivational interviewing may be a useful intervention in this regard (Wilhelm et al., 2006).

Goals and Needs

All behavior is goal oriented, and all goals derive from some form of need. Needs and goals are not static, however, but rather change in response to our physical condition, environment, experiences, and interactions with other people. We may actually be more aware of our goal than of the needs that lead us to seek that goal. In particular, we are usually more readily aware of our physiological needs than our psychological needs. The goals we select to pursue depend on our needs, personal experiences, cultural norms and values, self-images, physical capacity, and their accessibility within our physical and social environment.

The motivation for fulfilling needs can be either positive or negative. Positive drives take the form of needs, wants, and desires; negative drives take the form of fears and aversions. Likewise, goals can be either positive or negative. We may wish to direct our actions toward a positive goal (approach behavior) or away from a negative outcome (avoidance behavior). Even babies exhibit approach behaviors and avoidance behaviors that communicate their needs to parents and other caregivers. See Chapter 13 for more information about infant behavior.

A mother's desire to breastfeed based on her conviction that this practice offers her baby optimal health has a positive motivation. Her positive drive will help her persevere through initial soreness and engorgement to achieve her desired goal of a healthy, exclusively breastfed baby. By comparison, a mother who has internalized horror stories of painful childbirth and breastfeeding may wish to prevent pain and be quick to ask for a nipple shield, nipple creams, and a bottle.

Relationships

Relationships form the basis of our behavior with others. They are forged through work-related contacts, social interactions, and our involvement with groups and organizations. The ways in which we interact will take on different forms depending on the setting. Sociology studies relationships among people—within the economy, the family, education, organizations, religions, corporations, government, and ethnic groups. How individuals and groups interact can help predict social change and the ways in which people will respond to social change.

Attachment and Bonding

Childhood lays the foundation for adolescent and adult functioning. The first 2 years of life are vital in determining personality, social behavior, and the ability to form relationships. Experiences during this critical time can set the stage for the manner in which we approach future social situations.

Many social psychologists regard a child's first relationship to be a prototype for future relationships and believe it determines the way a person approaches and interacts with other people (Bowlby, 1982, 1975; Ainsworth et al., 1978). Understandably, the study of this first relationship focuses on the quality of attachment between a mother and her infant. An infant's bonding with his or her mother describes the baby's tendency to seek proximity to the mother, to be receptive to receiving care from her, and to feel secure in her presence. Strength of attachment is positively associated with the ability and sensitivity of the mother to respond to her infant's verbal and nonverbal signals.

Mothers who choose to breastfeed display enhanced sensitivity during early infancy that, in turn, may foster secure attachment. Among breastfeeding mothers, higher sensitivity is associated with longer duration of breastfeeding during the first postpartum year. These findings suggest a link between attachment security and breastfeeding (Britton et al., 2006).

Research on the physiology of the female brain has found that women are driven to connect from the earliest stages of fetal development through a strong communication connection network in the brain (Brizendine, 2006). Understanding how a mother responds uniquely to her own infant, when that child is smiling or crying, may be the first step in understanding the neural basis of mother–infant attachment. Research suggests that when first-time mothers see their infant's face, affective and cognitive information may be integrated and directed toward motivating behavioral responses in the mother (Strathearn et al., 2008). Significant areas of the brain become activated when mothers are shown happy faces of their infants compared to faces of unknown infants. This linkage raises questions about how brain responses predict maternal sensitivity and attachment and how the mother's responses affect the child's attachment.

Attachment is strong when mothers respond consistently, regularly, and promptly to their infants' actions. A parent's responsiveness to a baby's early hunger signs teaches the baby early trust. The child realizes, "I'm hungry and Mom feeds me; I'm warm; I feel safe; Mom's milk is good; I'm full." Conversely, when a parent ignores hunger cues and crying, the baby learns a very different lesson: "I'm hungry; I'm upset; I'm lonely. Where is Mom? Why doesn't she come?" These babies' attempts to self-soothe do not relieve hunger. The world does not feel safe and the baby does not feel secure. The mother is unpredictable; she sometimes answers and sometimes does not. In this scenario, the stage is set for fear, anxiety, helplessness, and hopelessness.

Group Behavior

We all belong to a variety of groups, both formal and informal. These groups—familial, work related, educational, religious, social, and recreational—influence how we communicate and interact with one another, how we perform tasks, and how we achieve goals. We are born into a social group, the family, where we gain our initial experiences. We grow and mature in social groups. We earn a living in a social group.

We have a defined role within each group structure, reflecting our own specific degree of status and power. We exhibit our own form of group behavior, and we communicate with one another by sending and receiving messages. We conform to group norms to one degree or another. We are aware of one another, interact with one another, and exert influence on one another. Generally, people join a group to attain a goal or otherwise satisfy a need. This kind of group participation addresses many social needs, such as approval, a sense of belonging, and friendship. Peer groups in similar life stages, such as those participating in young couples' Bible study classes in churches, play groups, or neighborhood associations, can form long-term friendships as they move through adult life stages together. Some groups share a common culture and economic status, which has implications for their behavior. In one study, for example, immigrant subgroups in a low-income, inner-city population had a higher likelihood of breastfeeding when compared with non-Hispanic white women (Lee et al., 2005).

In sociology, a "group" is usually defined as a collection consisting of a number of people who share certain aspects, interact with one another, accept rights and obligations as members of the group, and share a common identity. A group exhibits a degree of cohesiveness, but may either be loosely formed or have a formal structure. Like-minded people may form a formal association to accomplish a purpose based on shared interests and values. Most associations develop some kind of document that regulates the way in which they meet and operate; such an instrument is often called the organization's bylaws, regulations, or agreement of association. The group's policies guide the behavior and attitudes of its members. For instance, associations such as ILCA and IBLCE have codes of behavior that are expected and encouraged.

Primary and Secondary Groups

Some groups to which we belong are basic to our social development and have a significant impact on us as individuals. Members of these primary groups often know a good deal about one another and care about one another's welfare. The family is an example of a primary group. We have close, personal, and enduring relationships in a family. Members typically spend considerable time together and share many activities and experiences. In addition, the relationships within primary groups are deep because of the emotions invested in them.

In contrast, secondary groups tend to be temporary and may form for a specific purpose or task. Relationships are relatively impersonal, with little emotional investment. Interaction between members of secondary groups tends to focus on the activities that led the group to form rather than on the needs, desires, or concerns of the individual members. In fact, members of a secondary group often have little personal knowledge of one another.

Some secondary groups may evolve to take on the characteristics of a primary group. The critical difference between the two types of groups is the degree of emotional investment in the group and the degree of relationships among the members. The degree to which members feel bound to one another will determine the group's stability and the likelihood that members will conform to its norms. Members of cohesive groups like one another more and support common goals more strongly than members of less cohesive groups do. Cohesive groups enjoy interactions more and tend to be better problem solvers.

Since mothers have to surmount cultural obstacles to breastfeeding, breastfeeding support groups tend to be cohesive. These mothers swim against the cultural norm. The empowerment they receive from breastfeeding makes them strong advocates for other areas of their children's welfare as their children grow. Because of their strong beliefs, many mothers remain involved in childbirth, breastfeeding, and other educational issues long after their children have weaned.

The lactation profession is another example of a cohesive secondary group. La Leche League, ILCA, and IBLCE were all formed by women who were passionate about promoting healthy infant feeding practices. The strong beliefs and mutual commitment among the members of these groups have created a familial relationship of nurturing and loyalty.

Power and Empowerment

Power places controls within relationships. The center of power can shift in response to personal, interpersonal, and social changes. Power is dictated to a large degree by the social group within which the relationship exists.

Power occurs in various forms:

- Expert power derives from someone who has greater knowledge and skills than we do.
- Coercive power creates physical controls and coercion that is meant to limit our actions.
- Reward power takes the form of emotional or tangible rewards intended to alter our behavior.
- Legitimate power exists when another person or group has a genuine right to influence others.
- Referent power occurs when another person has attributes that we wish we had ourselves, which alters our behavior.
- Informational power has the ability to transform a non-expert into an expert.

Medical professionals possess expert power derived from their specialized and exclusive body of knowledge, extensive vocational training, monopoly of practice, and self-regulation. The medical profession itself helps to maintain the social order, which confers benefits on both society and the individual. The medical community has a wellspring of specialities, where each specialization possesses a unique body of knowledge, training, and area of practice. As a consequence, a single consumer may be under the care of a primary physician, endocrinologist, cardiologist, gynecologist, orthopedist, rheumatologist, dermatologist, and physical therapist. Owing to this multiplicity of providers, it has become increasingly important for consumers to coordinate their care and to assume informational power that enables them to control their outcomes.

With wider access to medical information through the Internet and other resources, today's consumers are better informed and more demanding than ever before. As a result, the social distance between patient and medical practitioner is narrowing. Patient rights, health-related support groups, alternative therapies, and homeopathic practices are all balancing forces that permeate the healthcare arena. Ultimately, power lies at the core of understanding a profession. Patients are transforming themselves from non-experts into experts through easy information access. The center of power is shifting, and the face of the medical profession has been forever altered—clear evidence that professions, as social organizations, mutate as a result of social and scientific developments.

Nurses, physicians, other caregivers, and patients all have and use power in their relationships with one another. It should be the goal of all healthcare providers to empower their patients and encourage them to take an active role in their relationships with practitioners. True empowerment occurs only when healthcare providers transform the ways in which they relate to patients.

Studies have demonstrated a strong correlation between perceived control and the duration of breastfeeding (Mistry et al., 2008). When healthcare providers relinquish coercive power and help mothers take more control over their health needs and the prevention of problems, mothers are empowered to gain mastery over their lives. This approach helps them develop a critical awareness of the root causes of their problems and a readiness to act on this awareness. Breastfeeding and mothering are empowering for women as well. Empowering a mother with breastfeeding confidence increases the likelihood that she will breastfeed (Mistry et al., 2008).

Feminism and Breastfeeding

From a feminist perspective, breastfeeding incorporates women's needs as biological and reproductive social beings (Smith, 2008). Feminist theory regards social expectations and roles as potentially oppressive to women. As a consequence, breastfeeding, which requires time with and access to the infant, is seen as compromising a woman's autonomy. Some feminists consider breastfeeding to be a gender difference that stands in the way of liberating women and, therefore, view bottle feeding as liberating. Hausman (2003) suggests a feminist health approach to breastfeeding advocacy. Van Esterik (2002, 1994) considers improvement of women's social and economic status as an important part of breastfeeding support and views it in the context of women's rights. A health-activist approach would create the social and economic conditions that make breastfeeding possible, successful, and valued for all women. Feminist health activism includes removing structural barriers to breastfeeding, such as economic barriers, lack of appropriate support from medical personnel, and work/family patterns (McCarter-Spaulding, 2008).

～ Knowledge and Culture

The culture and times in which we live influence the body of knowledge to which we subscribe. This knowledge may derive from folktales, religious and psychological beliefs, or science. Of these sources, scientific thought is currently the most predominant and successful premise for determining legitimate knowledge. Societal values, beliefs, and accepted wisdom often challenge the authenticity of scientific knowledge.

Science and Technology

Science and technology play central roles in the institutional structure of modern societies. Science is the systematic pursuit of reliable knowledge about the physical and social world. Through it, we obtain an understanding of the nature and operation of physical and social phenomena. The modern study of the natural and social world is rooted in the ancient Greeks' logical and rational attempts to comprehend the origins of disease (Goodman, 1992). These same Greeks viewed their gods as all-powerful, yet were the inventors of philosophy, mathematics, and science. A similar paradox exists for modern-day scientists who must reconcile Darwin's theory of evolution with their religious beliefs.

Although the sciences of sociology and anthropology can identify the origins of the family and anticipate future patterns from one generation to the next, the public is rarely consciously aware of this cause-and-effect relationship between social phenomena. Nor do most people understand how modern technology works. We fly from one city to another, we watch television, and we communicate with one another by cellular telephones and computers. The emergence of computer technology and the Internet has created profound social change and links individuals collectively through cyberspace in a mass society. Yet, for the most part, we lack even a basic understanding of the scientific principles that make this astonishing feat possible.

The Subjective Nature of Science

Not all science is objective. Much of what is studied depends on the availability of funding. Funding, in turn, is often contingent on whether there is a perceived commercial or political benefit to the research. For example, we would not expect a tobacco company to fund publicly available research that investigates the health risks of smoking. Likewise, a brewery is unlikely to subsidize research on fetal alcohol syndrome or teenage death rates from alcohol abuse. And, of course, manufacturers of artificial baby milk are not likely to fund research examining the superiority of human milk except in their efforts to isolate and patent human milk components. Of course, exceptions are possible. A company may perceive that such financial support will lessen criticism of its business practices, or it may wish to send a message that it promotes practices or products that seem to be contradictory to its interests. Artificial infant milk manufacturers have honed this practice to the highest levels imaginable in their "promotion" of breastfeeding.

Another complicating factor is that scientists do not always agree on how to collect and test data (Goodman, 1992). One scientist may believe that establishing constant truths should form the basis of science. A second scientist may approach science as an attempt to disprove apparent truths, believing that with good science it is possible to prove a hypothesis wrong. For example, a caregiver may recognize the importance of listening to patients and offering emotional support and find that patients who are listened to seem to have greater self-esteem. The question then becomes whether the variables of listening and self-esteem depend on each other and whether heightened self-esteem always results from listening to a patient. The first scientist would theorize that the two variables always appear together and, therefore, are connected to each other. The second scientist would test alternative suppositions to disprove the connection, perhaps testing whether self-esteem increases on occasions when there is no communication between the patient and the caregiver.

Sometimes, researchers seem to accept the conclusions their predecessors have reached and address only certain puzzles that are inherent in those conclusions. Those conclusions form the paradigm within which most scientists operate. Inevitably, however, evidence accumulates that repudiates accepted practice and thinking. The evidence eventually becomes so great that the paradigm begins to fall apart.

What an individual thinks and does affects how society is structured and, ultimately, what society accepts as reality. At the same time, society and the natural world create the circumstances through which we think and act. This illustrates the dynamic nature of the human condition. It continually changes in response to social influence and scientific fact, making it difficult to predict human behavior and social trends. Two hundred years ago, wealthy women were more likely to employ wet nurses and only the lower classes breastfed. More recently, that practice has changed in developed countries such as the United Kingdom, the United States, and Australia. Now the educated, upper-middle-class mother is more likely to breastfeed and lower-income and minority women disproportionately bottle feed (Wamani et al., 2005).

The pediatric profession arose in part from a desire to give artificial milk to infants whose mothers did not breastfeed. Mothers visited the new professional, a pediatrician, at periodic intervals in their babies' growth and acquired the appropriate recipe, or "formula" to sustain their children (Hess, 1923; Wolf, 2003). The age of infant formula feeding had arrived, with its set of rules and scheduled feedings. Nevertheless, despite the introduction of commercial proprietary infant formulas in the 1920s, most parents continued to breastfeed or use home recipes because they were easy to prepare and affordable. It was not until the 1950s that commercial formulas began to gain acceptance (Schuman, 2003).

The lactation profession arose several decades later, as part of a movement that sought to reverse the trend toward formula feeding and return infant feeding to its biological imperative. Researchers began to debunk the myths surrounding many unsubstantiated practices that had carried over from formula feeding to breastfeeding. Practitioners continue to correct misconceptions among the health profession and the public regarding breastfeeding care. As the paradigm continues to shift, previously accepted practices and thinking will change as well.

Evidence-Based Practice

A recent evolution in scientific thought has given rise to the pursuit of evidence-based practice. In an evidence-based society, scientific validation ultimately sways medicine. The media interpret research results, although these results are often couched in tentative terms, and the public relies on the media's interpretations rather than attempting to decipher the original research. As a lactation consultant, you may hear "sound bites" of information in the popular press that cast breastfeeding in a negative light. Careful examination of the original studies may show, however, that the conclusions, in fact, do support breastfeeding. More tools for critical thinking and discernment are discussed in Chapter 27.

Although an evidence-based approach has merit, it cannot be relied upon to the exclusion of caring, intuition, and other "nonscientific" variables. Medicine derives its credibility through science, but it is also an intuitive, humanistic, and behavioral discipline. Much of what we do in breastfeeding care is experiential, based on anecdotal reports. For example, the use of cabbage for engorgement was rediscovered from century-old practices that had been lost in a bottle feeding culture (Rosier, 1988). Although modern research may not convincingly validate the effectiveness of this practice, experience shows that many mothers have found it useful. Lactation consultants often observe trends among their clients that influence their care regimens. It is important that we balance such intuitive practices with evidence-based options.

∾ Decision Making

Personal knowledge and a flexible environment are the best predictors of women's satisfaction with their decision making about healthcare issues (Wittmann-Price, 2006). We make decisions concerning every aspect of our daily lives. Generally, we make these decisions without stopping to think about how we make them and what is involved in the process. A variety of factors—motivation, perception, learning, personality, and attitudes—influence our decision-making process.

We begin the act of making a decision by recognizing a need or a new circumstance. We search for information, we recall past experiences, and we evaluate alternatives. We judge the information against each alternative, select from among the alternatives, and make a final decision. Figure 3.6 illustrates the decision-making process.

whether they breastfeed or not, intuitively go through this process hundreds of times each day, with many fac-

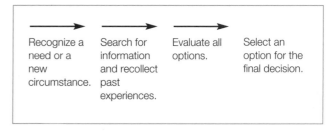

FIGURE 3.6   The decision-making process.

tors influencing their ultimate decisions. A Maori study found that women were diverted from breastfeeding by an interruption in a breastfeeding culture, difficulty establishing breastfeeding in the first 6 weeks, poor or insufficient professional support, perception of inadequate milk production, and returning to work (Glover, 2007). A decision to breastfeed in public is influenced by a mother's confidence, her ability to be discreet, her body image, previous experience, her child's age, the audience, her partner's feelings, the location, and perceptions of societal expectations (Hauck, 2004).

A breastfeeding mother may notice her 5-month-old is beginning to chew on her nipples, causing soreness. In response, she may call a lactation consultant or an experienced breastfeeding mother or consult her breastfeeding book. Through this process, she may learn that it is common for teething babies to change their nursing behavior. She evaluates the options, concluding that based on her baby's drooling and the buds in her baby's mouth that he is, indeed, teething. The mother may then try several comfort measures to minimize the baby chewing (e.g., breaking the latch herself or changing nursing positions). She will then select the one that best works for her and her baby. The same process occurs in deciding when to feed her baby, deciding whether to breastfeed in public, determining when she needs help with other breastfeeding issues, and a myriad of other parenting decisions. Recognizing the importance of validating a mother's decision making, a Swedish study suggested adding a new step to the Ten Steps to Successful Breastfeeding—namely, one that would address respect for mothers' individual decisions about breastfeeding (Nyqvist & Kylberg, 2008).

Influencing Decisions

Influencing someone's decision making begins with an appeal to the needs and interests of that person. Sometimes, objective, factual appeals are an effective method of persuasion. At other times, emotional appeals are more effective. In general, more-educated audiences respond better to factual appeals, and less-educated consumers respond better to emotional appeals. However, this is not always true. Healthcare professionals have been astounded and dismayed at the number of highly educated parents who embrace scheduled feeding programs despite the abundance of medical information advocating against these approaches (Rein, 2006; AAP, 1998; Aney, 1998).

Individuals are more likely to evaluate the pros and cons of a message when they are highly involved in the decision-making process. Making the message memorable and persuasive begins by arousing interest in it and giving the other person a reason to listen. The U.S. Ad Council uses this method effectively in its promotion campaigns. Asking questions generates involvement and helps to identify the points of interest and terminology that will be most effective. Interest ripens into desire only after we remove all lingering doubts from the other person's mind. Recognizing this relationship, many lactation consultants increase participation in prenatal classes by asking parents to voice their questions about breastfeeding at the start of the class. If no one volunteers, several "ice breaker" questions proposed rhetorically can draw out discussion.

It is important to be aware of any distractions that may impede the recipient's ability to receive and retain the key points of a message. If people are too engrossed in their thoughts or if they are emotionally unavailable, the message will not get through. The use of humor often increases the message's acceptance and persuasiveness: It attracts attention, increases comprehension, and enhances appreciation of the message. Consider demographic factors such as ethnicity and age when determining the appropriateness of using humor. Younger, better-educated, and professional people are generally more receptive to humorous messages. Lightening up your presentation, class, or other teaching with breastfeeding-related humor such as cartoons or anecdotes can both enliven the class and diffuse embarrassment.

The final step in influencing others' decision making is to involve them in forming a conclusion. You can ask them to voice their decisions; if the responses conflict with what you had hoped to convey, you can help them recognize the implications of their conclusion. When the consequences of a choice of action appear to be detrimental, people often begin to question the advisability of that decision. Verbalizing the implications of a positive decision can also serve to validate their choice and increase their self-confidence. Figure 3.7 illustrates the process of influencing a person's decision making.

If your message is to increase support for the use of human milk in the NICU and your audience consists of neonatologists, NICU nurses, and other neonatal healthcare professionals, you will need to use well-researched facts from respected sources to bolster your position. Hard data showing improved outcomes will arouse interest in your message (Sharpe, 2003). Detractors such as formula use need to be addressed and accounted for in your presentation. You can involve the audience by asking open-ended questions about what they would do or what they anticipate the results will be.

Compliance and Conformity

Social influence may be conscious or subconscious. It may be readily accepted, yielded to reluctantly, or resisted. Societal norms shape and influence our actions and result from social interaction. While the overall population appears to approve of breastfeeding in public, less-educated people are less likely to do so (Li et al., 2004). Society as a whole influences the decision to breastfeed, with cultural norms having a strong influence on feeding choice (Hernández & Callahan, 2008). Therefore, approaching the rest of the population in addition to pregnant women and mothers is an essential factor in breastfeeding promotion. Social influence is greatest in face-to-face interactions. Group behavior determines what is popular, fashionable, and normal; and perceived norms can influence behavior and effect social change.

Compliance

Acceptance is an internal process whereby we sincerely change because of social influence. In contrast, compliance occurs when we change our behavior or our expression of an attitude but do not accept the change completely. The degree to which we comply may depend in part on our self-esteem and our fear of "losing face." We may also be more likely to comply with a request from a person who has previously done us a favor. Thus building influence is an effective way of increasing compliance. When we begin with a small request and follow it with a

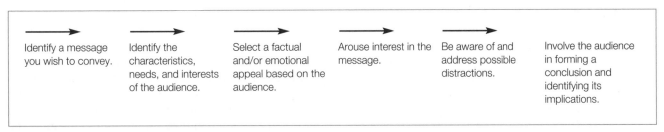

FIGURE 3.7   Influencing a person's decision making.

larger request, people will be more likely to comply with the larger request. Another popular approach is to begin with a large request that seems unreasonable and follow it with a more reasonable request with which we actually wish the person to comply.

If you practice in a hospital or healthcare provider's office, you will have many opportunities to use the skill of increasing others' compliance. Lactation consultants can help their facilities take "baby steps" toward becoming "Baby-Friendly" by using such approaches. Asking the purchasing department to no longer accept the "free" formula plied by marketing representatives may be too large a step initially. However, convincing the hospital to provide its own logo diaper bag as an advertising tool may enable you to remove the "free" formula gift bags as an interim step toward becoming a Baby-Friendly facility (UNICEF, 2009). Mapping out a strategy for gradual change will help you build one change at a time.

Despite recommendations to breastfeed exclusively for 6 months, many mothers fail to reach that goal. One reason women are no longer breastfeeding at 6 months was revealed in an Australian study, which found that many mothers had no intention to do so (Forster et al., 2006). Other reasons cited in the same study included smoking 20 or more cigarettes per day prepregnancy, not attending childbirth education, maternal obesity, having self-reported depression in the 6 months after birth, and the baby receiving infant formula while in hospital. Some of these reasons for noncompliance are within the power of lactation consultants and others who support breastfeeding women to influence.

Conformity

Whereas compliance primarily involves a request from an individual, conformity encompasses a wider range of influence. Conformity involves a change in attitude and behavior. It usually occurs in response to group pressure pushing individuals toward a social norm. People tend to conform to group norms when they find themselves in ambiguous or novel situations and lack prior experience that might serve as a frame of reference. Generally, the more ambiguous the situation and the less experience a person has, the more powerful the group influence will be.

The degree of attraction an individual feels toward the group and its perceived benefits affects conformity. People with high self-esteem tend to conform less following group pressure than do people who have low self-esteem. Groups we like and compare ourselves to are powerful sources of social influence. Conformity increases when the individual receives positive reinforcement, illustrating how the support of one person can have a considerable effect on another to comply with or to resist social pressure.

When this idea is translated into the context of breastfeeding, it becomes obvious why many mothers benefit from joining breastfeeding support groups. Identifying with and networking with other breastfeeding mothers provides emotional and subcultural support that these women may not receive from their extended family or friends. The moral support of mother-to-mother involvement encourages breastfeeding mothers to persevere through the predictable challenges of nursing a baby. It validates the importance of breastfeeding and the mother's choice to breastfeed.

Influence of Society

Social influence refers to a change in attitude or behavior that occurs because of interactions with others. Others attempt to influence the way we think, feel, and behave throughout our lives. Through our social interactions, we, in turn, attempt to influence others to think, feel, or act as we do. This encouragement of conformity is important in our society, which expects people to comply with requests and obey authority. At the same time, it is important for an individual to feel a unique sense of identity. Conflict can result from an attempt to maintain uniqueness and individuality while yielding to a certain degree of social influence.

A Glasgow study reported that knowledge and attitude predict breastfeeding initiation, and that social network members may influence mothers' feeding choices (Dungy et al., 2008). A study in Scotland assessed the influence of subjective norms—namely, the perceived influence of other people's views—on women's infant feeding decisions. The researchers found that subjective norms were important determinants for both breastfeeding and bottle feeding (Swanson & Power, 2005). They urged that future interventions to promote breastfeeding adopt a broad social approach, encouraging positive norms for existing and potential mothers and fathers, families, and people in general.

A U.S. Healthstyle Survey revealed regional variations in public knowledge, attitudes, perceptions, and support of breastfeeding (Hannan et al., 2005). This study addressed health benefits, breastfeeding in public, workplace breastfeeding policies, and breastfeeding duration. In another report, researchers noted that semiurban mothers in Malawi were more likely to practice optimal breastfeeding (Kamudoni et al., 2007). Still another investigation reported that country of origin is a significant predictor of breastfeeding intention (Bonuck et al., 2005).

Similarly, women in a U.K. population with high levels of socioeconomic deprivation identified society's negative attitude toward breastfeeding as a barrier to breastfeeding (McFadden & Toole, 2006). Concerns about feeding in public and the response of others were perceived as major obstacles to breastfeeding, as well as the challenge of living in a bottle feeding culture and attitudes of family and friends. Given these powerful environmental influences, it is unlikely that promoting breastfeeding solely to child-bearing couples will result in significant improvements in breastfeeding initiation or duration. Instead, infant feeding campaigns need to address changes at the societal level to reverse negative attitudes and increase acceptance of breastfeeding as a normal and natural feeding method (Tarrant & Dodgson, 2007).

Mothers who choose to bottle feed report that they would have been encouraged to breastfeed if they had received more information prenatally; more information from TV, magazines, and books; and family support (Arora et al., 2000). Based on a 2002 National Survey of Family Growth, U.S. mothers appear likely to choose the same feeding method for each of their children independent of the number of children they have (Taylor et al., 2008). Breastfeeding promotion efforts, therefore, need to target first-time mothers as they are making their infant feeding decision.

As mentioned earlier, society consists of a variety of subcultures, each of which interprets and responds to society's basic beliefs and values in a specific way. When a society undergoes constant change, as is the case in contemporary Western culture, this rapid change makes it especially difficult to monitor changes in cultural values. The existence of contradictory values adds another dimension of confusion. There is considerable pressure to conform to the values of family members, friends, and other socially important groups, but it is often difficult to reconcile these seemingly inconsistent values.

Influence of Family

Our family is often in the best position to influence our decisions. Because we generally have frequent contact with other family members, they are instrumental in establishing our values, attitudes, and behavior. The family serves as the primary agent for passing along basic cultural beliefs, values, and customs to society's newest members. Not surprisingly, then, a young mother's mother and her partner are most influential in the infant feeding decision (Morrison et al., 2008; Rose et al., 2004).

Research has shown that mothers participating in the U.S.-based WIC program primarily rely on experienced family and friends for advice. They perceive professional advice as credible when caregivers exhibit characteristics similar to those of experienced family and friends: confidence, empathy, respect, and calm (Heinig et al., 2009). Similarly, Australian women report moral and family influence in their infant feeding decision (Brodribb et al., 2007). Mothers in Ghana reported pressure from family as a barrier to exclusive breastfeeding (Otoo et al., 2009). Conversely, involving fathers in postpartum breastfeeding could significantly increase the rates of exclusive breastfeeding in the infant's first 6 months of life (Susin & Giugliani, 2008).

The role of grandmothers in infant feeding decisions needs to be understood and recognized. Breastfeeding often occurs within the context of an extended family in which grandmothers bring their own infant feeding practices and beliefs to their support of new mothers. While mothers often need and want grandmothers' support, their advice and concerns may reflect cultural beliefs that do not protect breastfeeding (Grassley & Eschiti, 2008). You can enhance grandmothers' knowledge and support of breastfeeding by including them in conversations about breastfeeding practices.

Paternal grandmothers in northern Malawi have a powerful role in the extended family and often favor tradition over conventional Western medicine in their ideas about early child feeding. In this part of Malawi, hospital personnel often hold disparaging and paternalistic attitudes toward "grannies" and their knowledge. Health education rarely involves grandmothers and, even if they are involved, their perspectives are not taken into consideration (Bezner et al., 2008).

Second to family, our friends are an important influence in our decisions. We are more likely to seek information from those friends whom we believe have values or outlooks similar to our own. The greater the similarity, the more likely we are to be influenced by their judgments. It is important to recognize these sources of influence when counseling mothers and considering what will be most helpful to them.

The increase in public awareness of the importance of breastfeeding has led to many mothers choosing to breastfeed for the first time in two generations of their families. A mother may experience intellectual pressure to breastfeed, yet struggle with negative feedback from family members. Lactation consultants deal frequently with the theme of regret versus guilt, and you can help the mother work through her feelings of being "disloyal" to her relatives if she breastfeeds.

Social Marketing

Behavior patterns determine our decisions and our responses to external influences. Marketing is a potentially powerful technology for bringing about socially desirable behaviors. This concept gave rise to the field of social marketing. The principles of social marketing can apply to a diverse set of social challenges, but the bottom line is influencing behavior. This type of marketing applies commercial marketing strategies toward improving the personal welfare of a particular population. Social marketers analyze, plan, execute, and evaluate programs designed to influence human behavior. The premise of social marketing is to help individuals consider and choose the strategy that best fits their readiness for action and their resources.

Product, price, place, and promotion—the "four P's"—are the primary variables that determine people's likelihood of changing their behavior. Within the context of social marketing, the product is a commodity, service, or health practice. Price involves the barriers or costs associated with adopting a particular behavior. Place encompasses either the location where the product or services can be accessed or the channels of communication and distribution points for the messages. Promotion constitutes messages that are memorable and persuasive. Designing programs that reflect what consumers truly want and that influence positive behavior change requires careful analysis of each of these factors and the ways in which they interact (U.S. Department of Health and Human Services [USDHHS], 2006).

An effective social marketing project for public or private health care typically begins with consumer-based research. A comprehensive social marketing plan is then designed, and specific strategies and materials are selected. An evaluation phase provides continuous monitoring and refinement of the plan. Ongoing monitoring allows social marketers and public health practitioners to modify products or services to meet consumers' expectations.

An example of social marketing for breastfeeding promotion is the National WIC Breastfeeding Promotion Project, "Loving Support Makes Breastfeeding Work," which was established by the United States Department of Agriculture (USDA), Food and Nutrition Service, Special Supplemental Nutrition Program for Women, Infants, and Children (WIC). The national campaign was developed as a social marketing program aimed at increasing breastfeeding initiation and duration rates among WIC participants, increasing public awareness of the importance of breastfeeding, and improving the environment of support for new mothers. The program began in 1997 following formative research into the barriers of WIC participants, their family members, and staff. It has since been implemented in all U.S. states. Program materials for clients, staff, and the media were developed to address key barriers to breastfeeding (embarrassment, time and social constraints, and lack of social support), and were expanded to target Spanish-speaking and Native American communities.

～ Summary

Society sets out boundaries for behavior and each structure within society is interconnected. Humans can and do direct their own lives and alter the social order around them. Tension from an unsatisfied need motivates us to take those actions that will fulfill the need and reduce the tension. Positive drives take the form of needs, wants, and desires. Negative drives consist of fears and aversions.

Our specific qualities, attributes, traits, and mannerisms both determine and reflect how we respond to our environment. Unconscious needs or drives lie at the heart of human motivation and personality. Personality types influence behavior; social relationships are fundamental to the formation and development of personality. Self-image influences our actions with different people and in different situations. Perception derives from sensory input and physical stimuli, as well as from our expectations, motives, and learning based on previous experience.

Learning is driven by four components: motivation, cues, response, and reinforcement. Through problem solving, we gain control over our environment. Processing information through a series of memory storehouses and repetition enables us to hold information in short-term storage long enough for encoding to occur, although information can be lost when the short-term store receives a great deal of input at once (information overload). Information in long-term storage is constantly reorganized as new links are forged between chunks of information. High involvement with an issue produces more extensive processing of information in both the right and left hemispheres of the brain.

The best predictor of behavior is the intention to act. Our feelings about what family, friends, and coworkers would think of the action we contemplate influence our intent. The formation of attitudes is strongly linked with personal experience, the influence of family and friends, direct marketing, and mass media. An effective strategy for changing attitudes is to make the individual's new needs prominent.

Motivation, perception, learning, personality, and attitudes all come together to influence the decision-making process. A person's level of involvement is pivotal to the degree of attention paid to a message and the care taken in decoding it. The use of humor often increases the acceptance and persuasiveness of a message. In addition, family, friends, and our position within our social class influence our decisions. Culture offers order, direction, and guidance by providing standards and rules of behavior.

Healthcare professionals and patients have and use power in their relationships with one another. The use of power places controls within these relationships. It should be the goal of healthcare providers to empower individuals and encourage them to be active in their relationships with practitioners. Nevertheless, true empowerment will occur only when healthcare providers transform the ways in which they relate to patients.

～ Chapter 3—At a Glance

Applying what you learned—

- Empower women both in their roles as mothers and in their career choices.

- Learn your area's demographics and characteristics to assist you in framing your interactions with families and enhancing your sensitivity to clients' cultural beliefs.
- Help breastfeeding mothers with the challenges of going against the societal norm of bottle feeding.
- Reinforce verbal instruction with written materials, demonstrations, lists of Internet resources, and other visual aids.
- Avoid making assumptions about teen mothers' motivations and goals.
- Empower mothers to make choices and to be accountable for their mistakes.
- Support the IBLCE Code of Ethics.
- Support the International Code of Marketing of Breastmilk Substitutes and subsequent resolutions.
- Incorporate ethics into your career and learn to integrate your internal personal needs with your external social needs.
- Respect cultural differences in foods, clothes, language, values, beliefs, and practices.
- Encourage parents to network formally and informally with other parents.
- Avoid overwhelming mothers with too much information.
- Elicit the best from mothers and colleagues.
- Make good first impressions.
- Use events or circumstances to help shape mothers' and colleagues' attitudes.
- Help mothers recognize infant signals to strengthen attachment and bonding.
- Respect the family as a mother's primary group.
- Help mothers connect with a breastfeeding support group.
- Empower mothers to take control over their health needs.
- Combine evidence-based practice with caring, intuition, and other "nonscientific" practices.
- Influence decision making by appealing to the needs and interests of mothers and colleagues.
- Build one influence upon another to increase compliance.
- Help parents sort through the myriad—and mixed—messages they receive from the media.
- Use humor to increase a message's acceptance and persuasiveness.

∾ References

Aiken TD. *Legal, Ethical, and Political Issues in Nursing.* 2nd ed. Philadelphia, PA: F. A. Davis Company; 2004.

Ainsworth M, et al. *Patterns of Attachment: A Psychological Study of the Strange Situation.* Hillsdale, NJ: Erlbaum; 1978.

American Academy of Pediatrics (AAP). *AAP Media Alert: AAP Addresses Scheduled Feedings vs. Demand Feedings.* April 20, 1998.

American Academy of Pediatrics (AAP), Subcommittee on Hyperbilirubinemia. Clinical practice guideline: management of hyperbilirubinemia in the newborn infant 35 or more weeks of gestation. *Pediatrics.* 2004;114(1):297-316.

Amir L, Donath S. Socioeconomic status and rates of breastfeeding in Australia: evidence from three recent national health surveys. *Med J Aust.* 2008;189(5):254-256.

Aney M. Babywise advice linked to dehydration, failure to thrive. *AAP News.* 1998;14(4):21.

Arora S, et al. Major factors influencing breastfeeding rates: mother's perception of father's attitude and milk supply. *Pediatrics.* 2000;106(5):E67.

Beauchamp TL, Childress JF. *Principles of Biomedical Ethics.* 5th ed. New York: Oxford University Press; 2001.

Bezner KRL, et al. We grandmothers know plenty: breastfeeding, complementary feeding and the multifaceted role of grandmothers in Malawi. *Soc Sci Med.* 2008;66(5):1095-1105.

Bonuck KA, et al. Country of origin and race/ethnicity: impact on breastfeeding intentions. *J Hum Lact.* 2005;21(3):320-326.

Bowlby J. Attachment. In *Attachment and Loss, Vol 1,* 2nd ed. London: Hogarth Press; New York: Basic Books; 1982.

Bowlby J. Separation: anxiety and anger. In *Attachment and Loss, Vol 2.* London: Hogarth Press; 1973. New York: Basic Books; Harmondsworth: Penguin; 1975.

Britton JR, et al. Breastfeeding, sensitivity, and attachment. *Pediatrics.* 2006;118(5):e1436-1443.

Britton JR, Britton HL. Maternal self-concept and breastfeeding. *J Hum Lact.* 2008;24(4):431-438.

Brizendine L. *The Female Brain.* New York: Morgan Road Books/Random House; 2006.

Brodribb W, et al. Identifying predictors of the reasons women give for choosing to breastfeed. *J Hum Lact.* 2007;23(4):338-344.

Chang JH, Chan WT. Analysis of factors associated with initiation and duration of breast-feeding: a study in Taitung, Taiwan. *Acta Paediatr Taiwan.* 2003;44(1):29-34.

Chen CH, Chi CS. Maternal intention and actual behavior in infant feeding at one month postpartum. *Acta Paediatr Taiwan.* 2003;44(3):140-144.

Dungy CI, et al. Infant feeding attitudes and knowledge among socioeconomically disadvantaged women in Glasgow. *Matern Child Health J.* 2008;12(3):313-322.

Ethics. *Encarta Online Encyclopedia.* Microsoft Network (MSN); 2009. www.encarta.msn.com. Accessed July 30, 2009.

Flacking R, et al. Effects of socioeconomic status on breastfeeding duration in mothers of preterm and term infants. *Eur J Public Health.* 2007;17(6):579-584.

Forster DA, et al. Factors associated with breastfeeding at six months postpartum in a group of Australian women. *Int Breastfeed J.* 2006;12(1):18.

Glover M, et al. Influences that affect Maori women breastfeeding. *Breastfeed Rev.* 2007;15(2):5-14.

Goodman N. *Introduction to Sociology*. New York: Harper Collins Publishers; 1992.

Grassley J, Eschiti V. Grandmother breastfeeding support: what do mothers need and want? *Birth*. 2008;35(4):329-335.

Gribble KD. Long-term breastfeeding: changing attitudes and overcoming challenges. *Breastfeed Rev*. 2008;16(1):5-15.

Hannan A, et al. Regional variation in public opinion about breastfeeding in the United States. *J Hum Lact*. 2005;21(3): 284-288.

Hauck YL. Factors influencing mothers' decision to breastfeed in public. *Breastfeed Rev*. 2004;12(1):15-23.

Hausman B. *Mother's Milk: Breastfeeding Controversies in American Culture*. New York: Routledge; 2003.

Heck KE, et al. Socioeconomic status and breastfeeding initiation among California mothers. *Public Health Rep*. 2006; 121(1):51-59.

Heinig MJ, et al. Sources and acceptance of infant-feeding advice among low-income women. *J Hum Lact*. 2009;25(1): 163-172.

Hernández PT, Callahan S. Attributions of breastfeeding determinants in a French population. *Birth*. 2008;35(4):303-312.

Hess J. *Infant Feeding: A Handbook for the Practitioner*. Chicago: American Medical Association; 1923.

Honeyball M. Maternity leave in the EU. *Eur Weekly, New Eur* April 20, 2009;830. www.neurope.eu/articles/94045.php. Accessed July 30, 2009.

Kamudoni P, et al. Infant feeding practices in the first 6 months and associated factors in a rural and semiurban community in Mangochi District, Malawi. *J Hum Lact*. 2007;23(4):325-332.

Kessler L, et al. The effect of a woman's significant other on her breastfeeding decision. *J Hum Lact*. 1995;11(2):103-109.

Kong SK, Lee DT. Factors influencing decision to breastfeed. *J Adv Nurs*. 2004;46(4):369-379.

Kronborg H, Vaeth M. The influence of psychosocial factors on the duration of breastfeeding. *Scand J Public Health*. 2004; 32(3):210-216.

Lee HJ, et al. Factors associated with intention to breastfeed among low-income, inner-city pregnant women. *Matern Child Health J*. 2005;9(3):253-361.

Li R, et al. Public beliefs about breastfeeding policies in various settings. *J Am Diet Assoc*. 2004;104(7):1162-1168.

Marrone S, et al. Attitudes, knowledge, and intentions related to breastfeeding among university undergraduate women and men. *J Hum Lact*. 2008;24(2):186-192.

McCarter-Spaulding D. Is breastfeeding fair? Tensions in feminist perspectives on breastfeeding and the family. *J Hum Lact*. 2008;24(2):206-212.

McFadden A, Toole G. Exploring women's views of breastfeeding: a focus group study within an area with high levels of socio-economic deprivation. *Matern Child Nutr*. 2006;2(3): 156-168.

McInnes RJ, Chambers JA. Supporting breastfeeding mothers: qualitative synthesis. *J Adv Nurs*. 2008;62(4):407-427.

Merewood A, Heinig, J. Efforts to promote breastfeeding in the United States: development of a national breastfeeding awareness campaign. *J Hum Lact*. 2004;20(2):140-145.

Mistry Y, et al. Infant-feeding practices of low-income Vietnamese American Women. *J Hum Lact*. 2008;24(4):406-414.

Mitra AK, et al. Predictors of breastfeeding intention among low-income women. *Matern Child Health J*. 2004;8(2):65-70.

Morrison L, et al. Determinants of infant-feeding choice among young women in Hilo, Hawaii. *Health Care Women Int*. 2008;29(8):807-825.

Noel-Weiss J, Walters G. Ethics and lactation consultants: developing knowledge, skills, and tools. *J Hum Lact*. 2006;22(2): 203-212.

Nyqvist KH, Kylberg E. Application of the Baby Friendly Hospital Initiative to neonatal care: suggestions by Swedish mothers of very preterm infants. *J Hum Lact*. 2008;24(3): 252-262.

O'Brien M, et al. The influence of psychological factors on breastfeeding duration. *J Adv Nurs*. 2008;63(4):397-408.

O'Brien M, et al. Exploring the influence of psychological factors on breastfeeding duration, phase 1: perceptions of mothers and clinicians. *J Hum Lact*. 2009;25(1):55-63.

Olson RG. *A Short Introduction to Philosophy*. Mineola, NY: Dover; 2003.

Otoo GE, et al. Perceived incentives and barriers to exclusive breastfeeding among periurban Ghanaian women. *J Hum Lact*. 2009;25(1):34-41.

Palmer G. *The Politics of Breastfeeding: When Breasts Are Bad for Business*. 3rd ed. London: Pinter & Martin; 2009.

Pedersen C, Boccia M. Oxytocin links mothering received, mothering bestowed and adult stress responses. *Stress*. 2002;5(4):259-267.

Persad MD, Mensinger JL. Maternal breastfeeding attitudes: association with breastfeeding intent and socio-demographics among urban primiparas. *J Comm Health*. 2008; 33(2):53-60.

Racine EF, et al. Individual net-benefit maximization: a model for understanding breastfeeding cessation among low-income women. *Matern Child Health J*. 2008;13(2):241-249.

Racine EF, et al. How motivation influences breastfeeding duration among low-income women. *J Hum Lact*. 2009;25(2): 173-181.

Rein S. Ezzo.info. Health care professionals and their concerns: health care professionals quoted in the news. 2006. www.ezzo.info/Articles/doctors-on-babywise.html. Accessed July 30, 2009.

Rose VA, et al. Factors influencing infant feeding method in an urban community. *J Natl Med Assoc*. 2004;96(3):325-331.

Rosier W. Cool cabbage compresses. *Breastfeed Rev*. 1988;1(12): 28-31.

Schiffman L, Kanuk L. *Consumer Behavior*. 9th ed. Englewood Cliffs, NJ: Prentice Hall; 2006.

Schuman A. A concise history of infant formula (twists and turns included). *Contemp Pediatr*, 2003;2:91.

Scott JA, et al. Factors associated with breastfeeding at discharge and duration of breastfeeding. *Paediatr Child Health*. 2001; 37(3):254-261.

Sharpe G. Milk banking: An investment in the future generations. Paper presented at: American Dietetic Association; October 24, 2003; San Antonio, TX.

Sideman A. American mothers to solve breast feeding problems with some help from India. Rediff on the Net; June 9, 1999. www.rediff.com/news/1999/jun/09us2.htm. Accessed July 30, 2009.

Smith P. Is it just so my right? Women repossessing breast-feeding. *Int Breastfeed J.* 2008;4;3(1):12.

Strathearn L, et al. What's in a smile? Maternal brain responses to infant facial cues. *Pediatrics.* 2008;122(1):40-51.

Susin L, Giugliani E. Inclusion of fathers in an intervention to promote breastfeeding: impact on breastfeeding rates. *J Hum Lact.* 2008;24(4):386-392.

Swanson V, et al. The impact of knowledge and social influences on adolescents' breast-feeding beliefs and intentions. *Public Health Nutr.* 2006;9(3):297-305.

Swanson V, Power KG. Initiation and continuation of breast-feeding: theory of planned behaviour. *J Adv Nurs.* 2005;50(3):272-282.

Tarrant M, Dodgson JE. Knowledge, attitudes, exposure, and future intentions of Hong Kong university students toward infant feeding. *J Obstet Gynecol Neonatal Nurs.* 2007;36(3):243-254.

Taylor JS, et al. Birth order and breastfeeding initiation: results from a national survey. *Breastfeed Med.* 2008;3(1):20-27.

Taylor SE, et al. Female responses to stress: tend and befriend, not fight or flight. *Psychol Rev.* 2000;107(3):411-429.

Tischler H. *Introduction to Sociology.* 9th ed. Florence, KY: Wadsworth; 2006.

United Nations Children's Fund (UNICEF). The Baby-Friendly Hospital Initiative. February 23, 2009. www.unicef.org/programme/breastfeeding/baby.htm. Accessed July 30, 2009.

United States Department of Health Human Services (USDHHS), Centers for Disease Control and Prevention (CDC).

Health marketing: Health marketing basics. June 27, 2006. www.cdc.gov/healthmarketing/basics.htm. Accessed July 31, 2009.

Van Esterik P. Breastfeeding and feminism. *Int J Gynaecol Obstet.* 1994;47:S41-S54.

Van Esterik P. Contemporary trends in infant feeding research. *Ann RevAnthrop.* 2002;31:257-278.

Wagner CL, et al. The role of personality and other factors in a mother's decision to initiate breastfeeding. *J Hum Lact.* 2006;22(1):16-26.

Walker M. *Still Selling Out Mothers and Babies: Marketing Breastmilk Substitutes in the USA.* Weston, MA: NABA REAL; 2007.

Wamani H, et al. Infant and young child feeding in western Uganda: knowledge, practices and socio-economic correlates. *J Trop Pediatr.* 2005;51(6):356-361.

Weber A. *Social Psychology.* New York: Harper Collins; 1992.

Wilhelm SL, et al. Influence of intention and self-efficacy levels on duration of breastfeeding for Midwest rural mothers. *Appl Nurs Res.* 2008;21(3):123-130.

Wilhelm SL, et al. Motivational interviewing to promote sustained breastfeeding. *J Obstet Gynecol Neonatal Nurs.* 2006;35(3):340-348.

Wittmann-Price RA. Exploring the subconcepts of the Wittmann-Price theory of emancipated decision-making in women's health care. *J Nurs Scholarsh.* 2006;38(4):377-782.

Wolf J. Low breastfeeding rates and public health in the US. *Am J Pub Health.* 2003;93(12):2001-2010.

Empowering Women to Breastfeed

Empowerment is a process that allows a person to gain the knowledge, skill sets, and attitudes needed to cope with new life circumstances. The focus of empowerment is on increasing confidence and eliminating the future need for assistance. This includes encouraging and developing the skills required for self-sufficiency.

People who demonstrate a sincere belief in breastfeeding as the natural and appropriate way to nourish an infant are the most effective in empowering breastfeeding mothers. Clinicians must move beyond a theoretical belief in breastfeeding, to instill practices that promote and support it among all members of the healthcare team. Unfortunately, some health workers are reluctant to promote breastfeeding for fear that they will create guilt in those mothers who choose not to breastfeed. A caregiver who appears to be ambivalent about breastfeeding sends mixed messages and creates personal doubts in mothers. By comparison, those who promote and support breastfeeding enthusiastically serve as powerful motivators for both mothers and the healthcare community.

A caregiver's approach with breastfeeding women is a significant factor in the effectiveness of that practitioner's support and advice. Establishing an empowering partnership increases mothers' confidence and self-esteem. These characteristics, in turn, foster parental independence and growth. Providing an effective learning climate will help lactation consultants achieve the goal of actively involving mothers in problem solving and decision making. Using humor in interactions with mothers helps them gain perspective during challenging times and increases teaching effectiveness. Understanding the components of communication that affect the messages sent will enhance those interactions as well.

∼ Key Terms

Adult learning	Informed consent
Body language	Learning climate
Consumer responsibilities	Learning style
Consumer rights	Mixed messages
Empowerment	Relinquishing control
Guilt	Self-efficacy
Health consumerism	Traits
Humor as a tool	Voice tone
Imagery	

∼ Health Consumerism

The healthcare system (at least in the United States) is a consumer-oriented operation concerned with attracting clients and keeping them satisfied and healthy. Those persons who participate as caregivers in this system must be alert to the needs and wishes of their clients and institute policies that will meet their needs. A decision-making partnership between parents and their caregivers, for example, empowers parents to accept responsibility for managing their lives.

As mothers learn about breastfeeding, they more clearly understand their options and develop the skills necessary to support breastfeeding. This approach, which builds confidence and self-esteem, promotes the mother's growth as both an individual and a parent. Personal knowledge and a flexible environment are the best predictors of women's satisfaction with decision-making about healthcare issues (Wittmann-Price, 2006). The process of each mother's education is a joint venture in which the mother helps determine what she needs to know. This philosophy of responsible and knowledgeable self-care forms the basis of the counseling approach promoted throughout this text.

Consumer Rights and Responsibilities

Caregivers have a responsibility to inform consumers of healthy practices and the consequences of their actions. As part of this interaction, consumers and providers share a two-way relationship of rights and responsibilities. Parents need information to grow as wise consumers. Those who have not been actively involved in their own health care may need guidance from their healthcare providers in taking more initiative in this area. As a lactation consultant, you can offer new mothers ways to help them communicate their desires to physicians and hospital staff. Healthy communication increases effective, positive interactions between caregivers and patients, which then leads to a healthy working relationship that is mutually respectful. The rights and responsibilities of mothers are summarized here.

The Mother's Rights

Every mother has the following rights:

- To understand what she is giving consent to
- To receive information concerning a drug or treatment prior to its administration
- To know about alternative methods of treatment
- To accept or refuse treatment or advice without pressure
- To know whether a procedure is medically indicated or elective
- To have access to her complete medical records
- To seek another medical opinion
- To be kept informed of the most up-to-date information
- To be treated as an equal partner in her health care
- To have her questions answered completely and courteously
- To be treated with respect
- To be provided with the best care possible, with a focus on prevention
- To make decisions regarding her treatment and that of her child
- To care for herself and her child to the maximum extent she is able

The Mother's Responsibilities

Every mother also has certain responsibilities:

- To learn what is available and make an informed choice
- To find caregivers who can help her reach her goals
- To listen to her caregivers with an open mind
- To let her preferences be known in a courteous manner
- To carry through on an agreed plan of care
- To learn the approximate cost of a procedure in advance
- To state why she changes caregivers, if applicable

Informed Consent

Informed consent means the consumer consents to treatment based on a foundation of sufficient information and education. An informed consumer has adequate preparation and education before treatment is administered. Of course, informed consent is possible only when the consumer takes the initiative for self-education and the responsibility for informed decision making. Consent given in an emergency is generally not considered informed consent, as the consumer has not had sufficient time to explore alternatives and to learn the implications involved in treatment. The majority of medical situations, however, allow adequate time for the consumer to achieve these goals. Even 20 or 30 minutes can permit time for consultation and research.

Informed consent benefits both the caregiver and the health consumer. By obtaining as much information as possible about a recommended treatment and by exploring alternatives and possible outcomes, the consumer is able to offer knowledgeable and responsible input into the decision-making process. Parents then can be actively involved in making decisions and in guiding the course of treatment for themselves and their families. For their part, healthcare providers benefit by having some of this responsibility shifted to the consumer. In this way, informed consent reduces the risk of malpractice suits in the event of an unfavorable outcome. It also enables providers to broaden their perspectives based on consumer input.

Informed consent is not a prerequisite for quality health care. However, it does increase the chances of a positive outcome for the consumer who has accepted the responsibility for becoming knowledgeable and actively involved in his or her own health care. The ultimate responsibility for informed decisions rests with the consumer, who should choose healthcare providers wisely and use them as resources. Consent forms protect both patients and healthcare providers. Parents can either decline or request procedures through consent forms (e.g., declining circumcision or vaccinations in the hospital or giving consent to the use of blood products in emergencies). To ensure that they fully understand their rights and responsibilities, mothers can check the patient's bill of rights in their hospital prior to admission, when possible.

You may encounter a wide range of understanding related to parental education and recognition of patient rights. For example, an educated, professional couple will likely have different expectations of health care than an expectant teen who does not speak the same language. The former couple has adequate intellectual, cultural, and financial resources to ensure that their desires are respected. The latter has no power and no voice in the healthcare system. Yours may be the only voice that helps advocate for such a young mother.

Suggestions for the Healthcare Consumer

An informed parent is an advocate for health consumerism, either consciously or unconsciously. Nevertheless, becoming an informed consumer can sometimes be confusing. When weighing the risks involved in medications and medical procedures, caregivers may at times interject subjectivity into the decision-making process. Based perhaps on tradition or accepted practice, this subjectivity is the cause, in part, of disagreements concerning the best course of treatment for a given situation. The fear of malpractice claims is a great motivator in such subjective approaches.

Following are some suggestions to share with parents who wish to become informed healthcare consumers:

- Acquire a medical vocabulary, subscribe to health electronic newsletters and magazines, access consumer-oriented medical references, research legitimate Internet medical sites, and use the public library.

- Attend courses for nonprofessionals, such as classes in first aid or home health care. Check local high schools, colleges, online classes, or civic organizations for such programs.

- Enlist the services of caregivers and hospitals that welcome and encourage patients to become actively informed.

- Select an independent prepared childbirth class that provides information on alternatives, enhances your understanding, and encourages active participation in medical decisions.

- Learn to recognize early symptoms of illness, and investigate appropriate methods of treatment before contacting the caregiver. This preparation will enable you to have an informed and concrete discussion of the situation with the caregiver.

- If you are unfamiliar with a medical term or do not understand what was told to you, ask to have the point clarified and explained in simpler terms.

- Discuss alternatives with your caregiver, and ask why one course of treatment was chosen over another.

- If the situation warrants, seek a second (and even third) opinion. As a healthcare consumer, this is your right and your responsibility.

- Learn the cost of a recommended treatment, as well as the costs of alternative treatments.

- If you are uncomfortable or dissatisfied with your caregiver's advice, you are not legally required to comply with it in most cases. However, you must be aware of the medical risks. You have the right to make your own choices. Even if it seems to the caregiver that you have made a wrong choice, the ultimate consequences and responsibilities are yours.

The Lactation Consultant's Role in Health Consumerism

In defining your role as a consultant to consumers in the healthcare system, it is important to keep in mind that one

of your primary goals is to encourage parents to take responsibility for their actions. This mandate applies to both health care and parenting. In your role as an advocate for health consumerism, you may wonder how to educate parents about options you know they cannot have with their present provider. You may be limited to simply preparing them to deal with the health care available within the framework of their current medical relationships. As a caregiver, it is not your role to suggest to parents that they change providers. Rather, it is the parents' responsibility to select and work with their medical services.

Mothers view lactation consultants as knowledgeable members of the healthcare team. As such, you need to be tactful in counseling mothers regarding their relationships with caregivers. Even so, you can help parents make choices after they have established their medical relationships. Recognize, too, that parents may sometimes choose a course of action with which you disagree either personally or professionally. You will need to examine your position and decide to what extent it is appropriate for you to become involved.

Helping Parents Become Better Health Consumers

Parents are responsible for the health of their children as well as for their own health; as a consequence, they have complicated consumer roles and interests. Your primary means of helping parents become good consumers is by educating the mother about breastfeeding through reading, conversations, classes, and meetings. Guide parents to the many reputable consumer-oriented books and Internet resources. Breastfeeding mothers can heighten awareness of the appropriateness of their choices within the larger healthcare system, too. Encourage a mother to tell her caregiver how increasing feeding frequency helped increase her milk production, for example. Suggest that she convey how the importance of breastfeeding goes far beyond the milk she feeds her baby.

When you answer parents' questions, first determine whether they are informed consumers. They may be unaccustomed to questioning statements made by their caregivers. Low-income, minority, teenaged, or single mothers are among the most vulnerable to patronizing attitudes of medical caregivers.

Often, the first time a mother realizes that she disagrees with a caregiver is when she is told to supplement her milk with artificial baby milk or to introduce solid foods into her baby's diet for no medical reason. Perhaps she merely voiced concern about whether her baby is receiving enough milk, or mentioned that the baby wakes at night to nurse. You can help a mother gain confidence in herself and her maternal instincts regarding her baby's needs. Emphasize to her that she is the one who knows her baby best. Help her tune into her baby's behavior and understand his or her needs. She may perceive a newborn feeding every 2 hours as a problem unless she understands why. When she understands, she will be less likely to ask her baby's physician, "Do I have enough milk?" By helping mothers further their education about breastfeeding, you can help develop their awareness of their larger rights and responsibilities as healthcare consumers. They can then help educate their healthcare providers on appropriate breastfeeding care.

You can also help a mother understand the difference between parenting issues and medical advice. Parents often turn to medical professionals for answers to parenting concerns. If a mother asks a caregiver what to do about her baby waking at night and her caregiver suggests letting the baby cry or giving supplemental foods, this is parenting advice, not medical advice. Most issues in the breastfeeding arena, in fact, are parenting concerns that do not require medical advice. What such concerns *do* require are informed parents who have faith in their abilities to determine what is best for their baby.

Presenting facts to parents will help them find those options that best suit their needs and goals. This need for education applies to all aspects of childbirth, breastfeeding, and parenting. When you teach parents about the benefits of family-centered maternity care, prepared childbirth, rooming-in, and exclusive breastfeeding for 6 months, you are not establishing goals for parents. Rather, you are educating them about health practices that will help them establish and achieve their own goals.

A healthcare delivery system that increases the incidence and duration of breastfeeding creates cost savings and better health outcomes over the life span of both the mother and the child. A system that does not actively support breastfeeding creates financial losses to the system, less optimal health outcomes, and costs to taxpayers and society as a whole. If the healthcare system does not meet the needs of parents, a change in caregivers may or may not be an option. In the years before managed care, U.S. consumers could express their dissatisfaction simply by changing providers or hospitals. In contrast, under the restraints of managed care, the option to change providers is often limited to once-a-year enrollment through the client's employer. Consequently, consumers continue to receive care within the system despite negative experiences. You can encourage positive change by urging parents to express their concerns and reinforce positive aspects of their care through written comments to their healthcare providers.

∽ Adult Learning Approach

A mother's control over her care increases when practitioners use an adult learning approach during consultations and discussions. The adult learning approach is one that engages the learner in actively learning rather than passively being taught. The role of the lactation consultant is to create circumstances that empower mothers to learn, acting as a "guide on the side" rather than a "sage on the stage." Instead of approaching mothers as a teacher, you serve as a facilitator who explores options and guides the mother in determining the course she will take. An adult learning approach enables you to develop a partnership with the mother and baby to form a problem-solving team. Simply telling a mother what to do and prescribing a course of care is not as effective as actively engaging the mother in the learning process. As an educator, your role is to provide choices and to encourage the mother to select those that will work for her. Doing so requires that she be an active participant in the learning.

Principles of Adult Learning

Adults have special needs and requirements as learners that are different from those of children and teens. Older learners bring with them an accumulation of life experiences, knowledge, and a belief system gained over their lifetime. Adults are practical, autonomous, self-directed, and goal oriented (Lieb, 1991). They need to be free to direct themselves and assume responsibility for their decisions and actions. A basic principle of adult learning is that people attach more meaning to those learnings they gain from experience than to those learnings they acquire passively. Adults have a deep psychological need to be generally self-directing, although they may be dependent in certain temporary situations (Knowles et al., 1998; Knowles, 1980). Your role as a facilitator is to guide new mothers in their learning and help them reach their goals rather than merely supplying them with facts. The key to self-directed learning is that learners have the primary responsibility for planning, carrying out, and evaluating their own learning (Merriam et al., 2006).

Readiness to Learn

Adults must be able to recognize the relevancy of what they are learning for it to have value. People generally become ready to learn something when they experience a need to learn it so that they can cope more satisfyingly with real-life tasks and problems. You can help mothers connect to their learning by drawing on previous knowledge and experience that is relevant and will add value to what they are learning. Adults, as do all learners, need to be shown respect. It is essential to treat them as equals in experience and knowledge, and to encourage them to voice their opinions freely. At the same time, it is natural for learners to be anxious or nervous when faced with a learning situation. They will respond positively to a rich, responsive, risk-free environment where new skills can be practiced and learned without judgment, where they have sufficient time for reflection and receive positive rein-forcement (Vella, 2002).

Learning is a continual process throughout life that results from stimulation of the senses. In some people, one sense is used more than others to learn or recall informa-tion. In addition, people tend to favor one side of the brain in their learning styles. Those with dominance in the left brain generally learn better from verbal instruction; thus they respond well to analytical and logical informa-tion. Right-brain learners respond more readily to images, symbols, intuition, and emotion. Matching your approach to the learner's style will achieve the best results.

Adults are generally willing to engage in learning expe-riences before, after, or during a life-changing event (Zemke & Zemke, 1995). They want to be able to apply whatever knowledge and skill they gain today to living more effectively tomorrow. The goals of any learning are to transfer new understanding and skills to a new setting, to use the behavior that was learned, and to refrain from other practices that were learned to be unhelpful. This transfer-ence is most likely to occur when the degree of learning is high and when learners can associate new information with something they already know. When they recognize that what they learned benefits them pragmatically, they will perform better, and the benefits will be longer lasting.

As an educator, you must also be sensitive to and respectful of generational differences in learning. Remain-ing a lifelong learner yourself will help you understand and meet the needs of the families with whom you work, regardless of any age differences. You will interact with parents and colleagues ranging from baby boomers (born in the period 1946–1964) to those born after 1995. Those in between include members of Generation X (born 1965–1979); Generation Y, also called Millennials (born 1980–1994); and Generation Z, also called Net Gen or the Internet Generation (born after 1994) (Raines, 2003). Most lactation consultants, like nurses and other health-care providers, are baby boomers—a generation whose members have passed their reproductive years.

As teen pregnancies continue to occur, caregivers will increasingly work with mothers who were born in the early to mid-1990s. The members of this newest generation are fluent in multiple media and in simulation-based virtual settings. They respond positively to communal learning that involves diverse, tacit, situated experience. An approach that balances experiential learning, guided mentoring, and collective reflection works well with these learners. They express themselves through nonlinear associations and favor learning experiences that are personalized to their individual needs and preferences (Dede, 2005).

An Effective Learning Climate

Learners perform best in a relaxed and nurturing envi-ronment. Through your body language and the effective use of communication and counseling techniques, you can create a climate that is relaxed, trusting, mutually respectful, informal, warm, collaborative, and support-ive. Establishing rapport helps motivate learners, as does a friendly, open atmosphere. People learn best under low to moderate stress; if the stress is too high, it becomes a barrier to learning. They also learn best when the degree of difficulty is not so high that they become frustrated by information overload. By recognizing that people learn at different speeds, you can sequence learning to match each learner's developmental readiness. An effective approach is to present information in a manner that stimulates as many senses as possible and with positive reinforcement.

Adult Learning Techniques

You do not need to teach everything to every mother. Assessing her needs and her readiness to learn will help you recognize what each mother needs to learn. Within a relaxed, trusting, collaborative, and mutually respectful learning environment, you and the mother can accom-plish planning, form a partnership, and explore issues together. This approach encourages self-direction and risk taking among mothers. When the mother takes an active part in setting her goals, she has ownership for the plan and is responsible for the outcome. She develops problem-solving skills and becomes more self-reliant.

Adults respond to a learning experience in much the same way as adolescents do. Nevertheless, older learners' expectations may be greater in some areas. In addition, the dynamics of interactions with adults is quite different from the dynamics with adolescents, largely because of the manner in which adults interact and the way they assess a facilitator's credibility. Figures 4.1 and 4.2 outline ways to enhance your interactions with adult learners.

Treat mothers as equals in life experience and knowl-edge, and demonstrate respect for their beliefs and opin-ions. As partners, you and the mother will mutually evaluate her needs and set objectives. Presenting choices

---

- Display self-confidence and a strong knowledge base.
- Project an ability to relate to people and a desire to share knowledge.
- Convey flexibility and a willingness to adapt.
- Maintain a sense of humor and a comfortable tone of informality.
- Project enthusiasm and respect for the learner.
- Project positive body language with frequent eye contact.
- Speak in a strong voice with carefully pronounced words.
- Dress in neat, clean, and stylish attire that is professional, but not distracting.

FIGURE 4.1   *Making positive impressions on learners.*

- Listen with empathy and understanding.
- Be flexible in your thinking and be willing to consider other options.
- Persevere when the solution to a problem is not readily apparent.
- Decrease the risk of being impulsive by thinking before you speak or act.
- Draw from past knowledge and apply it to new situations.
- Use descriptive language to communicate precisely.
- Use your ingenuity, originality, and insight.
- Be curious and learn to enjoy problem solving.

FIGURE 4.2   Increasing your effectiveness as a facilitator.

and asking what will work for her encourages self-direction as she practices techniques you have shown to her. Urging the mother to evaluate her learning will affirm that she understands what she has learned and that she knows what will work best for her. With this approach, the mother's competence and confidence increase, fostering greater self-esteem and independence.

Learning Styles

Adults learn through different modalities, primarily through visual, auditory and kinesthetic means. Tailoring your teaching strategies to each learning style will make you a more effective facilitator of a mother's learning. By engaging multiple senses, you can help visual, auditory, and kinesthetic learning to take place (Russell, 2006). This multisensory approach enhances the learning process.

Visual Learner   Visual learners prefer written instructions and will learn best when the educational process includes visual aids such as photographs, diagrams and illustrations. Such individuals respond well to carefully organized learning materials and may study by reading notes and organizing them in an outline form.

You can reach visual learners with well-organized and interesting visual materials presented in a variety of formats. Handouts, for example, should be visually appealing and easy to read. Capitalize on a variety of technologies such as computers, videos, and live demonstrations.

Auditory Learner   Auditory learners are very good at remembering what they say and what others say. These individuals learn best through verbal repetition and by repeating things aloud. They enjoy discussing ideas and express their interest and enthusiasm verbally. At the same time, they may be easily distracted by either too much or too little noise and can find it difficult to work quietly for long periods.

You can reach auditory learners by rephrasing points in several different ways. Writing down key points before verbally presenting them will help avoid confusion. Varying the speed, volume, and pitch of your voice will increase their interest. You may also want to incorporate sounds, music, and other oral technologies into your teaching for these individuals.

Kinesthetic Learner   Kinesthetic learners need to be physically involved in what they are learning. They enjoy handling learning materials and respond well to hands-on activities. Such individuals often take notes to keep busy, though they rarely use them. They typically have good motor coordination and can remember how to do something after doing it one time.

You can reach kinesthetic learners by allowing them to move around the room and providing lots of tactile activities where they can handle and practice with items. Encourage them to write down important points and ask for return demonstrations. Incorporate multimedia such as computers and video cameras to engage learners in active participation.

Levels of Learning

When embarking on an educational plan, you will want to select learning techniques that are appropriate to each situation in terms of heightening the mother's ability to learn and perform well. Involving the mother as an active participant in her learning will produce the best outcome. There are three levels of learning, each of which is appropriate depending on the circumstance. The three levels can be described as follows:

- Lowest level: I hear and I forget, or tell me and I may remember
- Middle level: I see and I remember, or show me and I may understand
- Highest level: I do and I understand, or involve me and I may master

Tell Me and I May Remember   The lowest level of learning occurs when information is shared verbally. There will be times in your interactions with mothers when verbal instructions are sufficient and appropriate. For example, you might approach a discussion of contraception, nutrition, or medications in this way. These types of information do not necessarily require visual or interactive reinforcement. Reinforcing the messages with printed materials will help the mother's recall of what she was told.

Show Me and I May Understand   Learning increases when something visual is added to verbal instruction. For example, visual demonstrations will enhance much of the

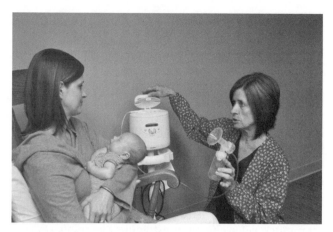

FIGURE 4.3   IBCLC demonstrating use of a breast pump.
Source: Printed with permission of Anna Swisher.

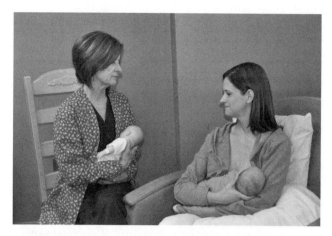

FIGURE 4.4   IBCLC demonstrating positioning while the mother practices.
Source: Printed with permission of Anna Swisher.

teaching you do with mothers. When you teach a mother how to position her baby at the breast, you can demonstrate the technique with a doll. A chart or computer animation showing the anatomy of the breast will help her to understand what is occurring in her breasts. Demonstrating manual expression with a cloth breast will help the mother see how to do it on her breasts. Demonstration is especially important when teaching mothers how to use a breast pump or other breastfeeding device. Discussions of topics such as engorgement, mastitis, nipple soreness, and thrush may also benefit from the use of a cloth breast, video clips, and photographs (see Figure 4.3). See Appendix H for sources of videos and bona fide Internet resources for teaching many aspects of breastfeeding, including positioning and hand expression.

Involve Me and I May Master   The level at which learning is most effective occurs when the learner is actively engaged in the learning process. Expanding on the demonstrations in the previous level, the mother enhances her learning by practicing along with the demonstration. For example, while you demonstrate positioning with a doll, the mother would put her baby to breast and follow along with the instructions. While you demonstrate manual expression or the use of a breast pump, the mother would follow along accordingly. In addition to heightening the mother's learning, this teaching method provides you with visual reinforcement that she understands and has mastered the technique. Such return demonstrations are essential to the mother's learning and growth (see Figure 4.4).

A Personal Approach

If you recognize that every mother and baby are unique, it becomes readily apparent that your approach will vary with each contact. Every mother you see brings with her a rich background of experiences, capabilities, resources, and beliefs that make her needs different from those of other mothers. Some women will appear confident and knowledgeable; others will have a greater need for increasing their self-esteem and confidence. Capitalize on each mother's strengths and build on her present capabilities, while being sensitive to those individuals who are anxious or nervous when faced with a learning situation. When she has learned a technique or overcome an obstacle, praise each mother for her accomplishment. Find something to praise about her baby as well—for example, "See how your baby looks at you!" or "Look at how your baby responds to your voice!"

Individualize your objectives and problem-solving technique with each mother and baby. This will help you avoid falling into the habit of approaching mothers with an established agenda. Respect the mother's background and tap into it. Mothers often offer rich resources for learning. In fact, you may find times when the mother is the teacher and you are the learner! Be the kind of learner you would have mothers be by demonstrating a willingness to learn from them. Increasing your own level of understanding and willingness to adapt your practices will improve your effectiveness as a facilitator. In addition, this openness will help you grow as a member of the healthcare team.

Keep pace with the mother and baby, recognizing that mothers will learn at different speeds and not all mothers and babies will be ready to learn on your schedule. Be alert to responses that suggest the degree of difficulty is causing the mother to become frustrated by information overload, and slow down if you sense that the mother is not taking in what you are saying. Using her language style and imagery will help you relate to each other. Matching her intensity and her sense of humor will help you adopt a receptive approach. Mothers typically respond well to being helped in such a personalized manner.

Relating to mothers individually and on a personal level will strengthen your helping relationship. Make it a point to use the mother's and baby's names. Focus on the mother as a whole person, rather than on her breasts or a particular condition. Consider every mother and baby to be a unique dyad, and broaden your scope beyond the immediate situation. This approach will enhance your effectiveness as their caregiver.

Hands in Your Pockets

Respect that mothers have a great need to be autonomous and self-directed as they settle in with their babies. While in the hospital, they lose a certain amount of autonomy and control, owing to the very nature of hospital procedures. You can help instill a feeling of greater control by approaching mothers and babies with respect for their self-direction. Make sure that any intervention is focused and that you have a good reason for becoming actively involved. Confine your interactions to guiding rather than directing, unless a need for intervention becomes clear.

Interest has grown in the role of "biological nurturing," or respecting the infant's innate ability to self-attach and feed (Colson et al., 2008). This approach stresses that caregivers minimize interventions and ensure the client's dignity and comfort, supported by a hands-off practice as appropriate (Colson, 2008).

Midwives in the United Kingdom learn this hands-off approach through a program that advocates teaching mothers about correct positioning and self-attachment without actually doing it for them. Studies have shown that mothers take greater ownership of their breastfeeding and have a higher rate of continuing to breastfeed when the midwife coaches them but does not touch them (Ingram et al., 2002; Fletcher & Harris, 2000). A hands-off approach puts the mother in control, actively involves her in the learning process, and contributes to her personal growth (Law et al., 2007).

Avoid a hands-off approach from becoming your mantra to the exclusion of times when appropriate intervention is required, however. Learn to recognize when you need to take a more active role to help the mother achieve a positive outcome.

Facilitating Learning

Childbirth and breastfeeding are both life-changing events. Lactation consultants can build on this optimal time for women's willingness to learn. First, be sure to assess each mother's learning needs by asking questions to help you determine what experience she brings to this life event. Is this her first baby, or is she an experienced parent? What exposure has she had to breastfeeding? Does she have relatives or friends who breastfed? Has she breastfed before? If so, what was her experience like? What has she read or heard about breastfeeding? Inquire

about her support system and resources. Does she have someone to help her with caring for her baby or with breastfeeding? How soon will she return to work or school? With this information in mind, you can engage the mother in helping to recognize what her learning needs are.

It is not always possible to determine the learning styles of all mothers in the brief amount of time you spend with them. By tailoring your approach toward characteristics of both right-brain and left-brain learning, an integrated style will emerge. Use of a variety of teaching methods will help you achieve this integration. Written instructions, verbal instructions, visual aids, multimedia (computer, video clips, podcasts, online learning, DVDs), and interactive learning in the form of demonstrations and verbal feedback are techniques you can use to reach parents from different walks of life.

Time for Practice

Create an environment where mothers can practice their new skills without judgment, with sufficient time for reflection, and with positive reinforcement. One of your most important functions is to observe at least one breastfeeding session with every mother and baby in your care, watching how they learn to respond to each other (see Figure 4.5). If you work with families in the immediate postpartum period, observe how the first feeding goes. Allow for the possibility that the baby may want only to nuzzle at the breast in the early hours after birth. There is usually no medical need to rush the first feeding. However, in a hospital setting, you must be aware that time constraints will exist. Optimally, you will be able to move at the baby's pace—not your pace, and not the mother's pace. The mother can hold her baby in skin-to-skin contact near her breast and watch for signs that the baby is interested.

If a mother needs to make adjustments in the way she holds her baby for feeding, you can model the correct

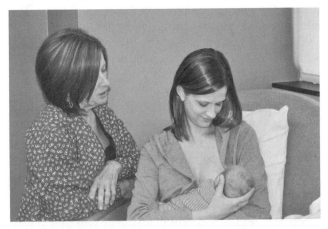

FIGURE 4.5   IBCLC observing a breastfeeding.
Source: Printed with permission of Anna Swisher.

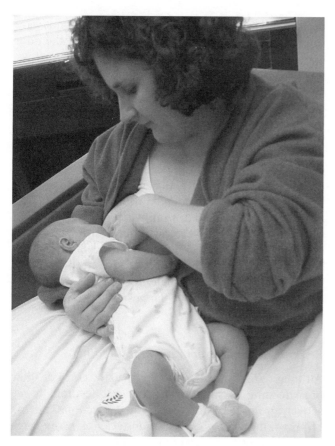

FIGURE 4.6   This mother needs help positioning her baby.
Source: Printed with permission of Anna Swisher.

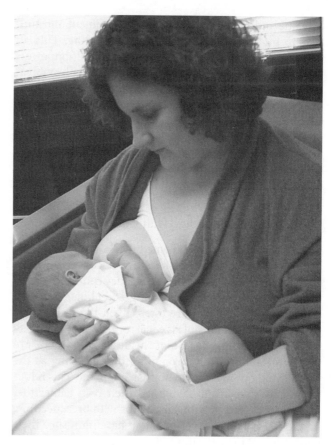

FIGURE 4.7   The same mother after being assisted with positioning.
Source: Printed with permission of Anna Swisher.

position with a doll while she moves her baby, rather than entering her space and touching her baby. Describe how she can make the necessary adjustment so her baby can get a good latch (see Figure 4.6 and Figure 4.7). This effort does not require that you take charge and put the baby to the mother's breast yourself. Rather, you can talk her through it while you model the correct technique.

Transferring Learning to Home

The goal of your work with mothers is for them to transfer what they learn about breastfeeding to their day-to-day lives. The degree to which a mother learns new skills will determine whether she will be able to put them into practice at home. For optimal learning to occur, it must take place at a time when the mother is most receptive and ready to learn. Numerous teachable moments occur throughout a mother's postpartum hospital stay, for example. Focus on those moments to maximize mothers' ability to learn and process information. Divide learning into several visits if time allows, avoiding overwhelming a mother with too much information. If the mother appears tired, distracted, or otherwise unable to focus her thoughts, suggest that you return at a later time. If she appears stressed, discouraged, or lacking in confidence,

help her talk through these emotional issues, if she is receptive, before attempting any new learning. The new mother will find it difficult to concentrate on learning or problem solving until she works through these concerns.

Many mothers appreciate help in accommodating breastfeeding to their lifestyles. Be attentive to circumstances that may create challenges in this regard. Will a return to work separate the mother from her baby for regular periods? Is she a single parent? Is she a teen mother? Does she live with her extended family? Does she have an active social life? Is she a professional woman with demanding work responsibilities? Considering these lifestyle factors will help you determine the educational approach best suited to each mother and baby. In addition, this sensitivity helps ensure that you provide the most effective learning opportunities to help parents blend breastfeeding into their daily lives.

⌒ Confidence in Breastfeeding

Confidence is a belief that something is correct or that a course of action is the best or most effective. Approaching breastfeeding promotion with confidence acknowledges its value and provides tangible encouragement and support to mothers who engage in breastfeeding. This, in turn, increases mothers' self-confidence and empowers them to reach their goals. An approach laced with ambivalence and mixed messages fails to support women in making informed feeding decisions for their babies. Self-confident people inspire confidence in others. When caregivers approach parents with a strong conviction in breastfeeding and a belief in the mother's ability to breastfeed, they help strengthen the mother's confidence in her decisions and capabilities.

Promoting Breastfeeding with Confidence

Research has clearly documented the health risks of not breastfeeding to mothers, babies, and society as a whole. Even so, many healthcare practices today continue to send the message that artificial feeding is a choice equal to breastfeeding. Mothers are often given the impression that feeding infant formula is equal to, and at times preferable to, breastfeeding. Some healthcare workers are uncomfortable actively promoting breastfeeding as the normal and optimal way to nourish an infant. This reluctance may stem from having fed their own babies formula, having had previous problems with breastfeeding, or another personal experience that has diminished their perception of breastfeeding.

Sending noncommittal messages compromises a mother's self-confidence and may cause her to question the wisdom of her decision. A noncommittal attitude by health workers also carries the danger of unwittingly promoting unhealthful practices. If parents do not learn the important differences between the two feeding methods, they will be unable to make the distinctions necessary to make an educated choice about feeding their infant. An ambivalent approach fails to teach parents about the health risks of providing formula to babies and the health risks to mothers from not breastfeeding. A positive and assertive approach to breastfeeding promotion conveys appropriate messages to parents and fulfills the responsibility of health workers to provide essential information for sound decision making.

Caregivers need to use language and adopt attitudes that send positive messages to parents about the superiority of breastfeeding and human milk, and the inferiority of artificial feeding. At prenatal visits and again at hospital admission, a pregnant woman is asked how she plans to feed her baby. This question is often phrased as "How do you plan to feed your baby?" or "Are you going to breastfeed or bottle feed?" Such an approach implies that two equal alternatives exist and that one is as good as the other. Given that infant formula is inferior to human milk, and given that breastfeeding is the optimal way to feed a baby, such an ambivalent approach does a disservice to parents. Unless you believe an alternative is equally healthy and an equally good choice, you would not want to phrase a question in a manner that leaves the door open for the less healthy choice.

By comparison, asking "What questions do you have about breastfeeding?" conveys the *expectation* that the woman will breastfeed to provide normal nutrition for her baby. This approach underscores the health imperative implicit in breastfeeding and conveys the expectation that mothers will breastfeed unless they respond otherwise. If a woman says she does not plan to breastfeed, you can tell her you'll be happy to help her if she changes her mind. If she is comfortable and confident with her choice, such a response should not cause a negative reaction. If she is unsure about her choice, however, she may start to question it and be open to discuss it further. She may have been unaware of the importance of breastfeeding to her baby's health and to her own health. Helping her become an informed consumer may empower her to make wise choices.

Rejecting Guilt in Promoting Breastfeeding

Although most health workers usually concede that breastfeeding is superior to artificial feeding, fewer actively promote breastfeeding with conviction. The fear of provoking guilt presents an obstacle for many caregivers—fear of creating guilt in mothers who choose not to breastfeed, fear of causing guilt in mothers who choose to breastfeed and fail, and fear of pressuring mothers to breastfeed. These reservations may call into question the appropriateness of influencing a mother's choice, but they disregard the responsibility to promote informed consumerism and informed choice. They also ignore the artificial infant milk industry's exploitation of parental misgivings to influence parents to bottle feed.

Parental rights and caregiver responsibilities are significant elements in informed choice. Parents have a right to the information necessary for making an informed choice about infant feeding. Caregivers have an equal responsibility to inform parents of their options so they can make responsible decisions. In teaching parents about the normalcy of breastfeeding and the risks of artificial baby milk feeding, caregivers are not making a choice for parents, but rather fulfilling their responsibility to share evidence-based health information. This sharing of information helps make parents aware of the issues involved in both feeding methods—including the health risks of not breastfeeding.

Guilt is not a factor when the medical community embraces the superiority of breastfeeding over artificial feeding and acknowledges its importance to the health of babies and mothers. Guilt does not prevent caregivers from promoting other healthy practices to their patients. When they advocate that parents use an infant car seat for their baby, caregivers do not worry about offending parents who elect to place their baby in danger by not using a car seat. Guilt is not a concern when informing parents about the need for immunizations. There is no guilt associated with advising against cigarette smoking or the use of drugs and alcohol for pregnant women. Likewise, guilt is not a consideration in recommending diets that are low in cholesterol and fat, or advising patients about good hygiene and dental care. Promoting the healthy practice of breastfeeding should be equally free of worry about making mothers feel guilty if they chose a less healthy alternative.

All members of the mother's healthcare team have a responsibility to educate her appropriately and to help her feel confident in her ability to breastfeed. A fear of instilling guilt cannot be allowed to prevent these providers from promoting breastfeeding and cautioning parents about the risks of not breastfeeding. Healthcare practitioners need to address women's knowledge, health beliefs and feeding intentions during antenatal care (Academy of Breastfeeding Medicine [ABM], 2009).

A U.K. study on infant feeding reported that parents of formula-fed infants had several misconceptions about breastfeeding. Parents of breastfed infants had more positive attitudes toward breastfeeding and were more knowledgeable about the health benefits and nutritional superiority of breastfeeding (Shaker et al., 2004). One factor that may influence parents in the United Kingdom and other European countries is the widespread availability of home health care. One survey found that caregivers are an important source of infant feeding information for parents (70 percent), followed by grandparents (53 percent). Ten percent of the surveyed mothers relied solely on health visitor advice (Gildea et al., 2009). Unfortunately, these kinds of home healthcare services are extremely limited in the United States. Caregivers have a responsibility to inform parents of artificial feeding risks without reserve, and parents have the right to the information necessary for making sound decisions.

The issue of guilt can be quite complex and confusing in the context of infant feeding. Many women feel a sense of personal failure at not breastfeeding—a response that does not always accompany the failure to stop smoking, the failure to use car seats, or the failure to meet immunization schedules. A woman assumes a risk in making her baby dependent on her ability to breastfeed. For some women, taking this risk can be more painful than the guilt of not breastfeeding. Consequently, even though choosing to feed artificial baby milk may cause her to experience guilt, the mother may continue with that choice.

Guilt in Not Promoting Breastfeeding

Naturally, parents want to feel they have done the best they can for their baby. Learning that their baby is experiencing a condition that was potentially avoidable

through breastfeeding will very likely produce guilt and anger. The parents may question why they were not told about the relationship between their child's health and breastfeeding, and their dismay may erode their confidence in the caregiver.

There are considerable consequences from failing to promote breastfeeding to mothers who elect to formula feed. Family finances suffer because of the cost of infant formula feeding and accompanying devices. Formula-fed babies have a higher incidence of illness, sudden infant death syndrome, emotional neglect, and child abuse. They are at a greater risk for developing allergies and asthma. The incidence of learning deficiencies is higher and IQ levels are lower in children who are not breastfed. In addition, the potential for contamination in artificial baby milk places an infant's health at risk. These realities are supported by scientific studies, as discussed in Chapters 1 and 9.

Women experience lack of breastfeeding as a loss at a conscious or subconscious level, regardless of whether the choice to not breastfeed is by decision or imposed (Labbok, 2008). A mother who wanted to breastfeed but was unable due to lack of support and encouragement may feel abandoned by her healthcare team. Omitting information does not contribute to a trusting relationship with mothers. It can also produce guilt in a mother whose child is diagnosed in later life with an illness for which breastfeeding affords protection. Perhaps, in an effort to spare a mother's guilt, her caregiver did not educate her about the risks associated with formula feeding, such as recurrent otitis media, diabetes, or Crohn's disease, which are known to occur more frequently in infants fed artificial milk. Through the course of her research into her child's condition, the mother may learn that breastfeeding decreases this risk. In such a case, in addition to feeling guilty, she is likely to regard her caregiver unfavorably for not helping her to make an informed decision.

Although breastfeeding may be instinctive on the baby's part, breastfeeding appears to be a learned skill for the mother. Women with a prenatal level of confident commitment are able to withstand lack of support and continue breastfeeding. Those who lack such confidence prenatally tend to lose their commitment to continue breastfeeding when challenged (Avery et al., 2009).

Guilt in the Context of Parenting

Guilt is defined as "the act or state of having done a wrong or committed an offense." A mother who feels guilty about her choice to not breastfeed most likely believes that she is failing to do what is in the best interest of her baby. Oski (1995) suggests that guilt can actually serve a positive purpose for families:

> "Guilt or no guilt is not the issue. The issue for me is what is best for babies. If the truth makes mothers feel guilty

and they develop some anxiety, perhaps the discomfort will tip the scales in favor of breastfeeding.

Parents who express feelings of guilt about their infant feeding choice can use this sense of guilt to become better parents. Appropriate guilt can be a positive emotion that leads to personal growth. It can serve as motivation for parents to change a particular behavior or action on behalf of their children. When you are open and honest with parents regarding the risks of artificial feeding, you will usually find that they appreciate learning what to watch for if they later introduce infant formula into their baby's diet. You can help parents make guilt work for them as a catalyst to become the best parents they can be. Make it work for you as well, helping you to provide the best advice and guidance possible.

Guilt About Past Actions

To be effective as a lactation consultant, you must also dispel any guilt you may feel about your own past actions. Your past practices may have included formula supplementation, frequent use of pacifiers, strict rules about frequency and length of feedings, unsupervised use of a nipple shield, or sending a mother home with gifts of formula. Perhaps in the past you presented breastfeeding as being complicated and reliant on a variety of gadgets and special techniques. You may have bottle fed your own children, either out of a lack of information or because you received little help or encouragement to breastfeed. Perhaps your effort to breastfeed was brief because of hospital practices that led to lactation failure.

Be kind to yourself, and recognize that you based what you did in the past on your existing knowledge and what you considered appropriate at the time. As we learn more about breastfeeding care and the negative consequences of past practices, we change the way we practice. Indeed, the lactation field as a whole continues to evolve in its recommended practices. You cannot expect more from yourself than being willing to learn and to change based on what you have learned. Allow yourself to grow and change free from guilt or regret associated with past actions. Help colleagues and other members of the mother's healthcare team recognize this growth in their practices as well.

Increasing Mothers' Self-Confidence

Self-confidence is extremely important in almost every aspect of our lives, and especially so for women who give birth to their first child and breastfeed. The degree to which we empower women to trust their bodies, their capabilities, their instincts, and their babies may significantly affect their breastfeeding satisfaction and duration. Lactation consultants, physicians, nurses, and other members of mothers' healthcare teams need to provide the teaching and support that will empower them to reach their breastfeeding goals. Self-confidence, image, and other emotional factors in women's perceptions are significant determinants of breastfeeding outcome. Some women continue to breastfeed despite extraordinary difficulties, while others give up when they encounter the slightest problem.

Having a realistic picture of what to expect in childbirth and in the early days and weeks of breastfeeding can be a factor in a woman's self-confidence. Idealistic expectations can set women up for emotional distress when their actual experience fails to meet their expectations. This distress may be further compounded by feelings of guilt and inadequacy for those who wean prematurely. Clinicians have a responsibility to accurately reflect the reality of breastfeeding and to support mothers when they experience difficulties (Hegney et al., 2008).

Self-Efficacy

Self-confidence is more aptly termed "self-efficacy," a belief in the ability to perform well. Each period of development brings with it new challenges. An optimistic sense of personal efficacy contributes to further competencies and a positive feeling of well-being. The experience of giving birth is a major turning point in women's lives, and breastfeeding is part of a woman's transition to motherhood (Marshall et al., 2007). Mothers often identify childbirth as their most significant learning experience. The act of creation brings to the woman a new awareness of her creative capacities. A new mother reassesses her capabilities and her capacity to assume a new role as parent. As one mother said, when she found that she could hear, understand, and remember the things she learned about breastfeeding, she began to think of herself as a learner for the first time (Belenky et al., 1997). Caregivers can capitalize on this powerful time in a woman's life by helping her gain skills, knowledge, and confidence in breastfeeding.

Interventions aimed at improving mothers' self-efficacy with breastfeeding are intended to result in longer and more exclusive breastfeeding (Nichols et al., 2009; Sisk et al., 2006). Acquiring self-efficacy begins with setting a goal and making a commitment to achieve it. In committing to breastfeed, a mother's confidence, and therefore her self-efficacy, will increase when she learns the skills necessary for achieving her goal. The most effective way of creating a strong sense of efficacy is through mastery of the necessary skills to achieve the desired outcome. In one study, mothers who contacted a breastfeeding support service primarily for problems with positioning, attachment, nipple pain, or mastitis reported greater comfort, knowledge, and confidence as a result of the support they received (Coffield, 2008). Mastering breastfeeding skills can increase a mother's belief in her abilities and feelings of competence—and the mother's healthcare team can be instrumental in helping her achieve these skills.

Our self-efficacy beliefs determine how we feel, think, behave, and motivate ourselves. People with high self-efficacy—that is, those who firmly believe they can perform well—are more likely to make more of an effort and persist longer as they strive to attain their goals (Bandura, 1994). Self-efficacy also affects how people respond to failure. Those with high assurance in their capabilities approach difficult tasks as challenges to be mastered and maintain a strong commitment to them. Further, people who receive recognition that they possess the capabilities to master a goal are likely to make a greater effort and sustain their goal. Educating mothers, supporting them in their attempts at mastery, and praising their accomplishments help empower these women to attain high levels of personal efficacy. In turn, this approach promotes optimal breastfeeding practices.

Women who receive prenatal education and postpartum support are twice as likely to initiate breastfeeding and to continue breastfeeding at least until the child reaches the age of 6 months (Gill et al., 2007; Su et al., 2007; Arora et al., 2000). Indeed, many mothers view breastfeeding as the one thing they can control in their immediate postpartum environment. The early weeks of breastfeeding are a pivotal time for establishing breastfeeding practices and confidence. Despite this fact, women typically receive less help with breastfeeding after hospital discharge, a time when interventions could increase self-efficacy and confidence to improve breastfeeding duration and exclusivity (Lewallen et al., 2006). Achieving a positive and rewarding breastfeeding experience produces feelings of power and accomplishment in a woman (Locklin & Naber, 1993). Lactation consultants can help to facilitate a mother's efforts to acquire this sense of control.

Use of behavioral and cognitive strategies that help women cope with the pressures linked to early mothering can increase breastfeeding duration (O'Brien et al., 2009). As a lactation consultant, you can help facilitate new mothers' stress management by encouraging them to increase their breastfeeding knowledge, to stay relaxed, to use positive self-talk, to challenge unhelpful beliefs, to learn problem-solving skills, to set goals, and to be mindful of their actions. Helping mothers set breastfeeding goals and providing the necessary education and support may enhance their self-perception and empower them to reach those goals (Betzold et al., 2007). Giving them the tools and support they need to identify and solve problems by themselves can improve breastfeeding self-efficacy (Kang et al., 2008) and increase their capability to transfer their skills beyond their learning environment.

Mothers who have a good self-image and feel confident in their parenting are more likely to form positive attachments with their children. Lactation consultants and others who care for these women prenatally and postpartum are ideally positioned to increase their self-efficacy and promote their growth as parents. Studies show that a mother who lacks confidence has difficulty establishing a relationship with her baby. Moreover, depressed parents may negatively affect the health and development of their children (McLearn et al., 2006). Self-confidence and the quality of the mother–infant relationship are strengthened when prenatal and postpartum parenting classes are combined with a parent support network (Ekström & Nissen, 2006). This combination of education, support, and networking with other parents typically proves empowering to a woman as she assumes the role of a breastfeeding mother.

A positive experience initiating breastfeeding can have a tremendous positive impact on a woman as she embarks on her passage into motherhood. Numerous studies cite the importance of supporting breastfeeding women and increasing their self-confidence. Empowering a mother with confidence in her ability to breastfeed increases the likelihood that she will breastfeed (Mistry et al., 2008; O'Brien et al., 2008) and extends her duration of breastfeeding (O'Brien et al., 2008). The availability of both lay and professional support extends breastfeeding duration significantly (Britton et al., 2002). Likewise, the availability of a telephone hotline relating to breastfeeding encourages greater empowerment in mothers (Wang et al., 2008). Studies of these and other issues cited throughout this text illustrate how pivotal the lactation consultant profession is in nurturing the growth of parents through our education, caring, and support. This growth extends far beyond the period of breastfeeding.

Trusting Mothers and Babies

When caregivers demonstrate confidence in the capabilities of mothers and babies, they also build on mothers' self-confidence and encourage them to engage in self-direction. Of course, empowerment of mothers requires caregivers to trust that mothers and babies are capable of assuming control. Newborns have amazing capabilities from the very moment of birth. When caregivers refrain from interfering with the process, and when mothers are taught how to read infant language, babies can communicate effectively to have their needs met. Further, when mothers can exercise legitimate control, they feel more independent, self-reliant, and confident.

Mothers who are treated in this way learn to trust themselves and their babies. Consequently, they find it easier to adjust to their maternal role and take responsibility for their learning. They develop problem-solving skills, accept the consequences of their decisions and actions, and control their outcomes.

You can help facilitate this growth by using words and actions that show you believe in the mother's abilities.

Facilitation skills that recognize the mother's expertise contribute to longer breastfeeding duration (Kruske et al., 2007).

Relinquishing Control The caregiver's goal should be one of empowering the breastfeeding mother to be independent and self-reliant. Trusting in the capabilities of mothers and babies enables caregivers to relinquish much of the control that has traditionally been associated with patient care. If a mother feels controlled, she may not recognize ways to help herself. She needs the opportunity to use her own inner resources to become self-sufficient. If she becomes dependent on others, she may lose sight of her own strengths. She may then expect others to solve her problems and find solutions, and she may blame those same people when they do not come through for her.

Many adults have experienced a hospitalization at some point in their life. The majority of hospitalized patients are ill or injured. This is not the case with a woman who enters the hospital to deliver her baby. Despite this distinction, however, the pregnant woman loses varying degrees of control the moment she passes through the hospital door. Her privacy is invaded, and she is placed in a dependent role during delivery and after she gives birth. Often, hospital and physician policies impose unnecessary controls over a mother and her newborn. Other people make decisions about the woman's care and that of her baby.

Many parents choose birthing centers and home births for the delivery of their children simply because of these factors. In many countries outside the United States, in fact, traditional midwifery is still the norm. In the United States, the medical community needs to recognize that a new mother should be regarded differently than an ill or injured patient. New mothers need greater control and options regarding their care and that of their infants.

Minimizing Interventions The loss of control that women experience during childbirth and postpartum care can undermine their confidence and sense of personal efficacy. As a member of the new mother's healthcare team, you can be instrumental in helping her to reestablish some of that control by avoiding unnecessary interventions. A gentle approach that minimizes interventions builds on the mother's confidence and self-direction. Medical intervention should never occur without a clear and specific purpose.

Breastfeeding advice often imposes too many rules—always hold the breast during a feeding, wear a bra that gives good support, avoid certain foods, watch the clock, always use both breasts at a feeding, use only one breast at a feeding, and on and on. These or other arbitrary rules about separating mothers and babies or giving supplements to breastfeeding babies are not well founded in science and interfere with establishing breastfeeding. A cavalier attitude about such practices is counterproductive to the goal of empowering the mother. London midwife Chloe Fisher (1996) tells us there is only one rule in breastfeeding: There are no rules!

Take care not to allow control issues to compromise the treatment that mothers and babies receive. As mentioned earlier, control is important to a new mother. She may need to reestablish control following birth and may lack control for a new venture such as breastfeeding. Even if this neonate is not her first child, it may be the first child she will breastfeed. The mother needs you and other caregivers to help her gain control or retain the control she has already established. Medical staff policies should model self-reliance and parental decision making from the very beginning. Doing so requires a negotiation of control between the caregiver and the patient. Caregivers need to become comfortable with the notion of relinquishing unnecessary control and placing control with babies and mothers—where it belongs.

～ Components of Communication

Communication—the most powerful tool we have—is a complex process that needs practice if it is to be used effectively. As lactation consultants, the communication we enter into with mothers differs greatly from casual conversation. Our therapeutic communication is calculated, deliberate, purposeful, and focused. It is intended to collect information, to assess and modify behavior, and to educate. The communication we use with mothers encourages them to interact in a manner that promotes their growth and moves them toward their goals.

Lactation consultants' success in communicating with mothers depends on effective interpersonal skills. Communication is influenced by culture, perceptions, values, relationships, context, and the content of the message. For therapeutic communication to be effective, caregivers must be aware of how we appear to the mother. If we appear rushed, speak quickly, and fail to establish eye contact, therapeutic communication may be hindered. Being aware of body language and other components of communication will enhance our effectiveness in our exchanges with patients.

The process of communication requires two basic elements: the delivery and the reception of a message. When delivering a message from one person to another, the way in which the message is received depends on three factors—body language, tone of voice, and the spoken message (Fast, 1988). Nonverbal language makes a far greater impression than the words that are actually spoken. Although you may be highly knowledgeable about every aspect of breastfeeding care and lactation, that knowledge will be lost if it is not transmitted effectively.

The Importance of the Spoken Word

The actual words you speak have a relatively low bearing on the message that the mother receives. Indeed, only 7 percent of the message that is conveyed is determined by the spoken word (Fast, 1988). To facilitate your effectiveness as a lactation consultant, you will inevitably study a variety of books, attend classes and conferences, and network with colleagues to learn all that is necessary about breastfeeding and lactation so that you can help mothers. Yet, the verbal communication of that information alone has relatively little impact on the mother's receiving the intended message.

This does not mean the words are not important. Obviously, the words and phrases you use can influence the mother's emotional reaction to what you say. Certain words and phrases may convey negative messages, even though that effect occurs unintentionally. It is important to avoid terminology that creates a negative impression or implies the mother is doing something incorrectly. Eliminating two specific words from your vocabulary can increase your effectiveness as a communicator.

Avoid the Use of "But"

Try to avoid using the word "but" to join two thoughts when you talk with mothers. When you say "but" you negate the first half of the thought and fail to achieve your intended outcome. Imagine how you would react if someone told you, "Your new hairstyle looks good on you, but it's a little outdated." You probably would not feel complimented. How might a child feel if his parent says, "Getting a B on your report is fine, but with a little more effort you can get an A next time." The parent may have thought he or she was complimenting the child on his performance and encouraging him to keep doing well. What the child heard, however, is that his performance wasn't good enough.

Suppose you tell a mother, "You are holding your baby in a good position, *but* if you turn him slightly toward you he can get a better latch." Without intending to do so, you have told the mother that she is not holding her baby correctly. The mother might think, "I'm not holding my baby right. I feel so dumb!" As soon as she hears the word "but," it creates a negative impression and she forgets the first part of the statement. Although your intention was to teach the mother how to hold her baby during breastfeeding, your phrasing has undermined her self-confidence as a new mother.

If you wish to connect two thoughts and at the same time correct the mother, you can simply replace the word "but" with "and." You could say, "You are holding your baby in a good position, *and* if you turn him slightly you will find that he can get an even better latch." Another way to phrase it is, "That's a good start. Now, you can turn him slightly toward you so that he can get a better latch." With

this choice of words, you succeed in your goal of helping the mother improve the manner in which she holds her baby. At the same time, you avoid any suggestion that she is doing something incorrectly. In so doing, you preserve her self-confidence and help her to grow as a mother.

Avoid the Use of "Should"

Try to eliminate the word "should" from your vocabulary as well. To state that a mother *should* do something implies that she was doing something she should not have done or that she is doing something incorrectly. Consider these statements by a caregiver who is attempting to teach the concept of need feeding and the avoidance of artificial nipples: "You should feed your baby whenever he wants." "You shouldn't give your baby a pacifier." Such phrasing, while intended to educate the mother in optimal practices, may sound judgmental to the mother. The implication is that the mother should breastfeed in the way you consider correct and appropriate.

You can offer the same advice in a more effective manner without diluting the message. For example, suppose a mother asks about supplementing her baby. You want to teach her to breastfeed exclusively and to refrain from the use of pacifiers. You can tell her, "Your baby needs nothing except your milk for the first 6 months. When you feed him in response to hunger cues, you will be meeting his needs. We discourage pacifiers because your baby needs to spend his sucking time at the breast." With this response, you teach correct practices and at the same time you educate the mother about the reasons for the advice. In addition, you avoid sending a judgmental message or undermining the mother's confidence.

Avoid Negative Imagery

Some words and phrasing create negative images and, therefore, should be avoided. Such terms abound in women's health—an *incompetent* cervix, *failure* to progress, *insufficient* milk production, a baby who *fails* to thrive. Even words intended to be positive can suggest the possibility of something negative. If you refer to a mother as being successful with her breastfeeding, you raise the possibility that she may be unsuccessful. Talking to a mother about establishing adequate milk production may suggest that her milk production might be inadequate. You can rephrase both of these messages by referring to the mother as reaching her breastfeeding goals and producing enough milk to meet her baby's needs.

Avoid Mixed Messages

Be certain that the words you use create the effect you want. Take care not to use phrases that create doubt in a mother's mind, send mixed messages, or compromise her self-confidence. Consider the message you may send to a mother with the following statements:

Statement: You need your rest. I'll take your baby to the nursery for you.

Message: You cannot get enough rest if you keep your baby with you. It does not really matter if you skip a feeding. We can give the baby a bottle of formula. Formula is just as good as your milk.

Statement: Are you going to try to breastfeed?

Message: You might not be able to breastfeed. A lot of mothers try and fail. You can go ahead and try, but do not be surprised if it does not work.

Statement: Do you have any milk yet?

Message: You might not have enough milk for your baby. We might need to give your baby a bottle. You should have more milk by now. Some women never establish milk production.

These messages clearly are not the ones you intend to send. You can tactfully help other caregivers recognize the effects of such phrases as well. Knowing that other elements of communication eclipse much of your spoken message, you can supplement your verbal messages with demonstrations, visual aids, written instructions, and careful attention to your voice tone and body language.

The Effect of Voice Tone

Tone of voice has a dramatic effect on the manner in which others respond to you. In fact, your voice tone is responsible for 38 percent of the message a mother receives (Fast, 1988). You can undoubtedly recall a time when you talked with someone on the telephone you hoped you would never confront again. You could tell by the tone of her voice and her speaking manner that she simply was not a pleasant person! Conversely, you can probably recall a time when the sound of another person's voice was so pleasant that it enhanced your exchange. You sensed you would enjoy interacting with her again.

Make sure your voice tone matches the message you want to send, both in exchanges with mothers and in conversations with colleagues. Your manner of speech can create a warm, friendly, even humorous atmosphere.

In evaluating your speech, also consider your volume. Many people speak either too loudly or too softly. Either extreme can irritate the other person and interfere with your message getting across.

Your rate of speech is another factor that influences the effectiveness of your communication. On the one hand, if you talk too quickly, you may appear rushed and the other person may become anxious or nervous. Remembering to stop and breathe can keep you from running out of breath and seeming rushed. On the other hand, talking too slowly can irritate others, who will wonder if you will ever get your message across.

Controlling the pitch of your voice may be a challenge. Often, our voices tend to get higher when we are angry or excited. Consciously trying to control this factor may help you to modulate the pitch and appear controlled.

Moderating the rate and pitch of your voice and talking slowly enough to pause and breathe will help you achieve an effective voice tone. All of these aspects of your speech can have a positive effect on the message you convey.

The Effect of Body Language

Of the three components in communication, body language has the greatest effect on the manner in which a message is received. Body language, which accounts for 55 percent of how the message is received (Fast, 1988), describes the behavioral patterns of nonverbal communication. It encompasses the mixture of all body movements, including smiling, eye contact, posture, space, and touching. Body language ranges from deliberate to unconscious gestures. It may apply in only one culture or span multiple cultural practices.

In addition to sending and receiving messages, body language can serve to break through defenses. Women tend to base their sense of self-worth on whether they feel accepted. They typically rely on visual communication cues such as facial expressions and eye contact to determine if they are accepted (Brizendine, 2006). The manner in which you capitalize on your nonverbal messages will determine your effectiveness in the care you give to mothers.

Smile

When we experience an emotion of any kind, our facial expression changes to reflect that feeling (Coon & Mitterer, 2008). This phenomenon has been described as "micro expressions"—facial expressions that flash across a person's face and last about one-fourth of a second. Micro expressions are beyond our control and express feelings of anger, contempt, disgust, sadness, surprise, and other human emotions (Ekman, 2007). Understanding this phenomenon may help you be aware of your reactions and the body language you exhibit.

A pleasant facial expression adds to a warm and inviting atmosphere. A calm, relaxed smile reflects that you enjoy your work and enjoy meeting people. That kind of smile will put mothers at ease. When you smile, you elicit a smile from the mother as well. It is almost impossible not to return a smile. The other person cannot help it—it is human nature to smile back! The warmth of a smile even comes through in your voice over the telephone.

Eye Contact

The eyes are the most important of all body parts in transmitting information. Eye contact has a powerful effect on your message. Establishing eye contact with a mother conveys your desire to communicate with her. It creates a warm, caring, and inviting climate. When you interact with another person, try to maintain eye contact at least 85 percent of the time. You can avoid too much intensity or the appearance of staring by blinking or by looking away and back again.

Eye contact can be a powerful tool for influencing others. The next time you are competing for a parking place or trying to merge into traffic, establish eye contact with the driver in the other car. The driver will probably bend to your wishes. If you are standing in line for a movie and another person tries to cut into the line, look the other person straight in the eye. Chances are the other person will turn away and go to the back of the line.

Be aware of the power your eye contact has on the messages you send. Failing to establish eye contact also sends a message. We all use this tactic to avoid talking with others or being seen by them. Consider, therefore, the message you send if you talk to a mother with your back turned or your eyes focused on what you are writing (see Figure 4.8).

In your eyes, you have a powerful communication tool—in fact, two of them! Consciously engaging in eye contact with mothers in your care will enhance your interactions and your effectiveness. At the same time, be aware that in some cultures, direct eye contact is considered rude. Develop cultural competence in caring for families from cultures and countries other than your own.

Posture

Posture is another aspect of body language that sends a strong message. To create a warm and inviting climate, you want your body to be relaxed and comfortable. Try to avoid crossing your arms or legs, which can convey an attitude of disinterest and emotional distance. Instead, sit or stand squarely with both feet flat on the floor. Rest your arms at your side or, when sitting, on your knees. This open body posture shows your intent to communicate on a meaningful level. Leaning forward further conveys your interest in interacting with the mother.

Body Position

We all have a certain amount of personal space that represents our "comfort zone." The amount of space people require to be comfortable varies. The ways in which we guard our personal zone and our reaction when others invade it affect how we relate to others. Be careful not to invade a mother's comfort zone and cause her to feel uneasy or awkward. At the same time, if you position yourself too far away, you may convey a message that you are too busy or uninterested in engaging the mother in a meaningful way. If you poke your head in the door and ask a mother how breastfeeding is going, you do not convey a willingness to help or an interest to interact (see Figure 4.9). Standing on the other side of the room has the same effect. Establish a position that is comfortable for both of you—not too far away and not too close.

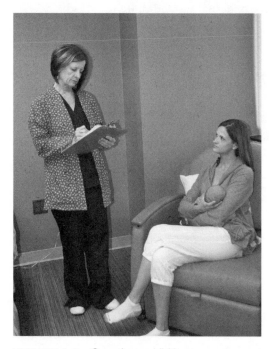

FIGURE 4.8   Caregiver exhibiting poor eye contact.
Source: Printed with permission of Anna Swisher.

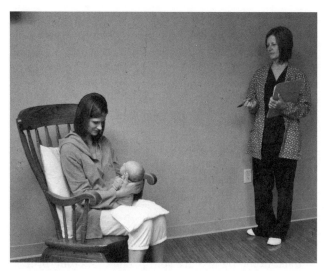

FIGURE 4.9   Caregiver too far from the mother to engage in meaningful dialogue.
Source: Printed with permission of Anna Swisher.

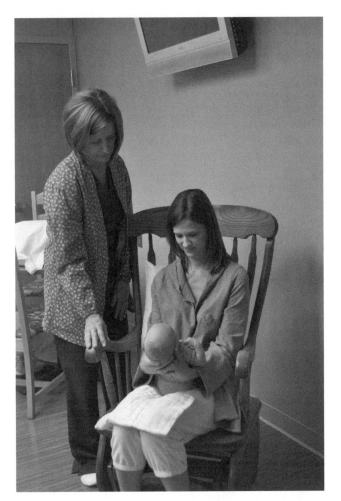

FIGURE 4.10 Caregiver positioned higher than the mother, suggesting a position of dominance and control.

Source: Printed with permission of Anna Swisher.

Another aspect of body position is altitude. When two people interact, the height that each person assumes in relation to the other creates a perception of importance or control. When the mother's caregiver looms over her, it can be intimidating to the mother and fails to empower her as the one in charge (see Figure 4.10). Placing the mother at an equal or greater height establishes that the mother is the person of greatest importance. It also leads to greater self-reliance, which is one of the goals of your consultation with the mother. To achieve this positioning, you can place a chair near the mother or even kneel on the floor next to her. Ask her permission and use her comfort as a guide.

Touch

Be judicious in your use of any posture that involves body contact. Some people are comfortable touching others; some are not. Some people will be receptive to being touched; some will not. The touch of a hand, or an arm placed around someone's shoulder, can convey warmth, caring, and encouragement. However, such a touch must

come at the appropriate moment and within the appropriate context.

On your first contact with a mother, she may respond favorably to your arm around her shoulder as you observe her baby at the breast. However, if you were to touch her breast immediately, she may react in an embarrassed or negative manner. When you need to examine a woman's breasts, be sure to ask her permission first—"May I examine your breasts?"—and explain the purpose (see Figure 4.11).

These same rules apply to touching the baby. If you would like to examine the baby's mouth or touch the baby in any other manner, explain this to the mother and ask permission before invading her space and taking her baby from her. Any oral exam or demonstration of feeding can usually be done with the parent holding the baby. Ask the parent to do as much as possible when you are performing assessments. If you are weighing the baby, have the parent put the baby on and off the scale. If the baby has a void

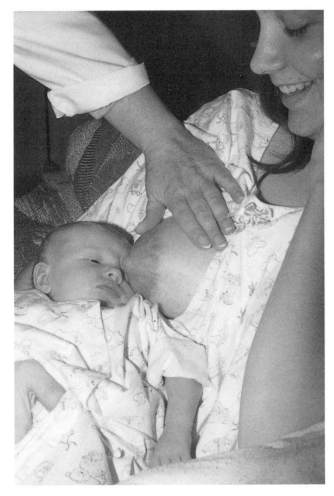

FIGURE 4.11 Ask permission before examining a mother's breasts.

Source: Printed with permission of Debbie Shinskie.

or stool, encourage the parent to change the diaper. Small steps like these convey respect for the parents' role, and reinforce the concept that the baby belongs to them, not the staff.

Cultural Differences

Be aware that a particular body gesture may send different messages in different cultures. In Western culture, for instance, shaking the head up and down indicates yes and shaking from side to side indicates no. In other societies, the opposite is true: Side to side means yes and up and down means no! Smiling, eye contact, personal space, touching, and posture may vary greatly from one culture to another. Learn about your clients' cultural backgrounds so that you are sure you send the intended messages and interpret their body language correctly.

Reading Body Language

In addition to gaining an awareness of your own body language, you need to be alert for nonverbal messages that the mother sends to you. As you continue to mature in your role and responsibilities as a member of the healthcare team, both your clinical knowledge and your understanding of human behavior will grow. This growth in knowledge and understanding will contribute to your ability to recognize and interpret many kinds of nonverbal communication.

Observing a mother's body language will help you determine whether she appears to be comfortable or in pain. Does she welcome eye contact, or does she avert her eyes? How is her tone of voice? Does she sound stressed or anxious (see Figure 4.12)? Is her facial expression animated or listless? Is she comfortable being touched? Does her body sag, or does she sit or stand with an erect posture? Does she have an air of self-assurance, or does she seem passive and unsure of herself? Does she shift her body and fidget? What is her posture while she is feeding her baby? Are her shoulders hunched and tense? If so, perhaps she needs some pillows to help her get comfortable. Does she curl her toes when her baby is feeding? This may indicate that she is in pain and needs to reposition her baby. Paying careful attention to all of these nuances of the mother's body language will help you gather impressions about her situation.

Humor as a Communication Tool

Humor serves as an indirect form of communication between caregivers and clients. It enhances learning (Cueva, 2006) by helping to open both sides of the brain, making it more likely that integrative learning will take place. Therefore, infusing humor into your interactions with mothers will enhance their learning. It also makes your job more enjoyable!

When a woman enters the hospital, clinic, or physician's office, many of the typical rules of society are suspended. She takes on a dependent role with her caregivers, who expect her to accept their concern and competency almost on faith. Humor can help the caregiver establish trust with the mother. With so little time to build a relationship in the healthcare setting, you will want to use any tools available to you to facilitate this process. The relaxed atmosphere created through humor will help you develop relationships in which mothers heed your advice and follow through with their plan of care.

As a lactation consultant, your goal is to make learning fun for breastfeeding mothers. This task sounds simple—yet mothers who lack self-confidence, who are anxious about their ability to breastfeed, or who have little support from family or friends may find it difficult to access their sense of humor and find enjoyment. Approach mothers in a friendly manner and, when they first initiate breastfeeding or when they confront challenges, help them see the humor in their situation so they can learn not to take it too seriously. Incorporating laughter into learning helps ensure that the mother learns the lesson well. Humanizing your interactions will help you achieve your ultimate goal of a happy mother and baby.

Using humor as a tool may not be as easy as it sounds. We adults—and especially those who work in the medical profession—tend to take ourselves far too seriously! As lactation consultants, we are often so intent on becoming better in our profession that we do not take the time to enjoy ourselves in the process. We need to become comfortable with having fun and incorporating humor in our work. Humor is something we choose, just as we choose to be in a foul mood or we choose to focus on the negative side of things. As members of the health profession,

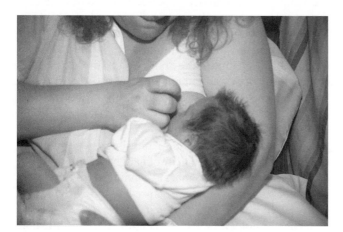

FIGURE 4.12 This mother's clenched hand conveys tension.

Source: Printed with permission of Judith Lauwers.

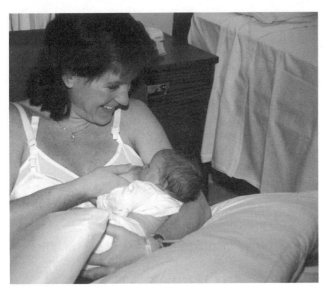

FIGURE 4.13   Mother laughing while she begins breastfeeding.

we need to be able to laugh at ourselves and learn to take ourselves more lightly. Learning to enjoy life and the challenges we face will help us keep perspective and find solutions. Humor can help our clients as well, particularly in terms of dealing with stress, tension, and frustration (see Figure 4.13).

The Role of Humor in the Healthcare System

To tap into our sense of humor, we first need to understand the nature of humor. Humor is more than an occasional witticism—it is a way of life, an attitude. Humor has a direct effect on both mental and physical health and, as such, it is important in all aspects of our life. A sense of humor helps you give the best of yourself to others. Humor as a component of the healthcare system is essentially humanism. A humanistic approach shows each mother that you accept her as a person. It indicates that you respect and care about her, and that you genuinely want to help her. You, in essence, are accepting the mother's humanity and offering your own in return.

Humor evolves naturally in a relaxed climate of support and acceptance. Such an atmosphere enhances a mother's self-concept and helps her remain tolerant and understanding of herself and her baby. The warmth and caring you transmit to the mother will help her use humor to relieve the stresses of learning how to be a mother and how to breastfeed her new baby. Armed with this attitude, she will be better able to laugh at herself and shake off missteps as she and her baby learn to respond to each other.

Big stresses are not always the ones that get to us. Life is full of minor daily irritations and obstacles that pile up.

We can choose to let those things make us miserable, or we can choose to use our humor and adopt a positive outlook to help us put it all into perspective. In health care, stresses may seem even more monumental, primarily because a loss of privacy and control often accompanies the stress. Traditionally, healthcare providers have intentionally avoided humor in their interactions with patients. Humor has many faces, however: It may come through in the form of a warm and friendly approach, a smile, or a light touch. Such pleasantries are a valuable use of humor in your work as a lactation consultant.

The Health Benefits of Humor

Two useful resources on the health benefits of humor are *Humor and the Health Professions: The Therapeutic Use of Humor in Health Care*, by Vera Robinson (1991), and *Anatomy of an Illness*, by Norman Cousins (1979). In *Anatomy of an Illness*, Cousins wrote about events in his life that were reported in 1976 in the *New England Journal of Medicine*. He used humor therapy to recover from a life-threatening disease that produced intense pain and paralysis. His health improved when he eliminated all medications, took heavy doses of vitamin C, and scheduled laughter sessions—watching videos of the television show *Candid Camera*, watching Marx Brothers movies, and reading humorous books. Cousins found that 10 minutes of genuine laughter had an anesthetic effect that gave him at least 2 hours of pain-free sleep. Gradually, he was able to regain movement and recover.

Humor actually causes a biochemical change in the body that is enormously healing and therapeutic. Eliciting laughter from a mother can produce positive effects in most of her body's major physiologic systems. Laughter speeds up heart rate, raises blood pressure, accelerates breathing, and increases oxygen consumption. It can stimulate muscles and relax muscle tension, thereby reducing pain and anxiety. Laughter stimulates the cardiovascular system, the sympathetic nervous system, and the production of catecholamines and endorphins, thereby boosting the immune system. It increases the amount of adrenaline in the brain, which stimulates alertness and memory and enhances learning and creativity. Following this arousal state, respiration, heart rate, and muscle tension actually return to below normal levels (Robinson, 1991).

This beneficial cascade of physiologic events may explain the growing popularity of Laughter Clubs in India and elsewhere. Members meet in a public place for a short period of sustained laughter before beginning the workday (Laughter Club International, 2009).

The physiologic benefits of laughter demonstrate that humor and a positive outlook can facilitate the healing process and disease prevention. Medical experts know that negative emotions can create organic changes within the body such as headaches and ulcers. It makes sense, therefore, that positive emotions can produce positive biochemical changes in the body as well.

Humor Enhances Learning

Humor can serve to establish relationships, relieve anxiety, release anger in a socially acceptable way, avoid or deny painful feelings, and facilitate learning (Buxman, 2008). When mothers have a positive outlook, they will be more likely to meet new challenges with enthusiasm and optimism. Humor and laughter reduce tension and anxiety, increase productivity, and contribute to learning enjoyment, interest, motivation, and creativity. In addition, they help us seek a more holistic appreciation of experience (Jenkins, 2007).

Integrating humor with learning promotes critical thinking and emotional intelligence (Chabeli, 2008). A humorous approach with mothers helps stimulate divergent thinking, increasing their willingness to look at a situation in a new way. This strategy frees the flow of ideas so that mothers can consider new alternatives and solutions. Humor stimulates both the right and left hemispheres of the brain at the same time, creating a level of consciousness and brain processing that enables the brain to work at its fullest capacity. When the right and left brain are integrated and functioning simultaneously, the capacity for learning is at its highest level. Humor helps achieve this goal.

As part of the mother's healthcare team, you can lighten the mood to facilitate a mother's learning and make the learning experience fun. Shared laughter will energize both of you and will increase the mother's ability to take risks. She will be more comfortable and, therefore, will feel more welcome to ask questions and offer input. She will also be more receptive to your advice. Humor gets people to listen. Humor is graphic. It creates images in the learner's mind and helps the learner to remember better and longer.

The appropriate use of humor can help mothers gain perspective and see that a situation is not so serious. When humor blends with the right atmosphere, timing, and style, it can enhance your interactions with a receptive mother. You can learn to determine the need for humor and your purpose in using humor with breastfeeding clients. Also be aware of a mother's personality and her level of receptiveness to your use of humor. Extroverted people tend to have a greater appreciation of humor (Mobbs et al., 2005). Even so, mild forms of humor can help even reticent mothers relax, which facilitates oxytocin release. Humor is as much a form of preventive medicine as breastfeeding. It increases a mother's self-confidence and improves her frame of mind and perspective. It helps the mother enjoy her baby. Your use of humor will teach her to see and use humor herself.

Using Humor to Relieve Stress

Laughter relieves stress and facilitates social bonding (Watson et al., 2007). Staff members in the emergency room of St. Christopher's Hospital for Children in Philadelphia, for example, have long recognized the value of humor. In June 1992, *Pediatrics* reported on a retrospective review of their most interesting chief complaints over a 20-year period:

> Some complaints that were charted and recorded in a notebook included "Needs circumcision because his tonsils and adenoids are so big"; "Can't find the baby's birthmark"; "Drank the dog's milk—from the dog's nipple"; "Lump down in his tentacle"; and "Swollen asteroids." Among the interesting telephone inquiries were "Hello, I would like to schedule an emergency" and "My little girl just kissed a dead chicken. Should I bring her in?" They keep a log of these statements to buoy the spirits of an emergency department staff stressed by long hours and a hectic work environment. (Nelson, 1992)

Lactation Humor

Lactation consultants, rightly or wrongly, have an image of being too serious. Novelist Sarah Bird's hilarious essay, "Lactation Nation," is a good antidote to this chacterization (Bird, 2008). She describes breastfeeding as "the last best hope for keeping our children from growing up with Joan Crawford intimacy issues and Bubble Boy immune systems."

In your own practice, you might develop a notebook or file describing humorous lactation situations. Using amusing terminology or a play on words may help you teach techniques to a mother. One lactation consultant makes it a point to use humor frequently with mothers. For example, she refers to the cross-cradle hold as the chicken hold: "I show the mother how her elbow is pointed out like the wing of a chicken. I wave it up and down and go 'cluck, cluck.' This gets the mother laughing and relaxes her (Kutner, 2009)." With such humorous imagery, the mother is also more likely to remember the technique she was being taught. People tend to remember stories more than any other form of teaching.

You can share an amusing anecdote that may have happened to another mother in similar circumstances. Keeping a humor diary will help you capture such moments. The humor is out there, just waiting for you to capitalize on it in your interactions with mothers.

- When a mother was asked, "Why aren't you going to breastfeed?" she answered, "It doesn't run in my family."
- A mother at a dinner party had her baby pull off just as her milk let down. Her dinner partner, mystified by the sudden droplets on his sleeve, brushed them off and gazed at the ceiling to find the leak.

• A mother and father were in the recovery room following a cesarean delivery. The father turned to the nurse and asked, "Did they pierce her nipples yet to let the milk out?"

When used appropriately, the use of humor in communication will enhance your effectiveness and enrich the lives of your clients and colleagues.

⌒ Summary

The caregiver's commitment, beliefs, attitude, and approach may be either a help or a hindrance to a mother's ability to reach her breastfeeding goals. The caregiver who presents breastfeeding as the natural way to feed babies and who demonstrates a sincere belief in the superiority of breastfeeding over artificial feeding helps increase the mother's self-image and confidence. As a lactation consultant, you serve as a facilitator for the mother's decision-making process, exploring options and developing a partnership with her in problem solving. This assistance helps the mother grow as an active health consumer who is informed and responsible concerning her own and her baby's health care. She will continue to grow within a climate that relinquishes medical control, limits interventions, and trusts in the abilities of mothers and babies. A personalized approach with every mother— one that assesses her needs, capitalizes on her strengths, and praises her accomplishments—helps lead to the mother's long-term satisfaction. Maintaining a sense of humor and using effective communication skills will help you establish an optimal learning climate and develop a meaningful rapport with mothers (Figure 4.14).

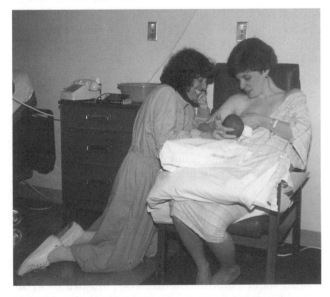

FIGURE 4.14   IBCLC using effective body language.

⌒ Chapter 4—At a Glance

Applying what you learned—

• Assume all mothers will breastfeed their newborns unless you are told otherwise.

• Recognize that your past actions were appropriate at the time and not a reason for guilt now.

• Recognize guilt as a positive emotion that leads to personal growth.

• Form a partnership with parents, and empower them to make decisions and accept responsibility for their actions.

• Help parents become informed health consumers.

• Place control and power with the mother and baby, not with the caregiver.

• Lobby for reducing unnecessary medical interventions.

• Help parents recognize their newborn's capabilities.

• Confine interactions to guiding rather than directing, unless intervention is needed.

• Create a learning climate that is relaxed, trusting, mutually respectful, informal, warm, collaborative, and supportive.

• Individualize your approach based on the mother's learning needs and readiness.

• Keep pace with the mother and baby.

• Actively involve the mother to heighten her learning and retention.

• Respond to the mother's learning style and use humor to enhance her learning.

• Avoid negative terminology that may undermine a mother's self-confidence or send a judgmental message.

• Use a smile and warm voice tone to appeal to mothers.

• Use body language that engages and empowers the mother.

• Recognize cultural differences in body language, personal space, and comfort with being touched.

• Read the mother's body language to determine her comfort and receptiveness.

⌒ References

Academy of Breastfeeding Medicine (ABM). Clinical protocol number #19: breastfeeding promotion in the prenatal setting. *Breastfeed Med.* 2009;4(1):43-45. www.bfmed.org. Accessed August 1, 2009.

Arora S, et al. Major factors influencing breastfeeding rates: mother's perception of father's attitude and milk supply. *Pediatrics.* 2000;106(5):E67.

Avery A, et al. Confident commitment is a key factor for sustained breastfeeding. *Birth*. 2009;36(2):141-148.

Bandura A. Self-efficacy. In: Ramachaudran VS, ed. *Encyclopedia of Human Behavior, Vol. 4*. New York: Academic Press; 1994:71-81.

Belenky M, et al. *Women's Ways of Knowing*, 10th anniversary ed. New York: Basic Books; 1997.

Betzold CM, et al. A family practice breastfeeding education pilot program: an observational, descriptive study. *Int Breastfeed J*. 2007;2:4.

Bird S. Lactation nation: how Austin's mobile mama made me a breast-feeding believer. *Texas Monthly*. August 2008. http://www.texasmonthly.com/preview/2008-08-01/bird.

Britton C, et al. Support for breastfeeding mothers. *Cochrane Database Syst Rev*. 2002;1:CD001141.

Brizendine L. *The Female Brain*. New York: Morgan Road Books/Random House; 2006.

Buxman K. Humor in the OR: a stitch in time? *AORN J*. 2008;88(5):714.

Chabeli M. Humor: A pedagogical tool to promote learning. *Curationis*. 2008;31(3):51-59.

Coffield K. The benefits of phone support and home visits: an evaluation of the City of Kingston's Breastfeeding Support Service. *Breastfeed Rev*. 2008;16(3):17-21.

Colson S. The nature–nurture debate and breastfeeding competencies: bringing nature to the fore. *Practising Midwife*. 2008;8(11):14-19.

Colson S, et al. Optimal positions triggering primitive neonatal reflexes stimulating breastfeeding. *Early Hum Develop*. 2008;84(7):441-449.

Coon D, Mitterer J. *Brain and Behavior. Psychology: A Journey*. Belmont, CA: Thomson Higher Education; 2008.

Cousins N. *Anatomy of an Illness*. New York: Norton; 1979.

Cueva M, et al. Healing hearts: laughter and learning. *J Cancer Educ*. 2006;21(2):104-107.

Dede C. Planning for neomillennial learning styles. *Educause Qrtly*. 2005;28(1). http://www.educause.edu/EDUCAUSE+Quarterly/EDUCAUSEQuarterlyMagazineVolum/Planning forNeomillennialLearni/157325. Accessed April 28, 2010.

Ekman P. *Emotions Revealed: Recognizing Faces and Feelings to Improve Communication and Emotional Life*. New York: Times Books; 2007.

Ekström A, Nissen E. A mother's feelings for her infant are strengthened by excellent breastfeeding counseling and continuity of care. *Pediatrics*. 2006;118(2):169-176.

Fast J. *Body Language*. New York: Pocket Books; 1988.

Fisher C. Breastfeeding basics. Paper presented at: The Annual Conference on Breastfeeding: Cross Cultural Connection; July 1996; Kansas City, MO.

Fletcher D, Harris H. The implementation of the HOT program at the Royal Women's Hospital. *Breastfeed Rev*. 2000;8:19-23.

Gildea A, et al. Sources of feeding advice in the first year of life: who do parents value? *Community Pract*. 2009;82(3):27-31.

Gill SL, et al. Effects of support on the initiation and duration of breastfeeding. *West J Nurs Res*. 2007;29(6):708-723.

Hegney D, et al. Against all odds: a retrospective case-controlled study of women who experienced extraordinary breastfeeding problems. *J Clin Nurs*. 2008;17(9):1182-1192.

Ingram J, et al. Breastfeeding in Bristol: teaching good positioning, and support from fathers and families. *Midwifery*. 2002;18(2):87-101.

Jenkins E. Using cooperative inquiry and clinical supervision to improve practice. *Br J Community Nurs*. 2007;12(2):63-69.

Kang JS, et al. Effects of a breastfeeding empowerment programme on Korean breastfeeding mothers: a quasi-experimental study. *Int J Nurs Stud*. 2008;45(1):14-23.

Knowles M. *The Modern Practice of Adult Education: From Pedagogy to Androgogy*. Chicago: Follett; 1980.

Knowles M, et al. *The Adult Learner: The Definitive Classic in Adult Education and Human Resource Development*. Houston: Gulf; 1998.

Kruske S, et al. The 'earlybird' gets the breastmilk: findings from an evaluation of combined professional and peer support groups to improve breastfeeding duration in the first eight weeks after birth. *Matern Child Nutr*. 2007;3(2):108-119.

Kutner L. *Certified Lactation Specialist Course*. Wheaton, IL: Lactation Education Consultants; 2009.

Labbok M. Exploration of guilt among mothers who do not breastfeed: the physician's role. *J Hum Lact*. 2008;24(1):80-84.

Laughter Club International. 2009. www.laughteryoga.org. Accessed August 1, 2009.

Law S, et al. Breastfeeding Best Start study: training midwives in a "hands off" positioning and attachment intervention. *Matern Child Nutr*. 2007;3(3):194-205.

Lewallen LP, et al. Breastfeeding support and early cessation. *J Obstet Gynecol Neonatal Nurs*. 2006;35(2):166-172.

Lieb S. Principles of adult learning. *Vision*; 1991. honolulu.hawaii.edu/intranet/committees/FacDevCom/guidebk/teachtip/adults-2.htm. Accessed August 1, 2009.

Locklin M, Naber S. Does breastfeeding empower women? Insights from a select group of educated, low-income minority women. *Birth*. 1993;20:30-35.

Marshall JL, et al. Being a "good mother": managing breastfeeding and merging identities. *Soc Sci Med*. 2007;65(10):2147-2159.

McLearn K, et al. The timing of maternal depressive symptoms and mothers' parenting practices with young children: implications for pediatric practice. *Pediatrics*. 2006;118(1):e174-e182.

Merriam S, et al. *Learning in Adulthood*, 3rd ed. San Francisco: Jossey-Bass; 2006.

Mistry Y, et al. Infant-feeding practices of low-income Vietnamese American women. *J Hum Lact*. 2008;24(4):406-414.

Mobbs D, et al. Personality predicts activity in reward and emotional regions associated with humor. *Proc Natl Acad Sci USA*. 2005;102(45):16502-16506.

Nelson DS. Humor in the pediatric emergency department: a 20-year retrospective. *Pediatrics*. 1992;89(6):1089-1090.

Nichols J, et al. The impact of a self-efficacy intervention on short-term breast-feeding outcomes. *Health Educ Behav*. 2009;36 250-258.

O'Brien M, et al. The influence of psychological factors on breastfeeding duration. *J Adv Nurs*. 2008;63(4):397-408.

O'Brien ML, et al. Strategies for success: a toolbox of coping strategies used by breastfeeding women. *J Clin Nurs*. 2009;18(11):1574-1582.

Oski F. In defense of guilt. *Contemp Pediatr.* 1995;12:9.

Raines C. *Connecting Generations: The Sourcebook for a New Workplace.* Fairport, NY: Axzo Press; 2003.

Robinson VM. *Humor and the Health Professions: The Therapeutic Use of Humor in Health Care.* Thorofare, NJ: Slack 1991.

Russell S. An overview of adult-learning processes. *Urol Nurs.* 2006;26(5):349-352, 370.

Shaker I, et al. Infant feeding attitudes of expectant parents: breastfeeding and formula feeding. *J Adv Nurs.* 2004;45(3): 260-268.

Sisk PM, et al. Lactation counseling for mothers of very low birth weight infants: effect on maternal anxiety and infant intake of human milk. *Pediatrics.* 2006;117(1):e67-e75.

Su LL, et al. Antenatal education and postnatal support strategies for improving rates of exclusive breast feeding: randomised controlled trial. *BMJ.* 2007;335(7620):596.

Vella J. *Learning to Listen, Learning to Teach: The Power of Dialogue in Educating Adults.* San Francisco: Jossey-Bass; 2002.

Wang SF, et al. Related factors in using a free breastfeeding hotline service in Taiwan. *J Clin Nurs.* 2008;17(7):949-956.

Watson KK, et al. Brain activation during sight gags and language-dependent humor. *Cereb Cortex,* 2007;17(2):314-324.

Wittmann-Price RA. Exploring the subconcepts of the Wittmann-Price theory of emancipated decision-making in women's health care. *J Nurs Scholarsh.* 2006;38(4):377-382.

Zemke R, Zemke S. Adult learning: what do we know for sure? *Training.* 1995;32(6):31-34, 36, 38, 40.

5

Counseling Skills: Learning How to Help Mothers

Helping mothers with breastfeeding goes far beyond book knowledge, research, scientific principles, and clinical practice. These considerations are all important—indeed, essential—to responsible health care. Nevertheless, if you lack effective communication and counseling skills, all of your knowledge and wisdom may fall on deaf ears. Whether you are a lactation consultant, other healthcare professional, or lay counselor, your primary role with breastfeeding mothers is that of a counselor. Counseling is the most basic element in the helping process. As a member of the healthcare team, you have a responsibility to acquire the skills and techniques that will maximize your effectiveness in helping mothers breastfeed. Because the focus of this chapter is counseling, the role referred to will be that of a "counselor," regardless of your professional credentials.

~ Key Terms

Active listening	Influencing
Attending	Informing
Building hope	Interpreting
Clarifying	Leading method
Emotional support	Open-ended questions
Empathetic listening	Passive listening
Evaluating	Physical comfort
Facilitating	Problem solving
Follow-up method	Reassuring
Focusing	Reflective listening
Guiding method	Self-efficacy
Identifying strengths	Summarizing

~ The Counseling Process

Basic counseling techniques provide the means for giving mothers the support they need to develop confidence in their mothering and breastfeeding abilities. Counseling skills involve encouraging the mother to express herself, educating her, and empowering her with problem-solving techniques. These skills are the essence of breastfeeding counseling. With effective counseling techniques, you can better communicate your breastfeeding knowledge, thereby increasing positive outcomes for the nursing dyad. The ultimate goal of each individual counseling contact is increased satisfaction for the mother. Talking through the mother's situation helps relieve her emotional stress and physical discomfort. This partnering helps the mother feel good about her participation in the outcome and increases her self-confidence.

The mother's increased self-awareness and understanding will lead to her personal growth, which in turn enables her to take responsibility for her situation and to develop self-sufficiency. Table 5.1 lists the general skills that will assist you in helping the mother reach her goals. Her satisfaction may depend in part on your perception of her needs, your use of counseling skills, and your personality traits. These factors are explored in the following sections.

Consider the variety of techniques described here to be part of your personal counseling "toolbox." It is neither expected nor appropriate to go through a rigid, prescribed process with every contact. Rather, you are encouraged to assess each contact and use those skills relevant to the situation. Practice the techniques presented in this chapter to learn which ones are compatible with your personality and approach. Use those that feel comfortable to you and that help you establish effective and supportive relationships with your clients.

The Counselor's Personal Traits

Your personality will have a direct effect on the rapport you establish with mothers. Mothers respond best to a

TABLE 5.1   Counseling Model to Meet the Mother's Needs

Mother's Needs +	Counseling Skills +	Counselor's Traits =	Satisfaction for Mother
• Emotional support	• Listening	• Empathy and warmth	• Reduced stress
• Immediate physical comfort	• Influencing	• Concern	• Increased self-confidence
• Understanding	• Facilitating	• Openness	• Personal growth
• Positive action	• Informing	• Positive regard and respect	• Acceptance of responsibility
	• Problem solving	• Clear, accurate communication	
		• Flexibility	

person who has a warm, caring attitude and who shows deep, genuine concern and empathy. Positive regard and respect, which acknowledge the mother's individuality and worth without judgment, give the mother freedom to open up and be her authentic self. It is important to accept mothers without judging their decisions based on your expectations. Show the mother that you value what she has to say. To reduce confusion and frustration, engage in clear, accurate communication. Maintaining flexibility will help ensure that you use your full range of skills to respond appropriately to the mother at different stages in the counseling process.

As part of your educational or work experience, you may have taken one or more personality assessment tests. If not, there are many tests you can use to determine your primary style of communicating and relating to people—for example, Myers-Briggs Type Indicator (Myers-Briggs, 2009), DiSC (Inscape Publishing, 2009), Birkman Method (Birkman International, 2009), and Wilson Social Styles (Wilson Learning, 2009). Many human resources departments use these tests in the hiring process. If you are presently working, check with your employer to see if these instruments are available to you. Community colleges and adult continuing education programs frequently offer them, and they are also available through the Internet and self-help books.

Gaining insight into your personality through such tests will help you identify both your strengths and your weaknesses as you work with mothers and babies. When you know your strengths, you can relax and enjoy your clients. When you know your weak areas, you can work toward modifying them. You can learn to accommodate your counseling skills to your personality in ways that will optimize your interactions with mothers.

If you are shy and quiet, for example, you may be overwhelmed by an encounter with a mother who has an extroverted, "Type A" personality. This type of person has a strong need to feel in charge and to see results. Understanding this preference may help you to not take the mother's forcefulness personally, or to feel as if she is being impatient and not listening to you. She may respond to your quiet assurance as calming, or she may get irri-

tated if you equivocate or appear hesitant. With this kind of person, direct statements of fact and plans of care phrased in terms of "results" may be better received.

If you are outgoing and talkative, your personality may be too forceful for a quiet, introverted mother. Such a client might be offended by jokes about breasts or breastfeeding, or by attempts at lighthearted humor. Take your cues from the mother, and from the family, if other family members are present. It is easier to tone down your chattiness than to overcome a perception that you are overbearing, insensitive, or "bossy." A more reserved mother might better appreciate ideas phrased as suggestions, with two or three options being presented, and her opinion being elicited at each step along the way.

The Mother's Needs

The counseling process helps fulfill the mother's needs for emotional support, understanding, and action. Making sure you address all three of these aspects of care during each contact will help ensure that the mother is satisfied. In addition, a mother who is experiencing physical discomfort may first need relief measures before proceeding with the counseling process. As shown in Table 5.1, you can use a variety of counseling skills as you interact with mothers (Brammer & McDonald, 2003). The skills presented in each category provide tools for your interactions with mothers. Use those that you find comfortable and natural so you can blend them with your personal communication style.

Emotional Support

Providing emotional support to a mother validates her feelings, emotions, and concerns. When a mother feels validated, in a calm atmosphere, she can take in information and join in problem solving. In contrast, if her emotions and frustrations are running high, she will not be receptive to teaching or addressing solutions to her problems.

Visualize preparing a stew in a pressure cooker. When the pressure cooker is put on a hot burner, it increases the pressure in the pot to cook the food quickly.

When the stew is cooked, you must slowly vent the steam to relieve the pressure before she removes the top of the cooker. If she opens it too soon, the stew will end up on the ceiling instead of on the dinner table!

Apply this same principle when you consider all the pressures and anxieties felt by mothers in your care. A flurry of emotions may be boiling and ready to explode. Just as with the pressure cooker analogy, you need to address these emotions before you work with the mother to resolve any problems she may have, such as engorgement, sore nipples, or her baby not latching well. Be careful not to become so focused on problem solving that you fail to first address a mother's emotional needs.

Your toolbox should include a variety of counseling skills that can be employed to help the mother lower her pressure and stress. Help her verbalize her feelings, and validate her concerns. Show acceptance, and praise her actions or attempts. Listen to what she is saying as well as what she is *not* saying. A mother who appears self-assured on the outside may have internal anxieties that reveal themselves through her body language or comments. Learn to read between the lines for any underlying messages. Make sure mothers are in a receptive state and able to process information before you begin the educating and problem-solving processes.

Over time, factors that cause distress can build up within a new mother. Your emotional support will help provide a sense of security and a climate that encourages the mother to express her feelings and anxieties. A classic principle in any helping profession is this: "People won't care how much you know until they know how much you care." To send the message that you genuinely care about a mother's well-being and concerns, provide her with emotional support. This assistance shows that you are interested in helping the mother achieve her goals. We all give support to those we love, unconsciously at times, simply as an outpouring of our care and concern for them. Emotional support is an essential tool in your counseling skills toolbox and will optimize the care you give to a mother. It helps her feel secure and at ease, reduces her anxiety, and gives her someone with whom to share her concerns.

Use of listening and influencing skills—attending, active listening, empathetic listening, reassuring, praising, and building hope—provide emotional support. All of these counseling tools are described in the next section. When you understand and become experienced in the use of these skills, you will find yourself giving support almost automatically. New mothers often feel inadequate at fulfilling all the demands made of them as a mother, wife, professional, student, and/or homemaker. To increase her self-confidence, frequently praise a new mother for how well she is handling all of her responsibilities. You may be the only person telling her that she is doing a good job! Your interest in the new mother and in her concerns, your enthusiasm for the things she is happy about, and your acceptance of her, her situation, and her decisions are all ways of showing support.

Immediate Physical Comfort

Often a mother requires some immediate action to reduce her physical stress before she will be in a state receptive to teaching. Perhaps she is tired, maybe her nipples are uncomfortable at the beginning of feedings, or perhaps her baby has slept through the night and her breasts are uncomfortably full or engorged. Before she can address ways to resolve her situation, she will first need immediate physical relief from her discomfort. In this case, you can first offer emotional support and then suggestions to help her feel better physically.

This approach temporarily deviates from the usual problem-solving process, in which you typically work toward defining the problem before suggesting any action. Intermediate actions to relieve the mother's discomfort will enable her to work with you to find the cause of the difficulty and eliminate it. After the mother is more comfortable, you can collaborate with her to develop a better understanding of the problem. Figure 5.1 shows how immediate physical comfort fits into the counseling process as a temporary measure. Giving physical comfort is not always necessary, of course. If a problem exists that is not urgent, or if the mother seems calm and relaxed, then you can follow the steps in the usual counseling process.

Understanding

The mother's understanding is basic to the success of the counseling process. To develop satisfaction from a contact with you, the mother needs to understand herself and her feelings about a problem or concern. She needs to define and understand the problem clearly, as well as the events or actions that led to it and the actions that will help resolve it. She also needs to understand her options so that she can make informed choices and assume responsibility for her actions. Such understanding comes from your use of listening, influencing, facilitating, informing, and problem-solving skills.

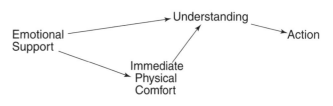

FIGURE 5.1   The counseling process.

Positive Action

After receiving the appropriate support and gaining an understanding of her situation, the mother will be better able to take positive action in dealing with her concerns. Even if a problem cannot be resolved immediately, she will gain satisfaction from actively working on it and can modify her action appropriately. You can initiate positive action by using the relevant problem-solving and decision-making processes and skills. By developing a plan together, you and the mother can mutually agree on what the mother will do.

~ *Methods and Skills in Counseling*

A systematic counseling process is used for meeting the mother's needs for emotional support, physical comfort, understanding, and action. In the context of breastfeeding support, counseling encompasses more than the typical definition of counseling as a "process of advising." Three distinct aspects characterize the counseling process used with mothers:

- The *guiding* method keeps the conversation going and helps you gather the information you need to assess the situation.

- The *leading* method encompasses the problem solving you will enter into with the mother.
- The *follow-up* method is the essential final portion of the counseling contact, in which you identify what needs to be done next.

These methods are described in the next section, followed by a discussion of the counseling skills incorporated into each method.

The individual skills used in each method of the counseling process are tools you can employ to create a climate of acceptance that makes counseling possible. The numerous examples in this chapter are intended to help you relate these skills to actual counseling situations. Of course, the most effective way to develop counseling skills and become proficient in their use is to practice them as frequently as possible. If you take the opportunity to practice your counseling skills in conversations with friends, colleagues, and family, you will quickly develop an appreciation of their effectiveness and make them a natural part of your communication style.

Table 5.2 outlines the skills used in each of the three counseling methods. It gives an overview of the counseling process and can serve as a reference for you as you read the individual discussions of the methods and skills.

TABLE 5.2 Counseling Methods and Skills

Method	Technique	Skills
Guiding	• Listening	• Attending • Active listening • Empathetic listening
	• Facilitating	• Clarifying • Interpreting • Asking open-ended questions • Focusing • Summarizing
	• Influencing	• Reassuring • Building hope • Identifying strengths
Leading	• Informing	• Presenting • Timing • Educating
	• Problem solving	• Listening to your first hunch • Looking for hidden factors • Testing your hunch • Exploring alternative hunches • Developing a plan
Follow-up	• Evaluating the session • Arranging the next contact • Researching outside sources • Renewing the counseling process	• Analyzing • Use skills listed above as needed

The Guiding Method

When time is at a premium, you may be inclined to jump into problem solving prematurely in an effort to help as many mothers as possible in the time available to you. This rush to judgment does a disservice to mothers and runs the risk of missing important clues about each mother's needs. It is better to give yourself totally to each mother in a calm and low-key atmosphere that provides emotional support and nurturing. Guiding skills will help you gather sufficient information and insights into the situation before you enter into problem solving. They are skills you will start a consultation with and will continue to use throughout your session with the mother.

The guiding method will help you truly listen to the mother and empathize with her by coming to understand her feelings, goals, and other factors that influence her actions. Guiding skills encourage the mother to express her ideas and concerns openly. She is able to listen to herself so that she (and you) understands the situation better. Guiding skills help you hear both what the mother is saying and what she is not saying—that is, the hidden messages she does not verbalize. The other purpose of guiding skills is to help transmit a message of acceptance of the mother's viewpoint and positive regard for her well-being. These skills help you say, "I care."

The guiding method is one in which the mother is helped through emotional support and limited direction from the counselor. Being aware of the mother's feelings, values, goals, and physical and emotional environments will enable you to discern her needs more clearly. The major responsibility for the direction of the discussion rests with the mother during this guiding process. As a consequence, she does most of the talking, which in turn allows you to concentrate on listening carefully to her message. To help you stay within your role in the guiding method, remember that you have two ears and only one mouth—your ears should do twice the work that your mouth does! During the guiding phase of your counseling contact, you should spend at least twice as much time listening as you do talking.

The aim of all counseling is self-help and self-efficacy, with the mother becoming skillful and self-sufficient through self-direction. By encouraging the mother to talk, reflecting her ideas, and clarifying her concerns, you help her see a clear picture of her situation. Ideally, the mother takes responsibility for what is happening and decides on her plan of care. Throughout the contact, continually evaluate the mother's capacity for independence and self-support. If she fails to take responsibility for herself, you may need to change your approach to encourage her to take the initiative while you continue to support her.

While giving the mother the opportunity to hear herself and to sort out her feelings and concerns, listening enables you to gather information. At times, you will need to be more actively involved in gathering information by directing the conversation so that the mother focuses on specific points. Facilitating the conversation in this way helps both you and the mother recognize and clearly define her situation. By engaging your facilitating skills, you act as a sounding board for the mother. As you gather information, you can use influencing skills to encourage her and give her emotional support if you feel the mother needs to increase her self-confidence or gain a new perspective. Influencing the mother's attitude in a positive way can help her view her circumstances more optimistically, thereby reducing her stress so that she is able to think more clearly and work toward a solution.

Listening

Listening skills that reinforce what the mother says will clarify her statements, show acceptance of her situation, and encourage her to arrive at solutions. Effective listening lets the mother know that you care about her enough to give her your total attention. Everyday listening usually takes place at one of four levels:

Level 1: The lowest level of listening is ignoring. No doubt, most adults have experienced this level of listening with a child or pet!

Level 2: The next level of listening is pretending, where the listener is trying to be polite but is not giving any attention to the speaker. It describes the noncommittal response you might receive if you interrupt someone who is deeply engrossed in reading or watching television.

Level 3: The third level is selective listening, in which the listener hears only certain parts of what is said. This can occur when you focus so much on how you plan to respond that you fail to listen carefully.

Level 4: The fourth level of customary listening is attentive listening, in which the listener actively focuses on the words and the message.

Learning to Listen Developing skills beyond everyday listening requires adoption of a consciously active process of responding to total messages and perceiving with your ears, eyes, and imagination. It means you must be silent much of the time and allow the mother to talk. We are all guilty of sometimes listening with half an ear to the speaker while busily figuring out what to say next or how to change the subject to something we would rather discuss. To help the mother, however, you need to listen carefully to what she is saying and avoid the temptation to interrupt. To do so, you must put your thoughts and interests aside for the moment so that you can give yourself more fully to the job of listening.

Listening requires time and patience, and often it means waiting until the mother develops an understanding of her feelings and concerns. Time is a valuable commodity for all of us. Few people take the opportunity to sit down with another individual and really listen to that person. For lactation counselors, failure to help a mother is often a result of snap judgments and not taking enough time to hear the whole story. You need to give the mother enough time to collect her thoughts. If you ask a new mother how everything is going, she may quickly reply, "Fine." Ten minutes later, after you have talked about increases in the frequency of feedings at particular stages in her baby's growth, she may say, "No wonder my baby is nursing constantly!" She may then tell you she has been under great stress because of this pattern and had begun to wonder if she has enough milk to satisfy her baby.

Many times a mother is not sure about how she feels and needs more time to talk and to feel at ease before you both communicate on the same level. When the mother has mixed feelings or several concerns, you will need time and ample conversation before you can be sure of how the mother really feels. Three listening skills that can help you gain this insight are attending, active listening, and empathetic listening.

Attending Attending is a passive listening skill that involves minimal responses intended to assure the mother that you are listening, without asking questions or making comments. Examples include "Yes," "I see," "I can appreciate that," "Oh," "Mmmmm," and "Really." The goal of attending behavior is to encourage the mother to continue talking freely. It has a strong reinforcing effect that helps the mother explore her way and be responsible for the course of the discussion. Attending minimizes your tendency to intervene unnecessarily. In fact, silence is another effective attending technique. At times, pausing in the conversation and waiting for the mother to fill the silence may encourage her to take a more active role.

Other aspects of attending include visual observation and the use of eye contact, posture, gestures, and listening in a non-interfering manner. The absence of any type of attending behavior, whether verbal or nonverbal, may discourage the mother from pursuing a topic and cause her to feel that you are not interested in what she has to say. Your use of eye contact and other nonverbal behavior, for example, sends strong messages to mothers. If you avoid eye contact with a mother, cross your arms or legs, or seem otherwise unapproachable, you may send a message that you are disinterested. You cannot alter such a message with any verbal attempt to show interest. You can transmit a positive nonverbal message and show that you are genuinely interested through direct eye contact, sitting at the mother's level, and leaning toward her with a natural relaxed posture, calm gestures, and a pleasant, engaged facial expression.

Active Listening Active listening, also called reflective listening, is a very useful technique for gathering information from the mother. Active listening lets the mother know you received her message completely and correctly. This is accomplished through clarifying, showing acceptance of the mother's viewpoint, and encouraging a response. With active listening, you paraphrase what the mother has said and reflect her message back to her. This type of exchange encourages the mother to respond and to feel free to explain her situation in detail. It provides an opportunity for the mother to recognize and solve her problem and creates an atmosphere in which she can grow and accept information.

In clarifying a message, active listening helps the mother hear what she is saying and think about it. Your response may involve some interpretation of her message, and her subsequent response lets you know that you understood correctly. This confirmation focuses the conversation and provides for better mutual understanding. Active listening is a skill that is particularly useful when talking to a mother who has only vague or as-yet-unspoken thoughts on a situation. It is also useful with a mother who is anxious or discouraged and not sure what her concern is or how she feels about it. Put simply, you cannot begin to offer suggestions until the mother is ready to accept them— and she will be ready only after her situation and her feelings are clear. Listening and encouraging the mother to continue talking are crucial steps in defining her concerns.

Active listening shows acceptance of the mother's viewpoint and goes beyond a more passive type of attending response such as "I see" or "Really." In active listening, your response indicates what you believe the mother's message meant. This confirmation of understanding encourages her to continue discussing the issue further. In this way, you let the mother know that you understand how she feels, that you are interested in what she is saying, and that you validate what she is feeling.

Using the mother's and baby's names helps personalize the exchange and enhances the helping relationship between you and the mother. Make a conscious effort to use both of their names frequently. It is especially important that you use the baby's name with a mother who continually refers to her infant as "the baby" and does not refer to her infant by name. This behavior could indicate that the mother is having difficulty bonding with her baby, and your use of the baby's name will help model bonding for the mother.

This first example illustrates this type of clarification:

Mother: My nipples hurt.

Counselor: Your nipples are sore when you feed Michael. [Some interpretation that the soreness occurs during a feeding; using the baby's name.]

Mother: Not just when I nurse, but after I wash them, too. [This is a correction, a clarifying message. Note that you have gathered some more information in her response that may help you in problem solving—namely, the fact that she washes her nipples after a feeding.]

The next example shows acceptance:

Mother: I'm not sure I can breastfeed much longer. My nipples are so sore that breastfeeding is really unpleasant!

Counselor: It's no fun to feed Christopher when it hurts. We talked about how enjoyable breastfeeding is, and this isn't fun at all. [This expresses understanding and validates the mother's concern.]

The final example encourages the mother to respond:

Mother: Molly is 4 months old now and always looks around the room instead of nursing. I guess she's ready to wean.

Counselor: You're wondering if Molly is ready to wean. [The mother's response will indicate whether she is considering weaning or wants to find ways to minimize distractions.]

With an active listening response, you first accept what the mother feels. This technique usually encourages her to relax and respond openly. It is a warm, sincere, and considerate way of talking that most people cannot resist. Instead of informing the mother right away that a 4-month-old infant does not usually self-wean and is probably just distracted, you first accept the mother's feelings, making no judgment. Later, after further discussion, you can offer the mother information about weaning and help her learn and grow. A mother may not feel comfortable sharing her personal feelings until you have talked for a while and trust develops. Active listening serves as an important means of developing trust and encouraging the mother to respond.

Empathetic Listening Listening as part of the counseling process goes beyond merely reflecting someone's words. The highest and most effective level of listening is empathetic listening. Simple, reflective or active listening conveys an intention to reply or to manipulate the conversation. The empathetic listener goes even further, listening with the intention to understand emotionally and intellectually. When using this skill, you listen with your ears, eyes, and heart, tuning in to the feeling, meaning, and behavior conveyed. You integrate your right brain and left brain to sense and feel what is being said. When you reflect the message back to the mother, you rephrase both the content and the feeling of what she said. Use of this skill will help you and the mother work through her feelings as well as her thoughts. When you reflect back what the mother seems to be saying, in your words, you reveal to her the emotions she has expressed.

Here is an example of an empathetic listening response:

Mother: I don't know whether I should nurse this baby. Molly is 2 years old and is very clingy. I'm afraid it might make her jealous and even clingier.

Counselor: You're afraid Molly will be more demanding if you nurse Juliette.

You may not be certain that this is the message the mother is sending. Hearing you say it back to her with your interpretation will help the mother know if she sent the intended message. She may say, "Yes, Molly already needs a lot of attention. I'm not sure how she'll react if I spend so much time nursing Juliette." If you misinterpreted her comment, she may say, "No, it's just that Molly is so sensitive and I don't want her to feel left out when I'm feeding Juliette." Her response to your comment will help you determine the direction to take with your next comment.

Empathetic listening helps you gain information that will clarify the mother's situation, which in turn makes it less likely that you will misinterpret her meaning. To illustrate the need to understand what the mother is saying before offering suggestions, Figure 5.2 contains a list of possible meanings for several statements. If you misinterpret the mother's initial statement, your explanation or suggestions will be inappropriate and unhelpful. The wide range of possible meanings reinforces the importance of coming to a common understanding with the mother. Be cautious when using empathetic listening, however, and keep your feedback statements tentative. You cannot be sure you know exactly what a mother is feeling. Watch your tone of voice and avoid sounding like a mind reader.

When using empathetic listening, sometimes you may find it difficult to think of words to express feelings. Figure 5.3 presents a list of "feeling words" to help you expand your vocabulary. You can add it to your counseling toolbox to assist you in reflecting the feelings of the mother you are counseling. Be specific in your responses. Avoid use of the general word "upset," which may communicate that you do not really understand the emotion the mother has expressed. When a mother sends you a "feeling" message, think to yourself, "What is she feeling?" Think of a word to describe the emotion she is expressing and then put that word into a sentence. If you concentrate on asking yourself this question, you will find that your empathetic listening responses come more easily and more spontaneously.

Facilitating

Facilitating skills actively encourage the mother to give more information and better define her situation. They also help focus the session on the mother's specific concerns. Facilitating requires you to direct the conversation so as to help the mother pinpoint issues and feelings that need to be expressed openly. While using these skills, in addition to asking open-ended questions, you clarify and

A mother says, "I think I'll have to give my baby a bottle in the evening so that my husband can do something for the baby."
Possible meanings:

- Mother wants to start a bottle.
- Husband wants to start a bottle.
- Husband feels left out.
- Mother wants father to take a more active role in child care.
- Mother wants baby to sleep through the night.
- Mother has other things to do in the evening and wants husband to care for baby.
- Husband doesn't think baby is getting enough nourishment.
- Mother is thinking of weaning her baby.
- Baby is fussy in the evening—mother thinks she doesn't have enough milk.
- Husband wants to help as much as possible.

A mother says, "My mother-in-law is here helping me these first 2 weeks, but she bottle-fed."
Possible meanings:

- Mother-in-law is not supportive of breastfeeding.
- Mother-in-law thinks baby isn't getting enough nourishment.
- Mother-in-law is helpful around the house but not with breastfeeding.
- Mother may be embarrassed breastfeeding in front of her mother-in-law.
- Mother-in-law envies her for being able to breastfeed.
- Mother-in-law is great. She wants to learn about breastfeeding and thinks it's wonderful.
- Mother-in-law is not familiar with differences between bottle feeding and breastfeeding, and mother needs information to pass on to her.
- Mother needs support and mother-in-law may not know how to provide it.

A mother says, "I have to wean to go to a wedding."
Possible meanings:

- Mother wants to wean, and the wedding is a convenient excuse.
- Mother does not want to breastfeed baby at wedding.
- Father wants mother to wean.
- Mother doesn't realize she can miss a feed.
- Mother doesn't know how to collect and freeze milk.
- Mother is not comfortable breastfeeding in public.
- Mother wants more freedom.
- Mother cannot wear her favorite dress due to increased breast size.
- Mother's favorite dress will not accommodate breastfeeding in public.

A mother says, "I don't know how long I'll be able to breastfeed. My sister had to wean at 10 days because her milk dried up."
Possible meanings:

- Mother is worried that her milk may dry up.
- Sister may be unsupportive of breastfeeding.
- Mother may not know about growth spurts.
- Mother is worried about her baby getting enough milk.
- Mother is not getting enough encouragement to breastfeed.
- Mother fears that if she breastfeeds, it may make sister look like a failure.
- Mother has a ready excuse if anything goes wrong.
- Mother is not sure how long she wants to breastfeed.

FIGURE 5.2   Possible meanings from a mother's statements.

interpret meaning and focus and summarize the conversation.

Clarifying Clarifying simply means to make a point clear. In counseling, you need to gather enough information from the mother to understand her message clearly and avoid miscommunication. One way you can clarify a point is by admitting your confusion about the mother's meaning and restating what you heard. You may also clarify what the mother has said by using other guiding method skills such as active listening, asking open-ended questions, and interpreting.

Here are some examples of clarifying responses:

- "Are you saying that . . . ?"
- "Let me see if I understand what you said."
- "Can you tell me more about . . . ?"

Asking Open-Ended Questions Asking open-ended questions is a useful skill for gathering information. It is the most direct way of finding out what you want to know. An open-ended question is one that cannot be answered with a simple "yes" or "no." Questions requiring only a yes/no response include those that begin with words such as "Are," "Is," "Do," and "Does." Such closed questions provide only minimal information and tend to shut down the conversation. In contrast, open-ended questions require answers that are more informative. They are the same questions a good reporter asks: "Who," "What," "When," "Where," "Why," "How," "How much," and "How often."

If you ask, "Are you eating well?" the mother will probably answer, "Yes," and you gain no helpful information. You can change that inquiry to an open-ended question by asking, "What did you eat today?" or "What

Words that reflect "upset"	Words that reflect "happy"
angry	accepted
anxious	appreciated
defeated	better
difficult	capable
disappointed	comfortable
discouraged	competent
disrespected	confident
doubtful	empowered
embarrassed	encouraged
feel like giving up	enjoy
frightened	excited
guilty	glad
hate, hated	good
hopeless	grateful
hurt	great
inadequate	happy
left out	love, loved
miserable	pleased
put down	proud
rejected	reassured
sad	relieved
stupid	respected
unhappy	satisfied
unloved	validated
worried	wonderful
worthless	

FIGURE 5.3 Words that reflect feelings.

do you usually eat for breakfast?" The mother's answers to these questions will tell you more about her diet and eating patterns.

As another example, suppose you suspect the baby is feeding infrequently and ask, "Does Samantha nurse often enough?" The mother can reply "Yes" or "No" and you will not have learned much. If you instead ask, "How many times does Samantha nurse in 24 hours?" you will learn more about Samantha's breastfeeding pattern. Think about what you want to learn and then create the question in your mind before asking it, so that you obtain more information than a simple "yes" or "no." As with many counseling skills, asking open-ended questions becomes easier and more natural with practice.

When you use open-ended questions, take care not to pose too many questions in sequence. In addition, avoid an interrogating manner that may cause the mother to feel threatened or irritated. Continually asking questions can establish a poor model for the relationship. The mother may learn to expect that when she describes symptoms and complaints, you will provide a solution from your wealth of information. You can discourage this pattern from the very beginning of a conversation by setting up a friendly atmosphere that encourages the mother to talk in a conversational style rather than answer a series of questions. Your goal is to encourage the mother to talk freely and to develop her own solutions whenever possible. Balancing open-ended questions with other guiding skills promotes the mother's self-sufficiency, builds her self-confidence, and discourages her dependence on you.

Interpreting Like active listening, the skill of interpreting clarifies, shows acceptance, and encourages a mother to respond. An interpreting response provides an analysis of what the mother says. It contains more of your thoughts and feelings than the simple rephrasing of what the mother said, such as "So you're saying that . . ." or "It sounds like you are saying . . ." or "That must mean. . . ." Drawing together several of the mother's statements and adding your tentative conclusions is a way to interpret what she said.

Make sure you leave the door open for the mother to process what you have said and to correct you if she believes you have misinterpreted her message. The goal of interpreting is to reflect the meaning of the conversation so the mother can see her situation in new ways and learn to interpret events in her life. You can use this skill to listen and respond empathetically. In the example in Figure 5.4, the counselor interprets each statement that the

Mother: I'm 7 months pregnant, and I'd really like to breastfeed my baby. Everybody in my family thinks I'm crazy.

Counselor: It sounds like the idea of breastfeeding is new and unfamiliar to your family.

Mother: My mother can't understand why I'd even want to. It's kind of hard for me to explain it myself. It's just kind of a feeling I have.

Counselor: So you're saying you would like to breastfeed this baby.

Mother: Yes, I do really want to. But my husband kind of thinks of breasts as something that belong in the centerfold of Playboy.

Counselor: Your husband doesn't want you to use your breasts to feed the baby.

Mother: No, it's not that exactly. I'm just not sure he understands what breastfeeding is all about.

FIGURE 5.4 Interpreting a mother's statements.

mother makes. This example is intended as illustration of the technique; in an actual counseling session, you would not interpret one statement after another. In the final response, the counselor misinterprets what the mother said and the mother corrects her.

Figure 5.5 presents additional examples that distinguish between interpreting and active listening. These examples illustrate the similarity between the two skills. Essentially, interpreting is a form of empathetic listening, which we learned earlier is the highest level of active lis-

---

Mother of a 4-week-old infant: "I can't get anything done during the day because I'm nursing all the time." [Frustrated]

- You feel your housework is getting away from you. [*Interpreting*]
- You're surprised a newborn needs so much time. [*Active listening*]
- You wish you had more time to do other things. [*Interpreting*]
- You seem to be nursing all day. [*Active listening*]

Mother of a 2-month-old infant: "Johnny is still waking up 2 times during the night, and I feel like a zombie most days." [Yawning]

- You're wondering if you'll ever get a good night's sleep. [*Interpreting*]
- You feel tired because your sleep is interrupted. [*Active listening*]
- It seems as if this will go on forever. [*Interpreting*]
- You're wishing Johnny would sleep longer at night. [*Active listening*]

Mother of a 2-month-old infant: "My physician said Jimmy was doing very well, but then he said it was time to start cereal twice a day." [Confused]

- You're wondering if Jimmy needs solid foods at this time. [*Active listening*]
- You don't feel Jimmy needs solid foods yet. [*Interpreting*]
- You're wondering why your doctor suggested cereal at this time. [*Active listening*]

Mother of a 1-year-old child: "Tommy and I enjoyed breastfeeding so much, and now all of a sudden he would rather do other things than breastfeed." [Disappointed]

- You seem to miss the daytime feedings. [*Interpreting*]
- Nursing times were such happy and warm times for you and Tommy. [*Active listening*]
- Tommy seems to prefer his toys and other activities. [*Active listening*]

Pregnant woman: "I want to breastfeed but I'm not interested in classes. Natural childbirth is horrible." [Fearful]

- You don't want to go through that. [*Active listening*]
- You think natural childbirth is painful. [*Interpreting*]
- It sounds as though you've heard about some unpleasant experiences. [*Interpreting*]
- Natural childbirth is not what you want. [*Active listening*]

FIGURE 5.5   Distinguishing between interpreting and active listening.

---

tening. Although you can use interpreting to analyze a conversation and to help a mother gain perspective, this skill should always be used with discretion. Take care not to cause the mother to feel annoyed or offended by your interpretations. Reserve this technique for situations in which you have a clear impression of what the mother is saying and when she seems to need help in sorting out her feelings.

Focusing   Focusing is useful when a mother seems to be rambling or changing the direction to an unrelated topic. Typically, a mother will raise several topics during a conversation. When you believe she has touched on her main concerns, you can focus the conversation by pursuing one aspect you believe could be useful to her. The goal of focusing is to pursue a more meaningful dialogue that increases understanding for both of you.

To focus the conversation, you could select one particular point to repeat or could condense a number of points into a selective summary to concentrate on issues such as how the mother feels and how the baby has been acting. Focusing is especially helpful with a very talkative mother, because if offers a way to bring her back to the important points that may really help her. You might say things like, "Tell me more about . . ." or "Can we talk about . . . again?" With focusing, you sort through the various issues to identify any topics you need to explore further. Consider the following conversation:

> Mother: Hi, Cathy. I really liked the book you recommended on breastfeeding and the family. I just wish my husband would have been willing to read it. I gave it to my neighbor. She's going to have a baby next month. . . .
>
> Counselor: You say your husband needs to learn more about breastfeeding?
>
> Mother: He sure could. He's really kind of uptight about what our two kids are going to think when they see me breastfeeding. They're getting older now. My son Matthew is going out for Little League, and he's really a pretty good pitcher for a kid his age. And my daughter who's in nursery school only knows about bottles.
>
> Counselor: Let's get back to your husband. He's afraid of how your kids will react when they see you breastfeeding the new baby?

In this example, the mother referred to her husband's attitude twice, and it was the first personal topic she mentioned. Often, the mother's first statement will provide a clue about her concerns, as will the number of times she brings up a topic.

You can use your feelings of confusion and sense of direction as a guide in deciding when and how to focus the conversation. With practice, this skill will become almost second nature. After you have focused the conversation, you can be alert to feedback from the mother to make sure that she considers the topic worth pursuing.

Summarizing Summarizing reassures the mother that you hear her message and that you understand her. It pulls together important points of a conversation. This skill is especially helpful when you and the mother have talked for a long time. It helps both of you to go over the highlights of the conversation and reinforce important aspects. The mother may need to hear the plan of care again, clearly and briefly, so that she is certain of what to try. When possible, urge the mother to do the summarizing. Her response will indicate her understanding, as well as help her assume responsibility. You may say, for example, "Let's see—to change your baby's schedule from daytime to nighttime sleeping, which things will you try?"

The following example illustrates a summarizing response:

> Counselor: You've been having trouble expressing your milk at work. We talked about finding a more private place to pump, playing some soothing music, and trying to schedule a longer break so you don't feel so rushed. I will e-mail you my information sheet on working and nursing. How does that all sound?

Influencing

Influencing the mother in a positive way can encourage her to continue to seek help and work toward solutions. A new mother often is unsure of herself. She may find that the reality of caring for her baby does not match her expectations, which may cause her to become discouraged or render her susceptible to poor advice. Heartening words from you will counteract these negative factors to give her reassurance, build hope, and identify her strengths.

Reassuring Reassuring is an influencing skill that gives the mother perspective and lets her know that many babies act like her baby—they have fussy periods, do not sleep through the night, do not nap when you want them to, nurse frequently, and so on. Use of this skill can help a mother see that her situation is normal.

Some limitations do apply with reassuring, however. Because this skill is easy to use, there may be a tendency to overuse it. Reassurance efforts sometimes come across as insincere sympathy or as a means of avoiding discussing the mother's concern. Be careful not to give the impression that you are minimizing the importance of her feelings or concerns. You can gently let her know that it is okay to feel the way she does and assure her that her situation will improve. Keep in mind that your goal is to build the mother's confidence. This will help you decide when reassuring is appropriate.

The following examples demonstrate reassuring responses from the counselor:

- "Even though breastfeeding in front of relatives can be difficult, it gets easier the more you do it."

- "You are really going through a rough period. The first 10 days of breastfeeding are the most challenging. It will get easier as you and your baby become more experienced."

Building Hope Hope is the mother's main antidote to discouragement and is a source of relief from tension and unmet expectations. It gives the mother who is experiencing a bad time the feeling that the future may bring relief.

Begin building hope by encouraging the mother to talk about her feelings. Help her see how her feelings relate to her present situation and how appropriate action can change those circumstances. Encouraging active participation helps the mother feel better and gets her functioning at an effective level. Mothers with such long-term conditions as persistent sore nipples, a fussy baby, or an unsupportive family, and those who have returned to work can usually benefit from your use of this technique.

Here are some examples of a counselor's responses that build hope:

- "Your aunt really discourages you by giving your baby a bottle, doesn't she? Would it help to give her some information on the importance of exclusive breastfeeding?"

- "Since you returned to work, you seem to feel like you are not giving your baby enough attention. Maybe you could set aside the first hour when you get home for just nursing and being together."

Identifying Strengths Identifying strengths is a form of praise that helps a mother focus on her positive qualities. It counteracts negative factors such as fatigue, a crying infant, or failure to meet preconceived expectations. Reminding the mother how well she handled a situation or how she can take advantage of a natural ability she has can encourage her to continue to work out an answer to her present concern. Reviewing past experiences from which the mother learned and grew can help her realize that she is capable of handling her present challenges. It encourages her to develop and rely on her resources and is a step in the direction of self-efficacy.

Discussing how past problems were resolved is the essence of this technique. Other growth experiences such as childbirth may be fruitful points from which to launch discussions. Be careful to select experiences that you know had positive outcomes so that the discussion is uplifting.

Recalling peak moments can be another way to identify strengths for the mother. Happy, exciting times such as her baby's first smile, a sibling's helpfulness, or an enjoyable evening with other new parents are pleasant memories for the mother. They can help her perceive her mothering experience as positive. She will see that she, her baby, and her family are special and that more memorable experiences will occur in the future. Recalling peak experiences is a type of praise that gives the mother a positive outlook and lets her know that you have taken an interest in her by the fact that you can recall important events in her life.

In the following examples, the counselor's responses identify strengths:

- "You handled that well."
- "You seem really tuned into your baby's needs."
- "You're the only one who can do that for your baby."

Practicing the Use of Guiding Skills

A variety of listening, facilitating, and influencing skills may be used in a given situation. The example in Table 5.3 illustrates the use of each of these skills. Table 5.4 presents less helpful responses to the same statement.

The next section contains statements that you can use to practice your use of guiding skills. First read the types of responses that would be least helpful or encour-

aging to the mother. These may even be comments you have heard others make to mothers. These statements are followed by more positive and helpful responses based on the skills discussed in this chapter.

My labor wasn't what I expected.
- Be glad you have a healthy baby.
- At least it's all behind you.
- That's why they call it labor!
- You're disappointed with the way it turned out.
- It didn't go the way you hoped it would.

I'm not sure what to do when the nurse brings my baby to me.
- Just hold him close to your breast and he'll figure it out.
- Haven't you read any books on breastfeeding?
- The lactation consultant will be here soon.
- You're unsure of yourself.
- You're feeling a bit overwhelmed.

TABLE 5.3   Effective Use of Guiding Skills

A pregnant woman says, "I'm afraid that breastfeeding might make my child too dependent."

Listening responses	• Attending	*Hmmm, you do . . .*
	• Active listening	*You're worried that breastfeeding will make your child too dependent.*
	• Empathetic listening	*You want your baby to grow into an independent child and you're not sure that breastfeeding will make that possible.*
Facilitating responses	• Clarifying	*What do you mean by "too dependent?"*
	• Interpreting	*You believe the dependency associated with breastfeeding will keep your child from exploring his world.*
	• Asking open-ended questions	*In what ways do you think breastfeeding will make your child too dependent?*
	• Focusing	*Let's get back to your concerns about . . . (This would be used later if it becomes necessary to focus on the mother's primary concern—dependence, or feelings of inadequacy as a prospective parent, or other concern.)*
	• Summarizing	*We talked about . . . . (This would be used later to go over the main points of this topic.)*
Influencing responses	• Reassuring	*Being a parent can be confusing. Many bottle-feeding mothers also wonder how the attention they give their baby relates to later independence.*
	• Building hope	*You know, research has actually shown otherwise. Babies given more attention and physical contact in the early years grow up to be more independent.*
	• Identifying strengths	*It's great that you are concerned about your baby's independence. How do you feel you can encourage him to become independent?*

TABLE 5.4 Unhelpful Responses to a Mother's Concern

A pregnant woman says, "I'm afraid that breastfeeding might make my child too dependent."

Unhelpful responses		
	• Disagreeing	*No, it makes him more independent.*
	• Criticizing	*That's because you don't know how babies learn to be independent.*
	• Ordering	*You need to read a book on parenting.*
	• Sharing experiences	*I used to think that way too. I remember when . . .*
	• Changing the topic	*I really wanted to talk to you about . . .*
	• Moralizing	*You really don't want your child to be so independent . . .*

I wish the doctor would spend more time with me.

- The doctor has a busy schedule.
- I can get you the doctor's telephone number.
- You have some unanswered questions.
- Are there any questions I can help you with?

I have to go back to work in 6 weeks.

- You're lucky to have a job.
- At least you can breastfeed until then.
- A lot of women combine breastfeeding and working.
- You're not sure you want to leave your baby.
- You're wondering how you can manage it.

My doctor says I have to give my baby formula.

- Your doctor knows best.
- A little formula won't hurt your baby.
- You don't want to give your baby formula.
- You don't understand why your baby needs formula.

My baby cries all the time.

- Try letting him cry himself to sleep.
- It will get better.
- You're worried you may not have enough milk.
- You're worried he doesn't want to breastfeed.

The Leading Method

The leading method requires you to take a more active role in directing the conversation. It is useful when the mother has identified a problem or concern that she is unable to solve with her available resources. The skills used in this method help both you and the mother see her situation more accurately and define the options open to her so that she can work with you to develop a plan of care. When you use these skills, you and the mother form a partnership in finding solutions.

The presence of a problem or concern that the mother is unable to solve with her existing resources distinguishes the leading method in counseling from the guiding method. Through educating and problem solving, you provide her with additional resources to lead her toward a solution. The use of leading responses changes the nature of the relationship between you and the mother from what it was during the guiding phase. In guiding, you encourage the mother to do most of the talking. In leading, more responsibility for the direction of the discussion falls on you rather than on the mother.

The goal of leading is for both you and the mother to understand her problem and to develop a plan of care. During the guiding phase, you will have gathered sufficient information and impressions from the mother, enabling you to enter into effective problem solving. You can move the mother toward greater understanding by educating her and offering her two or three possible solutions. The mother then will decide which suggestions she will try, based on her perception of the situation.

During the leading phase, it is important that the decision about the specific action to take rests with the mother, thereby allowing her to develop her self-efficacy. The mother may need this kind of reinforcement, especially at a time when she doubts her parenting abilities in other areas: "When do I pick up my baby?" "How warmly should I dress him?" "How do I care for him so that he will grow up to reach his potential?" Encourage mothers to make their own decisions on these issues.

The leading method works well when a mother clearly needs additional information or direction. When you have gathered enough information through listening and facilitating so that your conclusions are not premature or incorrect, your evaluation of the situation will be more accurate and you will be able to determine when leading is appropriate. You first need to take sufficient time to gain the mother's trust and clarify the situation so that you will know when leading will be helpful. Then you can intervene and educate the mother, working with her to overcome obstacles and find solutions.

Informing

Informing involves educating and explaining how something functions and why. It can range from stating a simple fact about nutrition to educating parents on the production of human milk. By providing a couple with the proper information at the appropriate time, you help them grow as parents. Parents learn about breastfeeding at childbirth preparation and breastfeeding classes, at support group meetings, and from caregivers, friends, and relatives. Some of what they hear may consist of cultural myths or fallacies. To ensure that they obtain the best and most accurate information, you can educate them and suggest appropriate reading material. Following up with discussions of parents' questions and ideas enhances the impact of what they learn and inspires parents to educate themselves further.

Explaining why things happen the way they do often makes basic facts more meaningful and more acceptable. For example, stating to a mother, "The more frequently you breastfeed, the more milk you will produce," may not convince her to feed her baby more frequently. By comparison, explaining briefly how nipple stimulation increases hormone production, which in turn increases milk production, will help her more fully understand this process. When the mother develops a richer, more in-depth understanding, she is more likely to institute changes that make her actions compatible with her new knowledge.

Before giving information to a mother, allow her enough time to explore her concerns and to determine what she needs to know. Ask yourself, "Does this mother need information?" If so, "How much information does she need?" Finally, "Is this the best time to educate her?" Determining the appropriate time for educating the mother—the teachable moment—can be critical to her accepting and processing the information. After you have determined which facts the mother needs, you can educate her, remembering to limit the amount of information so that it does not confuse or overwhelm her.

Here are examples of a counselor's responses that inform:

- "It might help to understand what happens when a baby has a growth spurt. As your baby grows . . ."
- "One way to tell if you are having letdown is by the leaking you're noticing from the other breast. When your baby sucks . . ."

Correcting a Misconception or Mismanagement

Sometimes you may need to correct a mother's perception of something or correct the way she is managing her breastfeeding. For example, if a mother is convinced that she will need to wean her baby when he gets teeth, you might first start with an active listening response such as "You're worried it will hurt when your baby has teeth." Then continue with something like this: "You will find that your baby's tongue covers his bottom teeth when he breastfeeds." With this twofold response, you have cleared up the mother's misconception and, at the same time,

given her support by accepting her statement. Moreover, you have corrected her perception without saying "but" or negating the importance of her concern.

Using a warm and friendly tone of voice, you can supply a mother with information without making her feel foolish or uninformed. Remember that you want to avoid telling a mother she "should" do something. Rather than saying, "You should . . ." or "I think . . . ," you can say, "You may want to . . ." or "You may find that when you. . . ." These types of responses will preserve the mother's self-confidence while you educate her.

The following example demonstrates a response to tactfully clear up a misconception:

Mother: Isn't it great the way you don't get your period while you're breastfeeding?

Counselor: Yes, that's true for some women. It doesn't always happen that way. There's a lot of variation among individuals. When you are lactating . . . [You can then go on to explain about the effect of lactation on menstruation and ovulation. The mother had the general idea and just needed some clarification.]

Problem Solving

An important element of your counseling role is helping the mother minimize problems and find solutions when they do arise. As you gather information, you can sort through the facts and help her clarify her situation. While guiding the mother, you may become aware that she has a problem. However, this is not always the case. Obtaining sufficient information and impressions will avoid your jumping in with irrelevant or unnecessary problem-solving advice.

To begin the problem-solving process, you first need to form a hunch about what the mother's problem may be. Based on that hunch, you can then look for additional factors to confirm that it is correct. To test your hunch, suggest to the mother what you consider her situation to be. If you both agree on the interpretation of the situation, you can go on to develop a plan of care together.

If the mother provides additional information that reveals your hunch to be incorrect, you will need to explore alternative hunches, reverting to guiding skills to gain more insights and information. After you and the mother have identified the problem, you are ready to develop a plan. Chapter 6 discusses each of the steps in the problem-solving process in more detail.

Combining the Guiding and Leading Methods

The most effective approach to counseling emphasizes the use of guiding skills. These skills best clarify the mother's message. You want to begin each contact with listening techniques that help "feel mothers out" and provide them with emotional support. Guiding skills encourage the mother to determine the direction of the conversation. They will produce the information and impressions you need before moving on to problem solving.

A conversation may reach a point where you realize the mother either has no problem or can handle her problem adequately on her own. You can then end the session with a summary of what you talked about and any plan of care. In contrast, if you determine that the mother needs further assistance, you can use your leading skills to educate and problem solve as needed.

When you avoid active participation early in the contact, the mother has the maximum opportunity to resolve her situation on her own, which encourages her emotional growth and increases her self-confidence. A conversation typically swings back and forth from guiding to leading as different topics arise. Achieving a balance between leading and guiding will help you develop a clear picture of the situation and build on the mother's self-efficacy.

The counseling conversation in Table 5.5 concerns a mother and her 3-month-old infant. In this example, the use of counseling skills enables the counselor and mother to define the problem and the counselor–mother pair to

TABLE 5.5   Counseling Examples of Guiding and Leading Skills

Mother	Counselor Response	Comments
(Sounding weary and discouraged) I'm so tired. My baby has been getting up three times a night for the last three nights	You really sound discouraged, Linda.	Counselor uses *active listening* to provide emotional support. She personalizes the exchange by using the mother's name.
Yeah. I thought we were really getting somewhere when Michael slept through the night last week. And now he acts starved at night. He eats and eats.	It seems to you like Michael is backsliding.	Counselor continues to give emotional support through *active listening*. She personalizes the exchange by using the baby's name.
I'll say. And just when my sister and her three kids have come for a week's visit.	Mmmm. That's a lot of company.	Counselor uses an *attending* response and *forms a hunch* that the mother is too active and her milk production has decreased. The mother did not say anything about her activities with her sister, whether she's doing too much, and so on. So the counselor cannot assume immediately that the mother is too tired and the baby isn't getting enough milk. She needs to wait for the mother's response to know if this hunch is correct.
It *is* a lot of people, but my sister is very helpful. She's doing most of the cooking, and she keeps my house in better shape than I do!	That's great for you, Linda. So she's really more help than work for you.	Counselor learns that her first hunch was incorrect. She uses *active listening* to encourage the mother to give her more information. She uses the mother's name to personalize the exchange.
Definitely.	Let's get back to Michael. What's he like during the day?	Counselor *focuses* the mother back on the baby and uses the baby's name to personalize the exchange. She uses an *open-ended question* to seek additional information. She is *looking for hidden factors* that will help identify the problem.
Well, he eats around 8:00 when he wakes up, then again around 10:30 before his nap. He sleeps until 1:00, then eats again. He eats again around 3:00, then takes another nap until about 6:00. Then he fusses and eats a couple of times during the evening and goes to bed about 10:00. At least that's what he's done the last couple of days.	Let's see, Linda, that's about 6 feedings during the day, that's 9 in 24 hours. How does each feeding go?	Counselor uses mother's name again to personalize the exchange. She *summarizes* what the mother has told her and asks an *open-ended question* to gain more information.

(Continued)

TABLE 5.5 Counseling Examples of Guiding and Leading Skills *(Continued)*

Mother	Counselor Response	Comments
Well, he fools around a lot, eating, looking around, and watching my sister's kids.	You know, Linda, this is the age when babies are easily distracted by people and motion and noise.	Counselor uses the mother's name and then responds with *interpreting* to test whether these distractions are the cause of the problem.
Michael is definitely distracted. Every time someone comes near he lets go and looks at them.	It's hard for Michael to pay attention to eating with so many people around.	Counselor uses the baby's name in an *active listening* response to voice an *alternative hunch*.
That's right.	So you're saying that Michael is distracted a lot during the day and seems really hungry at night.	Counselor uses the baby's name in an *interpreting* response to *test the hunch*.
Do you think he might be making up for not getting enough milk during the day? (This interpretation makes sense and she is pondering it.)	That seems to be a possibility.	Counselor uses an *attending* response to encourage the mother to add information that might shed more light on the situation.
That makes sense. When Michael and I were alone for a feeding yesterday, he ate for a long time and took an exceptionally long nap.	He seemed to sleep better when he ate with no distractions.	Counselor received confirmation that the *hunch* was correct and she uses an *interpreting* response.
Yeah. He did.	Linda, perhaps it might help if you breastfed Michael in a quieter place during the day.	Counselor uses the mother's and baby's names and *suggests an alternative action*.
I could go into the living room. The kids pretty much stay in the family room, and my sister and I could talk quietly.	Good idea. You might also try waking Michael sooner from his long afternoon nap and giving him an extra feeding in the afternoon.	Counselor uses the baby's name and *suggests an alternative action*. The mother has accepted the first suggestion and is trying to adapt it to her situation. The counselor will want to document this. It is the beginning of a *plan of action*.
Well, I could, but that would interfere with my making supper. I really like that quiet time to make supper, and I hate to work on supper in the morning.	It wouldn't work for you. Okay, so you're going to try to breastfeed Michael in a quieter place, to see if you can satisfy him during the day so he'll sleep better at night.	Counselor realizes the mother does not like the second suggestion and uses *active listening* as a graceful way to withdraw the rejected suggestion. By not pushing it, the counselor shows that she supports the mother and recognizes her right to make her own decisions on how to handle her situation. She uses the baby's name while *summarizing* what they have discussed and arriving at a *plan of action*. Although this example limits the plan to one option, there undoubtedly would be more suggestions in a real-life situation.
Yes.	Great, Linda! Please give me a call next week to let me know this has worked. Feel free to call me before then if you need to.	Counselor uses the mother's name and *arranges follow-up*.

progress through the problem-solving process. Guiding and leading skills are intermingled, with the counselor taking the lead only when the mother's conversation wanders away from the main concern or when she needs options pointed out to her. The nonassertive role played by the counselor encourages the mother to actively participate in the problem-solving process. It helps the mother understand and work out a solution that will suit her circumstance.

The Follow-up Method

To be fully aware of the mother's progress, you need to analyze the effectiveness of every contact. You can then determine how and when to plan the next contact and which preparation is needed for that encounter. Following up each counseling session with a subsequent contact will help you determine whether you have achieved your goal of increasing the mother's satisfaction and self-sufficiency. It will help you learn whether your suggestions have been useful and whether the mother needs further emotional support or assistance.

The follow-up method lets the mother know how actively concerned you are in helping her. It encourages you to review the situation and to research other sources of information as needed. If you practice in a fee-for-service setting, the mother's financial or insurance constraints may limit opportunities for follow-up. In such a case, appropriate referrals to community services or a breastfeeding support group can provide this component of follow-up and continuity of care.

Follow-up is an ongoing process that takes place during and after every counseling contact. By objectively analyzing the contact, you can determine what you and the mother accomplished and how to plan any subsequent contact so that it will be most beneficial to her. You can also research outside sources, such as literature and people and groups, to obtain information to meet the mother's special needs. You will then renew the counseling process with new information and a new perspective.

Generally, each individual contact requires some form of follow-up. The mother's level of need and the urgency of the situation will determine the nature of that ongoing care and dictate how soon and frequent it should be. The elements of follow-up—evaluation, planning and arranging for the next contact, researching outside sources, and renewing the counseling process—are discussed in the following sections.

Evaluating the Session

When evaluating a contact, ask yourself whether the session met the mother's needs for support, comfort, understanding, and action. Evaluate your use of counseling skills and the quality of information you gave to the mother. This approach enables you to determine those areas you need to explore further. The questions in Figure 5.6 will help you evaluate your contacts.

The evaluation process can be very encouraging for you as a counselor, too. It shows you how you have been helpful using counseling techniques such as supporting, clarifying, and educating. You will know that you have done a good job of counseling a mother if you can say some of these things to yourself:

- The mother freely talked about her concerns.
- She figured out what to do about her problem.
- She understood why her baby acted that way and what to do the next time.
- She seemed willing and eager to carry out the plan we developed.

It is equally important to evaluate yourself after you feel you have *not* helped a particular mother. Being open to this kind of self-examination will help you learn from your failures. You can plan how you will improve your future contacts and recognize that as you gain more experience, you will increase your effectiveness and success. Be kind to yourself! It is through our failures and mistakes

---

1. What support did I give? In what other ways could I have supported the mother?

2. Did the mother require immediate physical comfort? If so, what suggestions did I offer?

3. Did I gather enough information so that the mother and I both understood the problem? If not, what further information do I need?

4. Did I give appropriate information? Did the mother understand it? If not, what information do I need to give to the mother during the next contact?

5. Did the mother seem relaxed and talkative? If not, what skills can I use in a new approach for the next contact in order to encourage her to talk freely?

6. What plan did the mother and I make? Is it workable? If not, what alternative actions could I suggest?

7. Did the mother seem satisfied with the contact? If not, what areas should I explore in future contacts?

8. What follow-up did the mother and I arrange? Is it adequate, or should I contact the mother sooner?

9. Did I take usable notes during or after the contact? How were notes from previous contacts with this mother helpful? How can I improve my method of documentation?

10. Did I form a partnership with this mother and empower her to be self-sufficient in her problem solving?

11. Am I satisfied in my helping role with this mother? If not, what can I do to bring about greater satisfaction?

FIGURE 5.6   Questions for evaluating a counseling contact.

that we learn and grow. You might find it helpful to discuss a less than positive outcome with a colleague. Bear in mind that you cannot always "fix" a breastfeeding problem. The problem belongs to the mother, and she owns the responsibility for resolving it. You offer your expertise; the ownership needs to be hers.

Arranging the Next Contact

As the final step in your evaluation, you will want to plan for your next contact with the mother. Based on your analysis of the mother's satisfaction and needs, you will determine if further contact is needed and when it should occurs. This care may consist of a follow-up telephone call or a scheduled visit with you. Also decide who will initiate the contact and which additional information or assistance you will need to provide. Mother-to-mother peer counselors provide an important resource for many of these follow-up contacts. If you work in a postpartum setting, refer mothers to a community support group before they go home or to WIC-operated or public health clinic if they are enrolled in those services. This step will ensure that new mothers have adequate resources available to them after they leave you.

You can judge how soon you need to get back to a mother by the urgency of her situation. If she is having difficulty at every feeding, daily or even more frequent support and information from you would probably be helpful. Frequent contact is also important whenever the mother needs emotional support. Less critical or short-term problems usually require less frequent contact. For example, a mother who is becoming discouraged while trying to use an electric breast pump to get milk for her preterm infant in the hospital might benefit from your contacting her every day for a while. By comparison, a mother whose problem relates to a nonsupportive or interfering family member might prefer to talk with you periodically rather than daily.

Contact the mother any time you gain important new information, need to correct information you gave, or realize that you need to gather more information to help the mother resolve a problem. She will appreciate such concern about her welfare and that of her baby. Be sensitive to signals from her that she no longer feels the need for continued follow-up.

Always make sure the mother understands that she may call you before the next prearranged contact. If you asked a mother to call you and she does not, you may want to contact her. Many lactation consultants use e-mail communication with mothers, which minimizes missed calls. If you work in a busy practice and are unable to initiate frequent contact with mothers, a referral relationship with a support group in your community can provide the needed follow-up. You may then refer mothers to the support group or give mothers the name of a contact person.

Researching Outside Sources

At times, you may need to obtain further input and a fresh outlook on a problem. This is especially true if a situation lies outside the realm of your usual counseling. It is important that you recognize your own need for assistance. There may be issues you have overlooked. You are not required to have every piece of information about breastfeeding immediately available. You should, however, know where to find this information and when to use your resources.

Contacting another experienced lactation consultant to discuss the issue may provide you with a new perspective on a specific situation. Your colleague may suggest additional information you need to obtain from the mother, such as how the baby is acting between feedings or what the baby's physician says about the weight gain. You can also gain valuable support from a colleague. Internet resources such as Lactnet, an e-mail list for lactation professionals, and lactation websites are invaluable. It is important that you ask for help whenever you are involved in a situation that you are not able to resolve with your available resources.

Renewing the Counseling Process

The counseling process starts all over again with each successive contact. Begin with guiding skills and then progress to leading skills, just as in the original contact. You might start with an opening question such as "Hi, Ann. This is Heather. How have things been going since we last talked?" Then listen carefully to what the mother says. Perhaps everything you suggested worked and the problem is resolved. More likely, you can still help the mother work through a problem or concern.

～ Counseling Examples

The example scenarios in this section illustrate the use of counseling skills in a consultation. Pay particular attention to the caregiver's listening skills and provision of emotional support for the mother. Note the plan of care and follow-up arrangements between the mother and the caregiver. Guiding skills are interspersed throughout the contact. Abbreviations used to identify counseling skills are shown in Figure 5.7. The elements typically will progress roughly in the order in which they appear in the list.

Counseling Example with a Pregnant Woman

In Figure 5.8, Jan starts with open-ended questions to learn more about Kelly's situation. She then uses active listening to clarify Kelly's feelings. She focuses on Kelly's main concern by asking why she felt that some women

ES	Emotional support
AL	Active listening
I	Interpreting
OEQ	Open-ended question
IS	Identifying strengths
F	Focusing
E	Educating
PS	Practical suggestion
S	Summarizing
FU	Follow-up

FIGURE 5.7   Abbreviations for skills.

have difficulty breastfeeding. It becomes clear that a lack of information contributed to Kelly's hesitation to commit to breastfeeding. Jan begins to educate her and offer suggestions on how Kelly can learn more about breastfeeding.

Jan is careful not to overwhelm Kelly with information about the importance of human milk or reasons why she should breastfeed. Although that is certainly important information, she can address it another time. Together, Jan and Kelly form a plan of reading and attending the breastfeeding class. Jan summarizes the plan and arranges for follow-up.

Comparison of Two Caregivers

It is instructive to illustrate the differences between effective and ineffective counseling scenarios for the same mother. Figure 5.9 demonstrates the consequences of ineffective communication techniques. Figure 5.10 portrays the same scenario, this time with the caregiver using the counseling techniques effectively.

In Figure 5.9, Pam fails to provide emotional support and does not listen or respond to the mother's concerns about her emergency cesarean birth and failed birth plan. She does not pick up on Steph's feelings of inadequacy—

Kelly, a pregnant woman, arrives for an appointment with Jan, the lactation consultant, at her obstetrician's office.

Jan: Hi, Kelly! I'm glad you came to see me. When is your baby due? (OEQ)

Kelly: Oh, the baby's due in about 6 weeks. We are really getting excited!

Jan: It is exciting having a baby! (AL) Is this your first child?

Kelly: Yes, it is, and I wanted to talk to you about breastfeeding. I can't decide if breastfeeding is right for me.

Jan: You're not positive you want to breastfeed. (AL)

Kelly: Well, at first I kind of wanted to breastfeed, but my sister recently had a baby and she had so many problems that I just don't know. . . .

Jan: So you would like to breastfeed, and you want to make sure you don't have the same problems. (I)

Kelly: Yes, it seems like I have talked with so many people who had problems that I don't think I want to even try.

Jan: That's understandable. Why do you think your sister had difficulty breastfeeding? (F) [The lactation consultant is acting on the hunch that Kelly doesn't know much about breastfeeding.]

Kelly: I'm not sure. She didn't really know what to do.

Jan: It's true that many women have problems because they don't have the correct information about breastfeeding. (E) What kind of problems did your sister have? (OEQ)

Kelly: Oh, I can't exactly remember. It seems to me she had sore nipples, the baby was crying all the time, and she just didn't have enough milk. She just decided it wasn't worth it and then she quit. And then I have a friend who started breastfeeding and quit because her baby wanted to nurse all the time and she never could go anywhere. I really don't want to be tied down.

Jan: It's too bad your friend felt so hassled, because it is possible for a mother to do a number of things to fit breastfeeding into her life. Would you consider postponing your decision about breastfeeding until you learn a little more about it?

Kelly: Well, I've got time to make a decision, and I would like to try breastfeeding if I could be sure that it wouldn't be an ordeal like my sister had.

Jan: There is no way to guarantee that breastfeeding will be completely trouble free. Educating yourself will help you avoid most problems. You could start by reading some of our pamphlets on breastfeeding. Here's one on common questions mothers have and another one on how the breast makes milk. It would also help for you to attend a breastfeeding class. There is one scheduled next week on Thursday night that you could attend with your husband. I can also give you the number of a support group near you. (PS) Where would you like to start? (OEQ)

Kelly: Well, these pamphlets look interesting. Do they cover how to keep from having problems?

Jan: Some problems are covered. See, sore nipples and low milk supply are in here. If you read this information first, then we can talk about other concerns you have and I can suggest more reading if you like. What about the breastfeeding class? (OEQ/F)

Kelly: Yeah, that would probably be okay. I'll have to check with my husband and make sure he's free. Next Thursday night, did you say?

Jan: Yes. The class meets here in our office from 7:30 to 9:30, and because I'm teaching, we'll have an opportunity to talk again. There are several couples signed up for the class, so that will give your husband a chance to talk to some prospective breastfeeding dads, too. So, you are going to read the pamphlets, and then come to the class on Thursday night. (S) I will plan to see you then. If you have any questions before Thursday and you want to talk, don't hesitate to call me. (FU)

Kelly: Great. I'll see you next week. Thanks a lot!

FIGURE 5.8   Counseling example with a pregnant woman.

Steph is in her hospital room with her 2-day-old infant, Michael. Pam, her mother–baby nurse, comes to visit.

Pam: Hi, Steph! How are you doing today?

Steph: Oh, not very good.

Pam: Why? What's the matter?

Steph: I don't know. You know, I planned to have a natural childbirth with Bob in the delivery room, but I had to have an emergency c-section, and things just aren't going well.

Pam: You know the important thing is that you have a healthy baby. C-sections nowadays are almost as common as vaginal deliveries. It really isn't such a big deal any more.

Steph: I suppose. And I should just be grateful that he's healthy. But the other problem is that he isn't breastfeeding very well.

Pam: Really? Well, he sure looks content. Most c-section babies don't nurse very well the first couple of days anyway. He'll pick up.

Steph: All Michael wants to do is sleep all the time, and the nurses take real good care of him because I'm not moving around very well yet. His head is so floppy, and the nurses handle him so well. I'm afraid I might hurt him.

Pam: Isn't it great the nurses are so good with him! That saves you from having to do much, and you can get your rest. You'll have plenty of opportunity later on to take care of him.

Steph: I guess. I don't get a chance to hold him much, and he's always too sleepy to nurse.

Pam: It's probably all the pain medication you are taking and the anesthesia you had during the c-section. Don't worry about it. He'll wake up and start breastfeeding better when you get home. You just take care of yourself and get plenty of rest while you have people around who can help you.

Steph: I guess you're right. I hope he'll do better. I'm really worried about him. I'm afraid he's starving.

Pam: Don't worry; we can give him formula in the nursery. And he'll start nursing better. I'll be back later. Give me a call if you need anything else.

FIGURE 5.9   Ineffective counseling technique.

that the nurses did such a good job and Steph feels as though she cannot do anything right. Steph needs to know that her feelings are normal and that a sleepy infant is normal. Pam may inadvertently contribute to underlying feelings of guilt by saying that Steph's pain medication caused the sleepiness.

Steph needs help learning to respond to her baby's hunger cues and wakeful times. She needs to see that she is capable of caring for and breastfeeding her baby. Pam could have accomplished this goal by offering specific suggestions on infant care and breastfeeding. Most of all, in this example, Pam is very impersonal and dismissive, failing to respond to Steph as an individual.

In Figure 5.10, as with many breastfeeding issues, the mother's state of mind and self-esteem are the factors that

most influence her outcome. Pam listens to Steph and focuses on her concerns—disappointment over her birth experience and overall feelings of inadequacy. By building on Steph's ability to care for her infant and letting her know that awkwardness is common at first, Pam encourages Steph and helps her feel competent. By teaching Steph how to watch for Michael's cues and encouraging her to put Michael to the breast on her own, she shows that she believes Steph can resolve her problem.

Similar Counseling Strategies

Comparable approaches to counseling have been taught by Best Start Social Marketing and, more recently, by Every Mother, Inc. (2009). The Best Start Three-Step Counseling Strategy is divided into three components. The first step, asking open-ended questions and using appropriate probes, focuses on learning as much as possible about the client's concerns. The second step affirms the client's feelings and reassures her that she is not alone, which helps build a relationship with the client. Spending time on this step empowers the mother and helps to create an atmosphere of safety where she can feel confident sharing her concerns. It also serves as a bridge to the education the counselor will provide. The third step educates the client by using the principles of adult education and offering information in small bites.

The Every Mother approach, "Counseling with Both 'I's' Open," focuses on the concept of "connection before content," including building counselor communication skills in establishing rapport with clients before providing information. This approach includes rapport-building skills such as using appropriate body language and active listening principles such as validating feelings and asking open-ended questions to build an environment where clients feel safe sharing their concerns. It also highlights the need to understand and use emotion-based messages when providing solutions and options for addressing client concerns.

These counseling techniques share some similarities with the strategy presented in this chapter, including the use of active listening principles to build rapport before inundating a client with information or advice. Both techniques also emphasize the need for listening and affirmation, which are prominent elements of the technique described in this chapter. One difference is that the Best Start and Every Mother strategies begin with questions and then move to statements of affirmation. In contrast, the guiding method described earlier begins with emotional support (affirmation) before gathering information through guiding statements and limited use of open-ended questions; it then continues with affirming statements throughout the contact. All three systems include education and emphasize the need to avoid overwhelming the client with too much information. In addi-

---

Steph is in her hospital room with her 2-day-old infant, Michael. Pam, her mother-baby nurse, comes to visit.

Pam: Hi, Steph! How are you doing today?

Steph: Oh, not very good.

Pam: I'm sorry to hear that, Steph. (ES) What seems to be the problem? (OEQ)

Steph: I don't know. You know, I planned to have a natural childbirth with Bob in the delivery room, but I had to have an emergency c-section, and things just aren't going well.

Pam: What a disappointment! (ES) It is really hard when your birth experience doesn't go the way you planned. (AL).

Steph: I am disappointed. And I feel guilty for feeling disappointed, because Michael is beautiful and healthy, and that is all I should be concerned about. But I can't help wishing Bob could have been there to see him being born, and I feel as though both of us missed out somehow. To top it off, he isn't even breastfeeding well. He's too sleepy.

Pam: Steph, there is nothing wrong with feeling disappointed or even really angry. You need to have time to grieve your lost birth experience. Your feelings are part of the grieving process, and you need time to work them through. Being angry or disappointed does not make you a bad person or ungrateful for your beautiful little boy. Expressing your feelings is healing. And this is important. (E/S) You feel as though you can't do anything right because first of all you had to have a C-section, and now Michael won't even breastfeed! (I/AL)

Steph: That's right. Talk about being inadequate. And I feel so awkward with the baby. You nurses all know just what to do. You make it look so simple to hold up his floppy head, and change his diaper. And you wrap him perfectly in that blanket, just like a cute little mummy! When I do it, the blanket just falls apart.

Pam: You feel that because you are Michael's mom, you should be able to care for him better than anyone else. (I)

Steph: Yeah.

Pam: Learning all the best ways of caring for Michael takes time. Most first-time mothers feel inadequate at first. You and Michael just need time to adjust to each other, time to learn to communicate with each other. You can trust your intuition about how to care for him and respond to his needs. (IS/E) For example, you seem anxious about his sleepiness. Have you been wondering if you should wake Michael up to feed him?

Steph: Um-hm. I wondered if I should, if it would be okay. I wanted to try feeding him again, but then I wasn't sure how or when to go about it.

Pam: One of the best things to do is what you are doing right now, and that is keeping Michael with you as much as possible. That way, you can watch for his feeding cues, things like bringing his hands to his mouth or around his head, making little sucking motions, rapid eye movement, or rooting toward the breast when you hold him. Sometimes unwrapping him completely will rouse him out of a light sleep and remind him that it might be time to nurse. (IS/E)

Steph: But won't he get cold if I do that?

Pam: Your breasts are the warmest part of your body, and when Michael is snuggled up to you with skin-to-skin contact, he will stay warm and cozy. You can put his blanket over the two of you after he starts breastfeeding. (E)

Steph: Well, he's beginning to stir and looks as though he wants to suck on his hands. Should I try feeding him?

Pam: Super. Using a position like this [demonstrates] that holds your baby to the side is especially good so you can avoid putting pressure on your incision. Hold your breast so your fingers don't touch the dark part of your nipple. Now, gently touch his upper lip with your nipple. Look, there, he's opening his mouth really wide. Pull him gently to your breast nice and tight. Gently pressing on his back brings him in close without touching his head. He's got it! See, you know just what to do! Notice those long, drawing sucks? He's having a lovely lunch. (E/PS/IS)

Steph: It really helped having you here to get us started. How long should I let him nurse?

Pam: As long as he continues to breastfeed with those long nutritive sucks. After he's feeling pretty content, his hands will probably relax, and he'll drift off to sleep or come off your breast spontaneously. In either case, you can then put him to breast on the other side. If he wakes up and breastfeeds some more, that's fine. If he continues to sleep, that's okay, too. (E)

Steph: He's really nursing well now. I think we'll be okay. Thanks so much for your help.

Pam: I think you'll both be fine. Just trust your judgment, and if you can't figure out what to do, don't hesitate to ask for help. I'll stop in later to see how you're getting along. (FU)

FIGURE 5.10 Effective counseling technique.

tion, they share the common goals of empowering the mother, validating her concerns, and equipping her with problem-solving skills.

∼ Summary

Through your effective use of basic counseling techniques, you can provide mothers with the support and teaching that will help them develop confidence in their mothering and breastfeeding. Approaching each mother with a warm, caring attitude will show deep, genuine concern and empathy that helps her feel understood and empowers her to take positive action in dealing with her concern. Guiding skills help keep the conversation going while the counselor gathers information and provides emotional support. With leading skills, the counselor takes a more active role in directing the conversation and helps the mother work toward developing a plan of care. The final stage of a contact is arranging appropriate follow-up and analyzing the effectiveness of the counseling assistance and support. Developing and continuing to improve your use of counseling skills will enhance your effectiveness in communicating with parents.

～ Chapter 5—At a Glance

Applying what you learned—

- Recognize how your personality affects your rapport with mothers.
- Validate a mother's feelings, emotions, and concerns through attending, active listening, empathetic listening, reassuring, praising, and building hope.
- Help mothers with immediate physical comfort before attempting any problem solving when needed.
- Practice using counseling skills with family and friends to become proficient in their use.
- Avoid active participation early in the contact to allow maximum opportunity for the mother to provide information and insights.
- Develop listening skills that actively respond to both verbal and nonverbal messages.
- Perceive with your ears, eyes, and imagination.
- Use active listening to gather information, clarify messages, show acceptance, and encourage a response.
- Use empathetic listening to understand the mother's emotions and help the mother work through her feelings.
- Use clarifying, open-ended questions, interpreting, focusing, and summarizing to obtain more information, define the situation, and focus on specific concerns.
- Ask open-ended questions rather than closed questions to gather more information.
- Influence the mother positively by reassuring, building hope, and identifying her strengths.
- Gather enough information so your movement into the problem-solving phase of the counseling session is not premature or incorrect.

- Take time to gain the mother's trust and clarify the situation before engaging in problem solving.
- Give parents proper information at the appropriate time to help them grow as parents.
- Correct misconceptions or mismanagement with sensitivity.
- Form your first hunch based on information and impressions you gained earlier in the counseling session.
- Use a nonassertive approach to encourage the mother to be active in problem solving.
- Arrange appropriate follow-up after every contact by evaluating the session, planning and arranging for the next contact, and researching additional resources as needed.
- Make sure the mother knows when she may call or email you.

～ References

Birkman International. Birkman Method. 2009. www.birkman.com. Accessed March 13, 2009.

Brammer L, McDonald G. *The Helping Relationship: Process and Skills*, 8th ed. Boston: Allyn & Bacon; 2003.

Every Mother, Inc. Training programs. 2009. www.everymother.org. Accessed August 26, 2009.

Inscape Publishing. DiSC. 2009. www.inscapepublishing.com. Accessed March 13, 2009.

Myers-Briggs. Myers-Briggs Type Indicator. 2009. www.cpp.com. Accessed March 13, 2009.

Wilson Learning. Wilson Social Styles. 2009. www.wilsonlearning.com. Accessed March 13, 2009.

CHAPTER

6

Client Consultations

Women have more positive breastfeeding outcomes when they receive consistent encouragement, help, and guidance at appropriate times. Caregivers find a preventive approach to breastfeeding care to be a time-saving approach that is far more effective than crisis management. Some situations are suitable to counseling by phone or e-mail, whereas others require an in-person assessment. Sometimes a problem has advanced by the time contact occurs, requiring more intense problem solving. By collaborating with mothers, you will help them recognize problems, possible causes of those problems, and practical actions to resolve their situations. Using the counseling skills presented in Chapter 5 will help you determine the problem, gain insights into what caused the situation, and work toward a solution in tandem with the mother. This chapter describes a systematic approach to consultations, as well as several methods of documentation.

∽ *Key Terms*

Alternative hunches
Anticipatory guidance
Assessment
Breastfeeding descriptors
Consent
Crisis intervention
Documentation
Follow-up
Hidden factors
History
Hunch

Infant Breastfeeding
   Assessment Tool
   (IBFAT)
LATCH method
Mother–Baby Assessment
   (MBA)
Online help
Outreach counseling
Physician report
Plan of care
Problem solving
Telephone counseling

∽ *Reaching Out Through Anticipatory Guidance*

Anticipatory guidance is a proactive counseling technique. An outreach approach focusing on anticipatory guidance in the care of breastfeeding mothers is not a new concept, of course. Indeed, it forms the basis of breastfeeding counseling in support groups and breastfeeding programs throughout the world. All areas of the medical community engage in preventive medicine. Well-baby checkups, dental exams, routine breast exams, Pap smears, and routine eye exams are all examples of preventive care. Modern medicine clearly recognizes the benefits of early detection.

Anticipatory guidance is effective in preventing negative outcomes and enhancing positive experiences (Piotrowski et al., 2009; Barclay, 2008). Contact at key times can diminish problems or eliminate them entirely. It helps establish a foundation of knowledge that leads to optimal breastfeeding practices. This investment of time and energy pays off in terms of fewer problems and more positive outcomes for the mother and baby. An enjoyable experience for parents, coupled with less time spent in problem solving, makes this both a parent-friendly and time-saving approach.

When they receive practical information and support before significant milestones occur, parents can anticipate impending changes and identify their needs. For example, a mother may feel anxious and uncertain about breastfeeding. Anticipatory guidance prepares her psychologically so that she knows what to expect and feels more confident in meeting each new milestone. Research shows that the majority of parents do not discuss most standard topics with their healthcare providers. For this reason, clinicians need to take the initiative in providing information to parents through anticipatory guidance (Schuster et al., 2000).

The Timing of Anticipatory Guidance

Anticipatory guidance is just as important to routine health supervision as the history and physical examination. It is a fundamental part of preventive health care for the breastfeeding mother. This guidance needs to occur at a teachable moment, when retention of information is highest and when decision making takes place.

Women usually decide to breastfeed before the baby's birth, often prior to pregnancy (Guise et al., 2003; Earle, 2002). Therefore, earlier exposure to breastfeeding information is even more effective in supporting their decision-making process. Several studies suggest that adolescents are interested in learning about breastfeeding during their secondary school years (Nelson, 2009; Goulet et al., 2003; Ross & Goulet, 2002; Alnasir, 1992; Neifert et al., 1988). This is an ideal time for correcting misconceptions. Anticipatory guidance and education at this critical stage in an adolescent's development promotes positive attitudes and establishes a sound knowledge base. Early education can help students form healthy perceptions of sexuality and parenthood (Martens, 2001; Volpe & Bear, 2000; Yeo, et al. 1994). When adolescents reach adulthood, reinforcement of these early concepts will further guide them in making sound decisions.

It is easier to address specific needs after you and the mother have established a comfortable relationship. A climate characterized by acceptance, flexibility, and cooperation sets the stage for a positive breastfeeding experience (Finch & Daniel, 2002; Greenwood & Littlejohn, 2002; Parker & Williams, 2000). In particular, making contact with women during pregnancy helps build rapport and trust. The new mother is then likely to accept advice more readily from her support person during breastfeeding. After a program of comprehensive prenatal breastfeeding education, you can spend your valuable time with postpartum mothers and babies reinforcing and reviewing issues presented earlier.

A Mother's Need for Anticipatory Guidance

Breastfeeding mothers often lack role models, an experienced support person, practical and timely information, and the self-confidence to anticipate their own needs. For some mothers, their only source of breastfeeding information may be skimpy literature, formula company misinformation, or a brief discussion at a childbirth or postpartum class. At a time when the new mother's energies and concentration are centered on her infant's birth and her own changing role, retention of breastfeeding information may be minimal at best. She may combine half-remembered instructions with incorrect information from well-meaning friends and relatives, placing her breastfeeding at risk. In this sometimes chaotic environ-

ment, a knowledgeable caregiver becomes a key to the mother meeting her breastfeeding goals.

Anticipatory guidance can save both the mother and the infant from potential difficulties by guiding the mother one step at a time through her breastfeeding journey. When lactation consultation is done on a timely basis, you can teach and inform a mother well in advance of critical periods. Her preparedness and self-confidence will often be enough to prevent problems. Any problems, if they do occur, will also likely be of shorter duration, with the chances of recurrence being decreased.

Crisis Intervention

In contrast to anticipatory guidance, crisis intervention occurs after a problem already exists. It may seem to some that crisis intervention is less time-consuming than educating the mother before the delivery and supporting her throughout breastfeeding. Yet, the time spent later in problem solving negates any time saved. Even more important, the results for the mother are less positive. Although the mother may alleviate her immediate problem, the crisis might not have occurred at all had she been educated and supported adequately beforehand. Additionally, the situation has compromised her sense of well-being and self-assurance. Breastfeeding is a normal part of childbearing and family life. A problem-oriented approach must be replaced with one of prevention and preservation of the healthy normal phenomenon—the breastfeeding dyad of mother and baby.

Counseling Examples Contrasting Approaches

The value of anticipatory guidance is illustrated by two women who attend the same prenatal breastfeeding class. Compare the breastfeeding experiences for these two women over about a 3-week period. In Figure 6.1, Lynn receives help and support from both a lactation consultant and a mother-to-mother support counselor. In Figure 6.2, Denise receives the telephone number of a lactation consultant and understands that she may call if she has questions or problems. The log of each mother's contacts illustrates how timing and frequency of contact can affect their outcomes.

Lynn, who is equipped with information and support, is enjoying breastfeeding. She experiences a bit of nipple tenderness on the second day. Because her lactation consultant visited her the previous day, she feels comfortable calling her to ask for help. The soreness clears up after she is reminded about positioning her baby for a good latch and makes the necessary adjustments. Having learned about growth spurts and what to expect for her baby's first checkup helps Lynn anticipate these events. During her baby's growth spurt, the lactation consultant

8/15	Saw Lynn at 09:00 in hospital. Baby was born at 13:00 yesterday after a 3-hour labor. Apgars 9 and 9. Baby was put to breast within 1 hour. Feedings are unrestricted and going well. Baby has had 6 feedings. Reviewed feeding cues and what to look for with her baby's latch. Lynn stated a support counselor had called her several weeks ago. They discussed putting baby to breast as soon as possible after delivery. Suggested she obtain a book on breastfeeding and attend a breastfeeding class, which she did. Counselor had given her my name as the LC who would see her in the hospital. Will return when baby is ready for the next feeding.
8/15	Visited Lynn at 10:30. Observed a feeding. Baby had good feeding after initially helping mother with positioning and latch. Reviewed positioning options, frequency and duration of feedings, signs of milk transfer.
8/16	Lynn called from home. Her nipples are tender. We reviewed positioning and latch on again. Asked her to call me tomorrow if no improvement.
8/18	Lynn called. Nipples are less tender. She notices a difference with the way she positions baby. Realizes he wasn't getting a good latch before. Feels she finally can achieve an effective latch. Breasts seem fuller. Reminded her to rest and to follow baby's feeding cues. Discussed typical growth spurt at about 10 days to 2 weeks.
8/25	Lynn called. Is having rough day. Baby nurses constantly. She's ready to give a bottle. Reminded her about growth spurts and gave encouragement. Lynn says she will hold off one more day. Suggested she contact her breastfeeding counselor to find out when the next support group meeting will be held.
8/27	Called Lynn. Baby is nursing less frequently now. Nipples no longer tender. She spoke with counselor and plans to attend a support group meeting in 2 weeks. Discussed what to expect at baby's first checkup. Asked her to call after checkup.
9/1	Lynn called. Stated that baby's weight gain is good and breastfeeding is going great. Lynn in high spirits and enjoying breastfeeding.
12/6	Saw Lynn at the grocery store. Stated breastfeeding is going very well. She plans to become a counselor with her support group. Said, "I couldn't have done it without you!"

FIGURE 6.1   *Example of anticipatory guidance.*

8/12	Contacted by mother, Denise, who delivered her baby on 7/29 and began breastfeeding within 6 hours. She was given a lactation consultant's telephone number at hospital discharge. Baby was fussy at feedings for the first 2 days, and popped on and off the breast. Denise figured this was because she didn't have any milk yet. On day 3 Denise's nipples became very tender. She applied breast cream that was given to her by the hospital. Two days later, Denise's nipples were cracked and bleeding. Her breasts were full and uncomfortable. She remembered that she was given my phone number but could not find it. After another 5 days, baby wanted to nurse all the time. Denise began supplementing with formula two times a day, as she believed she did not have enough milk. Stated that nursing was still painful at this time. After another 3 days, baby began to prefer the bottle and was still fussy when Denise tried to nurse. Denise contacted the hospital to get my phone number. She called me in tears. Her baby is taking four bottles of formula a day. She wants to return to exclusive breastfeeding. Scheduled her for appointment today at 15:00.
8/12	Saw Denise and baby at office. Observed a feeding. Denise needed much help with positioning and attachment. Baby fussy; popped on and off frequently. Her nipples are red and tender. Evidence of thrush in baby's mouth. Advised her to contact her physician for appropriate treatment of nipples and baby's mouth. Gave her information sheet on treatment of thrush. Encouraged her to call me with questions or concerns.
8/15	Called Denise. She cannot detect any increase in milk production. Baby refuses the breast at most feedings. She is using medication for thrush on her nipples and in baby's mouth. Nipples are still tender but getting a little better. Denise is tired and frustrated at balancing bottle and breast. Discussed using nursing supplementer to increase milk production, but Denise did not wish to use it. Reviewed positioning and treatment of her sore nipples. Encouraged her to call me with questions or concerns.
8/18	Called Denise. She has decided to discontinue breastfeeding. She stated that she is disappointed, but resigned to bottle feeding.

FIGURE 6.2   *Example of crisis intervention.*

refers Lynn to the additional support of a breastfeeding counselor. Lynn is well on the road to long-term breast-feeding.

Denise's first contact with a lactation consultant is after her problems have advanced. Denise lacks the knowledge and self-confidence to persevere through the normal occurrence of a growth spurt and begins supplementing her baby with formula. She endures the discomfort of engorgement, sore nipples, and undiagnosed

thrush. By the time she contacts a lactation consultant, she is discouraged and her baby prefers bottle feeding over breastfeeding. Despite appropriate assistance, the lactation consultant is unable to help Denise return to her original plan of exclusive breastfeeding. Within 3 weeks after her baby is born, Denise is no longer breast-feeding.

With early contact, Denise might have felt comfortable calling her lactation consultant when she delivered.

Learning about effective positioning and latch would have increased her confidence and prevented prolonged nipple soreness. When she developed thrush, early treatment would have cleared the infection sooner. Having had no personal contact with the consultant before now, Denise put off placing a call until she was desperate. Unfortunately, this type of outcome is all too common. Incidents of untimely weaning can be reduced with appropriate anticipatory guidance by a lactation consultant or breastfeeding counselor.

Outreach Prevention

Prevention counseling requires more time during the early stages of breastfeeding. You can see from the counseling example that Lynn received twice the amount of assistance and support as Denise received during this period. Frequency of contact typically subsides, however, after the first several weeks, by which time mother and baby have developed together into a harmonious pair. You, the mother, and her infant will benefit from your guidance of the mother through her early stages, educating her in advance and increasing her self-efficacy.

Breastfeeding rates are higher when mothers receive consistent encouragement, help, and guidance prenatally, during their hospital stay, and throughout lactation (Gill et al., 2007; Su et al., 2007; Guise et al., 2003; Arora et al., 2000). A mother's breastfeeding education needs to be viewed in the larger context of a preventive approach to health care, much in the same way that dental checkups help prevent cavities. When she receives continuing support and information prenatally and throughout lactation, the mother becomes prepared and is knowledgeable in terms of her expectations. She is then better able to meet the challenges of mothering with confidence. Anticipatory guidance is especially crucial for mothers who will be returning to work or school (Angeletti, 2009).

When women receive necessary information and support, they have significantly longer breastfeeding experiences with fewer problems. Prenatal support is more effective than support given only after delivery; support both before and after delivery produces the best results. Lack of information is a key factor associated with reasons why mothers stop breastfeeding prematurely (Kishore et al., 2009; Rebhan et al., 2009; Sutton et al., 2007; Ummarino et al., 2003). Bottle feeding mothers report they would have felt encouraged to breastfeed if they had received more information through prenatal class, the media, and books. Family support is also a factor (Arora et al., 2000).

If extended outreach is not an option in your work setting, a hotline, warmline, or e-mail may be a practical method of facilitating contact with mothers. Occasionally, a mother may not desire contact as frequently as anticipatory guidance suggests. Your sensitivity to the mother's cues will establish an opportunity for a mother to gracefully make her wishes known. Some mothers prefer to handle the daily stresses of motherhood in a more private manner. In such a case, the most effective approach may be simply to let the mother know you are available and allow her to initiate any contacts.

Breastfeeding Support Counseling

Referral to a community support group will provide an avenue for anticipatory guidance. Before the advent of the lactation consulting profession, mothers received breastfeeding support primarily from volunteer lay counselors who developed relationships with mothers through a series of contacts. This form of support continues to provide mothers with day-to-day breastfeeding assistance. Today, lay counselors remain important partners in the mother's breastfeeding support team. Lactation consultants can be instrumental in helping support groups establish effective outreach to breastfeeding women in their community.

For the most part, contacts with breastfeeding counselors take place through phone or e-mail. A counselor contacts the mother several weeks or months before delivery and continues to contact her through weaning. Some mothers attend monthly support group meetings as well. The services provided by these lay counselors provide essential ongoing support for mothers.

The method used by lay counselors serves as a noteworthy model for anticipatory guidance and support. Mothers benefit from anticipatory guidance during their pregnancy as well as in the early months of breastfeeding. Some will welcome continued contact throughout their breastfeeding and weaning. If you do not incorporate such contact into your practice, clinic, or hospital, referral to a support group can provide this guidance. See Chapter 2 for a discussion of mother-to-mother support groups.

Prenatal Contact

Care providers and other support people need to make a concerted effort to reach women during pregnancy with messages that lay the groundwork for optimal breastfeeding practices. Encourage the expectant woman to educate herself about breastfeeding through reading, attending meetings or classes, observing other mothers breastfeeding, and voicing her questions and concerns. The use of listening skills will help you understand the mother's goals for breastfeeding, the extent of her breastfeeding knowledge, and her need for support. Be sure to give her an opportunity to ask questions and make certain that she does not have any unanswered questions or concerns.

Be sure mothers have your name, telephone number, e-mail address (if you provide e-mail consultation or support), and the best times to reach you. Remember that most mothers will be more comfortable receiving calls than initiating them. Initiating contact with a mother shows your interest and concern. You and the mother can establish the most convenient times for subsequent contacts, taking into consideration both parties' family, work, or school responsibilities and needs.

Continuing Regular Contact

Many mothers benefit from frequent contact in the early weeks of breastfeeding. Check that the mother under-stands the basic principles of breastfeeding management and the prevention of problems. Help her learn how to know when she is positioning her baby at the breast for optimal milk transfer and how to respond to hunger cues. Discuss ways to ensure ample milk production, respond-ing to her baby's periods of increased hunger (growth spurts), and typical nursing patterns for babies of differ-ent ages. Help her learn to trust herself and her baby as she observes her baby's behavior and reactions, Table 6.1 pre-sents guidelines for deciding how often to contact a mother and what to discuss at each stage.

TABLE 6.1   Anticipatory Guidance from a Breastfeeding Counselor

• During pregnancy	Contact the pregnant woman once or twice during her pregnancy. You can recommend books and videos, and urge her to begin acquainting herself with breastfeeding. Invite her to attend a support group meeting. This is an opportune time to begin building rapport with the mother, perhaps discussing her expectations and preparation for childbirth.
• When the baby is born	Hopefully you will be in close enough contact to know when the mother delivers. You can ask her to call and let you know when she has the baby. Ask if she would like you to visit her if there is no lactation consultant support in the hospital. If you are unable to visit her in person, a telephone call will be a second best option. Encourage her to talk about her labor and delivery. You may be the only person who shows an interest in helping her verbalize any disappointments or concerns regarding the birth. Find out how she feels and how her baby is doing. Ask her baby's name and start referring to her baby by name. Be sure that she knows when you will contact her again. Because most mothers spend a short time in the hospital, it may be impractical to schedule a contact during her stay. This makes close prenatal contact with her even more critical, because she will be more likely to let you know when she delivers.
• Just home from the hospital	Contact the mother within 2 to 3 days after she returns home, and more frequently for specific problems. You can first ask, "How do you feel?" and then inquire about the number of feedings, voids, and stools in 24 hours. Discuss, as necessary, common concerns such as fatigue, positioning the baby during feedings, how to know the baby is getting enough milk, and how to avoid problems such as sore nipples and engorgement. Try not to overwhelm her with too much information at one time.
• Baby 1 week old	Call to remind the mother that babies typically seem more hungry and increase feeding frequency at approximately 10 days old. Also remind her that her breasts will reduce in size around this time as she responds to her baby's increased feedings. Make sure she understands how milk production depends on supply and demand, and encourage her to continue to respond to her baby's feeding cues. Discuss typical breastfeeding patterns for this age, and assure her that you welcome calls from her.
• Before baby's 2-week checkup	You can help the mother understand what her baby's physician will be looking for at this checkup. Discuss normal weight patterns and normal feeding patterns, and help her form questions to ask the physician. Call the mother again after the checkup, and ask about weight gain and any recommendations the physician has made. Help her integrate the physician's suggestions into her breastfeeding and clarify any possible misunderstandings.
• Baby 6 weeks old	At about 6 weeks, the mother will be returning for her postpartum checkup. Discuss the possible effects of oral contraceptives on her breastfeeding. She may be interested in resuming her prepregnant activity level. Caution her about overdoing. Remind her that her baby may go through another hunger spurt at this time. This may be prolonged if the mother has been very active and has been missing some feedings.
• After the first month	Continue to keep in touch with the mother as the need arises. If you feel confident that the mother will call you whenever she has a question or problem, you could discontinue initiating calls. Some mothers will benefit from routine calls all the way through weaning.

Use of guiding skills in early contacts with a mother will help you determine when her confidence and knowledge will sustain her and your sessions can end. Your judgment and intuition, along with open communication and rapport with the mother, will help you and the mother decide when contact should subside. As the mother learns more about her baby and breastfeeding, the frequency of contacts can gradually diminish, unless she is experiencing problems. Initiating contact at times when the potential for problems typically occurs will give mothers the support and advice they need. Detailed records and thorough evaluations of each contact will help you determine appropriate follow-up.

⁓ Problem Solving with Mothers

You may not always be in contact with a mother at an early stage of a problem. In some cases, the mother may have received advice from various caregivers that was unhelpful, inappropriate, or contradictory. As a result, she may have lost hope about her ability to breastfeed when you see her for the first time. Although these conditions are less than ideal, the reality is that you will need to be prepared to enter into the problem-solving process at various levels. You also will need to be sensitive to the frustrations and anxiety the mother brings with her to the process. Sometimes a problem may advance to the point that your only recourse is to assist the mother in weaning and offer emotional support to her. When this happens, help the mother to recall with pleasure the positive aspects of her breastfeeding. She may need reassurance that breastfeeding can follow a more rewarding course for a subsequent baby.

Even when mothers practice sound breastfeeding techniques, problems may occur. You can help the mother recognize these situations, as well as the possible causes and practical actions she can take to resolve them. Problem solving involves more than simply offering a suggestion to the mother: It requires gathering information and comparing it to known patterns of problem development. This kind of troubleshooting often involves using your intuition to develop hunches. You can use these hunches to focus your thinking and select suggestions that will be most helpful to the mother in her particular circumstances.

No one universal solution is available that will solve every breastfeeding problem. Just as you have a toolbox full of counseling skills, so you need to have an even larger toolbox containing problem-solving skills. You will need the judgment, knowledge, and intuition to know which tools to pull from the box for a given situation. Suggestions may even contradict one another at different times! It is up to you to decide which action to offer first to a par-

ticular mother, based on your perception of her situation and her ability to cope. If your first suggestion does not lead to the solution of her problem, you will need to suggest other actions until she finds those options that work best for her.

Using Counseling Skills to Determine the Problem

Often, breastfeeding problems are complex issues with multiple causes and no specific "right" solution. The many factors that may affect breastfeeding—such as the infant's physical and medical status, the child's temperament and ability to suck, the frequency and length of feedings, the condition of the mother's breasts, hormonal disorders, and emotional influences—make it inappropriate to offer information without first clearly defining a mother's problem(s).

You can use the counseling skills presented in Chapter 5 to learn more about the relevant circumstances and to gather information about symptoms. By patiently listening and encouraging the mother to communicate openly, you show her that you value her perception of the problem and want to work with her conscientiously toward a solution. In taking this empathetic approach, you gain additional insight into what caused her situation and, therefore, can more easily determine her needs. Providing her with emotional support can reduce her anxiety and allow her to be more patient and objective in working toward a solution.

Sometimes a mother needs to take immediate action to reduce her physical discomfort before you can investigate the causes of her problem with her. In this case, you can first give her suggestions for physical relief and then continue with problem solving when she is more comfortable. If the mother does not receive comfort measures early in the contact, she may be unable to hear or accept the information you share with her.

The mother needs to understand her problem, the events and actions that led to it, and the steps that will help her resolve it. When she is armed with this information, you and the mother will be better able to develop a plan that produces the most satisfaction from her contact with you and decreases the likelihood of recurrences. The mother's understanding will come more readily when she is an equal partner in problem solving. By working with her to define her problem and explore possible actions, you help the mother understand her situation better and develop her confidence and skills.

Working Toward a Solution

When the nature of a problem takes shape through investigation with the mother, problem-solving skills will help you both move toward a solution. The problem-solving method should contain the elements that are essential to meeting the mother's needs. The consultation begins with gathering information and impressions before you enter into any intervention or active involvement. After gathering sufficient information and impressions, followed by taking a history and assessing the mother and baby, you can form a first hunch and begin to define the problem. While continuing to look for hidden factors, you can eliminate related causes and test your hunch. By comparing your ideas with the mother's suggestions, you can explore alternative hunches and look for other possible causes.

After you have defined the problem, you and the mother can examine the options, select one, and put it into action. Try to give the mother no more than two or three suggestions at a time to avoid overwhelming her. Ask the mother whether your suggestions suit her needs and how the two of you might adapt them to her situation. Be prepared to offer further suggestions as needed. Involving the mother in this way in developing a plan will increase the likelihood that she will follow it.

Step 1: Form Your First Hunch

When a breastfeeding problem arises, you will first want to determine how the mother views the situation. Ask what she thinks is the cause, and which actions she has already taken. From this basic information, you can form your hunch about the cause and come up with a possible solution to the problem. This step involves more of an unconscious reflex than a carefully reasoned analysis. Concentrating on this preliminary hunch is an essential first step to working toward a solution. It helps focus observations and reduces aimless thinking.

Your first hunch is only the beginning of the problem-solving process, however. Consider it a point of departure rather than a final destination. While forming your first hunch, continue to use your guiding skills to provide emotional support to the mother and to gather more information and impressions that further clarify and define the problem.

Step 2: Look for Hidden Factors

In many cases, hidden factors may contribute to a breastfeeding-related problem. An infant who nurses frequently at night may be sleeping for long periods during the day. A mother who thinks her milk is not rich enough may have expressed milk from her breasts and noticed the typical, thin, watery appearance of human milk. A mother who did not experience the sensation of her milk "coming in" and whose baby is not gaining weight may have significant endocrine problems. It is important to identify such hidden factors as early as possible in the process. Tuning in to the mother's needs, encouraging her to talk, and listening attentively will help you accomplish this goal. Guiding skills are essential to this process.

Step 3: Test Your Hunch

While gathering additional information, continue to evaluate your hunch to determine whether the situation is what you expected. New information may lead you to form a new hunch. Hidden factors and the mother's lack of breastfeeding information may obscure the problem until you explore all possibilities. A mother who first complained that it hurt whenever she nursed may have led you to believe she had sore nipples. By exploring the issue further, you might learn that she experiences discomfort when her milk lets down or that she interprets the typical tugging sensation of sucking as pain.

To test your hunch, you can use interpreting, focusing, and summarizing skills: "From what you're describing . . . ," "Let me see if I understand . . . ," "You seem to be. . . ." Help the mother hear what she is telling you so she can provide any further clarification necessary. When your hunch proves to be correct and the problem has been clearly identified, you are ready to develop a plan of care with the mother.

Step 4: Explore Alternative Hunches

The insights you gain in testing your hunch may alter your initial hunch. You then need to pursue other hunches to resolve the problem. Perhaps when you tested your hunch, the mother corrected you and led you in another direction. Exploring alternative hunches will help clarify the situation. Sometimes a problem may remain ill defined throughout several contacts with the mother, perhaps over several weeks. At such times, you and the mother might develop a trial plan that addresses the most obvious symptoms or concerns. When the mother recognizes which actions are most effective, she may begin to narrow down the cause of the problem. You can also network with other lactation consultants and healthcare team members about a situation that puzzles you.

Difficulty in determining the cause of and solution for a problem can be frustrating for both you and the mother. Acknowledge this frustration with the mother, and offer her your support and encouragement as you continue to work through the problem together.

Step 5: Develop a Plan

Throughout the problem-solving process, ideally you and the mother will function as a cohesive team to come up with workable alternatives. "Workable" means that the options fit the mother's situation and are specific to her problem. When you tell her *why* something is true, the mother will be better able to work out her plan of how to take action.

The way a mother responds to your facts and suggestions will give you important clues as to whether she feels they will help her. If she likes a suggestion and adapts it to her situation, you can be certain that she is likely to try it. If she seems noncommittal or replies with "Yes, but . . . ," she may be telling you that she does not believe that your suggestion will address her problem adequately. Gathering further information will continue to define the problem and possible solutions more clearly.

After you and the mother have discussed the possible actions to take, you can develop a plan together. Document any plan that you and the mother decide on. When you talk to her again, you can say, "Let's see, we talked about . . ." or "You were going to try. . . ." This recollection will show her that you are actively concerned about helping her and will help you keep the situation clear in your mind. (Appendix C presents the Standards of Practice for lactation consultants.)

To eliminate confusion and learn whether a particular action was helpful, it is best to develop a plan with only two or three actions for the mother. Asking her to summarize the plan will help you determine that she understands what you discussed. Be sure to follow up with her to learn if your plan worked. If it did not work, you can consider further suggestions.

Part of developing a plan is setting a time limit on the actions the mother will take and arranging for follow-up. Be sure to settle this arrangement with the mother: "So, you will try . . . for 2 days and will call me on Thursday afternoon to let me know how it worked. In the meantime, please call me if it gets worse or if something else develops." Make sure the mother knows she can contact you if she has further concerns.

⌒ *Consultation Methods*

It is important to recognize situations that require an in-person visit for assessment and advice and to distinguish them from those situations that lend themselves to a telephone contact. Today, many breastfeeding contacts occur over the telephone or via e-mail. Indeed, telephone counseling or e-mail contact is sufficient for a good deal of follow-up that occurs after hospital discharge or subsequent to a clinic or office visit.

It is important to establish parameters when using telephone or electronic communication. A lactation consultant's provision of telephone or e-mail services carries with it an implied contract to respond in a timely manner. Make sure the mother knows how soon she can expect to hear back from you. Establish with the mother the types of issues that are appropriate over the telephone or e-mail, and set limits for when a concern indicates a need to see her in person (Thomas & Shaikh, 2007). It is impor-

tant to keep a log of all such communication you have with mothers.

Circumstances frequently require that you see the mother and baby together. If such a situation occurs after hospital discharge, you may need to see the mother in her home or in your office. As mentioned earlier, hospital staff members have limited time to prepare mothers to care for their babies at home. As a consequence, many mothers will benefit from a visit following discharge to ensure that breastfeeding is getting off to a good start. In addition, counseling is easier, more personal, and much more pleasant when you and the mother can see each other face-to-face.

Telephone Counseling

Many breastfeeding contacts concern parenting issues that do not require a clinical assessment. If a mother voices concern that her baby is fussy or fails to sleep through the night, for instance, you can review her breastfeeding practices to determine if she is feeding frequently enough. If she describes engorgement, you can discuss adjustments in her breastfeeding routine. She may have questions about expressing her milk and returning to work or school. These issues generally do not require that you see the mother and baby in person to provide appropriate assistance.

Support for breastfeeding mothers after they leave the hospital is often inadequate in low-income, inner-city areas where few resources are available. A breastfeeding telephone support line can overcome this potential obstacle to continuing breastfeeding (Chamberlain et al., 2005). Telephone support, for example, increases exclusive breastfeeding among women who experience problems after hospital discharge (Coffield, 2008). Providing a telephone hotline in languages specific to the local client population can also increase the rate of breastfeeding exclusivity (Janssen et al., 2009).

Be aware of your telephone manner whenever you rely on a telephone contact to assist a mother. During face-to-face contacts, body language is a great determinant of how the mother will receive your message. In the absence of any visual cues such as body language, however, you must rely on your tone of voice and your spoken words to relay a message that will be most effective and helpful for the mother. A smile and soothing voice tone will convey warmth and sincerity and enhance the exchange.

Electronic Counseling

Computer-based communication is another form of assistance that often takes the place of face-to-face contact. Many women seek breastfeeding help on the Internet through health-related websites and online networking groups. Breastfeeding support groups and lactation consultants also take advantage of e-mail to communicate with mothers. Electronic communication potentially provides additional opportunities for caregivers to inform, reassure, encourage, and support breastfeeding families (Thomas & Shaikh, 2007). Of course, there is wide variability in the extent of information provided, usability of websites, and compliance with standards of medical Internet publishing (Shaikh & Scott, 2005). As a consequence, mothers need to be discriminating in the advice they find on these sites.

Patients are rightfully concerned about electronic health records' potential to result in breached privacy and misuse of health data (Simon et al., 2009). Loss and theft of private health information is a growing concern, especially with the widespread use of laptops and portable storage devices. Inform clients of privacy issues and include a disclaimer at the bottom of any electronic transmissions. Figure 6.3 shows some examples of such e-mail disclaimers.

Keep copies of all e-mail correspondence to and from mothers, just as you would paper documentation. Use of a Web-based server, such as Yahoo, Gmail, or Hotmail, keeps the e-mail on the server, which protects you against losing these messages in the event of a hard disk crash on your computer. If you download e-mails from your server to your hard drive, it is important to make backup copies on a flash drive or other storage device to protect the data over the long term. Guard your data securely and be diligent about client information storage (McEvoy & Svalastoga, 2009). See Chapter 26 for a discussion of patient/client confidentiality and privacy issues. Appendix A presents the Code of Ethics for the lactation consultant profession.

NOTE: The information contained in this document may be confidential. If you have received this information in error, please contact me at [put your contact information here]

NOTE: The information contained in this facsimile [or electronic mail] may be privileged and confidential and protected from disclosure. If the reader of this message is not the intended recipient, or an employee or agent responsible for delivering this message to the intended recipient, you are hereby notified that any dissemination, distribution, or copying of this communication is strictly prohibited. If you have received this communication in error, please notify the sender immediately at [put your contact information here].

FIGURE 6.3 E-mail disclaimers.

In-Person Visits

Many situations indicate a need to see a mother in person. Anytime you question whether you have sufficient insights into a mother's circumstances through phone or e-mail contact, inform her that you need to see her. You need to see the mother whenever you feel uneasy about a situation or unable to obtain sufficient insight during telephone or electronic communication. If a mother seems to be shy or has difficulty expressing her concerns by phone or e-mail, face-to-face interaction may be necessary. Clinical issues concerning the mother or the baby often require that you see them. Before the appointment, make sure the mother fully understands any fees associated with an in-person consultation.

If a mother reports sore nipples, or difficulties that imply latch problems or incorrect positioning, you will need to assess her breasts and observe a breastfeeding to gain sufficient insight into the problem. Likewise, severe engorgement will require a visit to gain further insight into the cause and treatment. Whenever a concern arises about poor infant weight gain, you will need to examine the baby, observe a feeding, and assess milk transfer. For your legal protection, as well as for the baby's safety, it is advisable to insist on a consultation or refer the mother to her physician for any poor or slow weight gain.

A mother who is using a breast pump of any type will need to learn how to operate the pump and receive help the first time she uses it. If the need for the pump stems from a problem with the baby or with getting breastfeeding established, the mother may need help in dealing with the situation. Thus mothers should acquire breast pumps from a person experienced in caring for breastfeeding mothers whenever possible, rather than from a pharmacy or other business that does not provide assistance and ongoing support.

∼ Elements in a Consultation

Consultations may take place in a variety of settings, including hospitals, clinics, caregiver offices, and mothers' homes. Begin the consultation by introducing yourself and using the mother's name—steps that will establish a personal tone for your exchange. Be aware of your body language, and focus on establishing eye contact and assuming a facial expression and posture that transmits an interest to engage with the mother in a meaningful way. Use of your guiding skills will help you gather information as you take a history and assess the mother and baby. Continue to use these guiding skills as you integrate them with problem solving in the logical flow of the consultation.

A study at the Vancouver Breastfeeding Centre in British Columbia illustrates a good model for the consultation process (Ellis et al., 1993). The Vancouver model progresses through a five-step process of assessment, analysis, diagnosis, care, and counsel. The assessment includes recording the mother's reason for the visit, a maternal and infant history, physical assessments of both the mother and the infant, and any additional problems the mother reveals during the visit. The mother then initiates breastfeeding with no intervention by the helper to provide baseline data. Impressions gained through observing the feeding, the physical assessment, and information obtained from the mother enable the helper to analyze the situation and factors that contributed to the difficulty. The helper then makes a diagnosis that provides direction for the appropriate care and counsel for the mother. The mother participates in developing a plan of care and returns for a follow-up visit to evaluate its effectiveness. When necessary, the helper adjusts the plan of care to address continuing concerns.

Obtaining Consent

In your helping role with mothers, many elements of your consultation will involve interactions that require the mother's consent, whether explicit or implied. Consent should encompass any areas in which you will work with the mother and the infant during the current and subsequent visits. This includes examining the mother's breasts, examining her baby and her baby's oral structure and sucking, and assisting with a breastfeeding. Consent considerations include the use of equipment and techniques that may be necessary to ensure an adequate caloric intake for the infant and to improve breastfeeding. Include a statement on the consent form that allows you to release information to the insurance carrier, to send reports to the mother's and infant's primary caregivers, and to consult with those caregivers regarding the pair's care. If you wish to use information obtained from the consultation for educational purposes, including photographs, include this consideration on the consent form as well. If mothers pay you directly for the consultation, consent should cover the receipt of payment as well as the rental or sale of any breastfeeding equipment.

It is good practice to obtain a signed consent form before initiating a consultation. If you practice in a hospital or a medical group where a consent form for all care provided within that setting has been signed, you may be covered by that general consent. It is wise to clarify this issue with your employer in such a work setting. A signed consent form protects the lactation consultant, and it is unwise to engage in a consultation without it. If a mother refuses to sign a consent form or crosses out significant parts, such as the sections allowing you to communicate with her or her baby's primary caregiver, you should not continue with the consultation. See Chapter 26 for further discussion regarding informed consent.

Health Insurance Portability and Accountability Act

In 1996, the U.S. Department of Health and Human Services instituted the Health Insurance Portability and Accountability Act (HIPAA). Healthcare practitioners are required to have signed HIPAA consent forms for all their patients. HIPAA provides federal protections that safeguard the privacy of health information and prohibits use or disclosure of such information unless authorized by the patient.

The legislation does recognize that certain incidental uses and disclosures may occur as a by-product of healthcare delivery, such as a third party overhearing the exchange. You can avoid such incidental disclosures by speaking quietly and avoiding the use of patients' names in public areas.

Locked file cabinets and computer passwords provide additional safeguards. If patients have participated in research, you can ensure their privacy and confidentiality by protecting identifiers from improper use and by destroying them at the earliest opportunity.

HIPAA does permit disclosure of patient's healthcare information without authorization, to public health authorities legally authorized to receive such reports for the purpose of preventing or controlling disease, injury, or disability, as in suspected child neglect or abuse.

Taking a History

When taking a history of the mother and baby, you will need to document exactly what the mother says and obtain an appropriate history relevant to the situation. The history needs to include all information relevant to the health of the mother and infant, both past and present, including significant illnesses, disorders, and surgeries. Using a standard history form or developing your own will help to ensure that you remember to ask all essential questions.

Skills in History Taking

Guiding skills will help you gather information and impressions while you record pertinent information on the history form. Of course, simply diving into a checklist of questions from your form will do little to put the mother at ease. Instead, use open-ended questions, active listening, and other guiding skills to validate her feelings and increase her comfort. Elicit the mother's story by asking her to describe how breastfeeding is going and which concerns or questions she has. Phrase open-ended questions so that they are directed toward any issues that need to be addressed. Encourage the mother to talk with your use of silence, as well as both verbal and nonverbal cues. Remember to listen to both what she says and how she says it. Be alert to her body language and take note of what she may not be saying.

You can help to focus the discussion by paraphrasing and summarizing the topics. If the mother has a problem, ask how she perceives it and when it began. Continue to provide feedback and give emotional support to the mother throughout the history taking. Build on the information the mother provides to flesh out any areas of the story you don't fully understand. Be as specific as possible and try to record what the mother says accurately, without interpretation (Rathe, 2000).

Items to Include in a History

Record any history of previous lactation and breastfeeding, as well as details about the current breastfeeding situation. Note any past or current medications taken by the mother and the baby. Be aware that people consume or use substances they do not recognize as "medications." For example, many mothers do not consider hormonal contraception to be of significance. Hormonal contraception includes birth control pills, depot drugs such as medroxyprogesterone acetate (Depo-Provera), and estrogen-emitting intrauterine devices, all of which can reduce a woman's milk production (see Chapter 19 for more discussion of contraception). Because mothers may not think of naming herbs, vitamins, or food supplements as medications, you may want to ask about these items individually. In addition, a mother may have been taking insulin or thyroid medication for most of her life and does not think to mention it. It is also important to ask about the mother's diet, including the amount and type of fluids consumed daily.

Question the mother about any previous surgeries, accidents, hospitalizations, or disorders. If you notice any scarring, ask her to clarify what caused it. A mother may not think to mention having a laparoscopic procedure, for instance. Tactful inquiries could lead to her mentioning that she had gallbladder removal or bariatric (gastric bypass) surgery. Other laparoscopic procedures may include treatment for ovarian cysts or other gynecological problems. Sufficient information gathering and active listening will help you identify any relevant information.

Explore issues related to the present situation by using open-ended questions and other guiding skills to gather as much information as possible. Be careful to word questions in such a way that will elicit the information you need. For example, you might ask, "How many times does your baby nurse in 24 hours?" rather than "How frequently does your baby nurse?" Try to *quantify* whenever possible (e.g., pain on a scale of 1 to 10 instead of "it hurts," number of days instead of "a while," number of hours rather than "all the time").

Include inquiries about the baby's feeding and growth patterns in the history taking, as well as a review of his or her sleeping, crying, and ability to socialize. Also record the infant's pattern of stools and voids and obtain an estimate of the amounts in the past 24-hour period. Ask the mother if there has been any change in this pattern and, if so, when the change occurred. Learn what the mother has tried and the results of her efforts.

If you choose to omit an item on your history form, inserting "NA" (not applicable) in the space will indicate that it is not pertinent to this specific mother and baby. Leaving a question blank could imply that you forgot to address that particular issue. Always think, "How would the court system view this entry?" and chart accordingly.

Institutional Settings

History taking for the lactation consultant practicing within a hospital or medical group may not require as much detail as that for a lactation consultant in private practice. However, The Joint Commission, previously called the Joint Commission on Accreditation of Healthcare Organizations (JCAHO), has established stringent guidelines for charting, including acceptable and non-acceptable abbreviations and acronyms (The Joint Commission, 2009; Kuhn, 2007). Your specific hospital, clinic, or practice should also have guidelines on charting. It is best practice to not use abbreviations unless they are understood by everyone who might refer to the records.

The medical charts kept for the mother and baby in a hospital, clinic, or physician practice will include much of the information you need for a lactation consultation. These data include the mother's medications and pregnancy complications and the baby's gestational age and types and amounts of feedings. Reading their charts before the consultation will familiarize you with the mother's and baby's histories. Any information relevant to lactation that is not already included on the charts can be noted in the appropriate place on the mother's and baby's charts after the consultation.

Performing an Assessment

If you practice in a hospital, staff will have assessed the baby prior to your consultation. Review that information, particularly the baby's daily weight status, intake, and output. In a private practice setting, you will need to perform a more detailed assessment that includes the baby's weight. In either setting, you will want to look for signs of the baby's hydration, caloric status, and general health, as well as the number of wet diapers and stools. (Chapter 13 discusses infant assessment in more detail.) Visual assessment of the mother's breasts and nipples will provide information for potential problem solving. If you need to physically examine the mother's anatomy, it is good practice to ask permission before initiating physical contact. Ask, "May I examine your breasts now?" Likewise, asking permission before examining her baby helps give the mother some control in the consultation process.

The assessment will usually include evaluating the mother and baby breastfeeding. If poor weight gain is the purpose for the consultation, you may need a full feeding assessment with pre-feeding and post-feeding weights (see the discussion in Chapter 18). Ensure the mother's privacy and help her move into a comfortable position to nurse her baby. Ask her to put her baby to her breast and allow her to demonstrate her technique without your intervention. Explain that you would like to observe what her baby does during the feeding. This focuses the assessment on the baby rather than on the mother, which is less threatening and intimidating to the mother and avoids the impression that you are judging her. Flexibility is fundamental to assessing a feeding, as you must be willing to move at the baby's pace.

Allow the feeding to proceed without any suggestions or interventions on your part until you have a clear picture of what is going on. If you perceive a problem, it is then appropriate to suggest to the mother some alternative methods or interventions. While you observe the feeding, you have an opportunity to visit with the mother and gain further impressions. You can incorporate the insights you gain into the plan of care you develop with the mother.

Use guiding skills to uncover details of the mother's economic and employment status, as well as her support network, cultural beliefs, and practices. Ask what her goals are for breastfeeding and what she has done to prepare for nursing her baby. Observe the interactions between mother and baby as well as the dynamics of the feeding process. Note the baby's and mother's temperaments, behavior, and emotional status. Observe the mother's and baby's positioning. Evaluate the baby's latch and be alert to evidence of milk transfer. Note the appearance and condition of the mother's breasts and nipples at the end of the feeding.

Once the physical and feeding assessments are complete, you will probably have developed a clearer idea of whether a problem exists and, if so, what the nature of the problem is. You can then begin to think about the overall goals for the mother and baby. If the mother has sore nipples, for example, the baby may not be receiving sufficient calories because the mother cannot nurse comfortably. Your overall goals will be to decrease the mother's pain while providing sufficient calories to the baby. From these general goals, you can develop a specific plan of care detailing the steps necessary to achieve the final goals of the mother nursing without pain and the baby nursing effectively and adequately.

Developing a Plan of Care

After you have clarified the mother's situation, you will be prepared to take a more directive role in the consultation. Based on the identified problem, you next want to determine what the mother needs to know. You cannot enter into a consultation with a prescribed agenda. What this particular mother needs relative to the problem may be different from what another mother with the same problem needs.

In developing a plan of care, begin with any essentials, such as a feeding plan for the baby, pain relief, and means of maintaining or increasing milk production. Help the mother understand what produced her situation and how she can avoid its recurrence. Brainstorm with her about some of the available options. Be mindful of the mother's reactions to your suggestions. Although you may sense what would be most effective for this particular situation, the mother must be able and willing to follow your suggestions. For example, you suggest cup feeding as a way to provide sufficient calories to the baby while allowing the mother's nipples to heal. If the mother does not embrace the idea of cup feeding, however, you will need to offer an alternative solution that she will find more acceptable. Your role is to provide choices and encourage the mother to decide what will work for her.

After you and the mother have decided on a plan, ask her to repeat the suggestions that she accepted, reviewing them as necessary. After she has recounted the plan, you can summarize it with her to avoid any confusion. If the baby's father is present for the consultation, be sure to include him in the discussion while developing the plan of care. Remember that your goal is to empower the parents and to increase their self-confidence and self-reliance. At the end of every consultation, ask yourself if you have accomplished this goal.

Mothers should receive instructions at hospital discharge that will help facilitate breastfeeding at home. For the mother and baby who are breastfeeding well upon discharge, a diary of the baby's feedings, voids, and stools, along with instructions regarding what is normal and where to get help, should suffice. Documentation for a problem-oriented consultation should include a written care plan based on the assessment of the mother's and infant's needs. A variety of care plans and other forms are readily available, so you do not have to develop your own unless you wish to. Having a standard form will help you remember to include all essential information.

Providing Follow-up

Before you end a consultation, discuss which kinds of support may be available from the mother's family and friends. Refer her to a community support group, especially if you sense that she will benefit from the emotional support and networking the group offers. Provide the mother with a written plan of care and, when appropriate, other materials, Internet/media resources, and breastfeeding devices. Mothers tend not to remember much of the discussion from these consultations, so they need written information for later reference.

As discussed in Chapter 5, follow-up is important to a mother's breastfeeding outcome. Depending on the situation, this follow-up may consist of another visit in the next day or so, or perhaps in a week or more. If it is a self-limiting situation, following up by phone or e-mail may be sufficient. The mother who sees you in preparation for her return to work, for example, may not require follow-up and could be asked to call with any concerns or questions. If you have arranged for the mother to call you and she does not call, you can try to contact her several times. Document each call and record whether you left a message on an answering machine or with a family member. If follow-up is critical, such as in the case of an infant who is failing to thrive, it would be wise to notify the baby's healthcare provider that the mother has not followed up as requested.

Writing Follow-up Reports

As a part of the mother's healthcare team, you will need to communicate regularly with other members of the team. These individuals usually include both the mother's caregiver (obstetrician, family practitioner, or midwife) and the baby's pediatrician or family practitioner. Regular communication is especially important if you work as an independent, community-based lactation consultant and do not have daily contact with other members of the mother's and baby's healthcare team. It is good practice to send reports to caregivers for both the mother and the baby. If you have immediate concerns, you may want to contact the caregiver directly to discuss them.

It is good practice to establish a routine of following up with documentation after every consultation. Send a physician report to all appropriate primary care or referring physicians within 24 hours of seeing a client. You may also want to send a brief report if you rent a breast pump, sell breast shells, or help a mother by phone or e-mail. Use all opportunities to inform other members of the healthcare team about your services. When you educate them through such reports, they will be more likely to provide continuity of care and refer patients to you.

Creating the physician report using computer software can ensure that your documentation has a professional appearance and provides you with a permanent record. Always use the spell-check feature on your computer and proofread the document carefully. A medical dictionary will aid you in this process and can be accessed online. Most caregivers take advantage of the timeliness, convenience, and cost savings of electronic communication by faxing or e-mailing reports rather than mailing them. Remember to include privacy notices on any report cover or e-mail to protect your client's confidentiality. Using the same format in your physician report as you do in your assessment forms will help you remember to include important elements. In addition, include contact information such as your name, credentials, address, telephone number, fax number, and e-mail address. Figure 6.4 identifies the elements that need to be included in a physician report. Table 6.2 demonstrates the steps in a counseling scenario.

1. Date the patient was seen.
2. Names and addresses of mother's physician and baby's physician.
3. Regarding: Mother's and baby's names and baby's date of birth.
4. Dear Dr. . . . ,
5. Patient was seen at your request, was self-referred, was referred by (include name if possible).
6. If you called the physician's office to give a verbal report or faxed in a short report, you can mention this in your letter.
7. Because of . . . (reason for referral).
8. Brief description of the mother's history (general health, conception, pregnancy, and birth).
9. Assessment of the mother's breasts and nipples.
10. Brief description of the baby's history (birth, Apgar scores, in-hospital feeding, current feedings, output, weights, behavior, etc.).
11. Assessment and present status of the baby (muscle tone, activity, skin turgor, oral cavity, behavior, weight, and so on).
12. Assessment of the feeding (include feeding weights, if possible).
13. Your assessment of the situation.
14. Suggestions you made to the mother and the action plan that was developed.
15. Arrangements for follow-up with the mother.
16. If the patient was referred to you, thank the physician for allowing you to participate in the care of her/his patient. If the patient self-referred, you may comment about working with the physician with this couple ("It was a pleasure . . .").
17. Sincerely yours, . . . (use all your credentials behind your name).

FIGURE 6.4 Elements of a physician report.

Evaluating the Consultation

An essential element of any consultation is an evaluation of the plan of care you and the mother established. As the situation changes, the plan of care may also need to change. If this plan does not bring about resolution of a problem, the situation may be more complicated than you first thought and may require another complete assessment. Determine whether the mother is adhering to the plan of care. Perhaps she was overwhelmed by too many suggestions or she was unable or unwilling to follow through with the plan. Sometimes family members may interfere with her attempts to adhere to the plan. Evaluate whether your approach was too rigid and determine whether other alternatives might work better. Remaining flexible, attending breastfeeding conferences, networking with colleagues, and reading current literature will help you offer the mother a variety of options. Following up with the mother will provide insights into the effectiveness of your consultation.

Critically assess your counseling skills to determine whether you are meeting the needs of mothers. Figure 6.5 identifies a series of questions asked of dieticians. It provides a useful model for crafting similar questions within your work setting (Isselman et al., 1993), and the responses indicate the quality of the consultation. The questions in Figure 6.6 combine the use of counseling skills with elements of a consultation to help you assess your effectiveness with mothers. Both sets of responses can be rated on a scale ranging from "strongly agree" to "strongly disagree."

∿ Documenting a Feeding

Use of a standard form for documenting feedings will help you remember to evaluate all essential elements of the breastfeeding process. It is recommended that some-

one knowledgeable in breastfeeding management observe and document at least one breastfeeding in each 8-hour period during the immediate postpartum period (International Lactation Consultant Association [ILCA], 2005). If you expect staff in a hospital setting to provide complete and useful information about every mother and infant, then you must use a method that is simple and does not seem daunting or time-consuming. In the hospital, you can also teach the mother to chart much of her own breastfeeding information. Giving her this responsibility is a step to her becoming self-sufficient and self-assured in her breastfeeding.

There are many methods for charting your assessment of mothers and babies during feedings. Whatever method you employ, avoid using terms such as "good," "fair," or "poor" to evaluate a feeding. When used alone, these terms give very little information about the mother's and baby's progress to another person who reviews the chart. Likewise, simply recording the duration of a feeding gives no indication of its quality. The remainder of this section describes various types of documentation; one of them will likely work for you.

Many hospitals use standard breastfeeding scoring forms, such as the ones described in this chapter. The use

TABLE 6.2   Main Parts of a Consultation

Situation: Nancy, the mother of a 2-week-old infant, says to you, "My son Justin just had his 2-week checkup. His doctor is concerned because his weight is still just under his birth weight. He thinks I may need to supplement with formula and I am so upset. I wanted to breastfeed exclusively and now I don't know what to do."

• Statement that shows emotional support	"You're upset because your pediatrician recommended that you supplement with formula."
• Consent	Ask Nancy to sign and date a consent form before proceeding with the consultation.
• Gather information through maternal–infant history and assessment	How often is Justin breastfeeding in 24 hours? Does he breastfeed during the day and night? What are his feeding cues to which Nancy responds? Does he swallow audibly during the feedings? Who ends the feedings? How does Justin react during and after feedings? How many voids and stools does he have in 24 hours? What does Nancy already know about breastfeeding? Did Justin's physician prescribe supplements now, or is that a future possibility if more immediate breastfeeding measures do not help Justin's weight gain? How is Justin's general appearance and hydration status? What is his present weight, birth weight, and hospital discharge weight? How are Nancy's breasts and nipples? What intake amounts do pre-and post-feed weights show? How are latch, position, and milk transfer? Your hunch: Nancy is unfamiliar with normal feeding cues, and therefore, Justin is not breastfeeding frequently enough for adequate milk intake and weight gain.
• Develop a workable plan with the mother	Be sure Justin is nursing 10 or more times in 24 hours around the clock. Teach Nancy feeding cues and baby-led feeding. Instruct her to watch and listen for audible swallows at feedings. Teach her how to do breast compression to enhance milk transfer. Help Nancy identify sources of support and household help through this time.
• Follow-up	Call the next day to evaluate how the changes in Nancy's breastfeeding routine are going. See Nancy and Justin for a weight check in 2 days.
• Physician's report	If Nancy is unsure about the physician's exact request regarding supplements, a call to the physician's office may be warranted to clarify that issue. A report outlining the plan of care should be sent within 24 hours.

1. My confidence in my counseling skills has increased over the past 6 months.
2. I have identified the counseling style in which I am most comfortable and effective.
3. I am able to adapt my counseling style to meet the needs of the patient.
4. I am now using more attending and listening skills in my counseling sessions.
5. I am now able to recognize when a patient is not attending or listening during the counseling process.
6. I am better able to acknowledge my feelings that arise during the counseling process.
7. I am better able to acknowledge the feelings of my patients during the counseling process.
8. I have altered the way I conduct the counseling session based on the recognition of my own or my patient's feelings.
9. I evaluate the counseling environment before beginning the counseling session.
10. I take steps to correct the environment before beginning the counseling session.
11. I have requested that management make changes in my work site counseling environment that will enhance the counseling process.
12. I need further instruction, encouragement, or evaluation to enhance my counseling skills.

FIGURE 6.5 Questions to measure the quality of a consultation.

of such forms is usually included in a hospital's policies and procedures. In this situation, if you wish to make any changes to a form, you will need to work with your unit's management and have any changes approved for use, usually by a forms committee.

Breastfeed Observation Aid

Figure 6.7 shows a form printed by the United Nations Children's Fund (UNICEF) and the World Health Organization (WHO) in their manual for training maternity staff throughout the world (UNICEF/WHO, 2009). The main categories to evaluate are observing the mother and baby, the breasts, the baby's position and attachment, and suckling. After having observed a complete breastfeeding, the clinician checks off (in the left column) the signs that breastfeeding is going well. The right column identifies signs of possible difficulty. Hospitals may find this method convenient for helping staff members recognize when a mother and baby need help. The intent of the checklist is for the elements to become ingrained in the clinician's memory so that noting the essential points when observing breastfeeding becomes second nature.

1. Understanding of the problem: LC understood the mother and helped her.
2. Breastfeeding information: Information was correct and appropriate. Not too much or too little.
3. Clarity of instructions: The mother understood the information and advice.
4. Good counseling skills: LC put mom at ease, encouraged her to share feelings.
5. Partnership with mother: Mother was drawn into the problem-solving process.
6. Encouraged mother's self-reliance: LC fostered greater self-assurance in mother.
7. Balance: LC achieved balance between listening, educating, and problem solving with no lecturing.
8. Arrangements for follow-up: LC made it clear when any further contact will take place and who will initiate it.
9. Overall impressions of mother's satisfaction with consultation.

FIGURE 6.6 Questions to evaluate counseling skills in a consultation.

Charting with Breastfeeding Descriptors

Table 6.3 outlines a documentation method that uses descriptors reflecting the level of achievement by the mother and baby (Barger & Kutner, 2009). When this method is used to document breastfeeding, it is important that all staff understand the definitions for the abbreviations. Each rating gives very specific information about the quality of the breastfeeding and is much more helpful than a vague term such as "good feed," where there is no definition of what a "good feed" entails. Use of these simple acronyms may be an attractive option for use by hospital staff in documenting effectiveness of feedings in the mother's hospital records.

The LATCH Method

Figure 6.8 shows the LATCH charting system (Jensen et al., 1994). Each letter of the acronym LATCH represents the scored item:

- Latch
- Audible swallowing
- Type of nipple
- Comfort (breast and nipple)
- Hold (positioning)

LATCH assesses the infant's ability to latch on to the breast and evaluates audible swallowing as a determinant of milk intake. Type of nipple indicates the shape, size, and texture of the nipple as an important factor in the baby's ability to latch. Comfort of the breasts and nipples

BREASTFEED OBSERVATION AID

Mother's name _____ Date _____

Baby's name _____ Baby's age _____

Signs that breastfeeding is going well: **Signs of possible difficulty:**

GENERAL

Mother: *Mother:*

☐ Mother looks healthy   ☐ Mother looks ill or depressed

☐ Mother relaxed and comfortable   ☐ Mother looks tense and uncomfortable

☐ Signs of bonding between mother and baby   ☐ No mother/baby eye contact

Baby: *Baby:*

☐ Baby looks healthy   ☐ Baby looks sleepy or ill

☐ Baby calm and relaxed   ☐ Baby is restless or crying

☐ Baby reaches or roots for breast if hungry   ☐ Baby does not reach or root

BREASTS

☐ Breasts look healthy   ☐ Breasts look red, swollen, or sore

☐ No pain or discomfort   ☐ Breast or nipple painful

☐ Breast well supported with fingers away from nipple ☐ Breasts held with fingers on areola

☐ Nipples protractile   ☐ Nipples flat, not protractile

BABY'S POSITION

☐ Baby's head and body in line   ☐ Baby's neck and head twisted to feed

☐ Baby held close to mother's body   ☐ Baby not held close

☐ Baby's whole body supported   ☐ Baby supported by head and neck only

☐ Baby approaches breast, nose to nipple   ☐ Baby approaches breast, lower lip/chin to nipple

BABY'S ATTACHMENT

☐ More areola seen above baby's top lip   ☐ More areola seen below bottom lip

☐ Baby's mouth open wide   ☐ Baby's mouth not open wide

☐ Lower lip turned outwards   ☐ Lips pointing forward or turned in

☐ Baby's chin touches breast   ☐ Baby's chin not touching breast

SUCKLING

☐ Slow, deep sucks with pauses   ☐ Rapid shallow sucks

☐ Cheeks round when suckling   ☐ Cheeks pulled in when suckling

☐ Baby releases breast when finished   ☐ Mother takes baby off the breast

☐ Mother notices signs of oxytocin reflex   ☐ No signs of oxytocin reflex noticed

FIGURE 6.7   UNICEF Breastfeed Observation Form.

Source: UNICEF/WHO Breastfeeding Promotion and Support in a Baby-Friendly Hospital: 20-Hour Course. 2009. www.unicef.org/nutrition/files/BFHI_2009_s3.slides.pdf. Reprinted by permission of the World Health Organization.

TABLE 6.3   Breastfeeding Descriptors for Documenting a Feeding

You may chart two types of feedings in one session. For example, a mother and baby may need considerable assistance with attachment. After the latch is achieved, the baby demonstrates nutritive sucking with audible swallows. This would be charted as *FBF → GBF*. Another example: You observe a baby that has some difficulty latching and the mom is poorly positioned. After offering assistance, the mother and baby overcome the obstacles and have an excellent feeding with lots of swallows. This would be charted as *Initial → PBF after assistance EBF*. Any rating below Excellent Breastfeed or Good Breastfeed will require further documentation that describes the problem and any help that is given.

Descriptor	Meaning	Elements observed
EBF	• Excellent breastfeed Note: It would be unusual to see an excellent breastfeed in the first 24 to 48 hours of life.	• Baby can latch on without difficulty • Sucks are nice and deep with a nice steady rhythm • Pauses are brief, and baby quickly resumes sucking again • Can hear baby swallowing frequently, sometimes with each suck • Mother does not need assistance positioning the baby or latching him on • No nipple discomfort
GBF	• Good breastfeed	• Baby can latch on without any difficulty • Sucks are nice and deep with a nice steady rhythm • Pauses are brief, and baby resumes sucking again without being moved or prodded • Some swallowing is hard • Mother requires a little help with positioning or latch-on • No nipple discomfort
FBF	• Fair breastfeed	• Baby is able to latch on to the breast and once on is able to stay on • Sucks are short and quick; only occasionally may there be a nice deep suck; no steady rhythm • Mother has to stroke or prod infant to resume sucking • An occasional swallow may be heard, but usually no swallowing is heard • Mother requires a lot of assistance with positioning and latch-on • Mother could be experiencing nipple discomfort
PBF	• Poor breastfeed	• Roots for the breast, licks the nipple • Latches on, but has difficulty doing it • Once latched-on he does not stay on the breast or if he does he does not suck • No swallowing is heard • Mother requires a lot of assistance with positioning and latch-on • Mother could have nipple discomfort or pain
ABF	• Attempted breastfeed	• Roots and licks at the nipple • Unable to latch on to the nipple • Mother requires a great deal of assistance
0BF	• No breastfeed	• No effort at the breast (too sleepy, lethargic, no interest) • Pushes away from the breast, fights or cries, or both • Despite lots of assistance, unable to accomplish a feed

Source: Jan Barger and Linda Kutner, Lactation Educational Consultants. Reprinted with permission.

	0	**1**	**2**
L Latch	Too sleepy or reluctant No sustained latch or suck achieved	Repeated attempts for sustained latch or suck Hold nipple in mouth Stimulate to suck	Grasps breast Tongue down Lips flanged Rhythmical sucking
A Audible swallowing	None	A few with stimulation	Spontaneous and intermittent <24 hours old Spontaneous and frequent >24 hours old
T Type of nipple	Inverted	Flat	Everted (after stimulation)
C Comfort (Breast/nipple)	Engorged Cracked, bleeding, large blisters, or bruises Severe discomfort	Filling Reddened/small blisters or bruises Mild/moderate discomfort	Soft Nontender
H Hold (positioning)	Full assist (staff hold infant at breast)	Minimal assist (i.e., elevate head of bed; place pillows for support) Teach one side; mother does other Staff holds and then mother takes over	No assist from staff Mother able to position and hold infant

FIGURE 6.8   LATCH method.

Source: Jenson D, Wallace S, Kelsay P. LATCH: a breastfeeding charting system and documentation tool. *JOGNN.* 1994;23(1):29. Reprinted with permission of John Wiley and Sons.

is an indicator of the possible need for adjustments in positioning or another aspect of breastfeeding care. Hold, the final component of the LATCH assessment, considers the breastfeeding position used by the mother and her ability to assume a comfortable position that enables her to achieve and maintain an effective latch.

The Mother–Baby Assessment Method

Figure 6.9 presents a tool modeled after the 10-point Apgar system. The Mother–Baby Assessment (Mulford, 1992) evaluates the progress of a mother and her baby as they learn to breastfeed. The five steps assessed are signaling, positioning, fixing, milk transfer, and ending. Signaling is the step in which the mother and baby reach agreement that a feeding will take place. Positioning refers to the placement of the mother's and baby's bodies in relation to each other. Fixing is the point at which the infant attaches to the breast and begins to suck. Milk transfer occurs when the baby's sucking releases milk and

the baby consumes the milk. The final step, ending, refers to the outcome of the feeding session. The caregiver evaluates the mother and infant on each of these steps, with 10 points being the highest possible score. The caregiver also documents any assistance the mother received.

The Infant Breastfeeding Assessment Tool

The Infant Breastfeeding Assessment Tool (IBFAT), shown in Figure 6.10, assesses the infant's behavior during a breastfeeding. A score of 0, 1, 2, or 3 is assigned to the level of stimulation required to coax the infant to the breast, the infant's rooting response, time lapsed from initiating the process until the infant latches, and the infant's sucking pattern. The mother also describes her baby's overall feeding behavior and the way she feels about the feeding. The total score for a feeding ranges from 0 to 12. The IBFAT instrument does not assess the mother's physical aspect of the feeding, nor does it specifically evaluate the baby's position and latch.

	M	B	HELP
Signaling	x	x	
Positioning	x	x	
Fixing	x		
Milk Transfer			
Ending			

Total Score 5 (With Help)

This is an assessment method for rating the progress of a mother and baby who are learning to breastfeed.

For every step, each person—both mother and baby—should receive an *x* before either one can be scored on the following step. If the observer does not observe any of the designated indicators, score 0 for that person on that step. If help is needed at any step for either the mother or the baby, check *Help* for that step. This notation will not change the total score for mother and baby.

1. SIGNALING

- Mother watches and listens for baby's cues. She may hold, stroke, rock, talk to baby. She stimulates baby if he is sleepy, calms baby if he is fussy.

- Baby gives readiness cues: stirring, alertness, rooting, sucking, hand-to-mouth, vocal cues, cry.

2. POSITIONING

- Mother holds baby in good alignment within latch-on range of nipple. Baby's body is slightly flexed, entire ventral surface facing mother's body. Baby's head and shoulders are supported.

- Baby roots well at breast, opens mouth wide, tongue cupped and covering lower gum.

3. FIXING

- Mother holds her breast to assist baby as needed, brings baby in close when his mouth is wide open. She may express drops of milk.

- Baby latches-on, takes all of nipple and about 2 cm (1 inch) of areola into mouth, then sucks, demonstrating recurrent burst–pause pattern.

4. MILK TRANSFER

- Mother reports feeling any of the following: thirst, uterine cramps, increased lochia, breast ache or tingling, relaxation, sleepiness. Milk leaks from opposite breast.

- Baby swallows audibly; milk is observed in baby's mouth; baby may spit up milk when burping. Rapid "call up sucking" rate (2 sucks/second) changes to "nutritive sucking" rate of about 1 suck/second.

5. ENDING

- Mother's breasts are comfortable; she lets baby suck until he is finished. After nursing, her breasts feel softer; she has no lumps, engorgement, or nipple soreness.

- Baby releases breast spontaneously, appears satiated. Baby does not root when stimulated. Baby's face, arms, and hands are relaxed; baby may fall asleep.

FIGURE 6.9 Mother–Baby Assessment (MBA) method.

Source: Mulford C. The mother–baby assessment (MBA): an "Apgar score" for breastfeeding. *J Hum Lact.* 1992;8:79-82. Copyright © 1992, International Lactation Consultant Association. Reprinted by permission of SAGE Publications.

Check the answer that best describes the baby's feeding behaviors at this feed.

1. When you picked baby up to feed was he/she

(a) deeply asleep (eyes closed, no observable movement except breathing)	(b) drowsy	(c) quiet and alert	(d) crying
____	____	____	____

2. In order to get the baby to begin this feed, did you or the nurse have to

(a) just place the baby on the breast as no effort was needed	(b) use mild stimulation such as unbundling, patting, or burping	(c) unbundle baby; sit baby back and forward; rub baby's body or limbs vigorously at the beginning and during the feeding	(d) baby could not be aroused
3	2	1	0
____	____	____	____

3. Rooting (definition: at touch of nipple to cheek, baby's head turns toward the nipple, the mouth opens, and baby attempts to fix mouth on the nipple). When the baby was placed beside the breast, he/she

(a) rooted effectively at once	(b) needed some coaxing, prompting, or encouragement to root	(c) rooted poorly even with coaxing	(d) did not try to root
3	2	1	0
____	____	____	____

4. How long from placing baby at the breast does it take for the baby to latch-on and start to suck?

(a) starts to feed at once (0–3 min)	(b) 3 to 10 minutes	(c) over 10 minutes	(d) did not feed
3	2	1	0
____	____	____	____

5. Which of the following phrases best describes the baby's feeding pattern at this feed?

(a) baby did not suck	(b) sucked poorly; weak sucking; some sucking efforts for short periods	(c) sucked fairly well; sucked off and on, but needed encouragement	(d) sucked well throughout on one or both breasts
0	1	2	3
____	____	____	____

6. How do you feel about the way the baby fed at this feeding?

(a) very pleased	(b) pleased	(c) fairly pleased	(d) not pleased
____	____	____	____

(Continued)

FIGURE 6.10 Infant Breastfeeding Assessment Tool (IBFAT) method.

Source: Matthews MK. Developing an instrument to assess infant breastfeeding behavior in the early neonatal period. Midwifery. 1988;4(4): 154-165. Reprinted with permission from Elsevier. http://sciencedirect.com/science/journal/02666138.

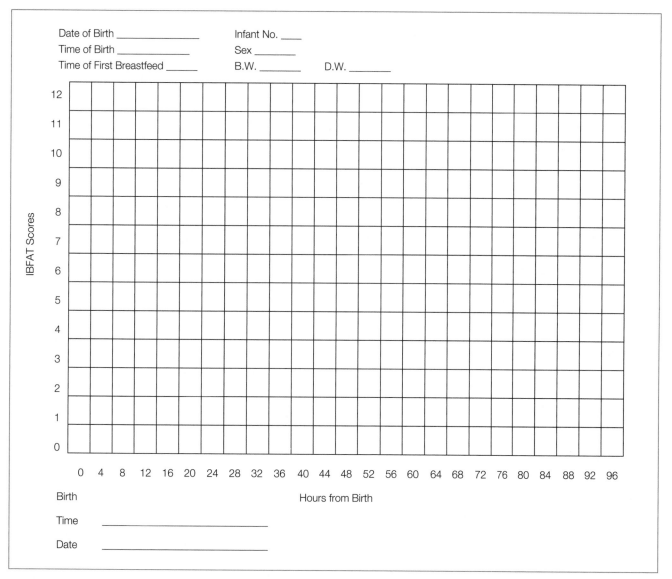

Date of Birth _____   Infant No. ____
Time of Birth _____   Sex _____
Time of First Breastfeed _____   B.W. _____   D.W. _____

FIGURE 6.10   Infant Breastfeeding Assessment Tool (IBFAT) method. *(Continued)*

Source: Matthews MK. Developing an instrument to assess infant breastfeeding behavior in the early neonatal period. *Midwifery*. 1988;4(4):154-165. Reprinted with permission from Elsevier. http://sciencedirect.com/science/journal/02666138.

∽ Summary

A preventive approach of anticipatory guidance helps parents achieve positive outcomes with breastfeeding and is ultimately a less time-consuming strategy for the healthcare staff. The most effective method of breastfeeding support focuses on early and continued contact so problems can be prevented or minimized. The nature of the situation determines whether it requires a face-to-face visit, or whether the issue can be handled through telephone or e-mail contact.

A breastfeeding consultation should begin with the caregiver establishing a receptive climate. After a supportive environment is in place and the mother has given her consent, the lactation consultant gathers information by taking the mother's and baby's histories, completing a physical assessment of both of them, and observing a feeding. The consultant then shares information, offers suggestions, and works with the mother to develop a care plan. Part of that plan will include follow-up to evaluate the mother's and baby's progress toward achieving her breastfeeding goals. Following the consultation, all necessary documentation is recorded appropriately, with a written report being submitted to the caregiver as indicated.

～ *Chapter 6—At a Glance*

Applying what you learned—

- Provide anticipatory guidance at times when retention will be high and decision making can occur.
- Encourage initial learning before delivery so postpartum teaching can focus on reinforcement.
- Provide a hotline, warmline, or e-mail access to ensure that mothers can contact you when necessary.
- Arrange for frequent contact with new mothers during the early weeks postpartum, either personally or through referral to a support group.
- Recognize when a problem requires an in-person consultation rather than telephone help.
- Check for hidden factors that may contribute to the problem before forming a hunch.
- Be open to new information that may lead you to form a new hunch, and explore alternative hunches until you and the mother define the problem.
- Obtain signed consent before initiating a consultation.
- Take a complete history of the mother and the baby.
- Assess the baby and the mother's breasts and nipples.
- Assess a breastfeeding, moving at the baby's pace and providing anticipatory guidance.
- Actively involve the mother in developing a plan of care.
- Give the mother a written plan of care and other necessary resources.
- Arrange appropriate follow-up and send reports to physicians for both the mother and the baby.
- Teach the mother to chart her breastfeeding information.
- Use documentation that provides sufficient information for evaluating the quality of the feeding.
- Assess your counseling skills for areas of improvement.

～ *References*

Alnasir F. Knowledge and attitude of secondary school-girls towards breast-feeding in Bahrain. *J Bahrain Med Soc.* 1992;4(1):6-10.

Angeletti MA. Breastfeeding mothers returning to work: possibilities for information, anticipatory guidance and support from us health care professionals. *J Hum Lact.* 2009;25(2): 226-232.

Arora S, et al. Major factors influencing breastfeeding rates: mother's perception of father's attitude and milk supply. *Pediatrics.* 2000;106:e67.

Barclay L. Nurse-administered anticipatory guidance may reduce ED visits for ear pain in toddlers. February 5, 2008. www.medscape.com/viewarticle/569720. Accessed March 12, 2009.

Barger J, Kutner L. *Certified Lactation Specialist Course.* Wheaton, IL: Lactation Education Consultants: 2009.

Chamberlain LB, et al. Calls to an inner-city hospital breastfeeding telephone support line. *J Hum Lact.* 2005;21(1):53-58.

Coffield K. The benefits of phone support and home visits: an evaluation of the City of Kingston's Breastfeeding Support Service. *Breastfeed Rev.* 2008;16(3):17-21.

Earle S. Factors affecting the initiation of breastfeeding: implications for breastfeeding promotion. *Health Promot Int.* 2002;17(3):205-214.

Ellis D, et al. Assisting the breastfeeding mother: a problem-solving process. *J Hum Lact.* 1993;9:89-93.

Finch C, Daniel E. Breastfeeding education program with incentives increases exclusive breastfeeding among urban WIC participants. *J Am Diet Assoc.* 2002;102(7):981-984.

Gill SL, et al. Effects of support on the initiation and duration of breastfeeding. *West J Nurs Res.* 2007;29(6):708-723.

Goulet C, et al. Attitudes and subjective norms of male and female adolescents toward breastfeeding. *J Hum Lact.* 2003;19(4):402-410.

Greenwood K, Littlejohn P. Breastfeeding intentions and outcomes of adolescent mothers in the Starting Out program: review. *Breastfeed Rev.* 2002;10(3):19-23.

Guise J, et al. The effectiveness of primary care-based interventions to promote breastfeeding: systematic evidence review and meta-analysis for the US Preventive Services Task Force. *Ann Fam Med.* 2003;1(2):70-78.

International Lactation Consultant Association (ILCA). *Clinical guidelines for the establishment of exclusive breastfeeding.* Morrisville, NC; ILCA; 2005.

Isselman M, et al. A nutrition counseling workshop: integrating counseling psychology into nutrition practice. *J Am Diet Assoc.* 1993;93:324-326.

Janssen PA, et al. Development and evaluation of a Chinese-language newborn feeding hotline: a prospective cohort study. *BMC Pregnancy Childbirth.* 2009;9(1):3.

Jensen D, et al. LATCH: a breastfeeding charting system and documentation tool. *JOGNN.* 1994;23:27-32.

The Joint Commission. The official "do not use" list of abbreviations. Updated March 5, 2009. www.jointcommission.org/PatientSafety/DoNotUseList/. Accessed August 1, 2009.

Kishore M, et al. Breastfeeding knowledge and practices amongst mothers in a rural population of North India: a community-based study. *J Trop Pediatr.* 2009;55(3):183-188.

Kuhn I. Abbreviations and acronyms in healthcare: when shorter isn't sweeter. *Pediatr Nurs.* 2007;33(5):392-398.

Martens P. The effect of breastfeeding education on adolescent beliefs and attitudes: a randomized school intervention in the Canadian Ojibwa community of Sagkeeng. *J Hum Lact.* 2001;17(3):245-255.

McEvoy F, Svalastoga E. Security of patient and study data associated with DICOM images when transferred using compact disc media. *J Digit Imaging.* 2009;22(1):65-70.

Mulford C. The mother–baby assessment (MBA): an Apgar score for breastfeeding. *J Hum Lact.* 1992;8:79-82.

Neifert M, et al. Factors influencing breastfeeding among adolescents. *J Adolesc Health Care.* 1988;9:470-473.

Nelson A. Adolescent attitudes, beliefs, and concerns regarding breastfeeding. *MCN Am J Matern Child Nurs.* 2009;34(4): 249-255.

Parker D, Williams N. *Lactation Consultant Series Two: Teens and Breastfeeding.* Schaumburg, IL: La Leche League International; 2000.

Piotrowski CC, et al. Healthy Steps: a systematic review of a preventive practice-based model of pediatric care. *J Dev Behav Pediatr.* 2009;30(1):91-103.

Rathe R. Medical history taking study guide. University of Florida. Updated December 19, 2000. medinfo.ufl.edu/year1/bcs/clist/history.html. Accessed March 13, 2009.

Rebhan B, et al. Infant feeding practices and associated factors through the first 9 months of life in Bavaria, Germany. *J Pediatr Gastroenterol Nutr.* 2009;4:467-473.

Ross L, Goulet C. Attitudes and subjective norms of Quebecian adolescent mothers towards breastfeeding. *Can J Public Health.* 2002;93(3):198-202.

Schuster MA, et al. Anticipatory guidance: what information do parents receive? What information do they want? *Arch Pediatr Adolesc Med.* 2000;154:1191-1198.

Shaikh U, Scott BJ. Extent, accuracy, and credibility of breastfeeding information on the Internet. *J Hum Lact.* 2005; 21(2):175-183.

Simon S, et al. Patients' attitudes toward electronic health information exchange: Qualitative study. *J Med Internet Res.* 2009;11(3):e30.

Su LL, et al. Antenatal education and postnatal support strategies for improving rates of exclusive breast feeding: randomised controlled trial. *BMJ.* 2007;335(7620):596.

Sutton J, et al. Barriers to breastfeeding in a Vietnamese community: a qualitative exploration. *Can J Diet Pract Res.* 2007;68(4):195-200.

Thomas JR, Shaikh U. Electronic communication with patients for breastfeeding support. *J Hum Lact.* 2007;23(3):275-279.

Ummarino M, et al. Short duration of breastfeeding and early introduction of cow's milk as a result of mothers' low level of education. *Acta Paediatr Suppl.* 2003;91(441):12-17.

UNICEF/WHO. *Baby-Friendly Hospital Initiative Training Materials* (updated 2009). www.unicef.org/nutrition/index_24850.html. Accessed March 1, 2010.

Volpe E, Bear M. Enhancing breastfeeding initiation in adolescent mothers through the Breastfeeding Educated and Supported Teen (BEST) Club. *J Hum Lact.* 2000;16(3):196-200.

Yeo S, et al. Cultural views of breastfeeding among high school female students in Japan and the United States: a survey. *J Hum Lact.* 1994;10:25-30.

The Science of Lactation

7

The Science of Lactation

The breast, a marvelously complex mechanism, has ensured the survival of the human race. Following our biologic imperative, we humans, as mammals, continue to feed and nurture our babies. Historically, mothers have instinctively nurtured their young, confident in their natural abilities to produce milk. It is only in recent decades that study of the anatomy and physiology of the breast has become an issue in lactation. Today, health professionals study every detail of the breast, both externally and internally. The growth of functioning breast tissue, milk synthesis (production), the letdown reflex, and types of nipples all receive intense scrutiny. The information presented in this chapter will help you, as a lactation consultant, understand the science involved in lactation. Our knowledge of the breast and lactation function has increased dramatically in recent years, thanks to ultrasound technology, computer imaging modalities, research, and increased public awareness of breast cancer and its prevention. Staying current on the ever-changing understanding of this amazing organ will assist you in your clinical practice.

∾ Key Terms

Acinus
Afterpains
Alveoli
Areola
Atresia
Atrophy
Autocrine control
Autonomic nerves
Axilla
Bactericidal
Blood and lymph systems
Capillaries
Colostrum
Connective tissue
Cooper's ligaments
Dermis
Duct system
Ductule
Edema
Epidermis

Epithelium
Estrogen
Evert
Exocrine gland
Fatty tissue
Feedback inhibitor of lactation (FIL)
Fibrocystic breast
Fistula
Foremilk
Galactocele
Galactopoiesis
Glandular tissue
Hindmilk
Hoffman technique
Hormonal imbalance
Hormone pathways
Hypopituitarism
Hypoplasia
Hypothalamus

Inhibited letdown
Innervation
Insufficient mammary tissue
Intercostal nerves
Intraductal papilloma
Inverted nipple
Inverted syringe
Involution
Keratin
Lactiferous sinus
Lactocyte
Lactogenesis
Lactose
Leaking
Letdown
Lobule
Lymph node
Lymphatic system
Lysozyme
Malignant
Mammary gland
Mammary ridge
Mammogenesis
Mature milk
Milk ejection reflex
Milk-producing tissue
Milk-transporting tissue
Milk synthesis
Montgomery glands
Myoepithelial cells

Nerves
Nipple pore
Nipple preference
Nipple shield
Oxytocin
Paget's disease
Parenchyma
Pinch test
Pitocin
Pituitary
Placenta
Plugged duct
Progesterone
Prolactin
Prolactin inhibitory factor (PIF)
Prolactinoma
Protractility
Reduction
Sebaceous gland
Secretory
Sheehan's syndrome
Sphincter
Supernumerary nipple
Supportive and sustaining tissue
Tail of Spence
Transitional milk
Whey
Witch's milk

∾ Anatomy of the Breast

The breast is part of the body's intricate system of reproduction. Although called a mammary gland, the breast is actually an organ. Each breast is an individual exocrine gland that functions and develops independently to extract material from the blood and convert it into milk.

Individuality in size and shape is especially evident during lactation, when a woman's breasts enlarge to accommodate milk synthesis. The rate of flow and the quantity of milk produced during lactation reveals the breast's uniqueness. The nipple, areola, and Montgomery glands are located within the surface layer of the breast. Knowledge of the components of the breast—skin, supportive tissue, and milk-producing and milk-transporting tissue—will enable you, as a lactation consultant, to help mothers understand the changes that occur in their breasts during pregnancy and throughout lactation.

Skin

Most human contact with the environment comes through the skin, which is the body's largest organ. Skin helps hold us together and acts as a defensive covering for deeper tissue. It is flexible and elastic to allow for changes in tissue size. Skin acts as a screen against the damaging effects of light and performs respiratory and excretory functions—in other words, it breathes and perspires. Skin contains hair, sebaceous glands, and sweat glands and is composed of cells with many distinct layers. Dead cells lie on the surface, while living cells reside underneath. The dermis and the epidermis make up two distinct layers within skin.

Skin Layers

The dermis, which is composed of connective tissue, is the inner layer of the skin. It contains nerve endings, capillaries (small blood vessels), hair follicles, lymph channels, and other cells. Muscle cells are located under this layer, except in the area of the areola and nipple, where the two intermingle.

The epidermis, which is made up of epithelial cells, is the outer layer of living cells. It covers and protects deeper skin layers from drying out and from invasion by bacteria. Over the course of their life, skin cells progress through the epidermis, from their initial growth in the germinating layer to their loss of fluid in the transitional layer and on to the surface layer of dead skin, called keratin (see Figure 7.1).

New cell growth in the germinating layer continually pushes dead cells outward toward the surface of the skin. As the cells move outward through the transitional layer, they undergo changes that cement them firmly together. This creates a tough, hard, waterproof barrier against bacterial invasion. The outer layer of the skin—the epidermis—protects the inner layer—the dermis—from abrasion and water evaporation.

Nipple

The nipple, the protruding part of the breast, extends and becomes firmer when stimulated, enabling the baby to

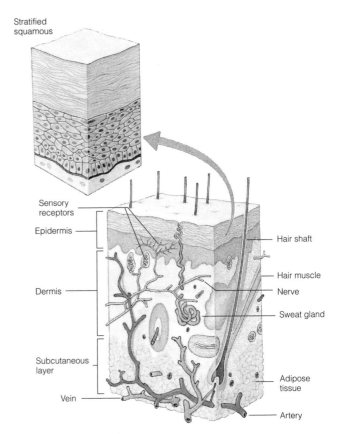

FIGURE 7.1 Skin layers.

latch onto the breast for nursing. The nipple is flexible and able to mold and elongate to conform to the baby's mouth during feeding. The tissue in the nipple is similar to the tissue in human lips, and is able to stretch and heal quickly. Sensory nerve endings in the nipple trigger milk release when the baby suckles.

The nipple is composed primarily of circular smooth muscle fibers that function as a closing mechanism for the milk ducts. Ductule openings, commonly called nipple pores, are located at the end of the nipple and enable the baby to receive the milk (see Color Plate 1). Ramsay and colleagues (2005a, 2005b, 2003) reported an average of 9 main nipple pores, with a range of 4 to 18. Love and Lindsey (2005) found an average of 5 pores, with a range of 1 to 17. Rusby and colleagues (2007) described multiple ducts sharing a few common openings, with the diameter and position of the duct being unrelated to whether it terminates close to the nipple or passes deeper into the breast. This variance in patent openings may explain why some women lactate more successfully after breast surgery than others (West & San Antonio Breastfeeding Coalition, 2009).

During the last trimester of pregnancy, changes within the ducts sometimes lead to a bloody discharge from the nipple (Lafrenier, 1990). This phenomenon occurs when epithelium spurs that extend into the ducts are traumatized, resulting in bleeding (Dewitt, 1985; Kline & Lash, 1964). It does not affect breastfeeding, and the bleeding often stops when the mother begins nursing. Known as "rusty pipe" syndrome because of the color of the blood, this condition typically resolves spontaneously (Virdi et al., 2001).The cause may be excessive use of breast shells or breast expression late in pregnancy, or the formation of edema during engorgement. Bleeding may also indicate an intraductal papilloma, a benign growth in the duct. Occasionally, bleeding can be a sign of intraductal carcinoma (Matsunaga et al., 2004; Sauter et al., 2004).

Areola

The areola is the dark circular area surrounding the nipple. Its size and color vary greatly from woman to woman. During puberty, menstruation, and pregnancy, the areola enlarges and becomes darker in color. There is little subcutaneous fat under the areola, and the underlying ducts are superficial and easily compressed (Ramsay et al., 2005a).

To nurse effectively, the baby's mouth needs to enclose a sizable portion of the areolar tissue. This enables the infant's tongue to compress a large amount of breast tissue against the palate to facilitate milk release. Many mothers will have heard that they need to get the entire areola into the baby's mouth. For mothers with especially large areolae, however, this is not a good marker. Suggest, instead, that the baby take in an area of areolar tissue that is approximately 1 inch in diameter, not just the nipple.

Montgomery Glands

The Montgomery glands, which have a "pimply" appearance, are sebaceous glands located around the areola. Also called Montgomery's tubercles, they secrete an oily substance that serves as a lubricant and a protective agent for the nipple. Because of this natural lubrication, the nipple and areola do not require creams and lotions to keep them soft and healthy. Montgomery gland secretions allow the skin to breathe and remain pliable. There is also some speculation that these secretions provide a taste and smell that enable the baby to find the nipple (Widstrom & Thingstrom-Paulsson, 1993). Because they are rudimentary mammary glands, Montgomery glands may secrete a small amount of milk as well (Smith, 1982).

Washing the nipples with any substance other than a gentle, unscented soap and plain water may remove this natural lubrication, dry out the breast skin, and reduce the scent. It is not usually necessary to use creams or oils on the nipples, and use of these items may reduce the amount of air reaching the tissue. Creams may also introduce a scent or taste that the baby dislikes or does not recognize.

Supportive and Sustaining Tissue

Other tissues that are vital to the function of the breast lie under the skin and between parts of the milk-producing and milk-transporting tissues. Connective tissues support the breast, and subcutaneous fatty tissues give it shape. Nerves provide a triggering mechanism for milk synthesis and release. The blood and lymph systems bring nourishment to breast tissue, supply the nutrients for milk, and filter out bacteria and cast-off dead cell parts.

Nerves

The breast contains sensory nerves that trigger breast function for lactation (see Figure 7.2). From the third, fourth, fifth, and sixth intercostal nerves, these sensory fibers innervate the smooth muscle in the nipples and blood vessels (Sarhadi et al., 1997; Silen et al., 1996). Intercostal nerves are located in the space between two ribs. Innervation is the distribution of nerve fibers or nerve impulses. Most sensation to the nipple and areola comes from the fourth intercostal nerve (Sun et al., 2004), although the second intercostal nerve may be involved as well (Sarhadi et al., 1996).

There is extensive innervation of the nipple and areola complex, involving both autonomic nerves and sensory nerves. Autonomic nerves have the ability to function independently, without outside influence. Innervation of the nipple differs from that of the areola. Although the areola has long been believed to be the more sensitive of the two, Godwin and colleagues (2004) suggest the opposite—that the nipple is more sensitive. He cites the higher

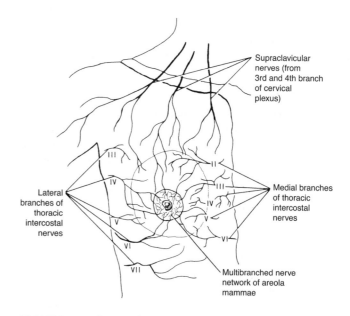

FIGURE 7.2 Innervation of the mammary gland.

Source: Printed with permission of the International Lactation Consultant Association.

density of the nipple as a possible explanation for this difference. Del Vecchyo and colleagues (2004) suggest that women with small breasts seem to experience more sensitivity than do those with large breasts.

A baby who grasps a good amount of breast tissue and sucks vigorously will stimulate the deeper nerves as well. This stimulation triggers oxytocin release and milk letdown. By comparison, a baby who is weak or tired or who sucks on the nipple alone may not provide adequate stimulation to the deeper nerves. Ultimately, this factor may result in less effective letdown and lower milk production.

Fatty Tissue

Fatty tissue within the breast cushions the organ and makes it comfortable and graceful. Fat cells are located throughout most of the breast, between lobuli (plural of "lobule") and milk ducts, and under the skin (Nickell & Skelton, 2005). Very little fat is deposited immediately beneath the areola and nipple, an area dominated by muscular tissue and duct branching (see Color Plate 1).

The amount of fatty and glandular tissue present determines breast size, but these tissues do not contribute to milk synthesis or transport. Therefore, the amount of fat or size of the breast is little indication of the quality or quantity of milk the mother will produce. Women with large or small breasts are equally capable of breastfeeding. Some women may have large breasts consisting of mostly fatty tissue and sparse alveolar growth (Ramsay et al., 2005a; Waller, 1957). Others may have smaller breasts containing ample alveolar lobes and little subcutaneous fat. Women with larger breasts may be more likely to have a larger storage capacity, explaining why some women deliver larger feedings to their infants at one time than other women (Kent, 2003; Cregan & Hartmann, 1999; Cox et al., 1996, 1998; Daly & Hartmann, 1995).

Connective Tissue

The breast contains fibrous connective tissue that supports and contains the fatty tissue and the milk-producing and milk-transporting tissues. Fibrous bands called Cooper's ligaments provide a framework to support the tissues of the breast. These ligaments attach the breast to the overlying skin and the underlying fibrous tissue enclosing the muscles. Fibrous tissue holds the segments of the breast together and supports the ducts as they fill with milk.

Sagging breasts and protruding abdomens most likely result from pregnancy and not lactation. Indeed, women who do not breastfeed their infants experience the same effects. Some caregivers believe that breast sagging can be lessened by the wearing of a good support bra during pregnancy and lactation, especially at times when the breasts are enlarged and full, although there is no research to support this belief. Mothers can wear a bra for comfort if they wish, but caution them against wearing bras that are tight or that have an underwire or other stiff part that can press on milk ducts.

Blood and Lymph Systems

Everything the breast cells need for nourishment—proteins, fats, carbohydrates, and other substances—is brought to them by the bloodstream. Fluids containing these nutrients pass through the capillaries to the tissue spaces, where they are absorbed. Capillaries are small blood vessels that link the arteries and veins. The body has amazing control over the amount of blood that flows into tissue, maintaining circulation at a level that meets the needs of each tissue. When the needs of the breast increase during menstruation and pregnancy, blood flow increases to this area to support tissue building. Later, when frequent suckling signals a need to increase milk production, more blood becomes available to provide the nutrients needed to make milk.

The lymphatic system—a complex network of capillaries, thin vessels, valves, ducts, nodes, and organs—functions like the bloodstream in reverse. Lymph is a thin, clear, slightly yellow fluid, consisting of approximately 95 percent water plus a few red blood cells and variable numbers of white blood cells. The lymphatic system absorbs excess blood fluids from the tissue spaces and eventually returns them to the heart (see Figure 7.3).

Lymph nodes function as filters in the lymph vessels to trap bacteria and cast-off cell parts. Each node is a potential dam that can, if necessary, arrest the spread of infection. At times, lymph nodes may swell and be painful. Most of the lymph produced within the breast flows into the nodes in the armpit. There, the lymph nodes trap bacteria that might otherwise travel up the ducts from the nipple or bloodstream. The swelling of a lymph node in the armpit could suggest that an infection is present in the breast, arm, or hand.

During breast engorgement (see Chapter 16), increased pressure from milk in the ducts decreases the flow of blood and lymph. This condition can cause fluids to accumulate in the tissues, referred to as edema (Cotterman, 2004; Hill & Humenick, 1994). With the lymphatic system at a standstill, the risk of local infection increases. In this scenario, the breast cannot remove bacteria and cell particles adequately, which leads to poor drainage of the ducts and alveoli.

Generally, bacteria multiply more effortlessly in stagnant fluids rather than moving fluids. This predisposes a poorly drained breast to mastitis (breast inflammation characterized by pain, swelling, redness, and fever). A mother with mastitis must remove milk as effectively as possible to reduce pressure within the breast. She can do so by feeding her baby more frequently and thoroughly,

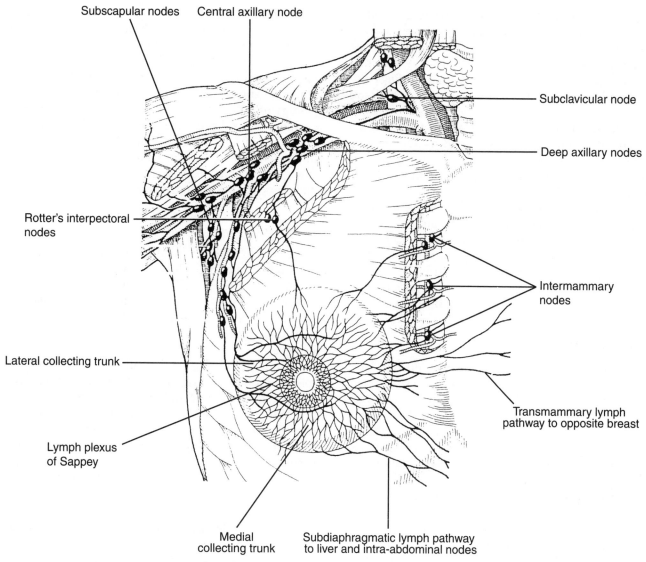

Subscapular nodes   Central axillary node

Subclavicular node

Deep axillary nodes

Rotter's interpectoral nodes

Intermammary nodes

Lateral collecting trunk

Lymph plexus of Sappey

Transmammary lymph pathway to opposite breast

Medial collecting trunk

Subdiaphragmatic lymph pathway to liver and intra-abdominal nodes

FIGURE 7.3   Lymphatic drainage of the breast.

Source: Printed with permission of the International Lactation Consultant Association.

or by expressing milk from the breast. See Chapter 16 for a discussion of mastitis.

Glandular Tissue

The breast contains highly efficient glands that take raw materials from blood and create new and essential nutrients for the baby. The breast parenchyma—functional parts of the organ—are composed of many smaller individual glands, or lobuli. These lobuli, in turn, consist of many milk-producing alveoli. Glandular tissue is the functional part of the breast that produces and transports milk. The lobuli connect to a system of ducts that provide a passageway for the milk to flow out of the breast and to the infant. Understanding the structure of the glandular tissue will help you, as a lactation consultant, assist mothers in preventing or treating breastfeeding difficulties.

Milk-Producing Tissue

The production of milk takes place in the breast in tiny individual glands called alveoli. (The singular form is "alveolus," also called "acinus.") Alveoli consist of epithelial cells (lactocytes) encased in a dense basketlike meshwork of smooth muscle, known as myoepithelial cells. Numerous capillaries surround the alveoli and bring nutrient-rich blood from which the alveoli make milk.

Through this same system, the alveoli receive the hormones oxytocin and prolactin, which signal them to release and produce more milk. Like other smooth muscle cells in the body, such as those in the uterine wall and nipple, myoepithelial cells contract when exposed to oxytocin released during suckling. The contraction of these cells in the alveoli results in a squeezing effect on the lobule, thereby forcing milk down the ducts. Myoepithelial cells multiply and greatly increase in size during pregnancy and lactation; conversely, they decrease in both size and number when breastfeeding ends. Color Plate 2 shows alveoli filled with milk, and Color Plate 3 shows the interior of a milk-filled alveolus and its surrounding myoepithelial cells. Color Plate 4 illustrates the constriction of the myoepithelial cells that forces milk from the alveolus into the duct.

Alveoli are grouped together to form lobuli, which are often compared visually to a cluster of grapes. The distribution of lobuli in the breast varies widely. Computer image research indicates that fewer lobes are present than previously believed, probably seven to ten per breast (Ramsay et al., 2003, 2005a). The tail of Spence denotes the breast tissue that extends into the axilla, or armpit.

Milk-Transporting Tissue

Milk flows through a system of mammary ductules, secondary ducts, and nipple pores, as shown in Color Plate 1. In the young girl, the duct system begins to form with a few small basic ducts in childhood. These ducts sprout and branch during puberty, forming tissue buds for the future development of alveoli and lobuli. With each ovulation, the ducts grow lengthwise as alveoli and lobuli develop. During the first 4 to 5 months of pregnancy, sprouting and growth of ducts and alveolar development intensify. In the second half of pregnancy, the duct and alveolar tissues become more specialized in preparation for their milk-related functions.

The mature lactating breast contains an intricate ductal system that transports milk out of the breast through an average of nine nipple pores. Each duct widens throughout the breast and in the area beneath the areola during the passage of milk through the ductule opening, then collapses when milk ceases to flow. The duct system is much more random and intricate than it has been presented historically in the literature (Ramsay et al., 2004). There is also great variance in its form from mother to mother (Ramsay, 2004). In all women, an intact duct system is necessary for milk transfer to the infant. For this reason, breast surgery or other interference with the milk-transporting system can compromise the mother's ability to transfer milk to her infant (see Chapter 25).

Texts published in earlier years referred to the ducts beneath the areola as lactiferous sinuses. This understanding evolved from cadaver work done by Sir Astley Cooper in 1840, in which he injected hot wax into the breast of a cadaver of a woman who had been lactating at the time of death. Scientists now hypothesize that the injection of the hot wax distended the cadaver's ducts, which led to the belief that lactiferous sinuses were larger than the rest of the ductule framework (Love & Lindsey, 2005; Ramsay et al., 2003). Real-time ultrasound computer imaging conducted in the modern era shows a temporary dilation of the ducts during letdown and the passage of milk through the ducts and out the nipple openings. After this passage, the ducts collapse until the next surge of milk (Ramsay et al., 2004, 2006). Unused milk actually flows backward through the ducts (Ramsay et al., 2004), which explains how bacteria can be introduced into the breast, sometimes causing mastitis.

Insufficient Mammary Tissue

Some women have very small, poorly developed breasts, a condition called hypoplasia. Unlike small breasts, these organs are widely spaced (more than 1½ inches apart), tubular, and thin—a marker for true insufficient glandular tissue. Color Plates 5–8 illustrate four common types of breasts (Huggins et al., 2000). Type 4 illustrates hypoplasia.

If a mother has great difficulty producing enough milk and you have ruled out breastfeeding technique as a cause, consider the possibility of underlying hormonal problems or true insufficient glandular tissue. If a mother tries all means of increasing milk production and is unable to maintain an adequate amount of milk, her baby may need supplements.

Signs of possible glandular insufficiency include the following conditions (Neifert et al., 1990):

- No noticeable change in breast size during pregnancy or lactation
- One breast appreciably smaller than the other
- Family history of lactation failure
- Inadequate milk production despite an appropriate feeding regimen
- Ductal atresia, where the lack of a milk duct opening prevents milk from being ejected from that particular duct

∼ Mammary Growth and Development

From the onset of puberty and throughout pregnancy, the mammary gland is in a stage of mammogenesis, when it develops to a functioning state. During the last trimester of pregnancy, it enters into lactogenesis, when milk synthesis and secretion are established. With the establishment of mature milk and throughout lactation, the breast is in a state of galactopoiesis. Involution occurs at the end of lactation, with the breast slowly returning to its prepregnant state. See Figures 7.4 and

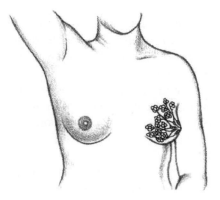

FIGURE 7.4 Breast before pregnancy.

Source: Illustration by Marcia Smith.

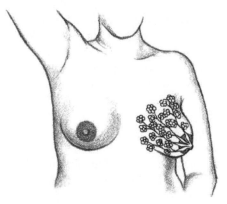

FIGURE 7.5 Breast during pregnancy.

Source: Illustration by Marcia Smith.

7.5 for a comparison of the breast before and during pregnancy.

Fetal Stage

The beginnings of breast development become noticeable in the fetus at 5 weeks of life. At this time, two mammary ridges (also called "milk lines") are detectable, extending from the armpits to the inner thighs. Because the milk lines appear before genitalia, breasts develop in males as well as females. The lower parts of the milk lines disappear after several weeks. By 20 to 32 weeks, the upper parts develop and form milk ducts. Sometimes the lower ends of the milk lines fail to regress, however, and the baby is born with one or more supernumerary nipples along this line. Toward the end of gestation, the ducts form openings in the nipples that are depressed below the surface of the skin. Just before birth, the nipples push outward and become level with the skin. In some cases, this step fails, resulting in a partially or completely inverted nipple.

Some babies (both male and female) are born with breasts that secrete a colostrum-like fluid, referred to as "witch's milk." This fluid consists primarily of shed epithelial cells and may result from an influx of hormones through the mother's placenta at birth. Babies who are born before term do not have this secretion. Left alone, witch's milk disappears in about 20 days.

Puberty

The majority of functional breast tissue development occurs during puberty and pregnancy, both of which are periods of increased hormonal activity. Although the structural growth of the breast is very apparent during puberty, only a small amount of alveolar development takes place at this time. Only slight development of functional breast tissue occurs during ovulatory cycles.

Because the breast covers the bony ribcage, it grows outward. Likewise, the skin that covers and contains the breast expands and grows to accommodate it. The result is an evenly rounded organ with a protruding nipple. With the onset of menstruation, the body's hormonal balance is altered by the increased production of estrogen, which promotes the growth of ducts and the connective tissue between them. A thick layer of fat is deposited under the skin and forms the firm and enlarged adolescent breast. The areola and the nipple grow and take on a deeper color during puberty (and again in pregnancy).

The initial major changes in functional breast tissue are typically complete approximately 12 to 18 months after the first menstrual period. The formation of fibrous connective tissue and the laying down of fat continue to increase breast size during each adolescent menstrual period. The mammary gland is relatively inactive between the events of puberty and pregnancy. Around 12 to 16 days before the onset of each menses, the ovaries release an egg, with estrogen levels increasing as well. The reproduction of ductule tissue and the formation of alveolar cells begin to prepare the breast for pregnancy at this time. However, this proliferation is not significant in terms of breast size.

The breast fullness experienced by women just before menstruation is attributable to the increased blood supply and excessive fluid retained in the tissues. After the end of each menstrual cycle, tissue growth regresses and glandular cells degenerate. In addition, loss of fluid from the tissues causes the breast to return to its previous size. Regression of tissue growth is incomplete, and the ovulatory cycle slightly enhances mammary growth for younger women (younger than approximately 30 to 35 years of age). In terms of overall breast development and preparation for lactation, breast tissue enhancement during pregnancy is far more significant than any gain that occurs during menstrual cycles.

Pregnancy

With the onset of pregnancy, the breast continues to progress through the stage of mammogenesis and further develops to a functioning state. It is at this time that hormonal changes cause a spectacular phase of growth and proliferation within the breast. During the first trimester of pregnancy (conception to 3 months), estrogen and progesterone levels cause the duct system to multiply. The skin begins to respond to internal enlargement with an increase in the circumference of the nipple and areola. Increased pigmentation or darkening may make this growth seem more apparent.

Glands of Montgomery, which often go unnoticed before pregnancy, now enlarge or elongate. These glands may become noticeable by the first missed menstrual period, alerting the experienced mother to an early sign of pregnancy. The area takes on a rough pimply appearance, which is most noticeable when the skin is cool. During this period, the Montgomery glands begin to secrete an oily substance that protects the nipple and areolar skin; this secretion of protective lubricant continues throughout pregnancy and lactation.

The duct system continues to develop throughout the second trimester (4 to 6 months). Alveoli begin to appear as a result of placental prolactin (see Color Plate 1). By the end of the second trimester, the blood supply and body fluids (lymph) that support alveolar growth and the multiplying number of alveoli may have increased the weight of the breast by as much as 1–1.5 pounds. Production of colostrum is established, and at this point, a woman would lactate were she to deliver prematurely (Hartmann et al., 2003).

General breast development continues throughout the third trimester (7 to 9 months). During this period, stretch marks may appear as evidence of stress on the skin. The nipple and areola continue to darken and enlarge, although their color may lighten somewhat when the mother gives birth and toward the end of lactation. This process is repeated with each succeeding pregnancy. The change in color and size often appears more pronounced in younger women whose breasts are not fully mature when pregnancy occurs.

From the time the alveoli begin to proliferate during pregnancy, alveolar cells constantly wear out and are replenished. This ongoing development explains why adolescent mothers are able to lactate despite their recent pubescent changes. The replenishment cycle continues throughout lactation.

Lactogenesis

Understanding the physiology associated with lactogenesis will help you guide mothers in their daily breastfeeding routine. Lactogenesis occurs in three stages to establish milk synthesis and secretion:

- *Stage I* lactogenesis starts at the beginning of the third trimester of pregnancy. At this time, epithelial cells are converted to a secretory state and plasma con-

centrations of lactose, total proteins, and immunoglobulin increase. Sodium and chloride decrease. Substances needed for milk synthesis are drawn from the maternal bloodstream.
- *Stage II* lactogenesis occurs at 2 to 5 days postpartum. It is referred to as the time when the colostral phase ends and transitional milk is produced. Blood flow within the breast increases, and copious milk secretion begins.
- *Stage III* lactogenesis, also called galactopoiesis, marks the establishment and maintenance of mature milk. It occurs 8 to 10 days postpartum.

For the lactation consultant, awareness of the various factors that influence milk synthesis will enable you to explain to mothers how frequent nursing increases milk production. Recognizing the factors that initiate letdown, the function of hormones in the letdown process, and their effects on breast tissue will help you identify problems with milk release and assist mothers to work out solutions.

Involution

Lactogenesis is followed by a period of involution, which is a normal process marked by the decreasing size—atrophy—of the breast. At this time, the breast slowly returns to its prepregnant state. The process takes about 3 months when accompanied by slow and gradual weaning. Abrupt weaning will cause marked involution in a matter of days or weeks.

After multiple pregnancies and extended breastfeeding, some women experience severe involution, in which

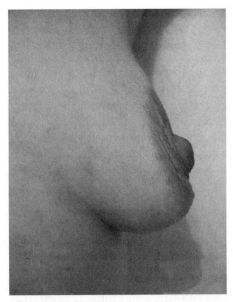

FIGURE 7.6   Involuted breast that has atrophied.

Source: Printed with permission of Anna Swisher.

fat deposits do not recur when the ducts regress (Figure 7.6). Normal breast shape usually returns within 3 years. Loss of fat and shape can also occur without breastfeeding. In the event of another pregnancy, the breast will regenerate and lactation will begin again (Lawrence & Lawrence, 2005). Some mothers with severe involution, in which fat deposits do not regenerate, may choose to have breast augmentation.

~ Hormonal Impact on Lactation

Hormones are chemical products of the endocrine glands that regulate functions of specific organs or tissues. A comprehensive understanding of lactation hormones and their function will help you identify problems with initiation and ongoing milk production. Lactation hormones affect letdown, milk production, breast tissue, and other aspects of a mother's physiology. The growth, maturation, and function of the breast are a result of stimulation by four major hormones—estrogen, progesterone, prolactin, and oxytocin.

Estrogen

Estrogen is produced in the ovaries, adrenal glands, and placenta. It stimulates growth of the uterus, vagina, and other reproductive organs. Estrogen is responsible for the development of female secondary sex characteristics, such as the distinctive female skeleton, body contour, and mammary glands. In the breast, this hormone causes the growth of mammary ducts and connective tissue between the ducts.

Progesterone

Progesterone is produced in the ovaries and placenta. The Latin word that is the origin of this term means "for gestation." Along with estrogen, progesterone works to maintain the reproductive tract and menstrual cycle. This hormone is essential for the maintenance of pregnancy and aids in the development of the milk-secreting cells in the breast. Progesterone inhibits prolactin's effects during pregnancy. A retained placenta following delivery and its accompanying progesterone can impair stage II lactogenesis.

Prolactin

Prolactin is produced in the placenta and in the anterior pituitary gland in the brain. The Latin word that is the origin of this term means "for lactation." Anterior pituitary prolactin stimulates alveolar growth in the breast during pregnancy. Prolactin levels in the mother's blood increase soon after initiation of the sucking stimulus. This hormone signals the breast to speed up milk synthesis. It both serves as a natural tranquilizer and stimulates feelings in the mother of restlessness and yearning for her baby. This physiologically conditioned response stimulates the mother to interact positively with her baby. Thus prolactin is often credited with inducing maternal behavior.

A mother can do several things to keep her prolactin levels high. She can position her baby for an effective latch, and avoid the use of artificial nipples or pacifiers that may cause nipple preference. She can give her baby unlimited access to the breast, breastfeeding as frequently as he or she wants, usually every 1 to 3 hours, and for as long as the baby wants at a feeding. Breastfeeding during the night, when prolactin release in response to sucking is greatest, will help to keep the mother's prolactin levels high as well.

Oxytocin

Oxytocin is produced in the hypothalamus and travels through nerve fibers to the posterior pituitary, where it is stored. The infant's suckling stimulates nerve endings in the nipple; nerve impulses then race through the hypothalamic region to the posterior pituitary and release oxytocin. The oxytocin is transported through the bloodstream to the breasts, where it causes smooth muscle cells to contract, thereby producing uterine contractions in childbirth, afterpains, and orgasm.

Oxytocin causes the muscle layer, or myoepithelial cell, around each milk-producing cell to contract during letdown. This phenomenon is called the milk ejection reflex, or letdown. In response, milk is pushed down the ducts and out through the nipple pores. The mother initially may need several minutes of stimulus to produce a high enough level of oxytocin to be effective in inducing letdown. She will notice when the milk begins to be ejected because the rhythm of her baby's sucking will change from rapid sucking (about 2 sucks per second) to regular deep, slow sucking (about 1 suck per second). Pitocin is a synthetic form of oxytocin, often used for induction or augmentation of labor.

Oxytocin is known as an affiliation hormone, or "mothering hormone." It plays a key role in the initiation of maternal behavior and the formation of adult pair bonds (Turner et al., 1999). Social stimuli may induce oxytocin release, and oxytocin may make positive social contact more rewarding. Some researchers believe oxytocin gives women a "tend and befriend" response to stress, encouraging their bonding with other women and the tending of children (Taylor et al., 2000).

Hormonal Imbalances

Because hormones in the mother's body regulate the lactation process, a disturbance in her hormone levels has the potential to affect milk production and release. Pituitary, thyroid, and adrenal imbalances can all alter a mother's hormone levels, as can certain medications. This imbalance may cause her to produce either too little or too much milk, to release milk at inappropriate times, or to fail to release milk at all. Women who have difficulty conceiving or who have become pregnant by the aid of reproductive technologies are at a higher risk for hormone imbalance and, consequently, milk insufficiency.

A mother who has breastfeeding problems accompanied by a vague feeling of physical discomfort or a history of previous thyroid problems or menstrual irregularities may have a hormone imbalance. Placental retention can inhibit the process of lactation by causing hormones to remain at pregnancy levels. The absence of breast fullness and changes in breast secretions can indicate the retention of placental fragments.

Hormone imbalances as a cause of breastfeeding problems are becoming more common, reflecting the increased number of women conceiving through infertility treatment, which typically manipulates hormonal levels. If a client fits the profile for hormone problems, refer her to her caregiver for a thorough hormonal screening—including measurement of progesterone, thyroid function, prolactin, and testosterone levels—to rule out hormone imbalance as a cause. Chapter 25 discusses hormonal issues, such as pituitary and thyroid dysfunction and polycystic ovarian (or ovary) syndrome (PCOS), in more detail.

Sheehan's syndrome—also known as hypopituitarism syndrome, postpartum hypopituitarism, and postpartum pituitary insufficiency—is a form of shock that can result from severe postpartum hemorrhage and hypotension. In this condition, the mother's blood pressure drops so low that blood fails to circulate to the pituitary gland. This causes some or all of the cells in the gland to stop functioning permanently. The mother may have produced some colostrum in her breasts before going into shock. Because of the malfunctioning pituitary gland, however, her breasts will remain soft after delivery and she may not be able to produce any milk. The damage to the pituitary gland is usually irreversible and may permanently rule out the prospect of breastfeeding.

~ Milk Synthesis

When the placenta is delivered, estrogen and progesterone levels in the mother's body drop sharply, and prolactin production in the anterior pituitary increases dramatically. The high level of prolactin combined with decreased levels of estrogen and progesterone signal the alveoli to start producing and secreting milk. When the infant has free access to the breast, the initial milk produced—colostrum—gives way to transitional milk. This is

followed by increased milk production and breast fullness beginning between the second and fifth days postpartum. With initial milk production, women typically experience a normal fullness in their breasts. Those who do not understand this normal physiologic response may mistake it for engorgement.

Colostrum Production

Colostrum is a unique substance that appears as a semitransparent, thick, and sticky liquid ranging in color from pale to deep yellow. It contains water, minerals, fat droplets, lymphocytes, and similar cells. It also contains cast-off alveolar cells, which offer a unique combination of nutrients designed to meet the nutritional and immunologic needs of the newborn. Colostrum acts as a natural lubricant and, because of its lysozyme content, is bactericidal (destroys bacteria).

Alveoli begin producing colostrum in the fourth month of pregnancy. At first, only small amounts are released into the center of the lobuli. As pregnancy advances, colostrum production continues to fill the alveoli. Some colostrum may leak out of the alveoli through the cell pores, and protruding portions of the alveoli may break away into the center of the lobule. Thus some women find that their breasts leak colostrum during the later months of pregnancy.

Role of Prolactin

Prolactin is the hormone that promotes milk synthesis. It is present in small amounts in all humans, both male and female. Prolactin levels increase gradually during pregnancy and reach a peak of 20 times the normal value near term. During pregnancy, estrogen and progesterone levels act locally on the alveoli to inhibit milk production and secretion. After delivery, when estrogen and progesterone levels have dropped, the high prolactin levels stimulate initial milk production. Levels increase again tenfold in response to sucking. After 3 months postpartum, prolactin levels range 3 to 5 times higher than the levels typically found in menstruating females. Continued stimulation results in doubling of the level above the baseline through the second year of lactation (Lawrence & Lawrence, 2005).

Autocrine Control

Milk synthesis does not rely entirely on endocrine (i.e., hormonal) control. Over time, milk production becomes dependent on the frequency and degree of drainage of each breast. Thus milk production changes from endocrine control to autocrine control. Frequent breastfeeding is necessary in the beginning to ensure an increase in the number and sensitivity of prolactin receptors as prolactin levels drop after delivery. As time passes, both prolactin receptors and frequent infant feeding are necessary for long-term milk production.

Autocrine control comprises local control within the gland. In the case of the breast, the control agent is a secretory product from one type of cell that influences the activity of that cell. This relationship suggests that milk remaining in the breast acts to inhibit the production of more milk. Thus the mother produces only what her baby needs and protects her energy expenditure during lactation (Peaker & Wilde, 1996; De Coopman, 1993). This theory helps explain why women are able to nurse with one breast exclusively through the course of lactation and not develop chronic engorgement or mastitis in the other breast (Ing et al., 1977). Research on lactating goats identified the apparent human whey protein, called feedback inhibitor of lactation (FIL), which enables autocrine inhibition of milk synthesis. Researchers believe a whey protein in humans provides a similar FIL function (Knight et al., 1998; Wilde et al., 1998).

Prolactin Inhibitory Factor

The prolactin inhibitory factor (PIF) prevents the release of prolactin at times when the baby is not nursing. Suckling inhibits PIF, thereby allowing the release of prolactin.

The frequency of feeding and stimulation of the nipple significantly affect the level of prolactin that is released. For this reason, it is important to encourage frequent feedings, to promote good positioning of the baby at the breast, and to avoid arbitrary use of nipple shields. In the absence of effective and frequent sucking to remove milk, prolactin production decreases and autocrine inhibition begins.

∽ Milk Ejection Reflex (Letdown)

Milk ejection, also referred to as letdown, is a reflex triggered by various stimuli. When the baby suckles, contact between the baby's tongue and the mother's nipple stimulates nerve endings to send a message to the hypothalamus. This message then goes to the mother's anterior pituitary, lowering levels of prolactin inhibitory factor and triggering prolactin release. As suckling continues, the posterior pituitary gland secretes oxytocin, causing the smooth muscles around the alveoli and the uterus to contract. The contraction forces milk down through the ducts to the duct openings of the nipple (Figure 7.7). The milk is then available to the baby, who obtains the milk through negative pressure generated by suckling.

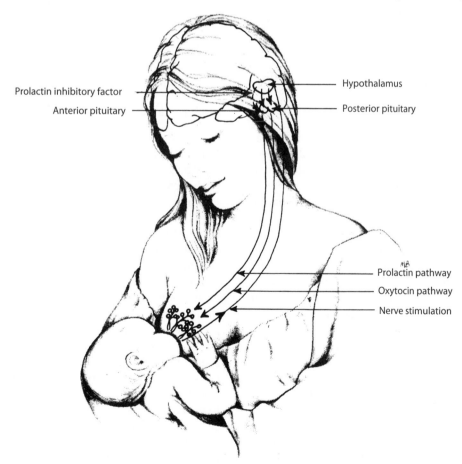

Prolactin inhibitory factor
Anterior pituitary
Hypothalamus
Posterior pituitary

Prolactin pathway
Oxytocin pathway
Nerve stimulation

FIGURE 7.7 Hormone pathways during suckling.

Milk ejection is bilateral—that is, occurring at the same time in both breasts. Sphincters at the end of the ducts prevent milk from flowing freely from the non-suckled breast, however. (A sphincter is a circular band of muscle fibers that narrows a passage or closes a natural opening in the body.) Letdown brings the milk into the ducts, thereby making it accessible to the baby through the activity of suckling. Initially, letdown causes active expulsion of milk through pressure within the ducts. This lasts for a very short time, and then the flow subsides. Positive pressure continues within the breast, and milk flow will continue with further suckling. Letdown provides free flow of milk, which is essential to move fat globules down through the ducts.

High-definition ultrasound shows that milk not removed from the breast flows back into the ducts. When milk does not flow freely in this manner, engorgement can develop, which could lead to a plugged duct or mastitis.

Signs of Letdown

Mothers experience several letdowns in a single feeding (Ramsay, 2004; Ramsay et al., 2004, 2006). The initial letdown is usually the only one the mother notices, however, owing to the large quantity of milk moved at this time. Some mothers may not recognize the letdown reflex consistently in the first days and weeks of breastfeeding. This is especially the case for women who are breastfeeding for the first time.

Some women notice that milk drips from one breast while the baby is nursing on the other breast. Because letdown occurs bilaterally, this leaking is a sign that milk has let down in both breasts.

Letdown may cause a tingling or tightening sensation as well. This feeling is the result of thousands of alveoli contracting and of the pressure of milk forced through the duct system. The mother may also experience increased thirst or sleepiness. In the first days postpartum, uterine contractions often accompany letdown due to oxytocin's action on the involuting uterus.

Some mothers experience no physical sensations to signal that their milk is letting down. They can be encouraged to look for signs in the infant that their letdown reflex is functioning. The baby may begin gulping or even gagging from the sudden rush of milk and the mother will hear more pronounced swallowing. In addition, she can monitor the number of wet diapers and stools her baby has during a 24-hour period to determine the effectiveness of letdown. From the end of the first week of life through the first 6 weeks, six or more wet diapers and three to five stools per day indicate that her milk is letting down and that her baby is well nourished. The mother's awareness of letdown may diminish as she and her baby become more experienced in breastfeeding and begin to focus on other aspects of their relationship.

A Functioning Letdown

A functioning letdown reflex is a necessary element in lactation. In its absence, the infant receives an inadequate amount of milk. Letdown enables the baby to receive the majority of the fat content of the milk, which tends to stick to the duct lining. As letdown occurs, it forces this creamy hindmilk down into the ducts. The infant then receives more fatty milk after letdown as the feeding progresses.

It is important that the infant nurse long enough on each breast to receive sufficient calories. Limiting nursing time on one breast to switch to the other breast could cause the infant to receive a large volume of foremilk, which contains fewer calories. This practice may cause gastric upset as well as low weight gain (Woolridge & Fisher, 1988). In human milk, 50 percent of the calories come from the fat content. Therefore, an inhibited letdown can result in underfeeding an infant even if the child consumes a fair amount of fluid.

Fat content correlates inversely with the amount of time between feedings (Kent, 2007, 2003; Kent et al., 2006; Cox et al., 1996, 1998; Daly et al., 1993). The percentage of fat is higher when feedings are frequent, thereby minimizing differences between hindmilk and foremilk. Conversely, restricting the number of feedings or limiting the baby's time at the breast can reduce fat intake. Because every baby's pattern of nursing is unique, it is advisable to encourage a mother to let her baby finish nursing on a breast rather than switching arbitrarily to the other breast.

Inhibited Letdown

Fatigue, anxiety, fear, and pain can all inhibit the letdown reflex. A new mother, for example, may be anxious about her breastfeeding and parenting. She may feel tense and pressured by work, family commitments, or unsupportive family and friends. She may be overtired due to lack of rest or overexertion. She may be in pain from childbirth or resulting surgery. Any of these circumstances could inhibit her letdown.

Stress or fatigue can inhibit the secretion of oxytocin and release adrenaline. This, in turn, can negate the effects of oxytocin on the myoepithelial cells. Letdown also can fail to occur when nipple stimulation is weak—for example, when the baby is not latching effectively.

If you suspect that a woman's letdown reflex is not functioning well, you can observe a feeding and suggest relaxation techniques like those presented in Chapter 14. You can also build the mother's confidence in her ability to nourish her baby by explaining that her body is able to sustain her baby now, just as it did during pregnancy. A consultation will allow you to discuss emotional factors that may be involved and ways the mother can cope with those stressors.

Conditioning Letdown

Mothers should be encouraged to relax both physically and mentally during the early weeks of breastfeeding. (Chapter 14 describes relaxation techniques.) The less tension a woman experiences, the more likely she is to let down her milk consistently during feedings. Nursing in a quiet location and a comfortable position and setting up a routine to begin each feeding will help ensure that letdown becomes a firmly established part of each feeding session. Development of such as pattern will condition the mother psychologically for her milk to let down. These conditioning techniques are especially helpful to a woman who is separated from her baby during the day and is providing milk through hand expression or pumping. She may notice that her milk lets down when she picks up her baby, when she hears a baby cry, or whenever she thinks about her baby.

〰 *Variations in Breast Structure and Function*

The ability to produce and release milk depends in part on the physical condition of the mother's breasts. A wide variety of breast sizes and nipple shapes will accommodate breastfeeding. Only a few variations in structure will create challenges with breastfeeding. Mothers can overcome some differences in structure, such as nipple inversion. Other circumstances, such as previous breast surgery that has severed milk ducts, may make it necessary to supplement breastfeeding with other nutrition or to rely totally on an alternative feeding method. In most circumstances, the size and shape of a mother's breasts are not usually indicators of how much milk she is able to produce, nor of how well her baby will thrive on her milk.

Examining the Mother's Breasts

It is not necessary to examine every woman's breasts and nipples. Nevertheless, if a difficulty arises that you suspect may be due to the mother's nipples or breasts, you should do an organized examination. A systematic breast exam can reveal the presence or absence of glandular tissue necessary for milk production. Some women associate breast examination with illness or cancer prevention, so make sure the mother understands why you are examining her breasts and what you are looking for. Use this opportunity to teach her about her breasts as well as techniques that will help her during breastfeeding such as breast massage, compression, and hand expression.

Before beginning a breast exam, ensure privacy to help the mother feel comfortable. Be aware of any customs of modesty that may make this procedure uncomfortable for her. Ask permission and explain your purpose before you begin the exam. If you practice in a nonhospital setting, be sure the mother has read and signed a consent form granting you permission to examine her and her baby.

History

The normal changes during pregnancy include breast growth and tenderness, darkening of the areolae, and increased Montgomery gland prominence, or "bumpiness." Ask the mother an open-ended question, such as "Which changes did you notice in your breasts during your pregnancy?," and listen to her responses. Use reflective listening to clarify what she says to you. If the mother reports breast growth, usually quantified by bra size, there is probably sufficient functioning tissue in both breasts. Be sure to question the mother more closely if she says no changes in her breasts occurred prenatally. Describing typical changes will help her recollect how her breasts changed. Often, the mother's partner or father of the baby is more observant about breast growth and can help clarify this issue.

Ask about any previous surgery or damage to the breast area. This may include breast reduction or augmentation. It could also include cardiac surgery or any other type of procedure that could affect breast function. Even an automobile accident in which the seat belt placed severe pressure on the breast could damage breast tissue.

Assessment

Examining both breasts at the same time will enable you to observe their symmetry. Note the skin's elasticity, the presence of normal glandular growth in the breast, and any engorgement, lumps, swelling, or redness. Look for evidence of past breast surgery that may have altered or severed some ducts (see Color Plate 9). Note the size and shape of the nipples and the size of the areolae.

Gentle compression of the nipple will help assess the ability of the nipple to evert into the infant's mouth during breastfeeding. How a nipple reacts with compression indicates to the lactation consultant what is happening inside the infant's mouth during breastfeeding. A nipple that retracts with compression is considered short shanked and may be the cause of sore nipples during breastfeeding (see the discussion of nipple inversion that follows).

Be sensitive and respectful when discussing the shape and size of a woman's nipples. If the message a woman hears seems negative, she may be unable to overcome that feeling to reach her breastfeeding goals. Reassure mothers that small and large breasts alike typically produce sufficient milk.

Differences in Nipples

Each woman's nipples are unique in shape, size, and the degree to which they protrude. Efficient milk transfer depends on a baby's ability to latch on to the breast, form it into a conical shape, and stretch it forward and then upward against the hard palate (roof of the mouth). A nipple that protrudes on stimulation aids the baby in finding and centering on the breast. It also provides tissue for the infant to grasp so as to draw sufficient breast tissue into his or her mouth.

Many differences exist in types of nipples. Size varies greatly, ranging from an average of 16 mm in diameter (Ramsay et al., 2005a) to more than 23 mm (Wilson-Clay & Hoover, 2008). Table 7.1 shows nipples classified into five types according to how they appear before and after stimulation. Stimulation such as touch, cold, or gentle compression can reveal whether true inversion is present. Color Plate 10 shows a nipple that appears normal and inverts, or retracts inward, when stimulated (Color Plate 11). The nipple in Color Plate 12 appears dimpled—yet after pumping to release the adhesions, it everts. A pinch test, as described in Chapter 21, will help test the protractility of the mother's nipples. Be aware that many variations of these types are possible, including bifurcated nipples, extremely long nipples, and thick, "meaty" nipples that are not truly inverted, but still difficult make it for babies to achieve a good latch.

Inverted Nipples

Estimates of nipple inversion range from 3.26 percent (Park et al., 1999) to 9 percent (Kalbhen et al., 1998) of women. The degree of inversion typically decreases with each subsequent pregnancy. Some mothers find that the skin's increased elasticity during pregnancy decreases the extent of inversion. Inverted nipples typically begin to respond to correction techniques during the last trimester of pregnancy. Some women may experience preterm labor if their nipples are stimulated, however. Because of this possibility, a woman should check with her caregiver before beginning any technique that involves nipple stimulation.

One study of suboptimal infant feeding behaviors included inverted nipples as a factor (Dewey et al., 2003). For the baby to receive milk, the infant needs to take in enough breast tissue to reach back almost to the hard palate. When the breast will not stretch to accommodate this pattern, the baby has difficulty maintaining suction. With a good latch, the baby takes in a large portion of the breast and forms it into a cone-shaped teat. Milk transfer, therefore, often depends more on the pliability of the entire breast than on the configuration of the nipple itself.

Methods to Decrease Nipple Inversion

Clinicians may try a variety of techniques to help evert nipples that are difficult for a baby to grasp, some of which are more effective than others. Mothers may have heard that wearing breast shells prenatally will improve nipple

protrusion, though no evidence exists to support this practice. Neither has the use of breast shells nor the practice of pulling the nipple to break adhesions (Hoffman technique) prenatally been proven to promote nipple elongation (MAIN Trial Collaborative Group, 1994).

Wearing breast shells between feedings has been suggested to improve nipple protractility by gently placing pressure on the skin, thereby stretching and pushing the nipple forward. A mother may be able to form the nipple by hand or with the aid of ice just before a feeding. Inverted syringes or devices marketed for this purpose, such as the LatchAssist, Nipplette, or Evert-It products, can help elongate the nipple as a preparation for breastfeeding (Arsenault, 1997; McGeorge, 1994; Kesaree et al., 1993). The same effect can be accomplished by applying suction via a breast pump. See Chapter 21 for detailed instructions on how to improve the graspability of the nipple with these methods. In using any of the techniques, mothers need to take care not to increase the suction to painful levels and to limit the frequency of their use to reasonable levels.

Nipple shields are often suggested as a potential solution to inversion (see Color Plate 13) and can be a useful transitional tool for breastfeeding when used appropriately and judiciously (Chertok, 2006; Meier et al., 2000; Wilson-Clay, 1996). Optimally, a lactation consultant would supervise use of a nipple shield to assure its appropriate use. However, nipple shields are readily available in stores and online, so mothers may buy them prenatally or without attention to size. Considerations when using nipple shields include selection of correct size and material (silicon, not rubber or latex), potential infant preference, possible breast tissue damage, adequate sucking stimulation, correct shield placement during feeding, and adequate milk transfer. Because nipple stimulation is reduced by a nipple shield, regular use should be accompanied by pumping to protect milk production. Chapter 21 discusses nipple shield use in more depth.

Lumps in the Breast

The general population usually associates lumps in the breast with breast cancer. In reality, many of the breast lumps associated with lactation are not a health risk. In fact, the normal state of the lactating breast is lumpy, due to the enlarged milk-filled alveoli distributed throughout the tissue. Other lumps may occur due to a plugged duct or breast infection (see Chapter 16). These two conditions are usually temporary, with the associated lumps disappearing after alleviating their cause.

If a lump does not move downward and begin to break up, consider a cause unrelated to breastfeeding. In this situation, the woman needs an examination by a caregiver to identify the cause of the lump. Lumps associated with fibrocystic breasts change with the menstrual cycle,

TABLE 7.1   Five Basic Types of Nipples

Type of Nipple	Before Stimulation	After Stimulation
Common nipple The majority of mothers have what is referred to as a common nipple. It protrudes slightly when at rest and becomes erect and more graspable when stimulated. A baby has no trouble finding and grasping this nipple in order to pull in a large amount of breast tissue and stretch it to the roof of his mouth.		
Flat nipple A flat nipple has a very short shank that makes it less easy for the baby to find and grasp. In response to stimulation, this nipple remains essentially unchanged. Slight movement inward or outward may occur, but not enough to aid the baby in finding and initially grasping the breast on center. This nipple may benefit from the use of a nipple everter to increase protractility.		
Inverted-appearing nipple An inverted-appearing nipple may appear inverted but becomes erect after stimulation. This nipple needs no correction and presents no problems with graspability.		
Retracted nipple A retracted nipple is the most common type of inverted nipple. Initially, this nipple appears to be graspable. However, on stimulation, it retracts, making attachment difficult. This nipple responds well to techniques to increase nipple protrusion.		
Inverted nipple A truly inverted nipple is retracted both at rest and when stimulated. Such a nipple is more difficult for the baby to grasp. All techniques used to enhance protractility of breast tissue can be used to improve attachment. Even if the nipple remains retracted, the baby should be able to latch on if the mother helps form her breast into his mouth.		

shrinking and becoming less noticeable after menstruation. Other types of cysts may also be present within the breast, as described in the following subsections.

Galactocele

A galactocele, caused by the closing or blockage of a milk duct, contains a thick, creamy milk-like substance that sometimes oozes from the nipple when the cyst is compressed. It can be aspirated, and some are removed surgically to prevent them from refilling. In a study of eight women with galactoceles, all resolved spontaneously (Stevens et al., 1997). This finding suggests that surgical intervention may not always be required. The presence of a galactocele is compatible with breastfeeding. If surgery is required, breastfeeding does not need to be interrupted. Case reports suggest that increased rates of galactoceles are observed after breast augmentation (Chun & Taghinia, 2009; Lin et al., 2008; Acarturk et al., 2005).

Intraductal Papilloma

Intraductal papillomas are the second most frequent cause of bloody discharge from the breast. An intraductal papilloma is a benign, nontender tumor within a milk duct. It is usually associated with a spontaneous bloody discharge from one breast. Breastfeeding may continue after serious disease has been ruled out and the discharge has stopped or surgeons have removed the involved duct.

Malignancy

When a breast lump is due to malignancy, breastfeeding may not be compatible with the treatments for cancer. In addition, a baby may refuse to nurse from a cancerous breast (Saber et al., 1996). You will, therefore, want to explore breast rejection by the baby whenever you find a lump. Be careful not to confuse such rejection with the common occurrence of temporary refusal to nurse for a few feedings. A baby may reject breastfeeding for a number of reasons, such as a plug of milk expelled from the breast or a physical condition in the baby.

Breastfeeding can continue if a biopsy is performed on a lump, as the procedure takes place under local anesthesia. In many cases, lumps are benign and breastfeeding is not interrupted. Mothers need to be aware that there is a small risk that a milk fistula (abnormal opening) may result from a biopsy; this complication can result in milk leaking from the biopsy incision site. Healing of the site may require temporary interruption of breastfeeding in that breast (Schackmuth et al., 1993).

Paget's disease is a rare form of malignancy of the breast that is usually unilateral (Color Plate 37). It produces a scaly, itchy skin condition on the nipple and areola that mimics eczema. The nipple may appear flattened, with a bloody discharge. In as many as 30 percent of cases, no visible skin changes occur. Almost half of all patients with Paget's disease have a lump in the breast felt at the time of diagnosis. It is important that mothers see a healthcare provider about any of these symptoms (National Cancer Institute [NCI], 2005).

Regular Breast Self-Examination

In the past, women were encouraged to check their breasts for lumps regularly and to notify their caregiver whenever they noticed unfamiliar lumps. More recently, studies have produced conflicting findings on the value of breast self-examinations in detecting breast cancer. Rather than recommending self-exams at only one time of the month (previously recommended on the 7 to 10 day after menses end), some clinicians now recommend self-examination at different intervals. The emphasis is on a woman becoming familiar with her breasts overall so that she can detect any changes over time (Love & Lindsey, 2005; Love & Barsky, 2004). Then, breastfeeding or not, women will develop a knowledge of their breasts and notice any changes more readily.

⌒ Summary

Although breasts vary from one woman to another in size and appearance, their basic anatomy makes it possible for the vast majority of women to nurture their babies in the manner nature intended. The breast is an intricate system of sensory nerves that trigger milk production, connective tissue that supports and contains fatty tissue, milk-producing glands, and milk-transporting tissues. Blood carries proteins, fats, sugar, and other substances needed for lactation to the breast. The breast, in turn, takes these raw materials from the blood to create nutrients for the infant. This nutrition travels through a system of lobuli and ducts to the nipple, where it is discharged through several nipple pores. Breast surgery that damaged the nerves or severed the ducts may compromise a woman's ability to lactate fully.

Although puberty triggers the development of functional breast tissue, hormonal changes during pregnancy produce the majority of growth toward lactogenesis. The areola undergoes changes in size and color, and the Montgomery glands become more pronounced. Throughout the 9 months of pregnancy, the breast experiences lactogenesis; this transforms the breast into a state characterized by milk production and secretion. Estrogen, progesterone, prolactin, and oxytocin all play a role in altering the hormonal balance to stimulate milk production and release. Stress and fatigue can upset this balance of hormones, and mothers may need to learn measures to lower their stress and stimulate milk letdown to facilitate successful breastfeeding.

∽ *Chapter 7—At a Glance*

Facts you learned—

Milk synthesis and breast development:

- The breast takes raw materials from blood and creates nutrients in the alveoli.
- Myoepithelial cells surround the alveoli, contract when an infant's suckling releases oxytocin, and force milk down the ducts to the nipple.
- Most functional breast tissue development occurs during puberty and pregnancy.
- Increased estrogen during menstruation produces growth of ducts and connective tissue.
- In the absence of pregnancy, tissue growth regresses and glandular cells degenerate.
- In the first trimester of pregnancy, the breast enters mammogenesis, during which the duct system multiplies, the skin stretches to accommodate internal enlargement, the nipple and areola increase in circumference, the areola darkens, and the Montgomery glands become noticeable.
- Colostrum is established by the end of the second trimester.
- Stage I lactogenesis: At the beginning of the third trimester of pregnancy, the breast begins to gather the nutrients needed for milk synthesis (including increases in lactose, total proteins, and immunoglobulin and a decrease in sodium and chloride).
- Stage II lactogenesis: Around the second to fifth day postpartum, transitional milk is produced, blood flow within the breast increases, and copious milk secretion begins.
- Stage III lactogenesis (galactopoiesis): About 8 to 10 days postpartum, establishment and maintenance of mature milk is achieved.
- Lactogenesis is followed by a period of involution, when the breast slowly returns to its prepregnancy state.

Hormones:

- Estrogen stimulates growth of the uterus, vagina, and other reproductive organs.
- Progesterone inhibits prolactin's effects during pregnancy.
- Prolactin stimulates alveolar growth and milk synthesis and induces maternal behavior.
- High prolactin levels can be maintained with unlimited, effective suckling and breastfeeding during the night.
- Oxytocin releases in response to suckling and causes myoepithelial cells to contract (milk ejection reflex).

- Pituitary, thyroid, and adrenal imbalances can affect milk production and release.
- Sheehan's syndrome (hypopituitarism) resulting from severe postpartum hemorrhage and hypotension can cause irreversible damage to milk-producing cells.
- Milk production depends on the frequency and degree of drainage of each breast.
- Autocrine control inhibits the production of more milk when milk is left in the breast.
- Suckling by the infant inhibits the production of prolactin inhibitory factor (PIF), thereby allowing prolactin release to occur.
- Letdown moves fat globules down through the ducts (hindmilk).
- Letdown can be inhibited by fatigue, anxiety, fear, or pain.

Breasts:

- Symmetry of the mother's breasts can be observed by examining both breasts at the same time.
- A small percentage of women have truly inverted nipples.
- An inverted nipple can be drawn out with an inverted syringe, commercial everter, breast pump, or nipple shield.
- The normal lactating breast is lumpy due to the enlarged milk-filled alveoli.
- A galactocele may resolve spontaneously or may be compressed, aspirated, or removed surgically.
- An intraductal papilloma produces a bloody discharge.
- Breast rejection by the infant may occur when malignancy is present.
- Paget's disease produces scaly, itchy nipples and areolas and sometimes bloody discharge.
- Widely spaced, tubular, asymmetric, and thin breasts are markers for insufficient glandular tissue.
- Women with a history of breast surgery should ask the surgeon if it involved functional tissue; their babies need to be monitored for appropriate intake and weight gain while they are nourished by breastfeeding.

Applying what you learned—

Teach mothers:

- To preserve the keratin layer and lubrication of skin on the nipple.
- That the baby needs to take in about 1 inch or more in diameter of areolar tissue.

- To ensure the baby grasps the breast well and sucks vigorously to stimulate the nerves.
- That breast size is related to the amount of fatty and glandular tissue present and does not predict how much milk can be produced.
- That breast sagging results from pregnancy, not lactation.
- That sucking stimulates milk production and that more blood becomes available to provide the nutrients needed to make milk when this signal is received.
- That engorgement decreases the flow of blood and lymph, causes edema, increases the risk of local infection, and leads to poor milk drainage.
- That frequent feedings, good positioning at the breast, avoidance of arbitrary use of nipple shields, and pumping in the absence of effective and frequent sucking are all measures that help protect milk production.

〜 References

Acarturk S, et al. An uncommon complication of secondary augmentation mammoplasty: bilaterally massive engorgement of breasts after pregnancy attributable to postinfection and blockage of mammary ducts. *Aesthetic Plast Surg.* 2005;29(4):274-279; discussion 280.

Arsenault G. Using a disposable syringe to treat inverted nipples. *Can Fam Physician.* 1997;43:1517-1518.

Chertok I. A pilot study of maternal and term infant outcomes associated with ultrathin nipple shield use. *JOGNN.* 2006; 35(2):265-272.

Chun YS, Taghinia A. Hyperprolactinemia and galactocele formation after augmentation mammoplasty. *Ann Plast Surg.* 2009;62(2):122-123.

Cotterman K. Reverse pressure softening: a simple tool to prepare areola for easier latching during engorgement. *J Human Lact.* 2004;20(2):227-237.

Cox D, et al. Blood and milk prolactin and the rate of milk synthesis in women. *Exp Physiol.* 1996;81:1007-1020.

Cox D, et al. Studies on human lactation: the development of the computerized breast measurement system; 1998; updated 2008. www.biochem.biomedchem.uwa.edu.au/page/69859. Accessed March 1, 2009.

Cregan M, Hartmann P. Computerized breast measurement from conception to weaning: clinical implications. *J Hum Lact.* 1999;15(2):89-96.

Daly S, et al. Degree of breast emptying explains changes in the fat content but not fatty acid composition of human milk. *Exp Physiol.* 1993;78:741-755.

Daly S, Hartmann P. Infant demand and milk supply. Part 2: the short-term control of milk synthesis in lactating women. *J Hum Lact.* 1995;11:27-37.

De Coopman J. Breastfeeding after pituitary resection: support for a theory of autocrine control of milk supply? *J Hum Lact.* 1993;9:35-40.

Del Vecchyo C, et al. Evaluation of breast sensibility using dermatomal somatosensory evoked potentials. *Plast Reconstr Surg.* 2004;113(7):1975-1983.

Dewey K, et al. Risk factors for suboptimal infant breastfeeding behavior, delayed onset of lactation, and excess neonatal weight loss. *Pediatrics.* 2003;12(3 Pt 1):607-619.

Dewitt JE. Management of nipple discharge by clinical findings. *Am J Surg.* 1985;149:789-792.

Godwin Y, et al. Investigation into the possible cause of subjective decreased sensory perception in the nipple–areola complex of women with macromastia. *Plast Reconstr Surg.* 2004;113(6):1598-1606.

Hartmann P, et al. Physiology of lactation in preterm mothers: initiation and maintenance. *Pediatric Annals.* 2003;32(5): 351-355.

Hill P., Humenick S. The occurrence of breast engorgement. *J Hum Lact.* 1994;10:79-86.

Huggins K, et al. Markers of lactation insufficiency: a study of 34 mothers. In: *Current Issues in Clinical Lactation.* Sudbury, MA: Jones and Bartlett; 2000:25-35.

Ing R, et al. Unilateral breastfeeding and breast cancer. *Lancet.* 1977;2:124-127.

Kalbhen C, et al. Mammography in the evaluation of nipple inversion. *AJR Am J Roentgenol.* 1998;170(1):117-121.

Kent J. Breastfeeding patterns: Variations on a theme. Paper presented at: Human Lactation Conference; June 10, 2003; Amarillo, TX.

Kent J. How breastfeeding works. *Midwifery Women's Health.* 2007;52(6):564-570.

Kent J, et al. Volume and frequency of breastfeedings and fat content of breast milk throughout the day. *Pediatrics.* 2006;117(3):e387-e395.

Kesaree N, et al. Treatment of inverted nipples using a disposable syringe. *J Hum Lact.* 1993;9:27-29.

Kline TS, Lash SR. The bleeding nipple of pregnancy and postpartum: a cytologic and histologic study. *Acta Cytolog* (Phila.). 1964;8:336-340.

Knight C, et al. Local control of mammary development and function. *Rev Reprod.* 1998;3(2):104-112.

Lafrenier R. Bloody nipple discharge during pregnancy: a rationale for conservative treatment. *J Surg Oncol.* 1990;43:228-230.

Lawrence R, Lawrence R. *Breastfeeding: A Guide for the Medical Profession.* 6th ed. St. Louis, MO: Mosby; 2005.

Lin W, et al. A late complication of augmentation mammoplasty by polyacrylamide hydrogel injection: ultrasound and magnetic resonance imaging findings of huge galactocele formation in a puerperal woman with pathological correlation. *Breast J.* 2008;14(6):584-587.

Love S, Barsky S. Anatomy of the nipple and breast ducts revisited. *Cancer.* 2004;101:1947-1957.

Love S, Lindsey K. *Dr. Susan Love's Breast Book.* 4th ed. Cambridge, MA: Da Capo Press; 2005.

MAIN Trial Collaborative Group. Preparing for breast feeding: treatment of inverted and nonprotractile nipples in pregnancy. *Midwifery.* 1994;10:200-214.

Matsunaga T, et al. Intraductal biopsy for diagnosis and treatment of intraductal lesions of the breast. *Cancer.* 2004; 101(10):2164-2169.

McGeorge D. The "Nipplette": an instrument for the non-surgical correction of inverted nipples. *Br J Plast Surg*. 1994; 47(1):46-49.

Meier P, et al. Nipple shields for preterm infants: effect on milk transfer and duration of breastfeeding. *J Hum Lact*. 2000;16(2):106-113.

National Cancer Institute (NCI). Paget's disease of the nipple: questions and answers. www.cancer.gov/cancertopics/factsheet/Sites-Types/pagets-breast June 27, 2005. Accessed March 1, 2009.

Neifert M, et al. The influence of breast surgery, breast appearance, and pregnancy-induced breast changes on lactation sufficiency as measured by infant weight gain. *Birth*. 1990;17:31-38.

Nickell W, Skelton J. Breast fat and fallacies: more than 100 years of anatomical fantasy. *J Hum Lact*. 2005;21(2):126-130.

Park H, et al. The prevalence of congenital inverted nipple. *Aesthetic Plast Surg*. 1999;23(2):144-146.

Peaker M, Wilde C. Feedback control of milk secretion from milk. *J Mammary Gland Biol Neoplasia*. 1996;1(3):307-315.

Ramsay D. Ultrasound imaging of the sucking mechanics of the term infant. Paper presented at: Human Lactation: Current Research and Clinical Implications; October 22, 2004; Amarillo, TX.

Ramsay D, et al. Breast anatomy redefined by ultrasound in the lactating breast. In: *Conference Proceedings of the Australian Society for Ultrasound in Medicine*. September 2003; Perth, Australia.

Ramsay D, et al. Ultrasound imaging of milk ejection in the breast of lactating women. *Pediatrics*. 2004;113(2):361-367.

Ramsay D, et al. Anatomy of the lactating breast redefined with ultrasound imaging. *J Anat*. 2005a;206:525.

Ramsay D, et al. The use of ultrasound to characterize milk ejection in women using an electric breast pump. *J Human Lact*. 2005b;21:421-428.

Ramsay D, et al. Milk flow rates can be used to identify and investigate milk ejection in women expressing breast milk using an electric breast pump. *Breastfeed Med*. 2006;1:14-23.

Rusby J, et al. Breast duct anatomy in the human nipple: three-dimensional patterns and clinical implications. *Breast Cancer Res Treat*. 2007;106(2):171-179.

Saber A, et al. The milk rejection sign: a natural tumor marker. *Am Surg*. 1996;62:998-999.

Sarhadi N, et al. An anatomical study of the nerve supply of the breast, including the nipple and areola. *Br J Plast Surg*. 1996;49(3):156-164.

Sarhadi NS, et al. Nerve supply of the breast specific reference to the nipple and areola: Sir Astley Cooper revisited. *Clin Anat*. 1997;10(4):283-288.

Sauter E, et al. The association of bloody nipple discharge with breast pathology. *Surgery*. 2004;136(4):780-785.

Schackmuth E, et al. Milk fistula: a complication after core breast biopsy. *Am J Roentgenol*. 1993;161:961-962.

Silen W, et al. *Atlas of Techniques in Breast Surgery*. Philadelphia/New York: Lippincott-Raven; 1996:18-19.

Smith D. Montgomery's areolar tubercle: a light microscopic study. *Arch Pathol Lab Med*. 1982;106:60-63.

Stevens K, et al. The ultrasound appearances of galactocoeles. *Br J Radiol*. 1997;70:239-241.

Sun J, et al. The neuro-vascular anatomical study of breast and its signification in reduction mammaplasty [Chinese]. *Zhonghua Zheng Xing Wai Ke Za Zhi*. 2004;20(4):277-279.

Taylor SE, et al. Female responses to stress: tend and befriend, not fight or flight. *Psychol Rev*. 2000;107(3):411-429.

Turner RA, et al. Preliminary research on plasma oxytocin in normal cycling women: investigating emotion and interpersonal distress. *Psychiatry*. 1999;62(2):97-113.

Virdi V, et al. Rusty-pipe syndrome. *Indian Pediatr*. 2001;38(8): 931-932.

Waller H. *The Breasts and Breast Feeding*. London: Wm. Heinemann Medical Books; 1957.

West D, San Antonio Breastfeeding Coalition. Breastfeeding after breast surgeries. Low Milk Supply Conference: February 21, 2009; San Antonio, TX.

Widstrom A, Thingstrom-Paulsson J. The position of the tongue during rooting reflexes elicited in newborn infants before the first suckle. *Acta Paediatr*. 1993;82:281-283.

Wilde C, et al. Autocrine regulation of milk secretion. *Biochem Soc Symp*. 1998;63:81-90.

Wilson-Clay B. Clinical use of nipple shields. *J Hum Lact*. 1996;12:279-285.

Wilson-Clay B, Hoover K. *The Breastfeeding Atlas*. 4th ed. Austin, TX: Lactnews Press; 2008.

Woolridge M, Fisher C. Colic, overfeeding, and symptoms of lactose malabsorption in the breast-fed baby: A possible artifact of feed management? *Lancet*. 1988;ii:382-384.

Maternal Health and Nutrition

A basic understanding of nutrition and its effect on health helps us make informed food choices and develop sound eating practices. A healthy diet is especially important to a pregnant woman and her developing fetus, and later as the mother breastfeeds her baby. Mothers will benefit from receiving nutrition information and guidance in selecting and preparing foods. You can help women understand the effects of their diets on breastfeeding and nutritional factors that may cause them to feel hungry or fatigued. Childbirth, breastfeeding and parenting classes offer excellent opportunities to discuss nutrition.

∼ Key Terms

Alcohol	Intrauterine growth
Allergen	retardation (IUGR)
Amino acids	Iron
Anemia	Kilocalorie (kcal)
Arachidonic acid	Macrosomia
Basal metabolic rate	Minerals
Body mass index (BMI)	Nutrients
Caffeine	Proteins
Calcium	Salt
Complex carbohydrates	Serum
Fat-soluble vitamins	Simple carbohydrate
Fat stores	Spina bifida
Fats	Sustainable farming
Food pyramid	Vegetarian diet
Foodborne disease	Vitamins
Genetically modified food	Water
Hemoglobin	Water-soluble vitamins

∼ Nutrition Education

Experiences we have in childhood relating to food consumption affect our perspective on food choices in later life. Habits that become firmly engrained are often difficult to change. Pregnancy and lactation are times in a woman's life when she is receptive to making changes in her eating habits so as to improve her health. A mother's body reserves, plus the food she eats, provide the energy and nutrients her baby needs to grow and develop. Inadequate nutrition due to improper diet can restrict healthy fetal growth by reducing the number or size of fetal cells, including brain cells. Severe maternal malnutrition due to critically low nourishment can contribute to fetal death. Those who care for women prenatally can help ensure the health of their babies by guiding them in sound nutrition principles.

Proper nutritional intake during pregnancy increases the likelihood that women will give birth to healthy, full-term babies. A healthy diet helps women keep their bodies in prime condition for labor, delivery, and lactation. Mothers often have questions about foods to eat or avoid when breastfeeding. An overly restrictive diet may put the mother or baby at nutritional risk. In addition, arbitrary dietary restrictions while breastfeeding may increase the risk of early weaning.

If you are the first person to notice possible dietary risk factors, you can refer the woman to a nutritionist or dietician for assessment. Referral is appropriate for women with a body mass index (BMI) of less than 19.8 (very underweight) or more than 26 (overweight), teen mothers who experienced menarche less than 4 years before giving birth, and women with medical conditions such as diabetes, bariatric surgery, or metabolic disorders (International Lactation Consultant Association [ILCA], 2007).

Increasing Obesity Rates

Research suggests that poor maternal nutrition during pregnancy increases the risk for the baby to develop chronic diseases later in life, such as obesity, hypertension, cardiovascular disease, and diabetes later in life (Zambrano, 2009; Pinheiro et al., 2008). Collectively, this cluster of diseases is called metabolic syndrome.

A lack of nutrition education combined with unhealthy practices has led to an increasing awareness of and alarm over the prevalence of obesity in Americans of all ages. During the past two decades, obesity rates have increased dramatically in the United States. In 2007, Colorado was the only state in which less than 20 percent of the population was deemed to be obese. Thirty states had obesity rates equal to or greater than 25 percent, and three of those states (Alabama, Mississippi, and Tennessee) had rates equal to or greater than 30 percent (Centers for Disease Control and Prevention [CDC], 2009a).

Obesity is a serious health concern for children and adolescents as well as adults. Obesity rates for children aged 2 to 5 years increased from 5 to 12.4 percent over the past 20 years. Rates for children aged 6 to11 years increased from 6.5 to 17 percent, and from 5 to 17.6 percent for those aged 12 to 19 years (CDC, 2009b; Ogden, et al., 2008). Obese children and adolescents are at increased risk to become obese adults (Whitaker et al., 1997). One study found that 25 percent of obese adults were overweight as children and that if overweight begins before 8 years of age, obesity in adulthood is likely to be more severe (Serdula et al., 1993). The American Academy of Pediatrics (AAP, 2007) calculates that an obese 4-year-old child has a 20 percent chance of becoming an obese adult, and an obese teenager has as much as an 80 percent chance of becoming an obese adult.

Healthcare costs of obesity-related diseases are estimated at $147 billion per year in the United States. America's First Lady, Michelle Obama, introduced an initiative in 2010 to combat obesity, noting that one-third of all children born in 2000 or later will develop diabetes. See Chapter 1 for more discussion on this initiative. Many others will develop obesity-related health problems such as heart disease, high blood pressure, cancer, and asthma (LetsMove.gov, 2010).

Counseling Women Regarding Their Nutritional Needs

Sound nutrition knowledge and effective counseling skills will help you counsel women about their nutritional habits with confidence. Nutritional education is frequently lacking in schools, although students typically are educated about fitness and diet. School cafeterias often display the U.S. Department of Agriculture's (USDA) "food pyramid"—a graphical depiction of the components of a recommended diet. All too often, however, children have few examples of healthy eating that might serve as good models to carry into adult life. In many cases, formal nutrition education ends in primary school, at a time when children do not have enough control over their diets to put the information into practice.

We learn much of what we know about nutrition through the media, and many of those messages consist of product marketing rather than independent analysis. An advertising campaign may tell us that a product has added vitamins, for instance, but does not explain that the additional vitamins replace the natural vitamins lost in processing. Newer issues, such as food content consisting of genetically modified or irradiated foods, may not be revealed (U.S. Department of Energy, Office of Science [USDEOS], 2008). The combination of marketing and limited nutritional education results in many people reaching adulthood with few skills to choose and prepare foods wisely. Health practitioners can help parents distinguish between marketing promotion and unbiased information.

Teachable Moments for Nutrition Counseling

Pregnancy and lactation are times when women are especially receptive to nutrition education. During these peak periods of interest, women typically want to provide their babies with the best nourishment possible. Many women wish to give birth without a lasting change in body image. Others may begin to recognize the close relationship between what they eat and how they feel. This period in a woman's life is a teachable moment—a time when she is most receptive to learning about nutrition. Tapping into mothers' motivating interests can influence a lasting change in their eating habits.

Recognize that every mother has a history of food choices, eating patterns, and cultural beliefs about food. Some women may be well educated in terms of nutrition, so it is important to make an effort to determine each mother's nutritional awareness before offering suggestions. Tap into your listening skills, and ask relevant questions so that you can offer information and suggestions based on each woman's needs and unique situation. As part of your counseling, you can encourage parents to assume responsibility for their health care and that of their children without lecturing mothers about what they "should" eat. Health and a feeling of well-being are closely related to nutrition, and education in this area can help parents make responsible decisions.

Of course, one person's definition of a "healthy diet" may differ from that of another person. You need to give mothers nutritional information based on sound, accurate principles. This educational content should not reflect your own individual preferences or dietary practices, fad diets, or unproven theories that can be detrimental to a woman's health, especially that of a pregnant or breastfeeding mother. By sharing basic nutritional information, you can minimize confusion or possible conflict and help mothers apply the information to their eating practices.

Dietary guidelines are jointly issued and updated every 5 years by the U.S. Department of Agriculture and Department of Health and Human Services. Current guidelines are available at www.dietaryguidelines.gov.

～ The Basic Nutrients

A basic understanding of nutrients and their function in the body is necessary for realizing the importance of good nutrition. All foods contain nutrients. A nutrient is any nourishing substance in food that is released by digestion and then absorbed and used to promote body function. Two types of nutrients are distinguished: macronutrients (protein, fats, and carbohydrates) and micronutrients (vitamins and minerals). When counseling a mother about her diet, concentrate on foods rather than the individual nutrients that make up those foods. Eating all of the nutrients required by the body in proper quantities leads to good nutrition. Each nutrient has a specific function and relationship to the body, and all nutrients must be present in the proper quantities to maintain health and a feeling of well-being.

Carbohydrates

Most foods contain carbohydrates, which the body breaks down into simple sugars. Carbohydrates are the main source of energy for all body functions and activity; they also help to regulate protein and fat metabolism. The body needs carbohydrates in sufficient quantity so that it can avoid relying on protein as an energy source, which in turn allows protein to perform other important body functions. The body converts excess carbohydrates in the diet into fat and stores it. Two major types of carbohydrates are found in foods: simple and complex.

Simple Carbohydrates

Simple carbohydrates include sugar, jams, honey, chocolate, and other sweets. They are a thin strip on the right side of the USDA food pyramid—a size that indicates we need very little of these foods in our diet. Sugary foods can cause a sudden rise in blood sugar level. After only a short time, the blood sugar level drops rapidly, which can create a craving for more food. When consumed in the absence of nutritional foods, food that contains large amounts of simple carbohydrates may cause fatigue, dizziness, nervousness, or headache.

Complex Carbohydrates

Complex carbohydrates include starches such as cereals, rice, breads, crackers, pasta, vegetables, and fruits. These foods are found on the bottom layers of the food pyramid, indicating that they are key components of a healthy diet.

Complex carbohydrates take longer to digest than simple carbohydrates and do not stimulate a craving for more food. In addition, complex carbohydrates such as whole-grain foods and unprocessed vegetables and fruits contain important vitamins and minerals that are often missing in processed foods. Fruits, vegetables, and whole-grain breads and cereals also provide needed fiber.

Proteins

Protein is the major source of building materials for all of the body's internal organs, as well as for muscles, blood, skin, hair, and nails. It is important to the formation of hormones that, among numerous other functions, control sexual development and the production of milk during lactation. Protein is also a source of heat and energy for the body. When the diet provides adequate energy from carbohydrates and fat sources protein can be used for functions other nutrients cannot perform.

Proteins are formed by combining, in many different ways, 22 building blocks called amino acids. The human body can synthesize 14 of these amino acids whereas the diet must supply the remaining 8 in proportions that allow the body to synthesize proteins properly. Foods that contain all 22 of the essential amino acids are known as complete protein foods, whereas those lacking or having extremely low amounts of any of the essential amino acids are called incomplete protein foods.

Dietary sources of protein include meats, eggs, nuts, grains, legumes, and dairy products such as milk and cheese. Most meats and dairy products are complete protein foods with high biological value. In contrast, most vegetable or plant proteins, such as beans and grains, are incomplete protein foods with low biological value. To provide for adequate nutrition, meals need a balance of foods that are weak in an essential amino acid and those that have adequate amounts of the same one. An incomplete protein food makes a complete protein complement when it is combined with other incomplete protein foods that fill in the missing pieces (i.e., the other amino acids). Peanut butter and bread, pasta and cheese, breakfast cereal and milk, and beans and rice are examples of such combinations.

The body constantly builds and repairs tissues. At times of stress, such as during surgery, hemorrhage, or prolonged illness, it is necessary to consume extra protein to meet the body's increased requirements for this function. The 2005 Dietary Reference Intake (DRI) guidelines recommend that women aged 19 to 70 consume 46 grams of protein per day, increasing to 71 grams during pregnancy and lactation (Institute of Medicine [IOM], 2005). In some countries, the official recommendations for protein consumption are slightly lower.

Most women may already be eating sufficient protein. In terms of food, the additional needs during pregnancy and lactation are quite low; a serving of baked beans with a slice of bread, for example, provides 10 extra grams of protein. Women should avoid high protein intake (intake more than twice the recommended amount), as it can overload the kidneys and increase loss of calcium through excretion (Diet-i.com, 2009).

Fats

Fats, the most concentrated source of energy in the diet, act as carriers for the fat-soluble vitamins A, D, E, and K. Fats prolong the process of digestion by slowing down the stomach's emptying, which in turn creates a longer-lasting sensation of fullness after a meal. Fatty acids, which give fats their different flavors, textures, and melting points, are either saturated or unsaturated. A healthy diet should contain a greater amount of unsaturated fats than saturated fats. Saturated fatty acids come primarily from animal sources, such as meat, milk products, and eggs. Unsaturated fatty acids come from vegetables, nuts, and seeds. Fish is a good source of omega fatty acids, although its benefit needs to be weighed against the potential for fish contamination (Guevel et al., 2008).

During digestion, two particular fatty acids—linoleic and alpha-linolenic, which are known as essential fatty acids (EFAs)—are converted into arachidonic acid (AA) and docosahexaenoic acid (DHA), respectively. Sufficient levels of AA and DHA are important for neural and visual development in the fetus. Foods containing large amounts of EFAs include vegetable oils; margarines and salad dressings made from unsaturated oils such as canola; soybean oil (for alpha-linolenic acid); and corn, sunflower, and peanut oils (for linoleic acid). AA is directly available from beef, pork, poultry, and eggs. DHA is available from fatty fish such as mackerel, salmon, and sardines. Encourage women to use a variety of types of oil in addition to animal sources of AA and DHA. A very-low-fat diet is usually not appropriate during pregnancy and lactation (World Health Organization [WHO], 2001).

Manufacturers of artificial infant milk aggressively market DHA supplement for pregnant and lactating women. Martek, the manufacturer of the DHA used in infant formula, sells this substance directly to the public through its consumer website (Martek Biosciences Corporation, 2004, 2009). This marketing plays on women's fears that their own milk is inadequate. You can reassure questioning mothers that, as long as they consume essential fatty acids in their normal diet, no additional DHA supplementation is necessary.

Vitamins

Vitamins are organic substances or groups of related substances that have special biochemical functions in the body. In particular, vitamins convert fats and carbohydrates into energy and help to form bone and tissue. The diet must provide necessary vitamins. Although the body can synthesize some vitamins, it needs adequate amounts of the precursor from the diet to do so. Table 8.1 lists the important functions of each vitamin during pregnancy and lactation.

Generally, breastfeeding women are advised to continue taking their prenatal vitamins throughout lactation. Mothers who regard their foods as being inadequate in vitamin and mineral content may consider taking other prescribed or over-the-counter supplements as well. Encourage women to consult their caregiver before taking supplemental vitamins and minerals during pregnancy or lactation, however. These supplements can be valuable additions to the diet, if needed in special circumstances such as anemia, food intolerance, or allergies. More generally, though, supplements should not replace the proper intake of foods rich in vitamins and minerals. They should be complements to—not substitutes for— good nutrition.

Consumption of excess amounts of some vitamins, such as vitamin A, can be harmful. High doses of vitamin B_6 (600 mg/day) have been reported in older studies to cause lactation suppression (Marcus, 1975; Foukas, 1973). However, a small study in 1976 did not find vitamin B_6 to be effective (Canales et al., 1976). A recent Cochrane Review found bromocriptine and cabergolines to be the most common lactation-suppression agents (Oladapo & Fawole, 2009).

Water-Soluble Vitamins

The body cannot store water-soluble vitamins (the B vitamins and vitamin C), so these nutrients need to be replenished on a daily basis. During lactation, water-soluble vitamins can move easily from maternal blood to milk, so maternal intake can affect the amounts found in milk for most of these vitamins. When mammary tissue reaches saturation in terms of water-soluble vitamin content, levels in the milk reach a plateau for vitamin C, thiamin (B_1), and biotin.

Folic acid contributes to cell growth and reproduction. It functions with vitamins B_{12} and C in the breakdown of proteins and the production of hemoglobin. Folic acid, for which adequate levels are especially important to pregnant women in preventing anemia, can be obtained from leafy green vegetables and whole grains. The U.S. Preventive Services Task Force advocates use of folic acid supplements during childbearing years for all reproductive-aged women to help prevent neural tube defects, including spina bifida (Wolff, 2009).

Excess water-soluble vitamins are excreted through the urine and are not stored in the body. In general, a varied diet that meets women's energy needs will provide sufficient amounts of water-soluble vitamins during lactation. Supplementation is unnecessary unless there is an

TABLE 8.1 Nutrition and Vitamin Chart

Key Nutrient	DRI for Ages 23–50	Important Sources	Important Functions
Water and liquids	N 4 cups P 6–8 cups L 8+ cups	Water, juice, milk	Carries nutrients to and waste products away from cells. Provides fluid for increased blood and amniotic fluid volume. Helps regulate body temperature and aids digestion. *Comments:* Often neglected. Is an important nutrient.
Protein amino acids	N 50 g P 60 g L 64 g	*Animal:* Meat, fish, eggs, milk, cheese, yogurt *Plant:* Dried beans and peas, peanut butter, nuts, whole grains and cereals, soy milk, meat substitutes	Constitutes part of the structure of every tissue cell, such as muscle, blood, and bone. Supports growth and maintains healthy body cells. Constitutes part of enzymes, some hormones, and body fluids. Helps form antibodies that increase resistance to infection. Builds and repairs tissues, helps build blood and amniotic fluid. Supplies energy. *Comments:* Fetal requirements increase by about ½ in late pregnancy as the baby grows.
MINERALS			
Calcium	N 800–1200 mg P 1200 mg L 1200 mg	*Animal:* Milk, cheese, yogurt, egg yolk, whole canned fish, ice cream *Plant:* Whole grains, almonds, filberts, green leafy vegetables	Combines with other minerals within a protein framework to give structure and strength to bones and teeth. Assists in blood clotting. Functions in normal muscle contraction and relaxation and normal nerve transmission. Helps regulate the use of other minerals in the body. *Comments:* Fetal requirements increase by about ⅔ in late pregnancy.
Phosphorus	N 1000 mg P 1200 mg L 1200 mg	*Animal:* Milk, cheese, lean meats	Helps build bones and teeth. *Comments:* Calcium and phosphorus exist in a constant ratio in the blood. An excess of either limits utilization of calcium.
Iron	N 18 mg P 30–60 mg L 18+ mg	*Animal:* Liver, red meats, egg yolk *Plant:* Whole grains, leafy vegetables, nuts, legumes, dried fruits, prune and apple juice	Aids in utilization of energy. Combines with protein to form hemoglobin, the red substance in blood that carries oxygen to and carbon dioxide from the cells. Prevents nutritional anemia and its accompanying fatigue. Increases resistance to infection. Functions as part of enzymes involved in tissue respiration. Provides iron for fetal storage. *Comments:* Fetal requirements increase tenfold in final 6 weeks of pregnancy. Supplement of 30–60 mg of iron daily recommended by National Research Council. Continued supplementation for 2–3 months postpartum is recommended to replenish iron.
Zinc	N 15 mg P 20 mg L 25 mg	*Animal:* Meat, liver, eggs, and seafood, especially oysters	A component of insulin. Important in growth of skeleton and nervous system. *Comments:* Deficiency can cause fetal malformation of skeleton and nervous system.
Iodine	N 150 μcg P 175 μcg L 200 μcg	*Animal:* Seafood *Mineral:* Iodized salt	Helps control the rate of body's energy use, important in thyroxine production. *Comments:* Deficiency may produce goiter in infant.

(Continued)

TABLE 8.1 Nutrition and Vitamin Chart *(Continued)*

Key Nutrient	DRI for Ages 23–50	Important Sources	Important Functions
Magnesium	N 400 mg P 450 mg L 450 mg	*Plant:* Nuts, cocoa, green vegetables, whole grains, dried beans, peas	Co-enzyme in energy and protein metabolism, enzyme activator, tissue growth, cell metabolism, muscle action. *Comments:* Most is stored in bones. Deficiency may produce neuromuscular dysfunctions.
FAT-SOLUBLE VITAMINS			
Vitamin A	N 800 RE P 1000 RE L 1200 RE	*Animal:* Butter, whole milk, cheese, fortified milk, liver *Plant:* Fortified margarine, green and leafy vegetables, orange vegetables, fruits	Assists formation and maintenance of skin and mucous membranes that line body cavities and tracts, such as nasal passages and intestinal tract, thus increasing resistance to infection. Essential in development of enamel-forming cells in gum tissue. Helps bone and tissue growth and cell development. Functions in visual processes, thus promoting healthy eye tissues and eye adaptation in dim light. *Comments:* Is toxic to the fetus in very large amounts. Can be lost with exposure to light.
Vitamin D	N 5 μcg P 10 μcg L 10 μcg	*Animal:* Fortified milk, fish liver oils *Plant:* Fortified margarine, sun on skin	Promotes the absorption of calcium from the digestive tract and the deposition of calcium in the structure of bones and teeth. *Comments:* Toxic to fetus in excessive amounts. Is a stable vitamin.
Vitamin E	N 8 mg P 10 mg L 13 mg	*Plant:* Vegetable oils, leafy vegetables, cereals *Animal:* Meat, eggs, milk	Tissue growth, cell wall integrity, red blood cell integrity. *Comments:* Enhances absorption of Vitamin A.
WATER-SOLUBLE VITAMINS			
B vitamins and folic acid	N 400 μcg P 800 μcg L 600 μcg	*Plant:* Liver, green leafy vegetables, yeast	Hemoglobin synthesis, involved in DNA and RNA synthesis, co-enzyme in synthesis of amino acids. *Comments:* Water-soluble vitamins are interdependent. Deficiency leads to anemia. Can be destroyed in cooking and storage. Supplement of 200–400 μcg/day is recommended by the National Research Council. Oral contraceptive use may reduce serum level of folic acid.
Niacin	N 13 mg P 15 mg L 18 mg	*Animal:* Pork, organ meats *Plant:* Peanuts, beans, peas, enriched grains	Co-enzyme in energy and protein metabolism. *Comments:* Stable; only small amounts are lost in food preparation.
Riboflavin	N 1.2 mg P 1.5 mg L 1.7–1.9 mg	*Animal:* Milk products, liver, red meat *Plant:* Enriched grains	Aids in utilization of energy. Functions as part of a co-enzyme in the production of energy within body cells. Promotes healthy skin, eyes, and clear vision. Protein metabolism. *Comments:* Severe deficiencies lead to reduced growth and congenital malformations. Oral contraceptive use may reduce serum concentrations.

TABLE 8.1   Nutrition and Vitamin Chart *(Continued)*

Key Nutrient	DRI for Ages 23–50	Important Sources	Important Functions
B$_1$-Thiamin	N 1.0 mg P 1.4 mg L 1.5 mg	**Animal:** Pork, beef, liver **Plant:** Whole grains, legumes	Coenzyme in energy and protein metabolism. **Comments:** Its availability limits the rate at which energy from glucose is produced.
B$_6$-Pyrodoxine	N 1.6 mg P 2.2 mg L 2.1 mg	**Plant:** Unprocessed cereals, grains, wheat germ, bran, nuts, seeds, legumes, corn	Important in amino acid metabolism and protein synthesis. Fetus requires more for growth. **Comments:** Excessive amounts may reduce milk production in lactating women.
B$_{12}$	N 2.0 μcg P 2.2 μcg L 2.6 μcg	**Animal:** Milk, cheese, eggs, meat, liver, fish **Plant:** Fortified soy milk, cereals, meat substitutes	Assists in the maintenance of nerve tissue. Coenzyme in protein metabolism. Important in formation of red blood cells. **Comments:** Deficiency leads to anemia and central nervous system damage. Is manufactured by microorganisms in intestinal tract. Oral contraceptive use may reduce serum concentrations.
Vitamin C	N 60 mg P 80 mg L 100 mg	**Plant:** Citrus fruits, berries, melons, tomatoes, chili peppers, green vegetables, potatoes	Important tissue formation and integrity. "Cement" substance in connective and vascular substances. Increases iron absorption. **Comments:** Large doses in pregnancy may create a larger than normal need in infant.

N–nonpregnant; P–pregnant; L–lactating; DRI–Dietary Reference Intake.

Source: Worthington-Roberts, B. Williams SR. *Nutrition in Pregnancy and Lactation*, 6th ed. New York: McGraw-Hill; 1996. Reprinted by permission.

The Recommended Daily Allowance (RDA) or Dietary Reference Intake (DRI) refers to the intake of a nutrient that fulfills the needs of 97.5 percent of healthy people in the population. It does not necessarily reflect the lowest acceptable intake for the majority of the population. In fact, it exceeds the actual requirements of most individuals within a population. As individuals have a range of requirements, these amounts must be used with care when referring to an individual's diet.

established nutritional risk for the mother. Further information on vitamin B$_{12}$ and vegetarian diets appears later in this chapter.

Fat-Soluble Vitamins

Unlike water-soluble vitamins, fat-soluble vitamins (A, D, E, and K) are stored in the body's fatty tissues. Vitamin A contributes to the growth of the skeleton and promotes healthy mucous membranes and vision. Vitamin K is essential for blood clotting. One form exists in green leafy vegetables, and another form is derived from bacteria in the gut. Although vitamin K deficiency in adults is rare, infants' stores at birth are low, which can lead to a risk of hemorrhagic disease in newborns. Maternal supplementation during the final weeks of pregnancy may reduce the risk. Infants usually receive vitamin K routinely at birth (Greer et al., 1997).

Vitamin D is unique in that diet is not its only source; that is, the body can manufacture vitamin D under the influence of sunlight. Low maternal levels of vitamin D during pregnancy, however, can result in a corresponding deficiency in the infant. Women at highest risk for this problem are those who do not consume milk or fortified margarine, who regularly avoid sunlight or spend little time outdoors, and who wear clothes that cover most of their skin. Women with dark skin coloring are at an even greater risk (Hirsch, 2007; Good Mojab, 2003). The baby's body stores accumulate during gestation; thus, if the mother has low levels of vitamin D, the baby will be born with low levels.

A regular short walk outdoors in sunlight, starting before or during pregnancy, can benefit both the mother and her baby in terms of their vitamin D level. Supplementing pregnant women and mothers who are deficient in this vitamin improves the nutritional status of both mother and baby as well. Supplementing the baby alone means the woman remains deficient, which places the next baby at risk for deficiency. Over-supplementation with vitamin D poses a risk to the baby, however, and can result in death. The AAP guidelines for infant supplementation with vitamin D have caused concern in the lactation community for this reason (Gartner, 2003).

Many recommendations for vitamin D were developed before scientists discovered that vitamin D is a pro-steroid, which the body converts into another form of steroid that circulates in the blood and is used in biological processes. Several researchers believe that the present DRI for vitamin D is inadequate, especially for dark-skinned populations and where body exposure to the sun is limited, such as in the Middle East. They call for much higher doses of 2000–4000 IUs per day, and still more during lactation (Saadi et al., 2009; Basile et al., 2006; Wagner et al., 2006; Hollis & Wagner, 2004a, 2004b). Given that the human body is meant to produce vitamin D through sunlight exposure, vitamin D deficiency is actually sunlight deficiency. See Chapter 9 for more information about vitamin D.

Minerals

When present in the body in appropriate levels, minerals contribute to a person's overall mental and physical well-being. They are involved in maintaining physiological processes, strengthening skeletal structures, and preserving the vigor of the heart, brain, muscles, and nervous system. In addition, minerals play important roles in the production of hormones and help maintain the delicate water balance essential to the proper functioning of mental and physical processes. The diet must supply essential minerals. A varied and mixed diet of animal and vegetable origin that meets the recommended energy and protein needs will typically furnish adequate minerals. Specific minerals and their functions are listed in Table 8.1. Three minerals—calcium, iron, and salt—are especially important during pregnancy and lactation, and are discussed here in more detail.

Calcium

Calcium is an important dietary mineral that gives bones their rigidity and teeth their hardness. This mineral also has a role in blood clotting and in controlling the action of the heart, muscles, and nerves. Consumption of adequate amounts of calcium will maintain the mother's bones and provide for fetal bone development. Increased maternal intestinal absorption during pregnancy provides the additional calcium needed at that time. Consumption of vitamin D along with calcium promotes optimal absorption and use of calcium.

Although pregnancy and lactation place high demands on the mother's body in relation to calcium, lactating women are no more prone to osteoporosis than those who have never been pregnant or have not lactated. Studies show that calcium is mobilized from the mother's bones during lactation, with a recovery of bone mass occurring after weaning (Chan et al., 2005). Overall, breastfeeding appears to increase the mother's bone mineral density, thereby helping to prevent osteoporosis (Sadat-Ali et al., 2005; Karlsson et al., 2001; Henderson et al., 2000). One study found a correlation between length of breastfeeding and decreased bone density (Dursun et al., 2006).

Pregnant women and mothers need adequate calcium intake, particularly women younger than the age of 25 who are still experiencing an increase in their bone content. Women who do not consume milk can obtain calcium through the sources listed in Table 8.2. Women who avoid all milk products must make up for the other nutrients available in milk—protein, vitamins, and calories—through consumption of other calcium-rich foods. Pregnant or lactating women who do not eat enough

TABLE 8.2 Good Sources of Calcium

Food	Calcium (mgs per serving)
Yogurt, plain (8 oz)	415
Cheddar cheese (2 oz)	408
Sardines, drained (3 oz)	372
American cheese (2 oz)	348
Yogurt, fruit-flavored (8 oz)	345
Milk, whole, low-fat, or skim (8 oz)	300
Watercress (1 cup chopped)	189
Chocolate pudding, instant (1/2 cup)	187
Collards (1/2 cup cooked)	179
Buttermilk pancakes (3–4 inches)	174
Pink salmon, canned (3 oz)	167
Tofu (4 oz)	145
Turnip greens (1/2 cup cooked)	134
Kale (1/2 cup cooked)	103
Shrimp, canned (3 oz)	99
Ice cream (1/2 cup)	88
Okra (1/2 cup cooked)	74
Rutabaga, mashed (1/2 cup cooked)	71
Broccoli (1/2 cup cooked)	68
Soybeans (1/2 cup cooked)	66
Cottage cheese (1/2 cup)	63
Bread, white or whole wheat (2 slices)	48

calcium-rich foods may need calcium supplements to provide the recommended 800–1200 mg per day. Calcium carbonate is the safest supplement. Several brands of bone meal and dolomite contain high levels of lead or other toxic metals, so urge women to avoid these products.

Iron

Additional iron is needed during pregnancy to support the growing fetus and placenta and to increase the mother's red cell mass. Low levels of iron can affect the oxygen-carrying capacity of the blood and cause a woman to feel tired constantly, even after adequate rest. An anemic woman has poor tolerance to blood loss and is at greater risk in the event of surgery. The effect of maternal iron deficiency on the fetus is unclear. Iron deficiency is most common in women with low socioeconomic status, multiple gestations, and limited education. These women are also at risk of poor pregnancy outcome, independent of iron deficiency.

When iron stores are low, the body absorbs more available iron. During pregnancy and the early months of breastfeeding when a woman is not menstruating, the reduction in blood loss partially offsets her additional needs. Recommended dietary intake of iron varies among different countries, as do practices regarding supplementation. Women who begin pregnancy with sufficient iron stores and eat a varied diet do not need iron supplements. Many doctors prescribe supplements routinely on the assumption that prepregnancy stores are low. If women were to have a blood test prior to conception, they could begin treatment for anemia before becoming pregnant.

Dietary iron exists in two forms. *Heme iron* comes from meat, poultry, and fish and is easily absorbed. *Non-heme iron* comes from vegetables, iron-enriched cereals, and whole grains. Adding small amounts of heme iron or foods containing vitamin C to the meal can improve iron absorption from non-heme sources. Iron absorption from non-heme food sources can be reduced with the consumption of tea and coffee; phylates in legumes and bran; and oxalates in spinach, beet greens, chard, rhubarb, and sweet potato. Excess calcium, both in food and supplements, can reduce iron absorption as well.

Some women avoid iron supplements due to gastrointestinal effects such as heartburn, nausea, constipation, and diarrhea. Effective dietary counseling can help these women improve their iron intake and absorption from foods. Supplements may be better tolerated when taken at bedtime and should be consumed with water or juice, and not with milk, tea, or coffee. During lactation, iron levels in the mother's milk remain steady and are unrelated to maternal iron status. Nevertheless, mothers should continue to pay attention to their iron intake to rebuild their stores.

Salt

As pregnancy progresses, the placenta needs increased blood flow to work efficiently. During a typical pregnancy, a woman's blood volume increases by more than 40 percent to meet this need. Although salt usually causes the body to retain fluid in the bloodstream, pregnancy is one condition in which the body actually requires *more* salt so that it can function well. In the past, physicians placed restrictions on pregnant women's salt intake in an attempt to control weight and reduce water retention. Such routine salt restriction during pregnancy is not beneficial and may even be harmful (Franx et al., 1999). Most pregnant women can continue to consume the same amount of salt as is recommended for the general population. It is not advisable that anyone have excessive salt intake, including pregnant women.

Water

Water is the most abundant—and by far the most important—nutrient in the body. It is responsible for and involved in nearly every body process. Most foods contain water, which is absorbed by the body during digestion. Fruits and vegetables are especially good sources of chemically pure water. The average adult female body contains 50–55 percent water (approximately 30 quarts) and loses about 2 quarts daily through perspiration and excretion.

A woman needs to consume adequate water to supply her fetus or breastfeeding infant with adequate fluids. Her consumption of additional water-containing foods as part of the normal increase in food amounts eaten during these periods, as well as her natural sense of thirst, will usually provide the additional water she needs. Sometimes lactating women fail to respond to their increased thirst. Having a beverage next to them when they nurse their baby will remind them to drink to satisfy their thirst. A woman needs approximately 6 to 8 cups of fluid per day during pregnancy and lactation, to ensure that her body has enough fluid to function and to avoid constipation (see Table 8.1). Thirst should dictate water consumption.

There are no data to support the suggestion that increasing a mother's fluid intake increases milk volume. In fact, women who consume excessive amounts of fluid actually produce less milk and their babies gain less weight (Dusdieker et al., 1985). Likewise, research does not support the contention that restricting fluids decreases milk volume (Illingworth et al., 1986). When fluids are restricted, the mother will experience a decrease in urine output, not in milk production (Lawrence & Lawrence, 2005). Mothers can monitor the adequacy of fluid intake by observing their urine. Except for the first morning void, the mother's urine should be clear to light yellow. If her urine appears more concentrated, she can increase her fluid intake throughout the day.

～ Nutrition in Pregnancy and Lactation

A woman's good nutritional status prior to conception and her continuing adequate nutritional intake during pregnancy contribute to a healthy pregnancy and delivery of a healthy baby. From infancy, the female body is developing toward childbearing. Under-nutrition as a child can result in short stature and a small pelvis, thereby increasing the risk of pregnancy complications. Throughout childhood, the body builds up its stores of contaminants such as pesticides and heavy metals, which in turn has implications when it comes time for childbearing. In an ongoing cycle, healthy babies need healthy mothers, and healthy mothers result from a healthy childhood. Thus, as a lactation consultant who performs nutritional counseling, your influence can extend to increase the overall health of the community, not just that of pregnant women, mothers, and infants.

Preconception Nutrition

When you see women prior to conception or between pregnancies, encourage them to eat a healthy, varied diet and to aim for the recommended weight range. Either a very low weight or a very high weight could decrease a woman's ability to conceive. Weight changes should be gradual—1 to 2 pounds per week—rather than the result of a crash diet. Similarly, an adequate and varied diet, correction of grossly abnormal body weight, and at most a moderate alcohol intake by the male partner can assist in conception and development of a healthy baby. In contrast, maternal alcohol intake can have serious effects on the baby, so women who are planning a pregnancy are encouraged to reduce or cease their consumption of alcohol. Healthcare providers often check iron levels before pregnancy, thereby ensuring that treatment for anemia can begin early if levels are low. A folic acid supplement is frequently recommended both prior to conception and during the first 3 months of pregnancy to reduce the risk of neural tube defects in the developing fetus.

Nutrition During Pregnancy

A woman needs an increased amount of most nutrients during pregnancy. Because there is potential for inadequate intake of folate, calcium, vitamin D, iron, and essential fatty acids in some groups of women, these nutrients need special attention during pregnancy. A woman who has been well nourished throughout her life may not need to make changes to her diet during pregnancy. By comparison, for a woman who has been poorly nourished prior to conception, pregnancy may provide an opportunity to improve her diet to promote a healthy outcome for her pregnancy.

Fetal growth may affect later adult health. For example, intrauterine growth retardation (IUGR) is associated with increased risk to the infant of coronary heart disease, stroke, diabetes, and high blood pressure in adult life. The underlying factor in this case may be restricted fetal growth followed by rapid postnatal "catch-up growth" (Barker, 2002; Robinson & Barker, 2002; Lumbers et al., 2001). Large size at birth, known as macrosomia, is associated with increased risk of diabetes and cardiovascular disease in later life and an increased risk of some cancers. Maternal insulin-dependent diabetes or gestational diabetes increases the risk for macrosomia and other infant health problems. Optimal birth weight and length affects both the child's health immediately after birth and a propensity to develop diet-related chronic disease (WHO, 2003).

Nutrition During Lactation

Sound nutritional practices will continue to enhance the well-being of the entire family long after pregnancy. Breastfeeding mothers, for example, need to recognize the effect their diet has on their health. An inadequate diet or irregular eating pattern can affect how a mother feels and acts and how she views herself and the world. This, in turn, may compromise her ability to cope with her baby and with other family members and friends.

Mothers do not need to consume special foods to maintain high-quality milk production. The normal healthy diet recommended for an average adult generally suffices to meet most needs. A very young mother, a woman who is carrying or nursing two or more babies, or a pregnant woman who is nursing another child may need to increase her food intake, however. These women can meet their needs by increasing their serving sizes, adding more foods at mealtimes, or eating extra foods between meals. Women in a wide variety of circumstances are able to produce milk of sufficient quantity and quality to support growth and promote the health of infants, even when the mother's supply of nutrients is limited (IOM, 1991).

Weight Changes in Pregnancy and Lactation

Attempts to restrict weight gain in pregnancy can be potentially harmful to the fetus and mother in some circumstances. There is a positive association between weight gain during pregnancy and fat concentration in the mother's milk. Therefore, when fat stores laid down in pregnancy are minimal, milk fat content may decrease. The study that reported these results developed no parameters to assess the minimum level of acceptable weight gain (Michaelsen et al., 1994).

Prepregnancy weight should determine a woman's target weight gain in pregnancy. Women older than 35 years of age may have a lower basal metabolic rate and may not require as great an increase in energy intake as younger women while pregnant. A woman's target weight gain based on prepregnancy weight (IOM, 1991) is:

- Underweight (BMI of less than 19.8): 28–40 pounds
- Normal weight (BMI of 19.8–26.0): 25–35 pounds
- Overweight (BMI of 26–29): 15–25 pounds
- Obese (BMI of more than 29): Approximately 13 pounds

Lactation uses energy from body stores and the mother's diet, with an average weight loss of 1–2 pounds per month for a mother with a healthy diet and normal physical activity. If the mother's intake exceeds her needs, or if she eats large amounts of sweet foods in place of more nutritious foods, she will likely gain weight during lactation. Such practices can also prevent a woman from consuming the vitamins, minerals, and other nutrients her body needs.

To reduce her energy intake, the mother can substitute skim milk for whole milk, unsweetened yogurt for other dessert-type foods, and low-calorie fluids for higher-calories options. Making choices of lean meat, fewer eggs, and less cheese will all help to reduce fat intake, thereby decreasing calorie consumption. A mother can add more foods to her diet if she begins losing weight too rapidly or if she becomes easily fatigued.

Dieting While Breastfeeding

Many women consider "going on a diet" while breastfeeding. Well-nourished women who reduce their caloric intake modestly can achieve gradual weight reduction and continued appropriate infant growth (Butte et al., 2005; McCrory, 2001; Lovelady et al., 2000). Well-nourished, healthy women can safely lose approximately 1.1 pounds (0.45–0.5 kg) per week. At this rate of weight loss, they should not experience any adverse effect on milk production, fat content in their milk, or infant growth (Dewey, 1993; Dusdieker et al., 1994). One study found that short-term dieting, coupled with aerobic exercise, did not affect milk production. A combination of exercise and diet to achieve weight loss is preferable to dieting alone because the latter reduces maternal lean body mass (McCrory et al., 1999). While this amount of weight loss is appropriate after lactation is established, caloric intake should not go below 1800 kilocalories (kcal) per day. In particular, liquid diets and diet medications should be avoided (Dewey & McCrory, 1994).

A healthy diet low in carbohydrates is compatible with breastfeeding. The mother should continue to eat fruits and vegetables and a limited amount of whole grains. To lose weight, she can eliminate high-carbohy-drate foods such as sugar, flour, breads, cakes, pasta, junk foods, desserts, potatoes, and rice. Limiting carbohydrates decreases appetite, however, so mothers need to ensure adequate caloric intake on this type of diet regimen.

Moderate, regular physical activity is part of a healthy lifestyle that can be incorporated into the postpartum period. An increase in physical activity can be achieved by using stairs instead of an elevator, parking farther from the building entrance when shopping, going for a walk with the baby, or participating in more structured exercise programs. Exercising four to six times per week, beginning 6 to 8 weeks postpartum, is safe for most women. The baby's acceptance of the mother's post-exercise milk does not appear to be a problem in most cases (Dewey et al., 1994). A mother who is considering a change in diet or exercise is encouraged to discuss her plans with her doctor or midwife prior to or at her postpartum check-up. Women who restrict their food intake may need multivitamin and mineral supplements.

Breastfeeding appears to contribute to a mother's postpartum weight loss, with one study noting larger reductions in hip circumference and greater weight loss at one month postpartum when mothers breastfed. At 6 months, changes were similar in all groups studied, regardless of infant feeding method (Kramer et al., 1993). Another study found that in the first three months after giving birth, breastfeeding mothers lose weight at the same rate as their formula feeding counterparts. In contrast, between 3 and 3 months postpartum, there was a significantly greater weight reduction when breastfeeding. Between months 1 and 12, the average weight loss was 4.5 pounds (2 kg) more in breastfeeding mothers than in formula feeding mothers. There was also a reduction in fat over the triceps area in breastfeeding mothers between months 9 and 12 that was not seen in formula feeding mothers (Dewey et al., 1993).

Postpartum weight loss occurs gradually and more easily in the normal course of breastfeeding and should not take place too quickly. Weight loss can be a significant issue for women, particularly in the postpartum period. Women above the normal range for BMI at 1 month postpartum were found to stop breastfeeding sooner, with no explanation for the early weaning (Rutishauser & Carlin, 1992). Overweight or obese women, especially first-time mothers, have a lower prolactin response to suckling and experience delays in stage II lactogenesis (Hilson et al., 2004; Rasmussen & Kjolhede, 2004). The higher progesterone levels contained in fat tissue may inhibit prolactin effects.

If you encounter women with eating disorders such as anorexia nervosa or bulimia nervosa, recognize your limitations and refer them for specialized help. Anorexia is the deliberate restriction of calories, to the point of starvation. A sign of this condition may be a very thin woman who complains about being "fat" even though she is clearly underweight. Women who are bulimic overfeed (binge) and then force themselves to vomit. They may use laxatives, diuretics, and extreme exercise to prevent gaining weight (National Eating Disorders Association [NEDA], 2009). These mothers may seem obsessed about their infants' feeding and elimination behaviors. If you observe these signs in your interactions with a mother, it may be appropriate to ask her about her eating habits and any history of an eating disorder.

∼ Making Healthy Food Choices

Women who receive practical, specific food suggestions are more likely to make healthy choices in their dietary practices. Basing their food selections and meal planning on nutritional guidelines will help improve their diets. In addition, an awareness of food labels, additives, and processing will help them to avoid unhealthy choices. Understanding the nutritional causes of hunger and fatigue can motivate them to choose dietary practices that will enhance their health and well-being. Healthy eating is compatible with limited budgets and special diets such as vegetarianism (USDA, 2007b). Sharing the information presented in this section will empower women to incorporate wise food choices into their lifestyles.

Industrialization has resulted in food being grown and processed in fewer locations and traveling farther to reach consumers (Sustainable Table, 2009). Moreover, there is growing concern about genetically modified food, irradiated food, environmental contaminants, bacteria outbreaks in food, and unhealthy practices in food processing. To counteract these trends, many families are increasingly consuming produce from local farmers markets, home gardens, and sustainable farms that maintain their productivity and usefulness to society indefinitely (Ikerd, 1990). The worldwide economic downturn in 2009 brought renewed interest in home gardening and local support for food growers as a means to save money and improve the quality of food in a family's diet. For counselors, educating and encouraging pregnant women and new mothers about a healthy lifestyle takes advantage of a unique teachable moment in their lives.

The Food Pyramid

The most widely used illustration of a healthy diet is the USDA's food pyramid, which groups foods with similar nutrient content (see Figure 8.1). The pyramid shows how much of each food group should be present in the diet, with proportions being depicted relative to their size on the pyramid. The USDA's MyPyramid tool enables users

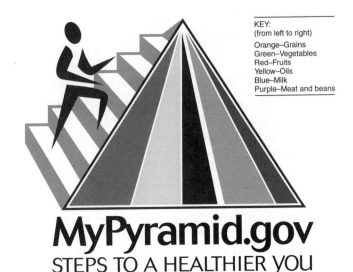

KEY:
(from left to right)
Orange—Grains
Green—Vegetables
Red—Fruits
Yellow—Oils
Blue—Milk
Purple—Meat and beans

FIGURE 8.1   The food pyramid.
Source: U.S. Department of Agriculture, www.MyPyramid.gov

to develop a personalized approach to healthy eating and physical activity. Proportions of foods and oils are shown by the different widths of the vertical food group bands, which are considered general guides rather than exact proportions. The plan calls for at least 30 minutes of physical activity per day, and discretionary calories to keep the body functioning and provide energy for physical activity. Mothers can visit www.mypyramid.gov for current dietary recommendations and to create their own personalized plans.

Total daily intake needs to contain a variety of foods from each group included on the food pyramid. While every meal may not contain foods from all of the pyramid groups, a balanced total daily intake will provide a nutritious, healthful diet. The pyramid food groups are especially helpful in planning daily food choices for meals. They can serve as a guide for evaluating diet and determining if a person is consuming enough of the right foods.

The food pyramid represents proportions of foods recommended for a healthy adult of normal weight. Pregnant and lactating women may need increased amounts—in the same proportions—to maintain an appropriate weight. Extremely overweight women will need to consume less food overall in the same proportions. Young adolescents who have not completed their growth cycle and women who are very active will require additional servings in each group to meet their energy needs. Mothers can personalize the amount of food needed for each stage of pregnancy at the MyPyramid website, using their age, height, and prepregnancy weight as input. The site also furnishes information on eating for breastfeeding and losing weight during breastfeeding (USDA, 2009).

Food Selection

Many women become more conscious of the foods they eat during pregnancy. In addition, their continuing nutritional awareness throughout lactation can lead to gradual improvement in the eating habits of the entire family. Wise selection of foods is an important factor in good nutrition. Of course, food preferences will affect a woman's food selection and she most often chooses foods that appeal to her, that are a part of her cultural heritage, and with which she is familiar. The person who does the shopping and cooking greatly influences the nutritional value of foods consumed by the family. Available storage and frequency of shopping also determine the variety and quality of the foods selected.

Giving considerable thought to grocery shopping promotes the selection of foods with the highest nutritive values. Fresh, unprocessed foods are the most nutritious and most desirable choices. Likewise, food served directly after purchasing or picking is the most flavorful and nutritious. If perishable foods are not consumed immediately, proper food storage will help to preserve their nutritional quality.

As a response to the increase in obesity rates, many communities require restaurants to list nutritional and caloric data on their menus. Restaurants often provide this information voluntarily, which can help parents to select healthy foods when they dine out.

Home gardening is an increasingly popular way to get the freshest vegetables and fruits. In addition, selecting fresh, crisp produce will ensure that it was stored properly to preserve its vitamins. Encourage mothers to select foods that are grown without, or with a minimum amount, of pesticides and heavy metals such as lead and mercury—substances that are stored in their fatty tissue and later enter into their milk. They can prevent this buildup of toxins by limiting their intake of freshwater fish and animal fats and by washing all fruits and vegetables thoroughly. Removing the skin of fresh fruits and vegetables robs them of much of their nutrients and fiber.

Reading Food Labels

Food labels provide nutritional information that assists shoppers in healthy food selection, with ingredients listed in order of weight. Assessing the nutritional quality of a can of chicken stew, for example, the contents should have chicken rather than water as the main ingredient. Food labels also identify additives such as sugar, salt, preservatives, flavoring, and coloring. In addition, they may state if a product is kosher, organic, or free from particular ingredients such as nuts or wheat.

Package labels offer information on the percentage of the recommended daily allowances of nutrients the food provides as well. Nutritional claims on the label may need extra attention. For example, a food marketed as low in fat could be high in sugar and, therefore, not a good food choice. Labels also give information on the food's preparation and storage. Learning to read labels will help women avoid additives such as corn syrup, sugar, and modified food starch, as well as large quantities of chemical preservatives and additives such as salt and fat.

Food Additives and Processing

Labels identify the foods and additives present in a product, with ingredients listed in descending order of quantity (weight). When comparing ingredients in several foods, the label for the most nutritious product will include fewer highly refined or artificial ingredients at the beginning of the list. Be aware that chemical additives that color the food, enhance flavor, or preserve freshness may alter the nutritional quality. While some changes may improve quality, it is important to weigh the benefits of each ingredient against its possible harmful effects.

Be aware that handling and preserving techniques can alter food quality. Foods such as fresh fruits and vegetables may contain additives that are not obvious to the consumer. For example, mushrooms may be bleached, and other vegetables may be treated with fungicides to retard mold growth. Some foods, such as peppers, cucumbers, and tomatoes, are waxed to preserve their freshness during long transport and storage times. Other foods, such as some oranges, are colored to enhance their visual appeal.

The methods used to treat foods often have distinct benefits, as they make it possible to store or ship the foods and make them available to the consumer throughout the year. It is nearly impossible for the consumer to avoid purchasing treated foods. By washing or peeling such foods, the consumer can reasonably avoid the consumption of undesirable ingredients. Washing with water and mild dish detergent can reduce pesticide residues in fruits and many vegetables.

A report on cumulative body burden found an average of 91 industrial compounds, pollutants, and other chemicals in the nine volunteers who participated in the study (Williams-Derry, 2004). Information on environmental contaminants and ways to avoid them can be found at the Environmental Working Group's website: www.ewg.org. See also ILCA's position statement on contaminants and breastfeeding at www.ilca.org. Additional information about toxins is presented in Chapter 10.

Effects of Processing on Nutritional Value

Processing foods can change their nutritional value either favorably or unfavorably. For example, a food's natural state may be changed through bleaching, removal of fiber, soaking, drying, heating, canning, or freezing. Because freezing preserves more nutrients than canning, frozen foods are a better choice than canned items. Nutritional differences are present among canned foods as well. For instance, fruits canned in heavy syrup contain many more empty calories than those canned in natural fruit juices. Fortifying some foods, such as enriched breads or cereals, replaces nutrients removed during processing. Fortification of other foods, such as iodized salt, provides nutrients needed by the general population that are difficult to obtain from other sources. Whole-grain products are richer sources of vitamin E, vitamin B_6, folic acid, phosphorus, magnesium, and zinc than are enriched refined products.

Some forms of processing can be especially beneficial. For example, popcorn that is "popped" is in a more digestible state than in its natural form. Home canning or freezing of fruits and vegetables makes it possible to store them safely for longer periods. Consumers need to be aware of both the benefits and the disadvantages of various methods of processing and try to select foods processed by methods that will provide the most nutrients at an affordable price.

Cooking food for as short a time and in as little liquid as possible—as with stir-frying and pressure cooking—helps preserve nutrients. Steaming is preferable to boiling, because the nutrients are not lost in the water needed for boiling. Raw food is even more desirable, as cooking destroys some vitamins. Raw spinach, for example, contains more B vitamins than cooked spinach. Nevertheless, some foods, such as meat, may contain harmful bacteria, which cooking can destroy.

Vegetarian Diets

Some families follow a vegetarian diet due to cultural, philosophical, ecological, health-related, or economic factors. As a consequence, it is very likely that you will encounter pregnant and lactating women who are on various forms of a vegetarian diet. Table 8.3 classifies several types of vegetarian diets based on the types of foods consumed.

A vegetarian diet that includes animal products such as milk and eggs can easily supply the pregnant or lactating woman with the nutrients needed to support her body functions and provide for the healthy growth of her baby. Indeed, the majority of the world's population consumes this type of diet. A rice-and-beans combination has been a staple in China, India, Africa, and South America for centuries. In some ways, a balanced vegetarian diet may be more healthful than a meat-based diet. Vegetarians consume more volume and fiber with fewer calories and fats, thereby aiding digestion and decreasing the likelihood of accumulating excess weight.

TABLE 8.3   Classification of Vegetarian Diets

Type of Vegetarian Diet	Types of Foods Consumed
Vegan	Foods from plant sources only (no animal products are consumed.)
Lacto-vegetarian	Milk and milk products, such as cheese and ice cream, in addition to plant foods.
Ovo-vegetarian	Plant foods and eggs.
Lacto-ovo-vegetarian	Plant foods, dairy products, and eggs.
Fruitarian	Fruits, nuts, olive oil, and honey.

Source: Higginbottom MC, Sweetman L, Nyhan W. A syndrome of methylmalonic aciduria, homocystinuria, megaloblastic anemia and neurologic abnormalities in a vitamin B12-deficient breast-fed infant of a strict vegetarian. *N Engl J Med.* 1978;299:317-323. Copyright © 1978 Massachusetts Medical Society. All rights reserved.

Balancing Foods in a Vegetarian Diet

Your guidance may be helpful to a woman who is new to a vegetarian diet, who has little nutritional knowledge, or whose access to food choices is limited. A teen mother living with her parents, for example, may eat the vegetables served at the family meal and avoid the meats. The key to successful management of a vegetarian diet is to plan combinations of foods that provide the essential amino acids. Without the proper balance of amino acids, the body is unable to synthesize the proteins essential for building tissues. A poorly managed vegetarian diet, or one that severely restricts the types of foods eaten, can be deficient in protein and minerals. This imbalance may result in inadequate growth of the fetus and breastfed infant and inadequate nourishment of the mother. A basic understanding of nutrition, careful meal planning, and selective food shopping are essential for a woman on a vegetarian diet.

Many vegetarians become well versed in nutrition through years of practice. They may be knowledgeable about balanced diets or may feel they are knowledgeable, yet not actually understand the basics of a healthful vegetarian diet. If you encounter a woman who you believe needs help with her diet, you may be able to motivate her to make changes by explaining the effect diet has on her well-being and on her baby's growth. You can build on her present knowledge of nutrition to help her understand which additional foods she needs. Open-ended questions will help you learn what she knows about nutrition and how she plans meals.

Table 8.1 will help you offer the mother practical suggestions for selecting foods to fulfill her nutrient needs.

Specific food suggestions are the most helpful to women. For example, combinations of bread or crackers with nut spreads or tofu (soybean curd) spreads are healthy snack foods. If dairy products are not traditionally part of the mother's diet, she can meet her calcium needs by adding large quantities of green leafy vegetables, broccoli, almonds, molasses, tofu, and fortified soymilk. Iron requirements can be the most difficult to meet. Foods containing vitamin C—citrus fruit or juice and fresh vegetables eaten at the same meal with legumes and whole grains—help the body absorb the iron from these foods. In contrast, drinking coffee or tea, including herbal tea, with the meal will decrease the amount of iron absorbed (Hurrell et al., 1999).

Be watchful for extremely strict vegetarian regimes such as a macrobiotic diet, raw foods diet, fruitarianism, or any other arbitrarily adopted pattern that may be harmful during pregnancy or lactation. These diets tend to be unbalanced, emphasizing one food group while neglecting others at the expense of needed proteins, vitamins, minerals, and calories.

Vitamin B$_{12}$ Intake

Vitamin B$_{12}$ is available primarily from animal sources. Women on vegetarian diets who avoid animal products such as milk, cheese, and eggs may, therefore, be deficient in this vitamin. A small amount of vitamin B$_{12}$ is present in fermented products and some seaweed. Unfortunately, these foods may not be incorporated into the vegetarian diet frequently enough to provide adequate amounts. Even mothers with low consumption of animal foods may be at risk for deficiency (Allen, 1994). Levels of vitamin B$_{12}$ are similar in both serum and human milk.

Low vitamin B$_{12}$ intake by the mother leads to low levels in her milk. Be alert for signs that suggest a deficiency in an infant between 4 and 8 months of age—namely, anemia, growth failure, neurological delay, tremors, and excess skin pigmentation. Vitamin B$_{12}$ supplementation during pregnancy and lactation is essential when the mother's diet limits or excludes sources of the vitamin (Kuhne et al., 1991). A caregiver who is knowledgeable about the woman's diet can prescribe these supplements.

Avoiding Feelings of Hunger and Fatigue

Food consumption should respond to hunger and understanding the causes of hunger may help a mother plan and control her selection of foods. An empty feeling in the stomach, discussing or seeing an appealing food, or a drop in the body's blood sugar level can activate hunger. The body absorbs foods at varying rates, and food affects blood sugar in different ways. It is, therefore, possible to feel hungry even after consuming a large amount of calories.

Refined sugar is absorbed directly and quickly, causing the blood sugar to rise and fall rapidly, and resulting in hunger soon afterward. The body converts complex carbohydrates such as potatoes and grains into sugar. These nutrients enter the bloodstream more slowly than when sugar is consumed alone, however, leading to a slower rise and more gradual fall in blood sugar.

Proteins and fats are digested even more slowly than carbohydrates. When these nutrients are consumed, blood sugar rises slowly and steadily, remains sustained for a longer period, and falls slowly. Therefore, although many foods will result in a full stomach, fluctuating blood sugar levels will continue to cause feelings of hunger and lack of energy in the absence of adequate protein and fat. A breakfast consisting primarily of refined carbohydrate foods such as presweetened cereal, doughnuts, or sweet rolls causes blood sugar to rise rapidly and then swoop downward. Fatigue will follow 2 or 3 hours later—hence the need for the traditional mid-morning break, with consumption of more sugar that continues the blood sugar swings.

Nonfood stimulants or suppressants may affect appetite as well. Caffeine and tobacco tend to suppress the appetite, whereas marijuana and alcohol stimulate appetite and promote indiscriminate snacking. Nevertheless, when it is consumed in large amounts, the empty calories from alcohol replace more nutritious foods and can result in nutritional deficiencies. Various over-the-counter and prescription medications can affect appetite as well, either suppressing or stimulating it, depending on the drug.

Consuming a sufficient amount of protein and complex carbohydrates at breakfast avoids mid-morning and mid-afternoon fatigue. Peanut butter on whole-grain toast, bread and cheese, yogurt and fruit, and whole-grain cereal and milk are breakfast meals that do not require much preparation. Breakfast should provide approximately one-third of the day's protein needs. This provides a feeling of well-being throughout the day as well as the highest degree of efficiency in terms of attentiveness, performance, and endurance.

Pregnant or lactating women need at least three well-balanced meals and two snacks daily, consisting of a variety of foods chosen from the food pyramid and distributed throughout the day. You can offer suggestions for high-quality foods that supply needed nutrients without excessive calories. You can also encourage women to read food labels carefully. The information on labels can help them make better decisions on healthy foods for their family.

Healthy Eating on a Budget

High-income, professional families have access to many healthy food options. When cost is not an issue, families may obtain gourmet organic meals from high-end grocery stores. Women in this socioeconomic class tend to be very aware of nutritional status. Organic, "green" (i.e., environmentally friendly and locavore), and "small carbon footprint" are buzzwords in food consumerism among this demographic group.

With food costs rising higher than the annual inflation rate—5.2 percent in 2007 alone (U.S. Department of Labor [USDL], 2009), eating healthy poses a greater challenge for low-income or "working poor" families. Women who are concerned about proper nutrition and who have a limited amount of money to spend on food can employ cost-saving methods in purchasing, storing, and preparing foods for their families. Supermarket sales and coupons can help control grocery costs, while advanced meal planning and use of a carefully itemized shopping list help to avoid impulse buys. Unit pricing labels can help reveal better buys, with store-brand items generally being the same quality as popular brand names at substantially lower prices. The U.S. Center for Nutrition Policy and Promotion offers USDA food plans based on low-cost, moderate-cost, and liberal budgets (USDA, 2007a).

Food in larger-sized packages is usually cheaper per serving and is practical when adequate storage is available and when the extra food in the house does not result in eating more. An alternative may be to shop with a friend and divide large packages. Convenience foods can be more expensive than the individual ingredients. In these cases, women can purchase individual items and make their own dishes. Wholesale cooperatives are popular ways to save money on food purchases, especially for large families. In addition, many charitable organizations and community food banks are available. Compiling a list of food resources in your community can help you guide mothers to them. Shopping wisely helps to limit spending and enables families to fit high-quality foods into their meals.

Proper storage and careful menu planning will help minimize food waste and fuel costs—both factors that are often overlooked when calculating food expenses. Stir-frying for a short time uses less fuel than boiling. Baking several items in the oven at the same time, such as a casserole, baked potatoes, and a dessert, minimizes fuel costs as well. In addition, careful storage of fruits and vegetables reduces bruising and waste.

Costs can be reduced further by basing meals on starchy foods such as pasta, rice, potatoes, or bread rather than building them around a higher-priced meat portion. Adding beans or vegetables to the main course stretches it to serve more people with less meat. Families who enjoy steak can purchase a beef chuck roast and slice it to half the thickness, making two steaks. When marinated and cooked with care, this option can be an appealing substitute for higher-priced cuts of beef. Canned fish is usually cheaper than fresh fish.

In addition to making these suggestions, you can direct women to a local health or welfare office for nutrition assistance. In the United States, the Supplemental Program for Women, Infants, and Children (WIC) provides supplemental foods and nutrition counseling to pregnant and postpartum women, breastfeeding mothers, and children from birth to age 5 if they meet basic requirements of low income or nutritional risk. Other U.S. food assistance programs include the food stamps program and Aid to Families with Dependent Children (AFDC). In Canada, the country's Prenatal Nutrition Program provides many of the same services as the U.S. WIC program. Check with the local health authority for similar programs in other countries.

Foods to Limit or Avoid

Many cultures include in their traditional diets a wide variety of foods that are thought to cause problems while breastfeeding. This list may include high-fiber foods, acidic fruits, gas-forming vegetables and beans, milk, spices, and chocolate. However, foods that one culture avoids may be highly valued for breastfeeding women in another culture. Pregnant and lactating women sometimes believe they must avoid certain foods that cause gas, or flatulence. In reality, foods that affect the mother do not necessarily have the same effect on the baby (Lust et al., 1996).

The essential oils found in foods such as garlic and some spices may have odors and smells that pass into the milk and are noticeable to the infant. Sensitivity to flavors in the mother's milk may increase acceptance of foods when the baby starts solid foods, as the baby is already accustomed to a variety of tastes (Forestell & Mennella, 2007; Mennella, 1995).

In general, most mothers find they can eat a wide variety of foods. If a mother suspects a particular food is causing a problem, she can omit that food for a week and then reintroduce it. A dietician can help determine whether exclusion of a major food such as wheat or milk is warranted and ensure replacement of the nutrients provided by the excluded foods.

Alcohol

Alcohol enters the bloodstream and quickly migrates to the milk. Human milk metabolizes alcohol at roughly the same rate as the body metabolizes it—$1\frac{1}{2}$ to 2 hours per ounce of absolute alcohol. Occasional alcohol use timed around breastfeeding does not seem to have any harmful effects on the breastfed infant (Hale, 2010). By comparison, moderate amounts of alcohol consumed regularly over time by the nursing mother may slow brain growth in her child. Consumption of large amounts of alcohol delays brain growth even more dramatically and limits parental effectiveness. Most ominously, use of excessive amounts of alcohol can cause life-threatening conditions in both the fetus and the breastfed infant. Chapter 10 further discusses alcohol consumption during lactation.

Caffeine

Caffeine passes to the infant through the mother's milk and very young infants cannot eliminate this toxin easily from the body. Infants who are particularly susceptible to caffeine's effects may experience fussiness or excessive wakefulness. Consult Chapter 10 for a more detailed discussion of substances found in human milk and their effect on the infant.

Allergens

Some evidence suggests that a fetus can be sensitized to allergens in utero and a breastfed infant sensitized through breastfeeding. A baby born to parents with a history of allergies has a greater possibility of developing the same allergies. Maternal avoidance of potentially allergenic foods such as cow's milk, eggs, and fish during late pregnancy and lactation has been associated with a lower incidence of allergy in children (Lovegrove et al., 1994; Sigurs et al., 1992). Nevertheless, most foods are considered to be acceptable in the mother's diet unless they cause allergic reactions in the parents or the mother consumes them in excessive amounts. Consult Chapter 10 for a more detailed discussion of substances found in human milk.

Foodborne Disease

Food poisoning can be a serious illness when it occurs during pregnancy. To reduce risks of such contamination, any reheated foods consumed by the pregnant woman should be hot all the way through. Raw eggs should not be consumed, and eggs should be cooked until both the white and the yolk are solid. Raw foods should be stored separately from cooked foods, and hands and utensils should be washed between preparing these foods. Food should be stored in a clean, dry, cool area away from flies, vermin, and household pets. In addition, pregnant women should drink only milk that is pasteurized and discard food not used prior to its expiration date. They can wear gloves when gardening or changing cat litter for further protection. All family members should wash their hands after using the toilet or changing diapers and before eating.

Pregnant women and women considering pregnancy should not eat shark, swordfish, king mackerel, or tilefish. These fish could contain enough mercury (a toxin) to harm a fetus's nervous system (USDHHS & EPA, 2004). Further, young children and nursing women also should avoid consuming those species of fish, which tend to live longer and have higher mercury concentrations in their tissues than other fish. Guidelines suggest it is permissible to eat as much as 12 ounces per week of shrimp, canned light tuna, salmon, pollock, and catfish. The FDA warns against eating more than 6 ounces of white albacore tuna, which contains more mercury than light tuna.

ᔕ Offering Nutrition Suggestions to Mothers

When you have a solid understanding of nutrition and its implications for pregnant and lactating women, you can incorporate nutrition suggestions in your counseling and educate women about the basic elements of proper nutrition. After a woman accepts what she has learned about nutrition, it is yet another step for her to realize that what she actually eats may conflict with her new beliefs. For example, many of us know that it is important to eat breakfast, yet we continue to skip this essential meal. Women need to recognize that where they eat out and shop, what they buy, how they plan meals, and what their snacking habits are all affect their eating habits.

Nutrition education can be a positive experience that promotes a continued interest in further education. Suggestions that result in an immediate improvement may catch a mother's interest. For example, women who are sensitive to the effects of caffeine may find that eliminating caffeinated beverages before bedtime will help them sleep better. Take care not to burden women with irrelevant information or unrealistic goals. For example, giving cooking tips to women who eat out frequently, suggesting expensive foods to a low-income family, or suggesting that a working mother avoid convenience foods altogether probably would not be practical or well received.

Some women fear they cannot breastfeed because they do not eat "well enough." Good nutrition need not become a barrier to breastfeeding. You can teach them that the human body is very flexible and can make good milk out of many combinations of foods. You can help mothers see the strengths in their diets and understand that small changes can lead to big improvements. They will learn how both they and their babies will be healthier.

Learn the Mother's Dietary Habits

Before suggesting diet improvements to a woman, you need to learn why she chooses certain eating patterns and which factors influence her food choices. You can tactfully investigate a woman's diet practices by finding out her usual eating habits. Remember that a closed question such as "Do you eat a good breakfast?" gives you very little information about what and how the mother eats. Few people would answer "No" to such a question! In contrast, open-ended questions or statements such as "What have you eaten today?" or "It sounds like you haven't had a chance to eat breakfast yet" provides you with information that is more specific. Taking enough time to gather information gives you insights into factors that influence the woman's dietary habits and enables you to offer meaningful and appropriate suggestions.

A woman's knowledge of nutrition and her attitudes about eating will affect her food practices significantly. She may eat impulsively, using food to try to satisfy other needs. If she is sensitive about her appearance, she may ignore her hunger in an effort to lose or control her weight. Alternatively, she may pay close attention to her eating practices so that she can look and feel her best. Some overweight and underweight women may not see themselves as others do and, therefore, lack motivation to change their eating habits. Providing accurate nutritional information may help women avoid fad diets and improve poor eating patterns such as skipping meals.

A woman's living situation and lifestyle affect the types of food that are available to her and the regularity of her meals. Women on limited incomes, and particularly those on assistance programs, may have a narrow selection of foods from which to choose. When new parents live with their relatives or others, other people may determine which foods they eat and how meals are prepared. A woman may eat in a desire to please someone who has prepared food for her, or she may eat with someone without really being hungry or needing to eat at that time. Work and school schedules often dictate whether family members share regular meals together and where they dine—at home, in restaurants, at fast-food chains, from vending machines, or as bagged meals. Even for the highly motivated woman, outside influences can make it difficult to achieve the well-balanced diet she needs for lactation.

A few women in your care may have health conditions that require special diet considerations. These may include food allergies or intolerances, diabetes, hypertension, anemia, ulcers, or weight problems. When these conditions exist, you can help the woman work within the guidelines suggested by her caregiver to plan a diet that is suitable for lactation. Referral to a dietician or nutritionist would also be appropriate in these circumstances.

Practical Suggestions for Diet

As you discover a mother's food practices, you can begin helping her to recognize the positive results of diet improvement. Women's interest in learning about nutrition may increase when they understand how they will feel better or how their lives will become easier with sound dietary practices. After you gain a general idea of a woman's eating patterns and the kinds of food she typically eats, you can begin suggesting diet changes. If she usually eliminates breakfast and consumes empty calories

the rest of the day, as a first step you can suggest a quick protein food such as peanut butter on toast and a glass of milk for breakfast. Later you may offer an additional suggestion of replacing white bread with whole-grain bread. Help her to change one step at a time, making sure she understands the purpose for each change.

A realistic goal is one of diet improvement in the direction of three well-balanced meals a day with snacks as needed. When such changes are gradual, the family may be more receptive and the woman is less likely to feel she must change her entire lifestyle to accommodate pregnancy and breastfeeding. After one change has become second nature, women will be more receptive to further change. Although you may move someone only a short way on the spectrum of food attitudes during the time she is in your care, even the slightest improvement is worth your efforts.

Pregnancy and Postpartum Nutrition

Pregnant women can be encouraged to begin working on good eating habits by learning the relationship of nutrition to the way they feel. Issues may include doing the best thing for the baby, having a healthy pregnancy, maintaining a safe weight during pregnancy, and losing pregnancy weight more easily after delivery. If a woman experiences morning sickness and nausea, she can eat a cracker or a protein such as a piece of turkey or a cube of cheese before getting out of bed. Following this "stomach settler" with a high-protein breakfast and continued access to simple and healthy foods throughout the day will help her avoid an empty stomach and the return of the nausea. Other tricks that help avoid nausea include opening a window or turning on a fan to remove food odors.

Encourage pregnant women to eat small, frequent meals, avoid fatty foods, and drink plenty of liquids. Some women may need to avoid highly spiced and very rich foods. Women who experience constipation can relieve it by engaging in regular exercise, drinking plenty of fluids, and consuming a sufficient amount of fiber in the form of fresh fruits and vegetables, whole grains, nuts, seeds, and bran. Avoiding refined foods may also help.

After the baby arrives, you can help the mother understand how a good diet will help her overcome problems with a fussy baby, recurring breast infections or nipple soreness, depression, and lack of energy. You can use the woman's problem or concern as a way of encouraging her to change her eating habits. It is important for the health of both mother and baby that a woman embrace good nutrition during pregnancy, and that she continue healthful habits throughout lactation.

Specific Food Suggestions

One of the most effective ways of encouraging healthful eating is to provide specific food suggestions to accompany the teaching of the basic principles of nutrition. Suggestions that mention specific foods are easier for people to accept and adapt to their eating practices. For example, you can translate the instruction, "You need 60 grams of protein each day," into a food practice with specific food selections that provide protein. Thus, you might say, "You can keep a couple of containers of yogurt on hand for mornings when you don't feel like making breakfast."

To help women limit their consumption of animal fats and trans-fats, suggest that they use vegetable and olive oils instead. All of the vitamins and minerals necessary for a balanced diet are made available by selecting a variety of foods from the food pyramid in forms as near as possible to their natural state. For example, a woman can eat whole-wheat bread rather than white bread, bake with whole-wheat flour mixed half and half with unbleached flour, use whole-grain cereals and crackers, and select brown or wild rice rather than polished, instant, or converted rice. See Table 8.1 for other suggestions.

Because many vitamins are water soluble, it is preferable to cook vegetables in a minimal amount of water, tightly covered, and until just tender. Cooking them in their skins will further help to preserve nutrients. Water saved from cooking vegetables can form the basis of soups and gravies. It is also good practice to serve something raw at every meal, such as carrots, celery, peppers, cauliflower, broccoli, spinach salad, cabbage, cucumbers, grapefruit sections, apple slices, or fresh pineapple.

Purchasing fruits canned in juice rather than in heavy syrup helps reduce sugar intake. One hundred percent fruit juices are superior to fruit drinks or other beverages that are high in sugar. Homemade popsicles consisting of fruit juice provide a nutritious substitute for commercial popsicles, which typically contain high levels of sugar. Other nutritious snack ideas include a bran muffin with cream cheese, cheese with crackers, yogurt dip with raw vegetables, fresh fruit, custard, popcorn, cottage cheese and fruit, and hard-boiled eggs.

Meal Planning

Giving forethought to meals during pregnancy can help a woman's meal planning for the first days or weeks after her baby arrives. Stocking up on staples in the last few weeks of pregnancy can help limit repeated trips to the store when the mother is home with her newborn. In addition, she can prepare meals and freeze them to reheat on days when time is at a premium. If the family has friends or other support systems to bring meals, they can suggest simple foods that can be frozen. Encourage the mother to avail herself of cultural foods believed to support pregnancy and enhance lactation. Many of these foods contain herbs now known to be galactagogues (Marasco, 2009).

Translating the number of servings required from the food pyramid into meals with the proper number of calories may seem challenging to a new mother. You can eliminate that step by offering her sample meal plans such as those shown in Table 8.4. The specific foods listed in the sample meal plans are suggestions for diet planning. They contain the proper number of calories and necessary nutrients to support the baby's growth and the mother's well-being. Substituting most sweets with more nutritious selections will provide ample amounts of food. A mother can substitute foods that suit her preferences; group foods into smaller, more frequent meals; or eat the lunchtime apple as a midmorning snack. In addition to the fluids suggested, remind her to drink water according to her thirst.

Group Instruction in Nutrition

Example is the best teacher, so any refreshments served at support group meetings and classes should be nutritious. You can encourage healthful snacking and eating habits either by bringing nutritious refreshments yourself or by requesting that volunteers bring specific foods to share. Nutritious snacks might include natural fruit juices, fresh fruit, raw vegetables and dip, wholesome cookies and breads, cheese and crackers, and other snacks discussed in this chapter. Figure 8.2 suggests topics on nutrition for group meetings.

∼ Summary

A responsible part of counseling is making sure that breastfeeding women have the opportunity and the necessary information to improve their health through nutrition. Unfortunately, poor dietary habits are widespread in today's often chaotic world, and are continually promoted by the advertising of nutritionally empty, high-calorie foods. Most mothers can benefit from sound practical suggestions. Becoming familiar with basic nutrition principles and the food practices of the women in your care will help you to understand influences on their diet. This, in turn, provides insight into helping them to institute changes.

You can be a positive force in helping women improve nutrition for themselves and their families. Educating them about their nutritional needs and the effects of their nutrition on their health and the way they feel helps to influence dietary changes. Offering practical food suggestions rather than theoretical dietary requirements makes it easier for women to embrace these changes. Pregnancy and lactation are milestones in a woman's life when she is most receptive to nutrition counseling. Helping families integrate sound nutrition gradually into their lifestyles increases the likelihood that these practices will continue to benefit family members for years to come.

TABLE 8.4 Sample Meal Plans

MyPyramid.gov
STEPS TO A HEALTHIER YOU

Sample Menus for a 2000 Calorie Food Pattern

Averaged over a week, this 7-day menu provides all of the recommended amounts of nutrients and food from each food group. (Italicized foods are part of the dish or food that preceeds it.)

Day 1

BREAKFAST

Breakfast burrito
1 flour tortilla (7" diameter)
1 scrambled egg (in 1 tsp soft margarine)
1/3 cup black beans*
2 tbsp salsa
1 cup orange juice
1 cup fat-free milk

LUNCH

Roast beef sandwich
1 whole grain sandwich bun
3 ounces lean roast beef
2 slices tomato
1/4 cup shredded romaine lettuce
1/8 cup sauteed mushrooms (in 1 tsp oil)
1 1/2 ounce part-skim mozzarella cheese
1 tsp yellow mustard
3/4 cup baked potato wedges*
1 tbsp ketchup
1 unsweetened beverage

DINNER

Stuffed broiled salmon
5 ounce salmon filet
1 ounce bread stuffing mix
1 tbsp chopped onions
1 tbsp diced celery
2 tsp canola oil
1/2 cup saffron (white) rice
1 ounce slivered almonds
1/2 cup steamed broccoli
1 tsp soft margarine
1 cup fat-free milk

SNACKS

1 cup cantaloupe

Day 2

BREAKFAST

Hot cereal
1/2 cup cooked oatmeal
2 tbsp raisins
1 tsp soft margarine
1/2 cup fat-free milk
1 cup orange juice

LUNCH

Taco salad
2 ounces tortilla chips
2 ounces ground turkey, sauteed in 2 tsp sunflower oil
1/2 cup black beans*
1/2 cup iceberg lettuce
2 slices tomato
1 ounce low-fat cheddar cheese
2 tbsp salsa
1/2 cup avocado
1 tsp lime juice
1 unsweetened beverage

DINNER

Spinach lasagna
1 cup lasagna noodles, cooked (2 oz dry)
2/3 cup cooked spinach
1/2 cup ricotta cheese
1/2 cup tomato sauce tomato bits*
1 ounce part-skim mozzarella cheese
1 ounce whole wheat dinner roll
1 cup fat-free milk

SNACKS

1/2 ounce dry-roasted almonds*
1/4 cup pineapple
2 tbsp raisins

Day 3

BREAKFAST

Cold cereal
1 cup bran flakes
1 cup fat-free milk
1 small banana
1 slice whole wheat toast
1 tsp soft margarine
1 cup prune juice

LUNCH

Tuna fish sandwich
2 slices rye bread
3 ounces tuna (packed in water, drained)
2 tsp mayonnaise
1 tbsp diced celery
1/4 cup shredded romaine lettuce
2 slices tomato
1 medium pear
1 cup fat-free milk

DINNER

Roasted chicken breast
3 ounces boneless skinless chicken breast*
1 large baked sweet potato
1/2 cup peas and onions
1 tsp soft margarine
1 ounce whole wheat dinner roll
1 tsp soft margarine
1 cup leafy greens salad
3 tsp sunflower oil and vinegar dressing

SNACKS

1/4 cup dried apricots
1 cup low-fat fruited yogurt

Day 4

BREAKFAST

1 whole wheat English muffin
2 tsp soft margarine
1 tbsp jam or preserves
1 medium grapefruit
1 hard-cooked egg
1 unsweetened beverage

LUNCH

White bean-vegetable soup
1 1/4 cup chunky vegetable soup
1/2 cup white beans*
2 ounce breadstick
8 baby carrots
1 cup fat-free milk

DINNER

Rigatoni with meat sauce
1 cup rigatoni pasta (2 ounces dry)
1/2 cup tomato sauce tomato bits*
2 ounces extra lean cooked ground beef (sauteed in 2 tsp vegetable oil)
3 tbsp grated Parmesan cheese
Spinach salad
1 cup baby spinach leaves
1/2 cup tangerine slices
1/2 ounce chopped walnuts
3 tsp sunflower oil and vinegar dressing
1 cup fat-free milk

SNACKS

1 cup low-fat fruited yogurt

TABLE 8.4   Sample Meal Plans (Continued)

Sample Menus for a 2000 Calorie Food Pattern

Averaged over a week, this 7-day menu provides all of the recommended amounts of nutrients and food from each food group.
(Italicized foods are part of the dish or food that preceeds it.)

Day 5

BREAKFAST

Cold cereal
1 cup puffed wheat cereal
1 tbsp raisins
1 cup fat-free milk
1 small banana
1 slice whole wheat toast
1 tsp soft margarine
1 tsp jelly

LUNCH

Smoked turkey sandwich
2 ounces whole wheat pita bread
1/4 cup romaine lettuce
2 slices tomato
3 ounces sliced smoked turkey breast*
1 tbsp mayo-type salad dressing
1 tsp yellow mustard
1/2 cup apple slices
1 cup tomato juice*

DINNER

Grilled top loin steak
5 ounces grilled top loin steak
3/4 cup mashed potatoes
2 tsp soft margarine
1/2 cup steamed carrots
1 tbsp honey
2 ounces whole wheat dinner roll
1 tsp soft margarine
1 cup fat-free milk

SNACKS

1 cup low-fat fruited yogurt

Day 6

BREAKFAST

French toast
2 slices whole wheat French toast
2 tsp soft margarine
2 tbsp maple syrup
1/2 medium grapefruit
1 cup fat-free milk

LUNCH

Vegetarian chili on baked potato
1 cup kidney beans*
1/2 cup tomato sauce w/ tomato tidbits*
3 tbsp chopped onions
1 ounce lowfat cheddar cheese
1 tsp vegetable oil
1 medium baked potato
1/2 cup cantaloupe
3/4 cup lemonade

DINNER

Hawaiian pizza
2 slices cheese pizza
1 ounce canadian bacon
1/4 cup pineapple
2 tbsp mushrooms
2 tbsp chopped onions
Green salad
1 cup leafy greens
3 tsp sunflower oil and vinegar dressing
1 cup fat-free milk

SNACKS

5 whole wheat crackers*
1/8 cup hummus
1/2 cup fruit cocktail (in water or juice)

Day 7

BREAKFAST

Pancakes
3 buckwheat pancakes
2 tsp soft margarine
3 tbsp maple syrup
1/2 cup strawberries
3/4 cup honeydew melon
1/2 cup fat-free milk

LUNCH

Manhattan clam chowder
3 ounces canned clams (drained)
3/4 cup mixed vegetables
1 cup canned tomatoes*
10 whole wheat crackers*
1 medium orange
1 cup fat-free milk

DINNER

Vegetable stir-fry
4 ounces tofu (firm)
1/4 cup green and red bell peppers
1/2 cup bok choy
2 tbsp vegetable oil
1 cup brown rice
1 cup lemon-flavored iced tea

SNACKS

1 ounce sunflower seeds*
1 large banana
1 cup low-fat fruited yogurt

* Starred items are foods that are labeled as no-salt-added, low-sodium, or low-salt versions of the foods. They can also be prepared from scratch with little or no added salt. All other foods are regular commercial products that contain variable levels of sodium. Average sodium level of the 7-day menu assumes no-salt-added in cooking or at the table.

(Continued)

TABLE 8.4 Sample Meal Plans

Sample Menus for a 2000 Calorie Food Pattern

Averaged over a week, this 7-day menu provides all of the recommended amounts of nutrients and food from each food group. (Italicized foods are part of the dish or food that preceeds it, which is not italicized.)

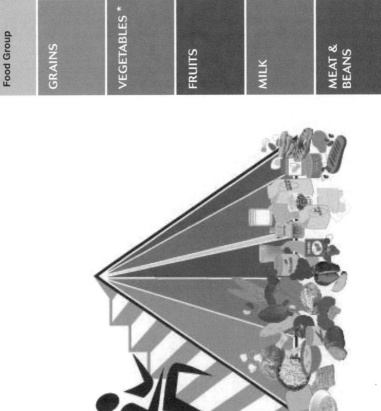

Food Group		Daily Average Over One Week
GRAINS	Total Grains (oz eq)	6.0
	Whole Grains	3.4
	Refined Grains	2.6
VEGETABLES *	Total Veg* (cups)	2.6
FRUITS	Fruits (cups)	2.1
MILK	Milk (cups)	3.1
MEAT & BEANS	Meat/ Beans (oz eq)	5.6
OILS	Oils (tsp/grams) 7.2 tsp/32.4 g	

*Vegetable subgroups	(weekly totals)
Dk-Green Veg (cups)	3.3
Orange Veg (cups)	2.3
Beans/ Peas (cups)	3.0
Starchy Veg (cups)	3.4
Other Veg (cups)	6.6

Nutrient	Daily Average Over One Week
Calories	1994
Protein, g	98
Protein, % kcal	20
Carbohydrate, g	264
Carbohydrate, % kcal	53
Total fat, g	67
Total fat, % kcal	30
Saturated fat, g	16
Saturated fat, % kcal	7.0
Monounsaturated fat, g	23
Polyunsaturated fat, g	23
Linoleic Acid, g	21
Alpha-linolenic Acid, g	1.1
Cholesterol, mg	207
Total dietary fiber, g	31
Potassium, mg	4715
Sodium, mg*	1948
Calcium, mg	1389
Magnesium, mg	432
Copper, mg	1.9
Iron, mg	21
Phosphorus, mg	1830
Zinc, mg	14
Thiamin, mg	1.9
Riboflavin, mg	2.5
Niacin Equivalents, mg	24
Vitamin B6, mg	2.9
Vitamin B12, mcg	18.4
Vitamin C, mg	190
Vitamin E, mg (AT)	18.9
Vitamin A, mcg (RAE)	1430
Dietary Folate Equivalents, mcg	558

* Starred items are foods that are labelled as no-salt-added, low-sodium, or low-salt versions of the foods. They can also be prepared from scratch with little or no added salt. All other foods are regular commercial products that contain variable levels of sodium. Average sodium level of the 7-day menu assumes no-salt-added in cooking or at the table.

Source: U.S. Department of Agriculture, www.MyPyramid.gov

There are many interesting and entertaining ways to present nutrition information during group discussions. It is hoped that those listed below will interest mothers in nutrition and help them understand how it relates to their daily food selection and preparation.

- At a discussion on the "First Days of Breastfeeding," you can emphasize good nutrition as a necessity for pregnant women and new mothers. Avoid overwhelming mothers with healthy food ideas. Stress two or three basic points, and explain why they are important.
- Diet recall: Ask mothers to record everything they have eaten that day. Have them analyze their diets according to food groups, or ask them to hand in their recall lists anonymously for the group to analyze. Look for foods that supply specific nutrients such as protein, vitamin C, iron, calcium, and so on.
- At a discussion on "Starting the Baby on Solid Foods," present a buffet of homemade infant foods, including finger foods for mothers to sample. For comparison, also provide a taste of the same food prepared commercially.
- To highlight a nutrition discussion, serve several complete protein dishes made with meat substitutes and show a variety of milk servings in nutritionally equal amounts (milk, cheese, yogurt, sesame seeds, soy products, and so on).
- Approach an old topic with a new point of view. For example, the health benefits of breastfeeding, delaying solid foods, and how to introduce solid foods can be approached from the perspective of avoiding food intolerances and entitled "Food Intolerances and Healthier Babies."
- Have a recipe swap, and ask everyone to bring a nutritious snack and recipe for all to sample and enjoy.

FIGURE 8.2 Nutrition topics for group meetings.

∾ *Chapter 8—At a Glance*

Facts you learned—

Nutrition in pregnancy and lactation:

- Pregnancy and lactation are times when women are often especially receptive to nutrition education.
- A mother's body stores and the food she eats provide energy and nutrients for her baby.
- Sugary foods may cause erratic blood sugar, fatigue, dizziness, nervousness, and headache.
- Complex carbohydrates take longer to digest and prevent cravings for more food.
- Protein is needed for formation of hormones and milk production during lactation.
- Fats create a longer feeling of fullness.

- Folic acid helps prevent anemia in pregnancy and neural tube defects.
- Vitamin B_{12} may help prevent neural tube defects and cardiac defects.
- A newborn's vitamin K levels are low and are typically supplemented.
- Low levels of vitamin D in a pregnant woman result in low levels in the baby.
- Pregnancy and lactation require increased calcium, iron, and water intake to ensure good health for both mother and child.
- Consuming excessive fluid can reduce milk production.
- A normal, healthy diet will meet the mother's nutritional needs during lactation.
- Lactation uses energy from body stores and from diet.
- Well-nourished, healthy women can safely lose about one pound (0.55 kg) per week after giving birth.
- Food additives and processing alter nutritional quality favorably and unfavorably.
- Vegetarian diets that include milk and eggs supply necessary nutrients.
- A mother's occasional consumption of alcohol timed around breastfeeding has not proven harmful to breastfed infants.
- Infants sensitive to caffeine may experience fussiness or excessive wakefulness.
- Most foods are acceptable during pregnancy, unless they cause allergic reactions in the mother or father or are consumed in excessive amounts.

Applying what you learned—

- Strive for diet improvement, where the ideal diet consists of three well-balanced meals a day with snacks as needed.
- Encourage pregnant women to eat small, frequent meals, avoid fatty foods, and drink plenty of liquids.
- Teach mothers about practical food choices rather than nutrients.
- Teach mothers to base their meal planning on the food pyramid.
- Teach mothers how to balance complete protein and incomplete protein foods.
- Teach mothers how to consume more unsaturated fats than saturated fats and to avoid trans-fats.
- Teach mothers to respond to their thirst as a signal to consume necessary additional fluids.
- Teach mothers that consuming protein and complex carbohydrates at breakfast help prevent later fatigue.

- Teach mothers to read food labels for nutritional information.
- Teach mothers that a healthy diet helps when they are coping with a fussy baby, and that it may reduce recurring breast infections or nipple soreness, depression, and lack of energy.

～ References

Allen L. Vitamin B$_{12}$ metabolism and status during pregnancy, lactation and infancy. *Adv Exp Med Biol.* 1994;352:173-186.

American Academy of Pediatrics (AAP), Committee on Nutrition: Prevention of pediatric overweight and obesity. *Pediatrics.* 2007;112(2):2003; reaffirmed *Pediatrics.* 2007;119(2):405. doi:10.1542/peds.2006-3222.

Barker D. Fetal programming of coronary heart disease: review. *Trends Endocrin Metab.* 2002;13(9):364-368.

Basile LA, et al. The effect of high-dose vitamin D supplementation on serum vitamin D levels and milk calcium concentration in lactating women and their infants. *Breastfeed Med.* 2006;1(1):27-35.

Butte N, et al. Energy requirements during pregnancy and lactation. *Public Health Nutr.* 2005;8(7A):1010-1027.

Canales E, et al. The influence of pyridoxine on prolactin secretion and milk production. *Br J Obstet Gynaecol.* 1976;83(5):387-388.

Centers for Disease Control and Prevention (CDC). Overweight and Obesity. NHANES Surveys (1976-1980 and 2003-2006); November 17, 2009a. www.cdc.gov/obesity/childhood/prevalence.html. Accessed March 8, 2010.

Centers for Disease Control and Prevention (CDC). Overweight and Obesity. U.S. Obesity Trends. Trends by State 1985-2008; November 30, 2009b. www.cdc.gov/obesity/data/trends.html. Accessed March 8, 2010.

Chan S, et al. Bone mineral density and calcium metabolism of Hong Kong Chinese postpartum women: a 1-y longitudinal study. *Eur J Clin Nutr.* 2005;59(7):868-876.

Dewey KG. Effects of maternal caloric restriction and exercise during lactation. *J Nutr.* 1993;128(2 suppl):386S-389S.

Dewey KG, et al. Maternal weight-loss patterns during prolonged lactation. *Am J Clin Nutr.* 1993;58:162-166.

Dewey K, et al. A randomized study of the effects of aerobic exercise by lactating women on breastmilk volume and composition. *N Engl J Med.* 1994;330:449-453.

Dewey K, McCrory M. Effects of dieting and physical activity on pregnancy and lactation. *Am J Clin Nutr.* 1994;59(suppl):446s-453s.

Diet-i.com. Diet information: How much protein do you need to eat in your daily diet? www.diet-i.com/protein-intake-in-daily-diet.htm. Accessed February 21, 2009.

Dursun N, et al. Influence of duration of total breast-feeding on bone mineral density in a Turkish population: does the priority of risk factors differ from society to society? *Osteoporos Int.* 2006;17(5):651-655.

Dusdieker LB, et al. Effect of supplemental fluids on human milk production. *J Pediatr.* 1985;106:207.

Dusdieker L, et al. Is milk production impaired by dieting during lactation? *Am J Clin Nutr.* 1994;59:833-840.

Forestell C, Mennella J. Early determinants of fruit and vegetable acceptance. *Pediatrics.* 2007;120(6):1247-1254.

Foukas MD. An antilactogenic effect of pyridoxine. *J Obstet Gynaecol Br Commonw.* 1973;80:718-720.

Franx A, et al. Sodium-blood pressure interrelationship in pregnancy. *J Hum Hypertens.* 1999;13(3):159-166.

Fukushima Y, et al. Consumption of cow milk and egg by lactating women and the presence of B-lactoglobulin and ovalbumin in breastmilk. *Am J Clin Nutr.* 1997;65:30-35.

Gartner L. Prevention of rickets and vitamin D deficiency: new guidelines for vitamin D intake. *Pediatrics.* 2003;111(4):908-910.

Good Mojab, C. Sunlight deficiency: a review of the literature. *Mothering.* 2003;117:52-55, 57-63. www.mothering.com/articles/new_baby/breastfeeding/sunlight-deficiency.html. Accessed February 20, 2009.

Greer F, et al. Improving the vitamin K status of breastfeeding infants with maternal vitamin K supplements. *Pediatrics.* 1997;99(1):88-92.

Guevel M, et al. A risk-benefit analysis of French high fish consumption: a QALY approach. *Risk Anal.* 2008;28(1):37-48.

Hale T. *Medications and Mothers' Milk.* 14th ed. Amarillo, TX: Hale Publishing; 2010.

Henderson P, et al. Bone mineral density in grand multiparous women with extended lactation. *Am J Obstet Gynecol.* 2000;182(6):1371-1377.

Hilson J, et al. High prepregnant body mass index is associated with poor lactation outcomes among white, rural women independent of psychosocial and demographic correlates. *J Hum Lact.* 2004;20(1):18-29.

Hirsch D. Vitamin D and the breastfed infant. In: Hale T, Hartmann P, eds. *Hale and Hartmann's Textbook of Human Lactation.* Amarillo, TX: Hale Publishing; 2007:425-461.

Hollis B, Wagner C. Assessment of dietary vitamin D requirements during pregnancy and lactation: Review. *Am J Clin Nutr.* 2004a;79(5):717-726.

Hollis B, Wagner C. Vitamin D requirements during lactation: high-dose maternal supplementation as therapy to prevent hypovitaminosis D for both the mother and the nursing infant. *Am J Clin Nutr.* 2004b;80(6 suppl):1752S-1758S.

Hurrell R, et al. Inhibition of non-haem iron absorption in man by polyphenolic-containing beverages. *Br J Nutr.* 1999;81(4):289-295.

Ikerd J. Quoted by: Duesterhaus R. Sustainability's promise. *J Soil Water Conserv.* 1990;45(1):4. NAL Call # 56.8 J822.

Illingworth PJ, et al. Diminution in energy expenditure during lactation. *Br Med J.* 1986;292:437.

Institute of Medicine (IOM). Dietary Reference Intakes for energy, carbohydrate. fiber, fat, fatty acids, cholesterol, protein, and amino acids (2002/2005). 2005. www.iom.edu/Object.File/Master/7/300/Webtablemacro.pdf. Accessed March 6, 2009.

Institute of Medicine (IOM), National Academy of Sciences. *Nutrition During Lactation*. Washington, DC: National Academy Press; 1991.

International Lactation Consultant Association (ILCA). Mannel R, et al., eds. *Core Curriculum for Lactation Consultant Practice*. 2nd ed. Sudbury, MA: Jones and Bartlett; 2007.

Karlsson C, et al. Pregnancy and lactation confer reversible bone loss in humans. *Osteoporos Int*. 2001;12(10):828-834.

Kramer FM, et al. Breastfeeding reduces maternal lower-body fat. *J Am Diet Assoc*. 1993;93:429-433.

Kuhne T, et al. Maternal vegan diet causing a serious infantile neurological disorder due to vitamin B_{12} deficiency. *Euro J Pediatr*. 1991;150:205-208.

Lawrence R, Lawrence R. *Breastfeeding: A Guide for the Medical Profession*. 6th ed. St. Louis, MO: Elsevier Mosby; 2005.

LetsMove.gov. First Lady Michelle Obama Launches Let's Move: America's Move to Raise a Healthier Generation of Kids. February 9, 2010. www.letsmove.gov. Accessed March 8, 2010.

Lovegrove J, et al. The immunological and long-term atopic outcome of infants born to women following a milk-free diet during late pregnancy and lactation: a pilot study. *Br J Nutr*. 1994;71:223-238.

Lovelady C, et al. The effect of weight loss in overweight, lactating women on the growth of their infants. *N Engl J Med*. 2000;342(7):449-453.

Lumbers E, et al. The selfish brain and the Barker hypothesis. *Clin Exp Pharmacol Physiol*. 2001;28(11):942-947.

Lust K, et al. Maternal intake of cruciferous vegetables and other foods and colic symptoms in exclusively breast-fed infants. *J Am Diet Assoc*. 1996;96(1):46-48.

Marasco L. Galactogogues and the ethics of their use. Paper presented at: San Antonio Breastfeeding Coalition, Low Milk Supply Conference; February 21, 2009; San Antonio, TX.

Marcus, RG. Suppression of lactation with high doses of pyridoxine. *S Afr Med J*. 1975;49:2155-2156.

Martek Biosciences Corporation. Mead Johnson launches prenatal and nursing supplement containing Martek DHA(TM) [press release]. Columbia, MD; October 6, 2004.

Martek Biosciences Corporation. www.martek.com. Accessed February 20, 2009.

McCrory MA. Does dieting during lactation put infant growth at risk? *Nutr Rev*. 2001;59(1 Pt 1):18-21.

McCrory MA, et al. Randomized trial of the short-term effects of dieting compared with dieting plus aerobic exercise on lactation performance. *Am J Clin Nutr*. 1999;69(5):959-967.

Mennella J. Mother's milk: a medium for early flavor experiences: Review. *J Hum Lact*. 1995;11(1):39-45.

Michaelsen K, et al. The Copenhagen Cohort study on infant nutrition and growth: breast-milk intake, human milk macronutrient content, and influencing factors. *Am J Clin Nutr*. 1994;59:600-611.

National Eating Disorders Association (NEDA). Eating disorders information index. www.nationaleatingdisorders.org. Accessed February 20, 2009.

Ogden CL, et al. High body mass index for age among US children and adolescents, 2003-2006. *JAMA*. 2008;299:2401-2405.

Oladapo OT, Fawole B. Treatments for suppression of lactation. *Cochrane Database Syst Rev*. 2009;1:CD005937.

Pinheiro A, et al. Protein restriction during gestation and/or lactation causes adverse transgenerational effects on biometry and glucose metabolism in F1 and F2 progenies of rats. *Clin Sci (Lond)*. 2008;114(5):381-392.

Rasmussen K, Kjolhede C. Prepregnant overweight and obesity diminish the prolactin response to suckling in the first week postpartum. *Pediatrics*. 2004;113(5):e465-e471.

Robinson S, Barker D. Coronary heart disease: a disorder of growth: review. *Proc Nutr Soc*. 2002;61(4):537-542.

Rutishauser L, Carlin J. Body mass index and duration of breastfeeding: a survival analysis during the first six months of life. *J Epidemiol Community Health*. 1992'46: 559-565.

Saadi H, et al. Effect of combined maternal and infant vitamin D supplementation on vitamin D status of exclusively breastfed infants. *Matern Child Nutr*. 2009;5(1):25-32.

Sadat-Ali M, et al. Effect of parity on bone mineral density among postmenopausal Saudi Arabian women. *Saudi Med J*. 2005;26(10):1588-1590.

Serdula M, et al. Do obese children become obese adults? A review of the literature. *Prev Med*. 1993;22:167-177.

Sigurs N, et al. Maternal avoidance of eggs, cow's milk and fish during lactation: effect on allergic manifestations, skin-prick tests and specific IgE antibodies in children at age 4 years. *Pediatrics*. 1992;89:735-739.

Sustainable Table. Introduction to sustainability: What is sustainable agriculture? www. sustainabletable.org/intro/whatis. Accessed March 6, 2009.

U.S. Department of Agriculture (USDA). The low-cost, moderate-cost and liberal food plans. Center for Nutrition Policy and Promotion; 2007a. http://www.cnpp.usda.gov/Publications/FoodPlans/MiscPubs/FoodPlans2007Admin-Report.pdf. Accessed February 21, 2009.

U.S. Department of Agriculture (USDA). National Nutrient Database for Standard Reference, Release 20. 2007b. www.ars.usda.gov/Main/docs.htm?docid=15869. Accessed March 6, 2009.

U.S. Department of Agriculture (USDA). MyPyramid for pregnancy and breastfeeding. Center for Nutrition Policy and Promotion; 2009. http://www.mypyramid.gov/mypyramidmoms/index.html. Accessed September 14, 2009.

U.S. Department of Energy Office of Science (USDEOS). Genetically modified food and organisms. November 5, 2008. www.ornl.gov/sci/techresources/Human_Genome/elsi/gmfood.shtml. Accessed February 21, 2009.

U.S. Department of Health and Human Services (DHHS), U.S. Environmental Protection Agency (EPA). What you need to know about mercury in fish and shellfish: 2004 EPA and FDA advice for women who might become pregnant, women who are pregnant, nursing mothers, young children. March 2004. www.cfsan.fda.gov/~dms/admehg3.html. Accessed February 20, 2009.

U.S. Department of Labor, Bureau of Labor Statistics. Consumer Price Index summary. www.bls.gov/news.release/cpi.nr0.htm. Accessed February 22, 2009.

Wagner CI, et al. High-dose vitamin D_3 supplementation in a cohort of breastfeeding mothers and their infants: a 6-month follow-up pilot study. *Breastfeed Med.* 2006;1(2): 59-70.

Whitaker R, et al. Predicting obesity in young adulthood from childhood and parental obesity. *N Engl J Med.* 1997;37(13): 869-873.

Williams-Derry C. Flame retardants in Puget Sound residents. *Northwest Environmental Watch.* 2004. www.northwest-watch.org. Accessed August 18, 2009.

Wolff T. Folic acid supplementation for the prevention of neural tube defects: an update of the evidence for the U.S. Preventive Services Task Force. *Ann Intern Med.* 2009; 150(9):632-639.

World Health Organization (WHO). *Healthy Eating During Pregnancy and Breastfeeding: Booklet for Mothers.* Geneva, Switzerland: WHO; 2001. www.euro.who.int/document /e73182.pdf. Accessed February 20, 2009.

World Health Organization (WHO). Diet, nutrition and the prevention of chronic diseases. Geneva, Switzerland: WHO, 2003. http://whqlibdoc.who.int/trs/WHO_trs_916 .pdf. Accessed March 8, 2010.

Zambrano E. The transgenerational mechanisms in developmental programming of metabolic diseases. *Rev Invest Clin.* 2009;61(1):41-52.

Properties of Human Milk

Human milk is a life-giving substance that provides more than enough nutrition for the newborn and infant child. The breast initially secretes protein-rich colostrum, which provides the infant with antibodies and other protection against disease. Colostrum is exactly what the newborn needs to make the transition to extrauterine life, both in amount and composition. During the first few days after birth, colostrum mixes with increasing quantities of newly formed milk and eventually transitions to mature milk. The composition of human milk is ideally suited to the human infant. Despite claims by the manufacturers of artificial baby milk substitutes (formula), no parallel exists for this perfect infant nutrition.

∼ *Key Terms*

Acrodermatitis
  enteropathica
Active immunity
Alpha-lactalbumin
Amylase
Antibacterial
Antibody response
Antigen
Antimicrobial
Antiparasite
Antiviral
Atopic dermatitis
Bifidus factor
Bioavailability
Calories
Carbohydrates
Casein
Centers for Disease
  Control and Prevention
  (CDC)
Cholecystokinin (CCK)
Colicky behavior
Colostrum
Cow's milk
Creamatocrit
Cytokines

Dehydration
Diarrhea
Donor milk
Dopamine
Eclampsia
Enteral feeding
Enzyme
Exogenous
Extremely low birth weight
  (ELBW)
Fat
Flora
Fluoride
Ghrelin
Glycan
Growth factors
Hemorrhagic disease
Human milk bank
Human milk fortifier
Humoral factors
Hypocalcemia
IgA
Immunologic properties
Iron
Lactobacillus bifidus
Lactoengineering

Lactoferrin
Lactose intolerance
Leptin
Leukocytes
Lipase
Long-chain
  polyunsaturated fatty
  acid
Low birth weight (LBW)
Lysozyme
Macrophages
Mature milk
Meconium
Mineral
Mucin
Myelin
Necrotizing enterocolitis
Neurological development
Neurotransmitter
Nosocomial
Nucleotide
Obestatin
Oligosaccharide
Otitis media

Passive immunity
Pathogen
Peptide
Phagocytic cells
Phthalates
Polysaccharides
Prebiotics
Probiotics
Product recall
Prostaglandin
Protein
Rickets
Rotavirus
Sepsis
Small for gestational age
  (SGA)
Vaccine
Very low birth weight
  (VLBW)
Virus
Vitamin D
Vitamin K
Whey

∼ *Colostrum: The Early Milk*

Colostrum can be secreted prenatally and for several days after birth. A thick, sticky, rich-looking substance, it comes in a range of colors and viscosity—from clear and thin, to orange and thick. The high concentration of protein found in this early milk is well suited to promote early rapid growth of the newborn. Colostrum is the residual mixture of materials present in the mammary glands and ducts, which started production at approximately 120 days' gestation. This substance mixes with the newly formed milk and is the thick, clear to golden-yellow fluid that the infant first receives.

In terms of its energy content, colostrum contains approximately 67 kcal/dL milk (18.76 kcal/oz). Compared with mature milk, it is richer in sodium, potassium, chloride, protein, fat-soluble vitamins, and minerals. It also contains less fat (2 percent) and lactose than mature milk (Czank et al., 2007a; Wagner et al., 1996; Jelliffe & Jelliffe, 1978), as well as the appropriate level and balance of the essential fatty acids required by the newborn (Ronneberg & Skara, 1992).

Colostrum has a laxative effect that eliminates meconium from the infant's bowels. Meconium is the thick, black, sticky substance that is present in the newborn infant's first stools. Stimulating bowel function is necessary for the infant's body to begin excreting waste products effectively. This elimination can be a critical factor in reducing the severity of jaundice.

In the first 24 hours, total infant intake of colostrum can range from 3 to 32 mL/kg body weight, or 10.2 to 108.8 mL based on a 7½-pound baby (Casey et al., 1986). This amount corresponds with the newborn's small stomach. A new mother may need to be reassured that her newborn is receiving nourishment in addition to other important health benefits until her milk production increases and changes to mature milk. The removal of colostrum by the infant stimulates further production of colostrum and milk in the breast. Any water or artificial milks the baby receives will dilute colostrum's effects. Additionally, a baby's kidneys are not capable of handling large volumes of fluid and are stressed by consumption of additional water; breastfed newborns do not need water.

Protective Qualities of Colostrum

Colostrum is considered a baby's first immunization against many bacteria and viruses. It makes valuable contributions to the infant's health that artificial baby milk cannot match, which makes it the baby's ideal first food. In particular, colostrum plays an important role in protecting the infant against infection. It contains many living cells that engulf and digest disease organisms. Colostrum is composed of approximately 70 percent leukocytes, compared to less than 10 percent leukocytes in transitional and mature milk (Hanson, 2007b). Leukocytes are white blood cells that defend the body against infectious disease and foreign materials; they also mediate pain. Colostrum aids in rapid gut closure (resistance of the baby's intestinal wall to penetration by disease organisms and antigens).

The mother produces antibodies to all the diseases to which she has already acquired relative immunity. Colostrum, in turn, contains many antibodies produced by her body in response to a threat by a particular microbial invader, or antigen. Thus the mother passes many antibodies both to her fetus through the placenta and to her newborn through her colostrum and milk.

Three specific antibodies that are highly concentrated in colostrum and human milk are immune globulin A (IgA), immune globulin G (IgG), and immune globulin M (IgM). An immune globulin (also known as immunoglobulin) is a group of proteins that provides immunity. Of these immunoglobulins, IgA occurs in the highest concentrations in colostrum and human milk and is the most biologically active. Secretory IgA is available only through the mother's milk and is not present in artificial baby milks. The baby cannot produce it until approximately 6 months of age.

The fetus receives most of its circulating antibodies from the placenta. The very high levels of IgA and other antibodies in colostrum provide further protection for the infant's gastrointestinal (GI) tract, guarding it against organisms that might otherwise invade it. Colostrum facilitates the establishment of bifidus flora (normal bacteria and other microbes) in the digestive tract. Bifidus flora promotes the growth of beneficial bacteria, primarily lactobacillus bifidus, and facilitates the passage of meconium.

Colostrum provides protection against a variety of pathogens (disease agents), including polio, Coxsackie B virus, several staphylococci, and *Escherichia coli*, the intestinal bacteria that can cause serious intestinal, urinary, and other infections in infants. Health professionals have found colostrum so effective in preventing disease that they give it to preterm infants and older children with compromised immune systems or metabolic disorders, including chronic renal failure (Arnold, 1995). Mature milk also is ideal for these needs (Tully et al., 2004).

~ Transition to Mature Milk

Colostrum changes to transitional milk by about the 6th day of life (Pang & Hartmann, 2007; Hartmann et al., 2003; Humenick et al., 1994; Viverge et al., 1990). During that time, volume increases until production typically ranges from 556 to 705 mL (14 to 19 oz) in a 24-hour period (Hartmann et al., 2003).

The color and consistency of human milk varies according to the type of milk and specific additives in the mother's diet. Transitional milk appears approximately 6 to 13 days postpartum and gradually changes to mature milk. As the baby's sucking stimulates the nipple, oxytocin is released and activates letdown. The milk then travels from the alveoli through the ducts, washing the fat from the walls of the ducts and ductules. This process results in hindmilk, which is much higher in fat and, therefore, richer looking than the initial milk, or foremilk.

Fat content varies from mother to mother and from feeding to feeding (Kent, 2007; Kent et al., 2006; Lai, 2004; Mitoulas et al., 2002). It is inversely proportional to the length of time between feedings and correlates with the degree of breast fullness. Although there is not a clear demarcation between foremilk and hindmilk, allowing a baby to finish at the first breast and not restricting feeding time ensures the baby has access to the fat available in that feeding (Kent, 2007; Kent et al., 2006; Daly et al., 1993a).

Appearance of Mature Milk

Human milk has a naturally watery appearance that looks even more diluted when the mother's milk volume is high. If the mother expresses milk at the end of a feeding when fat content is higher, she will note a thicker and denser consistency. Human milk has a typically bluish cast that results from the presence of casein, a component of the proteins in milk. It may take on other colors as well. A greenish color can result from additives in vitamins or iron supplements taken by the mother, or from her intake of deep green foods such as spinach and broccoli. Excessive amounts of vitamin A, either in foods or as a supplement, may color the milk yellow or orange. Black milk can result from use of the drug minocycline (Hunt et al., 1996). It is helpful to inform a mother about these variations so that she will not be concerned unnecessarily if they occur.

Milk Volume

The volume of a mother's milk depends on regular removal of milk from the breast, whether it be through nursing, manual expression, or pumping. It also depends on the degree of drainage at each feeding or pumping session. Volume does not decrease because of supplemental milk removal. In fact, it is more likely to increase under these circumstances, because removing milk signals the breast to make more milk. Removal of milk at one feeding signals the amount of milk that should be available at the next feeding (Kent et al., 2006; Daly et al., 1993b).

Minor variations may occur in the volume produced by each breast, on different days, or in response to the infant's sucking pattern. Milk often seems most plentiful in the morning hours, especially immediately after the mother awakens. She can express milk at that time and throughout the day without decreasing the amount of milk available to her baby.

Milk volume is most heavily dependent on the baby's removal of milk from the breast. Babies have the ability to self-regulate their feedings to meet their individual needs for optimal growth (Cox et al., 2008; Kent et al., 2006; Woolridge et al., 1990). They determine the amount they need from one feeding to the next through the amount of milk they remove. The average 1-month-old baby will take approximately 2 to 4 ounces per feeding (60–120 mL), or 24 to 32 ounces (720–960 mL) of milk over 24 hours. Reassure mothers that milk intake varies greatly from baby to baby. According to Kent and colleagues (2006), a daily average intake of 26.65 ounces (788 mL) may range from 16.17 to 45.86 ounces (478–1356 mL). Breastfed babies typically do not increase their milk intake to match the large volumes (8-ounce or 240-mL bottles) consumed by artificially fed babies.

Milk volume is influenced to a lesser extent by the mother's nutrition and water intake. Lactation consultants should not overemphasize the importance of diet during lactation, especially among first-time mothers who may be unsure of their bodies' ability to nourish newborn children properly (Greiner, 1994). When a woman's diet includes all nutrients in sufficient amounts—that is, the Dietary Reference Intake (DRI) of all nutrients—there is no significant decrease in milk volume. This helps explain why women worldwide are able to nourish their babies under varied nutritional conditions. Their babies have growth patterns similar to the baby of a well-nourished mother.

~ Composition of Human Milk

The composition of human milk changes throughout lactation as the child grows, and even during a given day or feeding. Scientists continue to study and make new discoveries about the many components in human milk, including fat, protein, lactose, carbohydrates, fatty acids, vitamins, and minerals. Each component has a specific function in ensuring optimal nourishment of the infant.

Human milk continually changes to meet the needs of the growing child from the first few days of colostrum to beyond the child's second year. The milk is high in immunoglobulins and protein during the first several weeks postpartum, though it assumes a relatively dilute state by the first month. Fat content decreases in the later months of lactation. From 6 to 12 months of age, babies receive three-fourths or more of their nutrient needs from human milk. During the second year of lactation, the output of human milk is equivalent to at least one 8-ounce glass daily. Thus human milk continues to be a valuable component in the toddler's diet in both quantity and composition.

Protein and fat content are usually higher at the end of a feeding, with 4 to 5 times more fat and 1.5 times more protein present in the milk at this stage of the feeding than at the beginning. The baby may consume nearly one-sixth of the available calories between minutes 11 and 16 of a feeding. For this reason, it is important that mothers place no limits on the amount of time the baby spends at each breast (Kent, 2007; Kent et al., 2006; Hall, 1997). For consumption of important fats, proteins, and calories, the mother should continue to nurse until the baby ends the feeding.

Human milk varies in sensory qualities in addition to undergoing appropriate changes in composition to meet the child's needs. Human milk provides the breastfed infant with richly changing experiences in taste and odor and provides a bridge in the transition from uterine nutrition to table foods. Flavor in the milk is affected by both what the mother eats and what she smells. As Mennella and Beauchamp (1991) noted in their research, babies demonstrate a preference for garlic-flavored milk. Variety in the infant's diet increases acceptance of foods later in life. These variations are not provided to the artificially fed child, whose formula has a consistent taste and smell. Artificial baby milk has a metallic taste, and the specialty formulas are especially distasteful. Table 9.1 compares the major elements in human milk with those present in other mammals' milk.

Calories

The caloric content of human milk is ideally suited to the human infant, so much so that formula companies design their manufactured products around the average calories found in human milk. Colostrum contains approximately 17 kcal/oz. By 2 weeks, the average caloric content of mature human milk is 20 kcal/oz., increasing to 26 kcal/oz. by 4 months. Differences in caloric content of

TABLE 9.1   Comparison of Components in Human Milk and Cow's Milk

Component	Human Milk	Cow's Milk
Water (ml/100 ml)	87.1	87.2
Energy (Cal/100 ml)	60–75	66
Total solids (g/100 ml)	12.9	12.8
Protein (%)	0.8–0.9	3.5
Fat (%)	3–5	3.7
Lactose (%)	6.9–7.2	4.9
Ash (minerals) (%)	0.2	0.7
Protein (% of total protein)		
Casein	40	82
Whey	60	18
Ash, major components per liter		
Calcium (mg)	340	1170
Phosphorus (mg)	140	920
Sodium (mEq)	7	22
Vitamins per liter		
Vitamin A (IU)	1898	1025
Thiamin (μg)	160	440
Riboflavin (μg)	360	1750
Niacin (μg)	1470	940
Vitamin C (mg)	43	1.1

mature milk result from variations in fat. If a feeding does not last long enough to reach the fatty hindmilk, the baby may not receive sufficient calories. In severely malnourished mothers, milk volume may be compromised (Bhutta & Haider, 2009; Ettyang et al., 2005; Kumar, 1989). In the vast majority of women, however, this is not an issue.

Fat

Human milk fat provides as much as 50 percent of the infant's energy needs. It is the main source of fat-soluble vitamins and essential fatty acids needed for growth and development of the infant's central nervous system, including brain growth and maturation of the immune system. Fat is an extremely variable constituent in human milk (Czank et al., 2007a; Mitoulas et al., 2002). The amount of available fat seems dependent on maternal body fat stores (Koletzko et al., 2001; Martin et al., 1993; Nommsen et al., 1991). Maternal fat stores laid down during pregnancy are easier to mobilize for lactation than other fat stores in the mother's body (Michaelsen et al., 1994). If the mother is severely malnourished, however, her milk fat levels may be lower (Bhutta & Haider, 2009; Ettyang et al., 2005; Kumar, 1989).

Fat content changes during a feeding as well. If a mother's milk fat content decreases, the baby will stay at the breast longer in an attempt to gain a higher fat yield. This yield is comparable to that available from a mother with higher milk fat (Tyson et al., 1992), which illustrates the importance of baby-led feeding (Perez-Escamilla et al., 1995). The amount of fat a breastfed infant receives depends on the length of sucking time at the breast. A baby who is not gaining sufficient weight may not be nursing long enough at each feeding or frequently enough throughout the day and night. If the mother ends feeding on one breast too early, the baby may fill up on foremilk from both breasts and receive no hindmilk. This could lead to behavior resembling colic and poor nourishment. Fat content decreases after 6 to 12 months and may be lower when the letdown reflex is inhibited.

Fatty Acids

Fatty acids are very important in the human diet. More than 200 types of fatty acids have been found in human milk (Jensen, 1999), including both saturated and unsaturated fatty acids (mono and poly), which are primarily medium and long chain in form. Like milk fat, the concentrations and types of fatty acids in human milk depend on maternal stores (Del Prado et al., 2001; Sauerwald et al., 2000). Arachidonic acid (AA) from linoleic acid and docosahexaenoic acid (DHA) from linolenic acid are essential for development of visual acuity (Innis et al., 2001; Williams et al., 2001; Carlson et al., 1996). Linoleic and linolenic acids, both of which are essential fatty acids, have significance in the quality of myelin laid down. One study showed that multiple sclerosis (MS) is rare in countries where breastfeeding is common. The development of myelin in infancy may be critical to preventing degradation later (Dick, 1976; Christensen, 1975). Another study described an increase in MS incidence in Mexico as breastfeeding rates decreased (Tarrats et al., 2002).

Fatty acids are affected by maternal diet (Czank et al., 2007a), an observation that formula manufacturers have exploited with their marketing of "supplements" for breastfeeding mothers. These companies highlight the addition of synthetic DHA and AA to their products, claiming that this supplementation makes them functionally similar to human milk, and implying equality of the natural and artificial milks (International Baby Food Action Network [IBFAN], 2007; Walker, 2007; Williams et al., 2001). (See the discussion of infant formula later in this chapter).

Carbohydrates

Lactose is present in human milk in high levels (7 percent) and accounts for almost all of the carbohydrate in the milk (Jelliffe & Jelliffe, 1978). Lactose provides 40 to 45 percent of the energy in human milk. Its concentration increases by approximately 10 percent over the first 6 months of lactation (Coppa et al., 1993). This component of milk is specifically designed to promote newborn growth and performs several unique functions that benefit the infant. For example, lactose enhances calcium absorption, thereby helping prevent rickets. It helps supply energy to the infant's brain and check the growth of harmful organisms in the intestine. It also is essential to development of the central nervous system (Czank et al., 2007b).

Lactose is the major sugar in mammalian milk and appears nowhere else in nature. Human milk has one of the highest levels of lactose among mammals. It is the most constant of all the constituents in human milk and remains constant throughout the day and in the face of dietary fluctuations (Jelliffe & Jelliffe, 1978). Lactose is digested slowly, producing a steady release of glucose into the bloodstream. Sucrose, the sugar often used in milk substitute formulas such as soy, is sweeter and splits rapidly, resulting in a high peak of glucose in the infant's bloodstream. Sucrose probably plays a significant role in tooth decay, whereas lactose does not (Erickson & Mazhare, 1999; Erickson et al., 1998). The consequences of feeding a human infant a food without lactose, such as soy formula or milk-based lactose-free formula, are not clear.

Human milk contains glycans, or polysaccharides. Polysaccharides are a class of carbohydrates (e.g., starch and cellulose) consisting of a number of monosaccharides joined by glycosidic bonds. Glycans are polysaccharides or oligosaccharides—that is, a type of complex carbohydrate. Oligosaccharides are the third largest solid in human milk, after lactose and lipids, and the most diverse component in breastmilk (LoCascio et al., 2007). To date, more than 130 have been identified in human milk (McVeagh & Miller, 1997).

Oligosaccharides protect the baby from pathogens by preventing these disease-causing agents from binding to receptor sites in the gut (Newburg et al., 2009; Newburg, 1996). They provide protection throughout the baby's digestive system (Morrow et al., 2005; Chaturvedi et al., 2001b), and specifically protect the baby against urinary tract infection (Hanson, 2004a; Pisacane et al., 1992; Coppa et al., 1990) and diarrhea (Coppa et al., 2006; Newburg et al., 2004). Oligosaccharides vary among mothers and over the course of lactation (Chaturvedi et al., 2001a).

The prebiotic and probiotic functions of human milk oligosaccharides have been studied extensively. Prebiotics are nondigestible food ingredients that stimulate the growth or activity of bacteria in the digestive system that are beneficial to the health of the body. Probiotics are dietary supplements of live microorganisms thought to be beneficial to the health of the body; lactic acid bacteria and bifidobacteria are the most common types of microbes used as probiotics, although certain yeasts and bacilli are also available for this purpose.

There has been explosive research and marketing of prebiotics and probiotics in artificial baby milks and other foods (Underwood, 2009; Moreno Villares, 2008; Westerbeek et al., 2008; Boehm & Moro, 2008). This research "continues the effort to mimic functional properties of human milk" (Nakamura et al., 2009). De Vrese and Schrezenmeir (2008) cite the report of unsuccessful attempts to make infant formula more like human milk by the addition of fructooligosaccharides and (primarily) galactooligosaccharides.

Protein

The growth and development needs of all animal species determine their milk composition. Within the animal kingdom, human milk contains the least amount of protein, which results in the slowest rate of growth. Protein in human milk is digested easily and readily absorbed into the bloodstream. The distribution of specific proteins in human milk is ideally suited to the growth of the human infant, as it enables the young child to use the proteins with extremely high efficiency. Colostrum contains approximately 3 times more protein than does mature milk. The protein content of human milk seems to remain relatively constant regardless of the mother's nutritional status or dietary practices.

Manufacturers of artificial baby milk substitutes have attempted to adjust their products so that they match the protein content of human milk as closely as possible. Infant formula, however, lacks certain proteins found in human milk, such as lactoferrin. The infant does not use lactoferrin completely and excretes some of these amino acids in the stool. Cow's milk curd is tough and rubbery, whereas the curd of human milk is soft, small, and less compact, making it easier for the infant to digest. Genetic engineering, also known as "transgenic" modification, seeks to place human milk components into dairy and the milk of other animals (Sabikhi, 2007; Yu et al., 2006).

Whey and Casein

Whey is the clear fluid in the milk, and casein is the curd portion. The ratio of these components changes from 90:10 in early milk to 60:40 in mature milk and to 50:50 in late lactation. Ratios in formula vary depending on the manufacturer. The ratio in Nestlé Good Start is 100:0, meaning there is no casein in this product (Nestlé, 2009). The ratio is 60:40 for Enfamil Lipil with iron (Mead Johnson, 2009). Similac Advanced with Iron has a ratio of 48:52 (Ross Products Division, 2009).

Lactoferrin

Lactoferrin, the iron-binding protein in whey, inhibits the growth of iron-dependent bacteria (such as *E. coli*) in the gastrointestinal tract. This action protects the baby against gastrointestinal infections. Lactoferrin renders intestinal iron unavailable to pathogens in the baby's gut, thereby protecting the infant from such infections as those caused by the *Salmonella*, *E. coli*, and *Candida albicans* bacteria. One study terms the elevated bifidobacterial count from lactoferrin "one of the greatest advantages that breastfed infants have over infants fed with milk formulas" (Chierici et al., 2003). Giving iron supplements to newborns can saturate lactoferrin, thus allowing proliferation of *E. coli*. Protection from lactoferrin is not present if the baby receives any other type of feeding.

Researchers have been exploring various methods to commercialize human lactoferrin. Lactoferrin, which is typically purified from human milk, costs more than $3600 per gram at 90 percent purity. One company markets recombinant human lactoferrin (rhLF), which is genetically engineered from fermented *Aspergillus*, a fungus (Agennix, 2009). Aggressive patenting of human milk components is just one more sign of the value of human milk—Agennix, for example, has 71 issued patents and many more pending for such components. A researcher funded by Nestlé states, "These recombinant human milk proteins may be incorporated into infant formulas, baby foods and complementary foods, and used with the goal to reduce infectious diseases" (Lonnerdal, 2006).

Lysozyme

Lysozyme, another whey protein, is one of the more than 20 active enzymes present in human milk. It provides an antimicrobial factor against enterobacteriaceae and gram-positive bacteria.

Taurine

Human milk contains eight essential amino acids, including taurine. Taurine is important for vision and general development and improves fat absorption in preterm infants.

Vitamins

Generally, all vitamins are available in sufficient quantities in human milk (note the following discussion of vitamins D and K). Excessive doses of vitamin B_6 (300–600 mg/day) have been reported to reduce milk production (Hale, 2010). Strict lacto-ovo-vegetarians may be deficient in vitamin B_{12}, which can result in megoblastic anemia and neurological malfunction in the newborn (see the discussion of vegetarian diets in Chapter 8). Colostrum is particularly rich in vitamin E, and mature milk levels are high in this nutrient as well. Because a deficiency in vitamin E in infancy can result in anemia, breastfeeding is considered to be a preventive measure against anemia in infancy.

Vitamin D

Vitamin D is a steroid hormone produced in the body from a pro-steroid that results from direct exposure of the skin to ultraviolet B (UVB) radiation in sunlight (Hirsch, 2007; Good Mojab, 2003a, 2003b). This vitamin is present in both the water- and fat-soluble portions of human milk (Lakdawala & Widdowson, 1997). Most pregnant women are deficient in vitamin D. Vitamin D deficiency in childhood can cause rickets, which is characterized by abnormal bone growth, muscle pain, and weakness. In infancy, it can lead to "developmental delays, failure to thrive, respiratory distress, tetany, and heart failure" (Good Mojab, 2002).

Supplementing the Infant There are no national data on the incidence of rickets in the United States (Scanlon, 2001). A recent Canadian study estimated an overall annual incidence in that country of 2.9 cases per 100,000 (Ward et al., 2007). Reports of increased rickets in breastfed infants prompted the American Academy of Pediatrics (AAP) to recommend that breastfed infants receive 200 IU/day of vitamin D. Note that the studies that led to the AAP's recommendation involved primarily non-Caucasian babies who rarely had sun exposure (Kreiter et al., 2000; Pugliese et al., 1998; Sills et al., 1994). In 2008, the AAP increased their recommendation to 400 IU/day beginning in the first few days of life (Wagner et al., 2008). Despite these recommendations, the majority of physicians fail to recommend vitamin D supplementation and most parents fail to comply (Taylor et al., 2010). There is an increased risk of vitamin D deficiency among those persons who have darkly pigmented skin, live in the northern hemisphere, receive little outside exposure to sunlight, or reside in an inner-city home, among other risk factors (Good Mojab, 2003a, 2003b, 2004; La Leche League International [LLLI], 2003; Bhowmick et al., 1991). Babies in day care often see very little sunlight, typically remaining indoors much of the day and arriving and leaving when it is already dark. Thus, rather than there being a vitamin D deficiency in human milk, the fault may lie with a lifestyle that does not allow for sufficient vitamin D production through sun exposure.

Exposure to Sunlight Previous studies have recommended exposing babies to adequate sunlight to promote production of vitamin D (Greer, 2001b; Specker, 1994). Specker and colleagues (1985) suggested the optimal exposure consists of 30 minutes per week wearing only a diaper, or 2 hours per week if fully clothed without a hat. A World Health Organization (WHO) recommendation states, "It is now understood that the optimal route for vitamin D ingestion in humans is not the gastrointestinal tract, which may permit toxic amounts to be absorbed. Rather, the skin is the human organ designed, in the presence of sunlight, both to manufacture vitamin D in potentially vast quantities and to prevent the absorption of more than the body can safely use and store" (Akre, 1989).

There are conflicting data on the appropriate amounts of sunlight for adults with varying degrees of skin pigmentation (Good Mojab, 2003a, 2004). Some studies show that adults with darker skin pigmentation require more UVB exposure to produce the same amount of vitamin D as adults with lighter skin pigmentation (Harkness & Cromer, 2005; Holick, 1995; Scragg et al., 1995; Clemens et al., 1982). Other studies suggest that skin pigmentation makes little difference in terms of vitamin D manufacture (Malvy et al., 2000; Matsuoka et al., 1991; Brazerol et al., 1988; Lo et al., 1986). There are no data available on the effect of skin pigmentation on vitamin D production in infants.

No research exists examining the relationship between the risk of skin cancer and a lifetime of minimal levels of sun exposure sufficient for endogenous production of adequate levels of vitamin D. Recommendations of small amounts of sun exposure are at odds with advice given by the Centers for Disease Control and Prevention (CDC) and the AAP, which recommends avoiding sun exposure for older babies and children by keeping them out of direct sunlight and by using sunscreen. Use of sunscreen, however, impedes the synthesis of vitamin D. The WHO currently recommends no sun exposure for babies younger than 1 year of age.

Supplementing the Mother Mothers can supplement their diet to increase the level of vitamin D in their milk. One study showed that supplementing the mother with 50 µg (2000 IU) of vitamin D per day was as effective for maintaining the baby's vitamin D levels as supplementing the baby with 10 µg (400 IU) per day (Ala-Houhala et al., 1986). Researchers increasingly contend that mothers need higher levels of supplementation to maintain adequate infant vitamin D levels. One study found that supplementing lactating mothers with 6400 IU daily for 6 months resulted in ample levels in both mothers and babies with no adverse effects (Wagner et al., 2006).

U.S. government health agencies consider levels of 1000 IU per day and greater to exceed human requirements. Other researchers believe that limited scientific methods and small sample sizes were used in the studies whose results form the basis for many vitamin D recommendations. Hollis and Wagner (2004a, 2004b) suggest that present guidelines for vitamin D requirements are very inadequate for adults deprived of sun exposure, especially for people with darkly pigmented skin and women during pregnancy and lactation. Holick (2007) suggests that approximately 800 IU of vitamin D or its equivalent daily provides sufficient amounts for children and adults unless there are mitigating circumstances.

In the absence of adequate exposure to UVB rays, vitamin D supplementation can increase vitamin D concentrations to be equal to those of people living in sun-rich environments. In one study, 18 lactating mothers received either 2000 IU or 4000 IU of vitamin D supplements daily for 3 months. The researchers concluded that the higher supplementation of 4000 IU safely increased vitamin D levels in both mothers and babies (Hollis & Wagner, 2004b).

Bone mineral content and markers for bone turnover are similar in breastfed and formula fed infants, even if breastfed infants have low vitamin D status. This finding suggests that mineral absorption may occur from a passive transport mechanism that is somewhat independent of vitamin D (Park et al., 1998). Hirsch (2007) suggests it is prudent to supplement both mother and child if vitamin D deficiency is present.

Vitamin K

Vitamin K is present in small amounts in human milk. Fetal stores of vitamin K protect the infant, as does the prophylactic dose usually given at birth, until the newborn receives sufficient milk from the mother and the child's intestine matures enough to manufacture its own. There has been much debate regarding the use of prophylactic vitamin K in newborns, as this practice raises the question of whether human milk is sufficient to provide adequate vitamin K for the newborn. Some experts question why supplemental doses of vitamin K are necessary, and if so, how they are given most effectively.

Protection from Hemorrhagic Disease Newborns routinely receive vitamin K to promote blood clotting and help them avoid hemorrhagic disease of the newborn (HDN). Presently, babies are not screened routinely for hemorrhagic disease. Lactation consultants should be aware that symptoms of hemorrhagic disease include convulsions, feeding intolerance and poor sucking, irritability, and pallor. This condition may also cause bulging or full fontanels, diminished or absent neonatal reflexes, and ecchymosis (bruising) (Bor et al., 2000).

Increasing the mother's dietary intake of vitamin K to more than 1 mg per day during the final weeks of pregnancy may reduce the risk of hemorrhagic disease (Greer et al., 1997). Breastfed infants may benefit from increased maternal vitamin K intake during lactation as well. A supplement of 5 mg of vitamin K to lactating mothers increases the concentration of this nutrient in human milk and significantly increases infant plasma vitamin K (Nishiguchi et al., 2002; Greer, 2001a).

Dosage Method Vitamin K is administered by either intramuscular (IM) injection or oral dose, though there is some debate about the best route to use with the newborn. Oral dosing is much less distressing to the newborn than an IM injection, which carries the added risk of nerve damage. Studies suggest that oral administration (initial dosing at birth, plus 2 to 4 follow-up doses) is as effective as an IM injection in providing protection (Arteaga-Vizcaino et al., 2001; Wariyar et al., 2000; Greer et al., 1997). The Danish practice of parents providing weekly oral doses of vitamin K for the first 3 months for primarily breastfed infants revealed high parental participation and no reports of hemorrhagic disease in an 8-year period (Hansen et al., 2003).

Minerals

The mineral balance in human milk meets the baby's needs perfectly. Human milk has a lower percentage of minerals, which minimizes the load placed on the baby's immature kidneys. The calcium in human milk is absorbed much more efficiently than the same nutrient in artificial milk (Rudloff & Lonnerdal, 1990). Indeed, the higher ratio of phosphorus to calcium present in cow's milk can interfere with calcium absorption. Therefore, artificially fed infants are more at risk for developing late neonatal hypocalcemia than their breastfed counterparts (Specker et al., 1991). In addition, under stressful situations such as hot weather or diarrhea, the higher mineral content of an infant formula based on cow's milk is a significant contributor to dehydration.

The higher solute load of infant formulas may require additional water intake by the infant to expel the solutes. Mothers often misinterpret the thirst induced by this type of food as hunger. Consequently, they feed more formula to their baby instead of the water the child needs. Babies who are breastfed exclusively require no water supple-

ments—not even in hot climates—because there is little waste to flush through the kidneys (Ashraf et al., 1993). Increased feedings will satisfy the infant's need for more fluids when it is hot. Part of the higher weight gains in artificially fed infants and set patterns for obesity in childhood and adulthood may result from greater sodium and water retention during infancy.

Iron

During the final 6 to 8 weeks of pregnancy, a healthy nonanemic mother lays down iron stores to provide her baby with enough iron through her milk for the first few months postpartum. Blood from the umbilical cord also contributes iron that is stored in the infant's liver. Although iron is present in human milk in only small quantities, this level is sufficient to meet the iron requirements of the exclusively breastfed full-term infant until the child is approximately 6 months old. A preterm infant may need iron supplementation due to receiving insufficient iron in utero.

The iron in human milk is absorbed more efficiently than the iron in cow's milk, partly because of the high vitamin C level present in human milk. Babies absorb 60 percent of the iron in human milk, compared with only 4 percent of the iron in artificial baby milk. Infants do not begin to deplete their iron stores until 4 to 6 months after birth, or even later. Routine supplementation of iron is of questionable value for this reason, and may even be detrimental to the breastfed infant. Lactoferrin loses its ability to inhibit the growth of bacteria when saturated with exogenous iron (Chan, 2003). A longitudinal study found that infants who were iron deficient at 12 months had been breastfed a shorter time than those who had sufficient iron levels (Thorsdottir et al., 2003).

Hemoglobin is the iron-containing portion of the red blood cell that carries oxygen to all parts of the body. The healthy infant's hemoglobin level is high at birth (18 to 20 g/dL), but then decreases rapidly as the child's body adjusts to extrauterine life. At 4 months of age, levels of hemoglobin typically range between 10.2 and 15 g/dL. Over this same period, there is also a change in the type of hemoglobin, from fetal to adult; the latter form is more efficient in delivering oxygen to the tissues. Therefore, although the actual amount (grams) of hemoglobin decreases, the efficiency of each gram increases as this change takes place.

Fluoride

Studies have shown conclusively that during the development of primary and secondary teeth, fluoride supplements ingested by the infant reduce cavities by 50 to 60 percent. In communities with fluoridated drinking water, breastfed babies receive fluoride through their mother's milk. If the family's water supply contains less than 0.3 ppm of fluoride, infant fluoride supplementation is recommended after the age of 6 months (CDC, 2001; Institute of Medicine, 1997).

Babies who receive supplementary fluoride may occasionally exhibit allergic reactions, described by mothers as taking the form of fussiness, irritability, refusal to take the fluoride, and spitting it up (Jelliffe & Jelliffe, 1978). Excessive fluoride may cause fluorosis, a condition in which teeth become mottled or discolored. Breastfeeding beyond 6 months may protect children from developing fluorosis in their permanent teeth (Brothwell & Limeback, 2003). One study concluded that infant formulas prepared with fluoridated water increase the risk of fluorosis in primary teeth (Marshall et al., 2004).

Other Constituents

Human milk contains more than 200 known components, including the trace elements copper, zinc, manganese, silicon, aluminum, and titanium. Scientists continue to study the significance of these components. Zinc deficiency in infancy, for instance, can cause failure to thrive and skin lesions. The increased bioavailability of the zinc in human milk can be life saving in the inherited zinc-deficiency disorder known as acrodermatitis enteropathica. Cow's milk formula has no effect on the development of this condition (Lawrence & Lawrence, 2005).

Researchers have identified more than 20 human milk enzymes, as well as prolactin and steroid hormones (Lawrence & Lawrence, 2005). One enzyme, lipase, is essential for digesting fat and making it available to the infant as energy. Another enzyme, amylase, is important for carbohydrate digestion (Dewit et al., 1993). Artificial baby milk lacks these digestive enzymes.

Nitrogen compounds in human milk are of key interest to researchers. Nucleotides, in the form of nonprotein nitrogen, are an integral part of the immune system. They act as the host defense against bacteria, viruses, and parasites, as well as various malignancies. Nucleotides are relatively absent in cow's milk and are now added to artificial baby milks (Inoue et al., 2008; Gil et al., 2007).

Other milk components under study include prostaglandins, bile salts, and epidermal growth factor. Epidermal growth factor (EGF), which is present in colostrum, preterm milk, and term milk, promotes the growth and healing of gut mucosa. In preterm babies, EGF may be significant in helping their guts mature more efficiently (Dvorak et al., 2003; Xiao et al., 2002). Artificial baby milks do not contain this growth factor.

Cytokines are proteins secreted by a variety of cells, but especially those found in the immune system, including granulocyte colony-stimulating factor (G-CSF). Concentrations of G-CSF are higher for 2 days postpartum and are lower in the milk of mothers with preterm infants. G-CSF receptor cells are present in the intestinal cells of breastfed infants (Calhoun et al., 2000).

Cholecystokinin (CCK) is a digestive hormone found in the digestive tract and brain. Triggered by the baby's sucking, CCK production may be responsible for the sleepiness mothers and babies experience while nursing. Release of this hormone also may create the feeling of satiety in babies (Marchini & Linden, 1992).

Ghrelin is a peptide hormone called the "hunger hormone." Researchers have found significantly high levels of ghrelin, but not CCK, in mothers. Ghrelin may be produced by the breast tissue (Kierson et al., 2006) or may come from the plasma (Aydin et al., 2006). Other peptide hormones identified in human milk include leptin and obestatin (Aydin et al., 2006). According to Aydin and colleagues, "Ghrelin, obestatin, and leptin in the milk may directly affect appetite and their levels may be related to the regulation of energy balance and the pathogenesis of obesity."

Studies of specific components also show that each mother's milk differs slightly due to individual genetic codes. In other words, each breastfed infant receives a unique product! One of the most interesting recent discoveries about human milk is the presence of nestin-positive putative mammary stem cells. These cells represent "a readily available and non-invasive source of putative mammary stem cells that may be useful for research into both mammary gland biology and more general stem cell biology" (Cregan, 2007). This possible alternative to embryonic stem cells for the purpose of research is of ethical interest to many researchers (Russo et al., 2006; Yoshimura, 2006).

⟡ Health Benefits of Human Milk

Human milk is a species-specific first food that offers biologically natural nutrition for the child as well as health protection to support the infant's developing immune system. The mother provides the specific protection her baby needs for the environment in which they live, both in terms of allergens and infection protection. Human milk further protects the infant through its packaging. It does not spoil, the temperature is always correct, it is not subject to mixing errors, there are no omissions of components, and there are no product recalls! Research continues to confirm new health benefits of human milk for the newborn, older child, and mother.

Intelligence and Neurological Development

Many studies demonstrate that human milk confers greater intelligence in human babies (Kramer et al., 2008; Horta et al., 2007; Elwood et al., 2005; Gomez-Sanchiz et al., 2004; Smith et al., 2003; Rao et al., 2002; Anderson et al., 1999; Horwood, 1998; Lucas et al., 1992). Because human milk is the biological norm, it is actually more accurate to state that artificially fed babies are statistically not as smart as breastfed infants. Noteworthy among these studies is Lucas and colleagues' seminal work with preterm infants fed human milk via tube feedings, away from the breast (Lucas, 1990; Lucas et al., 1990, 1992). These studies revealed a dose-related response, with the IQ of artificially fed babies being an average of 8.3 points lower at ages $7\frac{1}{2}$ to 8 years compared to their breastfed counterpoints. At 18 months, there was decreased neuromotor development, calculated as 15 motor development index points, and 23 points for infants born small for gestational age (SGA) in the artificially fed groups.

Spanish studies measuring infants at 18 months and 24 months found that breastfeeding longer than 4 months resulted in an average 4.6-point advantage (18 months) and 4.3 point advantage (24 months) on mental development scores (Gomez-Sanchiz et al., 2003, 2004). An IQ increase of as little as 3 points from 100 to 103 moves a person from the 50th to the 58th percentile of the population (International Lactation Consultant Association [(ILCA], 2007). Research continues to demonstrate that human milk provides children with an optimal start in terms of learning, abstract thinking, and complex problem-solving skills.

A study that examined breastfeeding and adult IQ found that breastfeeding is dose dependent. In this investigation, adults who had not been breastfed for 9 months or more as infants measured an average of 4.6 IQ points lower on the Weschler Adult Intelligence Scale (WAIS) and 2.1 points lower on the Borge Priens Prove (BPP), two standard intelligence tests than their breastfed peers (Mortensen et al., 2002). A meta-analysis of 11 studies found a difference in cognitive function of 3.16 points at ages between 6 and 23 months and years later. It was concluded that the cognitive developmental benefits of breastfeeding increase with duration of breastfeeding (Anderson et al., 1999). A study measuring verbal cognitive IQ found an adjusted score of 3.56 points lower for non-breastfed babies compared to babies breastfed beyond 6 months (Oddy et al., 2003a). A 2002 prospective study predicted an 11-point IQ disadvantage for SGA children compared to babies exclusively breastfed for 24 weeks (Rao et al., 2002).

In a study of children aged 6 through 8 years who had been very-low-birth-weight (VLBW) infants, artificially fed children scored 5.1 IQ points lower for visual–motor integration, 3.6 IQ points lower for overall intellectual function, and 2.3 IQ points lower for verbal ability than their breastfed counterparts (Smith et al., 2003). Another study found that at only 8.5 days old, artificially fed infants underperformed breastfed infants on orientation, motor, range of state, and state regulation dimensions on the Brazelton newborn assessment scale. Artificially fed infants had more subnormal reflexes, signs of depression, and withdrawal. It was concluded that lack of breastfeed-

ing hinders newborns' neurobehavioral organization (Hart et al., 2003).

The Promotion of Breastfeeding Intervention Trial (PROBIT) randomized trial study enrolled more than 17,000 infants and followed 81.5 percent of them to age 6.5 years. The artificially fed children had lower means on all of the Wechsler Abbreviated Scales of Intelligence measures. These students' academic ratings were significantly lower for both reading and writing (Kramer et al., 2008).

Dissenting research has also been produced, albeit frequently funded by formula companies. Jain and colleagues (2002) surveyed 40 studies on the link between breastfeeding and IQ. Although 68 percent of these studies concluded that breastfeeding increased intelligence, the "higher-quality" studies were less persuasive. The 40 studies in Jain et al.'s meta-analysis did not include the newer studies cited earlier.

Disease Protection

Human milk contains a wide variety of soluble, cellular, and humoral factors that affect maturation of the body's systems. The mother's milk protects the infant against a host of diseases and confers lifelong immunities. As infants grow, they develop their own active immunity as their bodies begin to produce antibodies. Through this means, children are protected against bacterial infections (Table 9.2), viral infections (Table 9.3), protozoans (Table 9.4), and allergies (Monterrosa et al., 2008; Bener et al., 2007; Turck, 2005; Newburg et al., 2004; Bachrach et al., 2003; Tellez et al., 2003; Van Odijk et al., 2003; Silfverdal et al., 2002). Perhaps the most spectacular disadvantage of artificial baby milk is the lack of protection against disease for the infants fed on it.

Studies show higher death rates for babies who are not fed human milk. Research from developed countries sometimes suggests that breastfeeding is not important for protection from infection for babies in wealthy nations (Rubin et al., 1990; Bauchner et al., 1986). In reality, these studies are flawed both methodologically and by improper grouping of partially breastfed and exclusively breastfed babies. Breastfeeding, in fact, could prevent an estimated 720 infant deaths per year in the United States (Chen & Rogan, 2004). Rates of preventable infant deaths in Brazil range from 33 to 72 percent of deaths from respiratory infections and 35 to 86 percent of deaths from diarrheal infections (Escuder et al., 2003). The longer an infant breastfeeds, the greater protection he or she receives (Chen & Rogan, 2004; Habicht et al., 1986). Chapter 27 discusses research and provides strategies to help you read and analyze all studies with discernment. These tools will be especially helpful when the popular media report on a study that sensationalizes a negative focus on breastfeeding.

In light of what has already been learned about human milk, the AAP (2005) recommends that all

TABLE 9.2   Antibacterial Factors Found in Human Milk

Factor	Shown in Vitro to Be Active Against
Secretory IgA	*E. coli* (also *pili*, capsular antigens, CFA1), *C. tetani, C. diphtheriae, K. pneumoniae, S. mutans, S. sanguins, S. mitis, S. agalactiae, S. salvarius, S. pneumoniae, C. burnetti, H. influenza, H. pylori, S. flexneri, S. boydii, S. sonnei, C. jejuni, N. meningitidis, B. pertussis, S. dysenteriae, C. trachomatis,* Salmonella (6 groups), *Campylobacter flagelin, S. flexneri* virulence plasmid antigen, *C. diphtheriae* toxin, *E. coli* enterotoxin, *V. cholerae* enterotoxin, *C. difficile* toxins, *H. influenza* capsule, *S. aureus* enterotoxin F, *Candida albicans*
IgG	*E. coli, B. pertussis, H. influenza* type b, *S. pneumoniae, S. agalactiae, N. meningitidis,* 14 pneumococcal capsular polysaccharides, *V. cholerae* lipopolysaccharide, *S. flexneri* invasion plasmid–coded antigens, major opsonin for *S. aureus*
IgM	*V. cholerae* lipopolysaccharide
IgD	*E. coli*
Free secretory component*	*E. coli* colonization factor antigen I (CFA1)
Bifidobacterium bifidum	Enteric bacteria
Growth factors (oligosaccharides, glycopeptides)	
Other bifidobacteria growth factors (alpha-lactoglobulin, lactoferrin, sialyllactose)	
Factor-finding proteins (zinc, vitamin B_{12}, folate)	Dependent *E. coli*
Complement C1-C9 (mainly C3 and C4)	Killing of *S. aureus* in macrophages
Lactoferrin*	*E. coli, E. coli*/CFA1, *Candida albicans*
Lactoperoxidase	Streptococcus, Pseudomonas, *E. coli, S. typhimurium*
Lysozyme	*E. coli,* Salmonella, *M. lysodeikticus,* growing *Candida albicans* and *Aspergillus fumigatus*
Unidentified factors	*S. aureus, B. pertussis, C. jejuni, E. coli, S. typhimurium, S. flexneri, S. sonnei, V. cholerae, L. pomona, L. hyos, L. icterohaemorrhagiae, C. difficile* toxin B, *H. pylori*
Nonimmunoglobulin (milk fat, proteins)	*C. trachomatis, Y. enterocolitica*
Carbohydrate	*E. coli* enterotoxin, *E. coli, C. difficile* toxin A
Lipid	*S. aureus, E. coli, S. epidermis, H. influenzae, S. agalactiae*
Ganglioside GM_1	*E. coli* enterotoxin, *V. cholerae* toxin, *C. jejuni* enterotoxin, *E. coli*
Ganglioside GM_3	*E. coli*
Phosphatidylethanolamine	*H. pylori*
Sialyllactose	*V. cholerae* toxin, *H. pylori*
Mucin (milk fat globulin membrane)	*E. coli* (S-fimbrinated) sialyloligosaccharides on sIgA(Fc), *E. coli* (S-fimbrinated) adhesion
Glycoproteins (receptor-like) + oligosaccharides	*V. cholerae*

(Continued)

TABLE 9.2 Antibacterial Factors Found in Human Milk *(Continued)*

Factor	Shown in Vitro to Be Active Against
Glycoproteins (mannosylated)	*E. coli*
kappa-Casein*	*H. pylori, S. pneumoniae*
Casein	*H. influenza*
Glycolipid Gb₃	*S. dysenterae* toxin, shigatoxin of shigella and *E. coli*
Fucosylated oligosaccharides	*E. coli* heat-stable enterotoxin, *C. jejuni, E. coli*
Analogues of epithelial cell receptors (oligosaccharides)	*S. pneumoniae, H. influenza*
Milk cells (macrophages, neutrophils, B and T lymphocytes)	By phagocytosis and killing: *E. coli, S. aureus, S. enteritidis*
	By sensitized lymphocytes: *E. coli*
	By phagocytosis: *Candida albicans*[†,‡], *E. coli*
	Lymphocyte stimulation: *E. coli,* K antigen, tuberculin
	Spontaneous monokines: simulated by lipopolysaccharide
	Induced cytokines: PHA, PMA + ionomycin
	Fibronectin helps in uptake by phagocytic cells

*Factors found at low levels in human milk can be antibacterial at higher levels, e.g., secretory leukocyte protease inhibitor (antileukocyte protease) has antibacterial *(E. coli, S. aureus)* and antifungal (growing *C. albicans* and *A. fumigatus*) activity.

[†]Fungi.

[‡]Contain fucosylated oligosaccharides.

Source: From Proceedings of Breast Milk and Special Care Nurseries: Problems and Opportunities Conference. August 1995. Melbourne. Copyright J. T. May and Australian Lactation Consultants Association Victorian Branch, 1995. Updated August, 1998.

Reprinted by permission of Department of Microbiology, La Trobe University, Bundoora Victoria 3083, Australia.

TABLE 9.3 Antiviral Factors Found in Human Milk

Factor	Shown in Vitro to Be Active Against
Secretory IgA	Polio types 1, 2, 3; Coxsackie types A9, B3, B5; echo types 6, 9; Semliki Forest virus; Ross River virus; rotavirus; cytomegalovirus; reovirus type 3; rubella varicella-zoster virus; herpes simplex virus; mumps virus; influenza; respiratory syncytial virus; human immunodeficiency virus; hepatitis C virus; hepatitis B virus; measles
IgG	Rubella, cytomegalovirus, respiratory syncytial virus, rotavirus, human immunodeficiency virus, Epstein-Barr virus
IgM	Rubella, cytomegalovirus, respiratory syncytial virus, human immunodeficiency virus
Lipid (unsaturated fatty acids and monoglycerides)	Herpes simplex virus, Semliki Forest virus, influenza, dengue, Ross River virus, Japanese B encephalitis virus, sindbis, West Nile, human immunodeficiency virus, respiratory syncytial virus, vesicular stomatitis virus
Non-immunoglobulin macromolecules	Herpes simplex virus, vesicular stomatitis virus, Coxsackie B4, Semliki Forest virus, reovirus 3, poliotype 2, cytomegalovirus, respiratory syncytial virus, rotavirus
alpha2-macroglobulin (-like)	Influenza haemagglutinin, parainfluenza haemagglutinin
Ribonuclease	Murine leukemia
Hemagglutinin inhibitors	Influenza, mumps

TABLE 9.3 Antiviral Factors Found in Human Milk *(Continued)*

Factor	Shown in Vitro to Be Active Against
Mucin (glycoprotein/lactadherin)	Rotavirus
Chondroitin sulphate (-like)	Human immunodeficiency virus
Secretory leukocyte protease inhibitor (colostrum levels)	Human immunodeficiency virus, *Bifidobacterium bifidum*, rotavirus
sIgA + trypsin inhibitor	Rotavirus
Lactoferrin	Cytomegalovirus, human immunodeficiency virus, respiratory syncytial virus, herpes simplex virus type 1, hepatitis C
Milk cells	Induced interferon: virus, PHA, or PMA and ionomycin
	Induced cytokine: herpes simplex virus, respiratory syncytial virus
	Lymphocyte stimulation: rubella, cytomegalovirus, herpes, measles, mumps, respiratory syncytial virus

Factors found at low levels in human milk, known to be antiviral at higher levels:

  prostaglandins E2, F2 alpha (parainfluenza 3, measles)

  gangliosides GM1-3 (rotavirus, respiratory syncytial virus)

  heparin (cytomegalovirus, respiratory syncytial virus)

  glycolipid Gb4 (human B19 parvovirus)

Source: From Proceedings of Breast Milk and Special Care Nurseries: Problems and Opportunities Conference. August 1995. Melbourne. Copyright J. T. May and Australian Lactation Consultants Association Victorian Branch, 1995. Updated August, 1998.

Reprinted by permission of Department of Microbiology, La Trobe University, Bundoora Victoria 3083, Australia.

TABLE 9.4 Antiparasite Factors Found in Human Milk

Factor	Shown in Vitro to Be Active Against
Secretory IgA	*Giardia lamblia*
	Entamoeba histolytica
	Schistosoma mansoni (blood fluke)
	Cryptosporidium
	Toxoplasma gondii
	Plasmodium falciparum (malaria)
IgG	*Plasmodium falciparum*
Lipid (free fatty acids and monoglycerides)	*Giardia lamblia*
	Entamoeba histolytica
	Trichomonas vaginalis
	Giardia intestinalis
	Eimeria tenella (animal coccidiosis)
Unidentified	*Trypanosoma brucei rhodesiense*

Source: From Proceedings of Breast Milk and Special Care Nurseries: Problems and Opportunities Conference. August 1995. Melbourne. Copyright J. T. May and Australian Lactation Consultants Association Victorian Branch, 1995. Updated August, 1998.

Reprinted by permission of Department of Microbiology, La Trobe University, Bundoora Victoria 3083, Australia.

mothers breastfeed their infants for at least 1 year. In making this recommendation, the AAP cites both the psychological value afforded the breastfeeding mother and infant and the protection against disease received by the maturing infant. WHO (2009b) recommends exclusive breastfeeding for 6 months and continued breastfeeding for 2 years and beyond. The American Academy of Family Physicians (AAFP, 2009) supports breastfeeding beyond infancy as well as tandem nursing.

Anti-infective Agents

At birth, the infant is suddenly exposed to a variety of microorganisms to which the mother is already immune. She passes this passive immunity to her baby, both across the placenta before birth and in her colostrum and milk after birth. When a new microorganism enters the environment, the mother most likely is able to produce corresponding antibodies to it. She passes these antibodies to the baby through her milk (Hanson, 2004b, 2007a).

In addition to this internal mechanism, it seems that the breast itself also produces antibodies to the organisms passed into it by the suckling infant. The mammary gland produces immunoglobulins locally and passes them to the infant in the mother's milk, thereby protecting the child from the harmful effects of disease organisms.

Although human milk is not sterile, it contains a number of anti-infective agents that maintain a very low bacterial level for many hours. As a consequence, breast-milk can destroy bacteria in the infant's GI tract before they affect the infant. Milk components also coat the GI tract, thereby preventing other offending organisms and molecules from entering the infant's system. Many researchers have reported a higher incidence of infection in artificially fed babies (Loland, 2007; Schack-Nielsen & Michaelsen, 2007; Jackson & Nazar, 2006; Paramasivam et al., 2006; Wold & Adlerbeth, 2000).

Immunoglobulin A The presence of IgA in colostrum and human milk protects the infant's GI tract against penetration by organisms and antigens. This immunoglobulin is probably the most important of the antiviral defense factors and is at its highest level immediately after birth. IgA binds to bacteria and prevents those pathogens from binding to receptor sites and invading the gut. While it does not kill the bacteria, IgA surrounds them and prevents these agents from attacking or attaching to receptor sites, thereby preventing their invasion of the body.

Levels of IgA remain relatively high for at least 6 or 7 months. IgA and sialic acid survive passage through the GI tract and are found in much higher concentrations in breastfed infants' stools than in artificially fed infants' stools (Kohler et al., 2002; Fernandes et al., 2001). Colostrum and human milk also contain living white cells—lymphocytes and macrophages—that engulf and digest bacteria and synthesize IgA and other protective substances.

Growth Factors and Enzymes Growth factors enhance the infant's development and the maturation of the immune system, the central nervous system, and organs such as skin. Two digestive enzymes, lactase and lipase, as well as many other important enzymes, protect babies born with immature or defective enzyme systems. Lactase is necessary for converting lactose into simple sugars that the infant can assimilate easily. A deficiency in lactase can result in lactose intolerance, a condition that generally occurs because of diminishing activity of intestinal lactase after weaning. A person who is lactose intolerant is unable to digest milk sugar (lactose). The condition is more prevalent in adults and is rare in children younger than 3 years of age. As discussed earlier, lactose helps prevent the development of rickets and aids in calcium absorption and brain development.

The enzyme lysozyme protects the breastfed infant by breaking down bacteria in the bowel. The bowel receives protection from lactoferrin, an iron-binding protein that acts together with specific antibodies to inhibit the growth of *E. coli*, the major cause of bowel infection in infants (Kelly & Coutts, 2000; Orrhage & Nord, 1999). Human lactoferrin is 100 times more resistant to breakdown than bovine lactoferrin (Van Veen et al., 2004). If a baby receives too much iron, either through supplements or enriched foods, the effectiveness of this protein will be diminished significantly (Chan, 2003).

Bifidus Factor Bifidus factor is a carbohydrate in human milk that discourages the growth of undesirable organisms such as *E. coli*. The factor, which is also known as *lactobacillus bifidus*, is present in high concentrations in both colostrum and mature milk. Human milk contains 7 times as much of this factor as does cow's milk. The bifidus factor works with the low pH of the stool to help beneficial bacteria grow in the infant's intestine while inhibiting the growth of harmful bacteria.

Thymus The thymus is a gland that is especially active in infancy and childhood. Its main function is to develop immature lymphocytes into immunocompetent T cells. The thymus in artificially fed babies is smaller than its counterpart in breastfed babies (Jeppesson et al., 2004; Hasselbalch et al., 1999). The smaller size of the thymus in artificially fed babies suggests that artificial feeding hinders the developing immune system.

Specific Protection

Human milk protects the infant and the breast by providing anti-infective agents and minimizing inflammation. It protects against infections outside the GI tract as well, including upper and lower respiratory infections (Ogbuanu et al., 2009; Mihrshahi et al., 2008; Brandtzaeg, 2007; Ip et al., 2007; Turck, 2005) including respiratory syncytial virus (RSV) (Oddy et al., 2003b; Levine et al., 1999; Bulkow et al., 2002); otitis media (see the separate discussion of this condition that follows); urinary tract infections (Marild et al., 2004); sepsis (Meinzen-Derr et al., 2004); rotavirus (Gianino, 2002; Mastretta et al., 2002); and meningitis (Hylander et al., 1998).

Artificial feeding increases the risk for childhood cancers (Smulevich et al., 1999), leukemia and lymphoma (Perrilat, 2002; Bener et al., 2001; Shu et al., 1999), Hodgkin's disease (Davis, 1998), and neuroblastoma (Daniels et al., 2002). Having been breastfed also lowers women's risk of breast cancer in adulthood (Potischman & Troisi, 1999; Freudenhim, 1994).

Not being breastfed increases the risks for a variety of chronic and autoimmune diseases, including inflammatory bowel disease such as Crohn's and ulcerative colitis (Thompson et al., 2000; Corrao et al., 1998), juvenile diabetes (Ip et al., 2007; Young et al., 2002; Kimpimaki et al., 2001; Monetinti, 2001), juvenile arthritis (Mason et al., 1995), multiple sclerosis (Tarrats et al., 2002; Pisacane et al., 1994), celiac disease (Ivarsson et al., 2002), hypertension (Singhal et al., 2001), and high cholesterol and heart disease (Owen et al., 2002, 2008; Singhal et al., 2004; Ravelli et al., 2000). Childhood and adult obesity is a major health problem worldwide. Breastfeeding protects against obesity (Butte, 2009; Griffiths et al., 2009; Rudnicka et al., 2007; Owen et al., 2005; Turck, 2005; Grummer-Strawn et al., 2004; Martin et al., 2004; Toschke et al., 2002), whereas artificial feeding increases obesity rates.

Otitis Media One of the most common infant infections—otitis media, or middle ear infection—occurs more frequently in the absence of breastfeeding. Aniansson and colleagues (1994) observed this link and noted that the first episode of otitis media occurs earlier in children weaned before 6 months of age. In their study, both mixed feedings and the absence of human milk in the diet increased the risk of infection.

Exclusive breastfeeding for at least 4 months appears to be the best protection against otitis media (Ip et al., 2007; Turck, 2005; Duncan et al., 1993). The longer the mother breastfeeds, the greater protection her baby receives. In one study, infants who were breastfed for at least 12 months had otitis media rates 19 percent lower than those for formula-fed infants (Dewey et al., 1995).

Even after weaning, the protection against otitis media afforded by human milk remains hard at work. Human milk stimulates the breastfed infant's immune system, reducing the risk of otitis media for several years after breastfeeding ends (Hanson et al., 2002). In a study conducted by the CDC, researchers found that "when compared with exclusively breastfed infants, infants who received only formula had an 80 percent increase in their risk of developing diarrhea and a 70 percent increase in

their risk of developing an ear infection" (Scariati et al., 1997).

Necrotizing Enterocolitis and Sepsis Artificial feeding increases the occurrence of necrotizing enterocolitis (NEC) among infants. NEC is characterized by inflammation of the intestinal wall, often causing the tissue to die. It is frequently associated with prematurity, respiratory disease, and early enteral feedings of formula in preterm babies (Lucas, 1990). NEC occurs in 2 to 7 percent of preterm babies (Buescher, 1994, 2004; Udall, 1990). It is 6 to 10 times more likely to occur in artificially fed babies than in those fed human milk exclusively (Ip et al., 2007; Lucas, 1990). Among babies born after 30 weeks' gestation, the risk of NEC is reported to be 20 times higher for the artificially fed babies. Furthermore, NEC is reportedly 3 times more likely to occur in babies who receive mixed feedings than in those who are fed only human milk (Dugdale, 1991; Lucas, 1990).

Research indicates that this same protection against NEC is found with pasteurized donor milk (Updegrove, 2004). A meta-analysis of four studies found infants who received donor human milk were 3 times less likely to develop NEC and 4 times less likely to have confirmed NEC (McGuire & Anthony, 2003). Researchers theorize that the secretory IgA and phagocytes found in breastmilk help protect infants against NEC (Buescher, 1994, 2004). Preventive therapy using human milk feedings has reduced NEC rates. Although probiotic and prebiotic supplementation is being tested in this population, caution is recommended (Caplan, 2009).

Another risk of artificial feeding to hospitalized babies relates to the higher incidence of nosocomial (hospital-acquired) sepsis observed among these infants. Researchers at George Washington University Hospital found that even though babies who received expressed human milk had bacterial colonies similar to those in formula fed babies, they nevertheless had a significantly lower incidence of infection (El-Mohandes et al., 1997). Although preterm infants may gain weight faster with artificial feeding, infants who are fed only human milk leave the hospital an average of 15 days earlier than the artificially fed infants because of reduced sepsis and reduced rates of NEC (Schanler et al., 1999).

Diarrhea In developing countries, 5 million children die each year from diarrheal disease. Human milk protects infants from digestive infections (Mihrshahi, 2008; Ip et al., 2007; Turck, 2005). Study data suggest that the risk of dying from diarrhea could decline 14 to 24 times if breastfeeding rates increased. Even babies in the industrialized world would benefit from the breastmilk-afforded protection against diarrhea (Brandtzaeg, 2003). A Brazilian study found non-breastfed infants were 82 percent more likely to experience diarrhea than infants who were exclusively breastfed for the first 6 months of life (Vieira et al., 2003). Exclusive breastfeeding also protects infants against diarrhea caused by *Giardia* (Tellez et al., 2003; Mahmud et al., 2001) and *E. coli* (Clemens et al., 1997).

Protection from Maternal Antigens Protection from human milk extends beyond common childhood illnesses and illnesses of the mother to the infant's immediate environment. Antibodies in human milk are highly targeted against infectious agents in the mother's environment—those to which the infant is likely to be exposed shortly after birth (Hanson, 2007a; Brandtzaeg, 2003). Whenever a mother contracts an infection, whether it be a cold, fever, or more serious illness, her body responds by producing antibodies in her milk that help protect her breastfed baby.

Although some viruses pass into the mother's milk, the presence of antibodies to counteract them offsets the potential harm to the baby. In fact, some evidence indicates that milk responds to and "remembers" for years specific infections it has encountered. In one study, Asian mothers in the United Kingdom showed antibodies to pathogens they had encountered in their home countries several years earlier (Nathavitharana et al., 1994). Researchers believe this transmission may confer passive immunity to the infant, as in the case of cytomegalovirus (Hamprecht et al., 2001).

A more likely mechanism of disease transmission from mother to baby is through close contact such as touching and through close mouth and nose contact, rather than through the mother's milk. When a breastfeeding mother contracts an illness, it is likely that her baby was exposed through contact during her most contagious period. Therefore, the most effective treatment for the infant is to continue breastfeeding while receiving any necessary medication. The mother can decrease the infant's exposure to the disease with careful hand washing before contact and, in extreme cases, by wearing a mask over her nose and mouth. A mother who develops a cold or fever need not worry about infecting her baby through her milk. Instead, she can practice good hygiene and limit facial contact with her baby during the infectious period. Urge her to rest and follow the treatment plan prescribed by her caregiver so that she can return to good health quickly and not compromise her milk production.

Immunization Response Human milk contains antibodies capable of enhancing infant antibody response (Van de Perre, 2003). Studies show lower immune responses to vaccines in artificially fed infants. Some researchers believe that breastfed and artificially fed infants have similar levels of protection after immunization (Scheifele et al., 1992). However, a variety of studies have concluded that breastfeeding offers both current and long-term immune-modulating effects on the child's developing cellular immune system (Jeppesen et al., 2004; Pickering, 1998; Pabst et al., 1997).

Other Immunologic Factors Countless unidentified factors in human milk aid in the protection of the infant from disease. Ongoing research continues to uncover more details about these protective factors. For example, mucins found in human milk play a role in protection against bacterial infections, including such severe illnesses as neonatal sepsis and meningitis (Schroten et al., 1992, 1993). They also are linked to protection against rotavirus, an acute GI infection (Gianino, 2002; Mastretta et al., 2002).

Human milk contains three essential thyroid hormones that are completely absent from cow's milk and conventional infant formulas. These hormones may be responsible for preventing hypothyroidism, masking diagnosis, and protecting the baby until he or she weans:

- Alpha-lactalbumin acts as a bactericide against *Streptococcus pneumonaiae*.
- A peptide in human milk inhibits bacteria and yeast growths (Hakansson et al., 2000).
- Xantine oxidase is an antibacterial enzyme that, when combined with nitrites, creates nitric oxide, which inhibits invasion of the body by Enterobacteriaceae, *E. coli*, and *Salmonella enteritidis* (Hancock et al., 2002).

Nucleotides are compounds derived from nucleic acids that are secreted by mammary epithelial cells. These agents play key roles in many biological processes, including promoting optimal functioning and growth of the gastrointestinal and immune systems. Human milk contains much higher amounts of nucleotides than cow's milk formulas (Carver, 1999). Formula manufacturers now add nucleotides to most artificial baby milks to compensate for this shortcoming.

Allergy Protection

There are almost no antibodies in the immature intestine of a newborn infant, which leaves the wall of the intestine susceptible to invasion by foreign proteins. Human milk contains high levels of antibodies, especially IgA, which provides antiabsorptive protection to the lining of the infant's intestine. This effect shields the surface from the absorption of foreign protein and from bacterial invasion. Increased gut maturation prevents foreign proteins from entering the infant's system. Human milk nutrients such as zinc and the long-chain polyunsaturated fatty acids aid in the development of the infant's immune response. The GI tract of infants develops more slowly when they do not receive human milk.

Cow's Milk Allergy

Giving babies even a single feeding of artificial baby milk in the first days of life can increase the rates of allergic disease. All formulas carry allergy risks, including soy formulas. Symptoms of allergy are more prevalent in infants fed cow's milk–based formula than in breastfed infants (Van Odijk et al., 2003; Tariq et al., 1998). And these effects are long lived: A Finnish long-term study revealed evidence of reduced allergy in a breastfed group at age 17 (Saarinen & Kajosaari, 1995). There is also the possibility that other food antigens may cause allergy responses in infants who are fed formula, because solid foods frequently are introduced at an earlier age in these infants. Exclusive breastfeeding for 4 months can postpone the onset of cow's milk allergy (Yinyaem et al., 2003).

Giving formula in the first week of life is the first of several factors in allergy development (Marini et al., 1996). Cow's milk is the most common food allergen in infants, with an estimated allergy rate between 3 and 5 percent in industrialized countries (Infante et al., 2003). One researcher suggests that 25 percent of colicky behavior occurs in response to cow's milk allergy (Lindberg, 1999). Most infants with cow's milk allergy develop symptoms before 1 month of age, often within 1 week after introduction of cow's milk protein-based formula (Host, 2002).

Cow's milk formulas do not contain the antibodies necessary to protect the infant's intestines. Instead, the foreign protein of cow's milk passes through the intestinal wall and causes allergic reactions in sensitive infants. These reactions may manifest themselves as colicky behavior, diarrhea, vomiting, malabsorption, eczema, ear infections, or asthma.

Atopic dermatitis, including eczema, is also much more common in artificially fed infants. One large meta-analysis of 18 studies found that exclusive breastfeeding during the first 3 months of life is associated with significantly lower rates of atopic dermatitis in children with a family history of this condition (Gdalevich et al., 2001a). By comparison, exclusive breastfeeding for 4 to 6 months and delaying supplemental foods reduces the incidence of atopic symptoms, especially eczema, as well as gastrointestinal symptoms attributable to cow's milk (European Society for Paediatric Gastroenterology, Hepatology and Nutrition [ESPGHAN], 2008).

Other Allergies

Human milk is best able to protect any infant, with or without allergic tendencies, until the child's intestinal tract and immune system mature. Although breastfeeding does not eliminate all possible food allergies, artificial feeding greatly increases their incidence and hastens their onset. In addition, this practice increases the incidence of asthma, a respiratory disease. Allergies cause half of all

asthma cases. One study showed that exclusive breastfeeding for less than 4 months was a "significant risk factor for recurrent asthma, with an odds ratio of 1:35" (Oddy et al., 2002). "A large cohort study found a dose-response effect, with a longer breastfeeding duration being protective against the development of asthma and wheeze in young children" (Dell & To, 2001). A meta-analysis of 12 studies found that exclusive breastfeeding during the first months of life is associated with lower asthma rates during childhood and especially benefits the child with a family history of allergy (Gdalevich et al., 2001b).

An infant is rarely, if ever, allergic to his or her mother's milk. At the same time, the infant may show allergic symptoms in response to foods ingested by the mother and passed through her milk (Hill et al., 2004; Saavedra et al., 2003). Allergens pass through the mother's milk and may cause reactions such as spitting, vomiting, gas, diarrhea, colicky behavior, or skin rash. Chapter 13 includes a discussion of the causes and treatment of colic.

Human Milk for the Preterm Infant

The medical community has become increasingly aware that human milk is vital to the preterm infant. The milk of women who deliver prematurely has special properties that are particularly beneficial to the infant (Hartmann et al., 2003; Butte et al., 1984). Such milk contains higher concentrations of sodium, chloride, and nitrogen, as well as immunoprotective factors. This composition may be of great significance in supporting the immature GI tract of the preterm infant.

Artificially fed preterm infants have an increased risk of NEC (Bisquera et al., 2002) as well as poorer neurodevelopment than their counterparts who are fed human milk (Lucas et al., 1994). Lack of human milk is also associated with lower IQ scores during childhood (Smith et al., 2003). Given these findings, many caregivers recommend that preterm infants receive their mothers' milk regardless of whether the mother had planned to breastfeed. Many mothers who intend to bottle feed will pump their milk for a baby in the neonatal intensive care unit (NICU). The next best choice is donor milk from a human milk bank (Wight, 2001).

Human Milk Fortifiers

Some debate remains over whether a mother's milk requires supplementation for her preterm infant. To date, the question of optimal brain growth has received little attention from researchers (Ebrahim, 1993). The main concern focuses on rectifying the missed intrauterine growth by providing increased protein and energy in the preterm infant's diet (Klein, 2002). Human milk has the ideal protein balance for babies who weigh 1500 g or more

(3 lb, 5 oz). For infants who weigh less than 1500 g, and especially those who weigh less than 1000 g (2 lb, 3 oz), the mother's milk is not considered adequate as the sole source of nutrition. Nevertheless, clinical practice guidelines in Canada encourage that breastmilk be used preferentially as food for these neonates (Premji et al., 2002). Human milk fortifiers (HMF) contain protein, calcium, potassium phosphate, carbohydrates, vitamins, and trace minerals. They may be necessary in these cases and can be added to the mother's milk for feedings of preterm infants.

Preterm infants who receive no supplementation may experience fractures of the long bones during rapid growth phases. Supplements are not without concern, however. Quan and colleagues (1994) found that some additives—particularly cow's milk–based infant formulas—have an adverse effect on the anti-infective properties of human milk. This effect was not seen in his study with soy-based infant formulas, nor was it observed with use of HMF. Soy-based formulas (discussed later) contain other problematic components for preterm infants. Preterm human milk protects against *E. coli*, *Staphylococcus*, *Enterobacter sakazaki*, and Group B *Streptococcus*, but this effect is absent when iron is added to the mother's diet (Chan, 2003).

Another study revealed lower lymphocyte counts in infants who were fed formula versus those who were fed either human milk alone or human milk containing HMF (Tarcan et al., 2004). A Cochrane Review found that preterm infants fed human milk with HMF had improved short-term weight gain and linear and head growth (Kuschel et al., 2004); there were insufficient data to evaluate long-term neurodevelopmental and growth outcomes. A 2007 Cochrane Review found that although preterm infants who received formula had greater short-term weight gains, they also had higher rates of NEC (Quigley et al., 2007). Another 2007 Cochrane Review reported major non-nutrient advantages for preterm or low-birth weight-infants who were fed breastmilk (Henderson et al., 2007).

Lactoengineering

Researchers have long proposed using mothers' hindmilk to increase the amounts of calories, carbohydrates, and proteins available to preterm infants—a process termed lactoengineering. One researcher added isolated human milk protein to mothers' milk for four babies with good results (Lindblad et al., 1982). NICUs are able to perform crematocrits, a test to measure fat and calories in human milk (Meier et al., 2002, 2006). A study in Nigeria found that low-birth-weight infants grew well without the addition of HMF to their feedings. The study, which did not include very-low-birth-weight infants, concluded that hindmilk feedings were effective and feasible for infants in developing countries (Slusher et al., 2003). Researchers are working to separate the crucial components of human milk for very preterm babies, including the fat, protein, and calcium, so that these infants can be supplemented with human—not bovine—milk fortifier (Kent, 2004; Lai, 2004).

⁓ Differences Between Human Milk and Infant Formula

Globally, a baby has an 80 percent higher risk of dying in the first year of life if not breastfed. Shorter breastfeeding is associated with higher risk as well (Chen & Rogan, 2004). Human milk contains a host of immunologic agents that protect the infant against infections and allergens until the child's internal defenses are more fully developed. Indeed, research has demonstrated that infant feeding has a lifelong effect on the immune system (Kelly & Coutts, 2000; Hanson, 1998; Hamosh, 1996). The individualized characteristics of each mother's milk provide her baby with nourishment that is ideally suited to the infant's specific needs for health and growth. Donor milk is always the best alternative for a baby whose mother cannot breastfeed or provide her milk.

During and after World War II, cow's milk formula came to be the routine source of infant nutrition in the United States and many other developed countries. With a growing reliance on scientific achievements and new technology, breastfeeding knowledge and skills decreased, especially in Western hospitals and the culture at large. Intense marketing of artificial milks by formula manufacturers ensued. Today, the United States is one of the largest markets for infant formula. More than half of all formula sold in the United States is obtained through the federally funded WIC program (Oliveira & Prell, 2004; Weimer, 2001).

Uncontrolled Marketing

Artificial baby milk feeding has been described as one of "the largest uncontrolled in vivo experiments in human history" (Minchin, 1998). Studies show that artificial baby milk carries with it serious health risks for infants, young children, and their mothers (Chen & Rogan, 2004; Raisler et al., 1999). In 1981, an awareness of these dangers prompted the World Health Organization to adopt the International Code of Marketing of Breastmilk Substitutes.

The Code, as it is referred to by breastfeeding advocates, aims to restrict the unethical marketing and promotion of food and drink, such as infant formula, used to feed babies inappropriately, as well as all associated paraphernalia, such as bottles and teats. When the World Health Assembly considered the Code, the United States cast the lone dissenting vote, which stirred a wave of controversy throughout the world. The United States finally approved the Code in 1994. (See Chapter 28 for more information.)

Composition of Artificial Baby Milk

Substantial differences exist between human milk and artificial baby milk. Put simply, the composition of artificial baby milk makes it far inferior to our species-specific milk. Nature has produced a product composed of hundreds of components, each with a specific function to ensure optimal nourishment of the human infant. Throughout breastfeeding, a mother's milk continually changes to meet her baby's needs.

Artificial formulas are deficient in many of the constituents that are essential for this optimal infant growth and health. They do not benefit from nature's consistency of quality and adaptability to the baby's age and unique needs. They provide no protection against allergies and confer no immunity to the baby. All formulas are slightly different, yet are intended to meet the universal needs of all infants. Logic dictates that nature's sole "formula"— human milk—eclipses any so called "ideal" substitute.

Individual companies compete with their rivals by advertising that their brand contains more of one element than that of another manufacturer. Their formula, they argue, is "closest to mother's milk" in that particular element. These pronouncements can be confusing to parents, who may worry that they must select one advantage over another. Try as they might, these companies will never replicate all the bioactive, immunologic, nutritional, and other health properties of human milk (Goldman, 1998; Hanson, 1998; Hamosh, 1996).

Too Little or Too Much

Artificial baby milk can contain micronutrients or macronutrients in either excessive or deficient amounts. It may also be completely lacking in essential elements. One of the more alarming deficiencies in infant formula involves the essential fatty acids that are important to proper brain development and visual acuity. No current formula has replicated human milk's complex pattern of fatty acids, even after adding fats derived from a variety of sources, including fish heads, egg yolks, and genetically engineered marine algae.

The benefits to the infant's brain development and visual acuity provided by these formulas remain controversial. One formula manufacturer removed those claims from its advertisements in Canada in response to pressure from Health Canada (Sterken, 2004). On the other side of the border, U.S. companies continue to stress their formulas' "enhancement" of brain and vision development.

The addition of these fatty acids has generated other concerns, such as those related to their effect on infant growth. In a study of human milk versus formula con-

taining added long-chain polyunsaturated fatty acids (LCPUFA), breastfed infants had significantly higher developmental scores at 9 and 18 months than the formula fed groups. They also weighed more and were taller at 18 months than the group fed LCPUFA formula (Fewtrell et al., 2002). Genetically modified and transgenic ingredients are not required to be labeled in the United States. The long-term effects of these ingredients are not known (ILCA, 2007).

These additives presently are made from algae and fungi (Agennix, 2009). In one study, lower levels of nervonic acid (NA), docosapentaenoic (DPA) acid, and DHA were found in all infants fed formula compared with infants fed human milk, regardless of the source of the formula supplement (Sala-Vila et al., 2004). In another study, formulas containing DHA resulted in higher DHA blood levels but did not result in significantly increased visual acuity (Horby, 1998). Current concentrations of DHA in infant formulas are considered inadequate (Sarkadi-Nagy et al., 2004). Moreover, there is concern about the potential for too much or an unbalanced intake of n-6 and n-3 fatty acids given the trend toward adding LCPUFA to other infant foods (Koo, 2003). The levels of palm olein needed to provide a fatty acid profile similar to human milk can lead to lower bone mineralization (Koo et al., 2003).

A 2008 Cochrane Review found that most of the well-conducted random-control studies failed to show significant beneficial effects of these additives on the physical, visual, and neurodevelopmental outcomes of infants born at term. According to the reviewers, "Routine supplementation of milk formula with LCPUFA to improve the physical, neurodevelopmental or visual outcomes of infants born at term cannot be recommended based on the current evidence" (Simmer et al., 2008b). Another review found similar results for effects on preterm infants, with the researchers citing no clear long-term benefits for infants receiving formula supplemented with LCPUFA (Simmer et al., 2008a).

Vitamin D, which is toxic in high doses, appears in excessive amounts in many formulas. Other formulas are deficient in chloride. Any formula that contains high levels of iodine could affect neonatal thyroid function. Some formulas are marketed as "hypoallergenic." One study found that these extensively hydrolyzed formulas are usually effective, but intolerance to hydrolysates has been observed (Smith et al., 2003).

Concerns About Soy Formula

Infants who consume soy formula receive the equivalent of 6 to 11 times the normal dose of isoflavones. This amount, if given to women, would change their menstrual patterns (Kumar et al., 2002). Congenitally hypothyroid infants receiving soy formula have demonstrated elevated levels of thyroid-stimulating hormone (TSH), even when taking thyroid medication (Conrad et al., 2004). In addition, soy milk contains approximately 80 times more manganese than human milk. Research on rats has shown that consumption of this type of formula may produce behavioral changes and lowered levels of the neurotransmitter dopamine, suggesting a possible correlation between heavy soy intake and neurological deficits (Tran et al., 2002).

Aluminum levels in soy formula are 36 times higher than those found in human milk. This is problematic because aluminum competes with calcium receptors and excess amounts are associated with renal problems. The AAP urges a reduction in the aluminum content of all formulas used for infants, and especially soy formulas and formulas tailored specifically for preterm infants (AAP, 1996).

The British Dietetic Association (BDA, 2003) discourages the use of soy formulas for infants. The European Society for Paediatric Gastroenterology Hepatology and Nutrition Committee on Nutrition reports that soy milk offers no nutritional advantage over cow's milk protein formulas, citing high concentrations of phytate, aluminum, and phytoestrogens (isoflavones) in the soy formulas. This organization suggests there are no data to support the use of soy protein formula in preterm infants and no evidence supporting its use for the prevention or management of infantile colic, regurgitation, or prolonged crying (ESPGHAN, 2006).

Infants may also experience additional hormonal effects from other estrogen-mimicking compounds known as phthalates, which are present in various plastics to which infants are exposed, often by artificial feeding (Densley, 1996). Specifically, bisphenol A (BPA), a chemical used in the manufacture of polycarbonate plastic, has raised concerns because it is found in many baby bottles and the internal linings of some formula cans. A national toxicology review found that BPA exposure is a concern for fetuses, infants, and children for effects on the brain, behavior, and prostate gland (U.S. Department of Health and Human Services [USDHHS], 2008).

Risks of Not Breastfeeding

Artificial feeding carries risks to infants, young children, mothers, and their families, regardless of where they live. In particular, the potential dangers of misuse of infant formula are especially worrisome in any impoverished community with substandard conditions and low education levels. Incorrect and inadequate use of infant formula accounts for approximately 1.5 million deaths each year worldwide (IBFAN, 2007; Walker, 2007). Some of these deaths occur even in affluent communities that have ample access to clean water and education, and in highly specialized intensive care nurseries.

It is intrinsically hazardous to deprive any infant of human milk (Lucas, 1990; Lucas et al., 1990). ILCA's (2007) *Core Curriculum for Lactation Consultant Practice* provides a comprehensive review of the risks associated with artificial feeding. Some of the key risks are summarized here:

- IQ levels may be 8 points lower in formula fed babies than in breastfed babies.
- Even one bottle of formula can change the baby's gut flora for 3 weeks.
- Formula sensitizes the baby to cow's milk protein and can provoke an allergy later in the first year if the baby is exposed again to cow's milk. Compounding the risk is the fact that formula fed infants are more likely to receive cow's milk at an earlier age than are breastfed infants.
- Bovine protein sensitivity can lead to serious malabsorption problems, even in affluent communities.

Table 9.5 shows some of the health risks of not breastfeeding.

Women who do not breastfeed experience an earlier return of fertility. This effect can result in shorter birth intervals, maternal depletion, and a higher number of pregnancies over their life span—all factors that may result in earlier maternal death. Women who do not breastfeed are also at increased risk for developing premenopausal breast cancer, ovarian cancer, and thyroid cancer, and they are more likely to develop osteoporosis in later life. Women who have gestational diabetes and do not breastfeed are at higher risk for converting to type 2 diabetes (Bentley-Lewis et al., 2008; Horta et al., 2007; Ip et al., 2007; Owen et al., 2006; Kjos et al., 1993). Gunderson (2008) finds this evidence insufficient to state a definitive relationship.

All too often, parents fail to learn of the health implications of not breastfeeding, in part because the media promote human milk substitutes as safe, acceptable, and the social norm (IBFAN, 2007; Walker, 2007; Hawkins, 1994; Sawatzki et al., 1994). Cultural conditioning and trust in the healthcare field foster the belief that "My doctor wouldn't recommend it if it weren't safe." Therefore, most bottle feeding parents do not question what they feed their babies. For parents to be responsible health consumers, they need all the facts. You can assist parents in acquiring necessary information so that they can make an informed decision about infant feeding.

Dangers in Manufacturing

Most parents are unaware of what is actually in the formula they give their babies. Such ignorance can be dangerous, as demonstrated by the tragedy in China that unfolded throughout 2008 when manufacturers added

TABLE 9.5   Health Risks Associated with Artificial Feeding

Health Risk as Identified in Studies	Study	Ratios Reported in Studies		
		Not Breastfed		Breastfed
Infant hospitalized more often	Study 1	15	to	1
	Study 2	10	to	1
Infant sick more often and to a greater degree	Study 1	21	to	8
Infant more likely to develop childhood cancers	Study 1	6	to	1
	Study 2	8	to	1
Infant more likely to develop gastroenteritis	Study 1	6	to	1
Infant more likely to develop ulcerative colitis and Crohn's disease	Study 1	3	to	1
Infant more likely to develop bronchitis and pneumonia	Study 1	5	to	1
	Study 2	2	to	1
Infant more likely to die from SIDS	Study 1	3	to	1
	Study 2	5	to	1
Premature infant more likely to develop necrotizing enterocolitis (NEC)	Study 1	20	to	1
Infant more likely to develop juvenile diabetes	Study 1	2	to	1
	Study 2	7	to	1
Women at greater risk for breast cancer	Study 1	2	to	1
Women at greater risk for ovarian cancer	Study 1	1.6	to	1

melamine to food products in an effort to decrease their costs and increase their profits. Melamine was added to infant formulas and foods, as well as adult and pet food products (resulting in thousands of pet deaths). More than 294,000 infants developed kidney stones. At least 6 of these infants died and more than 50,000 were hospitalized (Chen, 2009; WHO, 2008). Melamine and cyanuric acid were detected in two samples of formula in the United States as well. Health advocates question the U.S. Food and Drug Administration's statement that levels of melamine and cyanuric acid in U.S. formula are "safe" (USFDA, 2009).

In 2003, a series of tragedies involving formula resulted in the deaths of 15 infants within months of each other. The absence of vitamin B_1 (thiamine), which was mistakenly omitted from formula in Israel, resulted in brain damage in 17 infants and at least 2 deaths (Siegel-Itzkovich, 2003). The sale of bogus formula caused malnutrition in at least 171 infants and the deaths of at least 13 infants in China (Chinaview, 2008). One manufacturer was charged with relabeling animal feed containing dirt and flies as baby formula and selling it to Mexican food manufacturers (Gilot, 2004). Such questionable market-

ing tactics erode consumer confidence in food safety as a whole, and increase public and private health costs. These cases also demonstrate the lack of responsible oversight, lack of product assurance, and opportunity for unrestrained fraud in the infant formula industry.

The formula scandals in China have caused an upsurge in wet nursing, which in turn raises the question of whether the biological children of the wet nurses are being shortchanged. Many of these women move in with their employers, and some are not allowed to bring their own babies to work. This practice can result in the biological child being fed a human milk substitute so that the wet nurse can feed her employer's child (Fowler & Ye, 2008).

Product Recalls

There have been more than 50 formula or infant food recalls in the past 25 years in the United States alone. Recall reports are available at the U.S. Food and Drug Administration website (www.fda.gov). Manufacturing problems range from incorrect preparation to incorrect packaging. Contamination with bacteria, including

Enterobacter sakazakii, has occurred frequently (Walker, 2007; USFDA, 2002). *E. sakazakii* can cause severe illness and death, especially in preterm babies or babies with compromised immune systems (National Alliance for Breastfeeding Advocacy [NABA], 2009). Contamination with these bacteria is believed to have caused the death of one infant and led to the hospitalization of another (New Mexico Department of Health [NMDH], 2008). An updated list of recalls is maintained at www.naba-breast-feeding.org.

In an ironic twist, the most expensive formula, Nutramigen, was among Mead Johnson's recalls. The manufacturer's press release stated, "If not properly prepared, Nutramigen 16-oz. powder infant formula and Nutramigen 32-oz. ready-to-use infant formula have the potential to cause serious adverse health effects such as seizures, irregular heartbeat, renal failure or in extreme cases, death. Symptoms to look for include vomiting, diarrhea, decreased urine output, irritability, decreased activity or sunken eyes" (Mead Johnson, 2001). Chapter 28 discusses the unethical promotion of artificial baby milk in more detail.

Multiple Burdens with Formula Use

The use of artificial baby milks can have an adverse impact on all members of a family. It affects the family's time because they must always have infant formula available in sufficient quantity, along with the paraphernalia used to prepare and feed it. The preparation of the infant formula by the mother or other family member includes time for shopping, storing, preparing, and cleaning up—all time taken away from interacting with the baby or each other.

The impact of formula feeding on attachment between the mother and her baby has also raised concerns. A 14-year study found that, compared with babies breastfed for 4 or more months, non-breastfed babies were 4.5 times more likely to experience mistreatment from their mothers. Babies separated from their mothers for more than 20 hours per week had nearly a threefold increase in risk (Strathearn, 2009). It has also been reported that breastfed children have higher levels of parental attachment at ages 15 to 18 years (Fergusson & Woodward, 1999).

Drain on Family Finances

The family of a baby who is not breastfed will experience the economic burden of purchasing infant formula and feeding equipment—and the financial burden imposed by the need to purchase infant formula is significant. The San Diego Breastfeeding Coalition's 2001 study found an annual range in formula cost between $648 for a store brand and $2800 for Nutramigen, a hydrolyzed formula. Impoverished families could spend as much as 100 percent of their cash income for these products if they were to follow mixing instructions, especially in developing countries. All too often, in an attempt to stretch their supply of formula, parents may dilute it or supplement their baby's diet with inappropriate foods such as coffee, tea, sugared fruit drinks, and soy milk.

When formula feeding is used to nourish their children, women and other family members may be poorly nourished, with food money going toward infant formula and medications to deal with illnesses associated with formula feeding. Such malnutrition can have serious long-term consequences. Families also must bear the burden of increased medical expenses when the baby lacks the health protection of human milk. One study found that the average additional healthcare costs for a formula-fed infant ranged between $331 and $475 (Ball & Wright, 1999). Another found the average medical costs were $200 more for an artificially fed infant (Hoey & Ware, 1997). The Ban the Bags (2009) campaign calculated the additional cost to a formula feeding family to be more than $700 for name-brand formulas such as Similac and Enfamil than for a family that uses generic formula.

Drain on Community Resources

The effects on the community from the use of artificial baby milks are far reaching. The production and packaging of formula consume valuable land and resources. Production errors, such as contamination and mishandling, create a burden on society as a whole, as well as on the individual child. Once the formula is packaged, the distribution process takes additional resources for fuel and contributes to environmental pollution. Even the disposal of waste products, such as infant formula tins, taxes the environment. The ever-increasing need to improve infant formulas is a burden to research as well. It siphons off time and resources that might otherwise go toward mitigating unavoidable health concerns, helping women breastfeed, and making safe human milk available for infants whose mothers cannot provide it.

Drain on Health Care

Educating parents in the proper use of infant formula consumes valuable healthcare resources and time that healthcare workers could otherwise devote to other health issues. It is the healthcare industry's responsibility to make sure parents understand the nuances of purchasing, storing, mixing, and feeding formula. Additionally, the many errors, omissions, and purposeful rationing that occur with regularity impose harmful health consequences on the child, some subtle and some overt. Parents' time goes toward caring for children who are acutely and chronically ill due to the lack of human milk. The increase in healthcare expenses associated with formula use is a burden that is inevitably passed along to consumers and taxpayers.

Legitimate Needs for Formula

Step 6 of the Ten Steps to Successful Breastfeeding states that newborn infants should be given "no food or drink other than breastmilk, unless medically indicated." This recommendation recognizes there are circumstances in which a mother cannot breastfeed or feed her milk to her baby. If she is not a candidate for or does not wish to use donor human milk, she will need education regarding the use of human milk substitutes. There may be circumstances in which a mother simply rejects breastfeeding. She, too, will need instructions in the use of an alternative feeding method. Until the baby is 1 year of age, it is important that he or she receive infant formula rather than cow's milk. Infant formula should be the choice of last resort, used only after exhausting all other options to provide human milk. Unfortunately, this is usually not the case.

Maternal Circumstances That Preclude Breastfeeding

Some medical conditions prevent a mother from breastfeeding her baby. As discussed in Chapter 25, a mother with a physical condition such as Sheehan's syndrome, long-term drug therapy, severe congestive heart failure, or true insufficient milk production may need to feed her baby artificial milk if donor milk is not an option. In addition, because tuberculosis spreads through close contact, this condition in the mother may be dangerous to her breastfeeding infant. The mother can return to breastfeeding after she receives appropriate treatment for at least 1 week and is no longer infectious (Lawrence & Lawrence, 2005).

If a mother is infected with HIV prior to the birth of her baby and if she has access to a sanitary water supply, current health guidelines state she should not breastfeed her baby unless she can pump and pasteurize her milk to kill the HIV virus (WHO, 2009a; Jeffery et al., 2001, 2003; Black, 1996). If the mother's infection with HIV occurs after delivery, her baby has not been exposed to HIV in utero and it is believed breastfeeding would present an unnecessary risk (Leroy et al., 2007). The presence of HIV does not mean, however, that the baby cannot receive human milk. The mother's milk can be heat treated, or she can use banked human milk. The issue of HIV transmission through mother's milk continues to be debated by researchers. Refer to Chapter 25 for a more thorough discussion of the HIV debate.

A mother who has an active herpes lesion on her breast where the baby will come in contact with it should not breastfeed on the affected breast until the lesion heals. The baby may continue to nurse on the other breast, and the mother can express her milk and discard it from the affected side.

If a mother is severely ill with a condition such as psychosis, eclampsia, or shock, she may be unable to breastfeed until her healing is sufficient to begin or resume breastfeeding. Mothers who must take certain medications, such as cytotoxic or radioactive drugs, may need to stop breastfeeding while the drug is present and active (Hale, 2010). See Chapter 25 for more discussion of maternal circumstances that affect the ability to breastfeed.

Infant Circumstances That Require Formula

Human milk supplementation is required in situations such as hypoglycemia or dehydration, when the condition has not improved through increased breastfeeding or increased intake of colostrum or human milk. Babies with a very low or extremely low birth weight or who are born preterm (less than 1000 grams or 32 weeks' gestation) may require supplementation with human milk fortifier (Quigley et al., 2007; Landers, 2003; Morton, 2003; Klein, 2002). If it is determined that the baby needs to be supplemented, an alternative feeding method should be chosen that will interfere the least with the return to breastfeeding and fit most comfortably into the family's lifestyle.

Galactosemia is an extremely rare condition that requires the use of a special lactose-free formula such as soy formula. A baby with galactosemia is unable to metabolize lactose, which is the main carbohydrate in human milk. Therefore, the use of human milk (or even cow's milk) by any means is not possible. Be aware that babies with Duarte's variant, a variation of galactosemia, can breastfeed with precautions (see Chapter 25 for a further discussion of this issue). Although other inborn errors of metabolism, such as phenylketonuria (PKU) or maple syrup urine disease, require the use of milk substitutes, they also allow for carefully monitored intake of the mother's milk (Save Babies Through Screening Foundation, 2008).

Selecting a Brand and Type of Formula

The allergy history of the entire family—siblings, parents, and other close blood relatives—needs to be considered when selecting an artificial baby milk. In theory, parents should make the choice of a human milk substitute together with the baby's caregiver, mindful of the health implications for that particular family. The reality is that parents' brand choice often depends on which company left a case on their doorstep, which discharge pack they received at hospital discharge, and which cents-off coupons are available. The caregiver's choice may be a formula whose company sales representative is the best salesperson or gives the "best gifts." Some caregivers rotate brands. Consideration is not always given to which brand will agree best with a particular baby.

Formula is available in ready-to-feed, concentrated, and powdered forms. Family finances often dictate the choice of formula. As with other groceries, name-brand formulas such as Similac, Good Start, and Enfamil are much more expensive than generic or store-brand formulas. Frequent changes in artificial baby milk marketing, the continual so called "improvements" in existing products, and rebranding result in frequent changes in prices and names. Internet-savvy parents can easily compare the costs of formulas online from the manufacturer, discount websites such as www.discountformula.com, and retail giants such as Amazon.com.

Table 9.6 shows the annual costs for a range of artificial milks, based on a conservative estimate—consumption of 10,800 ounces for a baby's first year. The costs given in Table 9.6 do not include the cost of free formula or "toddler" milks that are heavily promoted for a baby's

second year and beyond in lieu of breastfeeding or plain cow's milk.

Powdered Formula

Powdered formula is the least expensive of the three types available. In 2009 dollars, the cost for standard cow's milk–based formula in the United States ranged from $540/year (generic) to $1667/year (Enfamil Lipil). Prices for "gentle" formula (partially broken-down whey) ranged from $788/year (generic) to $1695/year (Enfamil Gentlease). Hydrolyzed specialty formulas such as Nutramigen cost $2772/year. Powdered formula is the most portable form and has the longest shelf life. This option is also the most easily and most often contaminated and prepared incorrectly.

TABLE 9.6 Sample Artificial Baby Milk Brands (U.S.) and Annual Costs Based on 10,800 Ounces per Year

Artificial Baby Milk Brand	Product Size	Cost per Prepared Fluid Ounce	Total Annual Cost ($)
Member's Mark standard cow's milk formula	Powdered, 51.4 oz	$0.05/oz	$540
Member's Mark "Gentle" cow's milk formula	Powdered, 48 oz	$0.073/oz	$788
Enfamil Lipil cow's milk formula	Powdered, 38 oz	$0.115/oz	$1242
Enfamil "Gentlease"	Powdered, 12 oz	$0.157/oz	$1695
Enfamil Nutramigen (hydrolyzed)	Powdered, 16 oz	$0.2561/oz	$2772
Similac Advanced cow's milk formula	Powdered, 36 oz	$0.112/oz	$1209
Similac Sensitive	Powdered, 23.2 oz	$0.154/oz	$1668
Similac Organic	Powdered, 12.9 oz	$0.2105/oz	$2273
Earth's Best Organic milk or soy	Powdered, 13.2 oz	$0.1547/oz	$1670
Bright Beginnings Organic milk	Powdered, 25.7 oz	$0.1316/oz	$1421
Nestlé Good Start cow's milk formula	Powdered, 25.7oz	$0.145/oz	$1566
Nestlé Good Start (soy)	Powdered, 25.7oz	$0.1478/oz	$1922
Enfamil Lipil cow's milk formula	Concentrate, 13 oz	$0.192/oz	$2073
Enfamil ProSobee (soy)	Concentrate, 13 oz	$0.2027/oz	$2189
Nestlé Good Start (soy)	Concentrate, 13 oz	$0.2046/oz	$2209
Similac Isomil (soy)	Concentrate, 13 oz	$0.2548/oz	$2752
Similac Advanced concentrate	Concentrate, 13 oz	$0.2548/oz	$2752
Similac Sensitive concentrate	Concentrate, 13 oz	$0.231/oz	$2495
Enfamil Nutramigen (hydrolyzed)	Concentrate, 13 oz	$0.2885/oz	$3116
Similac Advanced cow's milk formula	Ready-to-feed, 192 oz	$0.2106/oz	$2275
Enfamil Lipil cow's milk formula	Ready-to-feed, 192 oz	$0.2142/oz	$2313
Nestlé Good Start soy	Ready-to-feed, 192 oz	$0.2135/oz	$2306
Similac Alimentum (hydrolyzed)	Ready-to-feed, 192 oz	$0.413/oz	$4460
Enfamil Nutramigen (hydrolyzed)	Ready-to-feed, 192 oz	$0.3125/oz	$3375

Sources: Online searches of manufacturers' websites, plus retail sites including Sam's Club, Wal-Mart, CVS, and discount retailer sites (March 2009).

Concentrated Formula

With annual costs in the range of $2072/year to $3116/year in the United States, concentrate is more costly than powdered formula but is easier to mix. As with powdered or ready-to-feed formula, parents should discard any unused portion within 1 hour after they have opened and mixed it.

Ready-to-Feed Formula

Ready-to-feed formula is the most convenient option. One of the advantages of this kind of formula is that the mother does not need to make decisions about whether to use tap water or bottled water to prepare the feeding. Nor would there be changes to the baby's system when traveling, as might occur when a variety of water supplies are used to reconstitute either powdered or concentrated formula. However, ready-to-feed formula is the most expensive of the three types, with annual costs ranging from $2275/year (Similac Advance) to $4460/year (Similac Alimentum) in the United States.

Homemade Formula

In light of increasing food contamination scandals, and as a means of saving money in the midst of a major worldwide recession, more and more families are making their own infant formula at home. Recipes abound online. Especially popular are formulas made with goat's milk and vegetarian recipes (Hall, 2008; Rockwell Nutrition, 2008). An advantage to parents who follow this course is that they avoid the worry about deliberate contamination of commercial formula with melanine, flour, and other production cost savers. Likewise, they need not worry about manufacturing contamination, and they know what is in the formula they are giving their children. The major disadvantage to homemade formula, as with commercial formula, is that it does not approximate human milk. These parents should be encouraged to let their healthcare provider know what they are feeding their child.

As can be expected, the infant formula industry does not want parents making their own formulas at home. Artificial baby milks are a highly profitable niche in the food industry—netting more than $8 billion for manufacturers annually. The USFDA website includes the following statement:

> Homemade formulas based on cows' milk don't meet all of an infant's nutritional needs, and cow's milk protein that has not been cooked or processed is difficult for an infant to digest. In addition, the high protein and electrolyte (salt) content of cow's milk may put a strain on an infant's immature kidneys. Substituting evaporated milk for whole milk may make the homemade formula easier to digest because of the effect of processing on the protein, but the formula is still nutritionally inadequate and still

may stress the kidneys. Today's infant formula is a very controlled, high-tech product that can't be duplicated at home. (USFDA, 1996)

Dangers in Preparation

In the past, a massive shift away from breastfeeding occurred partly due to aggressive marketing of infant formula, together with modeling of its use in wealthy countries where infant mortality is generally low (Palmer, 2009; Wolf, 2003; Michels & Baumslag, 1995). This change occurred both in developed countries and among women in developing countries who cannot use artificial baby milk safely and whose babies become ill and malnourished (Michels & Baumslag, 1995). In communities where the mother cannot afford to purchase sufficient quantities of infant formula, families may attempt to stretch the supply by diluting it. Unfortunately, these individuals may also lack access to refrigeration, clean water, or adequate waste facilities. Additionally, parents may not understand directions well enough to mix the infant formula properly (IBFAN, 2007).

Unsafe Water Supply

The AAP (2005) cautions mothers to check their water supply to make sure that it is safe for their babies to drink. Families who use well (or spring) water should have it tested. If there is any concern about unsafe water supply, they should purchase bottled water. When traveling, parents will want to consider the safety of the water en route.

If the mother is unsure about bacterial level in the water supply, she can use bottled water or boil the tap water for 5 minutes (boiling longer may increase the concentration of lead in the water). In older homes and in some newer ones, the water pipe joints contain lead solder, which leaches out more easily in hot water. Where lead poisoning is a concern, parents should obtain the water used for formula from the cold-water tap only. The AAP recommends that parents run the cold water for at least 1 minute before collecting it and longer if no one has run the water for several hours.

Another concern with the water used to mix formula is the extra fluoridation that occurs with the addition of fluoride to the community water supply. Excessive fluoride may cause fluorosis, a condition in which teeth become mottled or discolored. One study concluded that infant formulas prepared with fluoridated water increase the risk of fluorosis in primary teeth (Marshall et al., 2004).

The possibility that nitrites, sodium, bacteria, and parasites might be present in the water is another consideration. Babies are susceptible to methemoglobinemia from water containing nitrates.

Unsafe Mixing and Use

After a systematic review in the United Kingdom found that feedings often were not prepared accurately, the investigators stressed the urgent need to minimize the risk of incorrect preparation (Renfrew et al., 2003). Even when parents mix formula according to the directions, there may be wide variations in the final composition of the product. These discrepancies occur partly because the composition of formula in the can varies from season to season, depending on the cow's diet. In addition, powder can pack down in the can over time, so that a scoop of powder may contain a greater or lesser quantity by weight.

Powdered formula is the most prone to mixing errors. Parents may not follow package directions or use the specific scoop provided with the can. Each company has a particular set of instructions, and the size of the scoop is not uniform between manufacturers. Parents need to read the instructions carefully and use the scoop that came with that particular brand of formula. If a new mother indicates that she plans to use formula to feed her infant, caregivers should ask the mother to prepare the formula in the hospital as a return demonstration to ensure that she understands the correct procedure.

It is easy for parents to confuse concentrate with ready-to-feed formula. Even the most educated parents run the risk of misreading the label. For example, one college-educated father failed to read mixing directions carefully and fed his newborn concentrated infant formula. Additionally, the higher cost of ready-to-feed formula may tempt parents to save unused portions rather than discard them after the specified period. Furthermore, oral water intoxication resulting in seizures can occur when parents dilute expensive formula with more water than is called for (Keating et al., 1991).

Precautions for Parents

As with any food product, parents must monitor expiration dates regardless of which type of formula they use. They also need to consider how long the infant formula remains at room temperature and how long it may be stored in the refrigerator after the can is open. Because parents often mix several bottles at one time, they need to understand that artificial baby milk is an inert substance. Unlike human milk, it is not bacteriostatic and does not contain anti-infective properties to fight bacteria. The sugars in formula are an ideal growth medium for bacteria, and bacteria can multiply rapidly in formula that remains at room temperature. Formula should be refrigerated or chilled if it is stored in a diaper bag.

Parents should use a clean bottle and utensils for every formula feeding. They should wash the can opener and the top and bottom of the can with hot soapy water before opening the can. Suggest to mothers that they open the can from the bottom, because the bottom is less likely to have the same level of pesticide sprays from the warehouse as the top (Kutner, 2009). In addition, careful attention to expiration dates and label instructions is important. Some clinicians advise mothers to record the lot number of each can in the event of a later recall or class action lawsuit.

Parents should discard formula mixed from concentrate after 48 hours and discard formula mixed from powder after 24 hours. Formula removed from the refrigerator should be discarded after 1 hour. When a feeding is finished, parents should not save any unused portion for a later feeding.

❧ Summary

Human milk is the biologically normal nutrition for the human infant. The health benefits to the infant resulting from the immunologic properties of the mother's milk are irrefutable. Indeed, human milk is specific to the infant's age and its composition changes throughout lactation to meet the child's changing needs. Researchers continue to uncover new benefits of the many components in this rich and complex substance. There are also lifelong benefits to mothers who breastfeed; those who do not breastfeed risk significant health issues. For all these reasons, caregivers have a responsibility to promote the use of human milk for all babies. The American Academy of Pediatrics, World Health Organization, American Academy of Family Physicians, and American Dietetic Association, and others, translate this responsibility into strong statements in support of breastfeeding through the child's first year and beyond. Artificial baby milks are an inherently inferior substitute for mother's milk.

❧ Chapter 9—At a Glance

Facts you learned—

Colostrum:

- Consists of residual materials in the breast that mix with newly formed milk.
- Is richer than mature milk in terms of its sodium, potassium, chloride, protein, fat-soluble vitamins, and minerals content.
- Contains less fat and lactose than mature milk.
- Engulfs and digests disease organisms and aids in rapid gut closure.
- Has high concentrations of IgA, IgG, and IgM (as does mature milk).

Fat content:

- Varies from mother to mother and from feeding to feeding.
- Is inversely proportional to the length of time between feedings.
- Is related to the degree of breast fullness.
- Decreases in later months of lactation.
- At the end of a feeding may be up to four to five times higher than at the beginning.

Lactose:

- Enhances calcium absorption, thereby preventing rickets.
- Supplies energy to the infant's brain.
- Protects the infant's intestines from the growth of harmful organisms.
- Is essential to development of the central nervous system.
- Is the most constant among mothers of all the constituents in human milk.

Composition and volume:

- Composition changes throughout lactation as well as during a given day or feeding.
- Milk is high in immunoglobulins and protein during the first several weeks of breastfeeding.
- Milk often seems most plentiful in the morning hours.
- The volume of milk available depends on regular removal of milk from the breast.
- Three-fourths of an infant's nutrient needs through the first 12 months of life can be met by human milk.
- Daily output during the second year is at least 8 ounces.

Other properties of human milk:

- Oligosaccharides prevent pathogens from binding to receptor sites in the gut.
- Protein level is relatively constant, regardless of the mother's diet.
- The curd found in human milk is soft, small, less compact, and easy to digest.
- Lactoferrin inhibits growth of *E. coli*. Its effects decrease when it is saturated with exogenous iron.
- Lysozyme protects against enterobacteriaceae and gram-positive bacteria. Its level increases over the course of lactation.

- Long-chain polyunsaturated fatty acids promote optimal neural and visual development.
- Ghrelin, leptin, and obestatin—all appetite regulators—are found in human milk.
- All vitamins are present in sufficient levels in breastmilk, when combined with sun exposure to provide for manufacture of additional vitamin D.
- Healthy non-anemic mothers lay down sufficient iron stores to last for the first few months of breastfeeding.
- Suckling triggers the release of cholecystokinin (CCK) and causes sleepiness in mothers and babies.
- IgA protects the GI tract and is the most important of the antiviral defense factors.
- Lactase and lipase protect babies born with immature or defective enzyme systems.
- Lactase converts lactose into simple sugars that can be assimilated easily by the infant.
- A deficiency in lactase can result in lactose intolerance.
- Lysozyme breaks down bacteria in the bowel.
- Lactoferrin inhibits the growth of *E. coli*.
- Bifidus factor works with the pH of the stool to discourage the growth of *E. coli*.
- The antibodies found in human milk enhance the infant's antibody response.
- Mucins in human milk protect against bacterial infections.
- Thyroid hormones in human milk prevent hypothyroidism; receiving breastmilk protects the hypothyroid baby until weaning. Therefore, a breastfed hypothyroid baby may not be diagnosed until weaned.
- Alpha-lactalbumin inhibits bacteria and yeast growth.
- Xantine oxidase combined with nitrites inhibits infection with *E. coli* and *Salmonella enteritidis*.
- The nucleotides found in human milk promote optimal functioning and growth of the child's GI and immune systems.
- Human milk contains stem cells.
- High levels of antibodies provide antiabsorptive protection for the lining of the infant's intestine.

Specific health benefits of human milk:

- Leads to fewer dental caries and better dental health.
- Demonstrates dose-dependent effects in increasing IQ.
- Provides lifelong protection against disease.
- Destroys bacteria in the GI tract before they affect the infant.

- Protects the infant against upper and lower respiratory infections, otitis media, diarrheal disease, urinary tract infections, sepsis, rotavirus, meningitis, leukemia, lymphoma, Hodgkin's disease, and neuroblastoma.
- Lowers the infant's risk of breast cancer, chronic and autoimmune diseases, hypertension, high cholesterol, and heart disease.
- Decreases the child's risk of NEC and the incidence of asthma.
- Causes the child to produce antibodies against organisms passed into the breast by the suckling infant.
- Through passage of maternal antigens to the breastfed infant, protects against the common cold, fever, and more serious illness.

Milk of women who deliver prematurely:

- The milk of women who deliver prematurely is higher in sodium, chloride, nitrogen, and immunoprotective factors.
- Human milk fortifiers (HMF)—protein, calcium, potassium phosphate, carbohydrates, vitamins, and trace minerals—are used to supplement very-low-birth-weight (VLBW) infants.
- Lactoengineering offers an alternative to HMF by isolating hindmilk to increase calories, carbohydrates, and proteins for preterm infants.

Artificial formula:

- The composition of human milk makes it far superior to any artificial baby milk.
- Formulas are slightly different from one another, yet are intended to meet the universal needs of infants.
- Formula is deficient in many constituents essential for optimal infant growth and health.
- Formula has been found to:
  - Contain excessive or deficient amounts of micronutrients or macronutrients.
  - Completely lack certain essential elements.
  - Contain lower levels of nervonic acid (NA), docosapentaenoic acid (DPA), and docosahexaenoic acid (DHA).
  - Contain excessive amounts of vitamin D, which is toxic in high doses.
  - Be deficient in chloride.
  - Be contaminated with aluminum or bacteria.
- Soy formula can cause neurological deficits and renal problems.
- Formula use puts a burden on family finances, community resources, and healthcare dollars.

- Babies who are fed with formula are at health risk from contaminated water, mixing errors, and bacteria from formula left at room temperature for too long.
- Infants who are fed cow's milk are more likely to develop late neonatal hypocalcemia and dehydration.
- A single feeding of cow's milk in the first days of life can increase rates of allergy.
- Cow's milk is the most common food allergen in infants.
- Most infants with cow's milk allergy develop symptoms before 1 month of age, often within 1 week after introduction of cow's milk protein-based formula.
- Atopic dermatitis and eczema are more common in artificially fed infants.
- Babies should receive formula only if there is a legitimate need:
  - In the mother: Sheehan's syndrome, long-term drug therapy, severe congestive heart failure, insufficient milk production, tuberculosis (until after treatment), HIV (when safe alternatives exist), active herpes lesion, eclampsia, or use of cytotoxic or radioactive drugs.
  - In the infant: Hypoglycemia or dehydration if unimproved by increased breastfeeding and no donor milk is available, prematurity, galactosemia, phenylketonuria (PKU), or maple syrup urine disease.
- Homemade artificial baby milks are becoming increasingly popular.

～ References

Agennix, Inc. Recombinant human lactoferrin. 2009. www.rhlf.com. Accessed March 27, 2009.

Akre J. Infant feeding: The physiological basis. *WHO Bull Suppl.* 1989;67:29.

Ala-Houhala M, et al. Maternal compared with infant vitamin D supplementation. *Arch Dis Child.* 1986;61(12):1159-1163.

American Academy of Family Physicians (AAFP). AAFP policy statement on breastfeeding. 2009. www.aafp.org/x6633.xml. Accessed March 25, 2009.

American Academy of Pediatrics (AAP). Breastfeeding and the use of human milk. *Pediatrics.* 2005;115(2):496-506.

American Academy of Pediatrics (AAP), Committee on Nutrition. Aluminum toxicity in infants and children. *Pediatrics.* 1996;97(3):413-416.

Anderson J, et al. Breastfeeding and cognitive development: a meta-analysis. *Am J Clin Nutr.* 1999;70:525-535.

Aniansson G, et al. A prospective cohort study on breastfeeding and otitis media in Swedish infants. *Pediatr Infect Dis J.* 1994;13:183-188.

Arnold L. Use of donor milk in the treatment of metabolic disorders. *J Hum Lact.* 1995;11:51-53.

Arteaga-Vizcaino M, et al. Effect of oral and intramuscular vitamin K on the factors II, VII, IX, X, and PIVKA II in the infant newborn under 60 days of age. *Rev Med Child*. 2001;129(10):1121-1129.

Ashraf R, et al. Additional water is not needed for healthy breast-fed babies in a hot climate. *Acta Paediatr*. 1993;82:1007-1011.

Aydin S, et al. Ghrelin is present in human colostrum, transitional and mature milk [published online ahead of print September 26, 2005]. *Peptides*. 2006;27(4):878-882.

Bachrach V, et al. Breastfeeding and the risk of hospitalization for respiratory disease in infancy: a meta-analysis. *Arch Pediatr Adolesc Med*. 2003; 157(3):237-243.

Ball T, Wright A. Health care costs of formula-feeding in the first year of life. *Pediatrics*. 1999;103(4 Pt 2):870-876.

Ban the Bags. Hospitals should market health, and nothing else. www.banthebags.org. Accessed March 25, 2009.

Bauchner H, et al. Studies of breastfeeding and infections: how good is the evidence? *JAMA*. 1986;256:887-892.

Bener A, et al. Longer breast-feeding and protection against childhood leukaemia and lymphomas. *Eur J Cancer*. 2001;37(2):234-238.

Bener A, et al. Role of breast feeding in primary prevention of asthma and allergic diseases in a traditional society. *Eur Ann Allergy Clin Immunol*. 2007;39(10):337-343.

Bentley-Lewis R, et al. Gestational diabetes mellitus: postpartum opportunities for the diagnosis and prevention of type 2 diabetes mellitus. *Nat Clin Pract Endocrinol Metab*. 2008;4(10):552-558.

Bhowmick S, et al. Rickets caused by vitamin D deficiency in breastfed infants in the southern United States. *Am J Child Dis*. 1991;145:127-130.

Bhutta Z, Haider B. Prenatal micronutrient supplementation: are we there yet? *Canadian Med Assoc J*. 2009;180(12):1188-1189.

Bisquera J, et al. Impact of necrotizing enterocolitis on length of stay and hospital charges in very low birth weight infants. *Pediatrics*. 2002;109(3):423-428.

Black R. Transmission of HIV-1 in the breast-feeding process: review. *J Am Diet Assoc*. 1996;96(3):267-274.

Boehm G, Moro G. Structural and functional aspects of prebiotics used in infant nutrition. *J Nutr*. 2008;138(9):1818S-1828S.

Bor O, et al. Late hemorrhagic disease of the newborn. *Pediatr Int*. 2000;42(1):64-66.

Brandtzaeg P. Mucosal immunity: integration between mother and the breast-fed baby. *Vaccine*. 2003;24(21):3382-3388.

Brandtzaeg P. Why we develop food allergies. *Am Scientist*. 2007;95:28-35.

Brazerol W, et al. Serial ultraviolet B exposure and serum 25 hydroxyvitamin D response in young adult American blacks and whites: no racial differences. *J Am Coll Nutr*. 1988;7(2):111-118.

British Dietetic Association (BDA). Paediatric group position statement on the use of soya protein for infants. *J Fam Health Care*. 2003;13(4):93.

Brothwell D, Limeback H. Breastfeeding is protective against dental fluorosis in a nonfluoridated rural area of Ontario, Canada. *J Hum Lact*. 2003;19(4):386-390.

Buescher S. Host defense mechanisms of human milk and their relations to enteric infections and necrotizing enterocolitis. *Clin Perinatol*. 1994;21:247-262.

Buescher S. Anti-infective properties of human milk with special reference to the pre-term baby. Paper presented at: Human Lactation: Current Research and Clinical Implications; October 21, 2004; Amarillo, TX.

Bulkow L, et al. Risk factors for severe respiratory syncytial virus infection among Alaska native children. *Pediatrics*. 2002;109(2):210-216.

Butte NF. Impact of infant feeding practices on childhood obesity. *J Nutr*. 2009;139(2):412S-416S.

Butte N, et al. Longitudinal changes in milk composition of mothers delivering preterm and term infants. *Early Hum Dev*. 1984;9(2):153-162.

Calhoun D, et al. Granulocyte colony-stimulating factor is present in human milk and its receptor is present in human fetal intestine. *Pediatrics*. 2000;105:e7.

Caplan M. Probiotic and prebiotic supplementation for the prevention of neonatal necrotizing enterocolitis. *J Perinatol*. 2009;29 Suppl 2:S2-S6.

Carlson S, et al. Visual acuity and fatty acid status of term infants fed human milk and formulas with and without docosahexaenoate and arachidonate from egg yolk lecithin. *Pediatr Res*. 1996;39:882-888.

Carver J. Dietary nucleotides: effects on the immune and gastrointestinal systems: review. *Acta Paediatr Suppl*. 1999;88(430):83-88.

Casey C, et al. Nutrient intake by breast-fed infants during the first five days after birth. *Am J Dis Child*. 1986;140(9):933-936.

Centers for Disease Control and Prevention (CDC). Recommendations for using fluoride to prevent and control dental caries in the US. *MMWR*. 2001;50(RR-14).

Chan G. Effects of powdered human milk fortifiers on the antibacterial actions of human milk. *J Perinatol*. 2003;23(8):620-623.

Chaturvedi P, et al. Fucosylated human milk oligosaccharides vary between individuals and over the course of lactation. *Glycobiology*. 2001a;11(5):365-372.

Chaturvedi P, et al. Survival of human milk oligosaccharides in the intestine of infants. *Adv Exp Med Biol*. 2001b;501:315-323.

Chen A, Rogan W. Breastfeeding and the risk of postneonatal death in the United States. *Pediatrics*. 2004;113(5):e435-e439.

Chen J. A worldwide food safety concern in 2008: melamine-contaminated infant formula in China caused urinary tract stone in 290,000 children in China. *Chin Med J (Engl)*. 2009;122(3):243-244.

Chierici R, et al. Advances in the modulation of the microbial ecology of the gut in early infancy. *Acta Paediatr Suppl*. 2003;91(441):56-63.

Chinaview. China quality watchdog investigates baby milk powder scare. September 11, 2008. http://news.xinhuanet.com/english/2008-09/11/content_9920879.htm. Accessed March 25, 2009.

Christensen J. Multiple sclerosis: some epidemiological clues to etiology. *Acta Neurol Latinoam*. 1975;21(1-4):66-85.

Clemens J, et al. Breastfeeding and the risk of life-threatening enterotoxigenic *Escherichia coli* diarrhea in Bangladeshi infants and children. *Pediatrics.* 1997;100(6):E2.

Clemens T, et al. Increased skin pigment reduces the capacity of skin to synthesise vitamin D_3. *Lancet.* 1982;1(8263):74-76.

Conrad SC, et al. Soy formula complicates management of congenital hypothyroidism. *Arch Dis Child.* 2004;89(1):37-40.

Coppa G, et al. Preliminary study of breastfeeding and bacterial adhesion to uroepithelial cells. *Lancet.* 1990;335:569-571.

Coppa G, et al. Changes in carbohydrate composition in human milk over 4 months of lactation. *Pediatrics.* 1993;91:637-641.

Coppa G, et al. Human milk oligosaccharides inhibit the adhesion to Caco-2 cells of diarrheal pathogens: *Escherichia coli, Vibrio cholerae,* and *Salmonella fyris. Pediatr Res.* 2006; 59(3):377-382.

Corrao G, et al. Risk of inflammatory bowel disease attributable to smoking, oral contraception and breastfeeding in Italy: a nationwide case-control study. *Int J Epidemiol.* 1998; 27(3):307-404.

Cox D, et al. Studies on human lactation: The development of the computerized breast measurement system. 1998; updated 2008. www.biochem.biomedchem.uwa.edu.au/page/69859. Accessed March 1, 2009.

Cregan M, et al. Identification of nestin-positive putative mammary stem cells in human breastmilk. *Cell Tissue Res.* 2007; 329(1):129-136.

Czank C, et al. Chapter 4: Human milk composition: Fat. In: Hale T, Hartmann P, eds. *Hale and Hartmann's Textbook of Human Lactation.* Amarillo, TX: Hale Publishing; 2007a: 49-67.

Czank C, et al. Chapter 5: Human milk composition: Carbohydrates. In: Hale T, Hartmann P, eds. *Hale and Hartmann's Textbook of Human Lactation.* Amarillo, TX: Hale Publishing; 2007b: 69-73.

Daly S, et al. Degree of breast emptying explains changes in the fat content but not fatty acid composition of human milk. *Exp Physiol.* 1993a;78:741-755.

Daly S, et al. The short-term synthesis and infant-regulated removal of milk in lactating women. *Exp Physiol.* 1993b;78: 209-220.

Daniels J, et al. Breast-feeding and neuroblastoma, USA and Canada. *Cancer Causes Control.* 2002;13(5):401-405.

Davis M. Review of the evidence for an association between infant feeding and childhood cancer. *Int J Cancer.* 1998; 1(suppl):29-33.

de Vrese M, Schrezenmeir J. Probiotics, prebiotics, and synbiotics. *Adv Biochem Eng Biotechnol.* 2008;111:1-66.

Del Prado M, et al. Contribution of dietary and newly formed arachidonic acid to human milk lipids in women eating a low-fat diet. *Am J Clin Nutr.* 2001;74(2):242-247.

Dell S, To T. Breastfeeding and asthma in young children: findings from a population-based study. *Arch Ped Adolescent Med.* 2001;155(11):1261-1265.

Densley B. Phthalates in formula: a report. *ALCA Galaxy.* 1996; 7(3):34-37.

Dewey K, et al. Differences in morbidity between breast-fed and formula-fed infants. *J Pediatr.* 1995;126(5 Pt 1):696-702.

Dewit O, et al. Breastmilk amylase activities during 18 months of lactation in mothers from rural Zaire. *Acta Paediatr.* 1993;82:300-301.

Dick G. The etiology of multiple sclerosis. *Proc R Soc Med.* 1976; 69:611.

Dugdale A. Breast milk and necrotising enterocolitis. *Lancet.* 1991;337:435.

Duncan B, et al. Exclusive breastfeeding for at least 4 months protects against otitis media. *Pediatrics.* 1993;91:867-872.

Dvorak B, et al. Increased epidermal growth factor levels in human milk of mothers with extremely premature infants. *Pediatr Res.* 2003;54(1):15-19.

Ebrahim G. Feeding the preterm brain. *J Trop Pediatr.* 1993;39: 130-131.

El-Mohandes A, et al. Use of human milk in the intensive care nursery decreases the incidence of nosocomial sepsis. *J Perinatol.* 1997;17:130-134.

Elwood P, et al. Long term effect of breast feeding: cognitive function in the Caerphilly cohort. *J Epidemiol Community Health.* 2005;59(2):130-133.

Erickson P, et al. Estimation of the caries-related risk associated with infant formulas. *Pediatr Dent.* 1998;20:395-403.

Erickson PR, Mazhare E. Investigation of the role of human breast milk in caries development. *Pediatr Dent.* 1999;21: 86-90.

Escuder M, et al. Impact estimates of breastfeeding over infant mortality. *Rev Saude Publica.* 2003;37(3):319-325.

Ettyang G, et al. Assessment of body composition and breast milk volume in lactating mothers in pastoral communities in Pokot, Kenya, using deuterium oxide. *Ann Nutr Metab.* 2005;49(2):110-117.

European Society for Paediatric Gastroenterology, Hepatology and Nutrition (ESPGHAN), Committee on Nutrition. Complementary feeding: a commentary by the ESPGHAN Committee on Nutrition. *J Pediatr Gastroenterol Nutr.* 2008;46:99-110.

European Society for Paediatric Gastroenterology, Hepatology and Nutrition (ESPGHAN), Committee on Nutrition, Agostoni C, et al. Soy protein infant formulae and follow-on formulae: a commentary by the ESPGHAN Committee on Nutrition. *J Pediatr Gastroenterol Nutr.* 2006;42:352-361.

Fergusson D, Woodward L. Breast feeding and later psychosocial adjustment. *Paediatr Perinat Epidemiol.* 1999;139(2): 144-157.

Fernandes R, et al. Inhibition of enteroaggregative *Escherichia coli* adhesion to HEp-2 cells by secretory immunoglobulin A from human colostrum. *Pediatr Infect Dis J.* 2001;20(7): 672-678.

Fewtrell M, et al. Double-blind, randomized trial of long-chain polyunsaturated fatty acid supplementation in formula fed to preterm infants. *Pediatrics.* 2002;110(1 Pt 1): 73-82.

Fowler GA, Ye J. Got milk? Chinese crisis creates a market for human alternatives. *Wall Street Journal.* September 24, 2008. http://online.wsj.com/article/SB122220872407868805.html. Accessed March 13, 2010.

Freudenheim J. Exposure to breast milk in infancy and the risk of breast cancer. *Epidemiology.* 1994;5:324-331.

Gdalevich M, et al. Breast-feeding and the onset of atopic dermatitis in childhood: a systematic review and meta-analysis of prospective studies. *J Am Acad Dermatol.* 2001a; 45(4):520-527.

Gdalevich M, et al. Breast-feeding and the risk of bronchial asthma in childhood: a systematic review with meta-analysis of prospective studies. *J Pediatr*. 2001b;139(2):261-266.

Gianino P. Incidence of nosocomial rotavirus infections, symptomatic and asymptomatic, in breast-fed and non-breast-fed infants. *J Hosp Infect*. 2002;50(1):13-17.

Gil A, et al. Exogenous nucleic acids and nucleotides are efficiently hydrolysed and taken up as nucleosides by intestinal explants from suckling piglets. *Br J Nutr*. 2007;98(2):285-291.

Gilot L. Plant's baby formula called "filthy." *El Paso Times* (El Paso, TX). Borderland; p. 1 November 2, 2004. http://www.newsmodo.com/2004/11/02/plant%27s-baby-formula-called-%27filthy%27/display.jsp?id=3881923. Accessed March 13, 2010.

Goldman AS. The immunological system in human milk: the past—a pathway to the future. In: Woodward WH, Draper HH, eds. *Advances in Nutritional Research*. New York: Plenum Press; 1998:106.

Gomez-Sanchiz M, et al. Influence of breast-feeding on mental and psychomotor development. *Clin Pediatr (Phila)*. 2003; 42(1):35-42.

Gomez-Sanchiz M, et al. Influence of breast-feeding and parental intelligence on cognitive development in the 24-month-old child. *Clin Pediatr (Phila)*. 2004;43(8):753-761.

Good Mojab C. Sunlight deficiency and breastfeeding. *Breastfeeding Abstracts*. 2002;22(1):3-4.

Good Mojab C. Sunlight deficiency: a review of the literature. *Mothering*. 2003a;117:52-55, 57-63.

Good Mojab C. Sunlight deficiency: helping breastfeeding mothers find the facts. *Leaven*. 2003b;39(4):75-79.

Good Mojab C. Sunlight deficiency, vitamin D, and the breastfed baby: helping mothers make informed decisions. Paper presented at: Texas WIC 2004 Nutrition and Breastfeeding Conference; April 21, 2004; Austin, TX.

Greer F. Are breast-fed infants vitamin K deficient? *Adv Exp Med Biol*. 2001a;501:391-395.

Greer F. Do breastfed infants need supplemental vitamins? *Pediatr Clin North Am*. 2001b;48(2):415-423.

Greer F, et al. Improving the vitamin K status of breastfeeding infants with maternal vitamin K supplements. *Pediatrics*. 1997;99(1):88-92.

Greiner T. Maternal protein-energy malnutrition and breastfeeding. *SCN News*. 1994;11:28-30.

Griffiths L, et al. Effects of infant feeding practice on weight gain from birth to 3 years. *Arch Dis Child*. 2009; 94(8):577-582

Grummer-Strawn L, et al. Does breastfeeding protect against pediatric overweight? Analysis of longitudinal data from the Centers for Disease Control and Prevention Pediatric Nutrition Surveillance System. *Pediatrics*. 2004;113(2):e81-e86.

Gunderson E. Breast-feeding and diabetes: long-term impact on mothers and their infants. *Curr Diab Rep*. 2008;8(4):279-286.

Habicht J, et al. Does breastfeeding really save lives, or are apparent benefits due to biases? *Am J Epidemiol*. 1986; 123(2):279-290.

Hakansson A, et al. A folding variant of alpha-lactalbumin with bactericidal activity against *Streptococcus pneumoniae*. *Mol Microbiol*. 2000;35:589-600.

Hale T. *Medications and Mothers' Milk*. 14th ed. Amarillo, TX: Hale Publishing; 2010.

Hall A. Homemade baby formula. December 3, 2008. www.reliableanswers.com/med/homemade_baby_formula.asp. Accessed March 20, 2009.

Hall B. Changing composition of human milk and early development of appetite control: Keeping abreast. *J Human Nurtur*. 1997;12:3.

Hamosh M. Breastfeeding: Unraveling the mysteries of mother's milk. *Medscape Womens' Health*. 1996;1(9):4.

Hamprecht K, et al. Epidemiology of transmission of cytomegalovirus from mother to preterm infant by breastfeeding. *Lancet*. 2001;357(9255):513-518.

Hancock JT, et al. Antimicrobial properties of milk: dependence on presence of xanthine oxidase and nitrite. *Antimicrob Agents Chemother*. 2002;46:3308-3310.

Hansen K, et al. Weekly oral vitamin K prophylaxis in Denmark. *Acta Paediatr*. 2003;92(7):802-805.

Hanson L. Breastfeeding provides passive and likely long-lasting active immunity. *Ann Allergy Asthma Immunol*. 1998;5:178-180.

Hanson L. Protective effects of breastfeeding against urinary tract infection. *Acta Paediatr*. 2004a;93(2):154-156.

Hanson L. *Immunobiology of Human Milk: How Breastfeeding Protects Babies*. Amarillo, TX: Hale Publishing; 2004b.

Hanson L. Chapter 10: The role of breastfeeding in the defense of the infant. In: Hale T, Hartmann P, eds. *Hale and Hartmann's Textbook of Human Lactation*. Amarillo, TX: Hale Publishing; 2007a: 159-192.

Hanson LA. Session 1: Feeding and infant development breastfeeding and immune function. *Proc Nutr Soc*. 2007b;66:384-396.

Hanson L, et al. Breast-feeding: a complex support system for the offspring. *Pediatr Int*. 2002;44(4):347-352.

Harkness L, Cromer B. Low levels of 25-hydroxy vitamin D are associated with elevated parathyroid hormone in healthy adolescent females. *Osteoporos Int*. 2005;16(1):109-113.

Hart S, et al. Brief report: Breast-fed one-week-olds demonstrate superior neurobehavioral organization. *J Pediatr Psychol*. 2003;28(8):529-534.

Hartmann P, et al. Physiology of lactation in preterm mothers: initiation and maintenance. *Pediatr Ann*. 2003;32(5):351-355.

Hasselbalch H, et al. Breast-feeding influences thymic size in late infancy. *Eur J Pediatr*. 1999;158(12):964-967.

Hawkins N. Potential aluminum toxicity in infants fed special infant formula. *J Pediatr Gastroenterol Nutr*. 1994;19:377-381.

Henderson G, et al. Formula milk versus maternal breast milk or feeding preterm or low birth weight infants. *Cochrane Database Syst Rev*. 2007;4:CD002972.

Hill D, et al. Sensitivity to dietary proteins released in breast milk causing colic in infants. Paper presented at: AAAAI Annual Meeting; March 25, 2004; San Francisco.

Hirsch D. Chapter 23: Vitamin D and the breastfed infant. In: Hale T, Hartmann P, eds. *Hale and Hartmann's Textbook of Human Lactation.* Amarillo, TX: Hale Publishing; 2007: 425-461.

Hoey C, Ware J. Economic advantages of breast-feeding in an HMO: setting a pilot study. *Am J Manag Care.* 1997;3(6): 861-865.

Holick MF. Environmental factors that influence the cutaneous production of vitamin D. *Am J Clin Nutr.* 1995;1(3 suppl): 638S-645S.

Holick MF. Vitamin D deficiency. *N Engl J Med.* 2007;357:266-281.

Hollis B, Wagner C. Assessment of dietary vitamin D requirements during pregnancy and lactation. *Am J Clin Nutr.* 2004a;79(5):717-726.

Hollis B, Wagner C. Vitamin D requirements during lactation: high-dose maternal supplementation as therapy to prevent hypovitaminosis D for both the mother and the nursing infant. *Am J Clin Nutr.* 2004b;80(6 suppl):1752S-1758S.

Horby J. Effect of formula supplemented with docosahexaenoic acid and gamma-linolenic acid on fatty acid status and visual acuity in term infants. *Pediatr Gastroenterol Nutr.* 1998;26(4):412-421.

Horta B, et al. *Evidence on the Long-Term Effects of Breast-feeding: Systematic Reviews and Meta-analyses.* Geneva, Switzerland: World Health Organization; 2007.

Horwood L, Fergusson D. Breastfeeding and later cognitive and academic outcomes. *Pediatrics.* 1998;101(1):E9.

Host A. Frequency of cow's milk allergy in childhood. *Ann Allergy Asthma Immunol.* 2002;89(6 suppl 1):33-37.

Humenick S, et al. The maturation index of colostrum and milk (MICAM): A measurement of breast milk maturation. *J Nurs Meas.* 1994;2(2):169-186.

Hunt M, et al. Black breast milk due to minocycline therapy. *Br J Dermatol.* 1996;134:943-944.

Hylander M, et al. Human milk feedings and infection among very low birth weight infants. *Pediatrics.* 1998;102(3):E38.

Infante P, et al. Use of goat's milk in patients with cow's milk allergy. *Ann Pediatr (Barc).* 2003;59(2):138-142.

Innis S, et al. Are human long chain polyunsaturated fatty acids related to visual and neural development in breast-fed term infants? *J Pediatr.* 2001;139(4):532-538.

Inoue K, et al. Determination of nucleotides in infant formula by ion-exchange liquid chromatography. *J Agric Food Chem.* 2008;56(16):6863-6867.

Institute of Medicine (IOM). *Dietary reference intakes for calcium, phosphorus, magnesium, vitamin D and fluoride.* Washington, DC: National Academy Press; 1997:288-313.

International Baby Food Action Network (IBFAN); Kean YJ, Allain A, eds. *Breaking the Rules, Stretching the Rules 2007.* Penang, Malaysia: IBFAN; 2007.

International Lactation Consultant Association (ILCA); Mannel R, et al., eds. *Core Curriculum for Lactation Consultant Practice.* 2nd ed. Sudbury, MA: Jones and Bartlett; 2007.

Ip S, et al. *Breastfeeding and Maternal and Infant Health Outcomes in Developed Countries* (Report 153). Rockville, MD: Agency for Healthcare Research and Quality; 2007.

Ivarsson A, et al. Breast-feeding protects against celiac disease. *Am J Clin Nutr.* 2002;75(5):914-921.

Jackson K, Nazar A. Breastfeeding, the immune response, and long-term health. *J Am Osteopath Assoc.* 2006;106(4):203-207.

Jain A, et al. How good is the evidence linking breastfeeding and intelligence? *Pediatrics.* 2002;109(6):1044-1053.

Jeffery B, et al. Determination of the effectiveness of inactivation of human immunodeficiency virus by Pretoria pasteurization. *J Trop Pediatr.* 2001;47(6):345-349.

Jeffery B, et al. The effect of Pretoria pasteurization on bacterial contamination of hand-expressed human breastmilk. *J Trop Pediatr.* 2003;49(4):240-244.

Jelliffe D, Jelliffe E. *Human Milk in the Modern World.* New York: Oxford University Press; 1978.

Jensen R. Lipids in human milk. *Lipids.* 1999;34:1243-271.

Jeppesson D, et al. T-lymphocyte subsets, thymic size and breastfeeding in infancy. *Pediatr Allergy Immunol.* 2004; 15(2):127-132.

Keating J, et al. Oral water intoxication in infants: An American epidemic. *Am J Dis Child.* 1991;145(9):985-990.

Kelly D, Coutts A. Early nutrition and the development of immune function in the neonate. *Proc Nutr Soc.* 2000;59(2): 177-185.

Kent J. Breastmilk calcium for the pre-term baby. Paper presented at: Human Lactation: Current Research and Clinical Implications; October 22, 2004; Amarillo, TX.

Kent J. How breastfeeding works. *J Midwifery Women's Health.* 2007;52(6):564-570.

Kent J, et al. Volume and frequency of breastfeedings and fat content of breast milk throughout the day. *Pediatrics.* 2006; 117(3):e387-e395.

Kierson J, et al. Ghrelin and cholecystokinin in term and pre-term human breast milk. *Acta Paediatr.* 2006;95(8):991-905.

Kimpimaki T, et al. Short-term exclusive breastfeeding predisposes young children with increased genetic risk of type 1 diabetes to progressive beta-cell autoimmunity. *Diabetologia.* 2001;44(1):63-69.

Kjos S, et al. The effect of lactation on glucose and lipid metabolism in women with recent gestational diabetes. *Obstet Gynecol.* 1993;82(3):451-455.

Klein C. Nutrient requirements for preterm infant formulas. *J Nutr.* 2002;132(6 suppl 1):1395S-1577S.

Kohler H, et al. Antibacterial characteristics in the feces of breast-fed and formula-fed infants during the first year of life. *J Pediatr Gastroenterol Nutr.* 2002;34(2):188-193.

Koletzko B, et al. Physiological aspects of human milk lipids. *Early Hum Dev.* 2001;65:S3-S18.

Koo W. Efficacy and safety of docosahexaenoic acid and arachidonic acid addition to infant formulas: can one buy better vision and intelligence? *J Am Coll Nutr.* 2003;22(2):101-107.

Koo W, et al. Reduced bone mineralization in infants fed palm olein-containing formula: a randomized, double-blinded, prospective trial. *Pediatrics.* 2003;111(5 Pt 1):1017-1023.

Kramer M, et al. Breastfeeding and child cognitive development: new evidence from a large randomized trial. *Arch Gen Psychiatry.* 2008;65(5):578-584.

Kreiter SR, et al. Nutritional rickets in African American breast-fed infants. *J Pediatr.* 2000;137:153-157.

Kumar N, et al. The specific role of isoflavones on estrogen metabolism in premenopausal women. *Cancer.* 2002;94(4): 1166-1174.

Kumar S. Quantity and quality of breast milk in malnourished mothers. *Indian J Pediatr.* 1989;56(6):677-678.

Kuschel C, Harding J. Multicomponent fortified human milk for promoting growth in preterm infants. *Cochrane Database Syst Rev.* 2004;1:CD000343.

Kutner L. *Certified Lactation Specialist Course.* Lactation Education Consultants: Wheaton, IL; 2009.

La Leche League International (LLLI). *Sunlight deficiency, "vitamin D," and breastfeeding.* Schaumburg, IL: LLLI; April 2003.

Lai C. Variation in the composition of breastmilk and its fortification for pre-term babies. Paper presented at: Human Lactation: Current Research and Clinical Implications; October 22, 2004; Amarillo, TX.

Lakdawala D, Widdowson E. Vitamin D in human milk. *Lancet.* 1997;(8044):167-168.

Landers S. Maximizing the benefits of human milk feeding for the preterm infant. *Pediatr Ann.* 2003;32(5):298-306.

Lawrence R, Lawrence R. *Breastfeeding: A Guide for the Medical Profession.* 6th ed. St. Louis, MO: Elsevier Mosby; 2005.

Leroy V, et al. Acceptability of formula-feeding to prevent HIV postnatal transmission, Abidjan, Côte d'Ivoire: ANRS 1201/1202 Ditrame Plus Study. *J Acquir Immune Defic Syndr.* 2007;1;44(1):77-86.

Levine O, et al. Risk factors for invasive pneumococcal disease in children: A population-based case-control study in North America. *Pediatrics.* 1999;103(3):E28.

Lindberg T. Infantile colic and small intestinal function: A nutritional problem? *Acta Paediatr Suppl.* 1999;88(430):58-60.

Lindblad BS, et al. Blood levels of critical amino acids in very low birthweight infants on a high human milk protein intake. *Acta Paediatr Scand Suppl.* 1982;296:24-27.

Lo C, et al. Indian and Pakistani immigrants have the same capacity as Caucasians to produce vitamin D in response to ultraviolet irradiation. *Am J Clin Nutr.* 1986;44(5):683-685.

LoCascio R, et al. Glycoprofiling of bifidobacterial consumption of human milk oligosaccharides demonstrates strain specific, preferential consumption of small chain glycans secreted in early human lactation. *J Agric Food Chem.* 2007; 55(22):8914-8919.

Loland B. Human milk, immune responses and health effects. *Tidsskr Nor Laegeforen.* 2007;127(18):2395-2398.

Lonnerdal B. Recombinant human milk proteins. *Nestlé Nutr Workshop Ser Pediatr Program.* 2006:58:207-215; discussion 215-217.

Lucas A. Breastmilk and neonatal NEC. *Lancet.* 1990;336:1519-1523.

Lucas A, et al. Early diet in preterm babies and developmental status at 18 months. *Lancet.* 1990;335(8704):1477-1481.

Lucas A, et al. Breastmilk and subsequent intelligence quotient in children born preterm. *Lancet.* 1992;339:261-264.

Lucas A, et al. A randomized multicentre study of human milk versus formula and later development in preterm infants. *Arch Dis Child.* 1994;70:F141-F146.

Mahmud M, et al. Impact of breast feeding on *Giardia lamblia* infections in Bilbeis, Egypt. *Am J Trop Med Hyg.* 2001; 65(3):257-260.

Malvy DJ, et al. Relationship between vitamin D status and skin phototype in general adult population. *Photochem Photobiol.* 2000;71(4):466-469.

Marchini G, Linden A. Cholecystokinin: a satiety signal in newborn infants? *J Dev Physiol.* 1992;17(5):215-219.

Marild S, et al. Protective effect of breastfeeding against urinary tract infection. *Acta Paediatr.* 2004;93(2):164-168.

Marini A, et al. Effects of a dietary and environmental programme on the incidence of allergic symptoms in high atopic risk infants: three years' follow-up. *Acta Paediatr Suppl.* 1996;414:1-21.

Marshall TA, et al. Associations between intakes of fluoride from beverages during infancy and dental fluorosis of primary teeth. *J Am Coll Nutr.* 2004;23(2):108-116.

Martin J, et al. Dependence of human milk essential fatty acids on adipose stores during lactation. *Am J Clin Nutr.* 1993; 58:653-659.

Martin L, et al. Presence of adiponectin and leptin in human milk. Paper presented at: 2004 Pediatric Academic Societies' Annual Meeting; May 2, 2004; San Francisco.

Mason T, et al. Breast feeding and the development of juvenile rheumatoid arthritis. *J Rheumatol.* 1995;22(6):1166-1170.

Mastretta E, et al. Effect of lactobacillus GG and breast-feeding in the prevention of rotavirus nosocomial infection. *J Pediatr Gastroenterol Nutr.* 2002;35(4):527-531.

Matsuoka L, et al. Racial pigmentation and the cutaneous synthesis of vitamin D. *Arch Dermatol.* 1991;127(4):536-538.

McGuire W, Anthony M. Donor human milk versus formula for preventing necrotising enterocolitis in preterm infants: Systematic review. *Arch Dis Child.* 2003;88(1)SI:11-14.

McVeagh P, Miller J. Human milk oligosaccharides: only the breast. *J Paediatr Child Health.* 1997;33(4):281-286.

Mead Johnson, Inc. Nutramigen 16-oz. powder infant formula and Nutramigen 32-oz. ready-to-use infant formula recalled due to Spanish-language labeling error that could result in adverse health effects. 2001. www.meadjohnson.com/about/pressreleas/nutramigenengpr.html. Accessed March 17, 2009.

Mead Johnson, Inc. Product information descriptions. 2009. www.mjn.com/app/iwp/HCP/Content2.do ?dm=mj&id=/ HCP _Home/Product_Information/Product_Descriptions/ EnfamilLIPIL&iwpst=MJN&ls=0&cs red =1&r=3414930086# nutrientFacts. Accessed March 18, 2009.

Meier P, et al. Mothers' milk feedings in the neonatal intensive care unit: Accuracy of the creamatocrit technique. *J Perinatol.* 2002;22(8):646-649.

Meier P, et al. Accuracy of a user-friendly centrifuge for measuring creamatocrits on mothers' milk in the clinical setting. *Breastfeed Med.* 2006;1(2):79-87.

Meinzen-Derr J, et al. The role of human milk feedings in risk of late-onset sepsis. Paper presented at: 2004 Pediatric Academic Societies' Annual Meeting; May 1, 2004; San Francisco.

Mennella J, Beauchamp G. Maternal diet alters the sensory qualities of human milk and the nursling's behavior. *Pediatrics.* 1991;88:737-744.

Michaelsen KF, et al. The Copenhagen cohort study on infant nutrition and growth: breastmilk intake, human milk macronutrient content and influencing factors. *Am J Clin Nutr.* 1994;59:600-611.

Michels D, Baumslag N. *Milk, money and madness: The culture and politics of breastfeeding.* Westport, CT: Greenwood; 1995.

Mihrshahi S, et al. Association between infant feeding patterns and diarrhoeal and respiratory illness: a cohort study in Chittagong, Bangladesh. *Int Breastfeed J*. 2008;3:28.

Minchin M. *Breastfeeding Matters: What We Need to Know About Breastfeeding*. Victoria, Australia: Alma; 1998:360.

Mitoulas L, et al. Variation in fat, lactose and protein in human milk over 24 h and throughout the first year of lactation. *Br J Nutr*. 2002;88(1):29-37.

Monetini L. Bovine beta-casein antibodies in breast- and bottle-fed infants: their relevance in type 1 diabetes. *Diabetes Metab Res Rev*. 2001;17(1):51-54.

Monterrosa E, et al. Predominant breast-feeding from birth to six months is associated with fewer gastrointestinal infections and increased risk for iron deficiency among infants. *J Nutr*. 2008;138(8):1499-1504.

Moreno Villares JM. Probiotics in infant formulae: could we modify the immune response? *An Pediatr (Barc)*. 2008; 68(3):286-294.

Morrow A, et al. Human-milk glycans that inhibit pathogen binding protect breast-feeding infants against infectious diarrhea. *J Nutr*. 2005;135(5):1304-1307.

Mortensen E, et al. The association between duration of breast-feeding and adult intelligence. *JAMA*. 2002;287(18):2365-2371.

Morton J. The role of the pediatrician in extended breastfeeding of the preterm infant. *Pediatr Ann*. 2003;32(5):308-316.

Nakamura N, et al. Molecular ecological analysis of fecal bacterial populations from term infants fed formula supplemented with selected blends of prebiotics. *Appl Environ Microbiol*. 2009;75(4):1121-1128.

Nathavitharana K, et al. IgA antibodies in human milk: Epidemiological markers of previous infections. *Arch Dis Child*. 1994;71:F192-F197.

National Alliance for Breastfeeding Advocacy (NABA). Recalls of infant feeding products. www.naba-breastfeeding.org. Accessed March 25, 2009.

Nestlé. Supplementing your breastmilk. 2009. www.gerber.com/ Articles/Supplementing_your_ breastmilk.aspx. Accessed March 18, 2009.

New Mexico Department of Health (NMDH). Department of Health advises safe way to feed infants. November 25, 2008. http://www.health.state.nm.us/CommunicationsOffice/ documents/DOH%20Advises%20safe%20 way%20to%20 feed%20infants.pdf. Accessed March 26, 2009.

Newburg D. Neonatal protection by an innate immune system of human milk consisting of oligosaccharides and glycans. *J Animal Sci*. 2009;87(13 suppl):26-34.

Newburg D. Oligosaccharides and glycoconjugates in human milk: Their role in host defense. *J Mammary Gland Biol Neoplasia*. 1996;1(3):271-283.

Newburg D, et al. Innate protection conferred by fucosylated oligosaccharides of human milk against diarrhea in breast-fed infants. *Glycobiology*. 2004;14(3):253-263.

Nishiguchi T, et al. Improvement of vitamin K status of breastfeeding infants with maternal supplement of vitamin K_2 (MK40). *Semin Thromb Hemost*. 2002;28(6):533-538.

Nommsen L, et al. Determinants of energy, proteins, lipid and lactose concentrations in human milk during the first 12 months of lactation: The DARLING study. *Am J Clin Nutr*. 1991;53:457-465.

Oddy W, et al. The effects of respiratory infections, atopy, and breastfeeding on childhood asthma. *Eur Respir J*. 2002; 19(5):899-905.

Oddy W, et al. Breast feeding and cognitive development in childhood: a prospective birth cohort study. *Paediatr Perinat Epidemiol*. 2003a;17(1):81-90.

Oddy W, et al. Breast feeding and respiratory morbidity in infancy: a birth cohort study. *Arch Dis Child*. 2003b;88(3): 224-228.

Ogbuanu I, et al. The effect of breastfeeding duration on lung function at age 10 years: a prospective birth cohort study. *Thorax*. 2009;64(1):62-66.

Oliveira V, Prell M. Sharing the economic burden: who pays for WIC's infant formula? *USDA/ERS Amber Waves*. September 2004. www.ers.usda.gov/Amberwaves/September04/ Features/infantformula.htm. Accessed December 8, 2004.

Orrhage K, Nord C. Factors controlling the bacterial colonization of the intestine in breastfed infants. *Acta Paediatr Suppl*. 1999;88(430):47-57.

Owen C, et al. Infant feeding and blood cholesterol: a study in adolescents and a systematic review. *Pediatrics*. 2002; 110(3):597-608.

Owen C, et al. Does breastfeeding influence risk of type 2 diabetes in later life? A quantitative analysis of published evidence. *Am J Clin Nutr*. 2006;84(5):1043-1054.

Owen C, et al. Does initial breastfeeding lead to lower blood cholesterol in adult life? A quantitative review of the evidence. *Am J Clin Nutr*. 2008;88(2):305-314.

Owen C, et al. Effect of infant feeding on the risk of obesity across the life course: a quantitative review of published evidence. *Pediatrics*. 2005;115(5):1367-1377.

Pabst H, et al. Differential modulation of the immune response by breast- or formula-feeding of infants. *Acta Paediatr*. 1997;86(12):1291-1297.

Palmer G. *The Politics of Breastfeeding: When Breasts Are Bad for Business*. 3rd ed. London: Pinter & Martin; 2009.

Pang W, Hartmann P. Initiation of human lactation: secretory differentiation and secretory activation. *J Mammary Gland Biol Neoplasia*. 2007;12(4):211-221.

Paramasivam K, et al. Human breast milk immunology: a review. *Int J Fertil Women Med*. 2006;51(5):208-217.

Park MJ, et al. Bone mineral content is not reduced despite low vitamin D status in breast milk-fed infants versus cow's milk based formula-fed infants. *J Pediatr*. 1998;132(4):641-645.

Perez-Escamilla R, et al. Maternal anthropometric status and lactation performance in a low-income Honduran population: Evidence for the role of infants. *Am J Clin Nutr*. 1995; 61:528-534.

Perrilat F. Day-care, early common infections and childhood acute leukaemia: a multicentre French case-control study. *Brit J Cancer*. 2002;86(7):1064-1069.

Pickering L. Modulation of the immune system by human milk and infant formula containing nucleotides. *Pediatrics*. 1998;101(2):242-249.

Pisacane A, et al. Breast-feeding and urinary tract infection. *J Pediatr*. 1992;120(1):87-89.

Pisacane A, et al. Breastfeeding and multiple sclerosis. *Br J Med.* 1994;308:1411-1412.

Potischman N, Troisi R. In-utero and early life exposures in relation to risk of breast cancer. *Cancer Causes Control.* 1999;10(6):561-573.

Premji S, et al. Evidence-based feeding guidelines for very low-birth-weight infants. *Adv Neonatal Care.* 2002;2(1):5-18.

Pugliese MF, et al. Nutritional rickets in suburbia. *J Am Coll Nutr.* 1998;17:637-641.

Quan R, et al. The effect of nutritional additives on anti-infective factors in human milk. *Clin Pediatr (Phila).* 1994;33(6):325-328.

Quigley MA, et al. Formula milk versus donor breast milk for feeding preterm or low birth weight infants. *Cochrane Database Syst Rev.* 2007;(4):CD002971.

Raisler J, et al. Breast-feeding and infant illness: a dose-response relationship? *Am J Public Health.* 1999;89(1):25-30.

Rao M, et al. Effect of breastfeeding on cognitive development of infants born small for gestational age. *Acta Paediatr.* 2002;91(3):267-274.

Ravelli A, et al. Infant feeding and adult glucose tolerance, lipid profile, blood pressure, and obesity. *Arch Dis Child.* 2000;82(3):248-252.

Renfrew M, et al. Formula feed preparation: helping reduce the risks; a systematic review. *Arch Dis Child.* 2003;88:855-858.

Rockwell Nutrition. Can I use goat milk instead of infant formula? 2008. www.rockwellnutrition.com/Can-I-use-Goat-Milk-instead-of-infant-formula_ep_92-1.html. Accessed March 20, 2009.

Ronneberg R, Skara B. Essential fatty acids in human colostrum. *Acta Paediatr.* 1992;81:779-783.

Ross Products Division (Abbott Laboratories). Customer service response to inquiry. 800-227-5767. March 2009.

Rubin D, et al. Relationship between infant feeding and infectious illness: a prospective study of infants during the first year of life. *Pediatrics.* 1990;85:464-471.

Rudloff S, Lonnerdal B. Calcium retention from milk-based infant formulas, whey-hydrolysate formula, and human milk in weanling rhesus monkeys. *Am J Child Dis.* 1990;144:360-363.

Rudnicka A, et al. The effect of breastfeeding on cardiorespiratory risk factors in adult life. *Pediatrics.* 2007;119(5):e1107-e1115.

Russo J, et al. The concept of stem cell in the mammary gland and its implication in morphogenesis, cancer and prevention. *Front Biosci.* 2006;11:151-172.

Saarinen U, Kajosaari M. Breastfeeding as prophylaxis against atopic disease: Prospective follow-up study until 17 years old. *Lancet.* 1995;346:1065-1069.

Saavedra M, et al. Infantile colic incidence and associated risk factors: a cohort study. *J Pediatr (Rio J).* 2003;79(2):115-122.

Sabikhi L. Designer milk. *Adv Food Nutr Res.* 2007;53:161-198.

Sala-Vila A, et al. The source of long-chain PUFA in formula supplements does not affect the fatty acid composition of plasma lipids in full-term infants. *J Nutr.* 2004;134(4):868-873.

Sarkadi-Nagy E, et al. Formula feeding potentiates docosahexaenoic and arachidonic acid biosynthesis in term and preterm baboon neonates. *J Lipid Res.* 2004;45(1):71-80.

Sauerwald T, et al. Polyunsaturated fatty acid supply with human milk: physiological aspects and in vivo studies of metabolism. *Adv Exp Med Biol.* 2000;478:261-270.

Save Babies Through Screening Foundation, Inc. Galactosemia (GALT). www.savebabies.org/professionals/disease descriptions/galactosemia.html. Accessed March 28, 2009.

Sawatzki G, et al. Pitfalls in the design and manufacture of infant formulae. *Acta Paediatr.* 1994;402(suppl):40-45.

Scanlon K, ed. Final Report. Paper presented at: Vitamin D Expert Panel Meeting; October 11-12, 2001; Atlanta, GA. www.cdc.gov/nccdphp/dnpa/nutrition/pdf/Vitamin_D_Expert_Panel_Meeting.pdf. Accessed June 2, 2004.

Scariati P, et al. A longitudinal analysis of infant morbidity and the extent of breastfeeding in the US. *Pediatrics.* 1997;99(6):E5-E7.

Schack-Nielsen L, Michaelsen KF. The effects of breastfeeding I: effects on the immune system and the central nervous system. *Ugeskr Laeger.* 2007;169(11):985-989.

Schanler R, et al. Feeding strategies for premature infants: beneficial outcomes of feeding fortified human milk versus preterm formula. *Pediatrics.* 1999;104(6 Pt 1):1150-1157.

Scheifele D, et al. Breastfeeding and antibody responses to routine vaccination in infants. *Lancet.* 1992;340:1406.

Schroten H, et al. Inhibition of adhesion of S-fimbriated *Escherichia coli* to buccal epithelial cells by human milk fat globule membrane components: a novel aspect of the protective function of mucins in the nonimmunoglobulin fraction. *Infect Immun.* 1992;60:2893-2899.

Schroten H, et al. Inhibition of adhesion of S-fimbriated *E. coli* to buccal epithelial cells by human skim milk is predominantly mediated by mucins and depends on the period of lactation. *Acta Paediatr.* 1993;82:6-11.

Scragg R, et al. Serum 25-hydroxyvitamin D3 is related to physical activity and ethnicity but not obesity in a multicultural workforce. *Aust N Z J Med.* 1995;25(3):218-223.

Shu X, et al. Breast-feeding and risk of childhood acute leukemia. *J Natl Cancer Inst.* 1999;91(20):1765-1772.

Siegel-Itzkovich J. Police in Israel launch investigation into deaths of babies given formula milk. *BMJ.* 2003;327:1128.

Silfverdal S, et al. Long term enhancement of the IgG2 antibody response to *Haemophilus influenzae* type B by breast-feeding. *Pediatr Infect Dis J.* 2002;21(9):816-821.

Sills I, et al. Vitamin D deficiency rickets: reports of its demise are exaggerated. *Clin Pediatr (Phila).* 1994;33:491-493.

Simmer K, et al. Longchain polyunsaturated fatty acid supplementation in infants born at term. *Cochrane Database Syst Rev.* 2008a;1:CD000376.

Simmer K, et al. Longchain polyunsaturated fatty acid supplementation in preterm infants. *Cochrane Database Syst Rev.* 2008b;1:CD000375.

Singhal A, et al. Early nutrition in preterm infants and later blood pressure: two cohorts after randomised trials. *Lancet.* 2001;357(9254):413-419.

Singhal A, et al. Breastmilk feeding and lipoprotein profile in adolescents born preterm: follow-up of a prospective randomised study. *Lancet.* 2004;363(9421):1571-1578.

Slusher T, et al. Promoting the exclusive feeding of own mother's milk through the use of hindmilk and increased maternal milk volume for hospitalized, low birth weight infants (<1800 grams) in Nigeria: A feasibility study. *J Hum Lact.* 2003;19(2):191-198.

Smith M, et al. Influence of breastfeeding on cognitive outcomes at age 6–8 years: follow-up of very low birth weight infants. *Am J Epidemiol.* 2003;158(11):1075-1082.

Smulevich V, et al. Parental occupation and other factors and cancer risk in children: 1. Study methodology and non-occupational factors. *Int J Cancer.* 1999;83(6):712-717.

Specker B. Do North American women need supplemental vitamin D during pregnancy or lactation? *Am J Clin Nutr.* 1994;59(2 suppl):484S-490S; discussion 490S-491S.

Specker B, et al. Sunshine exposure and serum 25-hydroxyvitamin D concentrations in exclusively breastfed infants. *J Pediatr.* 1985;107:372-376.

Specker B, et al. Low serum calcium and high parathyroid hormone levels in neonates fed "humanized" cow's milk-based formula. *Am J Dis Child.* 1991;145:941-945.

Sterken E. Director, INFACT, Canada. Personal e-mail correspondence; April 27, 2004.

Strathearn L, et al. Does breastfeeding protect against substantiated child abuse and neglect? A 15-year cohort study. *Pediatrics.* 2009;123;483-493.DOI: 10.1542/peds.2007-3546.

Tarcan A, et al. Influence of feeding formula and breast milk fortifier on lymphocyte subsets in very low birth weight premature newborns. *Biol Neonate.* 2004;86(1):22-28.

Tariq S, et al. The prevalence of and risk factors for atopy in early childhood: a whole population birth cohort study. *J Allergy Clin Immunol.* 1998;101(5):587-593.

Tarrats R, et al. Varicella, ephemeral breastfeeding and eczema as risk factors for multiple sclerosis in Mexicans. *Acta Neurol Scand.* 2002;105(2):88-89.

Taylor JA, et al. Use of supplemental vitamin D among infants breastfed for prolonged periods. *Pediatrics.* 2010;125:105-111.

Tellez A, et al. Antibodies in mother's milk protect children against giardiasis. *Scand J Infect Dis.* 2003;35(5):322-325.

Thompson N, et al. Early determinants of inflammatory bowel disease: use of two national longitudinal birth cohorts. *Eur J Gastroenter Hepatology.* 2000;12(1):25-30.

Thorsdottir I, et al. Iron status at 12 months of age: Effects of body size, growth and diet in a population with high birth weight. *Eur J Clin Nutr.* 2003;57(4):505-513.

Toschke A, et al. Overweight and obesity in 6- to 14-year-old Czech children in 1991: protective effect of breast-feeding. *J Pediatr.* 2002;141(6):764-769.

Tran T, et al. Effects of neonatal dietary manganese exposure on brain dopamine levels and neurocognitive functions. *Neurotoxicology.* 2002;23(4-5):645-651.

Tully M, et al. Stories of success: the use of donor milk is increasing in North America. *J Hum Lact.* 2004;20(1):75-77.

Turck D. Comité de Nutrition de la Société Française de Pédiatrie. Breast feeding: health benefits for child and mother (article in French). *Arch Pediatr.* 2005;12S3:S145-S165.

Tyson J, et al. Adaptation of feeding to a low fat yield in breastmilk. *Pediatrics.* 1992;89:215-220.

Udall J. Gastrointestinal host defense and necrotizing enterocolitis. *J Pediatr.* 1990;117:S33-S34.

Underwood M, et al. A randomized placebo-controlled comparison of 2 prebiotic/probiotic combinations in preterm infants: impact on weight gain, intestinal microbiota, and fecal short-chain fatty acids. *J Pediatr Gastroenterol Nutr.* 2009;48(2):216-225.

United States Department of Health and Human Services (USDHHS), National Toxicology Program (NTP), Center for the Evaluation of Risks to Human Reproduction (CERHR). *Monograph on the Potential Human Reproductive and Developmental Effects of Bisphenol A* (NIH Publication No. 08-5994). September 2008. cerhr.niehs.nih.gov/chemicals/bisphenol/bisphenol.pdf. Accessed March 25, 2009.

United States Food and Drug Administration (USFDA). Second best but good enough. *FDA Consumer Magazine.* June 1996. http://www.fda.gov/Fdac/features/596_baby.html. Accessed March 27, 2009.

United States Food and Drug Administration (USFDA), Center for Food Safety and Applied Nutrition Office of Nutritional Products. Labeling and dietary supplements: Health professionals letter on *Enterobacter sakazakii* infections associated with use of powdered (dry) infant formulas in neonatal intensive care units. April 11, 2002; revised October 10, 2002. http://www.cfsan.fda.gov/~dms/inf-ltr3.html. Accessed March 25, 2009.

United States Food and Drug Administration (USFDA). Melamine contamination in China. January 5, 2009. http://www.fda.gov/oc/opacom/hottopics/melamine.html. Accessed March 25, 2009.

Updegrove K. Necrotizing enterocolitis: the evidence for use of human milk in prevention and treatment. *J Hum Lact.* 2004;20(3):335-339.

Van de Perre P. Transfer of antibody via mother's milk. *Vaccine.* 2003;21(24):3374-3376.

Van Odijk J, et al. Breastfeeding and allergic disease: a multidisciplinary review of the literature (1966-2001) on the mode of early feeding in infancy and its impact on later atopic manifestations. *Allergy.* 2003;58(9):833-843.

Van Veen H, et al. The role of N-linked glycosylation in the protection of human and bovine lactoferrin against tryptic proteolysis. *Eur J Biochem.* 2004;271(4):678-684.

Vieira G, et al. Child feeding and diarrhea morbidity. *J Pediatr (Rio J).* 2003;79(5):449-454.

Viverge D, et al. Variations in oligosaccharides and lactose in human milk during the first week of lactation. *J Pediatr Gastroenterol Nutr.* 1990;11:361-364.

Wagner C, et al. Special properties of human milk. *Clin Pediatr.* 1996;35:283-293.

Wagner C, et al. High dose vitamin D_3 supplementation in a cohort of breastfeeding mothers and their infants: a 6-month follow-up study. *BF Med.* 2006;1:59-70.

Wagner CL, Greer FR, and the Section on Breastfeeding and Committee on Nutrition. Prevention of rickets and vitamin D deficiency in infants, children, and adolescents. *Pediatrics.* 2008;122:1142-1152.

Walker M. *Still Selling Out Mothers and Babies: Marketing of Breast Milk Substitutes in the USA.* Weston, MA: NABA REAL; 2007.

Ward L, et al. Vitamin D–deficiency rickets among children in Canada. *CMAJ.* 2007;177(2):161-166.

Wariyar U, et al. Six years' experience of prophylactic oral vitamin K. *Arch Dis Child Fetal Neonatal Ed.* 2000;82(1):F64-F68.

Weimer J. *Economic benefits: A review and analysis.* Economic Research Service, USDA. Food Assistance and Nutrition Research Report 13. March 2001.

Westerbeek E, et al. Design of a randomised controlled trial on immune effects of acidic and neutral oligosaccharides in the nutrition of preterm infants: Carrot study. *BMC Pediatr.* 2008;8:46.

Wight NE. Donor human milk for preterm infants. *J Perinatol.* 2001;21(4):249-254.

Williams C, et al. Stereoacuity at age 3.5 y in children born full-term is associated with prenatal and postnatal dietary factors: a report from a population-based cohort study. *Am J Clin Nutr.* 2001;73(2):316-322.

Wold AE, Adlerbeth I. Breast feeding and the intestinal microflora of the infant: Implications for protection against infectious diseases. *Adv Exp Med Biol.* 2000;478:77-93.

Wolf J. Low breastfeeding rates and public health in the US. *Am J Pub Health.* 2003;93(12):2001-2010.

Woolridge MW, et al. Do changes in pattern of breast usage alter the baby's nutrient intake? *Lancet.* 1990;336:395-397.

World Health Organization (WHO). Executive summary. Presented at: WHO Expert Meeting to Review Toxicological Aspects of Melamine and Cyanuric Acid; December 1-4, 2008; Ottawa, Canada. www.who.int/foodsafety/fs_management/Exec_Summary_melamine.pdf. Accessed March 25, 2009.

World Health Organization (WHO). HIV and infant feeding. 2009a. www.who.int/childadolescent_health/topics/prevention_care/child/nutrition/hivif/en/index.html. Accessed March 25, 2009.

World Health Organization (WHO). Infant and young child feeding: model chapter for textbooks for medical students and allied health professionals. 2009b. www.who.int/nutrition/publications/infantfeeding/9789241597494/en/index.html. Accessed March 27, 2009.

Xiao X, et al. Epidermal growth factor concentrations in human milk, cow's milk and cow's milk-based infant formulas. *Chin Med J (Engl).* 2002;115(3):451-454.

Yinyaem P, et al. Gastrointestinal manifestations of cow's milk protein allergy during the first year of life. *J Med Assoc Thai.* 2003;86(2):116-123.

Yoshimura Y. Bioethical aspects of regenerative and reproductive medicine. *Human Cell.* 2006;19(2):83-86.

Young T, et al. Type 2 diabetes mellitus in children: prenatal and early infancy risk factors among native Canadians. *Arch Ped Adolescent Med.* 2002;146(7):651-655.

Yu Z, et al. Expression and bioactivity of recombinant human lysozyme in the milk of transgenic mice. *J Dairy Sci.* 2006;89(8):2911-2918.

Impurities in Human Milk

Concern and confusion may arise when a lactating woman takes medications or social toxicants, or when she is exposed to environmental contaminants. When impurities are present in a mother's milk, the most important consideration is the effect a particular substance will have on her breastfeeding infant. Drugs such as tobacco, caffeine, alcohol, marijuana, cocaine, and medications, when ingested by the mother, can travel through her milk to the baby. Environmental contaminants present in a mother's milk can pass on to her baby as well. Almost any substance that is present in the mother's blood will also be present in some amount in her milk.

～ Key Terms

Alcohol
Amphetamines
Bisphenol A (BPA)
Breast implants
Caffeine
Cocaine
Detoxify
Dichlorodiphenyldichloro
   ethylene (DDE)
Dichlorodiphenyltrichloro
   ethane (DDT)
Drugs of abuse
Environmental
   contaminants

Half-life
Heroin
Marijuana
Nicotine and tobacco
Over-the-counter
   medications
Persistent organic
   pollutants (POPs)
Phencyclidine
   hydrochloride
Polybrominated diphenyl
   ethers (PBDEs)
Social toxicant

～ Medications

Not long ago, experts believed that if a woman was breastfeeding, she should take no medications. If she needed medications while breastfeeding, she was told to wean until she no longer needed the medication. As experts have learned more about breastfeeding and human milk, they have adopted a more moderate approach toward medications and breastfeeding.

When reviewing the advisability of a particular substance, the degree to which it is excreted into the mother's milk and its possible effects on the infant are the primary considerations. The potential risk to the infant will depend on whether pediatric medicine uses the same drug as adult medicine. Additionally, a medication that is considered safe during pregnancy may not necessarily be safe during lactation. During pregnancy, the maternal liver and kidney detoxify and excrete substances for the fetus through the placenta. During lactation, however, the infant must handle the drug on his or her own (Lawrence & Lawrence, 2005).

Among the drugs on which information is available, few are contraindicated in breastfeeding (AAP, 2001). Generally, a relative infant dose of less than 10 percent of the adult dose is considered safe (Hale, 2010). Nonetheless, a breastfeeding mother should consult her baby's caregiver before taking any prescription drug, over-the-counter medication, or supplemental vitamins. A drug that is safe for the fetus and the breastfeeding infant may still affect the mother's letdown reflex, milk production, or milk secretion. The mother can remind the prescribing caregiver that she is breastfeeding and confirm the drug's advisability.

Drug Entry into Milk

In many cases, substances are excreted into the milk in low concentrations and pose no danger to the infant. Additionally, the molecular weight or binding capacity of some substances does not allow them to enter the mother's milk. When a substance passes into the milk, the infant's gastrointestinal (GI) tract often offers protection from it, either by not absorbing it or by altering it. The infant may experience some adverse effects, however, from substances that pass into the milk and are not altered or eliminated by the child's GI system.

Figure 10.1 shows the factors that influence the complex process by which a substance passes from the mother's bloodstream into her milk. Medications are transferred from the mother's plasma through the capillary walls, past the alveolar epithelium, and into the milk (see Figure 10.2). As illustrated in Figure 10.3, the gaps between alveolar cells are largest in the first 4 days postpartum, increasing the potential for drugs to enter the milk during that time span. As the alveolar cells enlarge, they shut off many of the gaps and reduce the amount of drug entry.

Infant Exposure

The potential effect of any substance on the breastfed infant is of primary significance when the mother needs medication. One consideration is whether the medication will pass into the mother's milk and be absorbed in the baby's GI tract. Another is whether the infant can be exposed safely to the substance as it appears in the milk.

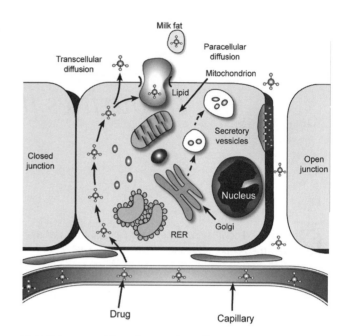

FIGURE 10.2   How drugs enter milk.
Source: Printed with permission of Thomas Hale, Hale Publishing.

Understanding the substance's characteristics can help resolve the dilemma faced by both healthcare worker and mother when the need for a medication arises. Many factors influence the level of a substance found in the infant's bloodstream, some of which relate to the infant and others of which reflect characteristics of the drug itself.

Timing: How Soon After Birth

One safety consideration for the infant is how soon after birth the mother takes a medication. Because the junctions

Factors to consider
- Size of the molecules in the substance (molecules over 800–1000 daltons have difficulty passing through alveolar cells).
- Solubility of the substance in water or fat (fat diffuses more easily into milk).
- Binding capacity of the substance with protein.
- pH of the substance.
- The milk/plasma ratio.
- Route of administration (oral, intramuscular, intravenous).
- Short- or long-acting version of the drug.
- Activity or inactivity of components of the substance.
- Rate of detoxification in the mother's system.
- Whether the substance accumulates in the mother's system.
- Duration of use.
- Time substance is ingested relative to a feeding.
- Number of days postpartum when substance is consumed.
- Age and size of the infant (preterm, full-term, older baby).
- Amount of milk the infant consumes (exclusively breastfed or supplemented).
- Absorption of the substance in the infant's gut.
- Safety in giving the substance to the infant directly.

FIGURE 10.1   Potential for infant exposure to substances in human milk.

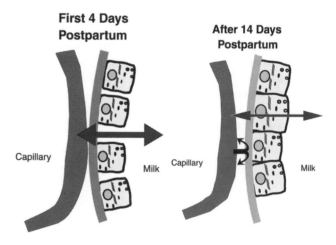

FIGURE 10.3   Alveolar cell gaps.
Source: Printed with permission of Thomas Hale, Hale Publishing.

between the alveolar cells in the mammary glands remain open for several days postpartum, more of a medication can penetrate the mother's milk at that time than in later weeks following the infant's birth (Hale & Hartmann, 2007; Hale & Ilett, 2002). The amount of a substance that passes to the baby relates directly to the amount of milk that is consumed. A newborn consumes small quantities of colostrum in the first few days, so the amount of other substances ingested would be small. Likewise, a baby who also receives artificial baby milk or solid foods will receive a lesser amount of a substance than will an infant who is breastfed exclusively. The volume of human milk consumed by a supplemented infant is less and possibly is diluted by the supplemental food in the infant's system.

Gestational Age

The baby's age and size are also factors in relation to the effects of medications taken by the mother. A preterm infant assimilates substances received through the mother's milk differently than does a full-term infant or older baby. An older and larger baby may be able to metabolize a substance more effectively; as a consequence, the substance will have less effect on the child's system. The baby's age will also determine the ability of the liver to detoxify a substance and excrete it in the urine or stool. Because an infant's liver is immature in the early days postpartum, it may be difficult for a neonate to excrete even small amounts of a substance. A drug that depends on the liver for detoxification could pose a risk if not metabolized effectively.

Resistance to Detoxification

On the one hand, if a substance is particularly resistant to being destroyed in the infant's GI tract, it would pose a danger to the infant as it accumulates to toxic levels. On the other hand, some drugs must be administered by injection because they are destroyed in the infant's GI tract when taken orally. These drugs may reduce the infant's systemic absorption of the drug but could cause GI symptoms such as diarrhea. Some substances compete for protein-binding sites, displacing other toxic substances that then can migrate to other parts of the body (Hale & Hartmann, 2007). For example, sulfadiazine, an antibacterial agent, may displace bilirubin and cause it to flow freely in the infant's blood during the first weeks postpartum; this effect increases the risk of jaundice for the baby.

Over-the-Counter Medications

Questions often arise about maternal use of over-the-counter medications such as pain relievers, cough medicines, cold remedies, suppositories, antacids, diarrhea remedies, and herbal preparations. Because these medications are more accessible than prescription drugs, there is a greater likelihood that mothers will use them. As a lactation consultant, you may receive calls questioning their potential risk to the baby and to breastfeeding.

Many cold remedies contain antihistamines to dry up nasal secretions. Products containing pseudoephedrine can lower mothers' milk production by as many as 24 percent (Aljazaf et al., 2003). Antihistamines also may enter human milk and produce sedation in the baby.

Any person taking over-the-counter medications needs to exercise caution in taking drugs and other substances when there is the possibility of interaction among prescription drugs, over-the-counter medications, herbs, and vitamins. Mothers are encouraged to discuss this potential with their baby's caregiver to determine the safety in taking an over-the-counter drug. Physicians need to know the mother's present consumption of drugs, vitamins, herbs, or other substances before they prescribe any additional medication.

Minimizing the Effects of Medications

Drugs present in the mother's milk may affect milk production or secretion. Some may lower production while others may stimulate it. These agents can also cause reactions in the infant. If she is taking medications, the mother should watch for unusual changes in her baby's behavior, feeding, and sleeping patterns such as fussiness, lethargy, rash, vomiting, or diarrhea. A mother can minimize the effects of drugs in her milk in a number of ways, as discussed in the following subsections.

Schedule Medications Around Breastfeeding

Mothers can adjust their schedule for taking a drug to achieve the least amount of drug possible entering the milk. In recognition of the usual absorption rates and peak levels of most drugs, the mother will want to take the medication toward the end of the dose cycle. A general rule may be to take the drug immediately after nursing or 3 to 4 hours before the next feeding. Depending on the drug, she may need to stop breastfeeding while the drug is at its peak level in her milk. She can take a fat-soluble drug at bedtime, after which the baby usually does not feed as often.

Avoid Drugs with a Long Half-Life

Urge mothers to avoid medications with long plasma half-life. This form is more difficult for the baby to eliminate and could build up over time to higher concentrations in the baby's plasma. Enzyme action in the liver is usually required to metabolize a drug with a long half-life, which in turn increases the possibility of its accumulation in a young baby.

Select the Least Offensive Drug

When possible, the caregiver should prescribe the drug that produces the least amount in the milk and has the least potential for causing problems. If a mother must take a medication that has not been tested for safety during lactation, she can discuss her options with her baby's caregiver. You can also provide her with information from a source such as *Medications and Mothers' Milk*, which rates drug safety on a scale of 1 to 5. See Table 10.1 for the safety of various families of drugs.

Medications Forum, a Web-based forum for healthcare professionals, is a key resource that provides information about new drugs on the market and their propensity for transfer into breastmilk. Information about new drugs is posted as soon as studies or anecdotal observations become available. The forum, which can be found at www.ibreastfeeding.com, is free and open to public access. If a mother is taking a medication that has not

been studied, or has been little studied, she can sign up for the lactation research registry at this same website.

Counseling Mothers About Medications

With medical issues such as medications, it is especially important to recognize that your role with mothers is to share information and point out options. Mothers will often contact you with questions and concerns about the safety of a particular medication while they are breastfeeding. Unless you have prescribing privileges, it is important that you confine your role to encouraging the mother to be an active health consumer. She needs to take responsibility for making decisions and taking specific action. You can help the mother pose questions and stimulate her thinking so that she will explore the facts and base her decisions on accurate and sound information.

A potential for conflict between specialties arises when lactation consultants have more education and information concerning lactation than do mothers' physicians. Lactation consultants have a responsibility to

TABLE 10.1   Safety of Medications with Breastfeeding

• Breastfeeding contraindicated.	• Anticancer drugs (antimetabolites). • Radioactive substances (stop breastfeeding temporarily).
• Continue breastfeeding: Side effects possible; monitor the baby for drowsiness.	• Psychiatric drugs and anticonvulsants.
• Continue breastfeeding: Use alternative drug if possible.	• Chloramphenicol, tetracyclines, metronidazole. • Quinolone antibiotics (e.g., ciprofloxacin).
• Continue breastfeeding: Monitor baby for jaundice.	• Sulphonamides, dapsone. • Sulfamethoxazole + trimethoprim (co-trimoxazole).
• Continue breastfeeding: Use alternative drug (may inhibit lactation).	• Estrogens (including estrogen-containing contraceptives). • Thiazide diuretics. • Ergometrine.
• Continue breastfeeding: Safe in usual dosage; monitor baby.	• Most commonly used drugs. • Analgesics and antipyretics—Short courses of paracetamol, acetylsalicylic acid, ibuprofen; occasional doses of morphine and pethidine. • Antibiotics—Ampicillin, amoxicillin, cloxacillin, and other penicillins. Erythromycin. • Antituberculars, antileporotics (see dapsone earlier). • Antimalarials (except mefloquine), anthelminthics, antifungals. • Bronchodilators (e.g., salbutamol), corticosteroids, antihistamines, antacids, drugs for diabetes, most antihypertensives, digoxin. • Nutritional supplements of iron, iodine, and vitamins.

Source: UNICEF/WHO. Breastfeeding and Maternal Medication: Recommendations for Drugs in the Eighth WHO Model List of Essential Drugs. Geneva, Switzerland: World Health Organization; 1995:3. http://www.who.int. Reprinted with permission of the World Health Organization.

educate mothers regarding practices that are supportive of breastfeeding, including the use of medications. See Chapter 2 for the discussion of scope of practice.

Several tenets in the IBLCE (2007) Code of Ethics address the lactation consultant's responsibility to educate parents. These include basing practices "on scientific principles, current research, and information" (Item 7), providing "sufficient information to enable clients to make informed decisions" (Item 11), and "providing information about appropriate products in a manner that is neither false nor misleading" (Item 12). These ethical responsibilities have contributed to IBCLCs choosing not to pursue licensing in states where licensure would fall under the administration of the state medical board. Instead, IBCLCs seek the independent licensure akin to that of occupational therapists, physical therapists, dieticians, and speech therapists.

The Internet provides a wealth of resources for researching medicines, including PubMed, the search engine for the National Library of Medicine (www.pubmed.gov). Many times, Internet savvy parents will have researched their options before they contact a lactation consultant for help. It is important that you present all drug information objectively and not in a manner that appears to be recommending or advising the mother about the safety of a particular medication. Encourage the mother to consult her physician regarding these questions and to share any concerns or questions she may have.

When a mother expresses doubts or fears about a medication, you can discuss the options available to her. Open-ended questions may help her identify her needs. After clarifying her situation, consider asking her the following questions:

- Is there an alternative course that would avoid any medication?
- Can the mother use other, safer medications or medical procedures?
- Do the benefits of the medication to the mother outweigh the possible risks to the baby?
- Does exposure to the medication pose less risk to the baby than the use of artificial baby milk?
- Is the mother's physician supportive of breastfeeding?

Locating Drug Information

Information about the advisability of taking a drug during breastfeeding needs to come from a reliable source. Become acquainted with each drug group and its potential risks and benefits. To locate a particular medication in a drug listing, you first need to determine the drug's generic name. Recommended sources include *Medications and Mothers' Milk*, by Hale (2010); *Clinical Therapy in Breastfeeding Patients*, by Hale and Berens (2002); *Drug Therapy and Breastfeeding*, by Hale and Ilett (2002); *Nonprescription Drugs for the Breastfeeding Mother*, by Nice (2007); and *Drugs in Pregnancy and Lactation*, by Briggs et al. (2008).

When presenting information to mothers, read the facts to them exactly as stated on the page, citing the reference for the information. Empower mothers to educate themselves about their condition and treatments for it. When you share studies and research in an appropriate, objective manner, mothers can use the information to make informed decisions. Encourage the mother to share her information and research with her physician. Responsive physicians welcome a partnership with their patients and other healthcare team members, including lactation consultants, to protect breastfeeding.

Critical Reading of Drug Studies

A legitimate evaluation of medical information must go beyond personal observation and withstand the test of scientific criticism. As part of this evaluation, the effectiveness of a drug or treatment should be compared with other treatments. Its safety should be determined after large numbers of observations over long periods. In all of these investigations, the burden of proof rests with the researcher—the one who is recommending a particular drug or treatment—especially if it involves a substance that is not well established in medical practice.

Many review articles written in both lay and professional publications are helpful in providing background information on lactation and impurities in human milk. When reading such articles, carefully consider each study's methods and conclusions. Figure 10.4 identifies factors to consider when reading literature about drugs. See Chapter 27 for an in-depth discussion of research methods.

~ Social Toxicants

Social mood-changing toxicants—tobacco, coffee, tea, alcohol, marijuana, and other drugs—are used in varying degrees in most cultures. It is important to recognize that the use of recreational drugs is not an issue of class, race, or economics. Caution mothers about any substances that can negatively affect the quality or quantity of their milk.

Nicotine and Tobacco

A breastfeeding mother who smokes cigarettes—even if only occasionally—may possibly affect her baby more by the smoke her baby inhales than by the amount of nicotine present in her milk. Researchers have found that smoking mothers are less likely to continue breastfeeding than nonsmokers (Rebhan et al., 2009; Giglia et al., 2006; Donath et al., 2004). Prior to 2001, the AAP classified nicotine, and therefore smoking, as incompatible with

Factor	Comments
Newness of the data	There is much case reporting of drugs used during breastfeeding that provides newer data, whereas most original data regarding drugs in human milk were published between 1920 and 1960.
Human versus animal data	Animal data may or may not apply to human lactation. The peer review process will assist in determining this relevance.
Completeness of screening	The reader should always look for whether the researcher mentions studying metabolites of the particular drug in question. If metabolites were not studied, justification is needed. Usually, researchers will justify that within their study. Consulting a pharmacologist will help you understand the significance and quality of a study about drugs.
Isolated cases	Much of the original data about a particular substance may be based on only 1 or 2 case reports, with insufficient controls. This results because ethics prevent experiments on humans. Clinicians are left to make decisions without complete data to guide them. If a mother needs a medication and wants to continue breastfeeding, physicians sometimes allow it, monitor it, and then write up the experience to share with colleagues. Such case reports have no control, but the medical community has at least a small amount of information instead of none. One cannot conclude universal safety from one case report. However, physicians who support breastfeeding even in difficult circumstances may be less reluctant to try a drug instead of stopping breastfeeding. You can encourage mothers taking newer or little-used medications to register at the International Registry for Lactation Research to benefit other mothers and babies by providing milk samples for research. Mothers can register at www.neonatal.ttushc.edu/lact.
Sampling technique	Older studies may show random sampling of milk rather than samples based on drug peak and trough levels. Trough is the lowest blood or milk level achieved by the drug during its dosing period. Women who are given gentamicin, for instance, are tested every 3 days or so to see what the highest and lowest levels of the drug are in the blood. This is done by testing an hour after a dose and an hour before the next dose is due. The timing of testing is different in different drugs. Some drugs have a narrow safety range, so it is important to keep the dose within that range. Although newer research is less problematic in this area, it is still important that you consider this when reading such research.
Personal correspondence	Although much personal correspondence is useful, the reader should be aware that the data may not be available for public inspection and could be biased. Often, personal correspondence is research in progress that lends support to the article at hand.
Speculation	Speculation by the author of the original article may be interpreted as fact after several review articles have been written. This can be a problem, and readers should always beware of speculation.

FIGURE 10.4   Factors to consider in drug literature.

breastfeeding. The AAP softened its position in order to be more supportive of breastfeeding. Nonetheless, another study found that 80 percent of mothers believed that women should not smoke any cigarettes if breastfeeding. Furthermore, only 2 percent of mothers in the study knew that nicotine replacements (the patch or gum) were acceptable when breastfeeding (Bogen et al., 2008). Although 84 percent of formula feeders in one study knew that breastmilk was better for their babies, smoking was one of the reasons they decided not to breastfeed (Noble et al., 2003). The periods before and during pregnancy are opportunities for educating smoking mothers and encouraging them to change their practices.

A mother who chooses to continue smoking should not smoke in the baby's presence. She can also time her breastfeeding to minimize the baby's exposure in her milk, smoking after a feeding rather than just before it. Smoking is not just an issue when a mother is breastfeeding, however. Babies who receive artificial baby milks are also exposed to undesirable chemicals in their parents' cigarette smoke without receiving the protective benefits of their mother's milk (Dorea, 2007; Minchin, 1991; Newman, 1990).

Effects on the Baby

Children whose parents smoke in the home have a greater susceptibility to respiratory ailments, including asthma, than do children of nonsmokers (Jang et al., 2004; Rizzi et al., 2004; Shiva et al., 2003). Exposure to secondhand cigarette smoke is linked to increased incidence of otitis media (Owen et al., 1993). Babies whose mothers smoke are at increased risk of sudden infant death syndrome (SIDS) (Daltveit et al., 2003; Kahn et al., 2003; L'Hoir et al., 1998). One review of sudden infant deaths found fivefold higher nicotine concentrations in nonbreastfed infants of parents who smoked. The reviewers concluded that nicotine intake by passive smoking is much more significant than intake of nicotine via breastfeeding (Bajanowski et al., 2008). Depressed autonomic cardiovascular control was observed in one study of the effects of smoking on infants (Dahlström et al., 2008). The mother and other members of the baby's household need to be discouraged from smoking inside the home, especially anywhere around the baby.

Nicotine in the mother's milk can cause fussiness, diarrhea, shock, vomiting, rapid heartbeat, and restlessness in an infant. Altered sleep patterns, including those involving less sleep, are correlated with smoking as well (Mennella et al., 2007). The mother may experience a decrease in milk production due to lowered prolactin levels, leading to poor infant weight gain. Smoking 20 cigarettes daily can lead to relatively high levels of fat-soluble nicotine in the mother's milk, which can be harmful to the baby and cause vomiting and nausea. It can also diminish the mother's milk secretion, lower the fat concentration in her milk, or inhibit her letdown reflex if the mother smokes immediately before feeding her baby (Hopkinson et al., 1992; Vio et al., 1991).

Any of these factors could be a cause of slow infant weight gain. For this reason, it is good practice to ask mothers of slow-gaining babies whether they smoke, if they have not already volunteered this information. Those who smoke should be encouraged to quit or to reduce the amount of cigarettes they smoke. Mothers who smoke will need twice the usual intake of vitamin C because smoking interferes with the body's ability to use that vitamin (Kim et al., 2004; Valachovicova et al., 2003).

Smoking cessation programs can be used by nursing mothers, including the use of a nicotine patch and chewing gum for nicotine withdrawal (Ilett et al., 2003; Hale & Berens, 2002). The nicotine level in patches and gums is approximately one-third that found in cigarettes. To continue nursing safely, mothers who follow such a program cannot smoke while using a nicotine patch or chewing gum, as this practice would further increase the baby's level of exposure to nicotine in addition to making the mother very ill.

Caffeine

Caffeine is present in coffee, tea, cola, and chocolate—substances often consumed in large quantities in Western culture. Breastfeeding mothers can safely ingest moderate amounts of these foods. The amount of caffeine present in human milk varies dramatically from mother to mother and according to the timing of ingestion. Some women appear to have low absorption and efficient metabolism and excretion, so that levels of caffeine in their milk remain low. Given these variations, each mother–infant pair is unique with respect to caffeine response. Acceptable levels of ingestion for the mother depend on her baby's reaction.

Effects on the Baby

Mothers can watch for signs of caffeine sensitivity in their babies, such as wakefulness, hyperactivity, and colicky behavior. These symptoms may indicate an excessive amount of caffeine in the mother's milk. Newborn and preterm babies are particularly susceptible to caffeine's effects, because their immature digestive systems take longer to eliminate caffeine from the body (Martin et al., 2007). A large prospective study researching the use of alcohol, nicotine, and caffeine found that caffeine consumption had a significant negative influence on breastfeeding duration (Rebhan et al., 2009).

Some breastfeeding infants have reacted to their mothers consuming 6 to 8 servings of caffeinated beverages daily; these symptoms disappeared within 1 week after caffeine was discontinued (Rivera-Calimlim, 1987). Ryu (1985b) found that daily consumption of as many as 5 cups of coffee with 100 mg of caffeine each did not result in detectable infant caffeine levels. In contrast, in another study in which mothers consumed 750 mg of caffeine, traces of caffeine persisted as long as 9 days after consumption (Ryu, 1985a). In one research study using rats, maternal caffeine consumption induced a series of subtle developmental alterations that may affect breathing in the newborn (Picard et al., 2008).

Sources of Caffeine

Table 10.2 identifies the most common sources of caffeine. Caution women against high intake of herbal tea as a substitute for caffeinated drinks, as herbal teas may contain active ingredients that can pass into human milk and cause toxic effects. Cathartics such as buckhorn bark and senna can cause cramps and diarrhea both in the infant and in the mother. Chamomile tea may sensitize the infant to ragweed pollen and cause an allergic reaction.

TABLE 10.2 Common Sources of Caffeine

Coffees	Service Size	Caffeine (mg)
Starbucks brewed coffee	16 oz. Grande	320
Dunkin' Donuts regular coffee	16 oz.	206
Starbucks vanilla latte	16 oz. Grande	150
Coffee, generic brewed	8 oz.	133
Coffee, generic instant	8 oz.	93

Teas	Service Size	Caffeine (mg)
Tea, brewed	8 oz.	53
Snapple, flavored	16 oz.	42
Snapple, Just Plain	16 oz.	18
Arizona Iced Tea, black	16 oz.	32
Nestea	12 oz.	26
Arizona Iced Tea, green	16 oz.	15

Soft Drinks	Service Size	Caffeine (mg)
Jolt Cola	12 oz.	72
Mountain Dew MDX	12 oz.	71
Mountain Dew	12 oz.	54
Pepsi One	12 oz.	54
Mellow Yellow	12 oz.	53
Diet Coke	12 oz.	47
TAB	12 oz.	46.5
Pibb	12 oz.	41
Dr. Pepper	12 oz.	42–44
Pepsi	12 oz.	35–38
Coca-Cola	12 oz.	35
Barq's Root Beer	12 oz.	22
7-Up, regular or diet	12 oz.	0
Fanta, all flavors	12 oz.	0
Fresca, all flavors	12 oz.	0

Soft Drinks	Service Size	Caffeine (mg)
Mug Root Beer, regular or diet	12 oz.	0
Sierra Mist, regular or free	12 oz.	0
Sprite, regular or diet	12 oz.	0

Energy Drinks	Service Size	Caffeine (mg)
Spike Shooter	8.4 oz.	300
Cocaine	8.4 oz.	288
Monster Energy	16 oz.	160
Full Throttle	16 oz.	144
Rip It, all varieties	8 oz.	100
Enviga	12 oz.	100
Tab Energy	10.5 oz.	95
SoBe No Fear	8 oz.	83
Red Bull	8.3 oz.	80
Rockstar Energy Drink	8 oz.	80
SoBe Adrenaline Rush	8.3 oz.	79
Amp	8.4 oz.	74
Glaceau Vitamin Water Energy	20 oz.	50
SoBe Essential Energy	8 oz.	48

Coffee Flavored Frozen Desserts	Service Size	Caffeine (mg)
Ben & Jerry's	8 fl. oz.	68–84
Haagen-Dazs	8 fl. oz.	58
Starbucks	8 fl. oz.	50–60

Over-the-Counter Drugs	Service Size	Caffeine (mg)
NoDoz (Maximum Strength)	1 tablet	200
Vivarin	1 tablet	200
Excedrin (Extra Strength)	2 tablets	130
Anacin (Maximum Strength)	2 tablets	64

Note: Most information was obtained from company websites or direct inquiries. Serving sizes are based on commonly eaten portions, pharmaceutical instructions, or the amount of the leading-selling container size.

Source: Modified from Center for Science in the Public Interest. *Caffeine Content of Food and Drugs.* Washington, DC: Center for Science in the Public Interest, 2007. http://www.cspinet.org/new/cafchart.htm. Accessed April 23, 2010.

Sage, parsley, and peppermint inhibit lactation; women often use them for weaning (Humphrey, 2003).

Alcohol

Alcohol rapidly enters a woman's bloodstream, and subsequently her milk, reaching the same level in the mother's milk as it does in her blood (Silva et al., 1993). Experts have not defined a safe level of alcohol consumption for the breastfeeding mother. Excessive amounts are known to block the release of oxytocin and affect letdown (Mennella & Pepino, 2008; Mennella et al., 2005). Generally, the consumption of one or two drinks socially is not considered to be a contraindication for breastfeeding.

A large prospective cohort study in Bavaria found that although nicotine and caffeine use were negatively correlated with breastfeeding duration, alcohol use was not (Rebhan et al., 2009). A mother may ask when it is safe to nurse again after having consumed alcohol. It is generally considered safe to breastfeed when she feels normal again—that is, when the effects of the alcohol have worn off. By this time, the levels in her bloodstream and her breastmilk will be quite low (Hale, 2010). Elimination guidelines for Motherisk, a Canadian maternal health program, recommend that mothers wait at least 2 hours per drink to avoid unnecessary infant exposure (Ho et al., 2001). One study found that the systemic availability of alcohol was diminished during lactation, although mothers still felt its effects (Pepino et al., 2007).

The mother's pattern of drinking is of greater concern than whether she has an occasional drink. Excessive alcohol consumption can limit parental effectiveness and result in life-threatening conditions for the infant. If the mother reports that she drinks frequently, consuming more than one or two drinks at a time, or if you suspect alcohol is a problem for her, she may need to be referred for help. Local alcohol and substance abuse treatment centers, drug abuse counselors, and Alcoholics Anonymous meetings are valuable resources in such cases. Impairment of the mother's judgment and her ability to care for her baby poses potentially more serious risks to the baby than the exposure to alcohol in her milk. Be aware that heavy alcohol use and maternal depression can be a sign of intimate-partner abuse (Sarkar, 2008). Familiarity with local resources for mothers in these situations is crucial.

Effects on the Baby

Alcohol consumption can cause sleepiness in the baby. It affects the infant's development and linear growth, and can result in lower weight gain (Flores-Huerta et al., 1992). One study found that babies of mothers who consumed the equivalent of four drinks daily had psychomotor scores one standard deviation below the mean (Little et al., 1989). A later study, although unable to repli-

cate these results, recommended studying older children to better determine outcomes (Little et al., 2002).

Alcohol consumption can cause sleepiness in the baby. The infant engages in significantly less active sleep after exposure to alcohol in the mother's milk (Mennella & Garcia-Gomez, 2001). Research has also shown that babies consume less milk after mothers ingest an alcoholic beverage (Mennella & Beauchamp, 1991).

Drugs of Abuse

Substance abuse is an ongoing concern for neonatologists, who see an increasing number of infants suffering from the damaging effects of drug exposure. Prenatal use of recreational drugs is associated with fetal distress, lower Apgar scores, impaired fetal growth, impaired neurodevelopmental outcome, and acute infant withdrawal (Wagner et al., 1998). Prenatal drug use is also associated with higher rates of sudden infant death (Aryayev et al., 2001). A case-control study of SIDS deaths found no association between maternal recreational drug use and SIDS, although paternal marijuana use during the periods of conception and pregnancy and postnatally were significantly associated with SIDS (Klonoff-Cohen & Lam-Kruglick, 2001).

Breastfeeding mothers should avoid all drugs of abuse. The AAP Committee on Drugs (2001) categorizes drugs of abuse as contraindicated during breastfeeding. These drugs include marijuana, amphetamines such as ecstasy, cocaine, heroin, and phencyclidine hydrochloride (angel dust). Drugs of abuse are hazardous both to the breastfeeding infant and to the mother.

Shortened breastfeeding duration is correlated with drug use in parents (Joya et al., 2009). One study showed that mothers intending to breastfeed were more likely to decrease or stop their substance abuse (Frank et al., 1992). Another study revealed that the fear of passing "dangerous things" to their babies through breastmilk prevented 25 percent of at-risk women in the study from breastfeeding (England et al., 2003).

Marijuana

Marijuana can lower or inhibit prolactin levels and compromise the mother's ability to produce sufficient quantities of milk. There are no documented long-term effects on breastfed babies whose mothers use marijuana (Djulus et al., 2005). Infants exposed to marijuana through their mothers' milk may test positive for as long as 3 weeks, however (Hale, 2010). The AAP categorizes marijuana as contraindicated in breastfeeding mothers.

Medicinal marijuana is used in Canada and in Europe to treat chronic pain and nausea. Lactation consultants in these countries may encounter breastfeeding mothers who are using the drug legitimately (Van der Meersch et al., 2006). Djulus and colleagues recommend that babies be monitored and that the risks of usage be weighed against the risks of artificial feeding in such cases.

Amphetamines

Amphetamines are stimulants that are quickly transferred from the mother's bloodstream into her milk. These agents include popular street drugs that go by names such as ecstasy, harmony, and love. Most studies on the effects of these drugs have been conducted in laboratory animals, primarily rats. One study on the levels of amphetamines in human milk found higher levels of amphetamine (taken prenatally) in the mother's milk than in her plasma for as long as 42 days after delivery. Small amounts were present in the baby's urine as well (Steiner et al., 1984). In another study, methamphetamine use in a breastfeeding mother was associated with a baby's death (Ariagno et al., 1995).

Hallucinations, extreme agitation, and seizures in the baby could occur from exposure to these drugs. If she chooses to use amphetamines, the mother should wait 24 to 48 hours after taking them before breastfeeding (Hale, 2010). As with all illicit drugs, the key concern is that a mother using these drugs may not be exercising prudent judgment and may not be aware enough to care for her baby appropriately. The AAP classifies amphetamines as contraindicated in breastfeeding mothers.

Medications to treat attention-deficit disorder and attention-deficit/hyperactivity disorder have exploded in popularity. These stimulants have amphetamine qualities. Young breastfeeding mothers may have been on these stimulants since childhood. Researchers have found that dexamphetamine is readily transferred into human milk. In one study, the relative infant dose was less than 10 percent and within a range that is generally accepted as being "safe" in the short term (Ilett et al., 2007). More research is needed to determine the long-term consequences of these agents on the developing child.

Cocaine

Cocaine is a powerful stimulant that acts on the central nervous system. Effects of cocaine intoxication in the infant include irritability, jitteriness, tremors, increased heart and respiratory rates, and convulsions or seizures (Schiller & Allen, 2005; Young et al., 1992). Although cocaine's "high" is brief, excreting the inactive metabolite from the body takes a long time. In fact, traces may be present in exposed infants' urine for more than a week.

Because cocaine is so easily absorbed and has a high milk/plasma ratio, significant passage of cocaine into breastmilk is probable (Hale, 2010; Dickson et al., 1994). Cocaine has a high capacity for binding to albumin, such that its concentration is likely to be higher in the mother's milk than in her blood (Bailey, 1998). In a case where one

mother used cocaine topically to relieve sore nipples, the baby suffered convulsions but survived (Chaney et al., 1988). The AAP classifies cocaine as contraindicated for use by breastfeeding mothers.

Heroin and Other Opiates

Heroin is a highly addictive drug that is converted to morphine once it enters the body. Although it is illegal in the United States, this drug is used for limited medical purposes in the United Kingdom and elsewhere. Heroin may pass to the infant through the mother's milk. It can cause increased sleepiness and poor appetite in the infant, resulting in an undernourished baby. An uncoordinated and ineffective sucking reflex may also result from heroin ingestion, as well as tremors, restlessness, and vomiting. The AAP categorizes heroin as contraindicated for use by breastfeeding mothers.

Methadone is an opiate that is sometimes given to heroin addicts in recovery. Research has shown that amounts of methadone in breastmilk appear to be small when mothers are participating in methadone maintenance programs; thus breastfeeding appears to be safe under these circumstances (Jansson et al., 2004; Begg et al., 2001). Infant levels are dependent on maternal dosage. The AAP has placed methadone in the approved category for breastfeeding women (Hale & Berens, 2002).

Buprenorphine is a newer treatment for heroin addiction. One case study found that the amount in the mother's milk was small and probably had little effect on the baby. The baby had no withdrawal signs when abruptly weaned later (Marquet et al., 1997). However, another study evaluating the use of buprenorphine for postpartum pain associated with cesarean section found a correlation with low infant weight gain and the amount of breastfeeding done, suggesting that this opiate has a suppressant effect (Hirose et al., 1997). The AAP has not reviewed buprenorphine for its safety with breastfeeding.

Phencyclidine Hydrochloride

Phencyclidine hydrochloride (PCP) is a powerful hallucinogen more commonly known as angel dust. Studies have found very high concentrations of this drug (10 times maternal plasma levels) in infant mice (Nicholas et al., 1982). PCP is stored in fat tissue and excreted very slowly from the body. The AAP categorizes it as contraindicated in breastfeeding mothers.

Counseling Implications

Regardless of the pharmacologic effects or safety of illicit drugs in regard to the infant, the overriding concern is the mother's ability to care for her baby when she is abusing drugs (Simmons et al., 2009; Donohue, 2004). Given the number of risks, both known and unknown, mothers should be educated whenever possible about the dangers of using such drugs, both prenatally and while breastfeeding. They also need to recognize the dangers involved due to the inhibition of effective parenting skills while under the influence of these drugs, whether they are breastfeeding or not.

Although you can educate a mother and warn her about harmful practices, you cannot take responsibility for her actions. If she chooses to ignore your advice, you can remind her of the potential danger to her baby and urge her to tell her baby's caregiver about the substance she is using. If a mother reports a history of drug abuse, or if a healthcare provider suspects drug use, a urine and or blood culture will be done if the mother gives birth to her baby in a hospital. If the mother tests positive for illegal drugs, referral to child protective services is mandated in most areas. If you witness signs of child endangerment, abuse, or neglect, most governments require that you report your observations to a child protective services agency. Familiarize yourself with the reporting requirements where you live, and add relevant contact information to your list of resources.

～ Breast Implants

Saline and silicone (made from silicon) are the two primary types of breast implants used for breast augmentation (i.e., to increase breast size). Of the two, saline implants are more likely to rupture. Perceived risks of silicone breast implants to the breastfeeding infant first made media headlines in the 1990s, although studies produced conflicting findings concerning their effects on an infant's swallowing dysfunction (Levine et al., 1996: Levine & Ilowite, 1994).

Berlin (1994) noted that the compound used in breast implants, polydimethylsiloxane (PDMS), was not present in the few samples of milk from mothers with implants. He also noted that Mylicon drops, which are frequently recommended as a remedy for infant colic, contain PDMS. A large cohort study of children of mothers with silicone implants and children of mothers with reduction surgery found no significant increases in connective tissue diseases or congenital malformations (Kjoller et al., 1998). Another study compared levels of silicon in cow's milk, cow's milk formula, milk from mothers with implants, and milk from mothers without implants. It found slightly higher silicon levels in the milk from mothers with implants (55.45 ng/mL) than in the milk from mothers without implants (51.05 ng/mL). Silicon levels were 10 times higher in cow's milk and even higher in infant formulas, however (Semple et al., 1998).

When Semple (2007) revisited his earlier study, he noted that he had looked only at silicon/silicone and did not address other potential contaminants that may be associated with silicone gel or the elastomer shell. One of these other potential contaminants is platinum. A 2006 study documented that women exposed to silicone breast implants have platinum levels that exceed those found in the general population. In this study, platinum was detected in both the mothers' milk and their plasma (Lykissa & Maharaj, 2006).

The incidence of capsular contracture is also higher with silicone implants than with saline. Capsular contracture is severe scar tissue formed in response to the presence of the implant. It may cause firmness, distortion, and pain (Gampper et al., 2007). The scarring can extend into the milk ducts and impair supply (see Color Plate 9).

In one study (Brown et al., 2006), researchers reviewed FDA adverse event reports for lactation difficulties, reproductive problems (spontaneous abortion, delayed conception), and medical conditions among offspring, including neonatal, infant, and childhood diseases and congenital defects that were attributed to breast implants. The researchers identified 339 reports that described maternal–child adverse events. Nearly half of these reports (46 percent) described actual problems with breastfeeding or expressed concern that implants would be unsafe or interfere with breastfeeding (Brown et al., 2006).

Another possible concern with implants may be an association with infertility (Zoccali et al., 2008). Women would be wise to delay implants until after they have their children and are no longer breastfeeding. See Chapter 18 for further discussion of the impact of breast surgery on breastfeeding.

～ Environmental Contaminants

While mothers can take measures to avoid the ingestion of social toxicants, they probably do not have much control over their exposure to contaminants in the environment. Many chemicals strongly resist breakdown into more benign components—a quality that has often led to environmental pollution. In the body, these toxins are primarily deposited in fat, and a mother's milk is naturally rich in fat. Therefore, human milk contains traces of many contaminants that pass on to the breastfeeding infant.

Hundreds of studies have documented the presence of contaminants in human milk. Indeed, maternal diet, especially the consumption of fish, is a major factor in levels of certain pollutants in breastmilk (Solomon et al., 2002). "The simple and natural truth is that women and their children have a fundamental right to clean breastmilk. The presence of chemical industry wastes in 'nature's first food' is a trespass on the most private parts of our lives" (Natural Resources Defense Council [NRDC], 2005).

The International Lactation Consultant Association (2001) issued a position statement on breastfeeding and environmental contaminants in human milk (available on the ILCA website at www.ilca.org). Mothers generally are not discouraged from breastfeeding because of exposure to environmental contaminants. Most studies conclude their reports by reaffirming the superiority of breastmilk. As the author of one study states:

> The findings of this study should not discourage women from breastfeeding. Women deserve the ability to choose to nourish and protect their children by breastfeeding, without having to fear that environmental pollution has compromised the value or safety of their milk. The real solution is to pass policies that will reduce the levels of these toxic chemicals in the environment to safeguard babies in the womb and protect breastmilk. (Williams-Derry, 2004)

Polybrominated Diphenyl Ethers

Flame-retardant chemicals—specifically, polybrominated diphenyl ethers (PBDEs)—are an ongoing environmental concern. Some of these chemicals, which are used in many computer plastics, foam cushions, textiles, and other products, accumulate in animals and people. In recent years, PBDE levels in people and the environment have risen dramatically, especially in Americans, who have levels 10 to 100 times those of Europeans. In studies conducted in laboratory animals, PBDEs are shown to cause learning, memory, and behavior problems. They also affect thyroid hormones and other bodily functions in laboratory studies (Schecter et al., 2003).

Persistent Organic Pollutants

Persistent organic pollutants (POPs) are organochlorine pesticides that include a class of chemicals known as polychlorinated biphenyls (PCBs). PCBs, which were banned internationally in the late 1970s, can impede a child's mental development and immune system. Scientists have found that PBDEs and PCBs work in similar ways and may even act together to impair development (Williams-Derry, 2004). It is unclear whether a relationship exists between postnatal PCB exposure through breastfeeding and neurological development (Ribas-Fito et al., 2001). An Inuit study calculated that 36 percent of the PCB traces in breastfed infants were due to breastfeeding and the remainder to prenatal exposure (Ayotte et al., 2003).

DDT and DDE

The potential for harm caused by dichlorodiphenyltrichloroethane (DDT) has been a concern for years. Restrictions on this pesticide's use have resulted in a decline in the levels of dichlorodiphenyldichloroethylene (DDE), the main breakdown product of DDT, in human milk since 1950. Despite this trend, a 1995 Australian study found DDT in nearly all samples of study milk. The study showed a number of infants had daily intakes above acceptable levels for chlordane, DDT, dieldrin, heptachlor epoxide, and PCB (Quinsey et al., 1995). Several studies have found that women with higher levels of DDE in their milk have more difficulty with milk production and are more likely to stop breastfeeding earlier, which implies that this chemical may interfere with lactation (Rogan et al., 1987). A Michigan study found that high levels of DDE in the mother's milk reduce protection against atopic disorders such as asthma, eczema, and hay fever (Karmaus et al., 2003).

Bisphenol A

Bisphenol A (BPA) has been used in plastics manufacturing for years, including baby bottles and the lining of metal cans holding infant formula. Levels of this chemical found in the liquid formula stored in these cans are likely to be far higher than those that leech from baby bottles (Environmental Working Group [EWG], 2007a, 2007b). BPA has been found in breastmilk (Ye et al., 2008; Kuruto-Niwa et al., 2007) in higher levels than in blood serum. The U.S. Food and Drug Administration cites concern about BPA exposure but fell short of banning its use in food containers, choosing instead to carry out "in-depth studies to answer key questions and clarify uncertainties about the risks of BPA" (USFDA, 2010).

BPA binds to estrogen receptors. In animal studies, it has been shown to damage reproductive, neurological, and immune systems during critical stages of development, including mammary gland development (Maffini et al., 2006; Markey et al., 2003). It has also been linked to breast cancer and to the early onset of puberty. Research has found that serum BPA concentrations are significantly higher in normal men and in women with polycystic ovary syndrome (PCOS) compared with normal women (Tsutsumi, 2005). Chapter 25 provides more information on PCOS (a condition that is related to low milk production).

Geographic Concentrations

Environmental contaminants vary depending on local pollution sources, diet, and occupation. Kazakhstan, for example, has the highest documented concentrations of tetrachlorodibenzo-p-dioxin (TCDD) in the world for women in their childbearing years, yet levels of many other toxins are lower in these women than in their counterparts in other regions of Europe (Lutter et al., 1998). Mothers in the Netherlands have 4 times the amount of PCBs and dioxins in their milk than mothers in Hong

Kong (Soechitram et al., 2003). Breastmilk contamination by lead and organochlorines such as PCB and DDT has actually declined by 50 to 70 percent or more in Germany (Schaefer, 2003). Where countries ban or regulate these chemicals, trends show a decline in pollutants such as organochlorine pesticides, PCBs, and dioxins in breastmilk (Solomon et al., 2002).

A link has been suggested between environmental contamination and hormonal development. Studies of girls in a valley with pesticide use revealed a lack of normal breast tissue development. This stunting has also been found in animal studies. It is thought that contaminants such as TCDD or DDE can bind to the body's hormone receptors, disrupting their normal function (West & Marasco, 2009; Markey et al., 2002; Fenton et al., 2002). These chemicals appear to affect lactation by stunting normal glandular growth.

Exposure at Home or at Work

Today, large numbers of women continue to breastfeed after returning to work. Some of these women have jobs that expose them to such chemical pollutants as lead, mercury, cadmium, pesticides, plastics, or solvents. Mothers need to be aware of these contaminants in the same way they are aware of drugs and alcohol. Offer anticipatory guidance to pregnant and new mothers by asking about any chemical exposure they may have at work or at home. Healthcare practitioners who suspect that a contaminant in the mother's milk may be the cause of illness in a child should ask about occupational exposure. Mothers sometimes inquire about having their milk tested. This is usually not necessary unless the caregiver suspects illness in the mother or baby that may be due to chemical exposure.

Reducing Exposure to Environmental Toxicants

Mothers can take precautions to reduce their exposure to contaminants and the potential for chemical pollutants to enter their milk—for example, by avoiding occupations that involve possible exposure to chemicals when possible. If such exposure is unavoidable, they may wish to consult with an expert in occupational medicine to evaluate whether the exposure is safe.

To reduce exposure to environmental toxicants within the home, mothers should avoid hobbies that involve the use of oil-based paints, paint or varnish removers, glues, and other solvent-based chemicals. Recommend avoidance of mothproofed garments, which may contain chemicals that can be inhaled or absorbed through the skin. Limiting the use of domestic sprays such as pesticides and household cleaners will also reduce chemical exposure.

Dietary precautions can also lower the risk posed by environmental contaminants. For example, limiting consumption of freshwater fish will reduce the mother's exposure to chemical wastes that wash into lakes and streams and become concentrated there. The U.S. Food and Drug Administration advises pregnant women, nursing mothers, and young children to avoid eating shark, swordfish, king mackerel, and tilefish to lower their mercury intakes. It also advises these groups to eat no more than 6 ounces per week of canned albacore tuna, or 12 ounces per week of a variety of other fish. Because toxins concentrate in fatty tissue, mothers should avoid fatty meats and remove excess fat when possible. They can also avoid eating organ meats (e.g., liver, gizzards, hearts, brains, intestines), where toxins are stored in greater concentrations. Thoroughly washing or peeling fresh fruits and vegetables will remove many chemicals that are present in these plant-derived foods. Mothers can also choose certified organic produce when practical and economically feasible. In recent years, a series of scandals and concerns about food safety have increased the popularity of organic gardening and the practice of buying local farmers' produce.

If you live in an area where contaminants are a concern, or if this is a key issue with the families you help, you may find the updated information available in the PAN Pesticide Database useful. This website (www.pesticideinfo.org) compiles toxicity and regulatory information related to pesticides.

∼ Counseling a Mother About Impurities

The guidelines in Figure 10.5 and Figure 10.6 will help you when you are counseling a mother concerning the potential for impurities in her milk. They can remind you of the proper procedures concerning these questions and guide

---

- Give well-documented facts in an objective manner.
- Make a mother aware of her options concerning potential impurities.
- Remind a mother that infant formula may sometimes be contaminated with impurities, as may water.
- Urge a mother to seek her caregiver's advice and to share her concerns openly.
- Urge a mother to remind her caregiver that she is breastfeeding.
- Cite references for facts that you give a mother.
- Discuss drug substitutes in a neutral manner, citing reliable sources.
- Suggest ways a mother can minimize the effects of drugs.
- Advise a mother to avoid unnecessary consumption of or exposure to contaminants.

FIGURE 10.5 Issues to address about impurities.

- Refrain from giving personal opinions.
- Do not interpret drug information for a mother unless you have prescriptive privileges.
- Do not advise a mother about a drug's safety; read straight from the literature.
- Do not indicate to a mother that you disagree with advice from her caregiver or other medical resource unless you are medically qualified.
- Do not suggest that a mother refuse a drug when it is needed.
- Do not encourage a mother to act against her caregiver's advice

FIGURE 10.6 Precautions in discussing impurities.

you when you are talking to a mother. These guidelines apply to any of the substances that may compromise the safety or quality of a mother's milk, and are especially important when discussing medications with a mother.

～ Summary

Almost any substance in the mother's blood will be present to some degree in her milk. The issue is whether it will be absorbed in the baby's GI tract and whether the infant's exposure to the substance as it appears in the milk is safe. Factors that influence the level of a substance found in the infant's bloodstream include how soon after birth the mother takes a medication, how the medication is metabolized, and what the baby's age and size are.

Drugs in the mother's milk may either increase or decrease milk production and secretion. They may also cause changes in the baby's behavior, feeding, and sleeping patterns such as fussiness, lethargy, rash, vomiting, or diarrhea. A mother can minimize the effects of drugs in her milk by selecting the least offensive drug, adjusting her schedule for taking the drug, and avoiding medications with long plasma half-life. When counseling mothers, drug information must be presented objectively from well-documented sources, and not in a manner that appears to recommend or advise the mother about the safety of a particular medication. Lactation consultants have an ethical responsibility to inform mothers about treatment options, which may include complementary medicine.

Environmental toxins are deposited primarily in fat and are excreted through the mother's milk. Maternal diet, especially fish consumption, is a factor in breastmilk levels of certain pollutants. Mothers can take precautions to reduce their exposure to contaminants and the potential for chemical pollutants in their milk. Silicone implants do not appear at this time to present a problem in terms

of breastfeeding. All recreational drugs are contraindicated for use by breastfeeding women.

～ Chapter 10—At a Glance

Facts you learned—

Medications:

- Few medications are contraindicated in breastfeeding.
- In general, a relative infant dose of less than 10 percent of the adult dose is considered safe.
- When counseling mothers, lactation consultants should use only drug information from well-documented sources.
- Lactation consultants should become acquainted with drug groups and their risks and benefits.
- Questions to ask about a particular medication:
  - Will it pass into the mother's milk and be absorbed in the baby's GI tract?
  - Can the baby safely be exposed to the substance as it appears in the milk?
  - How soon after birth will the medication be taken?
  - What is the baby's gestational age?

Social toxicants:

- Newborn and preterm babies are especially susceptible to caffeine because it takes them longer to eliminate this toxin.
- Generally, having one or two drinks socially is not a problem in relation to breastfeeding.
- A mother may breastfeed when the effects of alcohol have worn off.
- All recreational drugs are contraindicated.

Environmental contaminants:

- Silicone breast implants have not been proven dangerous when breastfeeding.
- Toxins are primarily deposited in fat and are found in breastmilk.
- The flame-retardant chemicals found in many modern-day products affect learning, memory, behavior, thyroid hormones, and other bodily functions when they are passed to children through breastmilk.
- PCBs affect the mental development of children.
- BPA has been found in human milk.
- DDE reduces protection against atopic disorders such as asthma, eczema, and hay fever.

- DDE affects protection against atopic disorders such as asthma, eczema, and hay fever.

Applying what you learned—

- Recommend that mothers minimize effects of a medication through the following steps:
  - Take the medication immediately after nursing or 3 to 4 hours before the next feeding.
  - Avoid breastfeeding when the medication is at its peak level in the milk.
  - Avoid drugs with a long half-life.
  - Select the least offensive drug.
- Recommend that mothers:
  - Consider alternatives that do not involve medication or substitute a safer medication.
  - Weigh the benefits of a medication against its possible risks to the baby.
  - Weigh the risks of a medication to the baby against the risks of artificial baby milk.
  - Avoid nicotine and tobacco, or time breastfeeding to minimize the baby's exposure to these substances through breastmilk.
  - Avoid excessive alcohol consumption.
  - Avoid all drugs of abuse.
  - Avoid occupations, hobbies, and fabrics that involve possible exposure to chemicals.
  - Avoid eating shark, swordfish, king mackerel, and tilefish.
  - Limit consumption of canned albacore tuna and other fish.
  - Avoid eating organ meats.
  - Wash or peel fresh fruits and vegetables.

See additional counseling tips in the tables found in this chapter.

∿ References

Aljazaf K, et al. Pseudoephedrine: effects on milk production in women and estimation of infant exposure via breastmilk. *Br J Clin Pharmacol.* 2003;56(1):18-24.

American Academy of Pediatrics (AAP), Committee on Drugs. The transfer of drugs and other chemicals into human milk. *Pediatrics.* 2001;108(3):776-789. pediatrics.aappublications.org. Accessed August 30, 2009.

Ariagno R, et al. Methamphetamine ingestion by a breastfeeding mother and her infant's death: *People v Henderson. JAMA.* 1995;274(3):215.

Aryayev N, et al. The significance of ante- and perinatal periods for formation of risk of sudden infant death syndrome. *Ginekol Pol.* 2001;72(12):931-939.

Ayotte P, et al. Assessment of pre- and postnatal exposure to polychlorinated biphenyls: lessons from the Inuit cohort study. *Environ Health Perspect.* 2003;111(9):1253-1258.

Bailey D. Cocaine and cocaethylene binding to human milk. *Am J Clin Pathol.* 1998;10(4):491-494.

Bajanowski T, et al. Nicotine and cotinine in infants dying from sudden infant death syndrome. *Int J Legal Med.* 2008;122 (1):23-28.

Begg E, et al. Distribution of R- and S-methadone into human milk during multiple, medium to high oral dosing. *Br J Clin Pharmacol.* 2001;52(6):681-685.

Berlin C. Silicone breast implants and breast-feeding. *Pediatrics.* 1994;4(Pt 1):547-549.

Bogen D, et al. What do mothers think about concurrent breast-feeding and smoking? *Ambul Pediatr.* 2008;8(3):200-204.

Briggs G, et al. *Drugs in Pregnancy and Lactation: A Reference Guide to Fetal & Neonatal Risk.* 8th ed. Baltimore, MD: Lippincott Williams & Wilkins; 2008.

Brown S, et al. Breast implant surveillance reports to the U.S. Food and Drug Administration: maternal–child health problems. *J Long Term Eff Med Implants.* 2006;16(4):281-290.

Chaney N, et al. Cocaine convulsions in a breast-feeding baby. *J Pediatr.* 1988;112:1345.

Dahlström A, et al. Nicotine in breast milk influences heart rate variability in the infant. *Acta Paediatr.* 2008;97(8):1075-1079.

Daltveit A, et al. Circadian variations in sudden infant death syndrome: associations with maternal smoking, sleeping position and infections. The Nordic epidemiological SIDS study. *Acta Paediatr.* 2003;92(9):991-993.

Dickson P, et al. The routine analysis of breast milk for drugs of abuse in a clinical toxicology laboratory. *J Forensic Sci.* 1994;39(1):207-214.

Djulus J, et al. Marijuana use and breastfeeding. *Can Fam Physician.* 2005;51:349-350.

Donath SM, et al. The relationship between maternal smoking and breastfeeding duration after adjustment for maternal infant feeding intention. *Acta Paediatr.* 2004;93(11):1514-1518.

Donohue B. Coexisting child neglect and drug abuse in young mothers: specific recommendations for treatment based on a review of the outcome literature. Review. *Behav Modif.* 2004;28(2):206-233.

Dorea J. Maternal smoking and infant feeding: breastfeeding is better and safer. Review. *Matern Child Health J.* 2007;11(3): 287-291.

England L, et al. Breastfeeding practices in a cohort of inner-city women: the role of contraindications. *BMC Public Health.* 2003;3(1):28.

Environmental Working Group (EWG). Expert panel warns of health risks from BPA. August 2, 2007a. www.ewg.org/node/ 22300. Accessed March 31, 2009.

Environmental Working Group (EWG). BPA levels in canned infant formula poses higher risk than baby bottles. December 5, 2007b. www.ewg.org/node/25642. Accessed March 31, 2009.

Fenton S, et al. Persistent abnormalities in the rat mammary gland following gestational and lactational exposure to 2,3,7,8-tetrachlorodibenzo-p-dioxin (TCDD). *Toxicol Sci.* 2002;67(1):63-74.

Flores-Huerta S, et al. Effects of ethanol consumption during pregnancy and lactation on the outcome and postnatal growth of the offspring. *Ann Nutr Metab.* 1992;36(3):121.

Frank D, et al. Cocaine and marijuana use during pregnancy by women intending and not intending to breast-feed. *J Am Diet Assoc.* 1992;92:215-216.

Gampper T, et al. Silicone gel implants in breast augmentation and reconstruction. *Ann Plast Surg.* 2007;5:581-590.

Giglia R, et al. Maternal cigarette smoking and breastfeeding duration. *Acta Paediatr.* 2006;95(11):1370-1374.

Hale T. *Medications and Mothers' Milk.* 14th ed. Amarillo, TX: Hale Publishing; 2010.

Hale T, Berens P. *Clinical Therapy in Breastfeeding Patients.* Amarillo, TX: Hale Publishing; 2002.

Hale T, Hartmann P. *Hale and Hartmann's Textbook of Human Lactation.* Amarillo, TX: Hale Publishing; 2007.

Hale T, Ilett K. *Drug Therapy and Breastfeeding: From Theory to Clinical Practice.* New York: Parthenon; 2002:4-6.

Hirose M, et al. Extradural buprenorphine suppresses breast feeding after caesarean section. *Br J Anaesth.* 1997;79(1):120-121.

Ho E, et al. Alcohol and breast feeding: calculation of time to zero level in milk. *Biol Neonate.* 2001;80(3):219-222.

Hopkinson J, et al. Milk production by mothers of premature infants: influence of cigarette smoking. *Pediatrics.* 1992;90(6):934-938.

Humphrey S. *The Nursing Mother's Herbal.* Minneapolis, MN: Fairview Press; 2003:229-230.

Ilett K, et al. Use of nicotine patches in breast-feeding mothers: transfer of nicotine and cotinine into human milk. *Clin Pharmacol Ther.* 2003;74(6):516-524.

Ilett K, et al. Transfer of dexamphetamine into breast milk during treatment for attention deficit hyperactivity disorder [published online ahead of print September 12, 2006]. *Br J Clin Pharmacol.* 2007;63(3):371-375.

International Board of Lactation Consultant Examiners (IBLCE). Code of ethics. 2007. www.iblce.org/codeofethics.php. Accessed March 25, 2009.

International Lactation Consultant Association (ILCA). Position on breastfeeding, breastmilk, and environmental contaminants. 2001. www.ilca.org. Accessed March 20, 2009.

Jang A, et al. The effect of passive smoking on asthma symptoms, atopy, and airway hyperresponsiveness in schoolchildren. *J Korean Med Sci.* 2004;19(2):214-217.

Jansson L, et al. Methadone maintenance and lactation: a review of the literature and current management guidelines. Review. *J Hum Lact.* 2004;20(1):62-71.

Joya X, et al. Unsuspected exposure to cocaine in preschool children from a Mediterranean city detected by hair analysis. *Ther Drug Monit.* 2009;31(3):391-395.

Kahn A, et al. Sudden infant deaths: stress, arousal and SIDS. *Early Hum Dev.* 2003;75:S147-S166.

Karmaus W, et al. Atopic manifestations, breast-feeding protection and the adverse effect of DDE. *Paediatr Perinat Epidemiol.* 2003;17(2):212-220.

Kim S, et al. An 18-month follow-up study on the influence of smoking on blood antioxidant status of teenage girls in comparison with adult male smokers in Korea. *Nutrition.* 2004;20(5):437-444.

Kjoller K, et al. Health outcomes in offspring of mothers with breast implants. *Pediatrics.* 1998;102(5):1112-1115.

Klonoff-Cohen H, Lam-Kruglick P. Maternal and paternal recreational drug use and sudden infant death syndrome. *Arch Pediatr Adolesc Med.* 2001;155(7):765-770.

Kuruto-Niwa R, et al. Measurement of bisphenol A concentrations in human colostrum. *Chemosphere.* 2007;66(6):1160-1164.

L'Hoir M, et al. Sudden unexpected death in infancy: epidemiologically determined risk factors related to pathological classification. *Acta Paediatr.* 1998;87(12):1279-1287.

Lawrence R, Lawrence R. *Breastfeeding: A Guide for the Medical Profession.* 6th ed. St. Louis: Elsevier Mosby; 2005.

Levine J, et al. Esophageal dysmotility in children breast-fed by mothers with silicone breast implants: long-term follow-up and response to treatment. *Dig Dis Sci.* 1996;41:1600-1603.

Levine J, Ilowite N. Scleroderma-like esophageal disease in children breastfed by mothers with silicone breast implants. *JAMA.* 1994;271:213-216.

Little R, et al. Maternal alcohol use during breast-feeding and infant mental and motor development at one year *N Engl J Med.* 1989;321:425-430.

Little R, et al. Alcohol, breastfeeding, and development at 18 months. *Pediatrics.* 2002;109(5):e72.

Lutter C, et al. Breast milk contamination in Kazakhstan: implications for infant feeding. *Chemosphere.* 1998;37(9-12):1761-1772.

Lykissa ED, Maharaj SV. Total platinum concentration and platinum oxidation states in body fluids, tissue, and explants from women exposed to silicone and saline breast implants by IC-ICPMS. *Anal Chem.* 2006;78(9):2925-2933.

Maffini M, et al. Endocrine disruptors and reproductive health: the case of bisphenol-A. Review. *Mol Cell Endocrinol.* 2006;254-255:179-186.

Markey C, et al. Endocrine disruptors: from wingspread to environmental developmental biology. Review. *J Steroid Biochem Mol Biol.* 2002;83(1-5):235-244.

Markey C, et al. Mammalian development in a changing environment: exposure to endocrine disruptors reveals the developmental plasticity of steroid-hormone target organs. *Evol Dev.* 2003;5(1):67-75. Erratum in: *Evol Dev.* 2004;6(3):207. [Dosage error in text.]

Marquet P, et al. Buprenorphine withdrawal syndrome in a newborn. *Clin Pharmacol Ther.* 1997;62(5):569-571.

Martín I, et al. Neonatal withdrawal syndrome after chronic maternal drinking of mate. *Ther Drug Monit.* 2007;29(1):127-129.

Mennella J, Beauchamp G. Maternal diet alters the sensory qualities of human milk and the nursling's behavior. *Pediatrics.* 1991;88:737-744.

Mennella J, et al. Acute alcohol consumption disrupts the hormonal milieu of lactating women. *J Clin Endocrinol Metab.* 2005;90(4):1979-1985.

Mennella J, et al. Breastfeeding and smoking: short-term effects on infant feeding and sleep. *Pediatrics.* 2007;120(3):497-502.

Mennella J, Garcia-Gomez P. Sleep disturbances after acute exposure to alcohol in mothers' milk. *Alcohol.* 2001;25(3):153-158.

Mennella J, Pepino M. Biphasic effects of moderate drinking on prolactin during lactation. *Alcohol Clin Exp Res.* 2008;32 (11):1899-1908.

Minchin M. Smoking and breastfeeding: an overview. *J Hum Lact.* 1991;7:183-188.

Natural Resources Defense Council (NRDC). Healthy milk, healthy baby: chemical pollution and mother's milk: chemicals in mother's milk. March 25, 2005. www.nrdc.org/breastmilk/envpoll.asp. Accessed March 31, 2009.

Newman J. Drugs and breastmilk [letter to the editor]. *Pediatrics.* 1990;86:148.

Nicholas J, et al. Phencyclidine: its transfer across the placenta as well as into breast milk. *Am J Obstet Gynecol.* 1982; 143(2):143-146.

Noble L, et al. Factors influencing initiation of breast-feeding among urban women. *Am J Perinatol.* 2003;20(8):477-483.

Owen M, et al. Relation of infant feeding practices, cigarette smoke exposure, and group child care to the onset and duration of otitis media with effusion in the first two years of life. *J Pediatr.* 1993;123(5):702-711.

Pepino M, et al. Lactational state modifies alcohol pharmacokinetics in women [published online ahead of print April 13, 2007]. *Alcohol Clin Exp Res.* 2007;31(6):909-918.

Picard N, et al. Maternal caffeine ingestion during gestation and lactation influences respiratory adaptation to acute alveolar hypoxia in newborn rats and adenosine A2A and GABA A receptor mRNA transcription [published online ahead of print July 25, 2008]. *Neuroscience.* 2008;156(3):630-639.

Quinsey P, et al. Persistence of organochlorines in breast milk of women in Victoria, Australia. *Food Chem Toxicol.* 1995;33(1):49-56.

Rebhan B, et al. Smoking, alcohol and caffeine consumption of mothers before, during and after pregnancy: results of the study "Breast-Feeding Habits in Bavaria." *Gesundheitswesen.* 2009;71(7):391-398.

Ribas-Fito N, et al. Polychlorinated biphenyls (PCBs) and neurological development in children: a systematic review. Review. *J Epidemiol Community Health.* 2001;55(8):537-546.

Rivera-Calimlim L. The significance of drugs in breast milk. *Clin Perinatol.* 1987;14:51.

Rizzi M, et al. Environmental tobacco smoke may induce early lung damage in healthy male adolescents. *Chest.* 2004;125 (4):1387-1393.

Rogan WJ, et al. Polychlorinated biphenyls (PCBs) and dichlorodiphenyl dichloroethane (DDE) in human milk: effects on growth, morbidity, and duration of lactation. *Am J Public Health.* 1987;77(10):1294-1297.

Ryu J. Caffeine in human milk and in serum of breast-fed infants. *Dev Pharmacol Ther.* 1985a;8(6):329-337.

Ryu J. Effect of maternal caffeine consumption on heart rate and sleep time of breastfed infants. *Dev Pharmacol Ther.* 1985b;8:355-363.

Sarkar N. The impact of intimate partner violence on women's reproductive health and pregnancy outcome. Review. *JOGNN.* 2008;28(3):266-271.

Schaefer C. Recreational drugs and environmental contaminants in mother's milk. Review. *Zentralbl Gynakol.* 2003; 125(2):38-43.

Schecter A, et al. Polybrominated diphenyl ethers (PBDEs) in US mothers' milk. *Environ Health Perspect.* 2003;111:1723-1729.

Schiller C, Allen P. Follow-up of infants prenatally exposed to cocaine. Review. *Pediatr Nurs.* 2005;31(5):427-436.

Semple J. Breast-feeding and silicone implants. Review. *Plast Reconstr Surg.* 2007;120(7 suppl 1):123S-128S.

Semple J, et al. Breast milk contamination and silicone implants: preliminary results using silicon as a proxy measurement for silicone. *Plast Reconstr Surg.* 1998;102(2):528-533.

Shiva F, et al. Effects of passive smoking on common respiratory symptoms in young children. *Acta Paediatr.* 2003;92(12): 1394-1397.

Silva DA, et al. Ethanol pharmacokinetics in lactating women. *Braz J Med Biol Res.* 1993;26:1097-1103.

Simmons L, et al. Illicit drug use among women with children in the United States: 2002–2003. *Ann Epidemiol.* 2009; 19(3):187-193.

Soechitram S, et al. Comparison of dioxin and PCB concentrations in human breast milk samples from Hong Kong and the Netherlands. *Food Addit Contam.* 2003;20(1):65-69.

Solomon G, et al. Chemical contaminants in breast milk: time trends and regional variability. *Environ Health Perspect.* 2002;110(6):A339-A347.

Steiner E, et al. Amphetamine secretion in breast milk. *Eur J Clin Pharmacol.* 1984;27(1):123-124.

Tsutsumi O. Assessment of human contamination of estrogenic endocrine-disrupting chemicals and their risk for human reproduction. *J Steroid Biochem Mol Biol.* 2005;93(2-5): 325-330.

U.S. Food and Drug Administration (USFDA). Bisphenol A (BPA)—Update on Bisphenol A (BPA) for Use in Food: January 2010. http://www.fda.gov/NewsEvents/Public HealthFocus/ucm064437.htm. Accessed February 5, 2010.

Valachovicova M, et al. Antioxidant vitamins levels: nutrition and smoking. *Bratisl Lek Listy.* 2003;104(12):411-414.

Van der Meersch H, et al. Medicinal cannabis: Review. *J Pharm Belg.* 2006;61(3):69-78.

Vio F, et al. Smoking during pregnancy and lactation and its effects on breastmilk volume. *Am J Clin Nutr.* 1991;54:1011-1016.

Wagner CL, et al. The impact of prenatal drug exposure on the neonate. *Obstet Gynecol Clin North Am.* 1998;25(1):169-194.

West D, Marasco L. *The Breastfeeding Mother's Guide to Making More Milk.* New York: McGraw Hill; 2009.

Williams-Derry C. Flame retardants in the bodies of Pacific Northwest residents. *Northwest Environmental Watch.* September 29, 2004. www.northwestwatch.org. Accessed March 25, 2009.

Ye X, et al. Automated on-line column-switching HPLC-MS/MS method with peak focusing for measuring parabens, triclosan, and other environmental phenols in human milk. *Anal Chim Acta.* 2008;622(1-2):150-156.

Young S, et al. Cocaine: its effects on maternal and child health. Review. *Pharmacotherapy.* 1992;12(1):2-17.

Zoccali G, et al. Silicone gel mammary prostheses: immune pathologies and breastfeeding. *Clin Exp Obstet Gynecol.* 2008;35(3):187-189.

3

Prenatal Through Postpartum

11

Prenatal Considerations

One who bears her children is a mother in part,
But she who nurses her children is a mother at heart.

—*Jacob Cats (1577–1660)*

Parents face many choices regarding the care of their new babies. Some choices, such as dress or daily routines, have little or no effect on the health of the child. Other healthcare choices directly affect the health and well-being of children in both the short term and the long term. Such choices include car seat use, whether to vaccinate, preventive well-child care, and breastfeeding. Just as there are serious risks to the child of parents who choose not to use a car seat, so there are also consequences in deciding to not breastfeed. Breastfeeding is the normal continuation of fetal life. Because breastfeeding often involves lifestyle adjustments, parents can benefit from guidance in blending it into their lives.

The healthcare profession has a moral and ethical obligation to provide true informed consent to women and their families before birth. To make a fully informed decision, parents need to understand the consequences of *not* breastfeeding. Lactation consultants can look for ways to educate parents before birth to help them make informed feeding decisions. Contacting local prenatal groups, childbirth educators, obstetricians, midwives, and family practice groups is an excellent start. If sound breastfeeding education is unavailable, you can provide breastfeeding classes to your clients. You might also provide breastfeeding updates to physicians, nurses, and other caregivers who see women prenatally.

ᕈ *Key Terms*

Caregiver
Cesarean birth
Continuing education
Decision to breastfeed

Hospital affiliation
Nipple correction
Self-efficacy
Standing orders

ᕈ *The Decision to Breastfeed*

A belief in breastfeeding is the underlying motivator in a woman's infant feeding decision. A variety of media, including brochures, books, the Internet, and DVDs, can provide information on this topic. Ultimately, however, they have little influence on the motivation to breastfeed. A search of the National Library of Medicine's database yields an explosion in the number of studies from around the world about intention to breastfeed. Whether it is Turkey (Camurdan et al., 2008), Taiwan (Kuo et al., 2008), Quebec (Semenic et al., 2008), India (Kumar et al., 2008), Greece (Ladomenou et al., 2007), the Netherlands (Gijsbers et al., 2006), China (Shi et al., 2008), Japan (Otsuka et al., 2008), or Nebraska in the heartland of America (Wilhelm et al., 2008), mothers around the world exhibit similar traits and needs. A positive attitude toward breastfeeding prior to pregnancy has the greatest influence on initiation. Avery et al. (2009) describe this attitude as a confident commitment that enables the mother to withstand both a lack of support and normal breastfeeding initiation challenges. The mother's intention to breastfeed and her self-efficacy are a common theme in these and myriad other studies as the greatest predictors of successful breastfeeding outcomes.

One study found that 63 percent of women made the choice to breastfeed prior to pregnancy, 26 percent during pregnancy, and 11 percent after delivery. A significantly greater number of experienced mothers decided to breastfeed prior to pregnancy compared with first-time mothers (Noble et al., 2003). In other studies, participants decided how to feed their baby either prior to conception or early in the pregnancy (Earle, 2000). Prenatal intention to breastfeed influenced both initiation rates and duration of breastfeeding in a study of 10,548 women in the United Kingdom. Women who intended to breastfeed for 1 month had a mean duration of 2.5 months, whereas women who intended to breastfeed for at least 5 months had a mean duration of 4.4 months (Donath et al., 2003). Of 341 mothers studied in the Netherlands, 73 percent started breastfeeding and 39 percent continued for at least 3 months. Those who continued had strong self-efficacy, whereas those who discontinued had social support for formula feeding from significant others (Kools et al., 2006).

Trends in Infant Feeding

Trends in infant feeding mirror trends in the management of labor and birth. Women often fear being totally responsible for their baby's weight gain and health, much as they fear embracing the responsibility of laboring and birthing. Specifically, many women describe a need to avoid pain in labor, or a need to have their caregiver "deliver" the baby. After giving birth, they may reject the next step of motherhood—breastfeeding—for fear of failure. Fear of failure may be due to the woman's lack of confidence that her body can produce sufficient food for her baby; it may also reflect an emphasis on breastfeeding "right" (Hall & Hauck, 2007). Women who view control as a priority are more likely to rely on bottle feeding.

A variety of issues can affect a woman's decision to breastfeed. Most educated women know breastfeeding is best for the baby. Thus health and nutrition benefits for her and her baby may motivate a woman to breastfeed. She may be concerned about the increased risk to her baby of substituting artificial milks. Nevertheless, you cannot assume a woman knows about the risks of artificial feeding, especially in a culture saturated with media and advertising that aggressively promote artificial feeding.

Because more than half of women make their infant feeding choices before pregnancy and 26 percent make the decision during pregnancy, public education is imperative. A Scottish study revealed that breast and bottle feeders had the same goals regarding infant feeding, but they differed in their perception of barriers to breastfeeding, including inconvenience and embarrassment at nursing in front of others (Shaker et al., 2004). During prenatal teaching, it helps to ask women to share their goals and concerns, and then to specifically discuss these barriers. Confidence with breastfeeding, the partner's feelings, the ability to be discreet, and maternal perceptions of societal expectations are all factors that may either empower mothers to breastfeed in public or dissuade them from doing so (Hauck et al., 2007).

Women who breastfeed their children perceive breastfeeding as more convenient, whereas those who bottle feed tend to perceive breastfeeding as less convenient, perhaps associating it with a loss of freedom. The latter women believe that with bottle feeding, someone else can feed the baby and they will be able to resume outside activities earlier than if they breastfeed. Among low-income women, other factors identified as barriers to breastfeeding include modesty, privacy, work or school conflicts, and lack of confidence. Lifestyle issues such as diet, stress, substance abuse, and inadequate sleep also present barriers to breastfeeding (England et al., 2003; Bryant, 1993).

Research shows that the women who are most likely to breastfeed are in their mid-thirties, college educated, white, married, and in the middle-income level. Statistically, African American and teen mothers are least likely to breastfeed (Ryan et al., 2002), although recently these groups have seen the largest increase in breastfeeding initiation. Hispanic mothers are more likely to initiate breastfeeding than African American or white mothers according to another study (Hurley et al., 2008). Hispanic women also breastfed their children on average for a longer time (5 months) than African American or white mothers.

A study of African American mothers found that those who breastfed were more educated, employed prior to birth, married, and using postpartum contraception. Breastfeeding was associated with a higher awareness of preventive healthcare measures (Sharps et al., 2003). Factors increasing the risk for not breastfeeding reported in an Australian study were being unmarried and currently smoking, with disadvantaged accommodations and lower educational levels (Yeoh et al., 2007). Maternal obesity is also a factor associated with lower initiation and shorter duration of breastfeeding (Amir & Donath, 2007). Conversely, a woman is more likely to breastfeed when she receives positive prenatal information about breastfeeding (Léger-Leblanc & Rioux, 2008; Semenic et al., 2008; Guise et al., 2003; Noble et al., 2003).

Influence from Other People

Significant people in a woman's life can exert a substantial influence over her decision to breastfeed. For example, a woman is more likely to breastfeed if other family members have either breastfed or are supportive of breastfeeding (Hill et al., 2008; Persad et al., 2008; Shi et al., 2008; Ekstrom et al., 2003). Friends and acquaintances who breastfeed provide additional role models. Support from the baby's father plays a pivotal role in the mother's decision as well. Likewise, the attitude and knowledge level of her healthcare practitioners influence a mother's choice (Clifford & McIntyre, 2008).

The Baby's Father

One of the strongest influences on the breastfeeding decision for many women is that of the child's father (see Figure 11.1). A father's involvement in nurturing a child is related to many positive outcomes for his child. These benefits include cognitive, developmental, and sociobehavioral gains such as improved preterm infant weight gain, improved breastfeeding rates, higher receptive

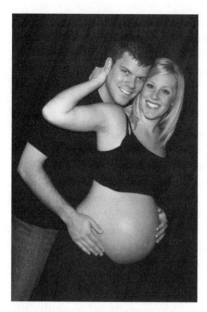

FIGURE 11.1   Expectant couple.
Source: Printed with permission of Leila Farber.

language skills, and higher academic achievement (Garfield & Isacco, 2006).

Pregnant women frequently say, "But if I breastfeed, my husband won't be able to feed the baby." Fathers want to be involved in caring for their infant, and they often see feeding as an important interaction. Despite both breastfeeding and bottle feeding parents "knowing" the benefits of breastfeeding, this understanding does not seem to outweigh the belief that bottle feeding is a means of paternal involvement (Earle, 2000). To overcome this obstacle, acknowledgment of the father's involvement in the baby's feeding choice needs to be included in breastfeeding promotion campaigns.

"Changing life" was the theme of one study with 20 first-time fathers, focusing on leaving bachelor life and becoming responsible for a child. For the participants in this study, being a father was "much more fantastic" than they could have imagined, and they felt they cared for the child equally when both parents were home. Nevertheless, fathers viewed the mother as the main parent, partly because the mothers breastfed the children. Fathers expressed ambiguity toward breastfeeding, describing it as necessary but causing them to feel insignificant (Fägerskiöld, 2008). In another study, fathers identified the process of postponing feeding the baby as a significant issue (Gamble & Morse, 1993). Such motivating factors in men's experiences can form the basis for the lactation consultant's prenatal education of parents.

A woman who perceives her husband to prefer breastfeeding is more likely to leave the hospital breastfeeding, and to exclusively breastfeed, than a woman who perceives her spouse to prefer formula feeding (Scott et al.,

2006). There is value in targeting interventions on the basis of parental attitudes rather than on sociodemographic factors. The father's approval of breastfeeding was the single most statistically significant indicator in one study of whether women breastfed (Littman et al., 1994). Other studies have revealed that fathers' approval and support are key influences in both breastfeeding initiation and breastfeeding beyond 4 months (Kong & Lee, 2004; Chang & Chan, 2003). Expectant mothers do not always correctly predict the attitudes of the father regarding breastfeeding (Freed et al., 1992).

The quality of a couple's relationship does not seem to be a factor in early breastfeeding termination. Even so, a good relationship is associated with more breastfeeding support and more involvement in the baby's care from the father (Falceto et al., 2004). As a lactation consultant, you can encourage more discussion of this issue by couples and more sharing of information with fathers. Educating fathers and encouraging their involvement with the baby leads to greater partner support and more positive attitudes about breastfeeding (Rose et al., 2004). Chapter 19 describes ways to ensure that fathers can be involved with their babies.

Caregivers

Caregivers exert a tremendous influence on a parent's choice of infant feeding method. Frequently, healthcare professionals are unaware of or may even openly dispute the value of breastfeeding despite the vast body of evidence supporting its benefits (Walker, 2007). The approach taken with women can move them in the direction of breastfeeding—or away from it. For example, asking a woman if she plans to breastfeed or asking how she plans to feed her baby implies equality between a mother's milk and substitutes. A more positive approach assumes that all pregnant women intend to breastfeed unless they indicate otherwise.

Hospital personnel are ideally positioned to promote breastfeeding at the time of admission, and to correct any misconceptions that may prevent mothers from breastfeeding their babies. If a woman indicates that she does not plan to breastfeed or if she seems ambivalent about her course of action, the hospital stay provides an opportunity to discuss concerns or misconceptions. For example, pumping and storing milk can be addressed with a woman who indicates she plans to return to work. Adding an informational brochure to the preadmission packet also gives mothers sound options (Texas State Department of Health and Human Services [TSDHHS], 2008). Helping with the breastfeeding decision conveys belief in the normalcy of breastfeeding.

In one study, breastfeeding duration increased after a combination of two prenatal visits, a postpartum hospital visit, and/or a home visit and phone calls (Bonuck et al., 2005). In contrast, Forster and colleagues (2006) found that two mid-pregnancy educational interventions had no significant effect on breastfeeding rates. The key determinants in this study were a strong desire to breastfeed, having been breastfed, being born in an Asian country, and older maternal age. Negative factors included having no intention to breastfeed for 6 or more months, smoking 20 or more cigarettes per day prior to becoming pregnant, lack of childbirth education, maternal obesity, self-reported depression in the 6 months after birth, and the infant receiving formula while in the hospital.

One study found that provider encouragement to breastfeed had a major effect on the segment of women least likely to breastfeed. There was a fourfold increase in breastfeeding initiation, a threefold increase in breastfeeding rates among low-income, young, and less-educated women, a fivefold increase among African American women, and nearly an 11-fold increase among single women (Lu et al., 2001).

A review of 20 trials involving more than 23,700 mother–infant pairs suggested that extra professional support increases exclusive breastfeeding and duration (Sikorski et al., 2002). Caregivers can help instill in women a belief in their ability to breastfeed and an understanding of breastmilk's superiority over artificial baby milk. A mother's confidence is determined in large part by her caregivers. At the same time, consistency in the message given to mothers is important. Five themes emerged in an extensive analysis of health service support for breastfeeding: the mother–health professional relationship, skilled help, time pressures, the medicalization of breastfeeding, and the hospital ward as a public place (McInnes & Chambers, 2008). It is incumbent on all who work directly with families to be a part of the solution in protecting breastfeeding, and not part of the problem.

There is a discrepancy between clinician perceptions that they speak about breastfeeding and mothers who believe their caregivers rarely discuss breastfeeding with them (Taveras et al., 2004a). Significant communication gaps also exist in terms of discussing breastfeeding duration and ways to breastfeed after returning to work. African American women were less likely to have received breastfeeding advice from counselors in the U.S. government's Women, Infants, and Children (WIC) program than white women were, and they were more likely to receive bottle feeding advice. Even so, African American women and white women were equally likely overall to report having received breastfeeding advice from medical care providers (Beal et al., 2003).

Prenatal parenting support and postpartum visits both increase the likelihood that families will continue breastfeeding, read to their 3-month-old child, and provide other appropriate parenting (Johnston et al., 2004). Concerns voiced by the prenatal focus groups centered on the realization that breastfeeding was both easy and diffi-cult, the importance and role of supportive others, the receipt of conflicting advice, the need for validating experiences, and modification of breastfeeding intention based on postpartum experiences (Moore & Coty, 2006).

Society

Many social barriers are in place in developed countries which, at best, fail to recognize breastfeeding as the natural way to nourish babies. At worst, barriers openly discourage breastfeeding. In prenatal contact with mothers, it is important that the caregiver is aware of these barriers and addresses them with clients. As a lactation consultant, you can help women verbalize and address the conflicting feelings that sometimes are involved in the decision to breastfeed (Hall & Hauck, 2007).

Separation of generations, frequent relocation, little experience caring for children, and lack of breastfeeding as the cultural norm can leave new mothers with little confidence in their ability to breastfeed or little understanding of how the process works. Few women have breastfeeding role models, often resulting in an attitude that the mother will "try" breastfeeding, but has an expectation of difficulties and even failure. When bottle feeding is widespread among family and friends, even a problem with just one aspect of breastfeeding may cause a mother to discontinue breastfeeding (Bailey et al., 2004). You can help women recognize the important contribution they make to society in their role as mothers and nurturers of the next generation.

Bottle feeding as the model in Western culture influences professionals and laypersons alike. When media and advertising portray the breast as a sexual object, they ignore nature's intended use of breasts for infant nutrition. Much of the healthcare system bases routines, policies, education, and even the facility's architectural layout on artificial feeding. Although the maxim "breast is best" is freely spoken, many infant feeding messages imply equality between human milk and artificial baby milk (Spear, 2006; Taveras et al., 2004b). When parents receive such mixed signals, they become even more confused.

Customs in the home environment may influence a woman to feed her baby artificially if that is what most women in her culture do. Her understanding of infant care or lack of knowledge about breastfeeding may cause her to question whether breastfeeding will fit into her lifestyle. Commercial messages about human milk substitutes and bottle feeding may convince her that there is little difference between breastfeeding and artificial feeding.

Mixed images of the breasts as sexual—as opposed to a means of nurturing babies—may prove confusing as well (Harris et al., 2003). An aversion to having her breasts touched may make it emotionally painful for a woman to breastfeed; such an aversion is common in women who are survivors of sexual or physical abuse (Sperlich & Yeng,

2008; Kendall-Tackett, 2005, 2007; Prentice et al., 2002). A woman may not even be aware of past abuse until birth and breastfeeding trigger memories. (Chapter 19 discusses abuse survivors in more detail.)

Greater employer support for breastfeeding employees is needed as well. In one study, mothers' expectations of returning to work in the first year did not deter them from initiating breastfeeding, although the return to work and quitting breastfeeding were closely and powerfully linked. Women in service occupations were able to breastfeed longer than women in administrative and manual occupations (Kimbro, 2006). Pumping options abound for women returning to work or school. For example, public aid programs (e.g., the WIC program) often provide pumps at no cost to low-income mothers. Chapter 24 offers a detailed discussion on ways that lactation consultants can help working mothers continue breastfeeding.

Realistic Expectations

Discussing the downside to failing to breastfeed with pregnant women can provide a sound basis for informed decision making. While breastfeeding, the mother has a free hand to attend to other needs or activities such as reading, snacking, and helping other children. Presenting the idea of traveling "with" the baby, instead of "away from" the baby can be very empowering and liberating for mothers whose cultural messages suggest they "need" to leave their baby. Because breastfeeding is possible almost anywhere, travel and other activities are more convenient when the baby accompanies the mother. You can help mothers with examples of how they can breastfeed modestly in front of others.

A breastfeeding mother need not purchase special equipment or incur daily expenses for infant formula. In addition, mothers are often pleased to find that their breastfed babies' stools and spit-up have a less offensive odor than those of formula-fed babies; the breastmilk spit-up and stools also do not stain clothing.

You can help a mother develop realistic expectations about breastfeeding by acquainting her with some of the realities. In the early days of breastfeeding, some women experience engorgement and nipple soreness. Because of the more frequent feedings required by a breastfed baby, a mother needs to be available to her young baby for nourishment. Bottle feeders often choose artificial feeding because they perceive breastfeeding as disagreeable in some respect. Fear of instilling guilt is not an acceptable excuse for failing to inform women of the potentially negative outcomes of formula use, because artificial milk falls far short of the biological norm of breastfeeding.

It is important to neither minimize nor dismiss a mother's concerns as she works through her infant feeding decision. You can encourage her to consider that breastfeeding is the normal, expected postpartum course.

Remind her, too, of the positive health, emotional, and financial features of breastfeeding. Help her see that there are ways to decrease discomforts and minimize inconveniences with this feeding approach. If she has specific concerns, address them by suggesting ways of coping and including her baby in her activities. This type of support may be all she needs to build her confidence and help her overcome perceived obstacles. Learning how to fit breastfeeding into their lifestyle will be the first of many accommodations parents will make as they blend their new child into their family.

Misconceptions That Influence Decision Making

A number of misconceptions about breastfeeding may cause a woman to choose not to breastfeed. You can help dispel these misunderstandings and increase a woman's confidence in her decision to breastfeed. Following is a list of some common misconceptions.

- *A breastfed baby will be too dependent on the mother.* Breastfed babies actually seem to display more independence because their needs are met (see Chapter 13).
- *Breastfeeding is too time-consuming.* There is actually less work involved for a mother in breastfeeding than in bottle feeding, if the mother is doing the bottle feeding. Breastfeeding frees the mother to spend valuable time with her baby and other family members (see Chapter 19).
- *My mother didn't have enough milk, so maybe I won't either.* A well-nourished woman produces the amount of milk her baby needs. The breastfeeding experience of the woman's mother or other female relatives has little bearing on her ability to breastfeed, barring genetic hormonal conditions. Between 1930 and 1980, healthcare practitioners gave women little effective advice or support to breastfeed, which led to many new mothers failing to breastfeed during those decades (see Chapter 1).
- *Maybe my milk won't agree with my baby.* Each mother's milk is ideally suited to her baby. Breastfed babies rarely experience negative reactions to their mother's milk. Conversely, many babies are unable to tolerate cow's milk (see Chapter 9).
- *My breasts are too small to breastfeed.* The size of a woman's breasts is determined primarily by the amount of fatty tissue, not functional breast tissue. Breast size usually has little bearing on her ability to produce sufficient milk (see Chapter 7).
- *I am too high-strung to breastfeed.* Breastfeeding can actually be calming to a high-strung woman because of the hormones (prolactin, oxytocin, and cholecystokinin) activated by nursing. The added skin contact with the baby can have a calming effect on a mother as well (see Chapter 7).

- *If I breastfeed, my diet will be too restricted.* Breast-feeding babies generally can tolerate the same foods the mother tolerates. The only foods a mother may need to restrict are those that seem to produce signs of intolerance in her baby (see Chapter 8).

- *If I have a cesarean birth, I won't be able to breastfeed.* The type of birth a mother experiences has no effect on her ability to breastfeed, although pain and sepa-ration may cause initial obstacles. Mothers who deliver by cesarean birth are able to breastfeed (see Chapter 12).

- *Breastfeeding will drain my energies too much.* All mothers find caring for a newborn tiring, regardless of which feeding method is used. Breastfeeding encourages a mother to relax during feeding times and helps her to get even more rest than a mother who bottle feeds her baby, if the mother is a sole care-giver. A mother can recoup her energies by making it a practice to rest while her baby is sleeping. Breast-feeding seems to be nature's way of ensuring that the mother gets the rest she needs in the postpartum period. A formula feeding mother spends more time purchasing and preparing formula and caring for the child, who will be sicker more often than a breastfed child. She also tends to get less rest from doing more household work while "freed" from resting as she nurses her baby (see Chapter 9).

- *Breastfeeding mothers lose their figures and get sagging breasts.* The sagging in a woman's breasts results from pregnancy and loss of muscle tone as a woman ages, not from having breastfed (see Chapter 7). Addition-ally, the caloric demands of breastfeeding can actually help mothers control their weight (see Chapter 8).

- *Artificial baby milk is just as healthy as human milk.* There are substantial differences between infant for-mula and a mother's milk. Human milk is a live sub-stance that provides immunity from disease to the child and has antibacterial properties. By comparison, formula is a growth medium for bacteria and is sus-ceptible to contaminants. See Chapter 9 for a detailed discussion about the properties and health benefits of human milk.

- *Breastfeeding is essentially an alternative to infant for-mula.* Breastfeeding is much more than the milk the baby receives: It is a dynamic process, a bonding rela-tionship between a mother and her baby. Breastfeed-ing involves people, not simply food for the baby (see Chapter 4).

- *I'll have to wean when I return to work anyway.* Moth-ers who are separated from their babies have many options, whether for a return to work, school, or other activity. They can express milk for the caregiver to feed to the baby or provide formula for the baby dur-ing the separation. Unrestricted breastfeeding at times when the mother and baby are together will help maintain milk production. Many employers and insurance companies support employees who breast-feed, as it lowers absenteeism and health insurance claims (see Chapter 24).

Conditions That Contraindicate Breastfeeding

It is extremely rare for a mother to be unable to breastfeed her baby, although a few conditions do contraindicate this method of feeding. Sheehan's syndrome, as discussed in Chapter 7, prevents the mother from producing milk. A few long-term drug therapies such as lithium or tamoxifen rule out breastfeeding, as the substance or treatment would be dangerous to the infant (Hale, 2010). Severe illness in the mother, such as unresolved congestive heart failure or chemotherapy treatment for cancer, may contraindicate breastfeeding as well. Mothers can breastfeed after at least 2 weeks of treatment for active tuberculosis (Lawrence, 1997). Women who test positive for the human immun-odeficiency virus (HIV) and live in a developed country with a sanitary water supply are advised not to breastfeed, although heat-treating expressed milk is a viable option. Chapter 25 discusses these conditions in more depth.

⌇ *Preparation for Breastfeeding*

Women throughout history have breastfed their babies without the aid of more recent scientific knowledge or special devices. Many modern women, however, benefit from learning about breastfeeding techniques and prepa-ration for breastfeeding. Although women historically have nurtured their babies primarily with their milk, the decades from 1930 to 1980 saw an increase in the popu-larity of bottle feeding and a decline in breastfeeding in the United States and many other industrialized coun-tries. Consequently, fewer family members may be knowledgeable enough about breastfeeding to offer today's mothers the practical breastfeeding information and sup-port they need.

An increased number of women began breastfeeding after 1980, however, and these women are now becoming grandmothers. They are the "wise women" elders whom expectant and new mothers need to solidify the world's cultural return to breastfeeding as the norm for babies. Mothers who were breastfed as children are more likely to exclusively breastfeed their own infants (Anderson et al., 2007). The educational process and the mother's active participation in planning for her breastfed baby are effec-tive means of preparing psychologically for breastfeeding. Her self-efficacy will increase through these activities, enabling her to overcome minor discomforts and obsta-cles she may experience that are associated with nursing her baby.

Learning About Breastfeeding

All women need to know the reasons to breastfeed as well as the risks of not breastfeeding so that they can make informed decisions about how they will feed their babies. Information helps dispel any misconceptions. A woman who plans to breastfeed will benefit from learning about this practice early in her pregnancy. The earlier she receives information, the greater the likelihood that she will breastfeed for a substantial period. Attentiveness and retention of the information may be greater in the later months of pregnancy, as she gets closer to her delivery date.

Early prenatal contacts can focus on the decision-making process, discussing individual goals for breastfeeding and the mother's vision of breastfeeding in everyday life. Explore how important feeding issues are to her and her partner and what they expect breastfeeding to be like. Answers to these questions provide a foundation for her breastfeeding education. You can then discuss the practical aspects of breastfeeding management closer to the time of delivery.

Pregnant women can develop a sound base for breastfeeding practices by attending a prenatal breastfeeding class and by seeking information through reading and the Internet. They may also begin attending meetings of a community support group for breastfeeding mothers. These meetings, which enhance women's confidence and increase their knowledge of breastfeeding, provide an opportunity for mothers to share common interests with others in the community.

Attending childbirth classes and practicing relaxation techniques can enhance a woman's awareness of her body and help her learn ways to overcome tension and discomfort. The information and skills she obtains during pregnancy will be especially useful to her when she and her baby go through the trial-and-error period of establishing a comfortable breastfeeding routine. She can familiarize herself with baby care and breastfeeding by associating with mothers of young babies and occasionally caring for babies during her pregnancy. In this way, she will develop proficiency in handling babies and build confidence in her mothering abilities. This kind of "practice mothering" will enable her to overcome worries she may encounter when her own baby arrives.

Give the mother information to help her blend breastfeeding into her life and assist her to avoid or minimize problems. Helping her identify aspects that will be useful to her personally leads to the development of useful strategies that she can apply postpartum. Such education is the most important tool for increasing breastfeeding rates (Rosen et al., 2008; Guise et al., 2003), and it helps the lactation consultant form an effective relationship with the mother (Pridham, 1993).

Figure 11.2 identifies questions that are helpful in gathering the information necessary to assess a woman's

---

Assessing a woman's need for breastfeeding education

- How does she feel about the prospect of breastfeeding?
- What practical knowledge does she have about breastfeeding?
- What prior experience or exposure does she have to breastfeeding?
- How many friends or relatives have breastfed?
- What reading has she done on breastfeeding? What videos has she seen?
- Has she attended a breastfeeding information class?
- Is she attending prepared childbirth classes?
- What has her physician discussed with her about breastfeeding?
- What has she done to prepare for breastfeeding?
- Has she checked for inverted nipples?
- What has she learned about breast care?
- What clothing does she have that will allow her baby easy access to her breast?
- What arrangements has she made for help at home?
- Has she arranged for rooming-in if she is delivering in a hospital?
- Is she interested in attending group discussions with other breastfeeding mothers?
- What are her specific questions or concerns?

FIGURE 11.2 Questions to ask prenatally about breastfeeding.

need for breastfeeding education and support. Open-ended questions such as these encourage mothers to respond with information that is more descriptive.

Don't forget to reach out to adolescents in your area. The birth rate for U.S. teens in 2007 was 22.2 per 1000 for teens aged 15–17, and 73.9 per 1000 for teens aged 18–19 (National Center for Health Statistics [NCHS], 2009). Many secondary school health classes welcome community speakers and health information. Chapter 19 offers more information on ways to encourage teen mothers to breastfeed.

Breastfeeding Classes

A large part of breastfeeding teaching occurs through group instruction. Given this fact, breastfeeding classes may be a significant part of your practice. One study examined three types of educational venues: (1) video and group teaching; (2) one-on-one prenatal instruction with a weekly postpartum support group led by a lactation consultant and a pediatrician; and (3) prenatal visits only. Women in all three groups had higher breastfeeding rates than members of the control group, who had no classes. There was no statistically significant difference in the outcomes produced by the three educational methods (Rosen et al., 2008).

Through classes, you can reach large numbers of women at various stages. The purpose of the class will determine its content. Ideally, the couple's childbirth classes will include breastfeeding discussions. Early in the series, couples tend to benefit from coverage of issues that help them make an informed decision regarding infant feeding. After they make their decision, a discussion of expectations and getting off to a good start with breastfeeding is helpful. A postpartum class after the baby begins breastfeeding provides continued support and information to parents.

Teaching a Breastfeeding Class

The most important rule in teaching a class is "Keep it simple." A prenatal breastfeeding classes may be 2 to 3 hours long. Classes that go longer than 3 hours are too much of a time commitment for busy parents-to-be, as most mothers continue to work or attend school until the baby's birth. Much of what you teach during the prenatal period will focus on the area of attitude and expectations. Expectant parents may remember little of the particulars for establishing breastfeeding. They will recall, however, the impressions they gained in class regarding the health benefits and long-term ease of breastfeeding, as well as the risks of not breastfeeding. These perceptions will reinforce their decision about how they will feed their baby.

There are no hard and fast rules in breastfeeding. All that is required is that the baby gains weight appropriately and that the mother is comfortable in the process. Encourage parents to trust their instincts and to respond to their baby's cues. Capitalize on teachable moments and tailor your teaching methods to adult learners. During a prenatal class, parents may focus on the imminent delivery of their baby and have difficulty projecting beyond that point. To engage them in the educational process, include activities that will involve them actively to enhance their learning. Use a variety of activities that appeal to different learning styles—visual, auditory, and kinesthetic (tactile). See Chapter 4 for a discussion of adult learning principles.

Recognize that much of what parents learn prenatally may not be retained after the birth. Reinforcing learning with handouts on specific issues will help overcome the tendency to forget. Visual learning from other breastfeeding parents and short videos may also help promote retention. Ideas from creative lactation consultants and breastfeeding support groups abound. For example, passing around a plate with appetizing homemade cookies and plain store-bought ones uses the sense of taste to drive home the point about the bland taste of infant formula compared to mother's milk that is flavored by foods the mother consumes. A tablespoon of water in a disposable diaper helps prospective parents (many of whom have never changed a baby's diaper) get a feel for what an ample void weighs. Concocting a breastmilk stool look-a-like from mustard and sesame seeds is a humorous teaching tool as well.

During a breastfeeding class, help parents to focus on the positive aspects of breastfeeding and to regard it as a learning and growth process for both the mother and the baby. Such education may help couples recognize that any challenges they encounter with breastfeeding are usually resolvable.

Infant Feeding Class

Advertising a class as an "infant feeding" class rather than a breastfeeding class will make it clear that the session is open to everyone regardless of whether they plan to breastfeed. Because fathers are instrumental in a mother's decision to breastfeed, be sure to encourage them to participate in classes. Often, couples express a concern that the father will feel left out if the mother breastfeeds. Help fathers recognize the importance of their participation in making the decision to breastfeed, and discuss ways they can be involved with the baby (see Chapter 19).

In this kind of early class, you may help some undecided couples choose breastfeeding. You can dispel any misconceptions the couples have and address information they will need for making their decision. Discuss the risks of not breastfeeding for both the mother and the baby, as well as the convenience, economics, and ease of travel with a breastfeeding infant.

Prenatal Breastfeeding Class

Many hospitals offer prenatal breastfeeding classes. If such a class does not exist in your hospital, you may be able to initiate one or refer families to community classes. You can also work in cooperation with childbirth education classes to ensure that information about breastfeeding is included and is consistent with what you teach; information delivered in such a forum may reach women who may not otherwise receive it. In addition, you may work with obstetric and family practice physicians and health clinics to increase correct and consistent information about breastfeeding during prenatal visits. See this chapter for more information on prenatal education.

In a prenatal class, you can address issues that will help parents prepare for establishing breastfeeding. Explain the importance of eating when hungry and drinking when thirsty without strict dietary regimens. Encourage the women to rest with their babies to facilitate recovery after childbirth.

Identify babies' behaviors as they relate to feeding, pointing out to parents that babies communicate through distinct cues before, during, and after feedings. Help them identify how these cues enable them to understand and best meet their babies' needs (Delight et al., 1991). Chapter 13 provides a more detailed discussion of infant hunger cues.

Use visual examples to demonstrate the positions that mothers commonly use for holding their babies for feeding, and give parents dolls with which to practice their own positioning. Show them through media and pictures how to recognize when their baby has a good latch and positioning at the breast. Explain how an effective latch is the key to milk transfer and avoiding nipple soreness.

Another goal of a prenatal class is to help couples learn how to determine when their baby is receiving enough milk. Discuss milk production in the context of supply and demand. Encourage them to watch for other signs of good intake, such as audible swallows and the number of wet diapers and stools. Provide them with a feeding diary to use during the first 2 weeks of breastfeeding to identify the appropriate number of feedings, voids, and stools.

The first 2 weeks after childbirth are a time of learning for both the mother and baby. To emphasize this point to expectant parents, you might suggest the analogy of the first time the couple danced together, awkwardly testing where to place their hands and feet. Help them see that the mother and baby are new dance partners learning how to fit together in the same way.

Open, honest discussion of these issues will help parents achieve a smooth transition to initiating breastfeeding. Figure 11.3 shows a sample outline for a prenatal breastfeeding class.

Postpartum Breastfeeding Class

Many mothers benefit from a postpartum class where they can receive support and information after they have begun feeding their babies. Pregnant women can be encouraged to attend this class as well. Such a program might even evolve into a mother-to-mother support group in which pregnant women have an opportunity to talk with breastfeeding mothers and to observe breastfeeding.

During a postpartum class, you can discuss what the new parents expect in the next several months. Help them anticipate typical infant behavior, growth spurts, crying, and teething. Discuss planning of activities, breastfeeding in public, and returning to work or school. You can also address complementary foods and weaning at this time.

Allow some time for group problem solving and prevention of problems such as engorgement, plugged ducts, and mastitis. Review the importance of exclusive breastfeeding and the question of supplementing with infant formula. In addition, make sure new parents understand that early supplementing with formula is a key predictor of not achieving breastfeeding goals (Bolton et al., 2009; Declercq, 2009; Camurdan et al., 2008; Otsuka et al., 2008; Semenic et al., 2008). Finally, make sure they know where they can go for help with questions or concerns. Figure 11.4 provides a sample outline for a postpartum breastfeeding class.

1. Couples raise questions about breastfeeding to address in class (list on board)—5 minutes
2. Why breastfeed? Couples' reasons for breastfeeding (list on board)—5 minutes
3. Breastfeeding as a biological norm—5–10 minutes
   A. Life-long "benefits" for baby and mother are actually just "normal"
   B. Breastfeeding is not just "a nice idea"-formula is a vastly inferior substitute with life-long implications
   C. What happened in U.S. Culture? From breast to bottle $8 billion U.S. annually
4. Anatomy and physiology of lactation (poster or draw on board)—10 minutes
   A. Colostrum: normal amounts and importance to baby
   B. Milk "coming-in"
      1. Avoiding engorgement
      2. Establishing a robust supply
   C. Supply and demand—10 minutes
      1. Real babies aren't TV babies
      2. Growth spurts
      3. The scoop on poop and pee (pass around diapers)
   D. Latch: avoiding difficulties (video)—6–12 minutes
   E. Positions: cradle hold, cross-cradle hold, side-sitting (football or clutch) hold, side-lying position (practice with dolls)—5 minutes
5. Knowing what's NOT normal—5 minutes
6. Factors that might affect milk supply—10 minutes
   A. Delayed onset of milk production: C-section, hypertension, edema, gestational diabetes, retained placenta, theca lutein cyst
   B. Hormonal issues for the mother: infertility, PCOS, hypothyroidism, androgen disorders
   C. Baby issues: prematurity, oral anomalies, difficult births, interventions
7. Coping strategies: reverse pressure softening and supplementing with colostrum—5 minutes
8. Going back to work—5–10 minutes
   A. Employers
   B. Pumping and storing milk
   C. Caregivers
9. Community resources and wrap-up (resource sheet)—5 minutes

FIGURE 11.3   Sample outline for a prenatal breastfeeding class.

Source: Printed with permission of Anna Swisher.

Prenatal Breast Care

Mothers often ask what kind of breast preparation is needed prenatally. During pregnancy, hormones act on the breast to prepare it for lactation. The skin stretches and becomes more pliable to accommodate internal breast development. Increasing pigmentation protects the nipple and areola, which may become enlarged; this pigmentation is due to increased content in melanin in the

I. Welcome and introductions (5 minutes)

II. Breastfeeding's continued importance (lecture and discussion—15 minutes)

    A. Review of risks of not breastfeeding

    B. AAP breastfeeding recommendations

III. Growing baby milestones and issues (lecture and discussion—20 minutes)

    A. Growth spurts

    B. Crying

    C. Sleep

    D. Baby's new abilities

    E. Teething

IV. New parents' issues (lecture, discussion, and video—20 minutes)

    A. Resuming activities, prioritizing, and not overdoing

    B. Ideas for including baby

    C. Staying healthy—rest, diet, and exercise

BREAK (10 minutes)

V. Returning to work or school (lecture, hands-on, and discussion—30 minutes)

    A. Options

    B. Planning ahead—talk with employer, prioritize needs

    C. How you will feed baby in your absence

    D. Pumps and other devices

    E. Troubleshooting and realistic expectations

VI. The family table and weaning (lecture and discussion—10 minutes)

VII. Where to find breastfeeding help (lecture—10 minutes)

FIGURE 11.4 Sample outline for a postpartum breastfeeding class.

Source: Printed with permission of Debbie Shinskie.

skin, which "toughens" the skin. The Montgomery glands lubricate the nipple and areola, thus protecting the keratin from drying out and flaking off.

Near the beginning of the third trimester, the mother can determine whether her nipples will need any assistance for a good latch. To do so, she can perform the pinch test (described in Chapter 21). A nipple that protrudes when stimulated makes it easiest for the baby to get a good mouthful of breast tissue, whereas a nipple that remains flat or inverts may require assistance to improve latch. The last trimester is the best time for a woman to manipulate flat or inverted nipples because at that time the skin has gained elasticity and stretches more easily than earlier in her pregnancy.

Nipple Correction

When a woman has flat or inverted nipples, she first needs to establish whether intervention is appropriate or necessary. A woman with a history of giving birth to premature children or a tendency toward miscarriage or false labor should discuss with her caregiver the advisability of nipple preparation, breast foreplay, or intercourse. Such stimulation could trigger oxytocin release and cause the uterus to contract and induce labor.

Some babies breastfeed on an inverted nipple without any difficulty; others experience difficulty when the inverted nipple prevents stimulation of the baby's palate to elicit a sucking response. Wearing breast shells in the first few weeks of breastfeeding may help to increase the nipple's eversion. Breast shells exert gentle pressure around the nipple, making the skin more pliable and the breast easier to grasp; the infant's suckling on the breast further increases skin elasticity. Recommendations for the use of breast shells are mixed, however. Some women use aids such as an inverted syringe or commercial products such as EvertIt or LatchAssist to pull out the nipple before a feeding. Chapter 21 discusses breast shells, including their drawbacks, and the use of nipple everters.

Colostrum During Pregnancy

Colostrum production begins during pregnancy, causing some mothers to leak copious amounts of colostrum while others experience no leaking at all. Prenatal leakage of colostrum is not a predictor of how much milk a mother will produce. Women whose breasts become uncomfortably full with colostrum can gently express it to the point of comfort.

Many women whose babies are at risk for supplementation at birth begin to express their colostrum during pregnancy, freeze it and take it to the hospital with them. These include women who have gestational diabetes, those who have type 1 or type 2 diabetes, and women who plan to have scheduled cesarean sections. Any baby that is large for gestational age (LGA) or who is separated from the mother due to a cesarean delivery is at high risk for being supplemented. In addition, LGA babies of mothers with diabetes are at higher risk for developing diabetes if exposed to bovine proteins and bovine insulin (Luopajärvi et al., 2008; Tiittanen et al., 2006). A mother can avoid formula by arranging with her physician for her colostrum to be used in the event of a need for supplementation.

Mothers who experience leaking and do not wish to collect their colostrum prenatally can blend the colostrum into the areola. If colostrum causes the bra to stick to the nipple, moistening the bra with warm water before attempting to remove it will prevent skin irritation.

Many mothers breastfeed during pregnancy and go on to tandem nurse their newborn and older baby. During the last trimester, the mother's milk changes to colostrum. Some toddlers wean when the taste of the milk changes and the quantity decreases, while others continue to nurse throughout pregnancy without incident. Chapter 14 discusses tandem nursing in more depth.

Practices to Avoid

Caution mothers against rubbing their nipples with a towel to toughen them—an old recommendation that damages breast tissue and should not be practiced. Mothers also will want to avoid wearing tight bras and other clothing that binds their breasts. Such localized pressure on breast tissue can cause discomfort and result in plugged ducts. In addition, urge women to avoid the following practices:

- Use of any drying agent on the nipples and areola
- Use of plastic liners in breast pads
- Use of artificial lubricants unless they are needed
- Use of lubricants that do not allow the skin to breathe or that must be washed off (read labels on lotions or creams carefully)

Practical Planning Suggestions

An expectant woman can prepare her family, home, and wardrobe for breastfeeding. This includes planning a quiet place for feedings, initial sleeping arrangements for the baby, and clothing that will accommodate breastfeeding. You can also encourage her to arrange household help for her early weeks at home with her newborn. These plans and preparations, as well as learning about breastfeeding, can be instrumental in building a woman's confidence about her feeding choice.

Nursing Area

Planning a convenient space for feedings will help the mother get a comfortable start with breastfeeding. Ideally, she will have a quiet spot where she can relax undisturbed for 20 to 30 minutes at a time. Whether she decides to nurse in a chair or on a sofa or bed, having several pillows available for support will help her relax and find a comfortable position. A comfortable chair with armrests will assist the mother in supporting her baby during feedings. A footstool will enable her knees to be high enough to provide additional support. In addition, placing a small table within arm's reach will provide a place for a beverage, snack, reading materials, laptop, cell phone, remote control, and any other items she may need. Just as planning for the baby's wardrobe helps a woman prepare mentally for the arrival of her baby, so planning a cozy nursing corner can help her feel confident and prepared for feeding her newborn at home.

Clothing Suggestions

Although many representations of breastfeeding women show their upper chest area uncovered, in truth, mothers can breastfeed discreetly with little of their body visible. Mothers usually have clothing that covers their upper torso while allowing the baby easy access to the breast. The baby covers the mother's lower chest and abdomen and keeps these body parts from view.

Because the wardrobes of most women already include many items suitable for breastfeeding, very few clothing purchases are actually necessary for breastfeeding. One type of clothing that is helpful is a loose-fitting item the mother can open midway from the bottom. Layered outfits, tank tops, blouses, pullovers, sweaters, and dresses with front or side openings are ideal. Blouses that button in the front can be unbuttoned from the bottom for good coverage. During feedings, the mother can drape any exposed area of the breast with an open sweater, jacket, blanket, or diaper. Nursing covers are an unnecessary expense and can make it difficult for the mother to see her baby's face.

Dark-patterned materials readily hide spots caused by milk leakage; and natural fiber materials are the most comfortable. Synthetic materials are less desirable because they tend to hold moisture and do not allow the skin to breathe. For nighttime feedings, the mother can select front-opening gowns, pajamas, or special nursing nightgowns with layered bodices.

Many nursing apparel manufacturers exist, including several that sell their wares on the Internet. Nursing fashions typically have openings such as flaps or zippers to make breastfeeding easy and discreet in public, but these clothes tend to be very expensive. Altering clothing the mother already has is a more cost-effective approach for most women. Expectant mothers can find good values for maternity and nursing clothes at resale stores and garage sales, especially those benefiting nursing mothers' groups.

Nursing Bra

The expectant mother may select a nursing bra during her last trimester of pregnancy, or she may choose to wait until after her mature milk has come in. Any woman who experiences significant breast growth during pregnancy will need new bras during that time. The ideal bra provides support, yet does not bind. A practical suggestion is to try on bras for proper fit before making a purchase and then buy only one bra initially. After she wears the new bra for a while, she can decide whether it meets her needs before purchasing another one. It will also save her money should the new bra not fit postpartum.

Mothers should avoid bras with underwires and elastic around the cups, as they can press on milk ducts and prevent sufficient drainage. For the same reason, the seams of the bra need to be well past the front of the breast, toward the underarm. Bra cups should be made out of cotton or a cotton–polyester blend. The mother can place a breast pad, handkerchief, or piece of diaper inside the bra cup to absorb leaking.

A bra with simple cup fasteners will allow easy access to the breast. Practicing unfastening and fastening the cup several times will help the mother determine if she can manage it easily with one hand. Velcro fasteners, although convenient, are sometimes noisy and may attract attention when breastfeeding in public.

Some mothers find that sports bras provide enough support while accommodating changes in breast size during the early days of lactation. Ultimately, however, mothers should try a variety of bras and decide which type best fits their unique needs. Nursing bras, being a niche market, are expensive. Those available at maternity resale shops or at large retail stores may meet women's needs more economically than the boutique bras touted on the Internet and in other parenting media.

Help at Home

New parents often receive many offers of help during the first several weeks after delivery. Although the individuals who are trying to help may be well intentioned, the family will want to clarify the roles of potential helpers before accepting any offers of assistance. Family and friends who wish to help can be encouraged to do household chores so the mother can relax, rest, and care for her baby. Perhaps the father can arrange for vacation time or family leave while the mother and baby settle in at home. It is important that helpers understand that the parents will be caring for and bonding with their baby. To assist in this process, the helpers can perform household tasks, run errands, shop for groceries, and ensure that the mother gets adequate rest and nutrition.

Some women arrange for the services of a *doula*—a Greek word referring to an experienced woman who helps other women either during the birth process or in the early postpartum period. Many times, a birth doula extends her services to the postpartum period as well, assisting the mother at home. A postpartum doula typically provides services to the mother in her home rather than attending the birth. She provides the care that the extended family optimally would provide, but that today's scattered families may not be able to give.

Sleeping Arrangements

Parents will need to consider sleeping arrangements for their breastfed baby, especially during the early weeks after delivery. Keeping the baby in the parents' bed or in a separate bed in the same room makes nighttime feedings easier. The mother then needs to make only minor adjustments for the baby to latch; limiting disruptions makes it more likely that both mother and baby quickly return to sleep.

Cosleeping is the norm in most of the world, and the practice has increased in the United States in recent years. Parents who do not wish for the baby to remain in their bed, however, can place an extra bed or mattress on the floor. This allows the mother to return to her bed and leave the baby undisturbed on the mattress (depending on

the child's age and degree of mobility) after the feeding ends. There are also commercial side-sleeper cribs that hook safely to the parents' bed. Some mothers prefer to place a rocking chair in the baby's room and to have nighttime feedings there instead of in the parents' room. See Chapter 13 for further discussion of cosleeping and other sleep issues.

～ Selecting a Physician or Midwife

The pregnant woman will need to select a caregiver for both herself and her baby. In the United States, the insurance company that provides coverage for the mother and child largely dictates the choice of caregiver. Low-income women are constrained by the number of providers who accept Medicaid. In contrast, women in other countries with single-payer or government-provided health care may not have these constraints. Women who establish a relationship with a gynecologist or midwife before pregnancy can decide whether that same caregiver will meet their needs for prenatal care and birth as well.

Perhaps an even more important decision than the prenatal care provider is the selection of a caregiver for the baby. This consideration is especially important for a woman who plans to breastfeed; she will want to know that her baby's caregiver supports her plans and will provide appropriate advice.

Factors to Explore with a Potential Caregiver

When parents select caregivers for the mother and her baby, they must investigate a number of issues to ensure that they are secure in their decision and have confidence in the caregivers' ability. Parents and caregivers must be able to develop a mutually respectful, adult working relationship. Not surprisingly, parents want a caregiver who listens, responds to questions, and demonstrates flexibility in decisions. Their goal is to form a long-term partnership with their caregiver for their baby's health. Bear in mind that many of the parents whom you encounter while working as a lactation consultant may be teens, from low-income families, or non-English speaking. It can be difficult for members of these groups to plan for long-term care. Although the discussion of key factors presented here assumes a certain level of social and educational attainment among parents, your family population may be quite different.

Background

Parents can check a caregiver's credentials and background by contacting the local hospital, the caregiver's office, or the area (county, province, or state) medical society. They may also question friends who use this caregiver's services. The Directory of Medical Specialists, available in any public library or online at www.abms.org, will indicate whether a physician graduated from a fully accredited medical school. Parents may also want to ask whether the caregiver is board certified and what his or her hospital standings are. These data serve as indicators of a physician's qualifications and professional standing. Another popular resource is Angie's List, an Internet subscription service that enables consumers to rate their providers (www.angieslist.com). As its existence suggests, the ever-present Internet has created a more educated consumer in many realms, including pregnancy, birth, and parenting.

Continuing Education

Parents can check the caregiver's office to see if current information about breastfeeding is available. They may also ask about any continuing education undertaken by the caregiver in relation to breastfeeding and other activities, such as teaching at a nearby hospital or medical school. In one survey, 4 out of 10 obstetricians suggested that their training in breastfeeding management was inadequate (Power et al., 2003). Other studies have found consistent deficits in practitioners' knowledge of breastfeeding (Saenz, 2000; Freed et al., 1995a, 1995b, 1995c). Saenz (2000) provides a helpful model for a lactation management rotation for medical residents. See Chapter 26 for further discussion of caregiver education.

Hospital Affiliation or Backup

Parents will want to know whether the caregiver has privileges at the facility where they plan to give birth. Is it family centered? Have they heard positive reports from people who have used the facility, including women who have breastfed? If a home birth or birth at a free-standing birth center is planned, what is the practice if a transfer to a hospital becomes necessary?

Accessibility

The caregiver should be readily accessible for both scheduled visits and emergencies. Many times, a nurse, medical assistant, or receptionist can answer parents' questions. However, when there is a pressing medical concern, parents have the right, after describing a problem to the nurse, to talk directly with the physician or midwife. They also will want to choose a caregiver who, when not on duty, provides coverage by someone who is acceptable to the parents. To determine whether there is a good fit, parents should ask how much time the caregiver allots for office visits, whether there are specific telephone hours, and how promptly calls are returned.

Standing Orders

Most physicians have standing orders—that is, orders the nursing staff follow unless directed otherwise—that apply to all patients under their care. Parents will want to learn their particular physician's standing orders relative to breastfeeding and postpartum care in the hospital. Such orders may concern the administration of certain medications, parameters for supplementing with formula, or other practices that parents may want to address before delivery.

In addition, the nursing staff will have special instructions, referred to as nursing protocol, in all areas, including breastfeeding. Parents will want to be alert to the possibility of scheduled feeding times as well as routine use of pacifiers, bottles, and formula supplementation. If the mother and physician develop a plan that is different from the standing orders or nursing protocol, suggest that they put it in writing. Both the parents and physician should sign this document and keep a copy. Hospital personnel also need a copy to help ensure compliance with the parents' wishes.

Relationship with the Patient

Parents will want a caregiver who genuinely listens to patients, gives understandable explanations, welcomes questions, and returns calls promptly. Will the caregiver openly discuss alternatives and welcome a second opinion? What is the caregiver's position on prepared childbirth and breastfeeding? To gain a sense of the caregiver's personality and capabilities, parents can also talk to friends who use this caregiver's services and discuss his or her strengths and weaknesses.

Selecting the Baby's Caregiver

Most parents in developed countries choose either a pediatrician or a family practice physician for their baby's care. A pediatrician specializes in health care for children from newborn through adolescence. A family practice physician, now considered to be a member of a specialty, is similar to the general practice or family doctor of the past and can treat the entire family. More information about each type of specialty is available at www.aap.org for pediatricians and at www.aafp.org for family physicians. Figure 11.5 contains a checklist for determining whether a physician—no matter what the specialty—is supportive of breastfeeding; the full text of this checklist appears in the article by Newman (2008).

Many pediatric offices have pediatric nurse practitioners (PNPs) on staff. These nurses have obtained extra education and certification in pediatrics, have prescribing privileges, and can handle routine well-child visits. One study found that although PNPs were more knowledgeable about lactation than pediatricians were, 38.2 percent reported they never counseled women about breastfeeding in their practices. Another 17.1 percent never assisted mothers with breastfeeding technique (Hellings & Howe, 2004). Many PNPs provide medical care for indigent or

☐ Gives you formula samples or formula company literature when you are pregnant or after you have had the baby.

☐ Tells you that breastfeeding and bottle feeding are essentially the same.

☐ Tells you that formula X is best.

☐ Tells you that it is not necessary to feed the baby immediately after the birth because you are (will be) tired and the baby is often not interested anyway.

☐ Tells you that there is no such thing as nipple confusion and you should start giving bottles early to your baby to make sure that the baby accepts a bottle nipple.

☐ Tells you that you must stop breastfeeding because you or your baby is sick, because you will be taking medicine, or because you will have a medical test done.

☐ Is surprised to learn that your 6-month-old child is still breastfeeding.

☐ Tells you that breastmilk has no nutritional value after the baby is 6 months or older.

☐ Tells you that you must never allow your baby to fall asleep at the breast.

☐ Tells you that you should not stay in hospital to nurse your sick child because it is important that you rest at home.

☐ Does not try to get you help if you are having trouble with breastfeeding.

FIGURE 11.5 Actions that indicate a health professional is not supportive of breastfeeding.

Source: Printed with permission of the Newman Breastfeeding Clinic and Institute.

welfare patients in clinics and are often the primary caregivers for these populations.

To ensure that the family–provider fit will be a good one, suggest that the parents arrange a prenatal visit with the caregiver to discuss the following issues:

- How soon after birth the first office visit will be scheduled
- Number of times the caregiver expects to see the baby for health maintenance
- The caregiver's staff privileges at the hospital where the baby will be delivered and, if none, how the caregiver refers patients to another pediatrician or family practitioner
- The degree to which parents are encouraged to make nonmedical decisions such as those related to feeding schedule, sleep patterns, supplemental foods, and weaning
- Treatment of jaundice in the newborn
- Viewpoint on circumcision

- Hospital policy regarding delay of antibiotic ointment in the baby's eyes, to enhance initial bonding between parents and baby
- Policy on vitamin, iron, and fluoride supplements
- Policy on initial vaccinations (such as immunization against hepatitis B)
- Percentage of breastfeeding babies in the practice and the average duration of breastfeeding
- Hospital policy regarding how soon the mother and baby can breastfeed after delivery
- Hospital's encouragement of rooming-in
- Breastfeeding protocol in the hospital
- Policy on water and formula supplementation
- Willingness to support the mother's breastfeeding practices
- Management of breastfeeding problems
- The person who answers breastfeeding questions
- Whether there are International Board Certified Lactation Consultants (IBCLCs) on staff and if mothers are referred to an IBCLC if none is on staff
- Criteria for starting solid foods
- Guidelines for weaning, including support for child-led weaning
- Relationship with breastfeeding support groups in the community

Communicating with Caregivers

When the mother and the caregiver have a plan, she can ask that the baby's chart reflect any change in that plan. Many times, the caregiver will be flexible when a mother explains her position with confidence and self-assurance. Make sure a mother knows that it is never too late to discuss a concern with her caregiver. If she has second thoughts after a visit, suggest that she call the provider's office. While in the hospital, if a mother has questions that cannot wait until the scheduled rounds, she can ask the nursing staff to contact the caregiver. If the staff is busy, they may not get to this task as quickly as the mother would like. In such circumstances, the mother may want to place the call herself rather than wait.

If a mother decides to contact her caregiver with a concern, you can help her formulate her questions and clarify the caregiver's response. Ask the mother exactly which words were used. Did her caregiver say, for example, "You *must* start solid foods now" or "You *can* start solid foods now"? Did her caregiver say, "You must supplement with formula" or "Your baby needs more food" (in which case she breastfeed more frequently). Encourage her to share any confusion tactfully.

Most caregivers enjoy educating receptive parents. Encourage the mother to communicate her commitment

to breastfeeding and to appeal for support through difficulties.

Conflicting Advice

When mothers are knowledgeable about breastfeeding,
they are more keenly attuned to advice from their caregiver that seems questionable. You can offer suggestions
to prepare a mother for times when questionable advice
seems detrimental to breastfeeding. To do so, provide her
with a solid basis of information and give her research and
resources, preferably in the physician's own field (e.g.,
pediatrics), to discuss with her caregiver. Encourage the
mother to work with and inform her caregiver about her
day-to-day breastfeeding. If she is under the care of a
medical team, suggest that she try to work with the most
supportive and knowledgeable member of that team.

Breastfeeding decisions are, for the most part, not
medical in nature. A caregiver's advice is simply that—
advice. When a caregiver advises a patient to have her
cholesterol checked, the patient decides whether to act
on the advice. If physician advice about breastfeeding
conflicts with what a parent has learned from other
informed sources, the parent chooses how to act. Parents
must comply only when the child faces a clear and well-
defined danger. Responsible parents will make responsible, informed decisions regarding the care of their baby.

Working Through Conflicts

If a mother experiences conflicts with her caregiver, you
can support her while respecting the primary relationship. Prepare her before a visit by reminding her of typical breastfeeding patterns at her baby's present stage of
development. Encourage her to write down specific questions prior to making her office visits.

When seemingly detrimental advice is given, urge the
mother to ask for the reason behind the advice and to
question whether alternative treatment is possible. Help
her work out solutions and adapt advice to her breastfeeding. If the caregiver advises that a baby receive formula supplements because of low weight gain, the mother
can first explore whether increasing the number of breastfeedings will be satisfactory in meeting this goal. If this is
not agreeable, you can suggest that the mother give the
supplements after first breastfeeding. You can further suggest that she use a device for supplementing at the breast
so her baby receives the supplement while nursing.

In the case of low weight gain, the caregiver may be
agreeable to a trial period during which the mother nurses
more frequently in an effort to increase her milk production. She could then schedule a weight check for a short
time later and postpone supplements until then. Another
alternative might entail a full feeding assessment with pre-
feed/post-feed intake measurements.

When a mother has successfully overcome breastfeeding challenges, such as low milk production or thrush,
encourage her to share her success with her caregiver.
This way, both the caregiver and the mother can learn and
benefit from her experience. The caregiver will then be
better able to help mothers with similar problems in the
future.

Recommending Caregivers to Mothers

If a mother finds she is always at odds with her caregiver,
she might consider changing to a new provider. In other
cases, a mother may be satisfied with her caregiver in
other areas and needs your help only with a specific
breastfeeding issue. Caregiver choices for women on public medical assistance may be very limited, whereas
women with adequate health insurance may have more
options available to them if they decide to change caregivers.

If a woman asks you to recommend a caregiver, try to
suggest the names of at least three local providers. When
you take this path, you are not recommending a particular individual, but rather providing the woman with a
choice of caregivers to suit her personality and her needs.
This practice also helps ensure that the breastfeeding
women in your community work with a variety of caregivers, which in turn increases the caregivers' practical
experience with breastfeeding care. In addition, it helps
you remain professional and objective in making recommendations and contacts with medical providers in your
community.

In addition to the caregivers' names, you can be prepared to give women factual information while avoiding
handing out any personal opinions. You may want to keep
accurate, up-to-date files on caregivers, including their
office hours, call hours, practices related to breastfeeding,
and standing orders for hospital and office procedures.
Most medical practices catering to this generation of new
parents have websites describing their practice, including
forms and online appointment setting capabilities. Practices that accept new patients will usually be happy to provide you with brochures and business cards as well.

To assist your clients in finding the right provider for
them, you can suggest pertinent questions they can ask a
prospective caregiver. You may also use your information
about caregivers to help prepare mothers for their hospital experiences and pediatric check-ups. ("Dr. _____ usually tells mothers to _____ at the first check-up. You may
want to think about this before you go so that you can
have any questions or concerns ready.") An informed and
prepared mother is more likely to be satisfied with the
outcome of her visit. She can then better understand and
follow recommendations and is less apt to need to call the
caregiver for clarification.

∽ Summary

The lactation consultant can be instrumental in helping parents make and be satisfied with their decision to breastfeed. Parents are entitled to facts that will enable them to make informed choices. Teaching and counseling parents prenatally will help them acquire this information at a time when they are considering a method of infant feeding. As a lactation consultant, you can help couples distinguish between breastfeeding facts and possible misconceptions that may cause confusion or concern. Provide practical suggestions prenatally regarding breast care and preparations at home. Be available to expectant parents who may need assistance in selecting a caregiver who is knowledgeable and supportive of breastfeeding.

If appropriate to your job function, consider offering a series of classes on breastfeeding to give prospective parents relevant information at key times. An early prenatal class on infant feeding will help in the decision-making process. A later prenatal class on practical breastfeeding management helps parents prepare for their baby's arrival, whereas a postpartum breastfeeding class reinforces effective practices and address questions parents may have as they continue breastfeeding. All of these early interventions lay a strong foundation of support for parents as they approach the birth of their baby and the beginning of breastfeeding. Helping to establish early breastfeeding and countering negative influences within the parents' social environment empower parents and increase their confidence.

∽ Chapter 11—At a Glance

Facts you learned—

Deciding to breastfeed:

- The women who are most likely to breastfeed have the following characteristics: in their mid-thirties, middle income, college educated, white, and married.
- Statistically speaking, African American and teen mothers are least likely to breastfeed.
- More than half of all women make their infant feeding choices before pregnancy.
- Support from the baby's father is pivotal to the infant feeding decision.
- The attitude and knowledge level of caregivers greatly influences parents' decision and confidence in breastfeeding.
- Prenatal support and postpartum visits increase the likelihood of continuing breastfeeding.
- Modesty, privacy, work or school conflicts, lack of confidence, diet, stress, substance abuse, and inadequate sleep create barriers to breastfeeding.

- Commercial messages about formula imply that there is little difference between artificial milks and breastmilk.
- Sexual images of breasts distort their biological function.
- Aversion to breasts being touched is common in survivors of sexual or physical abuse.

Prenatal preparation for breastfeeding:

- The last trimester is the best time for manipulating flat or inverted nipples.
- Discourage prenatal nipple stimulation when a woman has a history of premature delivery, miscarriage, or false labor.
- Cosleeping with the baby can make early feedings easier.
- Confidence in and a good working relationship with the physician are important to parents.
- To ensure compatibility of their views, parents can ask about physicians' background, breastfeeding knowledge, hospital affiliation, accessibility, and standing orders regarding breastfeeding.

Applying what you learned—

- Encourage discussion by couples and sharing of information with fathers.
- Explain the risks of not breastfeeding.
- Point out the health, emotional, and financial benefits of breastfeeding.
- Explain the convenience of caring for other children and traveling when breastfeeding.
- Acquaint mothers with the realities of breast fullness, nipple tenderness, and the need to be available to the baby for nourishment.
- Offer ways to cope with concerns and to include the baby in the mother's activities.
- Dispel misconceptions and increase confidence in the mother's decision to breastfeed.
- Be aware of circumstances in which a mother may not breastfeed her baby.
- Discuss practical aspects of breastfeeding closer to baby's due date.
- Encourage expectant parents to attend prenatal breastfeeding classes.
- Discuss individual goals for breastfeeding, and give mothers information that will help them blend breastfeeding into their lives.
- Teach infant feeding classes, and keep the message simple in these classes.

- Teach parents to trust their instincts and to respond appropriately to their baby's cues.

- Actively involve parents in learning, and reinforce their retention of knowledge by using visual aids and multiple learning modalities.

- Encourage fathers to participate in breastfeeding classes.

- Demonstrate multiple options for feeding positions, and have parents practice with dolls.

- Teach parents how to know when the baby is receiving enough milk.

- Discuss the basis of supply and demand in milk production.

- Offer a support group with time for problem solving and prevention of common problems.

- Talk with mothers about planning a nursing area, choosing clothing that allows easy access for feedings, selecting a nursing bra (how and when to do so), and arranging for help at home.

- Encourage mothers to be open with their physicians about their breastfeeding.

- Develop a collaborative, mutually respectful relationship with the mother and her physician.

- When recommending physicians, give at least three names and information about their breastfeeding practices and standing orders.

∿ References

Amir L, Donath S. A systematic review of maternal obesity and breastfeeding intention, initiation and duration. Review. *BMC Pregnancy Childbirth.* 2007;7:9.

Anderson A, et al. Differential response to an exclusive breast-feeding peer counseling intervention: the role of ethnicity. *J Hum Lact.* 2007;23(1):16-23.

Avery A, et al. Confident commitment is a key factor for sustained breastfeeding. *Birth* 2009;36(2):141-148.

Bailey C, et al. A "give it a go" breast-feeding culture and early cessation among low-income mothers. *Midwifery.* 2004;20 (3):240-250.

Beal A, et al. Breastfeeding advice given to African American and white women by physicians and WIC counselors. *Public Health Rep.* 2003;118(4):368-376.

Bolton T, et al. Characteristics associated with longer breastfeeding duration: an analysis of a peer counseling support program. *J Hum Lact.* 2009;25(1):18-27.

Bonuck K, et al. Randomized, controlled trial of a prenatal and postnatal lactation consultant intervention on duration and intensity of breastfeeding up to 12 months. *Pediatrics.* 2005; 116(6):1413-1426.

Bryant C. Empowering women to breastfeed. *Int J Childbirth Education.* 1993;8:13-15.

Camurdan A, et al. How to achieve long-term breast-feeding: factors associated with early discontinuation. *Public Health Nutr.* 2008;11(11):1173-1179.

Chang J, Chan W. Analysis of factors associated with initiation and duration of breast-feeding: a study in Taitung, Taiwan. *Acta Paediatr Taiwan.* 2003;44(1):29-34.

Clifford J, McIntyre E. Who supports breastfeeding? *Breastfeed Rev.* 2008;16(2):9-19.

Declercq E. Hospital practices and women's likelihood of fulfilling their intention to exclusively breastfeed. *Am J Public Health.* 2009;99(5):929-935.

Delight E, et al. What do parents expect antenatally and do babies teach them? *Arch Dis Child.* 1991;66:1309-1314.

Donath SM, et al. Relationship between prenatal infant feeding intention and initiation and duration of breast feeding: a cohort study. *Acta Paediatr.* 2003;92:352-356.

Earle S. Why some women do not breast feed: bottle feeding and fathers' role. *Midwifery.* 2000;16(4):323-330.

Ekstrom A, et al. Breastfeeding support from partners and grandmothers: perceptions of Swedish women. *Birth.* 2003;30(4):261-266.

England L, et al. Breastfeeding practices in a cohort of inner-city women: the role of contraindications. *BMC Public Health.* 2003;3(1):28.

Fägerskiöld A. A change in life as experienced by first-time fathers. *Scand J Caring Sci.* 2008;22(1):64-71.

Falceto O. et al. Couples' relationships and breastfeeding: is there an association? *J Hum Lact.* 2004;20(1):46-55.

Forster D, et al. Factors associated with breastfeeding at six months postpartum in a group of Australian women. *Int Breastfeed J.* 2006;1:18.

Freed G, et al. Accuracy of expectant mothers' predictions of fathers' attitudes regarding breast-feeding. *J Fam Pract.* 1992;37:148-152.

Freed G, et al. Breast-feeding education and practice in family medicine. *J Fam Pract.* 1995a;40(3):263-269.

Freed G, et al. National assessment of physicians' breast-feeding knowledge, attitudes, training, and experience. *JAMA.* 1995b;273(6):472-476.

Freed G, et al. Pediatrician involvement in breast-feeding promotion: a national study of residents and practitioners. *Pediatrics.* 1995c;96(3 Pt 1):490-494.

Gamble D, Morse J. Fathers of breastfed infants: postponing and types of involvement. *JOGNN.* 1993;22:358-365.

Garfield C, Isacco A. Fathers and the well child visit. *Pediatrics.* 2006;117(4):e637-e645.

Gijsbers B, et al. Factors associated with the initiation of breastfeeding in asthmatic families: the attitude–social influence–self-efficacy model. *Breastfeed Med.* 2006;1(4):236-246.

Guise J, et al. The effectiveness of primary care-based interventions to promote breastfeeding: systematic evidence review and meta-analysis for the US Preventive Services Task Force. Review. *Ann Fam Med.* 2003;1(2):70-78.

Hale T. *Medications and Mothers' Milk.* 14th ed. Amarillo, TX: Hale Publishing; 2010.

Hall W, Hauck Y. Getting it right: Australian primiparas' views about breastfeeding: a quasi-experimental study. *Int J Nurs Stud.* 2007;44(5):786-795.

Harris M, et al. Breasts and breastfeeding: perspectives of women in the early months after birthing. *Breastfeed Rev.* 2003;11(3):21-29.

Hauck Y, et al. Prevalence, self-efficacy and perceptions of conflicting advice and self-management: effects of a breastfeeding journal. *J Adv Nurs.* 2007;57(3):306-317.

Hellings P, Howe C. Breastfeeding knowledge and practice of pediatric nurse practitioners. *J Pediatric Health Care.* 2004;18(1):8-14.

Hill G, et al. Breast-feeding intentions among low-income pregnant and lactating women. *Am J Health Behav.* 2008;32(2):125-136.

Hurley KM, et al. Variation in breastfeeding behaviours, perceptions, and experiences by race/ethnicity among a low-income statewide sample of Special Supplemental Nutrition Program for Women, Infants, and Children (WIC) participants in the United States. *Matern Child Nutr.* 2008;4(2):95-105.

Johnston B, et al. Expanding developmental and behavioral services for newborns in primary care: effects on parental well-being, practice, and satisfaction. *Am J Prev Med.* 2004;26(4):356-366.

Kendall-Tackett K. *The Hidden Feelings of Motherhood.* 2nd ed. Oakland, CA: New Harbinger; 2005.

Kendall-Tackett KA. Violence against women and the perinatal period: the impact of lifetime violence and abuse on pregnancy, postpartum, and breastfeeding. *Trauma Violence Abuse.* 2007;8(3):344-353.

Kimbro R. On-the-job moms: work and breastfeeding initiation and duration for a sample of low-income women. *MCN J.* 2006;10(1):19-26.

Kong S, Lee D. Factors influencing decision to breastfeed. *J Adv Nurs.* 2004;46(4):369-379.

Kools E, et al. The motivational determinants of breast-feeding: predictors for the continuation of breast-feeding. *Prev Med.* 2006;43(5):394-401.

Kumar V, et al. Effect of community-based behaviour change management on neonatal mortality in Shivgarh, Uttar Pradesh, India: a cluster-randomised controlled trial. Saksham Study Group. *Lancet.* 2008;372(9644):1151-1162.

Kuo S, et al. Community-based epidemiological study on breastfeeding and associated factors with respect to postpartum periods in Taiwan. *J Clin Nurs.* 2008;17:967-975.

Ladomenou F, et al. Risk factors related to intention to breast-feed, early weaning and suboptimal duration of breastfeeding [published online ahead of print September 10, 2007]. *Acta Paediatr.* 2007;96(10):1441-1444.

Lawrence R. *A Review of the Medical Contraindications to Breastfeeding.* Technical Information Bulletin. Washington, DC: National Center for Education in Maternal Child Health, U.S. Department of Health and Human Services; October 1997.

Léger-Leblanc G, Rioux F. Effect of a prenatal nutritional intervention program on initiation and duration of breastfeeding. *Can J Diet Pract Res.* 2008;69(2):101-105.

Littman H, et al. The decision to breastfeed. *Clin Pediatr.* 1994;33(4):214-219.

Lu M, et al. Provider encouragement of breast-feeding: evidence from a national survey. *Obstet Gynecol.* 2001;97(2):290-295.

Luopajärvi K, et al. Enhanced levels of cow's milk antibodies in infancy in children who develop type 1 diabetes later in childhood. *Pediatr Diabetes.* 2008;9(5):434-441.

McInnes R, Chambers J. Supporting breastfeeding mothers: qualitative synthesis. Review. *J Adv Nurs.* 2008;62(4):407-427.

Moore E, Coty M. Prenatal and postpartum focus groups with primiparas: breastfeeding attitudes, support, barriers, self-efficacy, and intention. *J Pediatr Health Care.* 2006;20(1):35-46.

National Center for Health Statistics (NCHS). Births: preliminary data for 2007. *National Vital Statistics Reports.* March 18, 2009;57(12). www.cdc.gov/nchs/data/nvsr57/nvsr57_12.pdf. Accessed April 1, 2009.

Newman J. How to know a healthcare practitioner is not supportive of breastfeeding, revised. 2008. www.nbci.ca. Accessed August 8, 2009.

Noble L, et al. Factors influencing initiation of breast-feeding among urban women. *Am J Perinatol.* 2003;20(8):477-483.

Otsuka K, et al. The relationship between breastfeeding self-efficacy and perceived insufficient milk among Japanese mothers. *JOGNN.* 2008;37(5):546-555.

Persad M, Mensinger J. Maternal breastfeeding attitudes: association with breastfeeding intent and socio-demographics among urban primiparas. *J Community Health.* 2008;33(2):53-60.

Power M, et al. The effort to increase breast-feeding: do obstetricians, in the forefront, need help? *J Reprod Med.* 2003;48(2):72-78.

Prentice J, et al. The association between reported childhood sexual abuse and breastfeeding initiation. *J Hum Lact.* 2002;3:219-226.

Pridham K. Anticipatory guidance of parents of new infants: potential contribution of the Internal Working Model construct. *Image.* 1993;25:49-56.

Rose V, et al. Factors influencing infant feeding method in an urban community. *J Natl Med Assoc.* 2004;96(3):325-331.

Rosen I, et al. Prenatal breastfeeding education and breastfeeding outcomes. *MCN Am J Matern Child Nurs.* 2008;33(5):315-319.

Ryan A, et al. Breastfeeding continues to increase into the new millennium. *Pediatrics.* 2002;110(6):1103-1109.

Saenz R. A lactation management rotation for family medicine residents. *J Hum Lact.* 2000;16(4):342-345.

Scott J, et al. Temporal changes in the determinants of breastfeeding initiation. *Birth.* 2006;33(1):37-45.

Semenic S, et al. Predictors of the duration of exclusive breastfeeding among first-time mothers. *Res Nurs Health.* 2008;31(5):428-441.

Shaker I, et al. Infant feeding attitudes of expectant parents: breastfeeding and formula feeding. *J Adv Nurs.* 2004;45(3):260-268.

Sharps P, et al. Health beliefs and parenting attitudes influence breastfeeding patterns among low-income African-American women. *J Perinatol.* 2003;23(5):414-419.

Shi L, et al. Breastfeeding in rural China: association between knowledge, attitudes, and practices. *J Hum Lact.* 2008;24(4):377-385.

Sikorski J, et al. Support for breastfeeding mothers (Cochrane Review). *Cochrane Database Syst Rev.* 2002;1:CD001141.

Spear H. Breastfeeding behaviors and experiences of adolescent mothers. *MCN Am J Matern Child Nurs.* 2006;31(2):106-113.

Sperlich M, Yeng J. *Survivor Moms: Women's Stories of Birthing, Mothering and Healing After Sexual Abuse.* Eugene, OR: Motherbaby Press; 2008.

Taveras E, et al. Mothers' and clinicians' perspectives on breastfeeding counseling during routine preventive visits. *Pediatrics.* 2004a;113(5):e405-e411.

Taveras E, et al. Opinions and practices of clinicians associated with continuation of exclusive breastfeeding. *Pediatrics.* 2004b;113(4):e283-e290.

Texas State Department of Health and Human Services (TSDHHS). Nutrition Services Section. *Breastfeeding and Returning to Work.* Stock no. 13-06-11496 rev. 10/08.

Austin, TX: TSDHHS; 2008. www.dshs.state.tx.us/wichd/WICCatalog/PDF_Links/13-06-11496%20Breastfeeding%20and%20working%20English.pdf. Accessed March 24, 2010.

Tiittanen M, et al. Dietary insulin as an immunogen and tolerogen. *Pediatr Allergy Immunol.* 2006;17(7):538-543.

Walker M. *Still Selling Out Mothers and Babies: Marketing of Breast Milk Substitutes in the USA.* Weston, MA: NABA REAL; 2007.

Wilhelm S, et al. Influence of intention and self-efficacy levels on duration of breastfeeding for Midwest rural mothers. *Appl Nurs Res.* 2008;21(3):123-130.

Yeoh B, et al. Factors influencing breastfeeding rates in southwestern Sydney. *J Paediatr Child Health.* 2007;43(4):249-255.

Hospital Practices That Support Breastfeeding

Throughout much of the world, childbirth occurs within a midwifery model of family-centered care, with families giving birth in birth centers or at home. Recognizing breastfeeding as a continuation of the normal birth process, these cultures respect women's ability to give birth and minimize labor "management." In contrast, women in much of the industrialized world give birth in hospitals, which vary in practices that support or hinder the establishment of breastfeeding. For women who give birth in a hospital, the hospital's practices directly influence their breastfeeding. An environment that is supportive and accepting builds the mother's self-confidence in her ability to breastfeed her newborn child. Institutional routines need to reflect a belief in breastfeeding as the norm and to facilitate sound breastfeeding care. Policies must be evidence based, rather than based on personal experience or tradition.

∾ Key Terms

Analgesia
Artificial teats
Baby-Friendly Hospital
    Initiative (BFHI)
Bonding
Cesarean section
Cluster feeding
Clutch hold
Combined spinal-epidural
    anesthesia (CSE)
Discharge planning
Duarte's variant
Edema
Epidural anesthesia
Episiotomy
Finger-feeding
Football hold
Forceps
Galactose
Hunger cues
Hydration
Induction
Interventions

Kangaroo care
Mother-to-mother
    support group
Narcotic analgesia
Natural childbirth
Nipple shield
Nonnutritive sucking
Patient-controlled
    epidural anesthesia
    (PCEA)
Phenylalanine
Phenylketonuria
Phototherapy
Red flags
Rooming-in
Self-appraisal tool
Side-sitting position
Spinal anesthesia
Supplementary feeding
Ten Steps to Successful
    Breastfeeding
Vacuum extraction
Vernix

∾ Setting the Stage Prior to Birth

A supportive birth environment empowers parents at a time when they are most vulnerable. New mothers thrive in a climate of acceptance for breastfeeding, as evidenced by supportive policies and healthcare professionals. Almost 99.5 percent of U.S. women deliver their babies in hospitals (National Center for Health Statistics [NCHS], 2010). These rates are comparable to those found in Canada (Statistics Canada, 2008) and most other industrialized countries. Trends are changing in some countries, however. For example, the home birth rate in England increased from 1.0 percent in 1989 to 2.7 percent in 2007 (Office of National Statistics [ONS], 2008). Approximately 30 percent of babies in the Netherlands are born at home (de Jonge et al., 2009).

The high percentage of hospital births, the fear of litigation (in the United States), and the fractured U.S. healthcare system make normal birth an almost impossible challenge for parents (Declercq et al., 2006, 2002). Empowering childbearing families is the focus of nonprofit initiatives such as the Coalition for Improving Maternity Services (www.motherfriendly.org) and the Childbirth Connection (www.childbirthconnection.org).

Women typically view their caregivers as authority figures and value their opinions because of their extensive training and experience. Not surprisingly, then, caregiver attitudes about breastfeeding greatly influence mothers' attitudes and, indirectly, the quality of their breastfeeding experiences (Kutlu et al., 2007; Nakar et al., 2007; Lebarere et al., 2005). A 2004 survey conducted by the American Academy of Pediatrics (AAP) found that pediatrician support for breastfeeding has declined since a similar survey was carried out in 1995 (Feldman-Winter et al., 2008). Overall, pediatricians were less likely to believe that the benefits of breastfeeding outweigh the difficulties or inconvenience, and fewer believed that almost all mothers are able to breastfeed successfully. In 2004, more pediatricians reported reasons to recommend against breastfeeding. Although better prepared to support breastfeeding, their attitudes and commitment seem to have deteriorated.

Supportive Breastfeeding Policies

Hospital practices that support breastfeeding are at the heart of the Baby-Friendly Hospital Initiative (BFHI), a program that is discussed in depth in Chapter 28. Developing hospital policies based on the Ten Steps to Successful Breastfeeding (World Health Organization [WHO]/United Nations Children's Fund [UNICEF], 1989) is the first step to providing this kind of supportive environment. The Ten Steps to Successful Breastfeeding (Figure 12.1) form the basis of breastfeeding promotion throughout the world. Using the Ten Steps protocol has an extended positive impact on breastfeeding rates in a hospital setting as well as continued breastfeeding duration (DiGirolamo et al., 2008; Abolyan, 2006; Hofvander, 2005; Merten et al., 2005).

Developing a set of breastfeeding policies based on current scientific knowledge can help eliminate unnecessary and intrusive interventions that negatively affect the initiation of breastfeeding. Such policies do not need to be extensive. In fact, staff will follow policies more closely if they are brief and cover only salient points. When given the opportunity to develop or review breastfeeding policies, seek to establish policies that decrease obstacles that might otherwise hamper smooth breastfeeding initiation. In addition, make sure that policies are communicated to all healthcare staff who encounter breastfeeding mothers and infants. This audience extends beyond the nursing staff on the mother–baby unit, to include physicians, ancillary staff, patient care technicians, and administrative staff of all units that care for mothers and babies. For example, staff in the neonatal intensive care unit (NICU), labor and delivery, pediatrics, and, to a certain extent, the emergency room and medical–surgical units all have contact with breastfeeding mothers. To ensure that they are supported in their breastfeeding decision, parents need to receive consistent, accurate, and positive messages from all hospital employees and volunteers.

Knowledgeable Staff

It is important to educate healthcare staff in how to implement breastfeeding policies. Understanding the rationale and scientific basis behind these policies may increase their acceptance by the medical and nursing staff. In addition, training these personnel in basic breastfeeding care frees the lactation consultant to concentrate on cases that are more difficult. Basic instruction should include positioning and latch, evaluating the quality of a feeding, and knowing when and how to supplement infants. It should also include teaching and initiating pumping for mothers when the baby is not able to breastfeed, as when the baby is in a special care nursery. Having knowledgeable staff helps ensure that mothers receive appropriate and consistent help when the lactation consultant is not available. See Chapter 26 for further discussion of staff education.

∾ Supportive Labor and Delivery Practices

A woman's labor and delivery experience can affect early breastfeeding and determine whether she continues with this feeding method. Unfortunately, it may prove difficult to initiate normal postpartum breastfeeding after intrusive labor and delivery practices. Policies that routinely separate mothers and babies interfere with breastfeeding and are not in the best interests of families.

Many nurses in obstetrics support the normal physiological process of birth (Romano & Lothian, 2008; Curl et al., 2004; Lothian, 2004). Historically, however, nurses (primarily female) have had little power in the hospital hierarchy, which has long been dominated by male physicians' power and influence (Manojlovich, 2007). Change in this power structure has come slowly, prompted by evidence-based research and consumer demand. Of course, consumers are unlikely to demand change until they achieve awareness of what they are not being given. A warm, reassuring, and caring atmosphere supports the

---

Every facility providing maternity services and care for newborn infants should:

1. Have a written breastfeeding policy that is routinely communicated to all healthcare staff.
2. Train all healthcare staff in skills necessary to implement this policy.
3. Inform all pregnant women about the benefits and management of breastfeeding.
4. Help mothers initiate breastfeeding within a half hour of birth.
5. Show mothers how to breastfeed and how to maintain lactation even if they should be separated from their infants.
6. Give newborn infants no food or drink other than breastmilk unless medically indicated.
7. Practice rooming in—allow mothers and infants to remain together 24 hours a day.
8. Encourage breastfeeding in response to feeding cues.
9. Give no artificial teats or pacifiers (also called dummies or soothers) to breastfeeding infants.
10. Foster the establishment of breastfeeding support groups and refer mothers to them on discharge from the hospital or clinic.

FIGURE 12.1   Ten Steps to Successful Breastfeeding.

Source: World Health Organization (WHO/UNICEF). *Protecting, Promoting, and Supporting Breastfeeding: A Joint WHO/UNICEF Statement.* Geneva, Switzerland, WHO; 1989.

parents' goals and helps them develop self-confidence to make appropriate decisions concerning their baby.

Provide Labor Support

Women who receive support during labor are more likely to be breastfeeding at 6 weeks than are those who receive no support (Nommsen-Rivers et al., 2009). Ideally, hospitals will encourage women to have an experienced labor support person, often referred to as a doula, with them throughout the entire labor and delivery. Acceptance of doulas may vary depending on the hospital's philosophy of birth management. Doula help is associated with fewer medications, less anesthesia, and fewer complications. Babies are more alert and responsive after an unmedicated birth, which is a much more likely outcome when the mother has doula support. Alert and responsive babies, in turn, are better able to breastfeed within 1 to 2 hours after birth.

The presence of a doula during labor and birth provides the laboring woman with continuous physical, emotional, and informational support. The doula does not replace the baby's father or other support person chosen by the mother from her family or friends, but rather enhances the mother's support system. She is experienced in the use of comfort measures that will decrease the pain of labor without the use of medications or anesthesia. She provides ongoing support in a manner different from the baby's father.

Studies show that the presence of a doula results in fewer interventions for both mother and baby. Doula support can reduce the cesarean rate by 50 percent, labor length by 25 percent, Pitocin use by 40 percent, pain medication use by 30 percent, the need for forceps by 40 percent, and requests for epidural anesthesia by 60 percent (Klaus et al., 1992). These findings are supported by later studies that reveal significantly shorter length of labor, greater cervical dilation when epidural anesthesia is used, and higher Apgar scores at both 1 and 5 minutes after birth (Campbell et al., 2006). As documented in Table 12.1, a study in Mexico found that doula support lowered the cesarean rate, the average length of labor, and the use of epidurals and Pitocin (Trueba et al., 2000). Bruggemann and colleagues (2007) found that the presence of a companion of choice increased the mother's satisfaction with the birth and did not interfere with neonatal outcome or breastfeeding.

Limit Interventions

The use of medications, anesthesia, and other interventions during labor and birth can affect early breastfeeding and influence whether a baby is breastfed for a long period. Achieving normal and optimal postpartum breastfeeding management can be difficult after a labor and

TABLE 12.1 Outcome Differences with Doula Support

	Doula Supported	Not Doula Supported	Reduction (%)
Use of Pitocin	21 (42%)	48 (96%)	129%
Use of epidurals	4 (8%)	16 (32%)	300%
Mean labor length	14.5 hours. (±5.36)	19.38 hours (±7.3)	34%
Cesarean birth	1 (2%)	12 (24%)	1100%

Source: Adapted from Trueba G, et al. Alternative strategy to decrease cesarean section: support by doulas during labor. *J Perinat Educ.* 2000;9(2):8–13. Available at: http://www.pubmedcentral.nih.gov/articlerender.fcgi?artid=1595013&rendertype=table&id=tbl1. Printed with permission of Lamaze International.

delivery that involves intervention. Any policy that routinely and unnecessarily separates a mother from her baby interferes with breastfeeding and contradicts good medical care.

Nonessential Routine Interventions

Between 1975 and 1982, the United States experienced the peak of the "natural childbirth" movement. During that same period, breastfeeding initiation rates increased from approximately 25 percent to 62 percent. This span was followed by more than 2 decades during which birth interventions increased by more than 50 percent—interventions such as medications, epidural anesthesia, IVs, electronic fetal monitors, and cardiac monitors. Not surprisingly, in the same period, breastfeeding initiation declined from 62 percent to 51 percent.

Labor and birth, while normal biological processes, are not treated as such in most U.S. hospitals. Events that surround birth have a clear impact on breastfeeding (Smith, 2009). U.S. hospitals have increasingly come to rely on technology as a strategy to reduce litigation and decrease costs. As a consequence, there has been an unprecedented rise in the scheduling of births, including elective inductions and elective cesarean sections. In an ironic twist, women's fear of pain and loss of control during birth have resulted in a true loss of control for them during the childbirth experience. The cascade of events that begins with induction for dubious reasons (e.g., low amniotic fluid or a large baby) frequently ends in hours of stalled labor, an unplanned cesarean surgery, and a baby who does not feed effectively (Smith, 2007).

Limiting unnecessary technology surrounding their baby's birth helps parents get breastfeeding off to a good start. Taking this approach requires parents to educate themselves and advocate for their needs. Ideally, mothers should have the opportunity and assistance to put the baby to breast within 1 hour of birth unless there is a clearly identifiable medical reason for delaying the first feeding.

Elective Cesarean Section

The increased incidence of elective cesarean sections is especially troubling, especially in terms of the ethics of surgically removing a baby based on maternal request rather than medical necessity. Cesarean surgery increases the risk of neonatal death by 69 percent (MacDorman et al., 2008), maternal death by 100 percent (Clark et al., 2008), and postpartum stroke by 67 percent (Lin et al., 2008). The American College of Obstetrics and Gynecology (ACOG, 2008) has not taken a stand against this practice, but offers an equivocal opinion statement.

Despite the marked trend toward higher numbers of elective cesarean sections, there has been no improvement in perinatal mortality or morbidity with these deliveries. Much of the medical literature and media imply that consumer demand is driving this trend, although McCourt and colleagues (2007) assert that research between 2000 and 2005 actually shows evidence that only a very small number of women request a cesarean section. Rather, women's preference for a cesarean section appears to be influenced by cultural or social factors, or psychological factors such as perceptions of safety.

Another analysis of the increase in the rate of cesarean sections suggests that the power imbalance has shifted in favor of physicians, to the detriment of patients (Gamble et al., 2007). This imbalance of power and positional authority is particularly notable in terms of the care provided to economically disadvantaged women, teen mothers, or immigrants, many of whom do not speak English. These women typically have little or no power, and are bewildered and overwhelmed by the American approach to birth.

Studies using magnetic resonance imaging (MRI) on mothers delivering vaginally compared to mothers delivering surgically have revealed significantly different brain responses to their babies' cries. These findings suggest that mothers who deliver their children vaginally are more sensitive to their own baby's cry than mothers who deliver their children via cesarean section in terms of their sensory processing, empathy, arousal, motivation, reward, and habit-regulation circuits (Swain et al., 2008).

Interventions Used in Labor

Frequent and routine medical intervention during labor increases the risk of interference with breastfeeding. Many of these interventions result from the overuse of central nervous system depressants and epidural anesthesia. Women need to be empowered to birth their babies without the use of medications and anesthesia, and they should be given the cultural and emotional support to do so.

This complex issue needs to be addressed with young women long before pregnancy and childbirth, if we hope to ever recreate a culture of normalcy in a world of high-tech birth. Complications resulting from interventions tend to "normalize the abnormal" and lead to high volumes of sleepy, lethargic babies who cannot suck or feed robustly. Medications the mother receives during labor may cause her newborn to become drowsy and to have difficulty sucking (Hale, 2010). They may also make the mother less responsive to her baby. Optimally, expectant mothers would learn about those techniques and drugs that are least likely to interfere with breastfeeding, such as the use of support persons, walking, showers, bathing, birthing balls, and other comfort measures.

The issue of pain relief during labor is complex. An understanding of the medications a mother received during labor is an essential part of the lactation consultant's history-taking process. This issue is especially important when you encounter infants who are not sucking or who have other feeding difficulties. Analgesia dulls or reduces the sensation of pain but does not block total sensation. Anesthesia deadens the nerve, removing all sensation. The three types of anesthesia commonly used in labor and delivery are epidurals, spinals, and general anesthesia. Mothers may also receive combined spinal-epidural anesthesia (CSE).

Pitocin Pitocin is the trade name for oxytocin, the hormone excreted endogenously during labor. Pitocin, when used to induce or stimulate labor, has an antidiuretic effect. Edema may result from Pitocin use, particularly in extremities such as the breast and nipple tissue. The result can be "meaty" and "flat" nipples that make it difficult for the infant to latch until the edema is relieved. It can take as long as 2 weeks for the edema to resolve. To help soften the areolae and assist their babies in latching effectively, mothers can perform reverse pressure softening (RPS), a technique discussed further in Chapter 21 (Cotterman, 2004).

Clinicians have noted edema in women who receive many liters of IV fluids in conjunction with epidurals and Pitocin. These women often experience a delay in lactogenesis II, perhaps due to an overload of edema in the breast. Figure 12.2 shows severe edema in a mother's ankles and feet.

Concern has been expressed about what effect flooding the body with exogenous versus endogenous oxytocin might have on a woman acquiring the maternal role. Research shows that the more intravenous epidural analgesia received during labor, the lower the endogenous oxytocin measured during breastfeeding on the second day postpartum (Jonas et al., 2009). Interestingly, prolactin levels rose sooner in mothers receiving oxytocin infusion. Breastfeeding is associated with lower maternal stress hormone levels (adrenocorticotropic and cortisol).

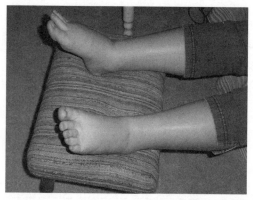

FIGURE 12.2 Edema resulting from excessive fluids.
Source: Printed with permission of Anna Swisher.

However, one study found higher cortisol levels in mothers who had epidural anesthesia and Pitocin (Handlin, 2009).

Analgesia Some mothers may receive analgesia such as nalbuphine, alphaprodine, butorphanol, and meperidine to "take the edge off" their labor pain. In recent years, these systemic medications have become less popular with the increased use of epidural anesthesia (discussed in the next subsection). Typically, a mother may receive systemic analgesia until she has dilated to 4 or 5 centimeters and can receive an epidural.

Pain relief medications diminish early sucking (Riordan et al., 2000). Consequently, mothers who receive such medications during labor are more likely to leave the hospital without having established breastfeeding. Mizuno and colleagues (2004a) demonstrated that sucking behavior during the early newborn period affects both breastfeeding initiation rate and duration. Thus any practice that delays early sucking can have long-lasting consequences.

Epidural Anesthesia Epidural anesthesia numbs the body from a certain point—for labor, optimally from the uterus down. There is usually a complete loss of sensation. To deliver this medication, a needle is passed through the ligamentum flavum (the bands that cover the spinal canal) and into the epidural space just outside the dura mater (the membrane surrounding the spinal cord). Anesthetic drugs such as morphine, fentanyl, or sufentanil are injected and a catheter is placed for additional infusion (American Society of Anesthesiologists [ASA], 2007). Patient-controlled epidural anesthesia (PCEA) is a newer pain management option in which the patient self-delivers a set amount of medicine. Self-administration has been associated with lower dosages and reduced hypotension (VanZandt, 2005).

Epidurals are used in both vaginal and cesarean section births. In recent years, the use of epidural anesthesia

has escalated in the United States and elsewhere. There were 4.3 million U.S. births in 2007 (NCHS, 2010), with an estimated 2.4 million women receiving epidural anesthesia during labor (Ruppen et al., 2006). Epidurals are perceived as easy, fast, and lucrative, which explains why they have become the labor pain management tool of choice (Macarthur & Ostheimer, 2008). Patients (and caregivers) often count the minutes until the birthing mother can receive her epidural. Unfortunately, epidurals can also affect breastfeeding ability, either directly through the medication (Hale & Hartmann, 2007) or through the chain of events triggered by anesthesia use. Table 12.2 presents extrapolated complications of epidural anesthesia.

A 2005 Cochrane Review found that epidural analgesia is associated with a 38 percent increased risk of instrumental delivery (forceps or vacuum) compared to opiate analgesia (Anim-Somuah et al., 2005). According to the findings from this meta-analysis, epidurals also increase the length of labor by an average of 25 minutes, and they lead to increased use of oxytocin.

A prospective cohort study found that epidurals using fentanyl (a powerful opioid) and type of birth were associated with partial breastfeeding and breastfeeding difficulties in the first week after birth. Mothers who received epidural anesthesia were more likely to stop breastfeeding than those who used nonpharmacological methods of pain relief (Torvaldsen et al., 2006). Other findings suggest that a dose-dependent response exists between fentanyl and artificial feeding (Jordan et al., 2005). The impaired sucking seen in these infants may constitute an "adverse drug reaction" for clinicians to consider (Jordan, 2006). Given this potential for complications women need to learn about the potential consequences of opioid use and other intrapartum medications.

A retrospective study of 351 mother–infant dyads found that significantly fewer babies of mothers receiving epidurals nursed within the first 4 hours of life. These babies were more often also given artificial milk during their hospital stay and fewer were fully breastfed at discharge (Wiklund et al., 2009). Another study refuted these findings, however, stating that "There is no good evidence that epidural analgesia causes reduced breastfeeding success" (Devroe et al., 2009).

Mothers who receive epidurals during labor have increased incidents of fever as well. Fernández-Guisasola and colleagues (2005) found that tests to rule out sepsis were ordered for 85 percent of the infants of mothers with fever after epidural analgesia. In such circumstances, the baby may receive antibiotics prophylactically or even be transferred to the NICU.

Spinal Anesthesia Spinal anesthesia, another common type of anesthesia used in deliveries, is typically administered during cesarean sections. A needle is passed through the dura mater into the cerebrospinal fluid (CSF), and an

TABLE 12.2   Complications of Epidural Anesthesia

Outcome	United States	Canada	United Kingdom	France	Switzerland
Births per year	4,019,280	330,000	646,000	761,464	72,905
Epidural rate, percentage of births	59	45	35	51	40
Number of injuries per country per year					
Epidural hematoma	13	1	1	2	0.2
Deep epidural infection	22	1	2	4	0.3
Persistent neurologic injury	9	1	1	2	0.1
Transient neurologic injury	603	50	98	114	11

For individual countries, information is from:

United States:

Service USDoHH: U.S. birth rate reaches record low. Available at: http://pregnancyabout.com/gi/dynamic/offsitehtm?site=http://wwwhhsgov/news/press/200. Accessed October 1, 2005.

Declercq E, Sakala C, Corry M, Applebaum S, Risher P: Listening to mothers: Report of the First National U.S. Survey of Women's Childbearing Experiences. Available at: www.maternitywise.org/pdfs/LtMreportpdf.2002.3pres/20030625html. Accessed October 1, 2005.

Canada:

Information CIfH: A regional profile, Giving Birth in Canada. 2005. Available at: http://dsp-psd.pwgsc.gc.ca/Collection/H118-22-2004E.pdf. Accessed October 1, 2005.

United Kingdom:

UNICEF: UNICEF Website UK. 2003. Available at: http://www.unicef.org/infobycountry/uk_statistics.html. Accessed October 1, 2005.

Markus Schneider, M.D., Professor, Universitäts-Frauenklinik Basel, Departement Anästhesie, Basel, Switzerland, personal communication by electronic mail, June 2005.

France:

France in facts and figures. 2005. Available at: http://www.insee.fr/en/ffc/chifcle_fiche.asp?ref_id=NATTEF02133&tab_id=237. Accessed October 1, 2005.

Switzerland:

Bundesamt für Statistik. Statistik Schweiz: Birth rate Switzerland 2002. 2004. Available at: http://www.bfs.admin.ch/bfs/portal/de/index/themen/bevoelkerung/stand_u_struktur/blank/kennzahlen0/natuerliche_bevoelkerungsbewegung/geburten.html. Accessed October 1, 2005.

Markus Schneider, M.D., personal communication by electronic mail, June 2005. Basel approximately 43 percent; Geneva about 80 percent. Forty percent is assumed.

Source: Ruppen W, et al. Incidence of epidural hematoma, infection, and neurologic injury in obstetric patients with epidural analgesia/anesthesia. *Anesthesiology.* 2006;105:394-399. http://journals.lww.com/anesthesiology/_layouts/oaks.journals/ImageView.aspx?k=anesthesiology:2006:08000:00023&i=TT2. Copyright © 2006, American Society of Anesthesiologists. Reprinted by permission of Wolters Kluwer Health and Dr. Wilhelm Ruppen.

anesthetic such as bupivacaine and a narcotic such as fentanyl are injected. From a technical perspective, spinal anesthesia is a stronger block than epidural anesthesia, is more evenly distributed, is easier to administer, and has a quicker onset of action. Nevertheless, this medication carries a risk of lowering the mother's blood pressure, which can distress the baby. There is also a higher incidence of nausea and vomiting, and a shorter duration of anesthesia. Complications can include a "high" spinal, affecting the mother's ability to breathe, cough, and swallow as well as loss of arm movement. A "total" spinal, in which the anesthesia extends into the brain stem, paralyzes the diaphragm and causes severe bradycardia, even cardiac arrest. The patient may remain conscious, blink, and move her lips, but is paralyzed. The medical team must then administer general anesthesia to intubate the patient.

Combined Spinal-Epidural Anesthesia Combined spinal-epidural (CSE) anesthesia is sometimes called a "walking epidural." It involves placing a needle into the epidural space, followed by passage of another, small-gauge needle into the spinal space. Smaller amounts of the drugs are required for this procedure. After the initial injection, a catheter is placed into the epidural space for additional drug administration (Camann & Alexander, 2006). CSE causes very rapid numbing, but the legs may maintain sensation, enabling the mother to walk and move during labor. The mother can still feel to push if the CSE is given in the late labor stages.

Hale and Hartmann's Textbook of Human Lactation (2007) provides a comprehensive, in-depth discussion of analgesic and anesthetic medications, including how they work and what effects they have on the mother and infant. It is important for you as a lactation consultant to be knowledgeable about pain management practices, even if you do not work in a hospital setting. Learning about labor medications and other interventions should become part of your detective work in helping mothers identify and overcome feeding difficulties after leaving the hospital.

Interventions Used During Delivery

Some routine medical intervention during delivery may increase the risk of breastfeeding difficulties. Episiotomies and mechanical devices are used to assist delivery. Interventions after delivery include suctioning and removing the baby from the mother before she has an opportunity to nurse her baby.

Episiotomy An episiotomy is a surgical incision through the perineum to enlarge the vaginal opening during delivery. This procedure increases the risk of a fourth-degree laceration—namely, a tear through the rectal mucosa. Women who have had an episiotomy often find it difficult to get comfortable, particularly when they sit upright. If the mother is uncomfortable sitting, it is difficult for her to relax enough to position the baby well at the breast. Although postpartum medications used to relieve this discomfort, such as hydrocodone and ibuprofen, pass through the mother's milk, they are approved for use in breastfeeding mothers by the AAP. It may reassure the mother to learn that because milk intake is low in the first few days, her baby will not be exposed to large quantities of these medicines if she needs to take them (Hale, 2010).

Suctioning In a vaginal birth, fluids in the baby's nose and mouth are normally squeezed out by labor and birth. In a cesarean birth, the baby needs some extra help and typically will have the nose and mouth suctioned to remove the fluids. Suctioning may also be necessary after a quick delivery. Hospital staff may be inclined to put a baby to the breast as a soothing measure immediately after deep suctioning. Unfortunately, this practice can cause some babies to appear to associate breastfeeding with the discomfort that preceded their first experience at the breast and react negatively whenever brought near the breast.

Mechanical Devices Complications with delivery can result in the use of forceps or vacuum extraction to help remove the baby from the womb. Forceps and vacuum extraction both carry increased risk of bruising, injury, and sensitivity to the infant's head. Such damage limits the positions in which the newborn will be comfortable when nursing. Bruising also increases the risk of jaundice, which can cause sleepiness and a lack of interest in feeding (Smith, 2007). Hospital lactation consultants have noted increased chomping and inability to suck in babies who have been subjected to forceps and vacuum extractions.

Removing the Baby to a Radiant Warmer Babies are placed in radiant warmers after delivery because of an inability to self-regulate their temperatures. Warmers are usually unnecessary, however, when a mother and baby remain together. Babies who are snuggled skin-to-skin with their mothers kangaroo-style ("kangaroo care") warm faster, stay warm longer, and have less risk of dehydration than babies placed under radiant warmers. Walters and colleagues (2007) found that skin temperature rose during kangaroo care in 8 of 9 infants, and temperature remained within a neutral thermal zone for all babies.

Skin-to-skin care has proved effective in reducing the risk of hypothermia as compared to conventional incubator care for infants weighing 1200 to 2199 grams (McCall et al., 2008). Skin-to-skin contact allows for adequate temperature maintenance without increased fluid loss. When the infant's nose is near the mother's skin, he or she breathes warm, humidified air, rather than dry hospital air. The heat from the mother's body is humid, unlike the dry air from artificial warmers.

Many studies support the benefits of skin-to-skin contact. A Cochrane Review of 30 studies found statistically significant and positive effects of early skin-to-skin contact on breastfeeding at 1 to 4 months postpartum. In particular, there were positive trends for maternal attachment behavior and affectionate touch during breastfeeding. Babies cried for a shorter length of time, and late preterm infants had better cardiorespiratory stability with early skin-to-skin care. No adverse effects were found from this practice (Moore et al., 2007).

A review of 17 other studies correlates skin-to-skin care with increased breastfeeding duration, maintenance of infant temperature, reduced infant crying, stable blood glucose levels, and expressions of maternal love and touch (Anderson et al., 2003). Furthermore, skin-to-skin contact for more than 50 minutes immediately after birth results in enhanced infant recognition of the mother's milk odor as well as longer breastfeeding duration (Mizuno et al., 2004b). Chapter 23 provides further discussion of skin-to-skin (kangaroo) care.

Delayed First Breastfeeding A delay of more than 6 hours before the first feeding is a factor in shorter breastfeeding duration than the mother intended (Chaves et al., 2007). The longer a mother waits to initiate breastfeeding, the more likely she will be to feed her baby infant formula in the first few days of life, and the more likely the hospital staff will be to give formula. Standard routines that delay breastfeeding for more than an hour after birth include weighing, measuring, bathing, warming, dressing, and wrapping the baby. Treatments include administration of antibiotic eye drops, vitamin K shot, hepatitis B shot (the first vaccination), and, frequently, pre-feeding blood glucose sticks.

Supplementing large for gestational age (LGA) babies is also common. In reality, these babies are at higher risk for diabetes, possibly triggered by early bovine protein exposure (Luopajärvi et al., 2008). Babies who are born by cesarean section and separated from their mothers are also frequently given formula as a first feeding. The labor and delivery staff can preserve and protect breastfeeding by avoiding these types of practices, which can hinder subsequent breastfeeding.

Promote Bonding Immediately After Birth

Ideally, parents will spend the initial moments after delivery with their baby engaged in hugging, smiling, loving, and nursing. They will flourish in their transition to parenthood in a supportive environment that enables them to begin their new family in privacy. After leaving the comfortable secure confines of the mother's womb, the newborn enters an unfamiliar and perhaps unsettling environment. When placed in the comfort of the mother's arms, the newborn responds to the warmth of her body and her familiar smell by nuzzling at her breast.

Infants are attuned to their mothers' smell, and it is believed that even the odor of the mother's milk reduces pain response (Nishitani et al., 2009). Research also has shown that a newborn prefers the mother's unwashed breast to a washed breast (Varendi et al., 1994). It may be that the infant actually locates the nipple through a pheromone-like effect rather than smell. An auxiliary olfactory sense organ, the vomeronasal organ (VNO) located in the bottom of the nasal cavity, detects pheromones. Perhaps this detection process—rather than the mother's scent—enables an infant to recognize and locate the nipple.

Bonding between the mother and her baby is strongest in the first 1 or 2 hours after birth. Skin-to-skin contact enhances bonding even further (Handlin, 2009; Charpak et al., 2005; Kennell & McGrath, 2005; Sinusas & Gagliardi, 2001). A newborn's rooting and sucking reflexes are particularly strong in the first hours following an unmedicated delivery. Placing the baby prone on the mother's reclined body in skin-to-skin contact has been shown to elicit newborn feeding behaviors (Colson et al., 2008). (Chapter 14 provides more discussion of these behaviors and the post-birth approach to care.) The mother's normal body bacteria will colonize her baby's body—but only

if she is the first person to hold the child, rather than a nurse, physician, or other caregiver. Keeping the mother and baby together will accomplish this immunoprotective goal.

Soon after birth, staff will observe and assess the baby and assign an Apgar score, which ranges from 0 to 10 (see Table 12.3). The Apgar score assigns up to 2 points each for heart rate, respiratory effort, body tone, grimace, and color. The score indicates the newborn's overall state of health and assists caregivers in determining if any intervention is necessary. It is performed at 1 minute of life and again at 5 and 10 minutes. This process need not interfere with bonding, as staff can perform the assessment while the mother holds her baby. The gestational age of the baby will also be determined using the Ballard score to evaluate neuromuscular and physical development (see Chapter 13).

U.S. state laws require treatment of all newborn infants' eyes with an antibiotic to safeguard against the effects of sexually transmitted disease. Staff can delay this procedure to allow the parents and baby at least 1 hour of uninterrupted time together. Postponing antibiotic treatment of the baby's eyes allows eye contact and enhances bonding between the parents and baby.

The Bonding Process

The term "bonding" was popularized in the classic book *Maternal–Infant Bonding* (Klaus & Kennell, 1982) and later in *Bonding: Building the Foundations of Secure Attachment and Independence* (Klaus et al., 2000). Bonding describes the close physical contact between the mother and baby soon after birth. Routine hospital practices that delay contact following birth, strict feeding schedules, and separation from the baby all discourage the development of attachment. This separation also delays acquisition of the parental role (see Chapter 19). The most favorable time to initiate bonding is in the first minutes after birth, when the baby is alert and the parents are most eager to see and touch their new child (Kennell & McGrath, 2005).

TABLE 12.3 APGAR Score

Five factors are used to evaluate the baby's condition and each factor is scored on a scale of 0 to 2, with 2 being the best score.

1. Activity and muscle tone
2. Pulse (heart rate)
3. Grimace response (medically known as "reflex irritability")
4. Appearance (skin coloration)
5. Respiration (breathing rate and effort)

The process of bonding begins with the first parent–infant contact in the hours following birth and continues as parent and infant interact to form a unique, lasting relationship. This close emotional tie develops through exchanging messages and feelings with all five senses—sight, touch, smell, taste, and sound. Parents often express attachment through touching, fondling, talking to, and kissing their babies while holding them face to face. Babies reciprocate through recognizing and responding to the parents' overtures. They smile, follow their parents' image with their eyes, and show signs of contentment and acceptance. The skin and eye contact, the pattern of the parent speaking, the baby responding, and other interchanges are essential to building a loving relationship. Time spent together soon after birth encourages affectionate contact between parent and child throughout the child's formative years.

The Positive Results of Bonding

Extended infant contact with the mother beyond regular feeding times during the first 3 days of life results in behavioral and developmental advantages during the child's early years (Klaus & Kennell, 1982). Mothers with extended contact, compared to limited early contact, show a higher incidence of breastfeeding and are more responsive to their children, with more fondling and face-to-face contact. At 3 months postpartum, these mothers perceived their adaptation to their infants to be easier. They expressed fewer problems with nighttime feedings, despite these feedings lasting almost twice as long as those in the control group, who did not have early extended contact. When observed during a 10-minute play period at 3 months of age, early-contact babies and mothers smiled and faced one another more. At 5 years, these children had significantly higher IQs and better-developed skills.

Paternal Bonding

Bonding encompasses the affectionate attachment of both mother and father to their newborn infant. Fathers who touch, fondle, and talk to their newborn babies form close emotional ties. The father's involvement with his baby promotes positive feelings about the birth experience as well, and strengthens the father's paternal role and family bonding (Pestvenidze & Bohrer, 2007). Fathers can experience a hormonal response to their babies' cries, as evidenced by a rise in their prolactin and testosterone levels (Muller et al., 2009; Gray et al., 2006, 2007). In addition, they are more responsive to infant cues than are nonfathers (Fleming et al., 2002). A father's fascination with his baby can mix with some jealousy about the more intimate relationship between the mother and her breastfeeding baby. Bonding and the building of

love for the baby helps the father adjust to new family relationships.

Help Mothers Initiate Breastfeeding

The duration of breastfeeding is higher for mothers who breastfeed immediately after giving birth (Merten et al., 2005). Initiating breastfeeding as early as possible confers many health advantages, in addition to assuring longer breastfeeding duration. For example, the increased oxytocin secretion from suckling contracts the uterus more quickly and controls bleeding immediately after delivery. Digestion of colostrum clears meconium from the baby's gut and provides immunological protection. Delaying the first bath until after the first breastfeeding allows the vernix to soak into the baby's skin, lubricating and protecting it. It also prevents temperature loss that could interfere with the first breastfeeding.

Routine use of synthetic oxytocin is not necessary when mothers breastfeed immediately after delivery. In fact, giving the mother additional Pitocin after delivery contributes to edema, which is associated with latch problems and delayed onset of milk production. Pitocin may be given prophylactically in U.S. hospitals without the mother's knowledge unless she knows to refuse it and has gained her physician's concurrence. She will need to include this refusal in her birth plan and be sure to remind the attendants.

Helping mothers maintain hydration during labor can support their early breastfeeding. Dehydration can deplete a woman's energy, which in turn may have a subtle impact on her birth and early feedings. Policies should allow women to labor in any position they choose, rather than requiring that women labor while lying down, which can produce more difficulty during second-stage labor because gravity is not assisting her. Following a difficult second stage and delivery, she could then experience further difficulty with the initiation of breastfeeding.

Let the Baby Lead the Way

It is unnecessary—and sometimes counterproductive—to rush or compel babies to breastfeed. A better approach is to leave a mother and her unwrapped baby together until they are ready to breastfeed. A warmed blanket placed over both of them will prevent heat loss. When left with their mothers quietly in skin-to-skin contact, babies typically will work through pre-feeding behaviors such as bringing their hands to their mouth, making sucking motions, and nuzzling and licking the breast (Righard, 2008). This is an optimal time to teach parents about hunger cues and encourage mothers to respond to them. See Chapter 13 for a discussion of infant hunger cues.

A classic study carried out in 1987, and then repeated in 1990, showed that unmedicated babies who remained undisturbed on their mother's abdomen accomplished breastfeeding on their own. They crawled up the mother's abdomen, searched out the nipple, latch, and sucked—all within about 1 hour of birth. In contrast, babies who were left with their mothers for 20 minutes and then removed to be bathed, suctioned, and have other procedures done had a great deal of difficulty remembering what to do (Righard & Alade, 1990; Widstrom et al., 1987). Research on biological nurturing also corroborates these observations (Colson et al., 2008).

Help with the First Breastfeeding

Birth attendants can help this natural process by placing the baby in skin-to-skin contact with the mother's abdomen or chest immediately after birth and covering mother and baby together with a warm blanket. The mother can make the breast available to allow the newborn to lick and explore the breast. The mother can initiate the rooting reflex by gently stroking her baby's mouth area with her nipple. In response, her baby will turn toward the nipple and open his or her mouth. A caregiver can be available to help with attachment if the baby wishes to breastfeed and has not started spontaneously within 1 hour. Mothers are who moved to a different room for the rest of their postpartum care should remain with their babies during transport to allow this continued contact.

Breastfeeding After a Cesarean Delivery

Cesarean delivery does not preclude early breastfeeding. A mother who delivers surgically can breastfeed as soon as she is in recovery. If the mother received general anesthesia during the course of the cesarean section, she may breastfeed as soon as she is awake and able to respond.

Cesarean sections increase the risk of supplemented breastfeeding in the hospital (as do lack of information about the importance of breastfeeding and not rooming-in. In turn, supplemented breastfeeding during hospital stay was the major factor associated with not breastfeeding at 1 month of age in one recent study (Asole et al., 2009). In another study, LATCH scores for mothers who underwent cesarean sections averaged 6.27 for the first breastfeeding and 8.81 for the third breastfeeding, out of a maximum possible score of 10. Scores averaged 7.46 for the first breastfeeding and 9.70 for the third feeding in mothers who delivered vaginally (Cakmak & Kuguoglu, 2007).

It is important to remain flexible in approaching each mother–infant dyad. What is comfortable for one postoperative mother may not be comfortable for another. Mothers who deliver by cesarean section often find it difficult to achieve a comfortable position for breastfeeding. Especially when dealing with breastfeeding after a cesarean, be open to new and inventive ways to help the baby settle at the breast. It is also important to be sensitive to the mother's emotional condition and to determine how much intervention she can tolerate. She has been through major trauma, and may be hearing only how "lucky" she is to have a "healthy baby." Research is beginning to recognize that post-traumatic stress disorder may occur after difficult births, although this understanding has not yet been translated into maternity-centered care in the United States (Beck, 2009; Beck & Watson, 2008; Alder et al., 2006).

Lying on her side with her baby lying next to her may help the mother avoid incision pain in the first hours. It also permits breastfeeding even if the mother's head must remain down because she received spinal anesthesia. She can place pillows behind her back and under her top knee to support her abdomen. Another possible reclining position is for the mother to lie on her back with the baby placed on top of her.

When the mother breastfeeds in a sitting position, she can place a pillow over the surgical incision to cushion it from the pressure of the baby's body. Pillows placed under her knees will provide further support if she is sitting in bed. Another useful position is with the baby along the side of her body with the arm closest to the breast, tucking her baby under her arm (side-sitting position, also known as a clutch hold or football hold).

A positive experience with initiating breastfeeding can help to normalize the postpartum experience for mothers who may feel a sense of failure or disappointment that they did not give birth vaginally. Putting the baby in skin-to-skin contact and encouraging closeness can assist the mother in connecting with her baby.

～ Creating a Supportive Postpartum Environment

Treating women as individuals and understanding their lifestyle and previous experiences regarding breastfeeding and parenting facilitates their learning. Parents are able to relax more when they have realistic expectations for the early days of breastfeeding. Although breastfeeding is instinctive by nature, it often requires learning and practice to accomplish. Especially in the early hours and days after childbirth, encourage mothers to be flexible and patient. Gentle humor can be relaxing.

First-time breastfeeding mothers are novices, as are their babies. They need time and patience to adjust to each other's idiosyncrasies as they learn to work together as a team. Although the mother may feel awkward and clumsy at times, in an accepting atmosphere her awkwardness will not deter her from continuing. A relaxed and supportive climate encourages a mother to seek help and laugh at any missteps as she and her baby learn together.

Taking time to instruct the mother and showing a willingness to listen to her concerns demonstrate the importance of breastfeeding. This emphasis encourages her to put forth extra effort to continue, ultimately making your role as a lactation consultant easier and more rewarding. Quality time spent instructing each mother is rewarded tenfold through her assuming responsibility for her baby's care and for her decisions. Your efforts in teaching and supporting the mother will help her reach her breastfeeding goals.

Eliminate Negative and Unnecessary Practices

Routines that inhibit interaction, practices that imply possible failure, and ineffective problem solving can all influence breastfeeding over both the short and long term. Such questionable practices often stem from tradition and misinformation. With some exceptions, the degree of knowledge regarding breastfeeding care is relatively low among the general population of nurses and physicians (Brodribb et al., 2008, 2009; Leavitt et al., 2009). As a consequence, their breastfeeding advice may derive from personal experience or misconceptions rather than being rooted in fact-based information. In the absence of sound knowledge of breastfeeding practices, erroneous and incorrect advice can lead to a bumpy start for the mother and baby.

Limit Interruptions

Limiting unnecessary interruptions during the mother's postpartum stay is a positive contribution to breastfeeding. All too often, hospital routines and procedures require continual interruptions from people entering the mother's room at any hour of the day or night. Morrison and colleagues (2006) reported an average of 54 interruptions (phone and in person) to the breastfeeding dyad on the first day postpartum. The mother's obstetrician will visit her daily to check on her progress. The pediatrician may come to her room to examine her baby or to report to her daily about her baby's progress. The nurse will enter her room periodically throughout the day and night to check her baby, monitor her temperature and blood pressure, examine any incisions and IV, check her uterus and breasts, provide medications and snacks, fill her water pitcher, and change her bed linens. These visits could occur as frequently as every hour.

Dietary personnel will bring meals. Housekeeping personnel will clean and empty trash. A photographer may stop by to take pictures. Someone will come for information for the birth certificate and billing. Other interruptions may occur from maintenance, media services, volunteer services, and clergy—not to mention friends and relatives who visit. Moreover, these interruptions are doubled if the woman shares her room with another new mother!

Encouraging mothers to request that visitors wait until the family goes home will help mothers get the rest they need. It also allows more time for teaching the mother about infant care and breastfeeding.

Avoid Babies Crying in the Nursery

Some hospitals still have centralized nurseries where nursing staff cares for babies most of the 24 hours, particularly at night. It is common for several babies to be crying in the nursery at any given time. "The belief that newborn infants need to cry is not true" (Anderson, 1989). In healthy full-term infants, an adequate functional reserve is present in the lungs after the first breath. The lungs have expanded as fully at 30 minutes post-birth as they are 24 hours later. Crying raises infants' levels of cortisol, a stress hormone. Continually elevated stress hormone levels are believed to contribute to infant illness (Mörelius et al., 2009; Shah et al., 2006).

Newborns who self-regulate their care by remaining with their mothers cry less than those whose care is controlled externally by hospital staff. In the first hour after birth, newborns in Anderson's (1989) classic study whose feedings were time controlled cried for 10 minutes and startled 12 times. They cried for 38 minutes during the first 4 hours after birth. In contrast, babies who self-regulated their care cried less than 1 minute in the first hour after birth and did not startle. They cried only 2 minutes during the first 4 hours after birth. Sucking pressures were 4 times as strong and blood pressure averaged 10 mm Hg lower than in the self-regulated infants compared to the babies who were under time-controlled care (Anderson, 1989). In addition, blood glucose levels stay higher when babies do not cry. Crying uses up glycogen stores, which results in a drop in glucose levels (Mazurek et al., 1999; Aono et al., 1993).

Place No Restrictions on Feedings

Breastfeeding-friendly health care imposes no rules or restrictions on feedings. Most hospitals state that they encourage breastfeeding in response to hunger cues. In reality, however, babies who remain in the nursery for most of the day customarily feed every 3 or 4 hours or when they cry. Feeding a baby on a rigid schedule or ignoring the child's natural hunger cues does not help the mother learn how to respond to those cues. It often does not allow the baby to begin feeding before he or she is frantic. Additionally, delayed or rigidly scheduled feedings slow milk production and increase the risk of breast engorgement. Perhaps not surprisingly, a Cochrane Review of three trials including 400 mother–infant dyads found that restricted feeding was associated with weaning by 4 to 6 weeks. It also found an increased incidence of sore nipples, engorgement, and the need to give supplemental formula feeds (Renfrew et al., 2000).

There is an increase in the incidence of jaundice and hypoglycemia in infants when feedings are limited (Johnson et al., 2009; Academy of Breastfeeding Medicine [ABM], 2006; Bhutani & Johnson, 2006). Clinicians refer to this effect as "lack of breastfeeding jaundice," indicating that the jaundice is a result of breastfeeding mismanagement. If the mother finds herself governed by a rigid schedule, she may not be breastfeeding often enough to stimulate milk production or satisfy her baby. Prenatal anticipatory guidance includes encouraging expectant parents to determine the hospital's infant feeding policy prior to delivery and to negotiate changes if needed. Baby-friendly hospitals place no rules or restrictions on feedings and keep babies with their mothers.

Give No Unnecessary Supplements

Babies often unnecessarily receive artificial formula or water to supplement colostrum because of a misconception that colostrum is insufficient for total nourishment. The only time breastfeeding babies should receive any type of supplement is for a specific medical need such as hypoglycemia, weight loss of 10 percent or more, signs of dehydration, prematurity, or lethargy. When a supplement is needed, the first choice should be the mother's colostrum. Chapter 21 describes the process of teaching hand expression to mothers.

Infants who are given supplements are at increased risk for early termination of breastfeeding (Asole et al., 2009; Pincombe et al., 2008; Chezem et al., 2003). Clear evidence indicates that breastfeeding infants do not need supplemental water (De Carvalho, 1981). Newborns who breastfeed frequently from birth, at least every 2 to 3 hours or in response to hunger cues, never need water and seldom need an artificial substitute. For this reason, routine use of glucose water or formula for breastfeeding babies should be discouraged. In addition, formula use can prime a child for development of long-term allergies. It also implies to the mother that her milk alone is not sufficient, which undermines her confidence in her ability to provide adequate nourishment for her baby (Li et al., 2008). In one study, mothers who intended to exclusively breastfeed, but whose babies were supplemented in the hospital, were less likely to do so by 1 week postpartum (Declercq et al., 2009). Even in a baby-friendly hospital, supplementation occurred 33 percent of the time—yet only 9 percent of these supplementations were found to be medically justified (Meirelles et al., 2008).

When there is a medical need for supplementation, a mother should never receive formula to give her baby without specific instructions. Staff should never send a mother home with vague instructions regarding supplementation such as "give the baby some formula after every feeding." She needs specific instructions, such as "Feed your baby 15 mL ($\frac{1}{2}$ oz) of formula after each time you breastfeed until you go to the clinic the day after tomorrow." The mother also needs to be taught how to bottle feed correctly (see Chapter 21 for more information on teaching paced bottle feeding). Such instructions give the mother specific guidelines and reassures her that supplementation, although it may be necessary at the moment, will not last long. In the absence of this guidance, she could fall into the trap of supplementing from the start and never establish full milk production.

Acceptable Medical Reasons for Supplements In light of the many risks associated with artificial baby milks, it is important to note that on rare occasions some babies will be unable to breastfeed. For the vast majority of babies, human milk is their normal and expected source of nourishment and protection. At the same time, it is crucial to understand situations in which a baby needs a supplement—either expressed mother's milk, donor human milk, or artificial baby milk. In some rare situations, breastfeeding must be avoided altogether. The 2005 AAP statement says that untreated active tuberculosis, human immunodeficiency virus (HIV)–positive status of the mother, use of a small number of drugs (mostly cancer chemotherapy agents), and use of illegal drugs contraindicate breastfeeding. Infection of the mother with human T-lymphotrophic virus 1 (HTLV-1) is usually a contraindication to breastfeeding as well (AAP, 2005).

The debate regarding preterm infants and their nutritional needs (discussed in Chapter 9) may continue for some time. Preterm infants who weigh as much as 1850 grams often receive human milk fortifiers. Babies who experience hypoglycemia that does not improve through increased breastfeeding need to receive additional human milk by an alternative means such as cup, dropper, or spoon until breastfeeding is established. If a baby is treated with phototherapy for jaundice, supplementation may be required. Because jaundice makes babies sleepy, the mother may need to pump her milk in such circumstances. If she cannot express enough milk, and if the institution does not provide donor milk, formula will be needed for calories and fluids.

Babies with certain inborn errors of metabolism, such as phenylketonuria (PKU), need supplementation of a low-phenylalanine formula in addition to breastmilk. Infants with galactosemia are unable to breastfeed (Ohura et al., 2007; Leung & Sauve, 2005; Thompson et al., 2003), except in the case of a form of galactosemia known as Duarte's variant. In the setting of this disease, it is possible to breastfeed, although the baby's galactose levels must be monitored carefully, with some nondairy formula probably provided (Ono et al., 1999; Ganesan, 1997). Galactosemia is discussed in detail in Chapter 25.

Sometimes a baby may be able to breastfeed, but the mother cannot. If the mother experiences a severe medical condition—such as psychosis, eclampsia, hemorrhage, or shock—her caregiver may delay breastfeeding or expressing milk. Advice to HIV-positive mothers in countries with sanitary conditions and a safe water supply is to not breastfeed (see Chapter 25), although they can express and heat-treat their milk to give to their infants. A mother who needs certain medications—such as cytotoxic, radioactive, or some antithyroid (other than propylthiouracil) drugs—will be unable to breastfeed while the drug remains in her body at a level that would harm the baby. This may necessitate temporary interruption of breastfeeding while the mother expresses her milk to maintain milk production. The mother might choose to wean and feed her baby donor milk or infant formula (WHO/UNICEF, 1993).

Give No Artificial Teats to Infants

Bottle use in the hospital is associated with shorter duration of exclusive breastfeeding and shorter overall breastfeeding duration (Rodriguez-Garcia & Acosta-Ramirez 2008). A baby sucks differently on an artificial nipple than on the breast. Consequently, the use of bottles and pacifiers appears to cause confusion for some babies. While some babies may not be confused when given an artificial nipple, they may prefer the smaller, longer, rigid latex or silicone nipple that fits in their mouth like their fingers.

Breastfeeding-friendly practices avoid the use of bottles unless there is a medical need for supplements. If a medical need for supplementary feedings arises, the mother can use a method other than a bottle and artificial nipple to feed her baby (see the discussion on alternative feeding methods in Chapter 21). If the mother is not rooming in with her baby, she can ask that the staff bring her baby to her when the child is hungry and at frequent intervals. She can also instruct the nursery to bring her baby to her during the night for feedings, which minimizes the possibility of others feeding the baby when separated.

Bottle feeding of preterm infants is a complex issue. A Cochrane Review found that although cup feeding significantly decreased "no breastfeeding or only partial breastfeeding" on discharge, it significantly increased the length of hospital stay (by 10 days). There was also a high degree of noncompliance in the largest study focusing on this issue. The one trial of tube feeding alone significantly reduced the number of "no breastfeeding or only partial breastfeeding" cases (Collins et al., 2008). A multidisciplinary approach is needed for these babies, in which occupational therapists, speech language therapists, lactation consultants, and other clinicians may use bottles as therapeutic transitional tools. See Chapter 23 for detailed discussion of the preterm infant.

A recent meta-analysis of studies from 1980 to 2006 found that the use of pacifiers was associated with shorter duration of breastfeeding (Karabulut et al., 2009). Kron-

borg and Vaeth (2009) found that pacifier use had an independent negative effect on the duration of breastfeeding. In contrast, O'Connor and colleagues (2009) found no correlation between pacifier use and shortened breastfeeding despite numerous observational studies; they suggested that this association may reflect breastfeeding difficulties or intent to wean.

Use Nipple Shields Wisely

A nipple shield is an artificial silicone nipple that is placed over the mother's nipple during breastfeeding (see Chapter 21). Nipple shields are available at retail stores, and many mothers buy them on their own. Some bring them to the hospital on the advice of friends or relatives who used them. Hospital personnel may give a mother a nipple shield to protect a sore nipple or to help the baby pull out a nipple that is difficult to grasp. Use of a nipple shield is usually not the first intervention recommended for nipple soreness, however. Sore nipples usually occur due to poor positioning, which the mother needs help correcting.

A nipple shield can be an effective tool when used appropriately (Chertok, 2009, 2006; Powers & Tapia, 2004; Meier et al., 2000; Wilson-Clay, 1996). If you sense a mother is fragile and overwhelmed, a nipple shield can buy some time to work with the baby before the stressed mother gives a bottle. When it is used, appropriate follow-up care by a lactation consultant is desirable, if the baby does not transition to breastfeeding easily without the shield.

Promote Practices That Support Breastfeeding

A strong set of supportive protocols enables the mother and baby to establish breastfeeding smoothly. Breastfeeding-friendly practices encourage the mother to be with her infant as much as possible; they transmit a belief in her ability to breastfeed and provide sound principles of breastfeeding care. As part of these practices, mothers and babies should remain together from the moment of birth, followed by rooming-in for the remainder of the hospital stay.

Encourage Rooming-in

Rooming-in is a component of family-centered maternity care that is a standard practice or option in most hospitals (see Figure 12.3). Parents may need to make prior arrangements for this accommodation if private rooms are not standard. Rooming-in provides maximum opportunity for the parents and infant to interact. Keeping the baby with the parents increases their self-confidence in handling their baby. Both parents can learn to diaper, clean, burp, and hold their baby. They can learn to recognize hunger cues, and the mother can feed her baby as frequently as the infant desires. It is also reassuring for the parents to have

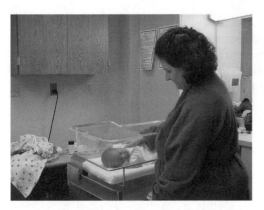

FIGURE 12.3 Mother and baby rooming in.
Source: Printed with permission of Anna Swisher.

their baby close, rather than in the nursery where they cannot see and respond to him or her. Encourage rooming-in as soon as a mother can care for her baby. If the mother had a cesarean birth, having a support person stay with her facilitates earlier rooming-in.

Variations in Rooming-in Policies The types of rooming-in arrangements vary from one hospital to another, although most hospitals in the United States now provide for rooming-in. This practice helps parents learn to care for their baby, and it reduces staffing needs. Expectant parents need to learn which rooming-in options are available to them, either through childbirth education classes or from their prenatal care providers. They can then locate a hospital that will meet their needs.

The 24-hour rooming-in option allows the baby to stay with the mother at all times. Some hospitals allow the baby to remain with the mother during the day except when she is sleeping or showering, during which the baby is taken to the nursery. Other hospitals require that the baby be taken to the nursery during visiting hours. Flexible rooming-in permits the mother to have her baby in her room and take her baby to the nursery if the need arises.

Many mothers find that flexible rooming-in, beginning from the moment of birth, is the most desirable arrangement. It offers new parents the chance to get acquainted with their baby and to learn childcare before assuming sole responsibility for caregiving at home. It also allows parents with older children an opportunity to get to know their new baby before returning home and dividing their time between the new baby and their other children.

Benefits of Rooming-in to Breastfeeding Hospital practices alone do not determine how long breastfeeding will continue. Nevertheless, there is clear evidence of a correlation between rooming-in and longer breastfeeding

duration (Bystrova et al., 2007; Merten et al., 2005). Positive breastfeeding results occur with rooming-in, especially when the mother receives guidance in infant feeding. Parents who know their babies' abilities are better able to notice them. Indeed, rooming-in offers physical and emotional benefits to the entire family: It allows for bonding and quick relief of fussiness and hunger and incorporates the baby into the family unit immediately after birth. The frequent feedings made possible by this arrangement encourage early milk production.

Mothers who care for their babies throughout the day and night in the hospital are more likely to have babies who are better breastfeeders. Optimal feeding occurs when the baby gives cues such as mouthing and hand-to-mouth activity. Rooming-in enables mothers to recognize and respond to their babies' hunger cues (Winberg, 2005). Thus babies who room in have more frequent feedings and greater weight gain. Because rooming-in promotes caregiver response, the baby experiences less crying and movement, thereby conserving energy (Braarud & Stormak, 2006). Such babies have less disorganized cries, startle less frequently, and feed more often than babies who are cared for in central nurseries.

Keeping mothers and babies together during their hospital stay promotes learning and enhances the mother's self-efficacy. In this supportive environment, she learns hunger cues and breastfeeding techniques in a setting where she can have her questions answered and her techniques evaluated. Additionally, mothers are able to provide antibodies to the microbes in the vicinity. If a baby remains in a nursery with its set of pathogens, the mother's milk will not reflect this.

Teach Mothers Hunger Cues

The ideal feeding pattern allows the baby to nurse whenever the infant demonstrates hunger cues, which in turn enables breastfeeding to get off to a good start. This practice ensures the early establishment of milk production through frequent breast stimulation and milk removal. Feeding in response to hunger cues also encourages bonding between the mother and baby and helps to avoid milk stasis, which can lead to problems such as breast engorgement or plugged ducts. There is a clear relationship between this type of responsive behavior and the establishment of sound breastfeeding practices.

Hospital policies that support responding to the baby will help mothers learn to recognize their babies' hunger cues. Newborns become hungry every $1\frac{1}{2}$ to 3 hours, and sometimes sooner. They may feed every 1 to $1\frac{1}{2}$ hours for 3 or 4 times in a row, and then sleep for 4 or 5 hours. To determine whether feedings are adequate, observing the number of feedings in 24 hours rather than timed intervals between feedings is easier for mothers.

Help mothers recognize that babies go to the breast for many reasons other than hunger. For example, infants may be uncomfortable and need to suck to relieve the discomfort. They may need to pass gas or have a bowel movement. They may simply want the nurturing comfort of the breast. Mothers sometimes worry that they do not have enough milk if their infants want to go to the breast frequently. It is important to help them understand how to know the baby is getting enough to eat and that nurturing at the breast is an important component of breastfeeding.

Frequent feedings day and night encourage early milk production and decrease uncomfortable breast fullness. Breastfeeding during the nighttime is essential for establishing milk production, and mothers need to respond to hunger cues at that time as well. A baby who wakes during the night needs to be breastfed—not offered pacifiers, water, or an artificial substitute. Many nursing mothers make up missed sleep by napping during the early postpartum period before they return to work or school.

Make sure parents understand that cue-based feeding does not mean responding to the baby's cries. Most babies show hunger cues (see Chapter 13) such as mouthing and hand-to-mouth activity for up to 30 minutes prior to engaging in sustained crying (Anderson, 1989). Babies who have been crying have difficulty breastfeeding because they are unable to organize themselves to focus on feeding. Crying compromises and disorganizes their suck, and their sucking strength drops. Recognizing that a baby's cry is a means of communication rather than manipulation will help parents understand that their baby's cry is signaling a need (Sears, 2009). Urge parents to watch for hunger cues before the baby progresses to crying.

Show Mothers How to Breastfeed

Nurses often cite lack of time as a barrier to providing adequate assistance to new mothers. This is a valid concern, especially in the era of managed care, staffing shortages, and minimal staff–patient coverage ratios. Although the problem is acute in the United States, staffing issues are found in other countries as well. Dykes (2005) found that the needs of breastfeeding women for emotional, esteem, informational, and practical support go largely unmet due to time constraints imposed on healthcare providers. These results call into question whether the hospital is the best place and space within which women should commence their breastfeeding journey.

The initial time taken by the maternity staff to ensure early breastfeeding initiation will help the mother establish sound breastfeeding practices. This investment, in turn, helps avoid difficulties later, which might require more time to be spent on problem solving. Every breast-feeding mother should receive basic instruction in day-to-day breastfeeding matters. A knowledgeable caregiver optimally will be present for the first feeding to assist, observe technique, and answer questions. Some mothers may require no help beyond that.

A breastfeeding mother has an important need for privacy during feedings, in a place that is quiet and where she and her baby can be uninterrupted. Mothers who are separated from their infants need special assistance with establishing milk production. They need to pump 8 to 12 times in a 24-hour period with a hospital-quality pump. Make sure they know where to obtain a pump and understand milk storage requirements, especially NICU storage protocols.

Some infants may have difficulty in their initial feeding attempts; others may latch and begin to suckle immediately. Many newborns sleep most of the time. It is common for a baby born in the hospital to show little interest in nursing in the first few attempts. It is also common for a baby to nurse regularly and eagerly on the first day and then appear sleepy or fussy on the second day postpartum. Make sure parents know these variations are all temporary and normal. Help them approach this time as an opportunity to practice their parenting skills and become acquainted with their baby.

A baby may lose as much as 10 percent of his or her birth weight during the first week after delivery. Generally, babies regain birth weight by 10 days to 2 weeks of life. It is important that the mother be aware of this pattern so that the initial weight loss does not concern her. A baby who has unrestricted access to the breast may experience little or no weight loss. When breastfeeding is going well, it is not uncommon for the baby to regain birth weight within 7 to 10 days after birth.

Teach Breast Care

Teaching mothers appropriate breast care will help them minimize the discomfort of nipple soreness. Healthy skin contains sufficient moisture to keep it soft and pliable. The nipples require no treatment unless they are tender or sore. In fact, a healthy nipple needs no special attention other than observing practices that will preserve the health of the skin. Primary among these practices is making sure the mother positions the baby to facilitate a good latch. Expressing a drop or two of colostrum and gently rubbing it into the nipple and areola after feeding will help with any initial tenderness.

Provide Effective Discharge Planning

Today's short hospital stays leave caregivers with little time for assessing breastfeeding knowledge, teaching basic techniques, and evaluating the mother–infant dyad for effective feeding. Internet sites, DVDs, and simple visual handouts can help to bridge this gap. At discharge, help the mother plan realistically to meet both the baby's and her own needs when she returns home. Although some mothers will have help at home for several days from relatives or friends, or through a postpartum doula service, the majority of mothers in the United States manage on their own.

Prior to hospital discharge, the postpartum nursing staff must ensure that the mother understands how to breastfeed and how to assess her baby's needs. Many women begin breastfeeding with no prior reading or instruction. Some may not even decide to breastfeed until after the baby arrives. Do not assume a mother will automatically know what to do, even if she has previously learned about breastfeeding. Once she is caring for her baby, a review of breastfeeding techniques will help her relate to the information more readily than she did before the baby arrived. The postpartum period is a time in a mother's parenting experience when she is eager to listen and learn what to do—a teachable moment.

Observing the mother and baby breastfeed on the day of discharge will provide a final opportunity to evaluate the mother's understanding of breastfeeding technique before she takes her baby home. It is also important that parents know how to tell when their baby is receiving sufficient nourishment at the breast. Given that worry about not having enough milk is the primary reason for supplementing with formula and for early weaning, teaching mothers the signs that the baby is transferring milk will allay their doubts about their ability to breastfeed. (Chapter 16 describes the signs of adequate milk production.)

Mothers need to leave the hospital with contact information for available resources, including local lactation consultants, breastfeeding support groups, and breast pump rental, if necessary. If concerns about potential feeding issues exist, the baby's caregiver needs to be informed and the mother needs to agree to a feeding plan that addresses the concerns. The mother will also need to schedule an appointment for her baby to be checked for weight and skin color. Many hospitals document the scheduling of this appointment by parents before discharge.

Refer Mothers to Resources for Support

Given that 24- to 48-hour stays for childbirth are the norm in most U.S. hospitals, breastfeeding families need resources for ongoing support. Most women find the first 2 to 6 weeks with a new baby to be the most difficult. A mother who is unfamiliar with typical newborn behavior may not know what to expect. Concerns related to sleep, crying, and sucking needs often are associated with breastfeeding because of its unique nature. Providing anticipatory guidance regarding these normal concerns will help prepare mothers for their occurrence. Because parents receive so much information in the hospital, they will benefit from having someone to call when concerns or questions arise.

Support encompasses more than providing necessary information and education. When women have identified qualitative aspects of the support they receive, the need for "sensitive individualized care" has ranked high on their lists of priorities (Sheehan et al., 2009). Learning about typical patterns of feeding and breastfeeding milestones will help a mother know what to expect, help to prevent problems, and aid her in continuing to breastfeed for as long as she desires. Mothers also need to learn about the risks associated with the use of infant formula and pacifiers (Karabulut et al., 2009; Kronborg & Vaeth, 2009; Dewey et al., 2003).

The Ten Steps to Successful Breastfeeding state that mothers should be referred to breastfeeding support groups. Online groups, breastfeeding forums, and Internet "breastfeeding cafes" are newer avenues for seeking ongoing breastfeeding support. As a lactation consultant, you may wish to compile a list of recommended sites for parents. Check the Web addresses frequently, as they often change. The mother may qualify for the local WIC program, so include WIC guidelines and contact numbers in your resource list. One-on-one peer support programs are also helpful (U.S. Preventive Services Task Force [USPSTF], 2008). If there are no local breastfeeding support groups, it would be advantageous for a hospital to develop its own.

A "warmline" can provide support to mothers after they go home. When mothers receive early contact and telephone follow-up from knowledgeable caregivers, the duration of breastfeeding significantly increases (Dennis & Kingston, 2008). In particular, mothers benefit from a follow-up telephone call made approximately 2 days after discharge. The baby should optimally have a weight and color check within 48 hours of discharge. Some hospitals provide this service only when markers for concern are noted at the time of discharge, such as weight loss of more than 10 percent of birth weight or early onset of jaundice. Other hospitals have no postdischarge services and simply refer the family to their community healthcare provider.

Mothers with insurance coverage can check whether their insurance plan includes a home health visit. If a mother qualifies, she may be able to arrange a home visit with the public health department. One study found that home health visits provided positive outcomes; only 6 percent of babies whose mothers received these kinds of visits had difficulties breastfeeding, compared to 34 percent of the group who did not receive visits (Mannan et al., 2008).

∾ Postpartum Care Plans

To provide continuity of care, postpartum staff need a clear understanding of breastfeeding technique. An informed staff can give breastfeeding mothers the tools that will enable them to breastfeed successfully at home. As a lactation consultant, you can assist the staff in developing a care plan that efficiently utilizes their time and talents. Make sure they know the signs to look for during a feeding that indicate breastfeeding is going well. A key sign in the baby is long drawing sucking, which indicates milk transfer; swallowing will not necessarily be audible. Signs in the mother include uterine cramping, thirstiness, and sleepiness—all of which indicate that the mother's milk is letting down. These indicators should all be observable by 2 or 3 days postpartum.

The AAP recommends that a breastfeeding be observed at least once every 8 hours during the hospital stay. In hospitals where lactation consultants see all breastfeeding mothers, at least one observation each day can be made by a lactation consultant. In some hospitals, lactation consultants see only first-time mothers; in other hospitals, they see only those patients referred by a nurse or physician. Lactation consultants can train staff to ensure that those who observe breastfeedings know what to look for and how to help with technique.

A 48-hour hospital stay leaves little time for teaching breastfeeding before the mother is discharged. Legislation passed in 1996 requires health insurance companies in the United States to cover 48-hour maternity hospital stays (Bradley, 1996). However, some hospitals have only a 24-hour stay as the norm for a vaginal delivery unless there are markers for concern, such as the mother testing positive for Group B strep or the baby not voiding or stooling.

Establishment of a care plan for breastfeeding during a 48-hour hospital stay will ensure that each hospital shift has assigned responsibilities to get breastfeeding off to the best possible start. Coordination of care and instruction helps ensure that families receive the information they need. Care plans should cover all areas in which the mother and baby receive care, beginning with labor and delivery and continuing through postpartum care. To assist in the development of such plans, the Academy of Breastfeeding Medicine provides evidence-based model protocols for peripartum breastfeeding management for the healthy mother and term infant (ABM, 2008), and for a model hospital breastfeeding policy (ABM, 2003).

Care Plan for a 48-Hour Hospital Stay

A 48-hour stay allows hospital staff numerous opportunities to observe and help mothers with breastfeeding. It permits teaching to be divided into several segments to avoid overwhelming the mother at any one time. Mothers have 2 days to practice breastfeeding with the support of knowledgeable staff, who can help them work through any difficulties prior to discharge.

Labor and Delivery

After delivery, a mother can learn about positioning her baby for the first feeding. Show the mother the hunger cues her baby is exhibiting at this time. A baby who is not interested in feeding can remain with the mother in skin-to-skin contact. Keep the room quiet, dim the lights, and reduce stimulation. Delay visitors for at least 1 hour to allow the parents quiet time alone with their baby.

Hours 1–8

Review positioning with the mother and stress the importance of a good latch. Observe a breastfeeding and point out to the mother the difference between nutritive sucking and nonnutritive sucking. Review hunger cues (see Chapter 13), and put the baby to the breast based on these cues. Keep the baby with the mother. Make the parents aware that their newborn may feed only once or several times during the first 8 hours of life.

If the baby has not fed at all by 6 to 8 hours post-birth, have the mother begin expressing milk by pump or manual expression. Hospitals usually have protocols for the length of time they will allow a baby to go without feeding before supplementing. If your hospital does not have a current protocol on supplementation, you may want to initiate adoption of the Academy of Breastfeeding Medicine's protocol on the use of supplementary feedings in the healthy term breastfed neonate (ABM, 2009).

Hours 9–16

Review basic nutrition with the mother, advising her to eat a normal healthy diet and to drink when she is thirsty. The baby should breastfeed 2 or more times during the next 8 hours. If the baby is not breastfeeding, teach the mother hand expression. Have the mother feed her expressed milk with an alternative feeding method such as a spoon, syringe, or finger-feeding. Review risk factors for breastfeeding problems (see Figure 12.4) and take appropriate action.

Hours 17–24

During hours 17–24 after birth, the mother should be able to demonstrate effective positioning and latch. Observe a feeding and ask the mother to point out nutritive and nonnutritive sucking. The baby should breastfeed 2 or more times during this period, with at least 6 feedings in the first 24 hours. If the infant is still not latching effectively, the mother should continue to express her milk 2 or 3 times during the shift and feed the milk to the baby.

Some issues have more of a negative impact on lactation than others. These issues have been set in bold.

In general, the more checkmarks the dyad has, the greater the risk they are for lactation problems or failure.[1]

If an issue that is set in bold or multiple issues are checked, it is suggested that the dyad be seen by lactation within 1–3 days of discharge.

Risk factors with which mother presents:

no breast changes with the pregnancy[2]

thyroid or pituitary problems[3]

breast abnormalities, e.g., hypoplastic breasts, wide angle, tubular, marked asymmetry[4,5]

prior lactation failure(s)[6]

flat or inverted nipples[7]

diabetic mother[8]

hypertension, essential or PIH[9]

eclampsia, preclampsia[10,11,12]

antenatal administration of betamethasone[13]

PCOS/other infertility problems[14,15]

maternal obesity (BMI > 29)[16,17,18,19,20,21]

adolescent mother[22,23,24]

advanced maternal age[25,26,27,28]

first time mother[29,30]

psycho/social stress/problems, e.g., depression, lack of support for breastfeeding[31,32]

smoking[33,34,35]

breast surgery or trauma including radiation[36,37]

states intention to both breast and bottle feed

states early intention to return to work[38]

Risk factors mother acquires while in the hospital:

stressful labor or delivery[39]

unscheduled C-section[40,41]

separated from her infant(s)[42,43]

delivery for multiples[44,45]

persistent sore nipples[46]

edema of extremities, therefore also of nipple/areolar complex[47,48]

Sheehan's syndrome[49]

anemia[50,51]

no signs of milk "coming in" by 72 hours[52]

breast pump dependent at the time of discharge[53]

Date: _____

Patient's Name _____

LC's Name _____

Risk factors with which the infant is born:

male infant[54,55,56,57]

stressful delivery[58]

birthed after a long running epidural[59,60]

one of a multiple[61]

oral anatomical abnormalities, e.g., tongue tie, clefts, macroglossia[62,63,64]

neurologic problems, e.g., Downs, hypotonia, hypertonia[65]

preterm[66,67]

born at 34 weeks gestation

born at 35 weeks gestation[68,69]

born at 36 weeks gestation

born at 37 weeks gestation

SGA or LGA[70,71]

Risk factors the infant acquires while in the hospital:

less than 2 hours of skin-to-skin with mother immediately after delivery[72,73,74]

separated from his mother, e.g., mother needed to rest without infant, septic work-up, blood work[75,76]

medical problems, e.g., jaundice, hypoglycemia, respiratory problems[77]

inadequate caloric intake[78]

using a pacifier[79,80,81]

requires a special feeding plan[82]

using a feeding device, e.g., nipple shield, SNS at the time of discharge[83]

weight loss of more than 7% on the 3rd day of life[84,85]

inability/refusal to latch to the breast and transfer breastmilk at the time of discharge[86]

receiving supplementation

been supplemented with an artificial bottle nipple more than 3 times[87]

getting less than 9 cc per feeding from the breast at 60 hours of life[88]

effective breastfeeding not established at time of discharge[89]

discharged from hospital in less than 48 hours[90]

1. Hurst NM. Recognizing and treating delayed or failed lactogenesis II. *J Midwifery Women's Health*. 2007;52(6):588–594.

2. Neifert M, et al. The influence of breast surgery, breast appearance, and pregnancy-induced breast changes on lactation sufficiency as measured by infant's weight gain. *Birth*. 1990;17:31–38.

3. Hapon MB, et al. Effect of hypothyroidism on hormone profiles in virgin, pregnant, and lactation rats and on lactation. *Reproduction*. 2003;126:371–382.

4. Huggins KE, et al. Markers of lactation insufficiency: a study of 34 mothers. In Auerbach KG, ed. *Current Issues in Clinical Lactation*. Sudbury, MA: Jones and Bartlett; 2000:25–35.

5. Hurst, 2007.

6. Hurst, 2007.

7. Riordan J. *Breastfeeding and Human Lactation*. 3rd ed. Sudbury, MA: Jones and Bartlett; 2005:247–248.

8. Hartmann P, et al. Lactogenesis and its effects of insulin-dependent diabetes mellitus and prematurity. *J Nutr*. 2001;131:3016S-3020S.

FIGURE 12.4   Red flags and risk factors for breastfeeding problems.

Source: Printed with permission of Jan Barger and Linda Kutner.

9. Hall R, et al. A breast-feeding assessment score to evaluate the risk for cessation of breast-feeding by 7 to 10 days of age. *J Pediatr*. 2002;141:659–664.

10. Lawrence RA, et al. *Breastfeeding: A Guide for the Medical Profession*. 6th ed. Sudbury, MA: Jones and Bartlett; 2005:560–561.

11. Walker M, Cox S. Pregnancy, labor and birth complications. In R. Mannel, PJ Martens, M Walker, eds. *Core Curriculum for Lactation Practice*. 2nd ed. Sudbury, MA: Jones and Bartlett; 2008:610–611.

12. Chen D, et al. Stress during labor and delivery and early lactation performance. *Am J Clin Nutrition*. 1998;68:335–344.

13. Henderson JJ, et al. Effect of preterm birth and antenatal corticosteroid treatment on lactogenesis II in women. *Pediatrics*. 2008;121(1):167–168.

14. Marasco L, et al. Polycystic ovary syndrome: a connection to insufficient milk supply? *J Hum Lact*. 2000;16:143–148.

15. Hale TW, Hartmann PE. *Textbook of Human Lactation*. Amarillo, TX: Hale Publishing; 2008:343–354.

16. Sebire NJ, et al. Maternal obesity and pregnancy outcome: a study of 287,213 pregnancies in London. *Int J Obesity*. 2001;25:1175–1182.

17. Kugyelka JG, et al. Maternal obesity is negatively associated with breastfeeding success among Hispanic but not black women. *J Nutr*. 2004;134:1746–1753.

18. Oddy WH, et al. The associated of maternal overweight and obesity with breastfeeding duration. *J Pediatr*. 2006;149(2):185–191.

19. Morin KH. The challenge of obesity. *JOGNN*. 2007;36:482–489.

20. Amir LH, et al. A systematic review of maternal obesity and breastfeeding intention, initiation, and duration. *BMC Pregnancy Childbirth*. 2007;7(9):1471–2393.

21. Rasmussen KM, et al. Prepregnant overweight and obesity diminish the prolactin response to suckling in the first week postpartum. *Pediatrics*. 2004;113:465–471.

22. Swanson V, et al. The impact of knowledge and social influences on adolescents breastfeeding beliefs and intentions. *Public Health Nutr*. 2006;9(3):297–305.

23. Volpe EM, et al. Enhanced breastfeeding initiation in adolescent mothers through the breastfeeding educated and supported teen (BEST) club. *J Hum Lact*. 2000;16(3):196–200.

24. Wambach KA, et al. Experiences of infant feeding decisions making among urban economically disadvantaged adolescents. *J Adv Nurs*. 2004;8(4):61–70.

25. Greenhill JP, Friedman EA. *Biological Principles and Modern Practice of Obstetrics*. Philadelphia: W.B. Saunders; 1974.

26. Soares D, et al. Age as a predictive factor of mammographic breast density in Jamaican women. *Clin Radiol*. 2002;57:472–476.

27. Jamal N, et al. Mammorgraphic breast glandularity in Malaysin women. *Am J Rosntgenol* 2004;182:713–717.

28. Cruz-Kochin N, et al. How much it is fat? *Plast Reconstr Surg*. 2002;109:6–68.

29. Hurst, 2007.

30. Crowell K, et al. Relationship between obstetric analgesia and time of effective breastfeed. *J Nurse Midwifery*. 1994;39:150–56.

31. McCarter-Spaulding D, et al. How does postpartum depression affect breastfeeding? *MCN*. 2007;32(1):10–17.

32. Hill P, et al. Primary and secondary mediators' influence on milk output in lactating mothers of preterm and term infants. *J Hum Lact*. 2005;21(2):138–150.

33. Amir LH, et al. Does maternal smoking have a negative physiological effect on breastfeeding? The epidemiological evidence. *Birth*. 2002;29:112–123.

34. Amir LH, et al. The relationship between maternal smoking and breastfeeding duration after adjustment for maternal infant feeding intention. *Acta Paediatr* 2004;93(11):1514–1518.

35. Law KL, et al. Parental smoking may affect newborn neurobehavior. *Pediatrics*. 2003;111:1318–1323.

36. Neifert, 1990.

37. Camune B, et al. Breastfeeding after breast cancer in childbearing women. *J Perinatal Neo Nurs*. 2007;21(3):225–233.

38. Arora S, et al. Major factors influencing breastfeeding rates: mother's perception of father's attitude and milk supply. *Pediatrics*. 2000;106:67.

39. Chen, 1998.

40. Hurst, 2007.

41. Chen, 1998.

42. Bergman NJ, et al. Randomized controlled trial of skin-to-skin contact from birth versus conventional incubator for physiological stabilization in 2100–2199 gram newborns. *Acta Paediatr*. 2004;93(6):779–785.

43. Hartmann PE, et al. Physiology of lactation in preterm mothers: Initiation and maintenance. *Pediartic Annals* 32(5) 351–355. 2003

44. Saint L, et al. Yield and nutrient content of milk in eight women breastfeeding twins and one women breastfeeding triplets. *Br J Nutr*. 1986;56:49–58.

45. Meier PP, et al. Increased lactation risk for late preterm infants and mothers: evidence and management strategies to protect breastfeeding. *J Midwifery Womens Health*. 2007;52:579–587.

46. Riordan, 2005.

47. Cotterman J. Reverse pressure softening. *Clinical Issues in Lactation*. 2000;4(3).

48. Miller V, et al. Treating postpartum breast edema with areolar compression. *JHL*. 2004;2:223–226.

49. Lawrence, 2005.

50. Renfree C. Anemia and the effects on the breastfeeding women. 2004. www.healthyconnections.ws/anemia.

51. Rioux F. Is there a link between postpartum anemia and discontinuation of breastfeeding. *Can J Dietetic Pract and Res*. 2006;67(2):72–76.

52. Dewey, 2003.

53. Hill, 2005.

54. Farber SG, et al. The effects of skin to skin contact (Kangaroo Care) shortly after birth on the neurobehavioral

(Continued)

FIGURE 12.4   Red flags and risk factors for breastfeeding problems. *(Continued)*

Source: Printed with permission of Jan Barger and Linda Kutner.

responses of term newborn: a randomized, controlled trial. *Pediatrics*. 2004;113(4):858–865.

55. Moore RE, et al. Randomized controlled trial of very early mother-infant skin to skin contact and breastfeeding status. *J Midwifery Women's Health*. 2007;52(2):116–126.

56. Morelius E, et al. Salivary cortisol and mood and pain profiles during skin to skin care for an unselected group of mothers and infants in neonatal intensive care. *Pediatrics*. 2005;116(5):1105–1113.

57. Moore E, et al. Early skin to skin contact for mothers and their healthy newborn infants. *Cochrane Database Syst Rev*. 2007;18(3):CD003519.

58. Chen, 1998.

59. Baumgarder D, et al. Effect of labor epidural anesthesia on breast-feeding of healthy full-term newborns delivered vaginally. *J Am Board Fam Pract*. 2003;16(1):7–13.

60. Lieberman E, O'Donoghue C. Unintended effects of epidural analgesia during labor: a systematic review. *Am J Obstet Gynecol*. 2003;186(5 Suppl Nature):S31.

61. Gromada KK. Breastfeeding multiples. *Core Curriculum for Lactation Practice*. 2nd ed. Sudbury, MA: Jones and Bartlett; 2008:465–482.

62. Ricke LA. Newborn tongue-tie: prevalence and effect on breastfeeding. *J Am Board Fam Pract*. 2005;18(1):1–7.

63. Griffiths M, et al. Tongue-tie treatment solves breastfeeding problems. AAP National Conference, *Abstract 39*. 2007.

64. Genna CW. *Supporting sucking skills in breastfeeding infants*. Sudbury, MA: Jones and Bartlett; 2008.

65. Walker M, Genna CW. Congenital anomalies, neurologic involvement, and birth trauma. *Core Curriculum for Lactation Practice*. 2nd ed. Sudbury, MA: Jones and Bartlett; 2008:623–635.

66. Meier, 2007.

67. Genna, 2008.

68. Meier, 2007.

69. Jain L, et al. Late Preterm pregnancy and the newborn. *Clin Perinatol*. 2006;33(4).

70. Bhutani VK, et al. Kernicterus in late preterm infants cared for as term healthy infants. *Seminars in Perinatology*. 2006;30:89–97.

71. Lawrence,2005.

72. Ferber, 2004.

73. Walters MW, et al. Kangaroo care at birth for full term infants: a pilot study. *MCN*. 2007;32(6):375–381.

74. Moores, 2007.

75. Bergman, 2005.

76. Genna, 2008.

77. Meier, 2007.

78. Meier, 2007.

79. Barger, J. Pacifiers—who's addicted? *Clinical Issues in Lactation*. 1997;1(2):5–6.

80. Barros FC, et al. Use of pacifiers is associated with decrease of breastfeeding duration. *Pediatrics*. 1995; 95:497–499.

81. Lawrence, 2005.

82. Engle WA. "Late-preterm" infants: a population at risk. Clinical Report of the AAP. *Pediatrics*. 2007;120(6);1390–1401.

83. Riordan, 2005.

84. Dewey, 2003.

85. Merry H, et al. Do breastfed babies whose mothers have had labor epidurals lose more weight in the first 24 hours of life? *ABM News and Views*. 2000;6(3):21.

86. Genna, 2008.

87. Howard CR, et al. Physiologic stability of newborns during cup and bottle feeding. *Pediatrics*. 1999;104:1204–1207.

88. Hurst, 2007.

89. Engle, 2007.

90. Hurst, 2007.

FIGURE 12.4   Red flags and risk factors for breastfeeding problems. *(Continued)*

Source: Printed with permission of Jan Barger and Linda Kutner.

The staff should refer her to a lactation consultant if lactation consultants do not automatically see all breastfeeding dyads.

Hours 25–32

Teach the mother the appropriate numbers of feedings, wet diapers, and stools in a 24-hour period. Give her a breastfeeding diary and information on how to know when breastfeeding is going well. Teach her about warning signs (see Figure 12.5) that indicate a problem, ways to prevent nipple soreness and engorgement, and reasons to call a lactation consultant. The baby should breastfeed 2 or more times during this shift.

Hours 33–40

Make sure the mother can position and latch the baby without help. Observe a feeding and document the findings. Teach the mother about her nutritional requirements (drink for thirst and eat when hungry), cluster feedings, role of the father, avoidance of artificial nipples, and risks of formula use. Discuss cosleeping and provide anticipatory guidance for the first few nights at home.

Hours 41–48

By now, the mother should be able to observe nutritive sucking and swallowing during feedings. Teach her that

Lactation Consultant Name & Phone:

_____

BREASTFEEDING IS GOING WELL IF:

- Your baby is breastfeeding at least 8 times in 24 hours.
- Your baby has at least 5–6 good wet diapers every 24 hours.
- Your baby has at least 3 tablespoon-size bowel movements every 24 hours.
- You can hear your baby gulping or swallowing at feedings.
- Your breasts feel softer after a feeding.
- Your nipples are not painful.
- Breastfeeding is an enjoyable experience.

Remember! If you go home from the hospital in 72 hours or less, your baby should be seen by a physician 2 or 3 days after discharge and again at 10 days to 2 weeks of age. It is your responsibility to contact the clinic or office to schedule these visits, and to notify them and/or your board certified lactation consultant if at any time you feel breastfeeding isn't going just right for either you or your baby.

WARNING SIGNS!
CALL YOUR BABY'S DOCTOR OR LACTATION CONSULTANT IF:

- Your baby is having fewer than 5–6 good wet diapers a day by the 4th day of age.
- Your baby is having fewer than 3 or 4 stools ("scoopable poops" of at least 1 tablespoon) by the 4th day of age, or is still having black tarry stools on day 5.
- Your baby is breastfeeding fewer than 8 times a day.
- Your milk is in but you don't hear your baby gulping or swallowing frequently during breastfeeding.
- Your nipples are painful throughout the feeding.
- Your baby seems to be breastfeeding "all the time," or consistently falls asleep within a minute or two at the breast.
- You don't feel as if your milk has come in by the 5th day.

Baby's birthdate and time _____

Your baby will be 4 days old on _____

Baby's birth weight _____

Baby's discharge weight _____

FIGURE 12.5 Signs that breastfeeding is going well.
Source: Copyright © Lactation Education Consultants. Used by permission.

crying is the last sign of hunger, that hunger cues are in place for 20 to 30 minutes before sustained crying, and that crying compromises and disorganizes the baby's suck. At this point in time, the baby should be latching and feeding well, and the parents should appear comfortable holding, dressing, and diapering their child.

Discharge

Make sure the mother understands the signs of adequate milk production. Give her contact information for resources and any necessary feeding plan. Notify the baby's caregiver of any potential problems based on risk factors, and ask the mother to confirm when she will have her baby checked for weight and skin color.

Care Plan for a 24-Hour Hospital Stay

The AAP has identified milestones for discharging families less than 48 hours after delivery. These milestones state that the infant must complete at least two successful feedings and be able to coordinate sucking, swallowing, and breathing while feeding. The mother must receive training and demonstrate competency feeding her infant. Prior to discharge, trained staff should assess the breastfeeding mother and infant for breastfeeding position, latch, and adequacy of swallowing (AAP, 2004). Because the brevity of 24-hour hospital stays requires abridged teaching, mothers should be encouraged to see a caregiver at 48 hours to compensate for the early discharge.

Labor and Delivery

After the birth, mothers can learn about positioning and management of the first feeding. Show the mother which hunger cues her baby exhibits at this time. If the baby is not interested in feeding, he or she can remain with the mother in skin-to-skin position. Keep the room quiet, dim the lights, and reduce stimulation. Refrain from visitors for at least 1 hour to allow parents quiet time alone with their baby.

Hours 1–8

Review positioning and observe the baby's latch. While observing a breastfeeding, point out to the mother the difference between a nutritive and nonnutritive suck. Review hunger cues, and guide the mother in putting the baby to the breast according to cues. Keep the baby with the mother. Make the parents aware that the child may feed only once or several times during the first 8 hours of life.

If the baby has not fed at all by 10 to 12 hours postbirth initiate milk expression by pump or manual expression. Hospitals usually have protocols for the length of time they will allow a baby to go without feeding before supplementing. Teach the mother the desired number of feedings, wet diapers, and stools in a 24-hour period. Give her a breastfeeding diary and information on how to know when breastfeeding is going well, and educate her about warning signs (see Figure 12.5) that indicate a problem.

Hours 9–16

The baby should breastfeed 2 or more times during the next 8 hours. If the infant is not breastfeeding, the mother should feed him or her expressed milk through an alternative feeding method such as a spoon, soft-feeder, syringe, or finger-feeding. Review risk factors for breastfeeding problems (see Figure 12.5) and take appropriate action.

Hours 17–24

The mother should now be able to demonstrate correct positioning and latch without help. The baby should breastfeed 2 or more times during this period, with at least 6 feedings in the first 24 hours. If the baby is not latching by mid-shift, discharge should be delayed until he or she has had at least two effective feedings. If the infant is still not latching well, the mother should continue to express her milk 2 or 3 times during the shift and feed the milk to the baby. The mother should be referred to a lactation consultant to develop a plan of care.

Teach the mother how to prevent nipple soreness and engorgement and when to call a lactation consultant. Review basic nutrition, and urge her to eat a normal healthy diet and to drink when she is thirsty. Teach parents that crying is the last sign of hunger, that hunger cues are in place for 20 to 30 minutes before sustained cry-

ing, and that crying compromises and disorganizes the baby's suck. The baby should be latching and feeding well before leaving the hospital.

Discharge

Make sure the mother understands the signs of adequate milk production. Give her contact information for resources and any necessary feeding plan. Notify the baby's caregiver of any potential problems based on risk factors, and ask the mother to confirm when she will have her baby checked for weight and skin color. Some hospitals have parents return on the day after discharge for weight and bilirubin checks if families leave within 24 hours after delivery. For those with no postdischarge services, it is the parents' responsibility to schedule postdischarge well-baby checks.

∽ Baby-Friendly Hospital Practices

To receive official Baby-Friendly status from the BFHI, hospitals undergo evaluation to determine the extent to which they promote and support breastfeeding. This chapter has explored elements covered by all Ten Steps to Successful Breastfeeding within the context of the mother's hospital experience. Figure 12.6 presents the

---

Step 1. Have a written breastfeeding policy that is routinely communicated to all healthcare staff.

1.1 Does the health facility have an explicit written policy for protecting, promoting, and supporting breastfeeding that addresses all Ten Steps to Successful Breastfeeding in maternity services?

1.2 Does the policy protect breastfeeding by prohibiting all promotion of and group instruction for using breastmilk substitutes, feeding bottles, and teats?

1.3 Is the breastfeeding policy available so all staff who take care of mothers and babies can refer to it?

1.4 Is the breastfeeding policy posted or displayed in all areas of the health facility that serve mothers, infants, and/or children?

1.5 Is there a mechanism for evaluating the effectiveness of the policy?

Step 2. Train all healthcare staff in skills necessary to implement this policy.

2.1 Are all staff aware of the advantages of breastfeeding and acquainted with the facility's policy and services to protect, promote, and support breastfeeding?

2.2 Are all staff caring for women and infants oriented to the breastfeeding policy of the hospital on their arrival?

2.3 Is training on breastfeeding and lactation management given to all staff caring for women and infants within 6 months of their arrival?

2.4 Does the training cover at least eight of the Ten Steps?

2.5 Is the training on breastfeeding and lactation management at least 18 hours in total, including a minimum of 3 hours of supervised clinical experience?

2.6 Has the healthcare facility arranged for specialized training in lactation management of specific staff members?

Step 3. Inform all pregnant women about the benefits and management of breastfeeding.

3.1 Does the hospital include an antenatal care clinic or an antenatal inpatient ward?

3.2 If yes, are most pregnant women attending these antenatal services informed about the benefits and management of breastfeeding?

3.3 Do antenatal records indicate whether breastfeeding has been discussed with the pregnant woman?

3.4 Is a mother's antenatal record available at the time of delivery?

3.5 Are pregnant women protected from oral or written promotion of and group instruction for artificial feeding?

FIGURE 12.6 Ten Steps to Successful Breastfeeding: Self-appraisal tool.

Source: WHO/UNICEF. *Protecting, Promoting, and Supporting Breast-Feeding: The Special Role of Maternity Services: A Joint WHO/UNICEF Statement.* Geneva, Switzerland: World Health

3.6 Does the health care facility take into account a woman's intention to breastfeed when deciding on the use of a sedative, an analgesic, or an anaesthetic (if any) during labor and delivery?

3.7 Are staff familiar with the effects of such medicaments on breastfeeding?

3.8 Does a woman who has never breastfed or who has previously encountered problems with breastfeeding receive special attention and support from the staff of the healthcare facility?

Step 4. Help mothers initiate breastfeeding within a half-hour of birth.

4.1 Are mothers whose deliveries are normal given their babies to hold, with skin contact, within a half-hour of completion of the second stage of labor and allowed to remain with them for at least the first hour?

4.2 Are the mothers offered help by a staff member to initiate breastfeeding during this first hour?

4.3 Are mothers who have had cesarean deliveries given their babies to hold, with skin contact, within a half-hour after they are able to respond to their babies?

4.4 Do the babies born by cesarean delivery stay with their mothers with skin contact at this time, for at least 30 minutes?

Step 5. Show mothers how to breastfeed and how to maintain lactation, even if they should be separated from their infants.

5.1 Does nursing staff offer all mothers further assistance with breastfeeding within 6 hours of delivery?

5.2 Are most breastfeeding mothers able to demonstrate how to position and attach their baby correctly for breastfeeding?

5.3 Are breastfeeding mothers shown how to express their milk or given information on expression or advised of where they can get help, should they need it?

5.4 Are staff members or counselors who have specialized training in breastfeeding and lactation management available full-time to advise mothers during their stay in healthcare facilities and in preparation for discharge?

5.5 Does a woman who has never breastfed or who has previously encountered problems with breastfeeding receive special attention and support from the staff of the healthcare facility?

5.6 Are mothers of babies in special care helped to establish and maintain lactation by frequent expression of milk?

Step 6. Give newborn infants no food or drink other than breastmilk, unless medically indicated.

6.1 Do staff have a clear understanding of what the few acceptable reasons are for prescribing food or drink other than breastmilk for breastfeeding babies?

6.2 Do breastfeeding babies receive no other food or drink (other than breastmilk) unless medically indicated?

6.3 Are any breastmilk substitutes including special formulas that are used in the facility purchased in the same way as any other foods or medicines?

6.4 Do the health facility and all healthcare workers refuse free or low-cost supplies of breastmilk substitutes, paying close to retail market price for any? (Low-cost = below 80% open-market retail cost. Breastmilk substitutes intended for experimental use or "professional evaluation" should also be purchased at 80% or more of retail price.)

6.5 Is all promotion for infant foods or drinks other than breastmilk absent from the facility?

Step 7. Practice rooming-in—allow mothers and infants to remain together—24 hours a day.

7.1 Do mothers and infants remain together (rooming-in 24 hours a day), except for periods of up to an hour for hospital procedures or if separation is medically indicated?

7.2 Does rooming-in start within an hour of a normal birth?

7.3 Does rooming-in start within an hour of when a cesarean mother can respond to her baby?

Step 8. Encourage breastfeeding on demand.

8.1 By placing no restrictions on the frequency or length of breastfeeding, do staff show that they are aware of the importance of breastfeeding on demand?

8.2 Are mothers advised to breastfeed their babies whenever their babies are hungry and as often as their babies want to breastfeed?

Step 9. Give no artificial teats or pacifiers (also called dummies or soothers) to breastfeeding infants.

9.1 Are babies who have started to breastfeed cared for without any bottle feeds?

9.2 Are babies who have started to breastfeed cared for without using pacifiers?

9.3 Do breastfeeding mothers learn that they should not give any bottles or pacifiers to their babies?

9.4 By accepting no free or low-cost feeding bottles, teats, or pacifiers, do the facility and the caregivers demonstrate that these should be avoided?

Step 10. Foster the establishment of breastfeeding support groups, and refer mothers to them on discharge from the hospital or clinic.

10.1 Does the hospital give education to key family members so that they can support the breastfeeding mother at home?

10.2 Are breastfeeding mothers referred to breastfeeding support groups, if any are available?

10.3 Does the hospital have a system of follow-up support for breastfeeding mothers after they are discharged, such as early postnatal or lactation clinic check-ups, home visits, telephone calls?

10.4 Does the facility encourage and facilitate the formation of mother-to-mother or health care worker-to-mother support groups?

10.5 Does the facility allow breastfeeding counseling by trained mother-to-mother support group counselors in its maternity services?

FIGURE 12.6 Ten Steps to Successful Breastfeeding: Self-appraisal tool. *(Continued)*

Source: WHO/UNICEF. Protecting, Promoting, and Supporting Breast-Feeding: The Special Role of Maternity Services: A Joint WHO/UNICEF Statement. Geneva, Switzerland: World Health Organization; 1989: iv. http://www.who.int. Reprinted by permission of the World Health Organization.

questions asked under each of the Ten Steps in the self-appraisal process.

You can be most helpful to the family during their early postpartum days by being alert to the potential for any complications. Make sure parents understand the importance of sound breastfeeding practices. Encourage them to view this time as a period of learning and adjustment and not to feel discouraged by any obstacles that they encounter. If parents receive conflicting advice from you and other caregivers, you can help them make appropriate compromises and decisions. You can also lead discussions among the postpartum and newborn staff about conflicting advice and the importance of explaining suggestions to mothers. Supporting the new family through this transitional time will help them settle into a relaxed atmosphere in their home.

◡ Summary

The course of a mother's breastfeeding takes root in her experience during and immediately after her baby's birth. Medications and other interventions in labor and delivery can affect the initiation of breastfeeding. Practices that unnecessarily interfere with breastfeeding need to be replaced. For the lactation consultant, it is important to advocate for policies that promote bonding, encourage breastfeeding within 1 hour of delivery, offer assistance with the first feeding, and create a climate of acceptance. Such policies encourage rooming-in, responding to hunger cues, and avoiding artificial nipple use. For new parents, it is important that they receive information about day-to-day breastfeeding and anticipatory guidance to prepare them for milestones. A sound breastfeeding policy and clear discharge guidelines provide the framework necessary for preserving and protecting breastfeeding for families and infants.

◡ Chapter 12—At a Glance

Facts you learned—

- Epidural medications diminish early suckling, lower blood pressure, and increase chances of intrapartum fever.
- Forceps and vacuum extraction increase the risk of bruising and pain in the infant.
- Pitocin and other IV medications may cause breast/nipple edema and delay milk production.
- Putting a baby to the breast immediately after deep suctioning is associated with breast aversion.

- "Kangaroo care" is usually as or more effective for maintaining a newborn's temperature than placing the infant in a radiant warmer.
- Delaying the first breastfeeding increases the risk that formula will be used.
- Bonding between mother and infant is strongest in the first 1 or 2 hours after delivery and is enhanced with skin-to-skin contact.
- Rooting and sucking reflexes are particularly strong in the newborn the first 1 or 2 hours after birth.
- Reverse pressure softening (RPS) may help soften the mother's areola and improve latch.
- Extended contact between the mother and baby in the first 3 days after delivery promotes behavioral and developmental growth in the infant, more exclusive breastfeeding, and more responsive behavior.
- Supplements should not be given routinely and should never be given to a mother without specific instructions.

Applying what you learned—

- Develop and communicate breastfeeding policies based on current knowledge.
- Teach healthcare staff how to implement breastfeeding policies.
- Teach physicians and nurses correct information about breastfeeding.
- Promote labor and delivery practices that support early breastfeeding.
- Advocate for limiting the use of medications, anesthesia, and other birth interventions.
- Promote delaying treatment of the infant's eyes for 1 hour to allow for better parent–child bonding.
- Teach hunger cues, and encourage mothers to respond to them.
- Help with the first breastfeeding in a non-interfering manner, and teach effective positioning and latch.
- Help mothers who underwent cesarean section find a comfortable position for breastfeeding.
- Create a relaxed and supportive learning climate that encourages mothers to seek help.
- Help mothers limit interruptions and visitors in the hospital.
- Teach staff to give supplements only for valid medical reasons.
- Teach staff to give no artificial nipples to infants unless requested by parents and to use nipple shields appropriately.
- Encourage rooming-in and place no restrictions on feedings.

- Provide effective discharge planning, and refer mothers to support groups.

～ References

Abolyan L. The breastfeeding support and promotion in baby-friendly maternity hospitals and not-as-yet baby-friendly hospitals in Russia. *Breastfeed Med.* 2006;1(2):71-78.

Academy of Breastfeeding Medicine (ABM). Clinical protocol #1: guidelines for glucose monitoring and treatment of hypoglycemia in breastfed neonates. 2006. www.bfmed.org. Accessed April 1, 2009.

Academy of Breastfeeding Medicine (ABM). Clinical protocol #3: hospital guidelines for the use of supplementary feedings in the healthy term breastfed neonate, Rev. 2009. www.bfmed.org. Accessed March 28, 2010.

Academy of Breastfeeding Medicine (ABM). Clinical protocol #5: peripartum breastfeeding management. 2008. www .bfmed.org. Accessed April 1, 2009.

Academy of Breastfeeding Medicine (ABM). Clinical protocol #7: model breastfeeding policy. 2003. www.bfmed.org. Accessed April 1, 2009.

Alder J, et al. Post-traumatic symptoms after childbirth: what should we offer? *J Psychosom Obstet Gynaecol.* 2006;27(2): 107-112.

American Academy of Pediatrics (AAP), Committee on Fetus and Newborn. Hospital stay for healthy term newborns. *Pediatrics.* 2004;113(5):1434-1436.

American Academy of Pediatrics (AAP). Breastfeeding and the use of human milk. *Pediatrics.* 2005;115:496-506.

American College of Obstetrics and Gynecology (ACOG). ACOG committee opinion, number 395, surgery and patient choice. January 2008. www.acog.org/from_home/ publications/ethics/co395.pdf. Accessed April 2, 2009.

American Society of Anesthesiologists (ASA). Practice guidelines for obstetric anesthesia: an updated report by the American Society of Anesthesiologists task force on obstetric anesthesia. *Anesthesiology.* 2007;106:843-863.

Anderson G. Risk in mother-infant separation postbirth. *Image.* 1989;21:196-199.

Anderson G, et al. Early skin-to-skin contact for mothers and their healthy newborn infants. Review. *Cochrane Database Syst Rev.* 2003;2:CD003519.

Anim-Somuah M, et al. Epidural versus non-epidural or no analgesia in labour. *Cochrane Database Syst Rev.* 2005; 19(4):CD000331.

Aono J, et al. Alteration in glucose metabolism by crying in children. *N Engl J Med.* 1993;329(15):1129.

Asole S, et al. Effect of hospital practices on breastfeeding: a survey in the Italian region of Lazio. *J Hum Lact.* 2009;25(3): 333-340.

Beck C. Birth trauma and its sequelae. *J Trauma Dissociation.* 2009;10(2):189-203.

Beck C, Watson S. Impact of birth trauma on breast-feeding: a tale of two pathways. *Nurs Res.* 2008;57(4):228-236.

Bhutani V, Johnson L. Kernicterus in late preterm infants cared for as term healthy infants. *Semin Perinatol.* 2006;30(2):89-97.

Braarud H, Stormark K. Maternal soothing and infant stress responses: soothing, crying and adrenocortical activity during inoculation. *Infant Behav Dev.* 2006;29(1):70-79.

Bradley W. Newborns' and Mothers' Health Protection Act of 1996. Pub L No. 104-204. 1996.

Brodribb W, et al. Breastfeeding and Australian GP registrars: their knowledge and attitudes. *J Hum Lact.* 2008;24(4):422-430.

Brodribb W, et al. Breastfeeding knowledge: the experiences of Australian general practice registrars. *Aust Fam Physician.* 2009;38(1-2):26-29.

Bruggemann O, et al. Support to woman by a companion of her choice during childbirth: a randomized controlled trial. *Reprod Health.* 2007;4:5.

Bystrova K, et al. The effect of Russian maternity home routines on breastfeeding and neonatal weight loss with special reference to swaddling. *Early Hum Dev.* 2007;83(1):29-39.

Cakmak H, Kuguoglu S. Comparison of the breastfeeding patterns of mothers who delivered their babies per vagina and via cesarean section: an observational study using the LATCH breastfeeding charting system. *Int J Nurs Stud.* 2007;44(7):1128-1137.

Camann W, Alexander K. *Easy Labor: Every Woman's Guide to Choosing Less Pain and More Joy During Childbirth.* New York: Random House; 2006.

Campbell D, et al. A randomized control trial of continuous support in labor by a lay doula. *JOGNN.* 2006;35(4):456-464.

Charpak N, et al. Kangaroo mother care: 25 years after. *Acta Paediatr.* 2005;94(5):514-522.

Chaves R, et al. Factors associated with duration of breastfeeding. *J Pediatr (Rio J).* 2007;83(3):241-246.

Chertok I. Reexamination of ultra-thin nipple shield use, infant growth and maternal satisfaction. *J Clin Nurs.* 2009;18(21): 2949-2955.

Chertok I, Schneider J, Blackburn S. A pilot study of maternal and term infant outcomes associated with ultrathin nipple shield use. *JOGNN.* 2006;35(2):265-272.

Chezem J, et al. Breastfeeding knowledge, breastfeeding confidence, and infant feeding plans: effects on actual feeding practices. *JOGNN.* 2003;32(1):40-47.

Clark S, et al. Maternal death in the 21st century: causes, prevention, and relationship to cesarean delivery, *Am J Obst Gyn.* 2008;199(1):91-92.

Collins C, et al. Avoidance of bottles during the establishment of breast feeds in preterm infants. *Cochrane Database Syst Rev.* 2008;8(4):CD005252.

Colson S, et al. Optimal positions for the release of primitive neonatal reflexes stimulating breastfeeding. *Early Hum Dev.* 2008;84(7):441-449.

Cotterman KJ. Reverse pressure softening: a simple tool to prepare areola for easier latching during engorgement. *J Hum Lact.* 2004;20(2):227-237.

Curl M, et al. Childbirth educators, doulas, nurses, and women respond to the six care practices for normal birth. *J Perinat Educ.* 2004;13(2):42-50.

De Carvalho M. Effects of water supplementation on physiological jaundice in breastfed babies. *Arch Dis Child.* 1981;56:568-569.

de Jonge A, et al. Perinatal mortality and morbidity in a nationwide cohort of 529,688 low-risk planned home and hospital births. *BJOG*. 2009;116:1-8.

Declercq E, et al. *Listening to mothers: Report of the first National U.S. Survey of Women's Childbearing Experiences*. New York: Maternity Center Association; October 2002. www.childbirthconnection.org/pdfs/LtMreport.pdf. Accessed April 2, 2009.

Declercq E, et al. *Listening to mothers II: Report of the second National U.S. Survey of Women's Childbearing Experiences*. New York: Childbirth Connection; October 2006. www.childbirthconnection.org/pdfs/LTMII_report.pdf. Accessed April 2, 2009.

Declercq E, et al. Hospital practices and women's likelihood of fulfilling their intention to exclusively breastfeed. *Am J Public Health*. 2009;99(5):929-935.

Dennis C, Kingston D. A systematic review of telephone support for women during pregnancy and the early postpartum period. *JOGNN*. 2008;37(3):301-314.

Devroe S, et al. Breastfeeding and epidural analgesia during labour. *Curr Opin Anaesthesiol*. 2009;22(3):327-329.

Dewey KG, et al. Risk factors for suboptimal infant breastfeeding behavior, delayed onset of lactation, and excess neonatal weight loss. *Pediatrics*. 2003;2(3 Pt 1):607-619.

DiGirolamo A, et al. Effect of maternity-care practices on breastfeeding. *Pediatrics*. 2008;122(suppl 2):S43-S49.

Dykes F. A critical ethnographic study of encounters between midwives and breast-feeding women in postnatal wards in England. *Midwifery*. 2005;21(3):241-252.

Feldman-Winter L, et al. Pediatricians and the promotion and support of breastfeeding. *Arch Pediatr Adolesc Med*. 2008;162(12):1142-1149.

Fernández-Guisasola J, et al. Epidural obstetric analgesia, maternal fever and neonatal wellness parameters. *Rev Esp Anestesiol Reanim*. 2005;52(4):217-221.

Fleming A, et al. Testosterone and prolactin are associated with emotional responses to infant cries in new fathers. *Horm Behav*. 2002;42(4):399-413.

Gamble J, et al. A critique of the literature on women's request for cesarean section. *Birth*. 2007;34(4):331-340.

Ganesan R. Borderline galactosemia. *New Beginnings*. 1997;14(4):123-124.

Gray P, et al. Fathers have lower salivary testosterone levels than unmarried men and married non-fathers in Beijing, China. *Proc Biol Sci*. 2006;273(1584):333-339.

Gray P, et al. Hormonal correlates of human paternal interactions: a hospital-based investigation in urban Jamaica. *Horm Behav*. 2007;52(4):499-507.

Hale T. *Medications and Mothers' Milk*, 14th ed. Amarillo, TX: Hale Publishing; 2010.

Hale T, Hartmann P. Chapter 27: Anesthetic and analgesic medications: implications for breastfeeding. In: Hale T, Hartmann P. *Hale and Hartmann's Textbook of Human Lactation*. Amarillo, TX: Hale Publishing; 2007:501-512.

Handlin L, et al. Effects of sucking and skin-to-skin contact on maternal ACTH and cortisol levels during the second day postpartum-influence of epidural analgesia and oxytocin in the perinatal period. *Breastfeed Med*. 2009;4(4):207-220.

Hofvander Y. Breastfeeding and the Baby-Friendly Hospitals Initiative (BFHI): Organization, response and outcome in Sweden and other countries. *Acta Paediatr*. 2005;94(8):1012-1016.

Johnson L, et al. Clinical report from the pilot USA Kernicterus Registry (1992 to 2004). *J Perinatol Suppl*. 2009;1:S25-S45.

Jonas W, et al. Effects of intrapartum oxytocin administration and epidural analgesia on the concentration of plasma oxytocin and prolactin, in response to suckling during the second day postpartum. *Breastfeed Med*. 2009;4(2):71-82.

Jordan S. Infant feeding and analgesia in labour: the evidence is accumulating. *Int Breastfeed J*. 2006;1:25.

Jordan S, et al. The impact of intrapartum analgesia on infant feeding. *BJOG*. 2005;112(7):927-934.

Karabulut E, et al. Effect of pacifier use on exclusive and any breastfeeding: a meta-analysis., *Turk J Pediatr*. 2009;51(1):35-43.

Kennell J, McGrath S. Starting the process of mother-infant bonding. *Acta Paediatr*. 2005;94(6):775-777.

Klaus M, et al. Maternal assistance in support in labor: father, nurse, midwife or doula? *Clin Consult Obstet Gynecol*. 1992;4(4):211-217.

Klaus M, et al. *Bonding: Building the Foundations of Secure Attachment and Independence*. New York: Perseus; 2000.

Klaus M, Kennell J. *Maternal-Infant Bonding*, 2nd ed. St. Louis, MO: CV Mosby; 1982.

Kronborg H, Vaeth M. How are effective breastfeeding technique and pacifier use related to breastfeeding problems and breastfeeding duration? *Birth*. 2009;36(1):34-42.

Kutlu R, et al. Assessment of effects of pre- and post-training programme for healthcare professionals about breastfeeding. *J Health Popul Nutr*. 2007;25(3):382-386.

Leavitt G, et al. Knowledge about breastfeeding among a group of primary care physicians and residents in Puerto Rico. *J Community Health*. 2009;34(1):1-5.

Lebarere J, et al. Efficacy of breastfeeding support provided by trained clinicians during an early, routine, preventive visit: a prospective, randomized, open trial of 226 mother-infant pairs. *Pediatrics*. 2005;115(2):e139-e146.

Leung A, Sauve R. Breast is best for babies. *J Natl Med Assoc*. 2005;97(7):1010-1019.

Li R, et al. Why mothers stop breastfeeding: mothers' self-reported reasons for stopping during the first year. *Pediatrics*. 2008;122(suppl 2):S69-S76.

Lin S, et al. Increased risk of stroke in patients who undergo cesarean section delivery: a nationwide population-based study. *Am J Obstet Gynecol*. 2008;198(4):391.e1-e7.

Lothian J. Promoting, protecting, and supporting normal birth. *J Perinat Educ*. 2004;13(2):1-5.

Luopajärvi K, et al. Enhanced levels of cow's milk antibodies in infancy in children who develop type 1 diabetes later in childhood. *Pediatr Diabetes*, 2008;9(5):434-441.

Macarthur A, Ostheimer GW. "What's New in Obstetric Anesthesia" lecture. *Anesthesiology*. 2008;108(5):777-785.

MacDorman M, et al. Neonatal mortality for primary cesarean and vaginal births to low-risk women: application of an "intention-to-treat" model. *Birth*. 2008;35(1):3-8.

Mannan I, et al. Bangladesh Projahnmo Study Group. Can early postpartum home visits by trained community health workers improve breastfeeding of newborns? *J Perinatol*. 2008;28(9):632-640.

Manojlovich M. Power and empowerment in nursing: looking

backward to inform the future. *Online J Issues Nurs*. 2007; 12(1):2.

Mazurek T, et al. Influence of immediate newborn care on infant adaptation to the environment. *Med Wieku Rozwoj*. 1999;3(2):215-224.

McCall E, et al. Interventions to prevent hypothermia at birth in preterm and/or low birthweight infants. *Cochrane Database Syst Rev*. 2008;1:CD004210.

McCourt, C et al. Elective cesarean section and decision making: a critical review of the literature. *Birth*. 2007;34(1):65-79.

Meier P, et al. Nipple shields for preterm infants: effect on milk transfer and duration of breastfeeding. *J Hum Lact*. 2000; 16(2):106-113.

Meirelles C, et al. Justifications for formula supplementation in low-risk newborns at a baby-friendly hospital. *Cad Saude Publica*. 2008;24(9):2001-2012.

Merten S, et al. Do baby-friendly hospitals influence breast-feeding duration on a national level? *Pediatrics*. 2005; 116(5):e702-e708.

Mizuno K, et al. Sucking behavior at breast during the early newborn period affects later breast-feeding rate and duration of breast-feeding. *Pediatr Int*. 2004a;46(1):15-20.

Mizuno K, et al. Mother-infant skin-to-skin contact after delivery results in early recognition of own mother's milk odour. *Acta Paediatr*. 2004b;93:1640-1645.

Moore E, et al. Early skin-to-skin contact for mothers and their healthy newborn infants. *Cochrane Database Syst Rev*. 2007;18(3):CD003519.

Mörelius E, et al. Stress at three-month immunization: parents' and infants' salivary cortisol response in relation to the use of pacifier and oral glucose. *Eur J Pain*. 2009;2:202-208.

Morrison B, et al. Interruptions to breastfeeding dyads on post-partum day 1 in a university hospital. *JOGNN*. 2006;35(6): 709-716.

Muller M, et al. Testosterone and paternal care in East African foragers and pastoralists. *Proc Biol Sci*. 2009;276(1655):347-354.

Nakar S, et al. Attitudes and knowledge on breastfeeding among paediatricians, family physicians, and gynaecologists in Israel. *Acta Paediatr*. 2007;96(6):848-851.

National Center for Health Statistics (NCHS). MacDorman M, Menacker F, Declercq E. Trends and characteristics of home and other out-of-hospital births in the United States, 1990-2006. National vital statistics reports; vol 58 no 11. Hyattsville, MD: NCHS; 2010.

Nishitani S, et al. The calming effect of a maternal breast milk odor on the human newborn infant. *Neurosci Res*. 2009;63(1):66-71.

Nommsen-Rivers L, et al. Doula care, early breastfeeding outcomes, and breastfeeding status at 6 weeks postpartum among low-income primiparae. *JOGNN*. 2009;38(2):157-173.

O'Connor N, et al. Pacifiers and breastfeeding: a systematic review. *Arch Pediatr Adolesc Med*. 2009;163(4):378-382.

Office of National Statistics (ONS). Birth statistics: births and patterns of family building England and Wales (FM1). Birth statistics 2007 series FM1 No. 36. December 2008. http://www.statistics.gov.uk/downloads/theme_population/FM1_36/FM1-No36.pdf. Accessed April 2, 2009.

Ohura T, et al. Clinical pictures of 75 patients with neonatal intrahepatic cholestasis caused by citrin deficiency (NICCD). *J Inherit Metab Dis*. 2007;30(2):139-144.

Ono H, et al. Transient galactosemia detected by neonatal mass screening. *Pediatr Int*. 1999;41(3):281-284.

Pestvenidze E, Bohrer M. Finally, daddies in the delivery room: parents' education in Georgia. *Glob Public Health*. 2007; 2(2):169-183.

Pincombe J, et al. Baby-Friendly Hospital Initiative practices and breast feeding duration in a cohort of first-time mothers in Adelaide, Australia [published online ahead of print January 2, 2007]. *Midwifery*. 2008;24(1):55-61.

Powers D, Tapia V. Women's experiences using a nipple shield. *J Hum Lact*. 2004;20(3):327-334.

Renfrew M, et al. Feeding schedules in hospitals for newborn infants. *Cochrane Database Syst Rev*. 2000;2:CD000090.

Righard L. The baby is breastfeeding—not the mother. *Birth*. 2008;35(1):1-2.

Righard L, Alade M. Effect of delivery room routines on success of first breastfeed. *Lancet*. 1990;336:1105-1107.

Riordan J, et al. The effect of labor pain relief medication on neonatal suckling and breastfeeding duration. *J Hum Lact*. 2000;16(1):7-12.

Rodriguez-Garcia J, Acosta-Ramirez N. Factors affecting how long exclusive

breastfeeding lasts. *Rev Salud Publica (Bogota)*. 2008;10(1):71-84.

Romano AM, Lothian JA. Promoting, protecting, and supporting normal birth: a look at the evidence. *JOGNN*. 2008; 37(1):94-104.

Ruppen W, et al. Incidence of epidural hematoma, infection, and neurologic injury in obstetric patients with epidural analgesia/anesthesia. *Anesthesiology*. 2006;105(2):394-399.

Sears W. Letting baby "cry-it-out" Yes, no! www.askdrsears.com. Accessed April 3, 2009.

Shah P, et al. Breastfeeding or breast milk for procedural pain in neonates. *Cochrane Database Syst Rev*. 2006;19(3): CD004950.

Sheehan A, et al. Women's experiences of infant feeding support in the first 6 weeks post-birth. *Matern Child Nutr*. 2009;5(2):138-150.

Sinusas K, Gagliardi A. Initial management of breastfeeding. *Am Fam Physician*. 2001;64(6):981-988.

Smith L. *Impact of Birthing Practices on Breastfeeding*. 2nd ed. Sudbury, MA: Jones and Bartlett; 2009.

Smith LJ. Impact of birthing practices on the breastfeeding dyad. *J Midwifery Women's Health*. 2007;52(6):621-630.

Statistics Canada. Births: 2006. Modified September 23, 2008. www.statcan.gc.ca/pub/84f0210x/2006000/5201662-eng.htm. Accessed September 13, 2009.

Swain J, et al. Maternal brain response to own baby-cry is affected by cesarean section delivery [published online ahead of print September 3, 2008]. *J Child Psychol Psychiatry*. 2008;49(10):1042-1052.

Thompson S, et al. Dietary management of galactosemia. *Southeast Asian J Trop Med Public Health*. 2003;34(suppl 3):212-214.

Torvaldsen S, et al. Intrapartum epidural analgesia and breast-feeding: a prospective cohort study. *Int Breastfeed J*. 2006;1:24.

Trueba G, et al. Alternative strategy to decrease cesarean section: support by doulas during labor. *J Perinat Educ.* 2000;9(2):8-13.

U.S. Preventive Services Task Force (USPSTF). Primary care interventions to promote breastfeeding: U.S. Preventive Services Task Force recommendation statement. *Ann Intern Med.* 2008;149(8):560-564.

Van Zandt S, et al. Lower epidural anesthesia use associated with labor support by student nurse doulas: implications for intrapartal nursing practice. *Complement Ther Clin Pract.* 2005;11(3):153-160.

Varendi H, et al. Does the newborn baby find the nipple by smell? *Lancet.* 1994;344(8928):989-990.

Walters M, et al. Kangaroo care at birth for full term infants: a pilot study. *MCN Am J Matern Child Nurs.* 2007;32(6):375-381.

Widstrom A, et al. Gastric suction in healthy newborn infants. *Acta Paediatr Scand.* 1987;76:566-572.

Wiklund I, et al. Epidural analgesia: Breast-feeding success and related factors [published online ahead of print November 5, 2007]. *Midwifery.* 2009;25(2):e31-e38.

Wilson-Clay B. Clinical use of nipple shields. *J Hum Lact.* 1996;12:279-285.

Winberg J. Mother and newborn baby: mutual regulation of physiology and behavior—a selective review. *Dev Psychobiol.* 2005;47(3):217-229.

World Health Organization (WHO)/United Nations Children's Fund (UNICEF). *Breastfeeding management and promotion in a baby-friendly hospital: An 18-hour course for maternity staff.* New York: UNICEF; 1993.

World Health Organization (WHO)/United Nations Children's Fund (UNICEF). *Protecting, promoting and supporting breastfeeding: A joint WHO/UNICEF statement.* Geneva, Switzerland: WHO/UNICEF; 1989.

13

Infant Assessment and Development

A newborn's behavior is linked closely to breastfeeding. Therefore, an understanding of newborn reflexes and characteristics is an important factor when assessing breastfeeding. The lactation consultant can identify and help parents learn to watch for and interpret their babies' behaviors. In particular, babies signal to their mothers through hunger cues. Patterns of behavior, growth, sleeping, crying, and digestion vary from one baby to another. Certain anatomic presentations may require a change in your approach to assisting a mother. A complete medical history and assessment of the mother and infant will help you identify situations that may affect lactation.

∽ Key Terms

Acrocyanosis
Alveolar ridge
Anoxia
Approach behaviors
Asymmetry
Average baby
Avoidance behaviors
Bauer's response
Bifurcated or bifid
Bovine IgG
Buccal pads
Candidiasis
Caput succedaneum
Cephalhematoma
Clavicle
Cleft lip
Cleft palate
Colic
Constipation
Cosleeping
Cow's milk intolerance
Cradle hold
Dancer hand position
Diaper rash
Diarrhea
Down syndrome
Erythema toxicum

Excoriated
Flexion
Fontanel
Food sensitivity
Frenulum
Frenum
Gastroesophageal reflux disease (GERD)
Grooming
Hirschsprung's disease
Hunger cues
Hydration
Hypertonic
Hypotonic
Infant acne
Infant states
Intravenous
Lactiferous ducts
Lactose overload
Leaky gut syndrome
Leukocytes
Macular
Molding
New Ballard Scale (NBS)
Palate
Perineum
Periosteum

Peristalsis
Placid baby
Projectile vomiting
Prone
Pustule
Pyloric stenosis
Rapid eye movement (REM)
Reflexes
Rooting
Sling
Soy milk intolerance
Spitting up

Stooling
Sucking
Sucking pads
Sudden infant death syndrome (SIDS)
Supine
Swaddling
Thrush
Turgor
Uvula
Ventral
Voiding
Yeast infection

∽ Assessment of the Newborn

Generally, the lactation consultant's initial contact with a breastfeeding mother should include an assessment of her baby. This guideline applies especially when there is concern about poor weight gain, food intolerance, irritability, lethargy, or sucking difficulties. To perform the assessment, the baby should be completely undressed and lying on a flat firm surface. Evaluate the infant's posture, skin, head, oral structure, clavicle, reflexes, color, elimination, and hunger cues. Be alert for any areas on the baby's body that cause pain or discomfort.

The New Ballard Score (NBS) is a gestational assessment tool that evaluates the tone of the infant's total body, wrist, biceps muscle, knee joint, shoulder girdle, and pelvic girdle. ("Girdle" refers to the bones that encircle the shoulder and pelvis.) The NBS reflects an expansion of the original scoring system in 1991 to include extremely preterm infants (see Table 13.1). A detailed description and free online illustration of the scale are available at www.ballardscore.com. If you are unfamiliar with assessing newborns, you will find the NBS helpful in assessing the normal newborn and identifying what is not normal. Chapter 23 covers preterm infants, and Chapter 25 discusses a variety of infant medical conditions.

TABLE 13.1   New Ballard Score (NBS) Maturational Assessment of Gestational Age

MATURATIONAL ASSESSMENT OF GESTATIONAL AGE (New Ballard Score)

NAME _____   DATE/TIME OF BIRTH _____   SEX _____

HOSPITAL NO. _____   DATE/TIME OF EXAM _____   BIRTH WEIGHT _____

RACE _____   AGE WHEN EXAMINED _____   LENGTH _____

APGAR SCORE: 1 MINUTE _____ 5 MINUTES _____ 10 MINUTES _____   HEAD CIRC. _____

EXAMINER _____

NEUROMUSCULAR MATURITY

	−1	0	1	2	3	4	5
Posture							
Square window (wrist)	> 90°	90°	60°	45°	30°	0°	
Arm recoil		180°	140°–180°	110°–140°	90°–110°	< 90°	
Popliteal angle	180°	160°	140°	120°	100°	90°	< 90°
Scarf sign							
Heel to ear							

RECORD SCORE HERE

PHYSICAL MATURITY

Skin	Sticky, friable, transparent	Gelatinous, red, translucent	Smooth, pink, visible veins	Superficial peeling and/or rash, few veins	Cracking, pale areas, rare veins	Parchment, deep cracking, no vessels	Leathery, cracked, wrinkled
Lanugo	None	Sparse	Abundant	Thinning	Bald areas	Mostly bald	
Plantar surface	Heel-toe 40–50 mm: −1 < 40 mm: −2	> 50 mm, no crease	Faint red marks	Anterior tranverse crease only	Creases anterior two-thirds	Creases over entire sole	
Breast	Imperceptible	Barely perceptible	Flat areola, no bud	Stippled areola, 1–2 mm bud	Raised areola, 3–4 mm bud	Full areola, 5–10 mm bud	
Eye/Ear	Lids fused loosely: −1 tightly: −2	Lids open; pinna flat, stays folded	Slightly curved pinna, soft, slow recoil	Well-curved pinna, soft but ready recoil	Pinna formed and firm, instant recoil	Thick cartilage, ear stiff	
Genitals (male)	Scrotum flat, smooth	Scrotum empty, faint rugae	Testes in upper canal, rare rugae	Testes descending, few rugae	Testes down, good rugae	Testes pendulous, deep rugae	
Genitals (female)	Clitoris prominent, labia flat	Clitoris prominent, labia minora small	Clitoris prominent, labia minora enlarged	Labia majora and minora equally prominent	Labia majora large, labia minora small	Labia majora cover clitoris and labia minora	

MATURITY RATING

Score	Weeks
−10	20
−5	22
0	24
5	26
10	28
15	30
20	32
25	34
30	36
35	38
40	40
45	42
50	44

RECORD SCORE HERE

GESTATIONAL AGE (weeks)

By dates _____
By ultrasound _____
By exam _____

Source: Ballard JL, Khoury JC, Wedig K, Wang L, Eilers-Walsman BL, & Lipp R. New Ballard score, expanded to include extremely premature infants. *J Pediatr.* 1991;119(3): 7. Reprinted with permission from Elsevier.

Posture

Babies favor the fetal position. Healthy, full-term newborns generally hold their arms and legs in moderate flexion. Their fists are closed and usually held near their face. When awake, the infant resists having the extremities extended and may cry at attempts to do so. As the baby matures, he or she will remain in the fetal position less often and will spend more time comfortably in semi-extension.

Observing the baby's body tone will give you clues about potential problems. When held in the ventral (abdominal) position, normal infants lie on their abdomen, draped over the examiner's hand, and alternate between trying to bring their head up and putting it down again. At extreme positions, a baby's body tone may be too loose (hypotonic) or too rigid (hypertonic).

Babies whose mothers have taken antidepressants in the selective serotonin reuptake inhibitor (SSRI) class may exhibit neonatal behavioral syndrome. This syndrome is characterized as one or more of the following signs and symptoms: jitteriness, irritability, lethargy, hypotonia, hypertonia, hyperreflexia, apnea, respiratory distress, vomiting, poor feeding, or hypoglycemia (Jordan et al., 2008; Ferreira et al., 2007). Note that these babies can exhibit either hypotonia or hypertonia.

Hypotonia

A hypotonic infant has very low body tone and tends to "droop" over the examiner's hand. With hypotonia, the baby's posture appears like a wet noodle. The extremities are in extension, and there is minimal resistance to passive movement. The baby appears floppy, sluggish, and flaccid (see Figure 13.1). A hypotonic baby may have difficulty staying latched to the breast due to a weak suck. He or she may find it difficult to maintain intra-oral negative pressure, even on the examiner's finger. The infant frequently nurses with the shoulders elevated to just beneath the ears in an effort to support the neck and chin. In the ventral position, the hypotonic baby lays over the examiner's hand with the head hanging down, unable to bring it up.

Hypotonia is a marker for certain syndromes and neurological disorders. In fact, ineffective sucking and hypotonia are often symptoms of an underlying problem, not the problem itself. For example, infant hypotonia and/or a poor suck were seen in 7 of 13 cases of Prader-Willi phenotype of fragile X syndrome; autism spectrum disorder (ADS) occurred in 10 of 13 cases (Nowicki et al., 2007). Hypotonia was found to be the most common motor symptom in one study of ASD (Ming et al., 2007). An infant who is preterm or who has Down syndrome will show some degree of hypotonia. Hypotonia can also be a symptom of botulism infection (Paty et al., 1987).

Hypertonia

A hypertonic infant has very rigid body tone. With hypertonia, the baby is often in hyperextension, arching away from the breast and the mother (see Figure 13.2). The mother may report that the child is difficult to comfort, pulls his or her head and face away from contact, and does not snuggle into her chest or neck, instead leaning back and away from her. Many hypertonic babies cannot tolerate anyone handling them and prefer to interact from a safe distance. They are often very alert and squirmy, and they will hold their heads erect from a prone (face-down) position or on the shoulder. When held in the ventral position, a hypertonic baby will be virtually straight, lifting both the head and buttocks, and maintaining them on a horizontal plane. A baby with neurological damage may be hypertonic (Scher, 2008a, 2008b). Hypertonia can also be a symptom of respiratory syncytial virus (RSV) infection (Kawashima et al., 2009; Millichap, 2009).

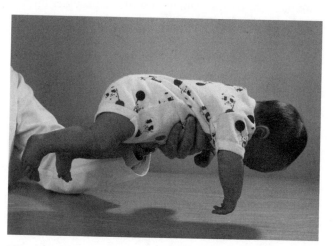
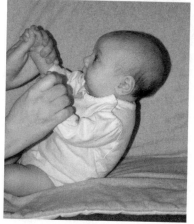

FIGURE 13.1 Hypotonic baby (left) and baby with good muscle tone (right).
Source: (left) © Saturn Stills/Photo Researchers, Inc. (right) Printed with permission of Anna Swisher.

Skin

A healthy newborn's skin is warm and dry, with a pink or ruddy appearance. The ruddiness is a result of increased concentration of red blood cells in the blood vessels, coupled with minimal subcutaneous fat deposits. Occasionally, a very large hemangioma may occur on or around the infant's lips or nose. If herniated or ulcerated, it can affect breastfeeding. The mother may need help with alternative feeding arrangements until treatment is obtained.

As many as 40 percent of babies are born with a birthmark (hemangioma) or mole (nevus). Small birthmarks (nevus simplex) typically comprise a flat, dark pink mark or series of marks usually occurring on the forehead, eyelids, or back of neck—hence, the term "stork bite," referring to the baby being carried by the stork. Birthmarks such as port-wine stains (nevus flammeus) can be quite large (McLaughlin et al., 2008). Many newborn birthmarks fade away by a few years of age. Others may respond to laser treatment later in life.

Lanugo

Lanugo is the Latin word for "down," meaning the fine small hairs found on some plants (Medterms, 2009). In newborns, lanugo describes the fine, downy hair covering the body. It usually appears in utero at about 5 months gestation and is shed at 7 to 8 months gestation. Lanugo is most abundant on preterm babies who are born at 5 to 6 months gestation.

Hydration

Hydration can be assessed by evaluating the turgor (resiliency) of the baby's skin. Turgor is the normal strength and tension of the skin, caused by outward pressure of the cells and the fluid that surrounds them. A good area on which to test skin turgor is the baby's chest, abdomen, or thigh. When gently grasped between your finger and thumb, the skin should spring back to its original shape when you release the tissue. It should not leave an indentation, fold, or wrinkled appearance. Loose skin that slowly returns to a position level with the tissue next to it is a sign of dehydration. The baby's skin may be dry, flaky, or peeling, especially by the end of the first or second week after birth. This appearance is normal, and not a sign of dehydration.

Color

Skin color will vary, depending on the baby's ethnic origin. A significant increase in the newborn's bilirubin level creates a yellowing in the skin color from jaundice, also called hyperbilirubinemia (see Color Plate 14). You can assess for jaundice in natural light by pressing the baby's skin with your index finger and noting the color when you lift your finger.

For a quick estimation, some caregivers use a method referred to as the "rule of fives" to estimate bilirubin levels in the infant. Jaundice becomes visible in the sclera (white portion of the eye) when the bilirubin level reaches approximately 5 mg/dL. Continuing down the body, the level increases progressively from the face to the feet by approximately 5 mg/100 mL. Jaundice to the level of the shoulders correlates to a bilirubin level of 5–7 mg/dL. Between the shoulders and umbilicus, levels will range from 7 to 10 mg/dL. Between the umbilicus and knees, levels are in the range of 10–12 mg/dL. Bilirubin levels are greater than 15 mg/dL below the knees.

Progression of color occurs only when the bilirubin level is rising. When it begins to fall, the skin color fades gradually in all affected areas at the same time (American Academy of Pediatrics [AAP], 2004). Be aware that visual assessment of jaundice is not consistently reliable (Moyer et al., 2000). If you see an infant with jaundice, refer the parents to the baby's primary healthcare provider immediately, so that levels can be measured precisely with a blood test if necessary. Chapter 22 provides an in-depth discussion of jaundice and its implications.

Acrocyanosis

Acrocyanosis describes a bluish tinge to the newborn's hands and feet (see Color Plate 15). It may be present after birth due to poor peripheral circulation, especially if the child experiences exposure to cold (Stanford School of Medicine, 2009). The bluish color should disappear after a few days. Parents often need reassurance that this condition is normal and not a sign that their baby is cold.

Erythema Toxicum

Erythema toxicum is a pink to red macular area with a yellow or white center (see Color Plate 16). It is the most

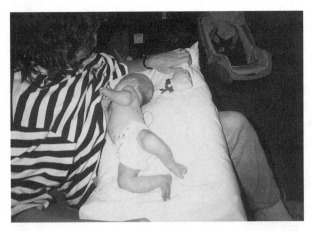

FIGURE 13.2 Hypertonic baby who arches away from the mother.

Source: Printed with permission of Linda Kutner.

common skin eruption in newborns, occurring in as many as 70 percent of infants. Full-term infants weighing more than 5.5 pounds (2500 g) are more likely to exhibit this rash (Carr et al., 1966). Erythema toxicum has no apparent significance and requires no treatment. It is common on the newborn's trunk or limbs and is temporary. It may be present at birth, but usually appears during the second or third days after birth and then disappears within 1 week.

Infant Acne

Infant acne resembles adolescent acne. It appears on the face, primarily on the nose, forehead, and cheeks (see Color Plate 17). The appearance changes depending on whether the baby is hot, cool, crying, or quiet. In most cases, infant acne starts at about 2 weeks of age and disappears at 8 to 10 weeks. It is believed to be the result of sebaceous gland stimulation by maternal or infant hormones. If a baby's newborn acne does not go away on its own, the baby's healthcare provider can rule out any underlying adrenal or endocrine problems (O'Connor et al., 2008).

Mottling

Mottling (cutis marmorata) is a white and reddish coloration of the skin on the baby's trunk and extremities (see Color Plate 18). This condition is a vascular response to cold and usually clears when the skin is warmed. Some babies' skin may mottle easily for several weeks, months, or even into early childhood. No treatment is needed (O'Connor et al., 2008).

Milia

Milia are very small "whiteheads" that are actually keratin deposits within the dermis (see Color Plate 19). As many as half of all newborns exhibit milia. They usually occur on the forehead, cheeks, nose, and chin, but may also occur on the trunk and diaper area (Paller & Mancini, 2006). Milia usually resolve by the end of the first month.

Diaper Rash

Diaper rash appears as a small, reddened, pimple-like rash. It should respond to careful washing of the buttocks combined with use of a zinc oxide ointment or cream. A diaper rash that does not clear up with appropriate treatment may indicate a yeast infection. If the skin is abraded or has pustules, the infant needs to be seen by a healthcare provider to rule out a bacterial infection.

Cradle Cap

Cradle cap (seborrheic dermatitis) is a thick, scaly dandruff, mostly found on the scalp (see Color Plate 20) and sometimes observed on the face, ears, neck, and even the diaper area. Cradle cap looks unattractive and can be dis-

tressing to parents. It may be caused by hormones, although a yeast infection should also be ruled out (Sheffield et al., 2007). The baby should be evaluated for immunodeficiency in the event of unresolved scaling with diarrhea and low weight gain or failure to thrive (Kim et al., 2001; Siegfried, 1993).

Head

The newborn's head is large, accounting for approximately one-fourth of the total body size. The skull bones are soft and pliable; they remain unfused at birth to accommodate the infant's descent through the birth canal during second-stage labor. After birth, the head may appear asymmetric due to the overlap of skull bones, referred to as molding. Severe molding can cause temporary difficulty with latch.

Caput Succedaneum

Caput succedaneum is a collection of fluid between the newborn's skin and cranial bone (see Figure 13.3). It usually forms during labor on the presenting area of the head in the cervical opening. The longer the head is engaged during labor, the greater the swelling can be. This condition occurs in 20 to 40 percent of vacuum extractions (Volpe, 2008). There may be red or bruised discoloration, and the baby may be sensitive to pressure on the affected area. Swelling begins to subside soon after birth. Vacuum extraction and the resulting caput have been associated with bald spots (alopecia) in a few cases (Lykoudis et al., 2007). Severe caputs and cephalhematomas (discussed in the next subsection) are associated with feeding difficulties (Genna, 2008).

Cephalhematoma

A cephalhematoma is a pool of blood between the bones of the head and the periosteum, the covering of the bone (see Color Plate 21). The resultant swelling may begin to form during labor and slowly become larger in the first few days after birth. It may take up to 6 weeks to resolve completely. Cephalhematoma is usually a result of trauma, often from forceps or vacuum extraction (Doumouchtsis & Arulkumaran, 2008; Goetzinger & Macones, 2008; U.S. Food and Drug Administration [FDA], 1998). Because the baby may be sensitive to touch on that area, the mother will want nurse in a position that avoids contact with the head. The bruising increases the risk for feeding difficulties and for jaundice as the blood is reabsorbed into the child's blood vessels.

Fontanel

The fontanel is a space between the bones of an infant's skull that is covered by tough membranes. The anterior

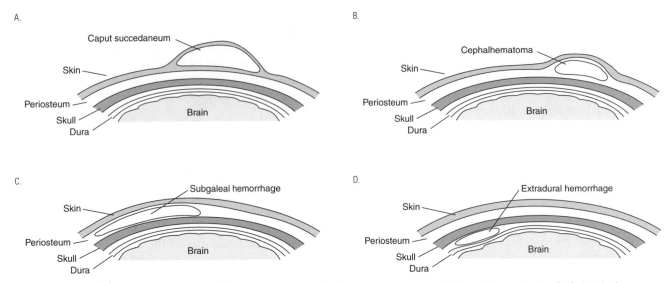

FIGURE 13.3   Common hematomas of the newborn scalp. A. Caput succedaneum. B. Cephalhematoma. C. Subgaleal hemorrhage. D. Extradural hemorrhage.

Source: Printed with permission of Anna Swisher.

fontanel remains soft until the baby reaches about 18 months. The posterior fontanel closes at about 2 months. Increased brain pressure may cause a fontanel to become tense or to bulge. If the infant is dehydrated, his or her fontanel may be soft and sunken, especially when the infant is supine.

Facial Asymmetry

Facial asymmetry may result from injury to the nerves due to birth trauma. If the baby's tongue is not centered in the mouth as a result, the mother can position her nipple over the center of the baby's tongue rather than the center of the mouth. Facial asymmetry may also occur in utero when the infant's face is wedged against his or her own body or the uterus. The asymmetry usually resolves over several days following birth, depending on the severity. Many parents find that babies with facial asymmetry respond well to chiropractic care (ICPA, 2010) or to physical or occupational therapy.

Eyes

Most babies' eyes are grayish blue at birth, with the final eye color developing when the child reaches 6 to 12 months of age. Sometimes babies will have broken capillaries in the sclera resulting from the birth; these resolve within the first 10 days postpartum. In addition, some infants may demonstrate swelling of the eyelids, which typically recedes in a few days after birth. Jaundice can cause a yellow staining in the sclera (the white portion) of the eye that appears when the baby's bilirubin level exceeds 5 mg/dL.

Neck

The neck surrounds the infant's esophagus and trachea. The epiglottis is the cartilage that overhangs the trachea and closes during swallowing to prevent food from entering the trachea (see Figure 13.4). An infant's neck is very short. Because it is too weak to provide head support, the newborn's head needs to be supported at all times. Supporting the baby's neck and shoulders at feedings will avoid the mother pushing on the child's head, which can be counterproductive.

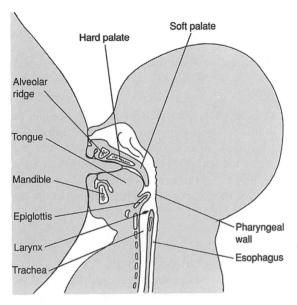

FIGURE 13.4   Swallowing anatomy.

Torticollis A baby whose head is continually turned to the side, usually to the right, may have torticollis—literally, "twisted neck" (see Figure 13.5). Torticollis in infants is caused by a shortening of the muscle that extends from the base of the ear down to the clavicle. The cause may be the baby's position or lack of space in the womb, birth trauma, or low amniotic fluid. Rarely, torticollis can be a marker for serious problems (Torticollis Kids, 2009), so the baby needs to be seen by the primary care practitioner for assessment.

A baby with torticollis may only be comfortable breastfeeding with his or her head turned to the side. Placing the baby in the side-sitting position (also called football or clutch hold) for feedings can provide better control over the infant's neck position. Some children with torticollis may feed well in the cradle hold for one side and not the other. In such a case, the mother can scoot the child over to the other breast without changing the angle of the neck. She can also try nursing lying down, with the bed providing postural support. The mother can try other nursing positions as her baby's range of motion improves through physical therapy or chiropractic care.

Jaw

The baby's jaw (mandible) is the part of the head that moves for feeding. All babies are born with degrees of receding jaws. Achieving a deep latch can be challenging when a baby's jaw is severely recessed or very small (micrognathia). A severely receding or small jaw is a

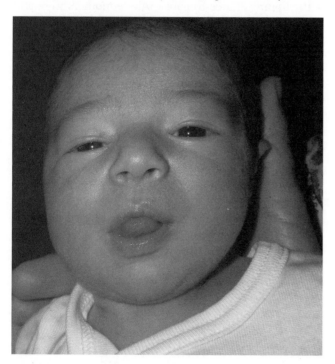

FIGURE 13.5 Baby with torticollis.

Source: Printed with permission of Catherine Watson Genna, BS, IBCLC.

marker for several genetic conditions, including Pierre Robin sequence (Cooper-Brown et al., 2008). (See Chapter 25 for more discussion of infant conditions.) As the baby grows, the jaw comes forward. Jaw (and later, dental) development is affected negatively by bottle feeding (Carrascoza et al., 2006; Raymond & Bacon, 2006; Page, 2001). Bottle feeding interferes negatively with oral facial development even after 6 months of breastfeeding (Carrascoza et al., 2006).

Oral Structure

Visual inspection of the mouth is an important element of the infant assessment. Look for gum lines that are smooth and a palate that is intact and gently arched. The tongue should be able to extend over the lower alveolar ridge (gum line) and up to the middle of the baby's mouth when it is open wide.

Lips

A baby's lips close around the breast and form a seal to create negative pressure. When assessing a baby's lips, look for friction blisters, which are typically seen on the midline of the top lip. Known as "sucking blisters," they can be signs that the baby is not generating enough negative pressure to keep the breast in the mouth, and is compensating by using the lip muscles (orbicularis oris) to compress the breast. If you see this condition in a newborn, ask the mother if the baby was born with the blister or whether it developed after birth. Babies can be born with sucking blisters from sucking on their hands in the womb.

The most noticeable defect involving the lips is a cleft lip. A baby may have a cleft lip combined with a cleft in the hard or soft palate, or a cleft lip with normal palatal development. A baby may also have a cleft palate with no lip defect. Chapter 25 discusses clefts in more depth.

Lip tone is an important consideration in nursing. In a baby, tight, pursed lips are a marker for impaired intra-oral pressure—a condition that is often seen in preterm infants. Soft, flaccid lips, with poor sealing and little resistance, can be a sign of low muscle tone. This type of deviation occurs in babies with neurological issues, such as Down syndrome, and in babies that have been affected by maternal drugs and medications or birth trauma such as facial nerve injury (Johnson et al., 2004; Ndiaye et al., 2001). Be aware that the philtrum—the midline space between the upper lip and the nose—has a slight dip. A flat philtrum can be a marker for neurological issues, especially fetal alcohol syndrome (Fetal Alcohol Syndrome Diagnosis and Prevention Network [FAS DPN], 2004).

Tongue

In breastfeeding, the baby's tongue draws the breast into the mouth and forms a groove or trough. When the infant suckles, a bolus of milk flows through the trough toward the back of the mouth and is swallowed. Observe the size and shape of the baby's tongue for any anomalies that could affect troughing or movement, especially if the mother complains of pain with breastfeeding. Assess whether the tongue is short or humped, unusually thick or thin, long or abnormally large. Macroglossia (large tongue) is a marker for genetic disorders, including Down syndrome and Beckwith-Wiedemann (also called EMG) syndrome. It is also associated with the low muscle tone found in children with neurological damage.

Alveolar Ridge (Gum Line)

The baby's alveolar ridge should be smooth and uniform. Occasionally, a baby will be born with a very bumpy gum line, from which it appears teeth are about to erupt. These bumps may be white or yellowish gingival cysts ("Epstein pearls"), a benign condition. Epstein pearls may also occur on the palate. These cysts resolve a few weeks or months after birth and no treatment is required. Rarely, a baby will be born with a baby tooth already erupted (natal tooth), or with a tumor on the gum pad (Eghbalian & Monsef, 2009; Kumar & Sharma, 2008).

Lingual Frenulum

The lingual frenulum is the fold of skin under the tongue that controls the tongue's motion. Frenula can vary in position, thickness, and length. If the baby is unable to extend the tongue over the alveolar ridge, this difficulty may be due to ankyloglossia—a tight frenulum, also referred to as tongue-tie (see Color Plate 22). Ankyloglossia may restrict movement of the tongue in several ways. For example, anterior restriction may cause the classic heart-shaped appearance when crying. Mid-tongue and posterior restriction may be more subtle. It is also possible to have a "hidden"—that is, sublingual—tongue restriction (Genna, 2008).

Ankyloglossia seems to be more common in males, with one study reporting 72 percent of cases occurring in males and 28 percent in females. Breastfeeding difficulties were the most common complaint in conjunction with this condition cited by the parents of infants younger than 1 year (Karabulut et al., 2008). A tight frenulum can make it difficult for the baby to stay attached to the breast during feeding and may result in poor weight gain. As a lactation consultant, you should be especially alert to the possibility of a tight frenulum as the cause of chronic nipple soreness, slow weight gain, long feedings, low milk production, mastitis, or plugged ducts. Clipping the frenulum (frenotomy) releases the lingual frenulum and improves tongue movement. Clipping is a simple procedure, in which a small cut is made at the anterior portion of the frenulum (see Figure 13.6). It usually enables the

baby's tongue to extend adequately for a good latch and milk transfer (Geddes et al., 2008; Ramsay, 2004).

Breastfeeding-supportive providers have observed the negative effects of ankyloglossia on breastfeeding for many years. Since the publication of the seminal study on this condition in 2002 (Ballard et al., 2002), the volume of medical research literature has exploded on the topic. Infants with a tight frenulum are significantly more likely to be exclusively bottle fed by 1 week of age (Ricke et al., 2005). One study reported that breastfeeding improved in 83 percent of 35 infants who had frenotomies. Parental satisfaction for this procedure was high, and no complications were reported (Amir et al., 2005). Another study reported that 27 of 28 babies whose frenula were clipped improved and fed well (Hogan et al., 2005).

Ultrasound imaging has provided new visual understanding of an infant's compensation when the ability to maintain a latch and suck is compromised (Ramsay, 2004). In a 2008 study involving 24 subjects, milk intake, milk transfer, LATCH scores, and mothers' pain scores improved significantly in all cases after the babies' frenula were clipped. Prior to the procedure, babies were shown on ultrasound to either compress the tip of the nipple or compress the base of the nipple with the tongue; these issues were either resolved or lessened in all except one infant after frenotomy (Geddes et al., 2008). Another study of 27 mother–baby dyads experiencing painful breastfeeding owing to ankyloglossia reported significant decreases in maternal pain and no complications with clipping. Three-fourths of these mothers were still breastfeeding when follow-up was undertaken 3 months

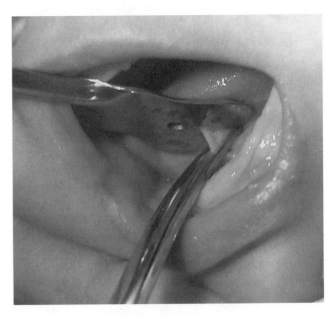

FIGURE 13.6   Frenotomy procedure.

Source: Printed with permission of Catherine Watson Genna, BS, IBCLC.

later and 92 percent were pain free (Srinivasan et al., 2006).

Ankyloglossia occurs in stages and varies in terms of its severity, including its effects on both form and function of the child's mouth (Genna, 2008; Hazelbaker, 1993, 2005; Ballard, 2002). Types 1 and 2 can be resolved by clipping (frenotomy or frenulotomy). More severe cases (types 3 and 4) may require frenuloplasty, a more invasive procedure that involves a V-shaped cut and stitches. Development and testing of a useful tool are ongoing to determine which babies with ankyloglossia will have difficulty breastfeeding (Madlon-Kay et al., 2008).

When you work with families whose babies have tight frenula, educating the parents is key to empower them to seek the appropriate help for their infants (Genna & Coryllos, 2009). Compiling a list of healthcare providers in your community who are knowledgeable about evaluating tongue-ties and who will clip them is also key to helping these families. Encourage the family to share the results of their child's evaluation and treatment with their primary care provider. Such sharing can help raise awareness and support in the medical community for treating ankyloglossia and other oral anomalies. Resources for healthcare providers include a protocol on neonatal ankyloglossia developed by the Academy of Breastfeeding Medicine (ABM, 2009) and a presentation on lingual frenulum (Palmer, 2003).

Frenum

The labial frenum is the fold of skin that anchors the upper lip to the top gum (see Color Plate 23). A large frenum results in a gap between the two top front teeth, although it does not usually interfere with the infant's latch. Some babies' frena are so prominent that it is difficult for them to flange the upper lip; in such cases, their mothers may report nipple compression and discomfort while breastfeeding. Clinicians report good results in having labial frena clipped when their constriction interferes with latch (Zeretzke, 2009; Wiessinger & Miller, 1995). Clipping and treatment are usually done for aesthetic reasons (Gkantidis et al., 2008). A presentation is available online that shows the appearance and treatment of labial frena (Palmer, 2001).

Buccal Pads

Buccal pads inside the cheeks (also called fat pads or sucking pads) add to the thickness of the cheek wall (see Figure 13.7). They help decrease the space within the infant's mouth, thereby increasing negative pressure and facilitating milk transfer. If the infant is malnourished or born preterm, buccal pads may not be present. To facilitate breastfeeding in such cases, it may be necessary to position the infant at the breast in such a way that the mother can use her finger against the cheeks to compensate for

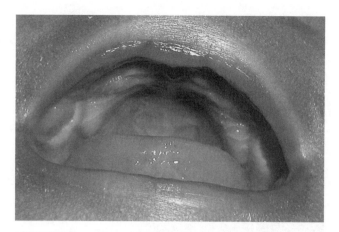

FIGURE 13.7   Buccal fat pads.
Source: Printed with permission of Catherine Watson Genna, BS, IBCLC.

the lack of fat pads, using the Dancer hand position. As the baby grows, the cheek muscles become stronger and provide more stability, and the size of the fat pads diminishes.

Palates

The roof of the mouth contains two palates: the hard palate and the soft palate. The hard palate is located in the front of the mouth; the soft palate lies behind it, in line with the end of the upper alveolar ridge. The condition and shape of the palate can become an issue in breastfeeding. When observing the palate, note whether it has a smooth slope, or is highly vaulted, grooved, or "bubble" shaped. If the palate is high, explore under the tongue for a tight frenulum. Some high palates may be caused by the baby's tongue not being able to reach the roof of the mouth to spread the palate during uterine development. Sometimes a palate is grooved, high, or channeled because of extended intubation with preterm or ill babies (Wilson-Clay & Hoover, 2008). Usually, however, high palates occur naturally.

A high, arched, or bubble palate can sometimes cause the mother's nipple to "catch" in the groove and, therefore, not elongate as it should during breastfeeding. This type of palate makes it more difficult for the infant's tongue to compress the breast tissue adequately so as to feed effectively. Mothers who have infants with such palates often complain of nipple soreness, long feedings, and an unsatisfied infant who needs to nurse frequently. Small protein-filled cysts (Epstein pearls), like those sometimes found on the gum lines, may also occur on the palate. They are not a cause for concern, as they typically resolve spontaneously after birth.

When an infant has a cleft lip, the condition is immediately obvious to everyone. Frequently, infants with cleft lips also have cleft palates. Occasionally, however, an infant may have a cleft of the soft palate that escapes initial

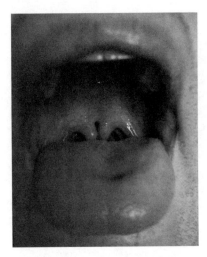

FIGURE 13.8   Bifurcated uvula.
Source: Printed with permission of Dr. Isidre Vilacosta.

diagnosis. Infants with a cleft palate may choke and gag while nursing. Milk can escape from the baby's nose when letdown occurs; stridor or wheezing may be heard. Changing positioning at the breast is often helpful to assess this kind of cleft palate. Some infants may have submucosal clefts, in which skin covers a cleft of the hard or soft palate. In this condition, a notched "V" shape may be observed on the hard palate. These babies often have a bifurcated (bifid, or split in two parts) uvula as well (see Figure 13.8), which may be a marker for a genetic disorder (Shprintzen, 2008). Babies with submucosal clefts may not feed effectively, resulting in low weight gain. See Chapter 25 for more information on breastfeeding an infant who has a cleft of the lip, palate, or both.

Thrush

Thrush is a yeast infection often characterized by white patches that cannot be removed without causing bleeding (see Color Plate 24). This kind of infection may occur between the baby's gums and lips, on the inside of the cheeks, and on the tongue. Thrush, which is most frequently caused by the organism *Candida albicans*, is also known as candidiasis. The infection may appear on the mother's nipples as well as in the baby's mouth, making it imperative that both mother and baby receive treatment at the same time. See the discussion in Chapter 16 on yeast as a cause of nipple soreness.

Clavicle

A fractured clavicle is a common birth trauma, usually identified during the baby's initial examination. In some cases, however, it may escape detection until later. In response to the damage, the baby may restrict the use of the injured arm and resist breastfeeding in a position that places pressure on the fractured area. For example, a baby with a fractured left clavicle may be uncomfortable feeding at the right breast in the cradle hold. An x-ray will confirm the fracture. Treatment typically consists of immobilizing the arm by pinning it in a T-shirt. A fractured clavicle heals quickly, usually within about 3 weeks. After healing, there may be a callus on the clavicle, which will disappear as the baby grows.

Chest

To assess the chest, observe it while the infant is breathing. Labored breathing—evidenced by marked retractions or observable indentations in the chest—may be a symptom of respiratory or cardiac problems. For this reason, a baby with difficulty breathing should always be seen by a physician.

Nipple appearance on the baby's chest is a sign of maturation. The more premature the baby is, the flatter the nipple bud will be. Supernumary nipples may be present either bilaterally or unilaterally (McLaughlin et al., 2008) and may be mistaken for moles. As discussed in Chapter 7, the infant breast may be swollen and even leak "witch's milk," a fluid thought to be caused by maternal hormones. This fluid disappears within the first 3 weeks after birth.

Reflexes

Reflexes in the newborn are present until the central nervous system has matured. They serve as a form of communication that tells us much about what the baby needs. Some reflexes are protective, such as blinking or gagging. Other reflexes indicate a need for more or different interaction. The Moro (or startle) reflex results when the infant is exposed to a loud noise, causing the infant's legs to draw up and arms to fling out. The grasp reflex is initiated by touching the palm of the baby's hand. If left unassisted after birth, the grasp reflex would help the baby move to the breast.

Arching indicates a need for different positioning or a pause from activity. It resembles the positioning of a hypertonic infant (Figure 13.2). If pressure exerted on the back of the head pushes the baby's face into a surface, as against the breast during a feeding, the baby may arch backward. Pressure on the soles of the baby's feet will elicit spontaneous crawling efforts and extension of the baby's head, referred to as Bauer's response. When positioning for a feeding, be careful not to press the baby's feet against the back or side of the couch or chair, as this pressure could cause the baby to arch away from the breast.

Rooting

A full-term healthy newborn has many reflexes that aid breastfeeding (see Table 13.2). At the forefront of these

TABLE 13.2 Gestational Development of Newborn Reflexes

Nutritive Sucking	
9 weeks	Move mouth and lower face
12 weeks	Swallow
18–24 weeks	Nonnutritive suck
32–34 weeks	Nutritive suck and swallow

Associated Reflexes and Responses	
26–27 weeks	Gag reflex with: tongue protrusion, head and jaw extension, contraction of the pharynx
28 weeks	Phasic bite—rhythmic opening and closing of the jaw in response to gum stimulation
28 weeks	Transverse tongue response—movement of the tongue toward the side of stimulation when its lateral surface is touched
32 weeks	Rooting reflex—searching response (progressively toward the side of facial stimulation)
40 weeks	Tongue protrusion response—protrusion when anterior tongue is touched (inhibited as infant grows)

Source: Printed with permission of the International Lactation Consultant Association.

reflexes are rooting and sucking. Stroking the baby's cheek lightly will cause the baby's head to turn in the direction of the stimulus. The mouth will open and the tongue will come forward. This rooting reflex, or response, is illustrated in Figure 13.9. Gently touching the baby's upper lip causes the mouth to open. The mother can initiate the rooting reflex by brushing her nipple against her baby's cheek, stimulating the baby to turn toward her breast and search for the nipple. She can also gently brush the baby's nose or philtrum (the midline spacing between the nose and mouth) to encourage a deeper, asymmetrical latch with the baby's head tilting back slightly.

Sucking

An object placed far enough back into the baby's mouth to reach the juncture between the hard and soft palate will elicit sucking. The increased definition of images produced through newer ultrasound technology suggests that the nipple does not necessarily extend to the juncture of the hard and soft palates, but rather extends to only a few centimeters before the hard and soft palatal juncture (Geddes et al., 2008; Ramsay, 2004). The nipple does not remain stationary during sucking, as movement is seen (Jacobs et al., 2007).

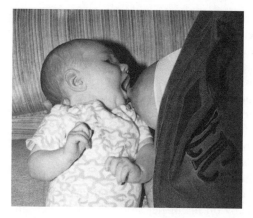

FIGURE 13.9 Rooting for the nipple is a feeding readiness signal from the baby.
Source: Printed with permission of Debbie Shinskie.

Babies demonstrate two types of sucking. A high-flow nutritive suck, characterized by a long, deep suck–swallow–breathe pattern, elicits about one suck per second. A low-flow nonnutritive suck, characterized by a light suck, almost a flutter, with short jaw excursions and little or no audible swallowing, elicits about two sucks per second. Chapter 15 provides a detailed discussion of sucking.

～ *Digestion*

Babies are unique individuals who exhibit their own growth and activity patterns. Patterns of digesting food and expelling waste are equally individualized. As a lactation consultant, you can help parents understand these characteristics and encourage them to observe and become familiar with their baby's digestive patterns and particular needs. Patterns of digestion need to take into account the baby's disposition, eating and sleeping patterns, and body temperature. A change in pattern can alert the parents to a problem or illness before it becomes serious. If the parents notice a change, encourage them to consider the baby's overall pattern before contacting the caregiver. This will help the parents determine whether the current issue represents one small change in the infant's habits or a more significant change. The parents also should observe the infant's skin color, changes in breathing, or other signs of illness such as glassy eyes or abdominal cramping. Four functions that occur during digestion—burping, spitting or vomiting, voiding, and stooling—are discussed in the following sections.

Burping

Breastfed babies need to be burped even though they usually do not take in as much air as bottle fed babies. Babies who suck vigorously may gulp air. If the mother watches for hunger cues and begins a feeding before her baby becomes ravenous, her baby will cry less, resulting in less air in the stomach. Burping increases comfort by decreasing gas pains and reducing spitting up. Gentle patting or rubbing helps air bubbles coalesce and rise to the top of the baby's stomach to be expelled. If a baby consistently spits up after nursing, the mother may not be taking enough time for burping.

The mother can rock her baby in her lap, and gently rub her baby's back. Another method is to hold the baby against her shoulder and massage or pat in the middle of the back with a firm pressure from the bottom up. She can also lay her baby on his or her stomach across her lap, turning the baby's head to one side so that the nose is free, and gently rub the back from the bottom up.

It helps some babies to remain at a 45-degree angle after feedings to bring up air before they are laid down for sleep. A baby sling, infant seat, or swing can accomplish this positioning. If the baby has been crying, the mother can try to burp the baby before putting him or her to the breast. If the baby is a vigorous feeder, he or she will need to nurse before becoming upset so as to cut down on the amount of air intake.

Spitting Up

The passage between the baby's stomach and mouth is very short. Additionally, the muscle valve at the upper end of the stomach (the cardiac sphincter, or lower esophageal sphincter) is not as efficient as it will be later in life. As a result, babies spit up quite often during the early months. Some infants spit up more than others do. Frequent spitting up could be a sign of overfeeding or overactive milk production. If the mother waits too long between feedings, the baby may be upset and gulp air with the milk. Mucus in the baby's stomach can also cause spitting up, especially directly after birth and when the baby has an upper respiratory infection.

Although spitting up is messy and inconvenient, it is not usually a reason for concern. Because cow's milk protein intolerance and nicotine can cause spitting up, however, the mother may want to consider adjustments in her lifestyle and diet. Her baby will benefit if she quits smoking or at least reduces the number of cigarettes smoked. She can burp her baby more often both before and during a feeding. More frequent feeding may also help to reduce spitting up. Occasionally, if the mother experiences an overproduction of milk, limiting the baby to one breast per feeding may help. Make this recommendation only after a complete feeding assessment to ascertain that the mother has overproduction.

Projectile Vomiting

Spitting up differs from vomiting in terms of the force with which the baby expels milk. The baby may dribble milk out with every burp, or may regurgitate with some force. A violent expulsion of milk is considered projectile vomiting and requires a physician's attention. Even breastfed babies can experience gastroenteritis or stomach flu. Babies become dehydrated much faster than older children or adults. Thus, if a baby vomits frequently, the parents need to contact their medical provider immediately.

If the baby suddenly begins vomiting when he or she is several weeks old, or if vomiting becomes progressively worse with a decreasing number of wet diapers, the baby may have pyloric stenosis. With pyloric stenosis, the outflow valve of the baby's stomach does not open satisfactorily to permit the contents of the stomach to pass through (Aspelund & Langer, 2007). This condition seems to be most common in firstborn white male infants.

Infant exposure to macrolides (a class of antibiotics that includes erythromycin, azithromycin, clarithromycin, and roxithromycin) through breastmilk may be associated with pyloric stenosis (Goldstein et al., 2009). Projectile vomiting is also associated with the use of the steroid prostaglandin for cyanotic congenital heart disease (Lacher, 2007). These side effects of other medications demonstrate the importance of taking complete histories on both the mother and the baby.

A sudden onset of vomiting can also indicate an obstruction of the intestines or a strangulated hernia. Both of these conditions require immediate medical evaluation and may result in surgery. Your role in supporting the family at that point changes to helping the mother protect her milk production. See Chapter 24 for more information on the lactation consultant's role with a baby who is ill or hospitalized.

Gastroesophageal Reflux

Some infants spit up only occasionally while others seem to spit up all the time. Spitting up multiple times in one day can be a sign of gastroesophageal reflux (GER). Reflux is also called gastroesophageal reflux disease (GERD), once clinically diagnosed as such. GER is a backflow of the contents of the stomach into the esophagus. It often occurs when the lower esophageal sphincter fails to close or is soft so that it does not stay securely closed. Because gastric juices are acidic, they produce burning pain in the esophagus.

Identifying Gastroesophageal Reflux   Infants with reflux may spit up several times after a feeding. Some spit up even during a feeding. Manifestations of GER include vomiting, poor weight gain, dysphagia, abdominal pain, substernal pain (below the sternum), retrosternal pain (behind the sternum), esophagitis, and respiratory disorders (Bhatia & Parish, 2009). Silent reflux may also occur, in which the stomach contents fail to come all the way back up. In such a case, the infant does not spit up but may experience burning and discomfort.

In a prospective study of 2642 children, 313 were found to have regurgitation. Only one child was definitively diagnosed with GERD with esophagitis. Another was diagnosed with cow's milk protein intolerance. Infants who were breastfed experienced a more rapid resolution of GER compared to artificially fed infants (Campanozzi et al., 2009).

Food allergy can contribute to GERD, colic, or constipation in infancy (Heine, 2006). Infants with these conditions often respond to a maternal elimination diet (or hypoallergenic formula if artificially fed). In an investigation into the specific role of cow's milk allergy in GER, researchers found an association in half the cases of infants with GER who were less than 1 year old (Salvatore & Vandenplas, 2002). In a high proportion of cases, GER not only was associated with cow's milk allergy, but also was induced by it. If a mother tells you her baby has reflux or if you see signs consistent with GER, cow's milk allergy could be a factor, with the offending protein coming either from the mother's diet or from supplemental formula.

Effects on the Infant The constant regurgitation of milk into the esophagus can cause severe irritation or pain for the infant. Some infants with GER learn to limit their intake, having made the association between a full stomach and the pain that accompanies reflux. Frequent spitting up and limited intake can lead to poor weight gain. If an infant with reflux has been self-limiting intake because of discomfort, the mother's milk production may be low because the baby removes only small amounts of milk at each feeding. Therefore, the infant with no or slow weight gain, whose mother has limited milk production, may experience an exacerbation of symptoms when she attempts to increase her milk production. Other infants with reflux may display signs of discomfort that look like hunger signs and so may actually be overfed, with excessive weight gain of 2 or more ounces per day. Because of this possibility, it is important to look for signs of reflux in any infant whose weight gain is outside the normal range in either direction.

Regurgitating human milk is not as irritating as regurgitating formula. Because infants digest human milk more quickly than infant formulas, they absorb more milk in the same amount of time. For these reasons, as well as because of the primary health risks of artificial feeding, it is not appropriate to switch a breastfed infant to formula as a treatment for GER.

Coping Strategies Infants who experience GER need to be fed in an upright position so that gravity can help the milk stay down. Holding the baby upright after a feeding will also help keep the milk down. In addition, these babies benefit from smaller, more frequent feedings. Another strategy is to nurse from only one breast at a feeding, provided the mother has adequate milk production. All of these actions will help limit the amount of milk the infant takes in at a feeding, yet ensure that the child gets the fattier hindmilk and is able to digest and retain more calories.

As another measure to counteract GER, parents might try putting the infant to sleep on an incline and using a pacifier after feedings. One study reported that these treatments do not appear to have a positive effect on this condition (Carroll et al., 2002). Other clinicians have found that they may be helpful and continue to recommend these interventions (Vandenplas et al., 2005). Each baby is different, and each will respond to strategies differently.

Carriers, seats, and positions that avoid pressure on the abdomen but keep the trunk supported and extended are preferred when the child has GER. This may mean limiting the use of car seats to car riding only, as well as limited use of burping positions that put pressure on the baby's stomach. Some parents find infant massage (Boekel, 2000; Huhtala et al., 2000) and chiropractic care (Alcantara & Anderson, 2008) to be helpful.

Mothers may be told they can mix their milk with cereal or a commercial thickener (such as Simply Thick) to see if the thicker fluid will stay down better. It is almost impossible to keep a mother's milk thick with rice cereal because the enzymes in human milk begin digesting starches almost immediately. When milk is thickened, some families have compensated for the slowness of feeding by using bottle nipples with larger holes, which defeats the purpose of thickening. Furthermore, the fact that the milk is not spit up does not mean that the actual reflux and pain have been treated effectively. Many women will abandon breastfeeding if they are told they must express their milk and feed it by bottle to provide thickening.

Having an infant with reflux can be very stressful for parents. It sometimes feels like having a baby with colic all day long. In some cases, the baby may be upset only at feeding time, which can feel like personal rejection to the mother. From a counseling standpoint, these parents need validation that reflux is stressful, that caring for their child is draining, and that their baby is not the pleasant, cooing, cuddly baby they envisioned. Acknowledging the parents' grief at the loss of this vision, and providing reassurance that they are not bad parents, can help them move forward and enjoy the moments when their baby does feel well. Support from other parents, friends, and relatives helps alleviate the sense of isolation parents may feel. Symptoms usually decrease in the second part of the first year of life and subside by the child's first birthday.

Medications If the case of severe reflux, the physician will need to be more involved in the child's care. For some infants, reflux can be severe enough to require medication. Some medications used for reflux decrease the acid level in the infant's stomach. Others encourage the infant's stomach to pass the milk more quickly into the intestines. Most babies who were prescribed anti-reflux drugs in one study were found to not meet the diagnostic criteria for GERD—a finding that calls into question whether anti-reflux medications are overprescribed for infants with regurgitation (Khoshoo, 2007).

Most physicians will usually try medications before resorting to a more invasive test such as a barium swallow, endoscopy, pH probe, or x-ray exam. These tests are indicated when the baby has poor weight gain or does not respond to medications (Wolf & Glass, 1992).

Elimination

Elimination patterns are significant indicators of a baby's intake. Keeping a diary of feedings, voids, and stools for the first week or two postpartum helps parents identify and assess patterns in their new baby's behavior. It also builds parents' confidence that exclusive breastfeeding provides sufficient nourishment for their baby. If concerns arise about intake, the diary provides a helpful record for medical care providers. There is wide variability in stooling and voiding among infants in the early days after birth, especially when there are differences in breastfeeding routine.

Voiding

A healthy newborn's urine is in the color range of pale yellow to clear. Newborns are characterized by small, frequent voids (Sillén, 2001). Voiding in full-term babies tends to occur when the baby is awake (Olsen, 2009). In the first week of life, the baby should have an increasing number of voids daily. Many hospitals correlate the number of voids and stools to the number of days old the baby is, up to day 4 or 5. By the time the baby is 4 or 5 days old, the baby should be voiding at least 6 times in 24 hours.

Urate Crystals Pink (copper or "brick dust") stains that appear with urination are urate crystals, whose presence indicates excess uric acid (see Color Plate 25). Urate crystals generally are not significant in the first 1 to 3 days of life. Assessment of the baby's hydration status is necessary if the stains appear after this time, however.

Stooling

A breastfed baby's stools differ greatly from those of a formula fed baby. The newborn's first stools are a black, tarry meconium, usually passed within the first 24 to 36 hours (see Color Plate 26). Transitional stools are greenish black to greenish brown, as the meconium gives way to brown and then to a golden or mustard yellow color

when the baby is approximately 48 to 72 hours of age (see Color Plate 27). The texture may range from watery to seedy yellow to a toothpaste consistency. There is no strong odor to the stools of a breastfed infant.

Infants in the first month of life should have a minimum of three or more soft, yellow, runny stools each day. An infant who has fewer than three stools in a 24-hour period may not be getting enough to eat and will need to be weighed, examined, and monitored for adequate intake. Encourage parents to become familiar with their baby's stooling patterns. Every baby's digestive system, and thus the pattern for expelling waste, is individual to that particular baby. One study found that the median number of stools per day is 6 in the first month of life and that stooling frequency is higher in breastfed infants (Tunc, 2008).

Babies' bowel habits change with age. A mother may find that at around 4 to 6 weeks of age, her baby will begin going for longer periods between bowel movements. Frequency of elimination in older breastfed infants can range from a baby having several stools every day to only stooling once every 3 days. Both patterns are acceptable. Stooling may decrease to once a day in the second month of life, a pattern that could continue until the end of 6 months, when supplemental foods are started (Tunc, 2008). The characteristics of healthy breastfed stools are described in Table 13.3, along with variations and their possible causes.

Infrequent Stooling When an infant is not stooling appropriately in the first month of life, the clinician needs to do a complete feeding assessment. Infrequent stooling in the first month may be due to insufficient milk intake. A baby who is voiding, but not stooling or gaining weight, may not be feeding enough, or may be feeding ineffectively. Such a child may not be receiving enough high-fat hindmilk, especially if the mother is limiting the frequency or duration of feedings. Moreover, infrequent stooling sometimes is the parents' first indication of low milk production. Stooling frequency usually corrects itself with additional feeding or longer feedings to assure the infant receives more hindmilk. This intervention works when the mother has adequate milk production and the baby is able to transfer milk well.

Infrequent stooling could be caused by Hirschsprung's disease, a condition in which a part of the infant's intestines lacks proper innervation and the stool cannot pass easily beyond that point. Symptoms in infants include difficult bowel movements, poor feeding, poor weight gain, and a large, bloated abdomen from the impacted stool and gas. Early diagnosis is important to prevent serious complications, including enterocolitis and colonic rupture (Kessmann, 2006). Breastfed infants with this condition may escape detection until the parents add solid foods to their diet and their stools become more

TABLE 13.3   Stool Patterns of a Breastfed Baby

Characteristics	Normal Stool	Variations	Possible Causes
Color	A newborn's stool is black, brown, or green in the first 3 days. This is meconium. Later, color ranges from brown or green to mustard yellow.	Unexplained color changes. Black, brown, or red spots.	Mother's or baby's diet. Mother's cracked nipples (possible bleeding—there is no harm to the baby). Bleeding from baby's rectum. If no known cause, the mother should consult the physician.
Consistency	Ranges from a toothpaste-like texture to a liquid with curds.	Very watery.	Foods in diet other than mother's milk, antibiotics, or illness.
		Hard pellets.	Foods in diet other than mother's milk, insufficient fluids, or baby tense or ill.
		Mucous.	Newborn mucus, cold, congestion, or allergy to mother's or baby's diet.
		Fibrous.	Bananas and cereal present in the baby's diet.
Odor	Very little, not unpleasant.	Unpleasant.	New foods in addition to mother's milk, antibiotics, or illness.
Frequency	Ranges from 1 with every feed to 4 a day under 1 month of age. Decrease in frequency after the first month of life.	Sudden change in frequency. Watch carefully and look for other symptoms.	Foods, maturity, or illness.
Volume	Varies with frequency. More frequent stools mean less volume per diaper.	Any sudden change. Watch carefully and be alert to other symptoms.	Foods, maturity, or illness.
Ease of expulsion	Easy and semicontrolled with some straining by the baby.	Flows out continually.	Foods other than mother's milk, illness, or antibiotics.
		Very difficult with extreme straining.	Foods other than mother's milk or insufficient fluids.

bulky and solid. Although this is a rare condition, any exclusively breastfed infant who is gaining adequate amounts of weight but not stooling frequently needs careful evaluation and monitoring. Cow's milk allergy has been shown to mimic Hirschsprung's disease (Kubota et al., 2006).

Constipation   Constipation is rare in breastfed infants. Lack of a daily bowel movement and straining at stooling do not indicate constipation in the infant, but rather are normal aspects of toileting. In infants, constipation is diagnosed by stool consistency and not by frequency. A soft stool indicates that the infant is not constipated. Con-

stipated stools are molded and firm to the touch like pellets or marbles. In young infants, nursing more frequently will resolve most infrequent stooling problems. Maternal iron supplements have been reported anecdotally to contribute to an infant's constipation. If this is the case, discontinuing these supplements for a few days may return the child's digestive system to normal.

Constipation sometimes occurs when parents add solid foods to the baby's diet. If the parents are giving large amounts of cereal, they can stop or decrease the cereal for several days until normal stooling is reestablished. They can then reintroduce the cereal in smaller amounts less frequently. The parents might also add more fruits and vegetables to the diet. If the baby is old enough to receive them, yogurt, oatmeal, or prune juice may help. Parents should not treat their infant with suppositories without consulting the baby's healthcare provider.

Diarrhea For new parents, it is important to teach them to distinguish between diarrhea and the typically loose stool of a breastfed baby. A mother who has been supplementing with formula and then returns to exclusive breastfeeding may mistakenly believe her baby has diarrhea. A mother whose other children were not breastfed might also need to recognize the difference. Likewise, grandmothers who did not breastfeed may worry that a normal breastmilk stool is diarrhea.

With diarrhea, the stool is much looser than normal, is very watery, and may be greenish and very foul smelling. It may indicate the beginning of an illness or a reaction to antibiotics taken by either the mother or the baby. If diarrhea is suspected, urge the mother to continue breastfeeding. Diarrhea removes valuable intestinal bacteria that aid in the digestion of food, and such bacterial colonizations can be restored with human milk feedings.

When a baby exhibits diarrhea, the mother should contact the baby's caregiver immediately, as babies can become dehydrated very quickly. Be sure the mother understands that human milk is not a dairy product; it is a clear fluid that provides all the electrolytes a baby needs. She should, therefore, continue breastfeeding and avoid supplementing with any electrolyte solution. Healthcare providers who are familiar with the artificial feeding (cow's milk–based formula) model for treatment may be unaware of this fact.

～ Infant Communication

Neurological research has increased our understanding that the full-term, nonmedicated human baby is exquisitely wired and very competent to breastfeed (Bergman, 2008; Moore et al., 2007; Bergman et al., 2004). Respecting the baby's innate ability to nurse capitalizes on the child's neurobehaviors and is empowering to mothers (Smillie, 2001, 2008). For these reasons, one of a lactation consultant's most important jobs is to help mothers understand, interpret, and respect their babies' communication and to respond accordingly. Attachment is important for developing maternal feelings. One study showed that women with anxiety or fear of attachment had higher rates of depression than those with feelings of security and attachment (Monk et al., 2008). Another study explored the link between postpartum psychological adjustment and feeding choice. In this investigation, a higher score on a depression scale at 1 month was correlated with quitting breastfeeding by 4 months after delivery (Akman et al., 2008).

Smiling is an important development in babies that appears to be dependent on interaction. Social smiling emerges out of attentive engagement with an interactive caregiver (Parlade et al., 2009). The concept of mutually responsive orientation (MRO), in which parental responsiveness elicits responses from infants, is associated with the development of self-regulation and self-representation (Kochanska et al., 2008). As a lactation consultant, you can play an important role by teaching parents to recognize infant signals and by giving positive feedback when they respond appropriately to their babies' cues. Smiling and other developmental milestones are addressed in Chapter 17.

Approach and Avoidance Behaviors

Infants exhibit specific behavior that indicates a willingness to be approached. This so-called approach behavior is integrated, stable, balanced, exploratory, and self-regulated. The signals illustrated in Figure 13.10 are characteristic of a more mature infant. Conversely, infants display avoidance behavior that indicates a desire to withdraw, as shown in Figures 13.11 and 13.12. Recognizing these behaviors will help parents know how to respond to their baby. Tables 13.4 and 13.5 describe infant approach and avoidance behaviors.

Hunger Cues and Stages of Alertness

Many infant approach behaviors signal an interest to breastfeed. For example, hunger cues may indicate hunger, thirst, or a need to be comforted at the breast. The infant will give cues the same way, regardless of the reason. An interest in feeding depends on the baby's level of alertness, as described in Table 13.6. Teaching hunger cues to parents will help them know when their baby is

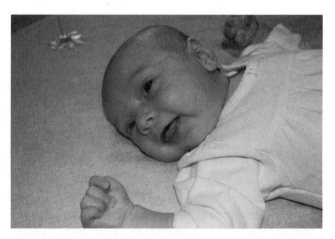

FIGURE 13.10   An infant exhibiting approach behavior.
Source: Printed with permission of Kori Martin.

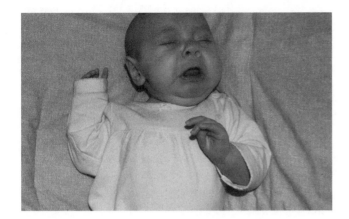

FIGURE 13.11 An infant exhibiting avoidance behavior.

Source: Printed with permission of Kori Martin.

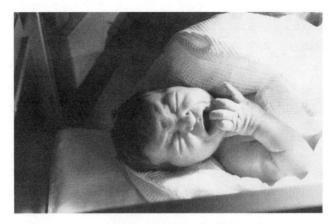

FIGURE 13.12 An infant exhibiting feeding avoidance.

Source: Printed with permission of Carole Peterson.

TABLE 13.4 Infant Approach Behaviors

Behavior	Description
Tongue extension	The infant's tongue either is extended toward a stimulus or it repeatedly extends and relaxes.
Hand on face	The infant's hand or hands are placed onto his face or over his ears, and are maintained there for a brief period.
Sounds	The infant emits undifferentiated sounds. At times, it may sound like a whimper.
Hand clasp	The infant grasps his own hands or clutches his hands to his own body. His hands each may be closed and touch each other.
Foot clasp	The infant positions his feet against each other, foot sole to foot sole. Or he folds his legs in a crossed position with his feet grasping his legs or resting on them.
Finger fold	The infant interweaves one or more fingers of each hand.
Tuck	The infant curls or turns his trunk or shoulders, pulls up his legs, and tucks his arms. He uses the examiner's hands or body to attain tuck flexion.
Body movement	The infant adjusts his body, his extremities, or his head into a more flexed position. He may turn to the side or attempt to attain a tonic neck response.
Hand to mouth	The infant attempts to bring his hand or fingers to his mouth. He does not have to be successful.
Grasping	The infant makes grasping movements with his hands. He may grasp either toward his own face or body, in midair, toward the examiner's hands or body, or toward the side of the bassinet.
Leg and foot brace	The infant extends his legs and/or feet toward an object in order to stabilize himself. He may push against the examiner's body or hands, the surface he is on, or the sides of the bassinet. Once touching, he may flex his legs or he may restart the bracing.
Mouthing	The infant makes mouthing movements with his lips or jaws.
Suck search	The infant extends his lips forward or opens his mouth in a searching fashion, usually moving his head at the same time.
Sucking	The infant sucks on his own hands or fingers, clothing, the examiner's fingers, a pacifier, or other object that he has either obtained himself or that the examiner has inserted into his mouth.
Hand holding	The infant holds onto the examiner's hand or finger with his own hands. He may have placed them there himself, or the examiner may have positioned them there. The infant then actively holds on.
"Ooh" face	The infant rounds his mouth and purses his lips or extends them in an "ooh" configuration. This may be with his eyes open or closed.
Locking visually and/or auditorily	The infant locks onto the examiner's face or an object or sight in the environment. He may lock on above or to the side of the examiner's face and maintains his gaze in one direction for observable periods. The sound component of an environmental stimulus may contribute to his locking.

Source: Adapted and printed with permission of Sarah Coulter Danner.

TABLE 13.5 Infant Withdrawal or Avoidance Behaviors

Behavior	Description
Spit up	The infant spits up, with more than a passive drool. However, the amount of vomit may be quite minimal.
Gag	The infant appears to choke momentarily or to gulp or gag. Swallowing and respiration patterns are not synchronized. This is often accompanied by at least mild mouth opening.
Hiccough	The infant hiccoughs.
Bowel movement grunting or straining	The infant's face and body display the straining often associated with bowel movements. He emits the grunting sounds often associated with bowel movements.
Grimace, lip retraction	The infant's lips retract noticeably. His face is distorted in a retracting direction.
Trunkal arching	The infant arches his trunk away from the bed or the mother's body.
Finger splay	The infant's hands open strongly, and the fingers are extended and separated from each other.
Airplane	The infant's arms either are fully extended out to the side at approximately shoulder level or the upper and lower arm are at an angle to each other and are extended out at the shoulder.
Salute	The infant's arms are fully extended into midair, either singly or simultaneously.
Sitting on air	The infant's legs are extended into midair, either singly or simultaneously. This may occur when the infant is lying flat on his back or upright.
Sneezing, yawning, sighing, or coughing	The infant sneezes, yawns, sighs, or coughs.
Averting	The infant actively averts his eyes. He may momentarily close them.
Frowning	The infant knits his brows or darkens his eyes by contracting his muscles.
Startle	The infant's limbs jerk once, occasionally followed briefly by a slight amount of jitteriness and possibly crying.

Source: Adapted and printed with permission of Sarah Coulter Danner.

TABLE 13.6 The Six Infant States

Infant state	Description
Deep sleep	Characterized by limp extremities, a placid face, quiet breathing, no body movement, and no rapid eye movement (REM). The baby lies very still, with an occasional twitch or sucking movement. He cannot easily be aroused.
Light or active sleep	Resistance in the extremities when moved, mouthing or sucking motions, body movement, and facial grimaces. The baby is awakened more easily and is likely to remain awake if disturbed. Most of the baby's sleep is spent in this state, with less regular breathing and rapid eye movement (his eyes flutter beneath the eyelids). Although he may stir and move about, he can return to sleep if left undisturbed.
Drowsy	The baby is aroused easily and may drift back to sleep. His eyes may open and close intermittently, and he may murmur, whisper, yawn, and stretch.
Quiet alert	The baby looks around and interacts with others. This is an excellent time to breastfeed. The baby is extremely responsive. His body is still and watchful, his eyes are bright, and his breathing is even and regular.
Active alert	The baby moves his extremities and plays. He is even more attentive, being wide-eyed, with rapid and irregular breathing. He may become fussy and is more sensitive to the discomfort of a wet diaper or excessive stimulation.
Crying	The baby is agitated and needs comforting.

ready to nurse. If parents wait until their baby cries to initiate feeding, the baby will already be exhibiting the final sign of hunger. Pointing out hunger cues during a breastfeeding assessment will help the mother recognize what to look for.

Knowing When to Initiate a Feeding

Hunger cues may be evident during the light sleep, drowsy, and quiet alert states. The baby will begin to wriggle, and tightly closed eyes may exhibit rapid eye movement (REM). Cues progress to passing one or both hands over the head, bringing a hand to the mouth (Figure 13.13), and sucking motions. If the cheek or mouth is touched at this stage, the baby will begin to root. Soon, more vigorous sucking begins. The baby then will settle back into a less active state.

The baby may exhibit hunger cues several times in the span of 20 to 30 minutes. If these signals remain unheeded, the infant could become frustrated and cry. Conversely, the child might become exhausted and fall back asleep without having received any nourishment. A missed feeding opportunity can have consequences for the next feed. This pattern is common in preterm infants, health-compromised infants, or infants who are fed by the clock or ignored.

Crying can cause a newborn to appear disorganized in terms of motor functions. It may take several minutes for the infant to settle enough to breastfeed. He or she may be unable to breastfeed at all until having slept again for a while. In either case, the mother has missed a feeding opportunity. If a mother needs to wake her baby for a feeding, she should do so when the baby is in a light sleep or a drowsy state. Most babies move from deep sleep to light sleep in approximately 20- to 30-minute cycles.

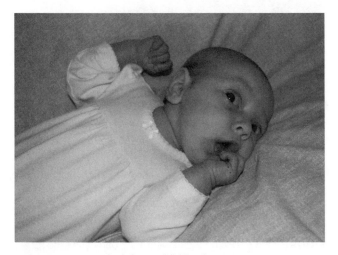

FIGURE 13.13   An infant exhibiting hunger cues.

Source: Printed with permission of Kori Martin.

∼ Infant Behavior Patterns

The first few weeks of a baby's life are a series of adjustments for everyone. For parents, it is a period when love, patience, and understanding for their infant are most important. Because newborns totally rely on their mothers to meet all of their needs, a mother may spend nearly all of her time and energies during the first month caring for her baby. At times, she may feel physically drained and emotionally frustrated by the infant's helplessness, while at the same time she enjoys the closeness and warmth of their growing relationship.

Infants' dispositions and patterns of sleeping and eating can affect the nourishment they receive. First-time mothers sometimes become concerned about their babies' dispositions. It helps them to know that babies experience a variety of behavior patterns, ranging from easygoing and undemanding to active and fussy. Studies show that an infant's temperament is inborn. As a lactation consultant, your specific guidance to a mother concerning breastfeeding may depend on the type of baby she has. Understanding the various behavior patterns, dispositions, and sleeping and eating patterns will help you offer appropriate suggestions. It may take some time for parents to discover all the variations and subtle nuances.

Average Baby

The average newborn who is exclusively breastfed will nurse anywhere between 8 and 12 times in 24 hours. Nursing more frequently is very normal, especially during times of cluster feeding. When a baby cluster feeds, the nursings may blend into one another, with few distinctions between starting and stopping. The newborn usually sleeps from 12 to 20 hours per day, possibly with one or two longer periods of sleep balanced by one or two fussy periods. Fussy periods typically occur in the early evening. Usually responsive when handled, the normal baby is generally quiet, alert, and listening while awake. The child soon may learn self-soothing by sucking on a fist or displaying some other type of comfort measure.

Easy Baby

Some babies have a breastfeeding pattern typical of an average baby, consisting of approximately 8 to 12 feedings in 24 hours, but have longer sleep periods and are less demanding, with relatively little or no fussiness. Mothers often refer to these babies as being "so easy." This mother may need to make a conscious effort to give her baby the tactile stimulation and attention needed for the child's emotional growth and physical development. Having an undemanding baby may allow her more free time, and she will want to take care not to overexert herself physically as a result. She can make good use of her free time by devoting some of it to her baby, even in the absence of many bids for attention.

Placid Baby

Some babies demonstrate placid behavior, requesting as few as 4 to 6 feedings in 24 hours. The mother will need to monitor her infant to guard against undernourishment. Because such a child sleeps as much as 18 to 20 hours per day, he or she is usually quietly alert and tranquil when awake. Although the infant makes few demands for attention, the infrequent feedings do not indicate a lack of hunger. The infant may wake, feel hungry, and need to nurse, yet not cry or demonstrate specific hunger cues to let the mother know he or she is awake and hungry. Rather, the infant soon falls back asleep until he or she awakes again and repeats the same pattern. The result can be an undernourished baby.

Lack of attention and stimuli for a placid baby can lead to poor emotional nourishment. Unlike with the easy baby, the mother does not meet the infant's needs for nourishment because the child does not know how to give the necessary cues. With such vital physical and emotional needs going unfulfilled, the infant may become withdrawn and lethargic. Mothers often describe a placid baby as being "such a good baby" who does not cry and sleeps through the night. You can discreetly ask the mother of a "good" baby about breastfeeding and elimination patterns. These babies may be slow weight gainers.

The mother of a placid baby must take care to meet her baby's needs without receiving the necessary cues. She can use a monitor or place a noise device in the crib, such as a safe rattle, bell, or squeaky toy, to alert her to movement in the crib. A placid baby will benefit from being carried in a sling or baby carrier and being kept close to the mother and other family members, even without bids for attention. The mother can take advantage of natural waking to pick up her baby and stimulate the baby to nurse. Parents of a placid baby should avoid pacifying techniques such as pacifiers, cradles, or swings. Babies who pacify themselves through thumb sucking can be encouraged to satisfy their sucking needs at the breast instead.

Active and Fussy Baby

Active, fussy babies may nurse more frequently than the average baby, perhaps because of a greater need to calm or comfort themselves. Such a child may seem insatiable at the breast and impatient for the milk to let down. The baby will have fewer sleep hours than average, and when awake, will be active and frequently unable to self-calm. In addition, the infant may have several periods of inconsolable crying during the day. The child may overreact to freedom and stimulation, and will need gentle, slow, and soothing movements from caregivers as a calming measure. The mother can keep her fussy baby warm and use swaddling to avoid startling. She and other family members can hold the baby often, close to their bodies.

An active, fussy baby may respond well to nursing, dozing, and playing at the breast for generous periods. The greater need to be comforted at the breast, combined with increased milk intake, may cause such an infant to spit up often from being overly full. The mother might try nursing on only one breast at a feeding to allow leisurely sucking on a drained breast without transferring more milk than the infant can handle. She may need to burp the baby often, as the over-eagerness at feedings can cause such a child to swallow more air. Some of these babies do well when the parents carry them in a sling and hold them upright after nursing (see Figure 13.14). When using a baby sling, parents are cautioned to make sure the baby's face is visible and is not pressed tightly against the wearer.

∾ Infant Growth

Lactation consultants regularly assess infant growth as part of their routine duties. Several factors need to be considered during this assessment. Note the infant's weight gain since the last weight check. Also look at the rate of weight gain since the lowest weight the child experienced (rather than birth weight). Record the baby's growth in length and head circumference. Monitor signs of adequate intake in relation to weight gain, including alert-

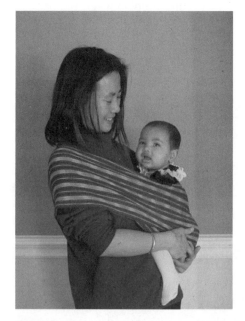

FIGURE 13.14   Parents can wear their baby in a sling for comforting.

Source: Printed with permission of Anna Swisher.

ness, skin turgor, moist mucous membranes, and adequate output.

Caloric Intake

The calorie content of human milk depends on its fat content, as 50 percent of the energy content of milk comes from the fat. Fat content varies between women, the time of day, the fullness of the breast, and even between breasts (Kent et al., 2006). Most women report one breast makes more milk than the other.

Energy needs for healthy, breastfed infants have been estimated as 9 to 39 percent lower than previously believed, with an average of 80 to 90 kcal/kg per day depending on infant age (Dewey, 2000). Whitehead (1995, 1985), using an average value of 69 kcal/kg per day, found that infants thrived on lower intake than theorized. Research demonstrates that breastfed infants are more metabolically efficient than artificially fed children (Whitehead & Paul, 2000). Mitoulas et al. (2002) found a range of 60 to 67 kcal/100 mL. Moreover, milk intake varies greatly from baby to baby. Kent and colleagues (2006) found an average intake of 788 mL (26.65 oz) with a range of 478 to 1356 mL (16.17 to 45.86 oz), a range similar to Dewey & Lönnerdal's (1983) findings of 341 to 1096 mL/day.

What these findings signify in practical terms is that a healthy baby is the best regulator of his or her own appetite. Ample evidence indicates that healthy, full-term infants self-regulate their food intake, provided no arbitrary scheduling or time limits are imposed on feeding. Giving babies water can affect their caloric intake, because the volume makes them feel full. Sterile water has no calories, and sugar (dextrose) water (D_5W) has only a limited amount of energy—6 kcal/29.57 mL (1 oz). Over the course of the day, the baby takes in the amount of milk needed for growth. Calorie content of the milk is an issue only when caring for preterm babies or babies with illness, low weight gain, failure to thrive, or disorders. See Chapter 23 for a discussion of these babies.

Babies utilize breastmilk very efficiently, such that breastfed infants have a leaner body mass than artificially fed infants (Heinig et al., 1993). These lower caloric (energy) intakes by breastfed infants explain their lower percentage of body fat beginning at 5 months (Dewey et al., 1993). Compared to formula fed infants, breastfed infants' energy intake is lower throughout the first 12 months of life (Heinig et al., 1993). At 1 month of age, formula fed infants consumed an average of 118 kcal/kg per day versus 101 kcal/kg per day for breastfed infants. This discrepancy persisted at 4 months, when energy consumption averaged 87 kcal/kg per day for formula fed infants versus 72 kcal/kg per day for breastfed infants (Butte et al., 1990a). Energy needs per day decrease as the baby gets older (Whitehead, 1995).

Breastfed infants have lower sleeping metabolic rates, rectal temperature, and heart rates, which may collectively account for the differences in energy intake and expenditure rates (Butte et al., 1991; Garza & Butte, 1990). A study of infants at 12 and 24 months revealed no difference in intake at these ages, suggesting that the different rates of growth and body composition do not persist into the second year of life (Butte et al., 2000). In recent years, however, evidence for a link between formula feeding and obesity into adulthood has been growing ever stronger (Palou & Picó, 2009; Patel et al., 2009), with a dose-dependent relationship being suggested (Weyermann et al., 2006; Harder et al., 2006). Other researchers question the validity of this link, citing parental and socioeconomic issues as confounding factors (Huus et al., 2008; Michels et al., 2007).

Weight Gain

A newborn initially may lose as much as 7 percent of his or her birth weight due to a loss of fluids and the passage of meconium. If the mother receives excessive intravenous fluids during labor, a fluid shift to the infant may occur that artificially increases the initial birth weight. Infants who experience fluid shifts typically void large amounts of urine in the first 24 hours of life and can lose more weight than a baby born without IV interventions. Exposure to medications during labor can depress the baby's central nervous system and lead to fewer feedings in the first days of life—another factor that will affect weight gain in the early days.

A weight loss of more than 7 percent of birth weight indicates a need for evaluation and perhaps assistance with breastfeeding. By day 3, a full-term infant should not lose any more weight, and the baby's weight should stabilize by the end of the first week. The baby should have regained his or her birth weight by 10 to 14 days after delivery. Infants who are not back to birth weight by this time require evaluation. Table 13.7 presents a typical weight gain pattern for a breastfeeding baby. It is important to recognize that this pattern may vary from one baby to the next.

From birth to about 3 months, breastfed infants tend to gain weight at similar or greater rates than artificially fed infants. Some studies show that breastfed infants gain weight faster during this time (Fawzi et al., 1997). Others reveal similar rates (Motil et al., 1997), statistically insignificant differences (Butte et al., 1990b), or even slower weight gain (Butte et al., 1990a). After 3 or 4 months, formula fed infants gain weight faster.

Breastfed infants follow the WHO standard for growth, whereas artificially fed infants deviate from this standard by exhibiting higher weight for age (Van Dijk & Innis, 2009). From 6 to 12 months, formula fed infants tend to weigh more than breastfed infants. Artificially fed

TABLE 13.7 Typical Weight Gain for a Healthy Infant

Birth Weight 7 lb 8 oz 3405 g	7% Loss at Day 4 6 lb 15 oz 3150 g	Gain per Day Days 4–10	Weight on Day 10
Slightly below birth weight at day 10, but with steady daily gain		0.7 oz 20 g	7 lb 4 oz 3290 g
Back to birth weight at day 10, with steady daily gain		1.2 oz 35 g	7 lb 8 oz 3395 g
Slightly above birth weight at day 10, with steady daily gain		1.6 oz 40 g	7 lb 9 oz 3688 g

Source: Printed with permission of the International Lactation Consultant Association.

babies weigh an average of 600–650 grams more than breastfed babies. Continued research has found no significant height differences between adults who were breastfed or artificially fed (Dewey, 2007).

Obesity

Assessing infant growth is of key interest in view of the obesity epidemic among youth, as discussed in Chapter 9. Researchers have correlated a lack of breastfeeding with an increased risk of obesity (Patel et al., 2009; Moreno et al., 2007). In fact, artificial feeding is a predictor of obesity in both infancy and adulthood (Dewey, 2007). The role of nutrition early in life is increasingly recognized as contributing to growth and metabolic changes in later life. Studies have established a strong correlation between early nutritional factors (reduced breastfeeding, increased formula feeding, and early introduction of carbohydrate-enriched baby foods) and adult-onset disorders in offspring, as well as the development of metabolic diseases in adulthood (Patel et al., 2009).

WHO Growth Charts

Many medical offices use weight charts published by formula companies, whose logos appear on the charts. These documents are based principally on 1977 growth charts from the U.S. National Center for Health Statistics (NCHS). The original charts were based on one ethnic and demographic group of primarily formula fed infants; as a consequence, they are not reliable for charting growth in breastfed babies. Although the U.S. Centers for Disease Control and Prevention (CDC) released new charts in 2000, there are notable differences between the typical growth pattern of breastfed infants and the expected growth pattern on the CDC charts as well.

The World Health Organization (WHO) compiled data at seven international study centers to develop a new set of international growth charts for infants and children through 5 years of age. These charts are based on the growth of exclusively or predominantly breastfed children (WHO, 2006). The 2006 WHO growth charts, which are printed in Appendix F, are the best indicator of growth for breastfed infants.

⁓ Sleeping Patterns

All babies require a great amount of sleep, although the specific amount of sleep each baby needs varies. Some babies sleep as few as 8 hours in a 24-hour period; others sleep as many as 20 hours per day. Understanding her baby's typical sleep patterns will help a mother adapt to the child's unique needs. The factors that cause variations among babies' sleep patterns may be developmental, environmental, or nutritional in nature. For example, over-tiredness or overstimulation can cause fretfulness before and during sleep. Sounds, lights, the temperature of the room and bedding, and low humidity (which causes difficulty in breathing) can all affect (and sometimes interfere with) sleep.

New research shows that the nucleotides in human milk play an important role in sleep homeostasis (Sánchez et al., 2009). Researchers found that these nucleotides exhibit significant circadian rhythms. The rise in nocturnal levels of these nucleotides could explain the "hypnotic" response to nursing at night in the infant.

Babies who sleep separated from their mothers may wake at night to seek nourishment and physical contact. The absence of the mother's body warmth and skin contact can make it more difficult for the infant to fall asleep and sleep undisturbed. A baby may also have trouble sleeping if the mother consumes too much caffeine, as this substance passes to the baby through her milk. See Chapter 17 for a discussion of developmental factors that affect sleep.

Encouraging the Baby to Sleep

Many parents voice concerns about their babies' sleep habits. You can help a mother determine whether she has realistic expectations. Perhaps she can keep a written record for several days of her baby's sleep patterns over a 24-hour period, including even 5-minute naps. Gaining a better understanding of her baby's behavior can help her relax and not allow sleep to be such an important goal. If the mother feels she is not getting enough sleep, you can encourage her to sleep when her baby does, especially in the early postpartum period. If she returns to work or school, the mother can retire early in the evening and take her baby to bed with her. Or, during the night, her partner can bring the baby to bed for nursing, allowing her to stay in bed.

Establishing a bedtime ritual can be enjoyable for both parents and baby. A routine helps the baby associate the ritual with going to sleep at an established time every night. Quiet, soothing activities directly before bedtime—such as a bath, story, rocking, and nursing—prepare the baby for sleep. The mother can warm the infant's sleeping area with a heating pad or hot water bottle before putting the child down (she needs to remove these items before laying the baby down). Flannel sheets may help keep the infant from waking because of the initial coolness of cotton sheets.

If a baby sleeps for longer periods during the day than at night, parents can try waking the baby more frequently during the day to discourage longer sleep periods. This practice enables the mother to nurse more often and helps the baby's rhythm come into harmony with the rest of the family.

Breastfeeding Issues with Sleep

An older baby who is well nourished is usually able to sleep for long periods at night. Nursing frequently during the day will accomplish this goal. Nursing directly before bedtime ensures a full stomach and helps soothe the baby. If the mother nurses while lying down in the middle of the bed, she can then move her baby to the crib when he or she is in a deeper sleep, or keep the baby in her bed until morning or until after the next feeding. (See the discussion of cosleeping in the next section.)

When the baby wakes in the middle of the night to nurse, avoiding stimulation will help the child return to sleep. For example, placement of a nightlight near the baby's bed eliminates the need to turn on a bright light. A soiled diaper can be changed before nursing on the second breast so the baby can nurse back to sleep on the second breast undisturbed. Keeping the baby and mother warm can help both return to sleep more easily.

With the emphasis in Western cultures on "sleeping through the night," it helps for parents to understand the

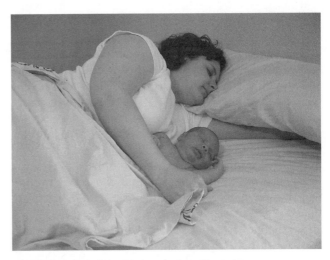

FIGURE 13.15   Mother cosleeping with baby.
Source: Printed with permission of Anna Swisher.

relationship between infant intake and their baby's need to nurse around the clock. In a study conducted by Kent and colleagues (2006), when infants nursed at night, the nighttime intake accounted for 20 percent of the total 24-hour intake. Babies who did not wake to nurse at night took larger feedings in the morning.

Cosleeping

The cultural expectation in many industrialized countries is that babies should sleep through the night and that independence (separation) is a good thing. In reality, this notion is at odds with human babies' biological need to be close to their parents for safety and development (McKenna et al., 2007). A human baby has an intense biological need to be close to his or her mother, including at night. A family bed shared by mother, father, and baby works for many parents to meet this need. Cosleeping helps babies fall asleep more easily, and babies wake easily when moved (Figure 13.15). Cosleeping is also helpful with a baby who wakes frequently during the night.

Cosleeping infants become aroused more often and in greater synchrony with their mothers than do separate sleepers (McKenna & Gettler, 2007). This relationship suggests that cosleeping may reduce the risk of sudden infant death syndrome (SIDS). The more frequent arousal also promotes nighttime breastfeeding. Mothers who cosleep with their babies nurse them 3 times more frequently than do mothers whose babies sleep in a separate room (McKenna & Gettler, 2007).

The AAP (2005a) recognizes the need for closeness to facilitate breastfeeding, and recommends that mothers and babies sleep in proximity to each other. At the same time, a statement released by the AAP Task Force on sudden infant death syndrome advises against parent–infant bed-sharing and supports the generic use of pacifiers (AAP, 2005b). The Academy of Breastfeeding Medicine (ABM, 2008) has issued revised guidelines for safe cosleeping in response to the AAP's statements (see Figure 13.16).

Contrary to popular thinking, breastfeeding mothers who routinely sleep with their infants receive more total hours of sleep than do those who routinely sleep separately, just not in one block of time. Moreover, routine bed-sharing mothers evaluate their sleep more positively than do solitary sleeping mothers (Mosko et al., 1997). As an alternative to sharing their bed with their child, parents can use a crib, or cosleeper, that attaches to their bed. For more information on this topic see the discussion of responsive parenting in Chapter 19.

Prevalence of Cosleeping

In most non-Western cultures and among many subgroups within Western cultures, an infant and mother remain together continually, both day and night. The warmth and familiar smell of the mother comforts the infant when sleeping in the parents' bed (the practice referred to as cosleeping). The infant can nuzzle at the breast and nurse ad lib, and the mother is not required to leave her bed to nurse her hungry infant. Thus the mother is able both to get the sleep she needs and to meet her infant's needs.

Cosleeping was the cultural norm in the United States until the twentieth century brought sweeping cultural changes to mechanistic, scientific, and behavioristic models of child development that defined "normal" behavior based on bottle feeding babies (Small, 1999, 2008; Sears et al., 2005). In recent decades, however, cosleeping has become more common and more widely accepted in Western culture.

In a survey of 2300 women, 85 percent of infants slept in the same room as their mother at 3 months and one-fourth of these babies slept in a nonsupine position. At 12 months, 29 percent continued to sleep in the same room and one-third of these babies slept in a nonsupine position. Bed-sharing rates were 42 percent at 2 weeks, 34 percent at 3 months, and 27 percent at 12 months. In the survey, the major reasons cited for bed sharing were to calm a fussy infant, to facilitate breastfeeding, and to help the infant or mother sleep better. The use of nonsupine infant sleep positions and bed sharing was highest among non-Hispanic black mothers (Hauck et al., 2008). In this study, the researchers focused on parents' "noncompliance" with the cultural prescription to not sleep with one's baby. Such an approach fails to respect parents' responsiveness to their babies and to recognize the need to increase infant sleep safety while protecting breastfeeding.

Precautions for cribs and adult beds:

- Use a firm mattress to avoid suffocation.
- Have no gaps between the mattress and the frame.
- Keep bedding tight around the mattress.
- Avoid strings or ties on baby's and parents' nightclothes.
- Avoid soft items such as comforters, pillows, featherbeds, stuffed animals, lamb skins, and bean bags.
- Keep the baby's face uncovered to allow ventilation.
- Put the baby on his back to sleep.
- Do not overheat the room or overdress baby.
- Do not place a crib near window cords or sashes.

Additional precautions for cribs:

- When baby learns to sit, lower the mattress level to avoid falling or climbing out.
- When baby learns to stand, set the mattress level at its lowest point and remove crib bumpers.
- When baby reaches a height of 35 inches or the side rail is less than three-quarters of his height, move the baby to another bed.
- Crib bumpers, if used, should have at least six ties, no longer than six inches.
- Hang crib mobiles well out of reach and remove when baby can sit or reach.
- Remove crib gyms when baby can get up on all fours.

Additional precautions for cosleeping:

- Parents pull back and fasten long hair.
- Do not use alcohol or other drugs, including over-the-counter or prescription medications.
- Have no head/foot board railings with spaces wider than allowed in safety-approved cribs.
- Use no bed rails with infants less than 1 year.
- Do not allow siblings or pets in bed with a baby less than 1 year old.
- Do not cosleep in a waterbed.
- Avoid placing bed directly alongside furniture or a wall.

Additional precautions regarding infant sleep:

- Do not sleep with baby on sofas or overstuffed chairs.
- Do not put baby to sleep alone in an adult bed.
- Do not place baby to sleep in car or infant seats.
- Obese mothers who are not breastfeeding avoid cosleeping.
- Refrain from cosleeping if mother smoked during her pregnancy or if mother or partner currently smoke.

FIGURE 13.16 Creating a safe infant sleep environment.

Source: Adapted from Donohue-Carey, P. *Solitary or shared sleep: what's safe? Mothering.* 2002;114:44-47. Updated 2009 by Patricia Donohue-Carey.

Concerns About Cosleeping

Some parents worry that it is emotionally unhealthy for an infant to share a bed with the parents or that this habit may be difficult to break once formed. Some fear the mother could inadvertently roll over onto the infant while she is asleep. You can reassure parents that most infants worldwide sleep with their parents. It has become a cultural norm in the United States for infants to sleep separated from their parents, not a biological norm.

Parents who cosleep with their infant can evaluate their sleep environment and make it as safe as possible for their baby. Both parents should feel comfortable with the decision to cosleep with their baby and be committed to following appropriate safety precautions. While no one sleep environment is guaranteed to be risk free, there are ways of reducing risks in both cribs and adult beds.

Sudden Infant Death Syndrome

Sudden infant death syndrome is the sudden death of an infant younger than 1 year of age that remains unexplained after an autopsy, examination of the death scene, and review of the clinical history (Willinger et al., 1991). In the typical SIDS case, parents find their seemingly healthy infant lifeless in bed. SIDS is the leading cause of death for infants 1 month to 1 year of age, with more than 2100 babies dying from this cause each year in the United States alone.

While SIDS occurs in all socioeconomic, racial, and ethnic groups, African American and Native American babies are 2 to 3 times more likely to die of SIDS than Caucasian babies. Most SIDS deaths occur when a baby is between 2 and 4 months of age, with 90 percent of all SIDS deaths occurring before the child reaches 6 months of age. Most babies who die of SIDS appear to be healthy prior to death. Sixty percent of SIDS victims are male and 40 percent are female (SIDS Alliance, 2009).

A baby who is not breastfed may be at greater risk for SIDS, both because of the lack of immunological protection and because of differences in breathing and arousal patterns (McKenna & Gettler, 2007; Horne et al., 2004). A German study found that exclusive breastfeeding at 1 month of age halved the risk of SIDS. Partial breastfeeding at the age of 1 month also reduced the risk, albeit not significantly. Breastfeeding reduced the risk of SIDS by approximately 50 percent at all ages throughout infancy (Vennemann et al., 2009).

Breastfed infants are aroused more easily from active sleep at 2 to 3 months of age than are formula fed infants. Given that this age coincides with the peak incidence of SIDS, this behavior may represent another protective mechanism of breastfeeding. Arousal from sleep, an important survival mechanism, may be impaired in victims of SIDS (Horne et al., 2004). Some researchers believe that infants' immature control mechanisms can be aggravated by environmental factors (Kahn et al., 2003).

The position in which the mother places her baby for sleep is a major factor in the risk of SIDS. Placing the baby in a supine position (on his or her back), rather than in a prone position (on his or her stomach), substantially reduces the incidence of SIDS (American SIDS Institute, 2009). Breastfeeding mothers who cosleep predominantly put their infants on their backs to facilitate reaching the breast. SIDS rates have declined by more than 50 percent in the United States since 1994, when the "Back to Sleep" public information campaign began.

Risks for SIDS are increased when parents smoke, put the baby to sleep in the prone position, and do not breastfeed. In fact, sleeping prone and maternal smoking are two significant risk factors for SIDS (Richardson et al., 2008, 2009; Adgent, 2006). Another risk factor is the baby's inhalation of passive smoke (Bajanowski et al., 2008; Bosdure & Dubus, 2006). Nicotine concentrations are 5 times higher in non-breastfed SIDS victims of parents who smoke compared to all other groups (Bajanowski et al., 2008). Parents who smoke around their baby need to be educated about the dangers to their baby.

Small-at-birth infants who sleep in a separate room are at increased risk for SIDS compared to similar infants who sleep in the same room with their parents (Blair et al., 2006). By comparison, researchers have not identified any excess risk from bed sharing with nonsmoking parents for infants born at term or at birth weight greater than or equal to 2500 grams. In one study, 36 percent of 745 deaths were attributable to the baby sleeping in a separate room (Carpenter et al., 2004). Furthermore, children who cosleep in their parents' room have lower cortisol levels, which translates to lower tension and stress (Waynforth, 2007).

An especially controversial aspect of the SIDS recommendation made by the AAP Task Force on SIDS suggested that using a pacifier to go to sleep may be protective against SIDS. The analysis, however, found that out of seven case-control studies of SIDS babies, babies who typically used pacifiers were more likely to have had SIDS if they did not use one. These cases of SIDS were compared to matched controls (i.e., babies without SIDS). The AAP Task Force expanded this finding to make a blanket recommendation that *all* babies (breastfed or not) be put to sleep with pacifiers. The irony of this recommendation is that the breastfed baby—the biologically normal baby—sucks to sleep at the breast, not on a plastic device.

∼ Crying and Colicky Behavior

Crying is an infant's first language, used to communicate distress and to elicit help from caregivers. New parents envision a smiling baby who smiles, coos, and snuggles, not one who is fussy and cries. As a consequence, they may worry that crying is a reflection of their parenting. You can help them recognize that babies fuss and cry because of their needs, not because the parents are doing anything incorrectly. Encourage them to focus on the positive attributes of this behavior—that a fussy baby is very alert, responsive to the environment, and a good communicator—rather than considering their baby to be difficult or spoiled. Table 13.8 describes several combinations of temperament that can affect a baby's disposition. Chapter 14 provides an extensive discussion of the baby who is fussy at the breast.

During pregnancy, the mother was in control and was the center of attention. Now it may seem that the baby has both the attention and the control. Mothers are vulnerable to negative reactions to their crying baby. When others stare at the parents of a crying baby or make rude or personal comments, the parents may feel out of control or judged. Many times the problem lies in the parents' expectations of what parenting will be like.

Parents are often advised not to pick up their crying infant and are encouraged to let the child "cry it out." (See Chapter 19 for a discussion of such "baby training" and its impact on breastfeeding.) In reality, infant crying is a powerful communication tool used by the baby to interact with the external environment. In a cause-and-effect relationship, the baby learns that he or she has the ability to make things happen through crying. By crying and eliciting the parents' response, the infant learns they will meet his or her needs. As a result, the child forms a greater attachment to his parents, develops trust more readily, and cries less. In contrast, a baby who is repeatedly left to cry alone learns that his or her needs will not be met. Failing to understand or respond to infants' mes-

TABLE 13.8   Influences on Baby's Disposition

Baby's Disposition	Mother's Disposition	Probable Outcome
Easy baby	Responsive mother	This is a predictable and cuddly baby whose mother is in tune with him. The mother feels good about her parenting based on the positive interactions with her baby.
Easy baby	Restrained mother	This baby is not very demanding, and such behavior may lead the mother to feel somewhat unnecessary. The mother initially may not develop comfort skills, believing they are unnecessary. She may divert her energies elsewhere, and her baby may, in time, exhibit more fussy behavior.
High-need baby with good attachment-promoting behaviors	Responsive mother	The mother cannot ignore the needs of her baby and responds to him. She is rewarded with occasional satisfied responses from her baby. She will continue to explore alternative responses until she finds one that reaches her baby. Because of his mother's responsiveness, the baby will also fine-tune his attachment-promoting skills, resulting in a parent–child relationship of mutual sensitivity.
High-need baby with poor attachment-promoting skills	Responsive mother	This type of baby often is referred to as slow to warm up. He shows little or no effort to respond to or be comforted by his mother's efforts. The mother's nurturing responses are fine-tuned by her baby's responses. When the baby's responsiveness is lacking, this may seriously jeopardize the mother–baby relationship. In some situations, it is helpful for the mother to seek assistance from a professional who is trained in interaction counseling.
High-need baby	Restrained mother	This situation places the mother–baby relationship at risk. Often, the mother has been advised to let the baby cry it out or to not spoil him. Continued lack of response to his needs will lead this baby to one of two outcomes. He will intensify his high-need behaviors, or he will give up. The baby who gives up essentially shuts down his communication and withdraws into himself. He is prone to attach to objects rather than persons.

Source: Adapted from Sears W, Sears M. *The Fussy Baby Book: Parenting Your High-Need Child from Birth to Age Five.* New York: Little Brown & Company; 1996.

sages can compromise their care as well as parental effectiveness, thereby undermining the budding relationship between parents and their baby (LaGasse et al., 2005).

One study found that parents with a restrained style had 50 percent less physical contact with their infants than those with proximal care (akin to attachment). The restrained parents had less contact when the infants were crying and when awake and settled. They abandoned breastfeeding earlier and their infants cried 50 percent more overall at 2 and 5 weeks of age. By comparison, proximal care parenting was associated with less overall crying per 24 hours and more frequent nighttime waking at 12 weeks (St. James-Roberts et al., 2007). Bouts of inconsolable crying occurred in all groups, and members of the groups did not differ in terms of their unsoothable bouts or their colicky crying at 5 weeks of age. You can encourage parents with crying babies by noting that sometimes parents do everything they can and the baby still cries.

Mothers may perceive infant fussiness as dissatisfaction with breastfeeding and conclude that supplementing with formula or cereal will provide a solution. To ensure that they do not give up on breastfeeding prematurely, parents need to be educated that crying is a baby's method of communicating with the world. Crying is meant to get their attention. The decibel level of a baby's cry is actually higher than street noise and can be 20 decibels louder than normal speech.

The crying pattern for a preterm infant is different from that of a full-term infant (Manfredi et al., 2008; Rautava et al., 2007). A preterm infant has a different rhythm, pause, and inhalation–exhalation pattern. His or her cry is a full octave higher than that of a full-term infant, signaling a greater urgency. Crying for a preterm infant requires great effort, which can cause distress and lower blood oxygenation. Preterm infants have been found to fuss and cry more frequently at 5 months of corrected age compared to their term counterparts (Maunu et al., 2006).

In response to her baby's cry, the mother's heart beats louder, her blood pressure increases, and the temperature in her breasts increases. The sound of a crying infant is disturbing and aggravating (see Figure 13.17); a sound designed to ensure that the newborn receives the attention he or she needs.

The Effect of Crying on the Infant

Babies who have been crying have difficulty breastfeeding. They are often unable to organize themselves and their behavior for a period after the crying spell. Sears and colleagues (2003) assert that, "Crying is good for the lungs like bleeding is good for the veins." When an infant cries or startles during the first 4 to 5 days of life, there is an

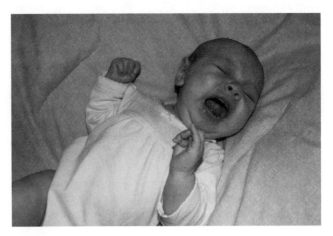

FIGURE 13.17   A crying infant needs to be settled before being put to breast.

Source: Printed with permission of Kori Martin.

increase in blood pressure, which in turn increases intracranial pressure. Poorly oxygenated blood flows back into circulation rather than into the lungs. Large fluctuations in blood flow increase cerebral blood volume and decrease cerebral oxygenation with respiratory problems (Brazy, 1988).

Crying significantly raises the baby's heart rate and blood pressure (Dinwiddie et al., 1979). It decreases the absorption of inhalant medications, which preterm babies frequently receive (Iles et al., 1999). The extreme pressure caused by crying is associated with pneumothorax and subcutaneous emphysema (Kadam & Kluckow, 2005). Metabolically, crying leads to increased glucose expenditure which, in the immediate postpartum period, could result in hypoglycemia. Crying also increases gastric distention and may result in a very discontented baby due to gas pain. Finally, crying increases levels of cortisol, a stress hormone (Ahnert et al., 2004).

Today, much neurological research focuses on the effects of early-life events on adult health. Neuroscience research indicates that the newborn infant brain is not an immature version of the adult brain, but rather is uniquely designed to optimize attachment to the caregiver (Moriceau & Sullivan, 2005). Adult learning and memory functions, as well as adult emotional and cognitive development, are strongly dependent on neonatal experiences (Sevelinges, 2008; Sevelinges et al., 2007). Clinical data suggest a correlation between traumatic attachments and adult mental illness, presumably through organizing brain development (Sullivan, 2003). In addition, some data support the hypothesis that early stress may be a critical factor in the development of chronic anxiety states. Pathological anxiety might then lead to syndromes such as panic and post-traumatic stress disorders (Shekar et al., 2005).

In one study, the quality of infants' attachment moderated the relationship between cognitive level and cortisol reactivity. Infants with low security scores had higher cortisol responses to the test stressors (van Bakel & Riksen-Walraven, 2004). In a similar repeat study, parents who were sensitive to their children's distress or uncertainty experienced elevated cortisol responses; no such response was observed in those who were less sensitive. These results indicate an important connection between behavior and physiology in parent–infant interactions (van Bakel & Riksen-Walraven, 2008). Sensitive response to their baby seems to wire parents for long-term sensitivity to their child's needs as the child grows.

Identifying the Cause of Crying

A baby's cry usually indicates some form of physical discomfort. As parents become accustomed to their baby, they will learn to distinguish among different types of cries. An infant's cry may indicate hunger, pain, or a reaction to the external environment. Too often, a mother immediately assumes that hunger is the cause and may blame low milk production or poor-quality milk for her baby's fussy disposition. You can encourage parents to investigate other causes for crying, especially if the baby has nursed recently and does not appear to be hungry. As parents become better acquainted with their baby's particular communication, they will learn to distinguish the causes of the crying.

Crying from Hunger

In the early weeks after birth, it is common for the baby to require frequent feedings and to sleep for short, frequent periods. As the mother tunes into her baby's pattern of sleeping and waking, she will learn to recognize a hunger cry. She will want to consider how long it has been since the last feeding and how much the infant nursed at that time. Other factors to take into account include the infant's general disposition, the ability to be soothed easily or with difficulty, and the hunger cues demonstrated by the infant.

A newborn may cry from hunger approximately $1\frac{1}{2}$ to 2 hours or more after a feeding. A hunger cry may be more prevalent in the evening hours when the mother's milk production seems lowest and the environment feels harried. As a result, cluster feeding is common in the early evening. Mothers who respond to hunger cries by nursing their babies will most likely have more contented babies. These infants will cry less frequently than those whose mothers maintain a strict feeding schedule and disregard their babies' cries. You can teach mothers to recognize and respond to hunger cues rather than waiting until the baby cries.

Crying from Body Discomfort

Wet or soiled diapers by themselves may not be sufficient to cause crying. However, when the diaper cools, the drop in temperature can cause discomfort, thus making the baby more responsive to stimulation and more likely to cry for other reasons. Babies also may cry from excessive heat. First-time parents tend to overdress a new baby even on the hottest summer day, fearing that the child may become chilled. In warm weather and cold weather alike, babies can be dressed in the same type of clothing that an adult would wear.

Even when temperature is controlled, babies may cry when they are undressed and lose the warm, secure feeling of clothing and blankets. A baby who is especially sensitive to this effect may benefit from swaddling. The texture of the cloth that touches the child's body is important. For example, plastic or rubber is more irritating than soft toweling or blanketing. Other skin irritations such as heat rash or diaper rash can be a cause of a baby's cries.

In addition to comfortable body temperature, swaddling, and avoidance of skin irritants, a baby may find comfort in close skin-to-skin contact with the parents. The mother can lie with her baby in bed or the bathtub; fathers can provide this contact as well.

A baby may cry from internal discomfort such as gas or overfullness. A baby who is constantly fussy during feedings may need to bring up a bubble of air. Gas in the intestines can cause discomfort and the mother can help her baby pass gas by using the techniques for comforting a colicky baby described later in this chapter. Additionally, some babies take in more milk than they are able to handle. Such overfeeding causes pressure, which in turn can produce discomfort. Mothers can encourage the baby to nurse long enough on one breast before offering the other one.

Crying from External Stimuli

When parents have tended to the physical needs of their baby and the child continues to cry, they will want to look for an external cause for the crying. Babies may startle and cry in reaction to sudden movement, touch, smell, light, noise, or excessive handling. This factor often accounts for the initial fussiness the baby demonstrates upon the transition from hospital to home. Constant, soft, soothing noise can be an effective comfort measure. The steady movement of being rocked is comforting, as is the motion of a car ride. Recreating the sounds and feeling of the womb comforts a newborn, as does swaddling (Karp, 2003, 2004). Swaddling reduces the amount of movement the baby can make and, therefore, the amount of stimulation experienced from movement. Confining the arms and legs prevents the infant from startling and provides a feeling of warmth, security, and constant touch stimulation. Although this practice may increase the time a baby sleeps and decrease time spent crying, it does not necessarily do so at the expense of time spent quietly awake.

Like all interventions, swaddling needs to be done appropriately. The increased popularity of swaddling has led to concern that it is associated with hip dysplasia and increased respiratory infection (Mahan & Kasser, 2008; van Sleuwen et al., 2007). Swaddling with full extension of the legs and adduction (open) of the hips with tight binding of the legs—a practice that is common in certain countries and among certain ethnic groups—is associated with hip dysplasia. In contrast, swaddling with the legs in normal flexion and abduction (together) shows no such association (Karp, 2008). Swaddling and putting a baby down to sleep in the supine position is associated with lower incidence of SIDS, whereas putting a swaddled baby to sleep prone raises the risk of SIDS.

Some babies dislike being swaddled and will cry or squirm when they are wrapped or held too tightly. Parents learn quickly what their baby prefers. Validating their knowledge of their baby helps reinforce parents' confidence in acquiring their parenting identity. Such a baby may push away from the breast when held too closely and need to nurse in a position that allows body movement. The mother can lie on her side to nurse while lightly supporting the baby from behind with her hand or a pillow. She could also lower her breast while leaning above her reclining infant. Figure 13.14 shows another comforting technique of "wearing" the baby in a sling. This practice provides the infant with the secure feeling of swaddling, with the added benefit of closeness to the person who wears the sling.

A baby receives important information about the surrounding world through touch. A mother whose touch is tentative and light may irritate the baby. With a firm touch, a mother communicates that she is confident, allowing her baby to relax and trust her. Gently stroking an infant's body during a feeding—called grooming—increases the mother's prolactin level. Such quiet, gentle touching does not usually interfere with feedings. However, poking or jiggling the baby during nursing could make it difficult for the baby to relax and result in crying.

Over-handling by well-meaning adults can cause a baby to cry as a plea to, "Please leave me alone!" Sometimes babies may prefer to lie quietly in their cribs and will react unhappily when picked up, especially if they have been overstimulated by lights, noise, interruptions to nursing or napping, and the attention of too many visitors. Some babies become very agitated when they are tired and might cry themselves to sleep.

If parents have ruled out hunger and discomfort, their baby may settle after a few minutes. They need to be encouraged to focus on the cues their baby gives in response to their parenting approach. If their baby is responding positively to a technique, it can be encouraged. If their baby exhibits withdrawal or avoidance behaviors, they will want to try a new approach.

Colicky Behavior

Much of the extreme infant fussiness that occurs is actually colic-like behavior, rather than true colic. The accepted research-based definition of colic focuses on the rule of threes (Wessel et al., 1954):

1. There is inconsolable crying for which no physical cause can be found and that lasts more than 3 hours per day.
2. This crying occurs at least 3 days per week and continues for at least 3 weeks.
3. The baby experiences spasmodic contractions of the smooth muscle, causing pain and discomfort.

This is quite different from the pattern of one or two fussy periods a day experienced by most infants. In defining colic, duration is more important than frequency.

The term "colic" derives from the Greek word *kolikos*, an adjective derived from *kolon*, meaning "large colon." Estimates of the incidence of infant colic range from 5 to 19 percent. Symptoms typically subside by 16 weeks of age in the majority of infants (Lucassen, 2007). Colic studies have not differentiated well between bottle fed and breastfed infants. Colic does seem to be more common when infants are fed solid foods while they are younger than 3 months of age.

A colicky baby exhibits unexplained fussiness, fretfulness, and irritability. Such a child appears to suffer from severe discomfort during the colicky period, with cries that are piercing, explosive attacks. A rumbling sound may be audible in the baby's gut. Excessive flatulence (gas) and apparent abdominal pain may cause the baby's legs to draw up sharply into the abdomen, or the baby's body to stiffen and twist. The infant may awaken easily and frequently, and appear intense, energetic, excitable, and easily startled—with clenched fists and a facial grimace. Continuous crying can cause the infant to swallow air and further aggravate the discomfort.

The exact cause of colicky behavior has not been determined medically. In fact, researchers do not even agree about the true incidence of colic. Some theories relate colic to stress and tension in the mother and child during pregnancy and lactation. Others believe the cause to be an immature digestive and intestinal system or allergies (Gupta, 2007). Pregnancies characterized by hyperemesis (marked by long-term vomiting, weight loss, and fluid and electrolyte imbalance), pelvic pain, and distress often correlate with infants with colic. A similar relationship exists for second-born infants and those with a family history of colic (Hogsdall et al., 1991).

Immature Gastrointestinal and Neurological Systems

Compared with other young mammals, a human baby is born in an extremely immature state—essentially neurologically incomplete. At 1 month, the infant's stomach capacity is one-tenth the size of an adult stomach. Moreover, a newborn has only 4 percent of the gastric glands that secrete digestive enzymes. The muscle layers surrounding the stomach and intestines are thin and weak, and the intestines lack the ridges and hair-like filaments that help process food.

Colicky infants transmit more macromolecules across the epithelium (lining) of the gut than those without colic symptoms (Lothe et al., 1990). In these children, peristalsis (wavelike rhythmic contractions of smooth muscle) may be irregular, faint, forceful, or spasmodic. Additionally, lack of muscle tone can cause food to move up out of the stomach as well as down into the intestines. The colons of colicky infants may contract violently during feedings. Whereas the colon in normal infants takes several hours to empty, for some colicky infants the colon may empty in less than 1 minute. One study found a correlation between colic and feeding disorders, including gastroesophageal reflux (Miller-Loncar et al., 2004).

Hormones

Babies have high levels of progesterone at birth, which helps relax the muscles of their intestines. The progesterone level drops 1 to 2 weeks after birth, which may account for the increase in colic symptoms at that time. Infants with colic-like behavior have high levels of motilin—a digestive hormone that stimulates muscle contractions—from the first day of life. Human milk has high levels of many enzymes that are necessary for digestion and, therefore, may aid in reducing the intensity of colic in some infants. Cholecystokinin (CCK), a digestive hormone abundant in milk, has been shown to be present in lower levels in infants suffering from colic (Huhtala et al., 2003). Cortisol, the stress hormone, is also thought to be a factor in the development of colic. A possible self-reinforcing loop of stress may lead to crying and to more stress.

Intrauterine and Birth-Related Problems

A notable increase in crying occurs in infants who are born prematurely, who are small for gestational age (SGA), or who experience birth trauma or anoxia (lack of oxygen). Increased excitability and fussiness are seen in infants whose mothers were hypertensive (high blood pressure). Maternal distress during pregnancy results in a threefold increased risk of infant colic (Sondergaard et al., 2003). To relieve infant colic, many parents seek help from chiropractic care, massage therapy, or craniosacral therapy. Referral by the family's primary care provider to occupational or physical therapy may also be helpful in reducing maternal distress by addressing the baby's symptoms.

Medications

Some women use opioids and other similar drugs on a long-term basis for pain management. Others are on methadone (synthetic heroin) maintenance therapy, to prevent relapse into heroin addiction (Dryden et al., 2009). If you work in a hospital setting, medical office, or clinic, you are likely to encounter these mothers and their babies. Many of the babies will exhibit neonatal abstinence syndrome (NAS) due to opiate withdrawal after birth. NAS may result in disruption of the mother–infant relationship as well as sleep–wake abnormalities, feeding difficulties, weight loss, and seizures in the infant. Treatments used for the baby include opiates, sedatives, and nonpharmacological comfort measures (Osborn & Sinn, 2005). Both the syndrome and the treatments (opiates and sedatives) can cause lethargy and feeding difficulties for the baby.

A careful feeding assessment and close coordination of care with the baby's healthcare provider are crucial for these mothers. Until the baby has been weaned off narcotics, the mother will need to pump her milk to protect milk production if the baby is not transferring milk effectively. Although methadone is considered safe for breastfeeding mothers, maternal use of any sedating medication requires monitoring of the baby (Hale, 2010). See Chapter 10 for more information on medications in mothers' milk.

Street Drugs

Prenatal maternal abuse of heroin, marijuana, barbiturates, or cocaine can result in colic-like behavior in the infant. Specifically, infants of substance abusers often exhibit signs of nervous system instabilities. Symptoms, which may not appear until a week or more after birth, may include excitability, trembling, restlessness, ravenous appetite, jitteriness, hyperactivity, shrill scream, feeding problems, and either hypertonia or hypotonia (Bläser et al., 2008). See Chapter 10 for more information on the effects of street drugs on the newborn.

Women who are currently using illegal drugs should not breastfeed and need a referral for counseling. If they deliver in the hospital, they will be referred to social services. If you encounter substance-abusing mothers in a community clinic or private practice, information about the risks to the baby needs to be shared kindly but honestly. If you suspect the baby is endangered, most states and provinces require mandatory reporting to child protective services. Your clinic, office, and hospital should have clear policies in place for helping these babies. If you are unfamiliar with these policies, talk with your organization's management. If you are in private practice, familiarize yourself with the social services available to drug-dependent families in your community, as well as legal reporting requirements.

Smoking Parent

Only 20 percent of women who smoke will initiate breastfeeding. As a variety of studies have shown, a clear correlation exists between infant fussiness and parental intake of nicotine. Canivet and colleagues (2008), for example, found an association between maternal smoking in pregnancy and subsequent colic. The same study also suggested that exclusive breastfeeding is protective against colic, including for infants of smoking mothers. Infants of smokers are more excitable and hypertonic than other infants. They require more careful handling and show more stress/abstinence signs, specifically in the central nervous system (CNS), gastrointestinal, and visual areas (Law et al., 2003). Even at 10–27 days postpartum, smoking-exposed infants demonstrate a greater need for handling, worse self-regulation, greater excitability, and arousal compared to unexposed infants (Stroud et al., 2009).

Smoking mothers have lower milk production (Hopkinson et al., 1992) and lower prolactin levels (Anderson et al., 1982) compared to mothers who do not smoke. No difference is apparent in milk production between women who smoke or who use a nicotine patch (Ilett et al., 2003). There is some debate about how nicotine affects prolactin levels. Some studies have shown lowered prolactin levels in women who smoke, whereas others show normal or increased prolactin levels, even in males (Hale & Hartmann, 2007).

Optimally, mothers who smoke will stop smoking or decrease the amount of cigarettes they smoke. They can also discuss the possible use of nicotine gum or patches with their physician. Acquaint yourself with smoking cessation programs available in your area. Discuss with both parents the need to refrain from smoking in the same room or automobile as the baby.

A mother who smokes may need help establishing and maintaining adequate milk production. If smoking lowers her milk production and she is unwilling to quit smoking, she may benefit from the use of galactogogues (see Chapter 18).

Food Sensitivity

An infant who reacts to something in the mother's diet is typically calm at the start of a feeding and then begins to pull off the breast, stiffens his or her body, cries, and then reattaches. The infant may repeat this pattern several times during the feeding. Symptoms can be continuous or can start after a feeding. It is rare for symptoms of a food sensitivity to show up before 3 weeks.

Signs of food sensitivity include the following findings:

- A stuffy or drippy nose without any other sign of having a cold
- Frequently pulling off the breast and arching and crying while feeding
- An itchy nose
- A red, scaly, oily rash on the forehead or eyebrows, in the hair, or behind the ears
- Eczema
- A red rectal ring
- Fretful sleeping or persistent sleeplessness
- Frequent spitting up or vomiting
- Diarrhea or green stools, perhaps with blood in them
- Wheezing
- Colic-like symptoms and behaviors

One study found that children who avoided exposure to a certain food allergen before the age of 3 to 6 months were less likely to become sensitized or develop food hypersensitivity. Women with a family history of allergic disease were more likely to breastfeed exclusively at 3 months and avoid including peanuts in the infant's diet at 6 months. Neither maternal dietary intake during pregnancy nor breastfeeding duration appeared to influence the development of sensitization to food allergens or food hypersensitivity (FHS). Weaning age, however, was thought to sometimes affect sensitization to foods and development of FHS (Venter, 2009). The authors found that a history of allergic disease did not seem to have much impact on these participants' dietary, feeding, and weaning practices. In line with these findings, you might want to give parents information prenatally about avoiding the early introduction of highly allergic foods.

Researchers whose work has been sponsored by Nestlé suggest that rising rates of food allergies in early childhood reflect increasing failure of early immune tolerance mechanisms. They assert that the practice of delaying complementary foods until 6 months of age may, therefore, increase the risk of immune disorders. Their recommendation is that complementary foods be introduced from approximately 4 months of age while maintaining breastfeeding for at least 6 months (Prescott et al., 2008). The researchers' funding source calls their results into question, however, underscoring the importance of critical discernment as you read and analyze research (see Chapter 26).

Cow and Soy Milk Intolerances

Cow's milk protein is a common cause of intolerance in infants. Almost all mammal milks contain some immunoglobulin G (IgG). According to researchers, the mean level of bovine IgG in colicky babies' mothers' milk is higher than the level found in the breastmilk fed to non-colicky babies (Clyne & Kulczycki, 1991). Study results found the range in human milk to be from 0.1 to 8.5 mg/mL, compared to 0.6 to 128 mg/mL in cow's milk formulas. The highest levels occurred in powdered formula; the lowest levels were found in formula concentrate. Bovine IgG levels can be so high or the half-life so long that trials of 2 to 7 days on a diet free of cow's milk may not be long enough to see results in a colicky child; instead, a 14-day trial may be necessary to obtain valid results. Note that there is no bovine IgG in soy or hydrolysate formulas.

Approximately 30 percent of colic-like behavior in breastfed infants is thought to be due to cow's milk protein intolerance. Some researchers have reported a decrease in the incidence of colic among breastfed babies when the mother omits dairy products from her own diet (Host, 2002; Lindberg, 1999). Thus a mother who suspects that her baby is intolerant to cow's milk might try eliminating dairy foods from her diet for 2 weeks. If cow's milk was the cause of her infant's colic-like behavior, she may see some improvement in 48 hours, although full resolution of the problem could take several days. The mother can then reintroduce dairy slowly into her diet after 2 weeks of a dairy-free diet. Ideally, she will start with hard cheeses or yogurt the 1st week, add soft cheeses in the 2nd week, butter and ice cream in the 3rd week, and cow's milk in small quantities in the 4th week. If the infant becomes fussy or other symptoms return, the mother can once again reduce her intake of dairy products.

In a completely milk-free diet, the mother takes in no milk, whey, caseinate, or sodium caseinate. Consumption of lactose is acceptable because it is a sugar and not a cow's milk protein. Caution mothers who use a dairy elimination diet to read food labels, because casein is used as a binder in many processed foods.

Mother's and Infant's Diets

Removal of possible sources of intolerance may provide relief to a colicky baby. Firstly, the mother should feed the infant nothing but her milk. Even vitamins, fluoride, and iron supplements can be a source of discomfort. Babies who receive antibiotics may be at a greater risk for developing food allergies. Antibiotics are linked to leaky gut syndrome, a condition in which the intestinal lining first becomes inflamed, and then thin and porous. Proteins that are not completely digested may cross from the intestines into the bloodstream. Leukocytes attack such

proteins and lead to an antigen–antibody reaction, which manifests itself as an allergic reaction upon subsequent exposure to that protein.

Babies usually are not bothered by foods in their mothers' diets. If the mother has a very sensitive baby, she may want to monitor her food intake, given that some of what she consumes may pass through her milk. Medications, vitamin supplements, caffeine, high-protein foods, milk, wheat, chocolate, eggs, and nuts are all potential sources of discomfort to an intolerant baby. Many mothers report that foods that make them gassy (e.g., cabbage, beans, and broccoli) also make their babies gassy, especially in the early days after birth. Because colicky babies can become food-intolerant children, there may be some validity to the theory of allergy as a cause of colic-like behavior.

Lactose Overload

Colic-like symptoms can occur when a baby consumes an unbalanced amount of milk, receiving too much lactose and too little fat. Levels of lactose (the sugar in human milk) are very high in human milk, which supports rapid brain growth in the infant. The amount of lactose in human milk is not dependent on the mother's diet. Although the amount of lactose is the same in both foremilk and hindmilk, fat concentrations are low in foremilk and high in hindmilk. If the infant receives an unbalanced feeding, he or she will get a higher percentage of lactose in comparison to the percentage of fat. The excess lactose then ferments in the baby's gut, which can lead to gassiness and fussiness.

Lactose overload should not be confused with lactose intolerance. Lactose intolerance arises when a person does not produce enough lactase—the enzyme required to digest lactose—and, therefore, cannot digest lactose. Primary (or true) lactose intolerance is an extremely rare genetic condition that requires medical intervention. Markers for this condition include dehydration, malabsorption, and failure to thrive (Anderson, 2006).

Lactose overload can result from an overactive letdown, overabundant milk production, or insufficient hindmilk intake (Anderson, 2006; Lawlor-Smith & Lawlor-Smith, 1998; Woolridge, 1988). When a mother places limits on her baby's time at the breast, she may end a feeding from one breast before letdown has occurred or before her baby has been able to obtain the amount of hindmilk needed. This practice results in the baby ingesting a larger ratio of foremilk on the first breast and then filling up on foremilk again on the second breast. Computer imaging research finds that fat intake varies between feedings, and that the emptier the breast, the higher the fat content (Kent et al., 2006).

In addition to typical colic-like symptoms, the infant with lactose overload may produce green, frothy, loose, and frequent stools. He or she may have poor weight gain, a bloated abdomen, and a great deal of gas. The symptoms of lactose overload are very similar to the symptoms of food intolerance.

Lactose overload can be a temporary problem when either the mother or the infant has been on prolonged antibiotic therapy. To avoid lactose overload, it is important that the mother to continue on the first breast until the infant has received the fatty hindmilk. Some babies may need to nurse repeatedly on the same breast before they switch to the other breast. If the mother has documented overabundant milk production, she can try nursing on one breast for several feedings before switching.

It is prudent to suggest to a mother that she feed on one side or reduce her milk production only after a full feeding assessment that includes before- and after-feeding (ac/pc) weights measured on a digital scale. This intervention may be combined with pumping residual milk. For example, a baby might present with the markers for overabundant milk production, but when ac/pc weights are done, the baby will have had an intake of only 2 or 3 ounces. In this case, the fussy behavior may be unrelated to nursing. If the mother were to down-regulate her milk production, breastfeeding could be harmed.

Treatment of Colic-like Symptoms

Many treatments for colic have been tried over the years, ranging from folk remedies to prescription medication. One study analyzed a general population of 617 couplets from birth to 1 year. Successful calming techniques for fussiness included holding, breastfeeding, walking, and rocking. Mothers who rated breastfeeding as highly effective had a higher frequency of breastfeeding. Mothers of infants with a diagnosis of colic were less likely to report breastfeeding as an effective method of infant comforting. In fact, a diagnosis of colic predicted shorter duration of full breastfeeding. Giving anticipatory guidance to parents about infant feeding, colic, and recommended breastfeeding duration may be helpful in ensuring that they maintain breastfeeding as long as possible (Howard et al., 2006).

One theory holds that colic indicates an over-reactive nervous system. According to this hypothesis, a colicky baby tenses easily and reacts with discomfort to most stimuli, including parental handling. The mother may feel that her baby's crying and pushing her away is a sign of rejecting her. She needs to learn that these reactions do not indicate rejection, but rather the need for soothing. Babies are better able to self-regulate when parents establish regularity and uniformity in their daily care. Predictability improves the baby's sleep–wake rhythm, thereby avoiding overtiredness and excessive crying (Blom et al., 2009).

Some parents find massage effective for soothing an infant with colic-like symptoms. Touch has relaxing effects on both the baby and parent. One effective technique includes:

- Hold the naked baby on the parent's lap, supine, with the baby's head resting on the parent's knees
- Gently massage the baby's stomach, shoulders, head, hands, and feet
- Turn the baby over and massage the back
- Hold and soothe the baby against the parent's shoulder until the crying ceases

Sometimes the baby will cry throughout the massage but be calm by the end. Other infants may respond immediately. Many resources for infant massage abound on the Internet, through community classes, and in the form of books. Resources from the International Association of Infant Massage (IAIM, 2009) can be helpful for parents.

A Cochrane Review found that 13 out of 23 studies on massage had high risks of bias. There was, however, some evidence of benefits from massage in terms of mother–infant interaction, infant sleeping and crying, and levels of hormones influencing stress levels (Underdown et al., 2006). The use of reflexology treatment (massage corresponding to specific organs) gave a "significantly better outcome" to a group of colicky babies compared to the observation group in one study (Bennedbaek et al., 2001). Massage on preterm babies in the NICU is linked to greater weight gain, earlier discharge, and increased developmental scores (Vickers et al., 2004; Beachy, 2003). Massage is calming for parents as well (Fujita et al., 2005).

Many cultures promote home remedies such as chamomile, catnip, fennel, dill, and anise for colic symptoms (Humphrey, 2003). An herbal tea containing chamomile, vervain, licorice, fennel, and balm mint was also found to be effective in a small random-control trial, but the volume necessary for treatment limits its usefulness (Crotteau et al., 2006). Another study found that fennel oil emulsion eliminated colic in 65 percent of the treatment group (Alexandrovich et al., 2003). Caution parents to discuss their options with their baby's caregiver before they use any over-the-counter, herbal, or folk remedy. Such treatments may even be dangerous: A blend of Chinese and Japanese types of anise resulted in two infant poisoning cases when used for treatment of colicky pain (Minodier et al., 2003).

Other parents try prescription medications to relieve their infants' symptoms, such as dicyclomine. This anticholinergic agent is used to treat the symptoms of irritable bowel syndrome and relieves muscle spasms in the gastrointestinal tract. Although some caregivers prescribe simethicone (Mylicon) drops for colic due to gas, these aids have not been proven effective.

Chiropractic care has provided drug-free relief for many babies (Jamison & Davies, 2006; Hipperson, 2004; Leach, 2002). In chiropractic care, gentle pressure is used to relieve nerve compression that impairs the affected system. A review of studies in which 697 children received a total of 5242 chiropractic treatments found that 85 percent of parents reported an improvement in their infants' symptoms. There were no serious reactions lasting more than 24 hours or severe enough to require hospital care (Miller & Benfield, 2008).

Although interventions can be of limited value, some parents find one that works much better for their baby, while others keep a repertoire handy for this purpose. When crying stops temporarily, parents cannot necessarily assume the cause is clear. Table 13.9 identifies some interventions parents may wish to try. One of the techniques, shown in Figure 13.18, is for the mother to place her baby across her lap. If all measures used to comfort the baby fail, the parents should consult their baby's caregiver to rule out a medical condition. The passage of time seems to be the best cure for colic-like behavior.

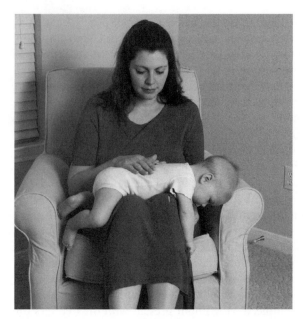

FIGURE 13.18   Placing the baby on his stomach across the parent's lap can help relieve colic symptoms.

Source: Printed with permission of Nelia Box.

TABLE 13.9   Measures for Comforting a Colicky Baby

Holding techniques	"Wear" the baby around the house in a cloth baby sling, walking and dancing in a soothing manner (make sure the baby's breathing is not blocked).
	Hold the baby upright against the parent's shoulder near the neck.
	Place the baby on his stomach across the parent's lap or knees.
	Carry the baby against the parent's hip.
	Lay the baby face down on the parent's chest.
	Lay the baby face down on the inside of the parent's forearm with the baby's head held in the crook of the parent's arm. The pressure on the stomach feels good and the parent can use the free hand to pat and rub the baby's back.
	Pick up the baby as soon as he starts to fuss. This will decrease the length of time he is fussy and prevent it from escalating.
Sounds and motion	Provide a steady noise from a vacuum, clothes dryer, music, humming, or tapes of the mother's heartbeat.
	Play a recording of the baby's own cry.
	Parents speak closely and softly in whispers.
	Position baby to look at the mother's and father's face.
	Provide an unexpected distraction to startle the baby to cease crying.
	Take the baby for a car ride to provide soothing, rhythmic motion.
	Bounce, swing, rock, and walk in slow, rhythmical movements.
Security and warmth	Place the baby in a warm bath.
	Check for any rashes that could indicate reaction to the fiber or detergent in clothing or blankets.
	Swaddle the baby to provide closeness and security, or unswaddle him if the blanket seems too constricting.
	Check the diaper for dampness and keep the baby warm with sweaters or blankets.
	Place a warmed hot water bottle against the baby's stomach area to help him release tension and thereby encourage the passing of gas.
	Fold his legs up to his stomach in a bicycle motion to help him eliminate gas.

Supporting the Parents of a Colicky Baby

When a baby experiences colic-like symptoms, parental stress and concern naturally increase. Colic seems severe enough to some parents that they visit the hospital emergency room. In fact, a crying child accounted for 19 percent of emergency room visits in one study (Perez Solis et al., 2003). An infant with persistent, intractable crying poses a challenge for the emergency physician (Horowitz, 2008). Parents of a colicky baby will need support, frequent contact, and reassurance. Depending on their reading level and desire, you can suggest appropriate resources to assist them in caring for their colicky child. For example, many Internet and parenting support forums are available. Breastfeeding support groups and online meetings can also provide a support network to help families get through this very intense and difficult beginning to their baby's life.

The mother of a colicky baby may experience frustration and guilt for resenting the child. Physical exhaustion is common from constantly trying to soothe and comfort a crying baby. A baby may react to the mother's emotional state and be comforted immediately when another person picks the child up, which can further add to the mother's feelings of guilt and inadequacy. She may feel that her baby is rejecting her and that she is the cause of her baby's colic-like behavior. During this time, the mother will need a great deal of emotional support. An association has been seen between postpartum depression symptoms, insecure maternal attachment style, and colic (Akman et al., 2006). Another study on maternal depression found that colic and prolonged crying were associated with high maternal depression scores; specifically, infantile colic at 2 months of age was associated with high maternal depression scores 4 months later (Vik, 2009).

Caring for an infant with unexplained, persistent crying is one of the most stressful events for new parents. Colic occurs in 10 to 25 percent of all infants and is the most common parental concern reported in the first year of life (Keefe et al., 2006a). In one study, a home-based nursing intervention proved helpful in reducing parenting stress and improving interactions between parents and their irritable infants (Keefe et al., 2006b). The findings suggest that infant colic may be a behavioral pattern that is responsive to environmental modification and structured cue-based care. Unfortunately, very few home health services are covered by insurance for families, especially low-income families on Medicaid in the United States. Other countries, such as the United Kingdom and Australia, have more robust home health support as part of their national health insurance.

One study suggested that colic has an emotional component, reporting that both parents of colicky infants had worse parent–child interaction compared with control parents. The interaction problems were most pronounced between fathers and infants in the severe colic group. Severely colicky infants did not interact as well as the controls. Interaction between the parents was more often dysfunctional in the severe colic group (Raiha et al., 2002).

Tension can aggravate a baby's colicky condition. The mother will need an avenue for venting her anger and frustration. She will benefit from the support of someone who is receptive, caring, and reassuring. Parents may need to take a break and spend some time away from the baby when necessary to keep their perspective. Encourage parents to get help if they feel they cannot cope with their baby's crying.

Shaking the baby in frustration or playing too roughly can cause shaken baby syndrome. Both parents and caregivers need to be educated about the causes of shaken baby syndrome, and know to never shake or handle their baby roughly. Shaking can cause brain damage, blindness, and death. It has been estimated that 53 percent of child traumatic brain injuries were inflicted from being shaken (Jenny, 2009; Keenan et al., 2003). Keenan and colleagues' (2003) study also found that children who incurred an increased risk of inflicted injury were born to young (less than 21 years), non-European American mothers or were products of multiple births. The National Center on Shaken Baby Syndrome has helpful information on recognizing and preventing this form of child abuse (Barr et al., 2009), available at www.dontshake.com.

∼ Summary

Infant assessment is a significant part of the lactation consultant's role with breastfeeding families. Recognizing deviations from normal in the infant's body, posture, skin, head, and reflexes provides important clues about the child's condition. In addition, assessment of the infant's oral structure and elimination patterns will help the lactation consultant determine whether changes are needed in the breastfeeding approach.

As a lactation consultant, you have the opportunity to educate parents about normal baby behavior. Many parents will have never been around babies or even held a baby until they hold their own child. Your experience with many healthy babies at different developmental stages will help you educate parents on normal healthy baby behaviors. Teaching parents how to recognize and interpret infant signals helps them tune into their baby's needs. As parents learn about normal infant behavior, growth, sleeping, crying, and digestion patterns, they become expert in interpreting their own babies' behaviors.

❧ *Chapter 13—At a Glance*

Applying what you learned—

Teach the mother:

- How to help her hypotonic baby stay latched.
- How to find a position for feeding her hypertonic baby.
- The Dancer hand position for a baby who lacks sufficient buccal pads.
- Rooting and other reflexes.
- How to recognize nutritive and nonnutritive sucking.
- What to do for frequent spitting up.
- The appropriate number of voids and stools.
- Approach and avoidance behaviors.
- Hunger cues.
- How to stimulate a sleepy baby and comfort a fussy baby.
- Expected weight patterns.
- Cosleeping and responsive parenting techniques.
- How to distinguish among different types of cries.

Evaluate the baby for:

- Skin turgor for breastfeeding adequacy.
- High palate or short tongue.
- Subtle defects, such as a cleft of the soft palate, a submucosal cleft, or a bifurcated (bifid) uvula.
- Body tone for clues about potential problems.
- Ability to extend the tongue over the alveolar ridge.
- Short frenulum or frenum.
- Fractured clavicle or sensitivity from forceps or vacuum.
- Severe caput succedaneum or cephalhematoma.

❧ *References*

Academy of Breastfeeding Medicine (ABM). Clinical protocol #6: Guideline on co-sleeping and breastfeeding revision. March 2008. www.bfmed.org. Accessed June 16, 2009.

Academy of Breastfeeding Medicine (ABM). Clinical protocol #11: Guidelines for the evaluation and management of neonatal ankyloglossia and its complications in the breastfeeding dyad. http://www.bfmed.org/Resources/Protocols.aspx. Accessed October 31, 2009.

Adgent M. Environmental tobacco smoke and sudden infant death syndrome: a review. *Birth Defects Res B Dev Reprod Toxicol*. 2006;77(1):69-85.

Ahnert L, et al. Transition to child care: associations with infant-mother attachment, infant negative emotion, and cortisol elevations. *Child Dev*. 2004;75(3):639-650.

Akman I, et al. Breastfeeding duration and postpartum psychological adjustment: role of maternal attachment styles. *J Paediatr Child Health*. 2008;44(6):369-373.

Akman I, et al. Mothers' postpartum psychological adjustment and infantile colic. *Arch Dis Child*. 2006;91(5):417-419.

Alcantara J, Anderson R. Chiropractic care of a pediatric patient with symptoms associated with gastroesophageal reflux disease, fuss-cry-irritability with sleep disorder syndrome and irritable infant syndrome of musculoskeletal origin. *J Can Chiropr Assoc*. 2008;52(4):248-255.

Alexandrovich I, et al. The effect of fennel (*Foeniculum vulgare*) seed oil emulsion in infantile colic: a randomized, placebo-controlled study. *Altern Ther Health Med*. 2003;9(4):58-61.

American Academy of Pediatrics (AAP), Subcommittee on Hyperbilirubinemia. Management of hyperbilirubinemia in the newborn infant 35 or more weeks of gestation. *Pediatrics*. 2004;114(1):297-316.

American Academy of Pediatrics (AAP). Policy statement on breastfeeding and the use of human milk. *Pediatrics*. 2005a; 115(2):496-506.

American Academy of Pediatrics (AAP). Policy statement: Task Force on Sudden Infant Death Syndrome. The changing concept of sudden infant death syndrome: diagnostic coding shifts, controversies regarding the sleeping environment, and new variables to consider in reducing risk. *Pediatrics*. 2005b;116(5):1245-1255.

American SIDS Institute. www.sids.org. Accessed on May 2, 2009.

Amir L, et al. Review of tongue-tie release at a tertiary maternity hospital. *J Paediatr Child Health*. 2005;41(5-6):243-245.

Anderson A, et al. Suppressed prolactin but normal neurophysin levels in cigarette smoking breastfeeding women. *Clin Endocrinol* 1982;17:363.

Anderson J. Lactose intolerance and the breastfed baby. August 2006. www.breastfeeding.asn.au/bfinfo/lactose.html. Accessed April 15, 2009.

Aspelund G, Langer J. Current management of hypertrophic pyloric stenosis. *Semin Pediatr Surg*. 2007;16(1):27-33.

Bajanowski T, et al. Nicotine and cotinine in infants dying from sudden infant death syndrome [published online ahead of print February 7, 2007]. *Int J Legal Med*. 2008;122(1):23-28.

Ballard JL, et al. Ankyloglossia: assessment, incidence, and effect of frenuloplasty on the breastfeeding dyad. *Pediatrics*. 2002;110(5):e63.

Barr R, et al. Do educational materials change knowledge and behaviour about crying and shaken baby syndrome? A randomized controlled trial. *CMAJ*. 2009;180(7):727-733.

Beachy J. Premature infant massage in the NICU: review. *Neonatal Netw*. 2003;22(3):39-45.

Bennedbaek O, et al. Infants with colic: a heterogeneous group possible to cure? Treatment by pediatric consultation followed by a study of the effect of zone therapy on incurable colic. *Ugeskr Laeger*. 2001;163(27):3773-3778.

Bergman N. Breastfeeding and perinatal neuroscience. In: Genna CW, *Supporting Sucking Skills in Infants*. Sudbury, MA: Jones and Bartlett; 2008:43-56.

Bergman N., et al. Randomized controlled trial of skin-to-skin contact from birth versus conventional incubator for physiological stabilization in 1200- to 2199-gram newborns. *Acta Paediatr*. 2004;93(6):779-785.

Bhatia J, Parish A. GERD or not GERD: the fussy infant. *J Perinatol.* 2009;29(suppl 2):S7-S11.

Blair P, et al. Sudden infant death syndrome and sleeping position in pre-term and low birth weight infants: an opportunity for targeted intervention [published online ahead of print May 24, 2005]. *Arch Dis Child.* 2006;91(2):101-106.

Bläser A, et al. Drug withdrawal in newborns—clinical data of 49 infants with intrauterine drug exposure: what should be done? [published online ahead of print February 7, 2008]. *Klin Padiatr.* 2008;220(5):308-315.

Blom MA, et al. Health care interventions for excessive crying in infants: regularity with and without swaddling. *J Child Health Care.* 2009;13(2):161-176.

Boekel S. Gastroesophageal reflux: The breastfeeding family's nightmare. Talk presented at: ILCA International Conference; July 27, 2000; Washington, DC.

Bosdure E, Dubus J. The effects of tobacco on children. *Rev Mal Respir.* 2006;23(6):694-704.

Brazy J. Effects of crying on cerebral blood volume and cytochrome aa3. *J Pediatr.* 1988;112(3):457-461.

Butte N, et al. Energy expenditure and deposition of breast-fed and formula fed infants during early infancy. *Pediatr Res.* 1990a;28(6):631-640.

Butte N, et al. Energy utilization of breast-fed and formula fed infants. *Am J Clin Nutr.* 1990b;51(3):350-358.

Butte N, et al. Sleep organization and energy expenditure of breast-fed and formula fed infants. *Pediatr Res.* 1991;32:514-519.

Butte N, et al. Infant feeding mode affects early growth and body composition. *Pediatrics.* 2000;106(6):1355-1366.

Campanozzi A, et al. Prevalence and natural history of gastroesophageal reflux: pediatric prospective survey. *Pediatrics.* 2009;123(3):779-783.

Canivet C, et al. Infantile colic, maternal smoking and infant feeding at 5 weeks of age. *Scand J Pub Health.* 2008;36(3):284-291.

Carpenter R, et al. Sudden unexplained infant death in 20 regions in Europe: case control study. *Lancet.* 2004;363(9404):185-191.

Carr JA, et al. Relationship between toxic erythema and infant maturity. *Am J Dis Child.* 1966;112(2):129-134.

Carrascoza K, et al. Consequences of bottle-feeding to the oral facial development of initially breastfed children [published online ahead of print September 21, 2006]. *J Pediatr (Rio J.)* 2006;82(5):395-397.

Carroll A, et al. A systematic review of nonpharmacological and nonsurgical therapies for gastroesophageal reflux in infants. *Arch Pediatr Adolesc Med Rev.* 2002;156(2):109-113.

Clyne P, Kulczycki A. Human breast milk contains bovine IgG: relationship to infant colic? *Pediatrics.* 1991;87:439-444.

Cooper-Brown L, et al. Feeding and swallowing dysfunction in genetic syndromes. *Dev Disabil Res Rev.* 2008;14(2):147-157.

Crotteau C, et al. Clinical inquiries: what is the best treatment for infants with colic? *J Fam Pract.* 2006;55(7):634-636.

Dewey K. Complementary feeding and breastfeeding. *Pediatrics.* 2000;106(5):1301.

Dewey K. Chapter 22: Nutrition, growth and complementary feeding of the breastfed infant. In Hale T, Hartmann P. *Hale & Hartmann's Textbook of Human Lactation.* Amarillo, TX: Hale Publishing; 2007; 415-423.

Dewey K, Lönnerdal B. Milk and nutrient intake of breast-fed infants from 1 to 6 months: relation to growth and fatness. *J Pediatr Gastroenterol Nutr.*1983;2(3):497-506.

Dewey K, et al. Breast-fed infants are leaner than formula fed infants at 1 year of age: the DARLING study. *Am J Clin Nutr.* 1993;57:140-145.

Dinwiddie R, et al. Cardiopulmonary changes in the crying neonate. *Pediatr Res.* 1979;13:900-903.

Doumouchtsis SK, Arulkumaran S. Head trauma after instrumental births. *Clin Perinatol.* 2008;35(1):69-83, viii.

Dryden C, et al. Maternal methadone use in pregnancy: factors associated with the development of neonatal abstinence syndrome and implications for healthcare resources [published online ahead of print February 10, 2009]. *BJOG.* 2009;116(5):665-671.

Eghbalian F, Monsef A. Congenital epulis in the newborn: review of the literature and a case report. *J Pediatr Hematol Oncol.* 2009;31(3):198-199.

Fawzi W, et al. Maternal anthropometry and infant feeding practices in Israel in relation to growth in infancy: the North African Infant Feeding Study. *Am J Clin Nutr.* 1997;65(6):1731-1737.

Ferreira E, et al. Effects of selective serotonin reuptake inhibitors and venlafaxine during pregnancy in term and preterm neonates. *Pediatrics.* 2007;119(1):52-59.

Fetal Alcohol Syndrome Diagnosis and Prevention Network (FAS DPN). Seattle, WA: University of Washington Center on Human Development and Disability; 2004. depts.washington.edu/fasdpn/pdfs/fasdpnbook.pdf. Accessed May 1, 2009.

Fujita M, et al. Effects of massaging babies on mothers: pilot study on the changes in moodstates and salivary cortisol level. *Complement Ther Clin Pract.* 2005;12(3):181-185.

Garza C, Butte N. Energy intakes of human milk-fed infants during the first year. *J Pediatr.* 1990;117(suppl):S124-S131.

Geddes D, et al. Frenulotomy for breastfeeding infants with ankyloglossia: Effect on milk removal and sucking mechanism as imaged by ultrasound [published online ahead of print June 23, 2008]. *Pediatrics.* 2008;122(1):e188-e194.

Genna CW. *Supporting Sucking Skills in Breastfeeding Infants.* Sudbury, MA: Jones and Bartlett; 2008.

Genna C, Coryllos E. Breastfeeding and tongue-tie. *J Hum Lact.* 2009;25(1):111-112. jhl.sagepub.com/cgi/reprint/25/1/111. Accessed April 24, 2009.

Gkantidis N, et al. Management of maxillary midline diastema with emphasis on etiology. *J Clin Pediatr Dent.* 2008;32(4):265-272.

Goetzinger KR, Macones GA. Operative vaginal delivery: current trends in obstetrics. *Women's Health (Lond).* 2008;4(3):281-290.

Goldstein L, et al. The safety of macrolides during lactation. *Breastfeed Med.* 2009;4(4):197-200.

Gupta S. Update on infantile colic and management options. *Curr Opin Investig Drugs.* 2007;8(11):921-926.

Hale T. *Medications and Mothers' Milk.* 14th ed. Amarillo, TX: Hale Publishing; 2010.

Hale T, Hartmann P. *Textbook of Human Lactation.* Amarillo, TX: Hale Publishing; 2007.

Harder T, et al. Differences between meta-analyses on breast-feeding and obesity support causality of the association. *Pediatrics*. 2006;117(3):987.

Hauck F, et al. Infant sleeping arrangements and practices during the first year of life. *Pediatrics*. 2008;122(suppl 2):S113-S120.

Hazelbaker A. *The assessment tool for lingual frenulum function (ATLFF): Use in a lactation consultant private practice* [thesis]. Pasadena, CA: Pacific Oaks College; 1993.

Hazelbaker A. Newborn tongue-tie and breast-feeding. *J Am Board Fam Pract*. 2005;18(4):326. Comment on *J Am Board Fam Pract*. 2005;18(1):1-7. Author reply 326-327.

Heine R. Gastroesophageal reflux disease, colic and constipation in infants with food allergy. *Curr Opin Allergy Clin Immunol*. 2006;6(3):220-225.

Heinig MJ, et al. Energy and protein intakes of breast-fed and formula fed infants during the first year of life and their association with growth velocity: the DARLING study. *Am J Clin Nutr*. 1993;58:152-161.

Hipperson A. Chiropractic management of infantile colic. *Clinical Chiropractic*, 2007;7(4):180-186.

Hogan M, et al. Randomized, controlled trial of division of tongue-tie in infants with feeding problems. *J Paediatr Child Health*. 2005;41(5-6):246-250.

Hogsdall C, et al. The significance of pregnancy, delivery and postpartum factors for the development of infantile colic. *J Perinat Med*. 1991;19:251-257.

Hopkinson J, et al. Milk production by mothers of premature infants: influence of cigarette smoking. *Pediatrics*. 1992;6:934-938.

Horne R, et al. Comparison of evoked arousability in breast and formula fed infants. *Arch Dis Child*. 2004;89(1):22-25.

Horowitz R. The crying game: Evaluation of the crying, irritable, afebrile infant. Talk presented at: Scientific Assembly: American College of Emergency Physicians; October 28, 2008; Chicago, IL.

Host A. Frequency of cow's milk allergy in childhood. *Ann Allergy Asthma Immunol*. 2002;89(6 suppl 1):33-37.

Howard CR, et al. Parental responses to infant crying and colic: the effect on breastfeeding duration. *Breastfeeding Med*. 2006;1(3):146-155.

Huhtala V, et al. Infant massage compared with crib vibrator in the treatment of colicky infants. *Pediatrics*. 2000;105(6):E84.

Huhtala V, et al. Low plasma cholecystokinin levels in colicky infants. *J Pediatr Gastroenterol Nutr*. 2003;37(1):42-46.

Humphrey S. *The Nursing Mother's Herbal*. Minneapolis, MN: Fairview Press; 2003.

Huus K, et al. Exclusive breastfeeding of Swedish children and its possible influence on the development of obesity: a prospective cohort study. *BMC Pediatr*. 2008;8:42.

Iles R, et al. Crying significantly reduces absorption of aerosolised drug in infants. *Arch Dis Child*. 1999;81(2):163-165.

Ilett K, et al. Use of nicotine patches in breast-feeding mothers: transfer of nicotine and cotinine into human milk. *Clin Pharmacol Ther*. 2003;74(6):516-524.

International Association of Infant Massage (IAIM). www.iaim.net. Accessed May 11, 2009.

International Chiropractic Pediatric Association (ICPA). Advancing the family wellness lifestyle. http://icpa4kids.org/finder.html?q=asymmetry. Accessed April 1, 2010.

Jacobs L, et al. Normal nipple position in term infants measured on breastfeeding ultrasound. *J Hum Lact*. 2007;23(1):52-59.

Jamison J, Davies N. Chiropractic management of cow's milk protein intolerance in infants with sleep dysfunction syndrome: a therapeutic trial. *J Manipulative Physiol Ther*. 2006;29(6):469-474.

Jenny C. Preventing head trauma from abuse in infants. *CMAJ*. 2009;180(7):703-704.

Johnson J, et al. Immediate maternal and neonatal effects of forceps and vacuum-assisted deliveries. *Obstet Gynecol*. 2004;103(3):513-518.

Jordan AE, et al. Serotonin reuptake inhibitor use in pregnancy and the neonatal behavioral syndrome. *J Matern Fetal Neonatal Med*. 2008;21(10):745-751.

Kadam S, Kluckow M. Subcutaneous emphysema of the posterior chest wall in a neonate. *J Paediatr Child Health*. 2005;41(8):456-457.

Kahn A, et al. Sudden infant deaths: stress, arousal and SIDS. *Early Hum Dev*. 2003;75:S147-S166.

Karabulut R, et al. Ankyloglossia and effects on breast-feeding, speech problems and mechanical/social issues in children. *B-ENT*. 2008;4(2):81-85.

Karp H. *The Happiest Baby on the Block: The New Way to Calm Crying and Help Your Newborn Baby Sleep Longer*. Bantam: New York; 2003.

Karp H. The "fourth trimester": a framework and strategy for understanding and resolving colic. *Contemp Pediatr*. 2004;21:94.

Karp H. Safe swaddling and healthy hips: don't toss the baby out with the bathwater [Letter to the editor]. *Pediatrics*. 2008;121(5):1075-1076.

Kawashima H, et al. Cerebrospinal fluid analysis in children with seizures from respiratory syncytial virus infection. *Scand J Infect Dis*. 2009;41(3):228-231.

Keefe M, et al. Effectiveness of an intervention for colic. *Clin Pediatr*. 2006a;45:123-133.

Keefe M, et al. Reducing parenting stress in families with irritable infants. *Nurs Res*. 2006b;55(3):198-205.

Keenan HT, et al. A population-based study of inflicted traumatic brain injury in young children. *JAMA*. 2003;290:621-626.

Kent J, et al. Volume and frequency of breastfeedings and fat content of breast milk throughout the day. *Pediatrics*. 2006;117(3):e387-e395.

Kessmann J. Hirschsprung's disease: diagnosis and management. *Am Fam Physician*. 2006;74(8):1319-1322.

Khoshoo V. Are we overprescribing antireflux medications for infants with regurgitation? *Pediatrics*. 2007;120(5):946-949.

Kim H, et al. Generalized seborrheic dermatitis in an immunodeficient newborn. *Cutis*. 2001;67(1):52-54.

Kochanska G, et al. Mother-child and father-child mutually responsive orientation in the first 2 years and children's outcomes at preschool age: mechanisms of influence. *Child Dev*. 2008;79(1):30-44.

Kubota A, et al. Cow's milk protein allergy presenting with Hirschsprung's disease-mimicking symptoms *J Pediatr Surg*. 2006;41(12):2056-2058.

Kumar B, Sharma S. Neonatal oral tumors: congenital epulis and epignathus. *J Pediatr Surg*. 2008;43(9):e9-e11.

Lacher M. Gastric outlet obstruction after long-term prostaglandin administration mimicking hypertrophic pyloric stenosis. *Eur J Pediatr Surg.* 2007;17(5):362-364.

LaGasse L, et al. Assessment of infant cry: acoustic cry analysis and parental perception. *Ment Retard Dev Disab Res Rev.* 2005;11(1):83-93.

Law K, et al. Smoking during pregnancy and newborn neurobehavior. *Pediatrics.* 2003;111(6 Pt 1):1318-1323.

Lawlor-Smith C, Lawlor-Smith L. Lactose intolerance. *Breastfeed Rev.* 1998;6(1):29-30.

Leach R. Differential compliance instrument in the treatment of infantile colic: a report of two cases. *J Manipulative Physiol Ther.* 2002;25(1):58-62.

Lindberg T. Infantile colic and small intestinal function: a nutritional problem? *Acta Paediatr Suppl.* 1999;88(430):58-60.

Lothe L, et al. Macromolecular absorption in infants with infantile colic. *Acta Paediatr Scand.* 1990;79:417-421.

Lucassen P. Infantile colic. *Clin Evid* [online]. July 1, 2007; pii: 0309.

Lykoudis E, et al. Alopecia associated with birth injury. *Obstet Gynecol.* 2007;110(2 Pt 2):487-490.

Madlon-Kay D, et al. Case series of 148 tongue-tied newborn babies evaluated with the assessment tool for lingual frenulum function. *Midwifery.* 2008;24(3):353-357.

Mahan S, Kasser J. Does swaddling influence developmental dysplasia of the hip? *Pediatrics.* 2008;121(1):177-178.

Manfredi C, et al. High-resolution cry analysis in preterm newborn infants. *Med Eng Phys.* 2008;31(5):528-532.

Maunu J, et al. Relation of prematurity and brain injury to crying behavior in infancy. *Pediatrics.* 2006;118(1):e57-e65.

McKenna J, et al. Mother-infant cosleeping, breastfeeding and sudden infant death syndrome: what biological anthropology has discovered about normal infant sleep and pediatric sleep medicine. *Am J Phys Anthropol.* 2007;45(suppl): 133-161.

McKenna J, Gettler L. Chapter 14: Mother-infant cosleeping with breastfeeding in the Western industrialized context: a bio-cultural perspective. In: Hale T, Hartmann P, *Textbook of Human Lactation.* Amarillo, TX: Hale Publishing; 2007: 271-302.

McLaughlin M, et al. Newborn skin: part II. Birthmarks. *Am Fam Physician.* 2008;77(1):56-60.

Medterms. 2009. www.medterms.com. Accessed April 27, 2009.

Michels K, et al. A longitudinal study of infant feeding and obesity throughout life course [published online ahead of print April 24, 2007]. *Int J Obes (Lond).* 2007;31(7):1078-1085.

Miller J, Benfield K. Adverse effects of spinal manipulative therapy in children younger than 3 years: a retrospective study in a chiropractic teaching clinic. *J Manipulative Physiol Ther.* 2008;31(6):419-423.

Miller-Loncar C, et al. Infant colic and feeding difficulties. *Arch Dis Child.* 2004;89(10):908-912.

Millichap JJ, Wainwright MS. Neurological complications of respiratory syncytial virus infection: case series and review of literature [published online ahead of print]. *J Child Neurol.* 2009;24(12):1499-503.

Ming X, et al. Prevalence of motor impairment in autism spectrum disorders [published online ahead of print April 30, 2007]. *Brain Dev.* 2007;9:565-570.

Minodier P, et al. Star anise poisoning in infants. *Arch Pediatr.* 2003;10(7):619-621.

Mitoulas L, et al. Variation in fat, lactose and protein in human milk over 24 h and throughout the first year of lactation. *Br J Nutr.* 2002;88(1):29-37.

Monk C, et al. The relationship between women's attachment style and perinatal mood disturbance: implications for screening and treatment [published online ahead of print May 21, 2008]. *Arch Women's Ment Health.* 2008;11(2): 117-129.

Moore E, et al. Early skin-to-skin contact for mothers and their healthy newborn infants. *Cochrane Database Syst Rev.* 2007;3:CD003519.

Moreno L, et al. Dietary risk factors for development of childhood obesity. *Curr Opin Clin Nutr Metab Care.* 2007;10(3): 336-341.

Moriceau S, Sullivan RM. Neurobiology of infant attachment. *Dev Psychobiol.* 2005;47(3):230-242.

Mosko S, et al. Maternal sleep and arousals during bedsharing with infants. *Sleep.* 1997;201(2):142-150.

Motil K, et al. Human milk protein does not limit growth of breast-fed infants. *J Pediatr Gastroenterol Nutr.* 1997;24(1): 10-17.

Moyer V, et al. Accuracy of clinical judgment in neonatal jaundice. *Arch Pediatr Adolesc Med.* 2000;154:391-394.

Ndiaye O, et al. Traumatic injuries of newborns after forceps delivery at the Abass Hospital Center Maternity. *Dakar Med.* 2001;46(1):36-38.

Nowicki S, et al. The Prader-Willi phenotype of fragile X syndrome. *JDBP.* 2007;28(2):133-138.

O'Connor N, et al. Newborn skin: part I. Common rashes. *Am Fam Physician.* 2008;77(1):47-52.

Olsen L. Urinary flow patterns of healthy newborn males [published online ahead of print February 23, 2009]. *J Urol.* 2009;181(4):1857-1861.

Osborn D, Sinn J. Formulas containing hydrolysed protein for prevention of allergy and food intolerance in infants. *Cochrane Database Syst Rev.* 2005;18(4):CD003664.

Page D. Breastfeeding is early functional jaw orthopedics (an introduction). *Funct Orthod.* 2001;18(3):24-27.

Paller A, Mancini A [Hurwitz S, original author]. *Hurwitz Clinical Pediatric Dermatology: A Textbook of Skin Disorders of Childhood and Adolescence.* 3rd ed. Philadelphia: Elsevier Saunders; 2006.

Palmer B. Frenums, tongue-tie, ankyloglossia. Paper presented at: Kansas City, MO; 2001. http://www.brianpalmerdds.com/frenum.htm. Accessed April 24, 2009.

Palmer B. Breastfeeding and frenulums. Paper presented at: Kansas City, MO; December 2003. http://www.brianpalmerdds.com/bfeed_frenulums.htm. Accessed April 24, 2009.

Palou A, Picó C. Leptin intake during lactation prevents obesity and affects food intake and food preferences in later life. *Appetite.* 2009;52(1):249-252.

Parlade M, et al. Anticipatory smiling: linking early affective communication and social outcome [published online ahead of print October 31, 2008]. *Infant Behav Dev.* 2009;32(1):33-43.

Patel M, et al. Metabolic programming: Role of nutrition in the immediate postnatal life [published online ahead of print

December 22, 2008]. *J Inherit Metab Dis.* 2009;32(2):218-228.

Paty E, et al. A case of botulism in an 11-month-old infant. *Arch Fr Pediatr.* 1987;44(2):129-130.

Perez Solis D, et al. Neonatal visits to a pediatric emergency service. *An Pediatr (Barc).* 2003;59(1):54-58.

Prescott S, et al. The importance of early complementary feeding in the development of oral tolerance: concerns and controversies. *Pediatr Allergy Immunol.* 2008;19(5):375-380.

Raiha H, et al. Excessively crying infant in the family: Mother-infant, father-infant and mother-father interaction. *Child Care Health Dev.* 2002;28(5):419-429.

Ramsay D. Ultrasound imaging of the sucking mechanics of the term infant. Paper presented at: Human Lactation: Current Research and Clinical Implications: October 22, 2004; Amarillo, TX.

Rautava L, et al. Acoustic quality of cry in very-low-birth-weight infants at the age of 1½ years. *Early Hum Dev.* 2007;83(1):5-12.

Raymond J, Bacon W. Influence of feeding method on maxillo-facial development. *Orthod Fr.* 2006;77(1):101-103.

Richardson H, et al. Sleep position alters arousal processes maximally at the high-risk age for sudden infant death syndrome. *J Sleep Res.* 2008;17(4):450-457.

Richardson H, et al. Maternal smoking impairs arousal patterns in sleeping infants. *Sleep.* 2009;32(4):515-521.

Ricke L, et al. Newborn tongue-tie: prevalence and effect on breast-feeding. *J Am Board Fam Pract.* 2005;18(1):1-7.

Salvatore S, Vandenplas Y. Gastroesophageal reflux and cow milk allergy: is there a link? *Pediatrics.* 2002;110(5):972-984.

Sánchez CL, et al. The possible role of human milk nucleotides as sleep inducers. *Nutr Neurosci.* 2009;12(1):2-8.

Scher M. Neonatal hypertonia: I. Classification and structural-functional correlates. *Pediatr Neurol.* 2008a;39(5):301-306.

Scher M. Neonatal hypertonia: II. Differential diagnosis and proposed neuroprotection. *Pediatr Neurol.* 2008b;39(6):373-380.

Sears J, et al. *The Baby Book: Everything You Need to Know About Your Baby from Birth to Age Two.* Boston, MA: Little, Brown; 2003.

Sears W, et al. *The Baby Sleep Book: The Complete Guide to a Good Night's Rest for the Whole Family.* New York: Little, Brown; 2005.

Sevelinges Y. Neonatal odor-shock conditioning alters the neural network involved in odor fear learning at adulthood. *Learn Mem.* 2008;15(9):649-656.

Sevelinges Y, et al. Enduring effects of infant memories: infant odor-shock conditioning attenuates amygdala activity and adult fear conditioning. *Biol Psychiatry.* 2007;62(10):1070-1079.

Sheffield R, et al. What's the best treatment for cradle cap? *J Fam Pract.* 2007;56(3):232-233.

Shekhar A, et al. Role of stress, corticotrophin releasing factor (CRF) and amygdala plasticity in chronic anxiety. *Stress.* 2005;8(4):209-219.

Shprintzen R. Velo-cardio-facial syndrome: 30 years of study. *Dev Disabil Res Rev.* 2008;14(1):3-10.

SIDS Alliance. January 2009. www.sidsalliance.org/advocacy/DayOnTheHill_Leave%20Behind.pdf. Accessed May 2, 2009.

Siegfried E. Skin manifestations of immune disorders in children. *Curr Opin Pediatr.* 1993;5(4):446-451.

Sillén U. Bladder function in healthy neonates and its development during infancy. *J Urol.* 2001;166(6):2376-2381.

Small M. *Our Babies, Ourselves: How Biology and Culture Shape the Way We Parent.* New York: Knopf; 1999.

Small M. Should babies be put on a sleep schedule? *LiveScience*'s human nature columnist. September 5, 2008. www.livescience.com. Accessed May 5, 2009.

Smillie C. How newborns learn to latch: a neurobehavioral model for self-attachment in infancy. *Acad Breastfeed Med News Views.* 2001;7:23.

Smillie C. How infants learn to feed: a neurobehavioral model. In Genna CW, *Supporting Sucking Skills in Infants.* Sudbury, MA: Jones and Bartlett; 2008:79-95.

Sondergaard C, et al. Psychosocial distress during pregnancy and the risk of infantile colic: a follow-up study. *Acta Paediatr.* 2003;92(7):811-816.

Srinivasan A, et al. Ankyloglossia in breastfeeding infants: the effect of frenotomy on maternal nipple pain and latch. *Breastfeed Med.* 2006;1(4):216-224.

St. James-Roberts I, et al. Individual differences in responsivity to a neurobehavioural examination predict crying patterns of 1-week-old infants at home. *Develop Med Child Neurol.* 2007;45(6):400-407.

Stanford School of Medicine. Newborn Nursery at LPCH. Acrocyanosis. 2009. www.newborns.stanford.edu/PhotoGallery/Acrocyanosis1.html. Accessed September 15, 2009.

Stroud L, et al. Maternal smoking during pregnancy and newborn neurobehavior: effects at 10 to 27 days. *J Pediatr.* 2009;154(1):10-16.

Sullivan R. Developing a sense of safety: the neurobiology of neonatal attachment. *Ann N Y Acad Sci.* 2003;1008:122-131.

Torticollis KidsInformation website for parents of children with torticollis. 2009. www.torticolliskids.org. Accessed April 24, 2009.

Tunc V. Factors associated with defecation patterns in 0-24-month-old children [published online ahead of print February 9, 2008]. *Eur J Pediatr.* 2008;167(12):1357-1362.

U.S. Food and Drug Administration (FDA). FDA public health advisory: need for caution when using vacuum assisted delivery devices. May 21, 1998. Updated May 11, 2009. www.fda.gov/cdrh/fetal598.html. Accessed September 18, 2009.

Underdown A, et al. Massage intervention for promoting mental and physical health in infants aged under six months. *Cochrane Database Syst Rev.* 2006;18(4):CD005038.

van Bakel H, Riksen-Walraven J. Stress reactivity in 15-month-old infants: links with infant temperament, cognitive competence, and attachment security. *Dev Psychobiol.* 2004;44(3):157-167.

van Bakel HJ, Riksen-Walraven JM. Adrenocortical and behavioral attunement in parents with 1-year-old infants. *Dev Psychobiol.* 2008;50(2):196-201.

van Dijk C, Innis S. Growth-curve standards and the assessment of early excess weight gain in infancy. *Pediatrics.* 2009;123(1):102-108.

van Sleuwen B, et al. Swaddling: a systematic review. *Pediatrics.* 2007;120(4)e1097.

Vandenplas Y, et al. The diagnosis and management of gastro-oesophageal reflux in infants. *Early Hum Dev.* 2005;81(12): 1011-1024.

Venneman M, et al. Does breastfeeding reduce the risk of sudden infant death syndrome? GeSID Study Group. *Pediatrics.* 2009;123(3):e406-e110.

Venter C. Factors associated with maternal dietary intake, feeding and weaning practices, and the development of food hypersensitivity in the infant. *Pediatr Allergy Immunol.* 2009;20:320-327.

Vickers A, et al. Massage for promoting growth and development of preterm and/or low birth-weight infants. *Cochrane Database Syst Rev.* 2004;2:CD000390.

Vik T. Infantile colic, prolonged crying and maternal postnatal depression. *Acta Paediatr.* 2009;98(8):1344-1348.

Volpe J. *Neurology of the Newborn.* 5th ed. Philadelphia: WB Saunders; 2008.

Waynforth D. The influence of parent-infant cosleeping, nursing, and childcare on cortisol and SIgA immunity in a sample of British children. *Dev Psychobiol.* 2007; 49(6):640-648.

Wessel M, et al. Paroxysmal fussing in infancy, sometimes called "colic." *Pediatrics.* 1954;114:421-434.

Weyermann M, et al. Duration of breastfeeding and risk of overweight in childhood: a prospective birth cohort study from Germany. *Int J Obes (Lond).* 2006;30(8):1281-1287.

Whitehead R. For how long is exclusive breastfeeding adequate to satisfy the dietary energy needs of the average young baby? *Pediat Res.* 1995;37(2):239-243.

Whitehead R. Infant physiology, nutritional requirements, and lactational adequacy. *Am J Clin Nutr.* 1985;41(2 Suppl): 447-458.

Whitehead R, Paul A. Long-term adequacy of exclusive breast-feeding: how scientific research has led to revised opinions. *Proc Nutr Soc.* 2000;59(1):17-23.

Wiessinger D, Miller M. Breastfeeding difficulties as a result of tight lingual and labial frena: a case report. *J Hum Lact.* 1995;11(4):313-316.

Willinger M, et al. Defining the sudden infant death syndrome (SIDS): deliberations of an expert panel convened by the National Institute of Child Health and Human Development. *Pediatr Pathol.* 1991;11:677-684.

Wilson-Clay B, Hoover K. *The Breastfeeding Atlas.* 4th ed. Austin, TX: Lactnews Press; 2008.

Wolf L, Glass R. *Feeding and Swallowing Disorders in Infancy: Assessment and Management.* San Antonio, TX: Therapy Skill Builders; 1992.

Woolridge M. Colic, "overfeeding," and symptoms of lactose malabsorption in the breast-fed baby: a possible artifact of feed management? *Lancet.* 1988;2:382-384.

World Health Organization (WHO). *WHO Multicentre Growth Reference Study Group: WHO child growth standards.* Geneva: World Health Organization; 2006. www.who.int/childgrowth/standards/en. Accessed May 10, 2009.

Zeretzke K. Personal email correspondence, May 12, 2009.

Getting Breastfeeding Started

Most mothers and babies are capable of easily mastering breastfeeding. Breastfeeding is a combination of instinct and learned skill for both mother and baby. Mothers have the desire to snuggle and cuddle with their newborns. Often they naturally hold their babies in positions that are very similar to breastfeeding even at nonfeeding times. Some babies have difficulty in their initial attempts at breastfeeding, while others begin nursing trouble free. Both mother and baby will learn the art of breastfeeding with time, patience, and gentle guidance as they learn to coordinate their natural behaviors with each other. Mothers who give birth to more than one baby require ingenuity and resourcefulness in managing breastfeeding. You also may encounter mothers who have another nursing child at home when they give birth to a new infant. You can assist these mothers as they balance the needs of both children.

∾ Key Terms

Assisted reproductive
   technology (ART)
Baby-led feeding
Biological nurturing
Calming techniques
C-hold
Clutch hold
Cradle hold
Cross-cradle hold
Dancer hand position
Dominant hand hold
Flanged
Football hold

Fussy baby
Latch
Lying down position
Modified side-sitting hold
Motility
Multiples
Posture feeding
Prone position
Rooting reflex
Rousing techniques
Searching response
Side-sitting hold
Tandem nursing

∾ Getting Ready to Nurse

Mothers typically look forward to their first breastfeeding session with anticipation and excitement. Ideally, a mother and baby remain together to begin nursing in the same bed where the baby was born. The earlier the mother begins to breastfeed, the earlier her baby will receive colostrum to promote stooling. This early sucking begins milk production sooner than for a woman whose first breastfeeding is delayed. Mothers and babies should be kept together and not subjected to unnecessary separation that interferes with this process. Delays in initiating breastfeeding can contribute to engorgement and low milk production. Some evidence also indicates that a delay can affect the duration of breastfeeding (Wiklund et al., 2009; Chaves et al., 2007).

Establishing a Breastfeeding Routine

Mothers who are breastfeeding for the first time may feel awkward initially while the baby settles onto the breast. Reassuring mothers that this feeling of awkwardness is common and to be expected helps them view breastfeeding as a new venture. It requires time to learn the nuances of positioning the baby for feedings. These first sessions are ideal practice times for the mother and her baby as they both learn how to fit together.

Nursing a baby usually becomes second nature very quickly. A few simple preparations can help the mother develop self-confidence, increase the ease with which she breastfeeds, and ensure effective breastfeeding. These preparations include attending to her physical needs before a feeding. The mother can use the bathroom, wash her hands, and gather whatever she will need during the feeding. These items may include pillows to help position herself and her baby, a beverage, a cloth for burping her baby, her laptop, cell phone, remote control, reading material, breast pads, diapers, wipes, and a change of clothes for her baby. If she gathers a basket of the items she will want, she can carry it anywhere in her house. She can keep similar items in her diaper bag for when she is on the go. She might also want to silence her phone so that she and her baby will be undisturbed during the feeding. Suggestions for relaxing and creating an optimal climate for feedings appear in Table 14.1.

Encouraging Baby-Led Feedings

Full-term, healthy newborns have an innate ability to tell their parents when they need to eat and when they are finished. Imposing time restrictions on feedings can lead to

TABLE 14.1   Creating a Relaxing and Effective Climate for Nursing

Issue	Suggestions for the Mother
Relaxation techniques	• Spend a few minutes before going to sleep to analyze your own relaxation techniques, e.g., movements, positions, and room darkness. Repeat these techniques at other times for relaxation. • Remove distractions, e.g., find a quiet spot and take the phone off the hook. • Get comfortable, e.g., empty your bladder; find a cozy chair or bed; get pillows for support; remove eyeglasses, shoes, or tight clothing; adjust room temperature. • Listen to relaxing music. • Take a deep breath and let it out slowly. Repeat this several times. • Breathe steadily and rhythmically, noting the faint movement of your body, and breathe slowly to relax further. • Tense your entire body and relax the tension slowly. Concentrate on one muscle at a time, starting from your toes, and progress up to the facial muscles, until your limbs, eyelids and all body parts feel heavy. • Use massage or warm compresses on tense parts of your body. • Take a warm shower or bath. • Close your eyes and move them back and forth or up and down. Then rest your eyes and feel the release of tension. Relax your eyes by thinking about a ship sailing away from you and disappearing over the horizon. • Allow your mind to drift into a sleepy state and think pleasant thoughts, e.g., enjoyable moments, pleasures, or dreams. • Think about your baby, of milk flowing, or of water rushing. • Think about, write down or talk with someone about your fears, stresses, tensions, and what you feel causes them. Then let your mind drift or think of pleasant thoughts and feel the release of tension. • Visualize some strenuous or precarious activity, such as walking across thin ice, and then pretend it has ended and you are at ease. • Pray. • Meditate on a passage of a text from a favorite author.
Creating an optimal climate	• Nurse in a quiet spot away from distractions. • Avoid embarrassing or stressful situations for feeding. • Drink juice, water, or noncaffeinated tea before and during feeding. • Set up a routine for beginning a feeding.
Recharging your batteries	• Nap or rest when the baby rests. • Simplify daily chores and establish priorities around the baby. • Get help with household, child care, and other responsibilities. • Take a break from the daily routine with an evening out, shopping, a walk, or lunch with a friend.
Feeding-related techniques	• Use warm compresses before feeding. • Express a little milk and gently stimulate the nipple. • Use breast compression while the baby is nursing. • Lie down to nurse. • Nurse the baby in bed at night. • Hold the baby skin to skin during feeding.

engorgement for the mother and underfeeding for the baby. This practice also alters a baby's natural intake of foremilk and hindmilk. Switching breasts without cues from the baby overrides this natural ability to self-regulate feedings. Such overriding of a baby's freedom can set up negative reactions and behaviors that may lead to breast refusal. Interference with the intake of foremilk and hindmilk can lead to colic-like symptoms in babies, as discussed in Chapter 13. Specifically, limiting nursing time on one breast so that the infant can nurse on the other breast can result in less hindmilk intake; this increased foremilk intake coupled with less hindmilk may result in lactose dumping into the infant's small intestine (Anderson, 2006). Lactose overload in the small intestine causes fermentation and, consequently, increased gas and gut motility in the gastrointestinal tract. This can lead to a very uncomfortable, fussy baby (see Chapter 13 for a discussion of colic).

Babies have the ability to self-regulate their feedings to meet their individual needs for optimal growth (Van Dijk & Innis, 2009; Dewey, 2007; Kent et al., 2006). Confusing a mother and baby by specifying exact times for spacing and length of feedings will lead to frustration for both. Such restrictions impose an unnecessary burden at a period when the mother is becoming acquainted with her new baby. After all, no adult eats a meal in exactly the same amount of time as all other adults; nor do adults enjoy having their meals regulated by a clock. The same is true with babies.

Mothers need to be encouraged to watch their babies for cues—not the clock. Their babies cannot tell time: They just know that they are unhappy when they are hungry and content when they are full. The hunger cues described in Chapter 13 tell parents when their baby is ready for a feeding. When parents learn how to recognize hunger signs, they are able to let their baby lead the way. Help mothers learn how to observe their baby's feeding readiness. Being placed in a position for feeding at times when the baby is not ready to nurse can produce frustration and cause the baby to be wary of the whole process. A healthy, full-term baby knows when it is time to nurse and exhibits a progression of signs that indicate a desire to feed.

The baby is equally able to let the mother know when the feeding is finished. Encourage mothers to begin a feeding on the side that received the least stimulation at the previous feeding and to continue nursing on that breast until the baby releases it. If the baby unlatches after only a short time, the mother can try burping or addressing any other discomfort her baby may have, and then resume nursing on the same breast. If the feeding on one breast seems especially lengthy, the mother can observe the sucking pattern and switch her baby to the other breast if sucking has become non-nutritive. Not all mothers need to use both breasts at every feeding. In the early days of nursing, however, it is good practice to encourage mothers to stimulate both breasts equally, to assure optimal milk production in both breasts.

Exceptions to Baby-Led Feedings

There are some instances when a mother needs to be diligent in monitoring the time between feedings rather than relying on her baby to determine frequency. The first occurs in the case of a medicated birth, as discussed in Chapter 12. Many babies born after long medicated labors have depressed central nervous systems (CNS), latching problems, and sleepiness (Smith, 2009). Encourage the mother of a sleepy, medicated baby by reassuring her that the sleepiness will pass. The baby will soon exchange this sleepiness for fussiness, most frequently in the evening hours. Other occurrences that can result in incompetent feeders in the immediate postpartum period are babies born very preterm, babies with birth trauma, and babies with neurological or congenital issues such as Down syndrome, Turner syndrome, or cerebral palsy.

Babies with these conditions are sleepy, difficult to rouse, and ineffective at the breast, and they often appear "content to starve." They frequently develop jaundice, which increases the sleepiness even further. These babies need a lot of stimulation to nurse. They need frequent feedings and often require supplementation with alternative feeding methods (see Chapter 23). Mothers of these babies need to "watch the clock" temporarily and be vigilant about getting calories into them. Very early preterm babies often have significant health problems, such as cardiac or respiratory issues, that require continual monitoring and care by the parents. See Chapter 23 for more discussion on very preterm babies.

Late preterm babies born at 34 to 36 weeks gestation need to be monitored carefully as well. They do not always demonstrate strong hunger cues and often go home without competent breastfeeding skills (Academy of Breastfeeding Medicine [ABM], 2004; Wight, 2003). The mother of a late preterm infant can focus on three goals: feeding the baby, protecting her milk production, and transitioning the baby to full feeding at the breast. Usually, as the due date approaches, the baby suddenly seems to "wake up" and begins to nurse robustly.

～ Beginning the Feeding

The manner in which the mother brings her infant to her breast sets the stage for the quality of the feeding. The mother must be in a comfortable position to support her baby, and her baby's position needs to facilitate an effective latch that the baby can maintain. The baby can usually be placed in a position to easily accommodate breastfeeding. In most cases, the baby's mouth will work correctly if the mother's and baby's body positions do not interfere with the process, and if helpers are not overly intrusive. Skin-to-skin contact for the first few feedings after birth facilitates breastfeeding and has been found to influence the duration of exclusive breastfeeding (Vaidya et al., 2005). It also helps in the event of crying or other avoidance or stress behaviors, and calms the baby to facilitate nursing.

Biological Nurturing

Neurological research confirms the innate abilities of the baby to root, and to find and self-attach to the mother's breast after birth if given time and the respect to do so. Babies are neurologically primed to achieve their innate goal of nursing (Bergman, 2008). As feedings begin in the postpartum period, both mother and baby need time to interact without the interference of rapid interventions.

Although much research has focused on rooting, sucking and swallowing, other reflexes are now thought to play important roles in robust breastfeeding behavior. These individual reflexes, termed "primitive neonatal reflexes" (PNRs), include 20 feeding behaviors and positions. Biological nurturing allows these reflexes to facilitate nursing. The reflexes—which are classified into four types (endogenous, motor, rhythmic and anti-gravity) and two functional clusters (finding/latching and milk transfer)—either stimulate or impair nursing. For example, rather than the newborn preferring to lie on a side with pressure along the back, researchers postulate that the newborn is an abdominal feeder and, like some other animals, displays anti-gravity reflexes that aid latch.

The belief that breastfeeding initiation is an innate behavior for both mother and baby, rather than a learned practice, challenges the routine skills-teaching currently central to breastfeeding support. Researchers have observed significantly more PNRs as stimulants in semi-reclined postures associated with biological nurturing than when mothers were upright or side-lying (Colson et al., 2008; Colson, 2007a, 2007b). They hypothesize that when mothers lie semi-reclined and the infants lie prone on the mothers' chest, instinctive maternal behaviors and PNRs are triggered, thereby stimulating breastfeeding.

Biological nurturing recognizes that because all mothers' bodies are different, no one posture can possibly fit all needs. Mothers will easily find the right posture for their own needs and comfort when routine suggestions are avoided. Comfortable, sustainable postures will change and evolve throughout the breastfeeding time span. Initially, they may change from feed to feed or on a daily basis (Colson, 2005). Biological nurturing research validates the importance of intuition and instinct to the mother–baby dyad. It also testifies to the importance of healthcare givers respecting this time, and not interrupting or taking over the process.

Lobbying for this uninterrupted time can be challenging in hospitals with time constraints on deliveries, especially within the U.S. healthcare system. Another factor driving the trend toward more interventions in breastfeeding is the high incidence of medicated babies and mothers whose instinctive behaviors may be blunted by drugs. Every healthy mother and baby should be given the time to initiate these innate reflexes. If you observe a lack of robust nursing initiation on the part of the newborn, gentle help may be appropriate to avoid the cascade of supplementation endemic in many U.S. hospitals.

Mothers need to understand the principles of effective positioning that will provide the optimal circumstances for their baby to feed. They also need to recognize situations where a biological nurturing position would be impossible or inappropriate. Healthcare professionals can incorporate a biological nurturing approach within a framework of care that provides women with a range of skills to enable them to adapt their breastfeeding to a variety of situations (UNICEF, 2009).

The Mother's Positioning

The mother needs to find a comfortable position, with her back and arms supported by pillows where necessary, as illustrated in Figure 14.1. When she is positioned well, her

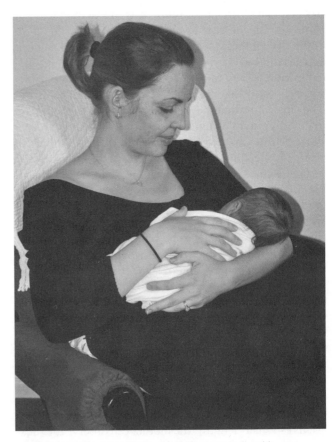

FIGURE 14.1   A mother using pillows to help with positioning and comfort.

Source: Printed with permission of Anna Swisher.

posture will be relaxed, with her shoulders resting comfortably against the back support. When sitting, her feet can rest comfortably on the floor or a footstool, with her knees higher than her hips. This encourages the baby to remain close to the mother's chest rather than falling away from her. Placing her knees higher than her hips also helps prevent the mother from leaning over her baby to breastfeed. If she is lying down, reclining enables the baby to rest prone on her torso, helping to trigger searching responses.

Typical postpartum discomforts need to be addressed in the early breastfeeding sessions, particularly in the perineal and incision areas. Positioning should place the least stress on any sore areas. A mother who delivers by cesarean section can place a pillow on her lap to protect her abdominal incision. Alternatively, she can position the baby at her side in the side-sitting (also football or clutch) hold, with pillows to raise the infant to a level near the breast and protect her abdomen. If the mother is in pain, you may see her toes curled, facial grimacing, or hunched shoulders. She may also become uncomfortable if she remains in the same position for a long time. Helping mothers find ways to become positioned comfortably in early feedings sets them on a course for extended breastfeeding.

Supporting the Breast

In the early weeks of breastfeeding, breast support is often helpful in preventing nipple soreness and facilitating a good latch. This is especially the case when the mother's breasts are large. The weight of a large breast can cause it to pull slightly from the baby's mouth and interfere with maintaining a good latch. To deal with this issue, the mother can cup her free hand to form the letter C—referred to as the C-hold—with her thumb on top and her fingers curved below the breast well behind the areola, as

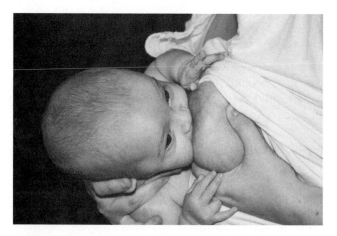

FIGURE 14.2   Using the C-hold to support the breast during a feeding.

Source: Printed with permission of Kori Martin.

in Figure 14.2. She can then gently guide her baby to the breast centering the nipple in the baby's mouth. After the mother and baby have mastered positioning and latch, the mother may no longer need to support her breast.

The purpose of the C-hold is to support the weight of the breast. It should not be so pronounced that it compresses the breast vertically to the baby's mouth. The mother's hold should parallel the angle of the baby's mouth, with her thumb opposite the baby's nose so that the shape of the breast is parallel to the shape of the baby's mouth. Consider this analogy, which most mothers can readily picture: She should hold the breast just as she would hold a taco or sandwich—that is, parallel to her mouth, not vertically (Wiessinger, 1998). Mothers who have trouble with tactile input may respond better to word pictures or visual handouts. Others need kinesthetic learning, where you might gently put your hand around her hand to help if she is receptive.

A slight variation of the C-hold works well with preterm infants and other babies who have weak muscle development and find it difficult to hold the jaw steady while they suck. This position, which is known as the Dancer hand position, begins in the C-hold. The mother brings her hand forward to support her breast with the first three fingers. She supports the baby's chin by resting it in the area of her hand between her thumb and index finger, as illustrated in Figure 14.3. The mother then bends her index finger slightly so that it gently holds the baby's cheek on one side, with her thumb holding the other cheek. This hold helps decrease the available space in the baby's mouth and increases negative pressure. When the mother uses steady, equal pressure while holding her baby's cheeks, she avoids interfering with the rooting reflex. As the baby's muscle tone begins to improve, she can place her thumb back on top of the breast, leaving the index finger to support the baby's chin.

The Baby's Positioning

One of the most exciting areas of neonatal research focuses on the newborn's intrinsic ability to breastfeed. As mammals, human babies are wired to nurse. The newborn uses a series of neurosensory cues to search for and independently find the mother's teat, grasp it with the mouth, and initiate feeding (Smillie, 2008). Many feeding problems may be due in part to the short circuiting of this newborn dance through the interruptions of Western birthing practices.

Newborn behaviors include the stepping response to scoot up the mother's body to the breast, rooting to find the breast, grasping to achieve latch, and commencing suckling (Righard & Alade, 1990). Thus the bobbing and bouncing thought by many caregivers to signal immaturity is now seen as a purposeful reflex termed the searching

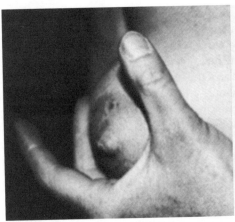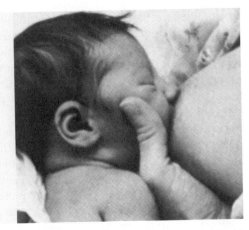

FIGURE 14.3   The Dancer hand position supports the baby's mouth and gently compresses his cheeks.

Source: Printed with permission of Sarah Coulter Danner.

response (Smillie, 2001, 2008). This series of behaviors is not confined to the newborn period, but rather can extend as long as the stepping reflex lasts.

Improper positioning of the baby at the breast is the major cause of nipple soreness. When the baby's positioning avoids pulling on the nipple, the potential for pain is lessened. That is not to say that mothers will not react with surprise at the sensation of the first latch, as evidenced in Figure 14.4. It is common for mothers to describe a certain amount of discomfort when they first begin breastfeeding. This sensation should subside after time and should not escalate to prolonged pain. Note the helper in Figure 14.4, who is holding the baby's head. Pushing the baby's head toward the breast is not recommended, as it can result in the baby's chin being flexed to his or her chest, making opening wide and swallowing more difficult.

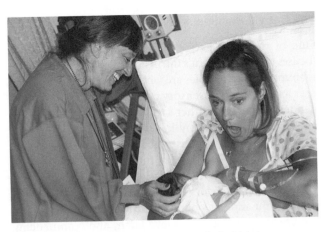

FIGURE 14.4   The surprise of a baby's first latch.

Source: Printed with permission of Tammy Arbeter.

Postural stability is important for a baby to initiate feeding behaviors. When positioned properly, the baby will be well supported and cuddled around the mother. The mother holds the baby in chest-to-chest contact, level with her breast. When self-attaching, the baby may respond best when held vertically between the mother's breasts, with his or her head below or at the same height as her breasts. As the baby reaches for the breast, the mother continues to provide postural support from her torso and/or arms. The infant's ear, shoulder, and hip should be in alignment, and his or her body should be flexed. The baby's cheeks should both be the same distance from the breast. With a close hold, the baby's chin presses deeply in the breast. If the breast obstructs breathing, she can pull the baby's back and shoulders in toward her body. This will usually angle the infant's head slightly away from the breast and allow the child to breathe freely. Note that mothers with soft or "squishy" breast tissue may need to use their thumb to depress the breast slightly away from the baby's nose.

The Baby's Mouth

The mother can encourage nursing by establishing eye contact, speaking, and stroking the infant. Allowing the baby to find the nipple independently will provide the signal to open his or her mouth wide enough to get a large mouthful of breast tissue. Color Plate 28 shows the baby's mouth beginning to open. If the mother were to attempt a latch at this point, the baby would fail to get far enough back on the breast. Chapter 15 discusses latch in detail.

The baby's mouth should be positioned slightly below the center of the breast so that he or she reaches up to it. Lining up the baby's nose with the mother's nipple is often a helpful visual reference, as this positioning will result in the lower lip covering more of the areola than the upper lip. Some babies latch better with the nipple angled up toward the hard palate; this helps trigger the baby's suck reflex and encourages the infant to take in more of the areola below the nipple. The baby's tongue will extend over the lower gum (alveolar ridge), many times far enough to extend out to the lower lip. If the baby's head turns away from the breast, stimulating the rooting reflex entices the infant to turn back toward the breast with an open mouth.

Rooting Reflex (Response)

It is the contact of the breast on the baby's face that signals rooting. When eliciting the rooting reflex or response, the mother will want to take care not to stimulate any other part of her baby's face. The child will instinctively root toward the source of the stimulation and may become confused and frustrated. Widstrom and colleagues (1993) demonstrated that eliciting the rooting reflex by touching the cheek with the nipple causes the infant's head to turn toward the stimulus, with mouth opened wide and tongue extended. Licking movements precede rooting when the infant was in an alert state.

Forcing the baby to the breast can disturb the rooting–tongue reflex system. When crying, the baby's tongue moves up toward the palate. If forced to the breast (even with gentle force), a crying infant may remember the forced situation and defensively place the tongue up toward the palate at subsequent feedings. This reaction may also occur if a mother forces her baby to the breast when the child is not hungry.

∼ *Assisting at a Feeding*

During the early postpartum weeks, becoming acquainted with their baby is the most important adjustment for parents. The newborn may prefer quiet at one time and stimulation at another time. During these early weeks in the child's life, parents learn the many things that make their baby unique. They learn to become sensitive to their baby's physical needs, disposition, and behavior at the breast. Acquainting parents with typical infant patterns will help them adapt their routines to meet the needs of their baby.

Learning the baby's patterns of behavior can be challenging in the early days after birth. Help parents understand that it will become easier and feel more natural with time. Let them know, too, that learning to interpret their baby's signals may occur more slowly with babies who demonstrate ambiguous signals than with babies who give clear signals. You can explore with the mother ways to modify her baby's patterns, when necessary, and adapt to her baby's nuances. Being available to assist her at early

feedings will help build her confidence and put the parents on the road to long-term enjoyment of their parenting experience.

Observing a Feeding

After the baby has latched on is an ideal opportunity for the lactation consultant or other helper to sit back and watch the mother and baby. Observe the mother's posture, noting whether she is comfortable and has her back supported. Watch how she holds the baby, and identify whether she needs to hold her breast to assist with latch. Note the position of the baby's body, the position of the mouth on the breast, the placement of the tongue, and the position of the baby's head and hands. The baby should appear comfortable, with his or her body in good alignment. The child's lips should flange out, and the cheeks should be smooth, with each being an equal distance from the breast.

The baby should settle into long, deep sucks, in a rhythmic suck–swallow–breathe pattern. When the mother has more copious milk, swallowing will be heard. When a large quantity of milk is flowing, a baby sucks about once per second. Conversely, an infant sucks about twice per second when there is little milk flow. A faster sucking pattern may indicate the time between milk ejections or signal the end of the feeding on that breast. If the baby exhibits the faster pattern throughout an entire feeding, he or she may not have a good latch or there may be little milk available. If clicking is heard when the baby sucks, repositioning will help the baby attain a better latch.

Assisting a Reluctant Nurser

In the early days of breastfeeding, a baby's reluctance to nurse is frequently a result of something unrelated to feeding. The mother and baby may simply need time to learn how to respond to each other. Observe the mother and baby at a feeding to assess what may be happening. Learn from the mother and baby, and trust that they will work out any difficulties. Do not be in a hurry to do or say anything until you have determined that they need help. If the baby's reluctance continues for several hours or days, the mother will need to express milk to maintain production and prevent engorgement.

In the early days after birth, it is common for a baby to seem unresponsive to the mother's attempts to breastfeed. The infant may be sleepy or medicated from the delivery or from the mother's pain medication during her postpartum recovery. In some cases, the baby simply may not be hungry at the time the mother attempts a feeding. Watching her baby for hunger cues will help her determine the most receptive times for feeding. When the mother needs to stimulate her baby to nurse, she can try the rousing techniques listed in the following section. She can use these techniques both before and during a feeding when necessary.

The Baby Who Is Sleepy

Sleepiness in newborns is common in the early days after birth, perhaps from labor medications, or simply because of the immaturity of the baby's system. Given that the mother needs to nurse frequently enough to establish milk production, it may sometimes be necessary to wake the baby for feedings to establish a good pattern. Many newborns sleep for longer periods during the day and nurse more at night. Waking these babies periodically during the day will help turn their schedule around and encourage longer sleep periods at night. Parents will need to be patient, because it may take several weeks to reverse the baby's rhythm.

Possible Causes of Sleepiness

You can help the mother explore possible causes for her baby's sleepiness. These causes may include the following:

- The mother received medications during labor.
- A traumatic birth resulted from a long labor or long second-stage labor.
- The baby is preterm.
- It is the baby's usual sleepy period.
- The first feeding was delayed.
- The mother overlooked hunger cues.
- The baby has sensory overload, as in a loud nursery.
- Sleepiness is in response to interventions, particularly circumcision.
- The baby is jaundiced.
- A schedule was imposed on feedings.
- The mother had a cesarean delivery.
- The baby is experiencing hypothermia.

Care Plan for a Sleepy Baby

After exploring causes for the baby's sleepiness, the lactation consultant and the mother can determine a plan of care. In the hospital, 24-hour rooming-in with skin-to-skin contact enables parents to observe and respond to hunger cues. Help them distinguish between deep sleep and light sleep. The mother can attempt to put her baby to breast every half-hour to hour, when the child shows signs of a light sleep state.

Until feedings are well established, the mother will need to pump or hand express her milk to feed to her baby. Using an alternative feeding method will avoid the potential for the nipple preference that may result if the baby receives a bottle. If her milk or donor milk is not available, she will need to feed the baby artificial baby milk. It is important that the mother monitor her baby's output and watch for symptoms of dehydration or hypoglycemia. A protocol for appropriate supplementation of healthy, full-term breastfed infants can be found at www.bfmed.org.

Parents can try a number of rousing techniques to interest the baby in feeding. Of course, initiating a feeding when the baby demonstrates hunger cues will achieve better results than trying to feed a baby who is in deep sleep. The first step, on picking the infant up, is to loosen the blankets to provide air exposure. Because the baby will likely be in need of a diaper change anyway, this can be the next step.

Skin-to-skin contact often facilitates an interest in nursing. Therefore, the mother can unclothe and cuddle her baby upright between her bare breasts. If the baby still does not awaken, she can continue the skin-to-skin contact between her breasts while talking quietly to her baby. Dimming the lights will encourage the baby's eyes to open. If the infant still does not waken, the mother can allow him or her to sleep for another half to 1 hour and then try again.

Rousing Techniques

- Talk to the baby and try to make eye contact.
- Loosen or remove blankets.
- Hold the baby upright in a sitting or standing position.
- Partially or fully undress the baby.
- Change the baby's diaper.
- Stimulate the baby through increased skin contact, such as massage or gently rubbing the baby's hands and feet.
- Stimulate the baby's rooting reflex.
- Stimulate the baby's sense of smell by bringing the child close to the breast so that he or she can detect the scent of the mother's skin.
- Stimulate the baby's sense of taste by expressing milk onto the nipple or into the baby's mouth.
- Wipe the baby's forehead and cheeks with a cool, moist cloth.
- Manipulate the baby's arms and legs by playing pat-a-cake, doing baby exercises, and so on.
- Give the baby a bath or, better yet, take a bath with the baby to provide increased skin-to-skin contact.
- If the baby takes the breast but does not maintain a rhythmic suck–swallow–pause pattern, try stroking under the baby's chin from front to back. Also, compress the breast, as with manual expression.
- Express colostrum onto a finger and elicit sucking with the finger.

The Baby Who Cries and Resists Going to Breast

At times, a baby may seem to resist when put to breast. When moved toward the breast, such an infant cries loudly instead of starting to suck. The longer the mother tries, the more the baby cries and fights against it. Some babies seem to be more fussy and irritable during the first month of life, being easily stimulated and excited. They may cry frequently and require continuous attention during their waking hours. In addition, they may be especially sensitive to being handled or become frightened by their flailing arms and legs. Swaddling the baby to restrict startling and movement may provide a sense of security and calm (Karp, 2008, 2004).

The mother will need to soothe her fussy baby before beginning a feeding. A crying baby has difficulty coordinating breathing and swallowing, and may choke or swallow air. Similarly, a baby who is overly hungry may choke and gag due to over-eagerness to nurse. The mother can prevent these problems by carefully observing her newborn's behavior and beginning the feeding before the baby becomes too upset or overly hungry. The mother may not always be able to prevent such hunger or fussiness, however, and will benefit from suggestions for calming her fussy baby. She can try these suggestions before and during the feeding, as well as at other times during the day.

When a sensitive baby is fussy, the mother may become tense and frustrated by the behavior. If the baby responds to this tension by crying even more, the mother needs to break the cycle by changing her behavior in some way. She can leave the room for several minutes and use relaxation and breathing techniques to calm herself. Enlisting the help of the father, another relative, or a friend to care for the baby will help the mother get relief away from the baby for longer periods. Talking with you or someone close to her about her feelings of anger, frustration, and inadequacy may help relieve her tension. She may also benefit from a walk outdoors or a soothing bath or massage.

A mother can improve her outlook by keeping her body in good condition and eating nutritious foods. Suggest that she plan easy meals and snacks that include sufficient protein to ensure a feeling of well-being, as well as adequate B vitamins to promote calm nerves. She can rest whenever possible, nurse while lying down, and enlist the help of others to care for the baby while she naps. See Chapter 13 for further discussion on crying and care of a fussy or colicky baby.

Possible Causes of Fussiness

- Caregivers have handled the baby too much.
- The baby is in pain or has experienced pain.
- The mother received medication during labor or postpartum that passed to the baby.
- The baby has discomfort from forceps, vacuum extraction, internal monitor lead, or cephalhematoma.
- The baby has oral aversion because of deep suctioning or other invasive procedures.
- The baby is irritable.
- The baby received an artificial nipple or pacifier, which resulted in nipple preference.
- The mother's lack of confidence causes her to hold her baby tentatively.
- The baby needs to be swaddled to provide boundaries or to be soothed by being cuddled in skin-to-skin contact with the mother.
- The baby has shut down from too much intervention, such as someone attempting to push the child on the breast.
- The mother and baby were separated, resulting in missed hunger cues and missed imprinting.
- Rarely, fussiness in a baby can be a sign of serious problems, such as neurological disorders.
- The baby is withdrawing from nicotine or other drugs.

Care Plan for a Fussy Baby

Encourage the mother to hold her baby calmly in skin-to-skin contact at the breast. Limit latching attempts to no more than a few minutes at a time. If latching attempts cause resistance or crying, stop and try again 10 or 15 minutes later, after the baby is calm. Avoid placing pressure on a potentially painful site or holding the baby in a feeding position when administering medical treatment.

As with a sleepy baby, it is important for the mother to express or pump her milk and feed it to a fussy baby until regular feedings are established. The baby should not receive any unnecessary bottles or pacifiers. If medication is prescribed to calm the baby, encourage the mother to ask questions about its possible side effects.

Calming Techniques

- Limit invasive procedures to minimize crying.
- Provide skin-to-skin contact.
- Cuddle without pushing the baby to breastfeed.
- Work with the baby for short periods.
- Be sensitive to and respect the baby's cues.
- Build the mother's confidence.
- Use slow, calm, deliberate movements in caring for the baby.
- Cuddle, hold, and walk with the baby.
- Talk or sing to the baby in a soft voice.
- Swaddle the baby.

- Nurse in a dark, quiet room.
- Rock in a rocking chair to relax both mother and baby.
- Burp the baby often (unless burping seems upsetting). Burp before switching to the other breast at a feeding.
- Carry the baby in a position that puts gentle and firm pressure on the child's abdomen—for example, on the mother's hip or shoulder.
- Play music, create a monotonous noise by running a vacuum cleaner or dishwasher, or play a recording of such sounds.
- Change the baby's diaper when it becomes damp or soiled.
- Mother and baby sleep or nap together so the baby is comforted by her body warmth and heartbeat.
- Massage the baby for 10 to 15 minutes (the baby may fuss during the massage and then become quiet afterward).
- Use a sling to carry the baby close to the mother's body.
- Use a baby swing for times when individual attention is not possible.
- If the baby was born at full term and has established good temperature control, remove the infant's clothes to provide air exposure for limited amounts of time.
- Lay the baby on his or her stomach on the mother's lap while she gently bounces her knees or moves them back and forth.
- Have the mother and baby take a bath together.
- Get help from others—father of the baby, grandparents, or other support person. Sometimes the baby will calm when held by someone who is calm.
- Provide monotonous movement with a stroller or car ride.
- Remove allergens from the mother's diet.

Ending a Feeding

A baby who nurses robustly and effectively usually will gently release the breast when finished feeding. If the mother needs to interrupt the feeding before this point is reached (i.e., to achieve a better latch), she can break the suction by inserting her finger gently into the corner of the baby's mouth between the gums. Color Plate 36 illustrates this technique. In addition, the mother can press a finger against her breast near the corner of the baby's mouth, allowing her breast to slip easily out of the child's mouth.

If the mother notices her baby chewing on tugging on her nipple toward the end of a feeding to the extent that it causes discomfort, she may need to end the feeding. When the mother's finger touches the baby's lips to begin breaking suction, the baby will instinctively begin to suck faster—a reflexive response to having the lip touched while at the breast. The mother can gently continue her efforts to remove her baby.

Generally, urge the mother to continue a feeding until the baby releases the breast spontaneously. She can then put the baby to the other breast and continue to nurse at both breasts, one after the other, for as long as the baby wants. There is always milk in the breast except in case of maternal problems, as discussed in Chapter 20. Unless the mother feels pain or discomfort, there are milk transfer problems, or the child experiences medical problems such as reflux, babies can stay at the breast for as long as nutritive sucking and swallowing are observed.

〜 Breastfeeding Positions

Once a baby has achieved effective breastfeeding (defined as latching, suckling, and transferring milk without pain for the mother), mothers typically hold their babies in a variety of positions at the breast. The most common positions are the cradle hold, side-sitting hold, cross-cradle hold, and side-lying position. Posture or prone feeding and some other variations are also useful in particular circumstances. If a mother achieves an effective latch using a less traditional position, there is no reason for anyone sto interfere. Avoid saying anything negative and avoid touching the mother or baby when she first positions her baby. Such intervention could undermine the mother's confidence or increase her anxiety.

For a visual representation of how to position her hand or her baby, you can use the analogy of the breast as a clock with the hour hands identifying the position you are describing (see Figure 16.2 in Chapter 16). This analogy can serve as a general guide while she learns different ways to hold her baby for nursing. When offering advice to mothers, always remember to account for variations in anatomy between mothers, as well as comfort and self-efficacy levels. If a particular analogy does not resonate with a mother, change it to something that works. The following sections describing breastfeeding positions assume that a mother is nursing her baby at her right breast.

Cradle Hold

The cradle hold is the traditional position in which the mother sits with her baby's body across her abdomen. With her baby at the right breast, she places the child's head in the crook of her right arm and supports his or her body with her right hand, as shown in Color Plate 29. Using the clock analogy, the mother's left index finger would be at about 6:00 and her left thumb at 1:00. She might cup her left hand around her breast to facilitate latch, with her index finger between 10:00 and 11:00 and her thumb between 2:00 and 3:00.

This position may not be optimal if the mother and baby are experiencing any problems with latch or milk transfer. When using this hold, the mother has limited control over the movement of her baby's head. Thus she cannot assist or guide the baby to a better latch. Even so, the cradle hold is the position most mothers instinctively use, and you should not interfere with it unless it is clearly ineffective. Sometimes a baby's latch can be adjusted by gently realigning the baby's body, without breaking the latch.

Side-Sitting (Also Football or Clutch) Hold

In the side-sitting (also called football or clutch) hold, the mother holds her baby under her arm much in the same way she clutches a purse to her side or a football player holds the ball while running. She places her baby's body along her right side with his or her feet toward her back. Pillows can be used to help support the baby and the mother's arm. Holding the baby's head in her right hand, she supports the child's body with her right forearm and raises his or her head to breast level, as shown in Color Plate 30.

This position is especially effective for nursing a preterm baby, who fits snugly under the mother's arm. It is also useful for full-term infants who have difficulty latching. The mother is able to hold her baby's entire body on her arm and can respond to the child's body movements better. She can hold and form her breast with her left hand and can perform breast massage easily. This hold is helpful in tricking a baby into nursing on a breast that the infant refuses in the traditional sitting position. In addition, it may be effective with babies who have a short tongue or ankyloglossia, for nursing multiple children (e.g., twins, triplets), for mothers with a cesarean incision, or for mothers with very large breasts. A woman with large breasts may also benefit from use of a firm pillow or folded blanket, resting the weight of her breast on the pillow like a "table."

Many times mothers have difficulty seeing their baby's body in a side-sitting hold. A modified version of the hold keeps the baby off the mother's stomach, while enabling the mother to see her baby better. It may also provide better postural support for the baby and avoid the feeling that the baby is slipping or falling. In the modified side-sitting hold, the baby is placed on the side of the mother with the top of the baby's head toward the middle of her chest and the feet facing away from her. The mother holds the baby with her left arm for nursing on the left breast (see Figure 14.5) and can use her right hand as needed for support. If she cups the breast, her thumb will be at the 3:00 position and her index finger between 8:00 and 9:00.

Cross-Cradle (Dominant Hand) Positions

The cross-cradle hold combines the side-sitting hold and the cradle hold, so that the mother rests her baby's head

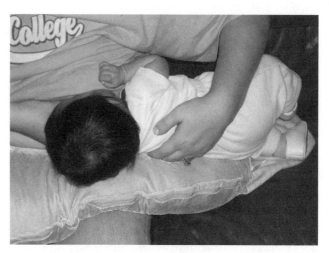

FIGURE 14.5 Modified side-sitting hold.
Source: Printed with permission of Anna Swisher.

in her hand. It is sometimes referred to as the dominant hand position, although the mother can use either her dominant or less dominant hand. In the dominant hand position, the right-handed mother supports her baby's neck and shoulders with her right hand and supports the child's body with her forearm. She then moves her arm with the baby across her body to the opposite breast, as shown in Color Plate 31. She can support her left breast with her left hand, with her thumb at 3:00 and her left index finger at 9:00.

Holding the baby with the dominant hand is especially helpful in early feedings, or with a baby who is not self-attaching well. This position allows the mother to exert better control over her baby's movements. Feedings are easier to manage, which increases the mother's self-confidence. Some mothers find it more comfortable to begin a feeding in a cross-cradle position and then bring the other arm around to hold the baby in a cradle position after the infant has secured a good latch.

Side-Lying Position

Lying down to nurse helps the mother get needed rest. It is also a position that allows the baby to self-attach. To use this position, the mother lies on her side, with her knees slightly bent. Pillows placed under her head, between her legs, and behind her back will help her achieve a comfortable position. She can position her lower arm under her head and use her top arm to support the baby's head and back. Alternatively, she can place her lower arm under the baby's head or along the back of the child's body, using that arm to provide support. She can put her baby to breast first and then raise or lower the breast by rolling her body. Placement of a pillow or rolled towel or blanket behind the newborn's back will help to keep the child lying on his or her side for an effective latch.

To nurse on the top breast, the mother can roll toward the baby so that her top breast is level with the baby's mouth. She may need to rearrange the pillows to provide necessary support. Another method for changing breasts is for the mother to hug her baby against her chest so they roll together to the opposite side, as shown in Color Plate 32.

Prone Position (Posture Feeding)

If the mother has overabundant milk production that causes excessive amounts of milk to gush into her baby's mouth, the prone position—also called posture feeding—may be useful. In this position, the mother places her baby above the breast to achieve better control over milk flow. The mother lies on her back, or semi-reclined, with her baby lying in stomach-to-stomach position on top of her (see Color Plate 33). To get into this position easily, the mother can begin in a sitting position, put her baby to breast, and then lean back.

This position is essentially the one described in the biological nurturing approach. Prone feeding may be useful at times when letdown seems strongest, such as in the early morning. It also is useful for babies who bite or retract their tongues, as gravity encourages the infant's jaw to fall forward.

Other Creative Breastfeeding Positions

Over the millennia of human existence, women have devised some creative positions to nurse their babies. Perhaps conventional nursing positions would aggravate a sore spot on the nipple or the mother has a plugged duct that would benefit from a different nursing position. One alternative feeding method is to place the baby on the bed, as shown in Color Plate 34, and lean over the child on hands and knees. The mother can then position the breast in the baby's mouth by rotating his or her body. To avoid back strain, she can raise the baby with pillows or blankets. This position is useful for babies who are in traction or who have undergone surgery. As an alternative, the mother can lie on her back and place the baby on his or her stomach with the feet over her shoulder, as shown in Color Plate 35. Such variations demonstrate that there is no one correct position for nursing. As long as the baby is able to manage an effective latch, and the mother is comfortable and enjoying her baby, mothers can continue to be creative in their approaches.

It is important for the lactation consultant to affirm what works for a mother and her baby, and to offer alternatives only when something is *not* working. Some mothers become frustrated that there is no one "right" answer for their questions. In reality, parenting is an ongoing process that continually unfolds. Encourage the mother to recognize that she has the capacity and the capability to discover what works for her baby today. Tomorrow may be different, and next month will definitely change. Enjoying the process of being in the moment is a part of the mothering journey.

❦ Breastfeeding Multiples

Mothers of multiples (twins, triplets, and so on) can attain the same breastfeeding outcomes as the mother of a single baby. Although there may be more demands on her time and she faces some special challenges, such a mother will find that breastfeeding brings a calming element to an otherwise hectic life. It is certainly a more pleasurable expenditure of time than preparing formula and heating bottles while listening to the cries of hungry babies! It also saves parents the expense of buying double or triple the amount of infant formula and the increased medical expenses associated with more frequent illnesses from not being breastfed (Bartick & Reinhold, 2010).

When a woman learns she is expecting more than one baby, she may be told that she cannot breastfeed or that she will have to feed her babies on a schedule. You can help her sort through conflicting advice and find which arrangement will work best for her. The greatest gift you can give to the prospective mother is reassurance that she can make enough milk for her babies. Records from 1900 reveal that wet nurses in France were able to furnish 2230 grams (78 oz) of milk per day. One woman yielded as much as 2840 grams (100 oz) in 1 day (Budin, 1907)!

The few possible exceptions to ample milk production include a woman with hormonal problems, one who has had breast surgery or trauma to the breast, or one with true insufficient glandular development. Lactation consultants have noted that some infertile women who conceive through reproduction technology have difficulty with milk production. See the discussion on insufficient milk production in Chapter 25.

Prevalence of Multiple Births

The number of multiple births has more than doubled over the past 2 decades. In 2005, 133,122 twin babies and 6,208 triplet babies were born in the United States alone. Women are increasingly having babies after age 30, an age when multiples occur more frequently. In addition, more women are using fertility treatments to help them conceive. Fertility treatments—also known as assisted reproductive technology (ART)—increase the likelihood of multiple births (U.S. Department of Health and Human Services [USDHHS], 2009).

Most women with multiples will face all of the same issues that mothers of preterm babies encounter, but often with the complication of significant health problems in their children. Twins are at substantially greater risk for illness and death than singletons, albeit to a lesser extent than triplets or higher-order multiples. Notable risks include low birth weight, preterm birth, and neurological impairments such as cerebral palsy. Twin and triplet-or-more births are significantly more likely to occur with ART births than with births resulting from natural conception (CDC, 2008). In 2005, among women who conceived through ART, 13 percent of singletons, 63 percent of twins, and 95 percent of triplets or more were born preterm (Centers for Disease Control and Prevention [CDC], 2008).

Breastfeeding Prevalence

Not surprisingly, mothers of multiples are far less likely to breastfeed (2.44 times) than mothers of singletons. The duration of breastfeeding is also significantly shorter for these infants (Yokoyama et al., 2006; Yokoyama & Ooki, 2004). Although feeding choice does not appear to be associated with prematurity or low birth weight, the decision to bottle feed is almost 2 times higher for women whose husbands were not cooperative in childrearing. The degree of anxiety mothers felt when informed about a multiple pregnancy also played a role, with mothers who felt greater anxiety being 1.73 times more likely to bottle feed their children.

Nevertheless, women who experience multiple birth increasingly desire to breastfeed their babies. Families using ART to achieve pregnancy tend to be highly educated and have higher income—the key demographic of families who breastfeed in industrialized countries. Breastfeeding of preterm and even full-term multiple-birth infants is complex and demanding for these families, however, and just as challenging for healthcare givers who want to help them (Leonard & Denton, 2006). Families with multiples require ongoing help from healthcare providers who are committed to the provision of human milk for these children.

The Council of Multiple Birth Organisations (COMBO, 2007), an advocacy coalition, has outlined a declaration of rights and statement of needs for twins and higher-order multiples. One of its proclamations advocates for education regarding the nutritional, psychological, and financial benefits of breastfeeding for preterm and full-term infants. It cites the need for encouragement and coaching in breastfeeding techniques, and simultaneous bottle feeding of co-multiples. In addition, it advocates for adequate resources, support systems, and family work leave for parents of multiples. Another COMBO statement cites the need for specialized education and assistance to promote and encourage bonding and breastfeeding for families with medically fragile multiples.

Breastfeeding Routine

A mother of multiples will probably need to pay closer attention to her breastfeeding schedule than a mother of a single baby, at least until the babies reach their "full-term" date and are robust feeders. With creative planning and flexibility, she will find the routine that works best for her. Breastfeeding encourages a mother to regard each baby's needs individually. It promotes more time in close physical contact with her babies, enabling her to provide a maximum amount of skin contact with each one. Nursing her babies separately at least once every day, and spending other time alone with each baby, enhances bonding and the emergence of individuality in each baby (Gromada, 2007).

While in the hospital, having the babies together for feedings will enable the mother to learn the practical aspects of feeding them. She may need plenty of pillows to help her position her babies. Having the help of another person to keep one baby positioned at the breast will help her latch the second baby onto the other breast. If she has more than two babies, she can feed the other baby with an alternative method while two are nursing. Rotating babies at each feeding will give all of them equal time at the breast. If one baby must remain in a special care nursery, the mother can nurse the baby who is able to be with her and express her milk for the other one. Some hospitals find that keeping multiples together in the same bed, referred to as "co-bedding," is beneficial to the babies.

Simultaneous Feedings

Many mothers prefer to nurse their twins simultaneously rather than separately. The mother can enjoy nursing times more if she does not hear the hunger cries of her other baby. Otherwise, she may rush through the first feeding and find it less relaxing. She may also have less opportunity to interact in a meaningful way with her babies. Figure 14.6 illustrates three positions for nursing both babies simultaneously.

A variety of options for managing simultaneous feedings exist. The mother may confine each baby to one breast only and always reserve the same breast for the same baby. One drawback to this practice is that one baby may have a stronger suck, which can cause the mother to develop a larger breast on that side because of greater stimulation and milk production. Another drawback is the baby's visual development. Feeding a baby from two different sides stimulates different parts of the infant's body and provides equal vision stimulation to both eyes. Alternating babies between breasts at each feeding or every few feedings will ensure equal stimulation of both breasts and coordinated visual development. Alternatively, each baby may nurse on one breast each day and switch to the other breast the next day.

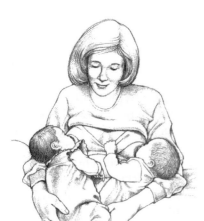 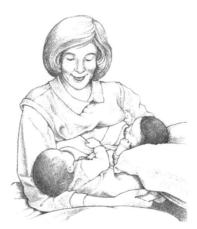 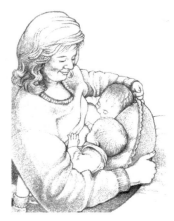

Babies are crisscrossed, with each one in the cradle hold, with support from the mother's hands under their buttocks and pillows placed under the mother's elbows.

Babies are placed with one in the cradle position and one in the side-sitting (football or clutch) position, with pillows supporting the mother's arms. A pillow on her lap may also help.

Both babies are placed on a pillow in the side-sitting (football or clutch) position. A footstool can add to the mother's comfort.

FIGURE 14.6 Positions for nursing multiples.

Source: Illustrations by Marcia Smith.

On some occasions, one baby may exhibit hunger cues at a time when the other baby is not interested in nursing. The mother might choose to delay feeding the hungry baby until the other one is willing to nurse so that she can economize on the time she spends feeding them. It is important that healthcare providers not add to the mother's dilemma by causing her to feel guilty about taking this step. Each mother must work out her own routine and will appreciate your support in her decision. At another time, you can discuss with her each baby's individual needs and the importance of responding to them. Perhaps she can breastfeed the hungry baby and keep the second one close by, in hopes that letdown and proximity will stimulate that child's interest in feeding. She can also try to awaken the second baby to feed at that feeding.

Feeding Higher-Order Multiples

Breastfeeding higher-order multiples requires even more creativity than breastfeeding twins. In the early days after their births, the mother will most likely need the help of another person at feedings. It is very time-consuming to nurse each baby separately. The mother can nurse two babies at one time, while she or someone else feeds the other baby or babies with an alternative feeding method. Alternatively, she can nurse the first two babies simultaneously and place the others on both breasts afterward.

The mother will eventually become adept at managing feedings on her own. As with twins, she will want to be sure that all babies receive the same amount of time at the breast and that both of her breasts receive equal stimulation. The mother should be sure to offer the breast to all babies throughout the day so that they all receive milk from the breast. It may be helpful to keep a log of each baby's diapers and feeds to help monitor the children's growth.

Challenges with Parenting Multiples

Initial bonding may be complicated with multiples. It may be even more complex when one baby remains hospitalized longer than the other(s). In such a case, the parents will have bonded with one baby and may find it difficult to establish the same attachment with the other(s) after the delay in coming home. Parents may need to focus on developing a close relationship with both or all of their babies. As each baby arrives home, they can make arrangements that will allow them to spend more time bonding with the new arrival. Sometimes this dilemma is never resolved, however.

Parents' reactions to having multiples can range from delight to dismay. The quality of their support system is a major factor in their coping abilities. Both parents' emotions—but especially the mother's feelings—are likely to fluctuate, depending on how each day goes. The mother may feel more stressed by the constant demands on her time and energy. The father may feel shunted aside, wondering what happened to their identity as a couple. In addition, household priorities will need to change to accommodate the demands of more than one baby. Time-saving techniques will be essential in establishing a new daily routine. Good nutrition can help safeguard both the mother's health and sense of well-being.

Higher-income mothers may hire others to help with child care, or use shopping and cleaning services to assist them with tasks of daily living. Mothers who do not have these options may be able to find teenagers to help them for a few hours during the day. Seasoned mothers of older multiples may be happy to be resources for new mothers. You can help in forging these bonds by asking these mothers if they would like to help other mothers and give their permission to be contacted.

Breastfeeding Challenges

Mastitis may be more common among mothers of multiples, due to both fatigue and the mother's abundant milk production. A missed feeding by one or more babies can result in engorged breasts more quickly than in the case of a mother with one baby. Given this possibility, a mother with multiples will need to be accessible to her babies for feedings or able to pump easily. When she is away, she must be sure to express milk to avoid engorgement and the possibility of plugged ducts. A manual pump or a car adapter for her electric pump may prove handy in case of travel or appointments.

Multiples develop and grow at varying rates, just as other siblings do. Although growth spurts may occur simultaneously, it is more likely that these events will come at slightly different times for each baby. The babies may be ready for solid foods and weaning at different times as well. Mothers of multiples are more likely to supplement their babies early. They may feel pressured by well-meaning friends and family to begin supplemental foods earlier than usual or to wean at an earlier age.

Some mothers of multiples may breastfeed exclusively for several months, whereas others may elect to supplement their children every day. Occasional supplements given by another person allow the mother to have some time alone for a few hours if she wishes. This kind of a breather will help her keep a perspective on her mothering and can provide a workable compromise. Supplemental feedings are typically needed with higher-order multiples, mostly from a time management standpoint. You can provide support to these mothers by affirming that any breastmilk is better than none.

A case study of quintuplets described the breastfeeding journey of a highly motivated mother to provide human milk to all five of her babies (Szucs, 2009). The mother provided approximately half of their intake with her own milk and supplemented with donor milk (see Figure 14.7). At 5 to 6 months postpartum, she usually breastfed each baby once and one baby twice daily, while continuing to pump 6 to 7 times per day. Plugging parents of higher-order multiples into these support systems of volunteers will assist their long-term efforts after the babies arrive. Web resources for coordinating care

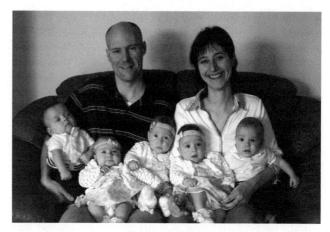

FIGURE 14.7　Quintuplets exclusively on breastmilk.
Source: Szucs KA, et al. Quintuplets and a mother's determination to provide human milk: it takes a village to raise a baby—how about five? *J Hum Lact.* 2009;25:79. Reprinted by permission of SAGE Publications.

abound, which enables groups of helpers to sign up for duties online and avoid duplication.

When multiples are born preterm, the family may have success obtaining insurance coverage for donor milk for a longer period of time. Many families do not have insurance, however, and they may not qualify for government health programs such as Medicaid. Even so, these families may be able to receive donor milk from other sources. As a lactation consultant, you can provide information about the safe heat treatment to home-pasteurize donated milk, which may help this practice become a more attractive alternative for families.

Although exclusive breastfeeding is the optimal choice, breastfeeding does not have to be an "all or nothing" proposition for mothers of multiples. Breastfeeding enables babies to bond with their mother, a rewarding and comforting element in the lives of babies whose individual personalities are emerging. There is a tendency to regard multiples as a single entity, a group. Nurturing at the breast and feeling the close special attention of the mother is reassuring to each individual baby in the group (Gromada, 2007).

Support for Mothers of Multiples

Most mothers know before delivery that they are carrying multiples, especially when the pregnancy results from infertility treatment. Anticipatory guidance and information are especially helpful to such women. Success stories from mothers who have breastfed triplets and quadruplets are very empowering and can help reassure expectant mothers about their abilities. In addition, online forums, websites, and Internet breastfeeding cafés can provide emotional and practical support. Table 14.2 provides some suggestions for counseling mothers of multiples.

Support from the lactation consultant and other significant people in her life will be important in helping the mother accommodate breastfeeding to the busy routine of parenting multiples. Mothers of Multiples clubs, which offer excellent support and advice about caring for multiples, are available in many communities. The primary purpose of Mothers of Multiples clubs is not to provide breastfeeding support, however, and many mothers in these groups choose to bottle feed. Help in this area can occur simultaneously with support from a lactation consultant or breastfeeding support group, preferably one that includes other mothers nursing multiples.

∼ Tandem Nursing

Tandem nursing is the term used to describe the breastfeeding of two or more children of different ages. It can occur if a mother is still breastfeeding when she begins another pregnancy. She may choose to continue nursing throughout the pregnancy and to nurse both babies when the new baby arrives. Tandem nursing may also occur when a child who had previously weaned shows a renewed interest in breastfeeding when he or she sees the new baby at the mother's breast. A very warm relationship can develop between nursing siblings and their mother. Breastfeeding can provide a good lesson in sharing and touching and encourages affection and close friendships between siblings.

Breastfeeding During Pregnancy

Women have been advised for years to wean their nursling when they become pregnant with another child. The reasoning behind this advice is that oxytocin released during breastfeeding stimulates uterine contractions. The concern is that breastfeeding during a new pregnancy could, because of oxytocin's effect on the uterus, lead to abnormal uterine contractions, unintended abortion, impaired placental blood flow in later pregnancy, intrauterine growth retardation, preterm contractions or

TABLE 14.2   Counseling Mothers of Multiples

Mother's Concern	Suggestions for Mother
Lack of time for all tasks	• Plan nursing schedule. • Carefully evaluate priorities. • Use time-saving methods for household chores. • Prepare simple nutritious meals. • Enlist help from others.
Bonding with more than one baby	• Breastfeed separately at least one time every day. • Spend time alone with each baby every day.
Bonding with a baby who has a delayed homecoming	• Regard babies as individuals and meet their separate needs. • Obtain help with babies who are already settled in, and spend more time with the new arrival.
Nursing two babies at the same time	• Let each baby nurse exclusively on one breast. • Put babies on alternate breasts at each feeding. • Let each baby nurse on one breast for the entire day and alternate breasts daily.
Spending too much time nursing babies separately	• Whenever one baby is hungry, nurse both.
Nursing three or more babies	• Nurse two at a time and get help from another person to feed the other baby. • Alternate babies so a different one is fed with alternate means at each feeding. • Nurse two babies simultaneously and the other baby on both breasts afterward.
Greater susceptibility to mastitis	• Avoid long periods away from the babies. • Remove milk from your breasts when feedings are missed.

labor, low birth weight, or even fetal death (Onwudiegwu, 2000). Two researchers reported a case of placental abruption associated with breastfeeding during pregnancy (Eckford & Westgate, 1997) that resulted in emergency delivery and death of the newborn. However, Flower (2003) notes that high levels of progesterone block the uterus from sensitivity to the effects of oxytocin until the end of the pregnancy, which suggests that the risk for heavy contractions due to nursing is slight.

A mother who becomes pregnant while still nursing a previous child may be reluctant to give up the special relationship that she and her nursing child enjoy. Additionally, her child may be reluctant to give up nursing and may resist attempts at weaning. The American Academy of Family Physicians (AAFP, 2001) has voiced strong support for "extended" breastfeeding, recommending that breastfeeding continue beyond infancy and that women receive ongoing support and encouragement for doing so. It also acknowledges that women commonly continue nursing when they are pregnant with another child.

Moscona (misspelled as "Moscone" in the original article) and Moore (1993) surveyed 57 women who were still breastfeeding while pregnant. Most of these mothers gave the main reason for continued nursing as meeting the child's emotional needs or allowing the child to self-wean. Forty-three percent of these children nursed through the pregnancy and continued to tandem nurse after the new baby's arrival. The babies born to this cohort were healthy and were of normal size for gestational age.

Health of the Fetus

A concern about tandem nursing is that the developing baby may be undernourished. One study found no significant differences in fetal growth, although mothers had reduced maternal fat stores when less than 6 months had elapsed between pregnancies (Merchant et al., 1990). In another study, 17 percent of children were weaned during a new pregnancy, which resulted in higher mortality rates for the weaned child in non-industrialized countries (Jakobsen et al., 2003). Other studies have found a correlation between the mother breastfeeding during pregnancy and lower weight gains for the new baby (Marquis et al., 2002). The main reason for early weaning (defined as taking place before the infant reached 15 months of age for this study) in Senegal was found to be either maternal death (41 percent) or a new pregnancy (27 percent). Twenty-six percent of these children died before the age of 2, especially those weaned because of maternal death (Mané et al., 2006).

The Mother's Health

Another concern with continuing the nurse during pregnancy is the nutritional status of the mother. In addition to the lower fat stores reported by Merchant and colleagues (1990), researchers question whether mothers' bodies recover nutritionally when there is short spacing between children. A literature review suggests that longer spacing is associated with lower child malnutrition risk in some populations but not all (Dewey & Cohen, 2007). Breastfeeding was not included as a factor in the analysis, however. Maternal outcomes were mixed, which the researchers suggested might be partly due to the hormonal regulation of nutrient portioning between the mother and the fetus when the mother is malnourished.

Short intervals between pregnancies, among other factors, are associated with maternal malnutrition among African women (Lartey, 2008). Supplementing infants with high-energy, nutrient-dense food from 4 to 7 months of age, twice daily, is associated with greater maternal weight gain (Ly et al., 2006). The supplemented infants were breastfed for significantly longer-duration periods than controls, and their mothers had a lower risk of a new birth.

Siega-Riz and Adair (1993) found that lactating women gained less weight during the first trimester of pregnancy than nonlactating women did. While the former group gained more during the third trimester, suggesting a rebound effect, their weight for the total pregnancy was still less than that of the nonlactating prospective mothers. The authors recommended that the mothers consume more energy and nutrients to meet the demands of pregnancy and breastfeeding—a nutritional recommendation that seems appropriate for all pregnant breastfeeding mothers.

If the mother continues to nurse during a pregnancy, she will want to be sure that she is eating nutritiously. One review found moderate to strong evidence linking weight gain that fell short of the Institute of Medicine's recommendations to preterm birth, low birth weight, small for gestational age (SGA) birth weights, and failure to initiate breastfeeding (Viswanathan et al., 2008). As a lactation consultant, you should encourage mothers to consume enough nutrients to meet their nutritional needs as well as those of the fetus and the nursing child. Although the nursing child will receive additional nourishment from supplemental foods, he or she will still be depleting the mother's nutritional stores.

Preterm Labor

The exception to the recommendation to continue breastfeeding a nursling during pregnancy may be a woman who has experienced a preterm birth or who is at true risk for premature labor. In this situation, the concern is that the oxytocin released during breastfeeding might trigger preterm labor. Thus it may be necessary for the expectant mother to wean her child to avoid the possibility of miscarriage. These mothers may need to abstain from sexual relations as well. Encourage the mother to discuss her specific circumstances with her caregiver, and be available to help the mother with weaning.

Effects During Pregnancy

Because nipple tenderness is common in early pregnancy, the mother who continues breastfeeding during pregnancy may experience discomfort when her child touches her breasts. Some pregnant women feel nauseated when the older child nurses. These discomforts may discourage some women from nursing when they are pregnant. The older child may react as well. Hormones of pregnancy alter the composition and taste of the mother's milk; this difference in taste and consistency causes some children to self-wean. Some mothers experience a decrease in milk yield about the 4th or 5th month of pregnancy, which causes some children to lose interest in breastfeeding and wean themselves. One study reported that 57 percent of the children weaned during pregnancy (Moscone & Moore, 1993). In another study of 503 pregnant nursing mothers, 69 percent of the nurslings weaned during pregnancy (Newton & Theotokatos, 1979).

If the woman's baby is younger than 1 year old when she conceives, frequent weight checks can be used to monitor the child for adequate intake. If her milk production decreases to the point that it does not meet the infant's needs, supplements may be necessary. Remind the mother that children younger than 1 year of age should not receive whole cow's milk. They should not have goat's milk either, despite the perception in some circles that goat's milk is a "closer" match to human milk than bovine milk. As discussed in Chapter 1, more families are using donated breastmilk or creating their own homemade formulas. A family that who plans to use donor milk needs to learn how to safely heat-treat the milk if the donor has not been tested. If the parents supplement with homemade formula, they should review the ingredients with the baby's healthcare provider.

Breastfeeding Siblings

Mothers may worry that they will not have sufficient milk to sustain both an older child and a new infant during tandem nursing. In reality, adequate milk production is rarely an issue, as the increased sucking will continue to increase the mother's milk production. The important factors are the emotional needs of the older child and the mother's own comfort. If a mother believes that her older child will benefit from the emotional nurturing of breastfeeding, she may choose to continue nursing. If she is uncomfortable with her child nursing, it may be better to wean the older child rather than feel resentment when the toddler nurses.

Toddlers who continue to nurse can position themselves at the breast easily, making simultaneous feedings with an older child and a newborn manageable. Such a

child may be old enough to understand the need to wait to nurse and the concept of taking turns, which can facilitate separate feedings. Each child will indicate a preference to nurse at a particular time of day. The mother may want to nurse each of them separately at this special time to give them each close individual attention.

Because the older child is receiving additional nutrients from other foods, the mother needs to put her younger baby to breast first, when milk production and release are greatest. The older child can then nurse on the less full breast, thereby obtaining less milk. The mother needs to let the baby finish a feeding first to obtain adequate hindmilk. Another option is to reserve a particular breast for each child and to alternate breasts daily to equalize production.

Because the toddler is a more efficient nurser whose feeding will increase the mother's milk production, the mother may find that she produces so much milk that her younger baby receives too strong a flow of milk and chokes when attempting to nurse. In this event, she can allow her older child to nurse briefly before putting her baby to breast. A recommended resource for pregnant nursing mothers is *Adventures in Tandem Nursing: Breastfeeding During Pregnancy and Beyond* (Flower, 2003).

If the mother weans her older child, she will want to do so gradually, as in any other weaning situation. It can be more difficult when she is still nursing her young baby because the older child may want to nurse whenever he or she sees the baby at the breast. The mother can try to nurse her baby at times when the older child is not present or when that child is happily occupied with other things. Substituting other special activities and snacks in place of breastfeeding can help her older child move easily toward total weaning. The father can take over evening rituals such as baths and bedtime stories. Encourage the mother to substitute an ample amount of hugs, cuddles, and touching to help the older child feel included.

～ Summary

Learning to recognize their baby's instincts, reflexes, and responses will guide parents in meeting their baby's needs. The mother's early days with her baby are important in the establishment of a strong foundation for breastfeeding. Establishing a routine for feedings will help the mother become comfortable with the process. Lactation consultants and others who care for them in the early days can teach mothers how to recognize hunger cues and to trust their instincts in nurturing their babies. They can also ensure that mothers understand the principles of positioning and attachment. Make it a goal to observe every mother and baby at a breastfeeding to assess technique and offer any necessary assistance. Be available to assist with babies who have difficulty latching. Provide support for mothers whose babies are sleepy or fussy, and offer suggestions for rousing or calming the baby. The time spent by caregivers assisting mothers in these early feedings will influence the course of the mother's long-term breastfeeding. Assure the mother that the learning process passes quickly.

∽ Chapter 14—At a Glance

Applying what you learned—

- Create a relaxing and effective climate for mothers.
- Enable a mother to nurse her baby directly after birth and offer help as necessary to assist her with this process.
- Keep mothers and babies together after birth.
- Limit unnecessary interventions.
- Protect the mother's milk production.
- Allow the baby to pace his or her feedings.
- Make sure no time-related rules are imposed on feedings.
- Observe an entire breastfeeding for effective technique.

Teach mothers:

- Exclusive breastfeeding in response to hunger cues.
- Positioning of the baby's body for feedings.
- Common nursing positions.
- C-hold for early feedings when necessary.
- Typical infant patterns.
- How to stimulate a sleepy baby to nurse.
- How to comfort a fussy baby for an effective feeding.
- How to watch the baby for signs that he or she wants to end a feeding.
- Signs of good attachment:
  - The baby's mouth is open wide.
  - The baby's chin is touching the breast.
  - The baby's lower lip is curled outward.
  - The baby sucks, pauses, and sucks again—in slow, deep sucks.
  - The mother hears the baby swallowing.
- Signs of poor attachment:
  - The nipple looks flattened or striped as it leaves the baby's mouth at the end of the feeding.
  - The mother experiences nipple pain during and after feedings.
  - The mother's breasts are engorged.
  - There is inefficient removal of milk from the breast.

Teach mothers of multiples:

- Breastfeeding babies separately at least once every day.
- Spending nonfeeding time alone with each baby.
- Co-bedding.
- Options for positioning, scheduling, and simultaneous feedings.
- Responsive parenting and support groups.

If nursing during pregnancy:

- Ensure adequate nutrition.
- Consult the caregiver in pregnancies at risk for preterm labor.
- If weaning older child, do so gradually.
- Delay supplementation with cow's milk until the child reaches 1 year of age.
- Ways to substitute nursing and include an older child.
- If tandem nursing, put younger baby to the breast first, but let the infant end the feeding on his or her own.

∽ References

Academy of Breastfeeding Medicine (ABM). Protocol #10: Breastfeeding the near-term infant (35 to 37 weeks gestation. 2004. www.bfmed.org/Resources/Protocols.aspx. Accessed May 5, 2009.

American Academy of Family Physicians (AAFP). AAFP policy statement on breastfeeding. Breastfeeding: Position paper. 2001.

Anderson J. Lactose intolerance and the breastfed baby. August 2006. www.breastfeeding.asn.au/bfinfo/lactose.html. Accessed April 15, 2009.

Bartick M, Reinhold A. The burden of suboptimal breastfeeding in the United States: a pediatric cost analysis. *Pediatrics.* 2010;125(5):e1048-e1056. Epub ahead of print Apr 5, 2010.

Bergman N. Breastfeeding and perinatal neuroscience. In: Genna CW. *Supporting Sucking Skills in Infants.* Sudbury, MA: Jones and Bartlett; 2008:43-56.

Budin P. *The Nursling: The Feeding and Hygiene of Premature and Full-Term Infants.* Paris; 1907. Lecture 3. Malony WJ, trans. London: Caxton. www.neonatology.org/classics/nursling/nursling.html. Accessed May 15, 2009.

Centers for Disease Control and Prevention (CDC). assisted reproductive technology report: Section 5: ART trends, 1996-2006. December 3, 2008. http://www.cdc.gov/art/ART2006/section5.htm. Accessed May 16, 2009.

Chaves R, et al. Factors associated with duration of breastfeeding. *J Pediatr (Rio J).* 2007;83(3):241-246.

Colson S. Maternal breastfeeding positions: have we got it right? (2). *Pract Midwife.* 2005;8(11):29-32.

Colson S. Biological nurturing (1): a non-prescriptive recipe for breastfeeding. *Pract Midwife.* 2007a;10(9):42, 44, 46-47.

Colson S. Biological nurturing (2): the physiology of lactation revisited. *Pract Midwife.* 2007b;10(10):14-19.

Colson S, et al. Optimal positions for the release of primitive neonatal reflexes stimulating breastfeeding. *Early Hum Dev.* 2008;84(7):441-449.

Council of Multiple Birth Organisations (COMBO). Declaration of rights and statement of needs of twins and higher order multiples. June 2007. www.ists.qimr.edu.au/Rights.pdf. Accessed May 17, 2009.

Dewey K. Nutrition, growth and complementary feeding of the breastfed infant. In Hale T, Hartmann P. *Hale & Hartmann's Textbook of Human Lactation.* Amarillo, TX: Hale Publishing; 2007:415-423.

Dewey K, Cohen R. Does birth spacing affect maternal or child nutritional status? A systematic literature review. *Mat Child Nutr.* 2007;3(3):151-173.

Eckford S, Westgate J. Breastfeeding and placental abruption. *J Obstet Gyn.* 1997;17(2):164-165.

Flower H. *Adventures in Tandem Nursing: Breastfeeding During Pregnancy and Beyond.* Schaumburg, IL: La Leche League International; 2003.

Gromada K. *Mothering Multiples: Breastfeeding and Caring for Twins or More,* 3rd ed. Schaumburg, IL: La Leche League International; 2007.

Jakobsen M, et al. Termination of breastfeeding after 12 months of age due to a new pregnancy and other causes is associated with increased mortality in Guinea-Bissau. *Int J Epidemiol.* 2003;32(1):92-96.

Karp H. The "fourth trimester": a framework and strategy for understanding and resolving colic. *Contemp Pediatr.* 2004; 21:94.

Karp H. Safe swaddling and healthy hips: don't toss the baby out with the bathwater [Letter to the editor]. *Pediatrics.* 2008; 121(5):1075-1076.

Kent J, et al. Volume and frequency of breastfeedings and fat content of breast milk throughout the day. *Pediatrics.* 2006; 117(3):e387-e395.

Lartey A. Maternal and child nutrition in sub-Saharan Africa: challenges and interventions. *Proc Nutr Soc.* 2008;67(1): 105-108.

Leonard L, Denton, J. Preparation for parenting multiple birth children. *Early Hum Dev.* 2006;82(6):371-378.

Ly CT, et al. Early short-term infant food supplementation, maternal weight loss and duration of breast-feeding: a randomised controlled trial in rural Senegal. *Eur J Clin Nutr.* 2006;60(2):265-271.

Mané NB, et al. Early breastfeeding cessation in rural Senegal: causes, modes, and consequences. *Am J Public Health.* 2006;96(1):139-144.

Marquis G, et al. Postpartum consequences of an overlap of breastfeeding and pregnancy: reduced breast milk intake and growth during early infancy. *Pediatrics.* 2002;109(4): e56.

Merchant K, et al. Maternal and fetal responses to the stresses of lactation concurrent with pregnancy and of short recuperative intervals. *Am J Clin Nutr.* 1990;52(2):280-288.

Moscone [sic] S, Moore MJ. Breastfeeding during pregnancy. *J Hum Lact.* 1993;9(2):83-88. [Author's name, Moscona, was misspelled in original article.]

Newton N, Theotokatos M. Breast-feeding during pregnancy in 503 women: does psychobiological weaning mechanism exist in humans? *Emotion Reprod.* 1979;20B:845.

Onwudiegwu U. Is breastfeeding during pregnancy harmful? *J Obstet Gyn.* 2000;20(2):157.

Righard L, Alade M. Effect of delivery room routines on success of first breastfeed. *Lancet.* 1990;336:1105-1107.

Siega-Riz A, Adair L. Biological determinants of pregnancy weight gain in a Filipino population. *Am J Clin Nutr.* 1993; 57(3):365-372.

Smillie C. How newborns learn to latch: a neurobehavioral model for self-attachment in infancy. *Acad Breastfeed Med News Views.* 2001;7:23.

Smillie C. How infants learn to feed: a neurobehavioral model. In Genna CW. *Supporting Sucking Skills in Infants.* Sudbury, MA: Jones and Bartlett; 2008:79-95.

Smith, L. *Impact of Birthing Practices on Breastfeeding,* 2nd ed. Sudbury, MA: Jones and Bartlett; 2009.

Szucs K, et al. Quintuplets and a mother's determination to provide human milk: it takes a village to raise a baby—how about five? *J Hum Lact.* 2009;25(1):79-84.

UNICEF. The Baby Friendly Initiative's position on biological nurturing. Statement 18. February 2009. www.babyfriendly.org.uk/items/item_detail.asp?item=558. Accessed May 16, 2009.

U.S. Department of Health and Human Services (USDHHS), National Women's Health Information Center. Healthy pregnancy: twins, triplets and more. March 5, 2009. www.womenshealth.gov/pregnancy/you-are-pregnant/twins-multiples.cfm. Accessed May 1, 2009.

Vaidya K, et al. Effect of early mother-baby close contact over the duration of exclusive breastfeeding. *Nepal Med Coll J.* 2005;7(2):138-140.

van Dijk C, Innis S. Growth-curve standards and the assessment of early excess weight gain in infancy. *Pediatrics.* 2009;123(1):102-108.

Viswanathan M, et al. Outcomes of maternal weight gain. *Evid Rep Technol Assess.* 2008;168:1-223.

Widstrom AM, et al. The position of the tongue during rooting reflexes elicited in newborn infants before the first suckle. *Acta Paediatr.* 1993;82:281-283.

Wiessinger D. A breastfeeding teaching tool using a sandwich analogy for latch-on. *J Hum Lact.* 1998;14(1):51-56.

Wight N. Breastfeeding the borderline (near-term) preterm infant. *Pediatric Ann.* 2003;32(5):329-336.

Wiklund I, et al. Epidural analgesia: breast-feeding success and related factors. *Midwifery.* 2009;25(2):e31-e38.

Yokoyama Y, et al. Breastfeeding rates among singletons, twins and triplets in Japan: a population-based study. *Twin Res Hum Genet.* 2006;9(2):298-302.

Yokoyama Y, Ooki S. Breast-feeding and bottle-feeding of twins, triplets and higher order multiple births. *Nippon Koshu Eisei Zasshi.* 2004;51(11):969-974.

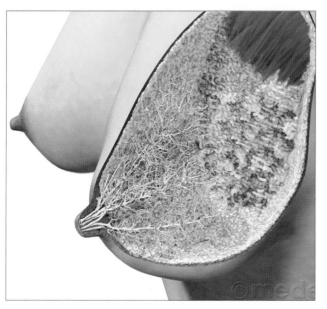

COLOR PLATE 1. System of ducts and ductules in the lactating breast. *Source:* © Medela, Inc., 2010.

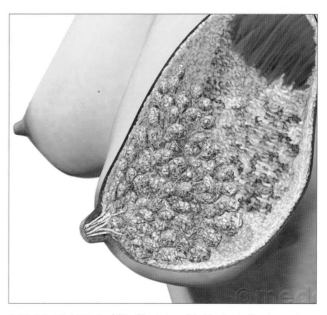

COLOR PLATE 2. Milk-filled alveoli in the lactating breast. *Source:* © Medela, Inc., 2010.

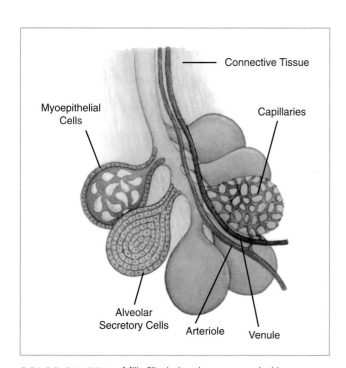

COLOR PLATE 3. Milk-filled alveolus surrounded by myoepithelial cells. Illustration by Ka Botzis.

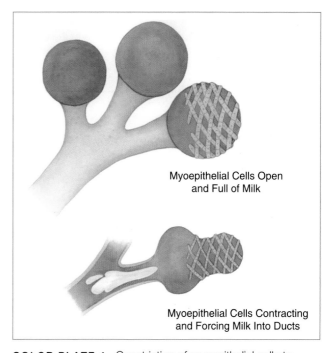

COLOR PLATE 4. Constriction of myoepithelial cells to force milk from the alveolus. Illustration by Ka Botzis.

Common Types of Breasts

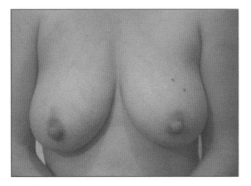

COLOR PLATE 5. Type 1: Rounded breasts with normal lower medial and lateral quadrants. *Source:* Printed with permission of Anna Swisher.

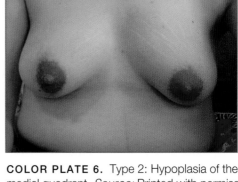

COLOR PLATE 6. Type 2: Hypoplasia of the lower medial quadrant. *Source:* Printed with permission of Anna Swisher.

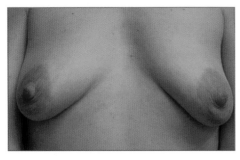

COLOR PLATE 7. Type 3: Hypoplasia of the lower medial and lateral quadrants. *Source:* Printed with permission of Anna Swisher.

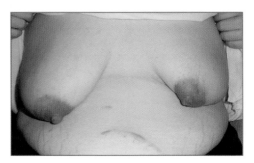

COLOR PLATE 8. Type 4: Severe constrictions with minimal breast base; areolae may be very bulbous. *Source:* Printed with permission of Anna Swisher.

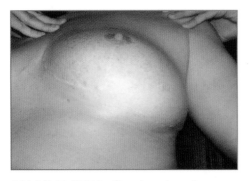

COLOR PLATE 9. Scar from breast surgery can be a marker for severed ducts. *Source:* Printed with permission of Anna Swisher.

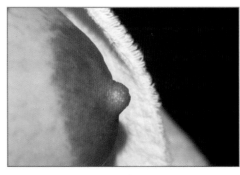

COLOR PLATE 10. Nipple appears normal. *Source:* Printed with permission of Kay Hoover.

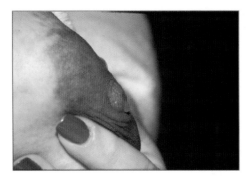

COLOR PLATE 11. Nipple from Color Plate 10 inverts when stimulated. *Source:* Printed with permission of Kay Hoover.

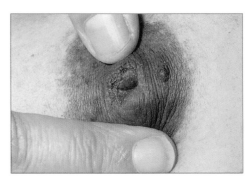

COLOR PLATE 12. Nipple appears dimpled. *Source:* Printed with permission of Jan Riordan.

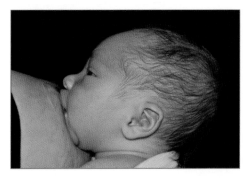

COLOR PLATE 13. Baby latching onto the breast with the aid of a nipple shield. *Source:* Printed with permission of Anna Swisher.

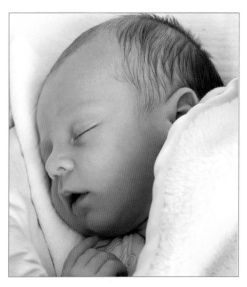

COLOR PLATE 14. Baby with hyperbilirubinemia. *Source:* © Marcin Okupniak/Dreamstime.com.

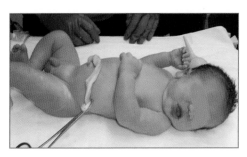

COLOR PLATE 15. Baby with acrocyanosis. *Source:* Printed with permission of Dr. Charlie Goldberg.

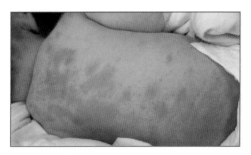

COLOR PLATE 16. Baby with erythema toxicum. *Source:* Printed with permission of Dr. Jeffrey Hull.

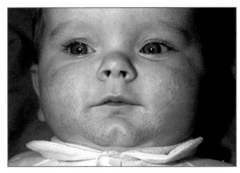

COLOR PLATE 17. Baby with infant acne. *Source:* Printed with permission of Dr. Kenneth Greer.

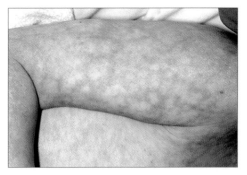

COLOR PLATE 18. Baby with mottling. *Source:* Printed with permission of Dr. Kenneth Greer.

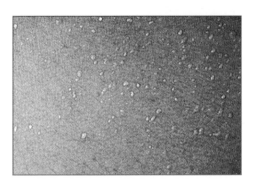

COLOR PLATE 19. Milia on the baby's skin. *Source:* Printed with permission of Dr. Kenneth Greer.

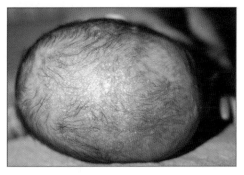

COLOR PLATE 20. Cradle cap on the baby's scalp. *Source:* © Biophoto Associates/Photo Researchers, Inc.

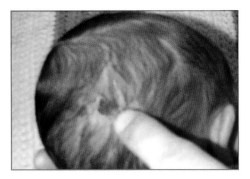

COLOR PLATE 21. Baby with a cephalhematoma. *Source:* Printed with permission of Anna Swisher.

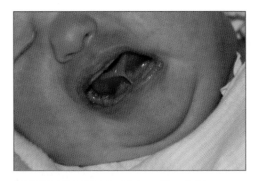

COLOR PLATE 22. Baby with a tight frenulum. *Source:* Printed with permission of Anna Swisher.

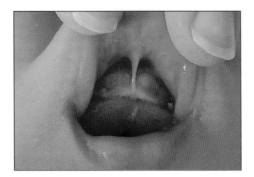

COLOR PLATE 23. Baby with a tight frenum. *Source:* Printed with permission of Anna Swisher.

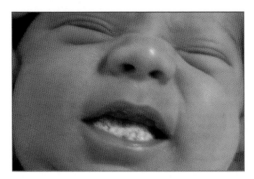

COLOR PLATE 24. Baby with thrush in his mouth. *Source:* Printed with permission of James Heilman, MD, and Wikipedia.

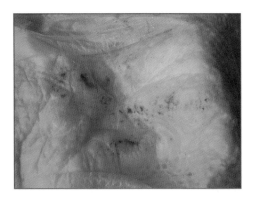

COLOR PLATE 25. Urate crystals in the baby's diaper. *Source:* Printed with permission of Judith Lauwers.

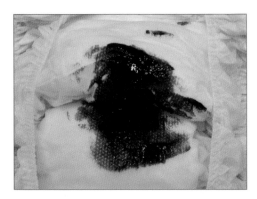

COLOR PLATE 26. Newborn meconium stool. *Source:* Printed with permission of Anna Swisher.

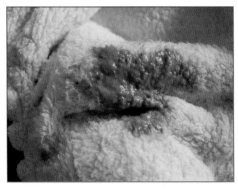

COLOR PLATE 27. Typical breastmilk stool. *Source:* Printed with permission of Kori Martin.

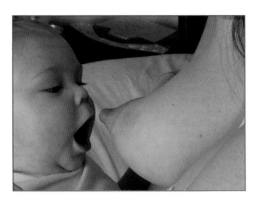

COLOR PLATE 28. The baby begins to open his mouth for a good mouthful of breast tissue. *Source:* Printed with permission of Nelia Box.

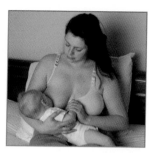

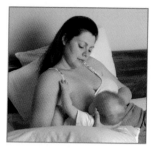

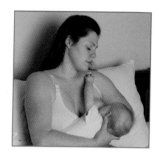

COLOR PLATE 29. Cradle hold nursing position. *Source:* Printed with permission of Nelia Box. *Source:* Printed with permission of Nelia Box.

COLOR PLATE 30. Side-sitting (also called football or clutch) nursing position. *Source:* Printed with permission of Nelia Box.

COLOR PLATE 31. Cross cradle (dominant hand) nursing position. *Source:* Printed with permission of Nelia Box.

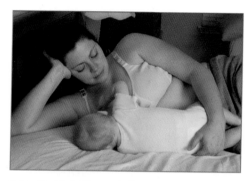

COLOR PLATE 32. Lying down nursing position. *Source:* Printed with permission of Nelia Box.

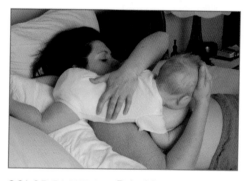

COLOR PLATE 33. Prone position (posture feeding). *Source:* Printed with permission of Nelia Box.

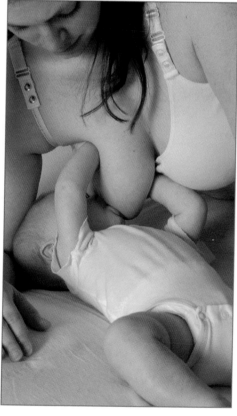

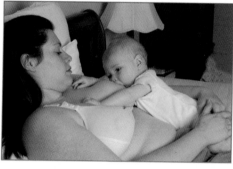

COLOR PLATE 35. Baby lying over the mother's shoulder. *Source:* Printed with permission of Nelia Box.

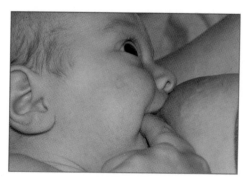

COLOR PLATE 34. Leaning over the baby to nurse. *Source:* Printed with permission of Nelia Box.

COLOR PLATE 36. A finger placed in the corner of the baby's mouth helps to break suction and remove the baby gently. *Source:* Printed with permission of Anna Swisher.

Breasts Conditions

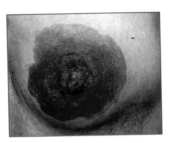

COLOR PLATE 37.
Paget's disease on the nipple.
Source: Printed with
permission of S.J. Parker.

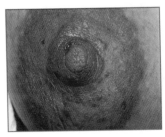

COLOR PLATE 38.
Yeast infection on the nipple.
Source: Printed with
permission of Kay Hoover.

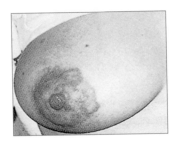

COLOR PLATE 39.
Psoriasis on the nipple.
Source: Printed with
permission of Karen Foard.

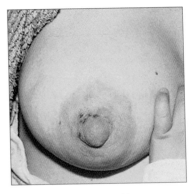

COLOR PLATE 40. Herpes on
the nipple. *Source:* Printed with
permission of Chele Marmet.

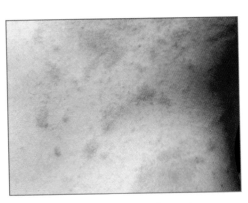

COLOR PLATE 41. Poison ivy rash.
Source: © Joy Brown/ShutterStock, Inc.

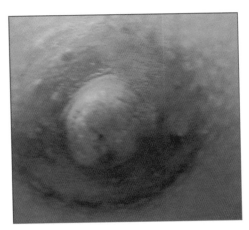

COLOR PLATE 42. Stage I nipple trauma—
superficial intact. *Source:* Printed with
permission of Anna Swisher.

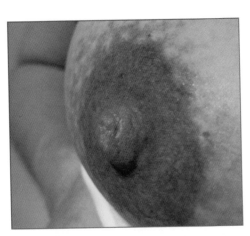

COLOR PLATE 43. Stage II nipple trauma—
superficial with tissue breakdown. *Source:* Printed
with permission of Anna Swisher.

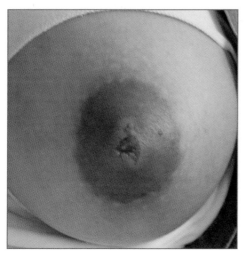

COLOR PLATE 44. Stage III nipple trauma—partial thickness erosion. *Source:* Printed with permission of Anna Swisher.

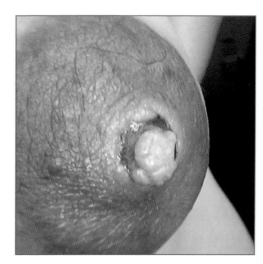

COLOR PLATE 45. Stage IV nipple trauma—full thickness erosion. *Source:* Printed with permission of Linda Hill.

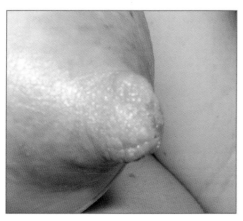

COLOR PLATE 46. Cracked nipple. *Source:* Printed with permission of Catherine Watson Genna, BS, IBCLC.

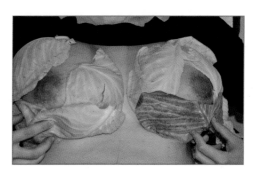

COLOR PLATE 47. Mother with cabbage on her breasts to relieve engorgement. *Source:* Printed with permission of Anna Swisher.

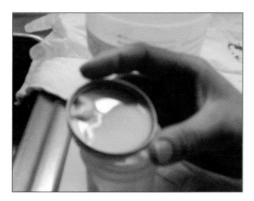

COLOR PLATE 48. Lump in milk released from a breast infection. *Source:* Printed with permission of Judith Lauwers.

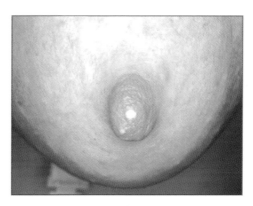

COLOR PLATE 49. Milk blister on the nipple. *Source:* Printed with permission of Jan Riordan.

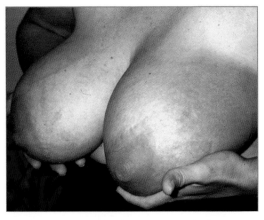

COLOR PLATE 50. Mother with mastitis. *Source:* Printed with permission of Sarah Coulter Danner.

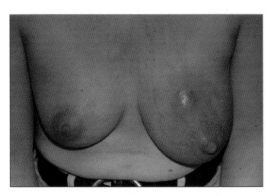

COLOR PLATE 51. Breast abscess before surgery. *Source:* Printed with permission of Kay Hoover and Barbara Wilson-Clay.

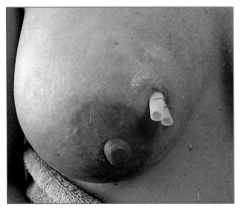

COLOR PLATE 52. Breast abscess after surgery. *Source:* Printed with permission of Kay Hoover and Barbara Wilson-Clay.

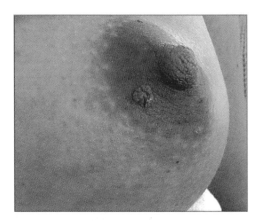

COLOR PLATE 53. Scar on breast (bottom left) from childhood injury. *Source:* Printed with permission of Anna Swisher

15

Infant Attachment and Sucking

An awareness of the mechanics of infant sucking will help caregivers understand the transfer of milk from the breast to the baby. The mechanics of breastfeeding are substantially different from those of bottle feeding. The way a baby sucks at the breast, the baby's sucking needs, and the feeding pattern established all affect milk transfer. Although some infants have difficulty sucking, most attachment and sucking difficulties can be resolved with minor adjustments to latch and positioning. This chapter explores infant sucking related to breast attachment and milk transfer.

∾ *Key Terms*

Bolus
Carpal tunnel syndrome
Chiropractic care
Craniosacral therapist
Intervention levels
Intubation
Latch
Masseter muscle
Milk ejection reflex (MER)
Milk transfer
Neuromotor dysfunction
Nutritive sucking (NS)
Nonnutritive sucking
(NNS)

Oral structure
Orbicularis oris muscles
Pharynx
Small for gestational age
(SGA)
Soft palate
Suck training
Sucking
Sucking needs
Sucking pattern
Suckling
Syringe feeding
Trough

∾ *Sucking and Suckling*

The terms "sucking" and "suckling" are often used interchangeably, and different disciplines assign different meanings to them (ILCA, 2007). Definitions of suckling range from describing the mother, to active nursing, to the act of nursing. Genna (2008) defines suckling as the act of feeding at the breast, and sucking as the oral motor activity that transfers milk. Those same distinctions are used in this text.

Sucking is both physically and emotionally pleasurable, and the means by which a baby derives comfort and nourishment. Sucking stimulates saliva, which contains enzymes that help predigest food. It also stimulates gastrointestinal secretions, hormones (including cholecystokinin), and gut motility. In particular, these digestive hormones promote satiety and sleepiness in the baby.

Sucking is calming and helps the baby pass gas and stool. It activates prolactin release in the mother, stimulating milk production and yearning for her baby. As sucking continues, oxytocin is released, promoting maternal and protective feelings in the mother. Oxytocin release triggers milk ejection and helps the uterus return to its prepregnancy state (Geddes, 2009a).

Sucking needs vary from one baby to another. Many babies are born with red marks or blisters on their hands or wrists from sucking in utero. Babies use their thumbs, fingers, and hands as a means of soothing and calming themselves. The need for sucking is usually greater in the first 3 months after birth than at any other time. As a lactation consultant, you can encourage mothers to be sensitive to this important aspect of their babies' health. Satisfying a baby's sucking needs enhances the infant's physical growth and well-being.

The Infant's Sucking Pattern

Sucking and feeding develop in a predictable and organized way after birth (Delaney & Arvedson, 2008; Arvedson, 2006). Sucking and swallowing are coordinated in a rhythmic pattern of repeated bursts of suck–swallow–breathe. By pausing between bursts of sucking, babies are able to regulate their breathing. In functional suck–swallow–breathe sequencing, swallowing does not occur simultaneously with breathing. Swallowing while breathing results in aspiration—that is, taking foreign matter into the lungs. A pattern of increased sucks per minute is associated with fewer swallows. Therefore, a higher sucking frequency correlates with more breaths and higher oxygen saturation.

Research shows that an infant's respiratory rate is lower during sucking than during a pause in breastfeeding (Geddes et al., 2007). The respiratory rate during sucking is related to both the duration of the suck burst and the rate of sucking. The respiration rate is lower during active sucking bursts and is more marked with longer sucking burst duration. Sucking develops on a continuum, with preterm infants demonstrating fewer sucks per burst and longer pauses than full-term infants and older children.

Bottle feeders breathe less often than breastfeeding babies during feedings (da Costa & van der Schans, 2008). The sucking associated with bottle feeding produces lower oxygen rates and higher heart rates. A study of healthy, full-term breastfeeding babies found that their oxygen levels were higher at 2 months after birth than at 1 week postpartum. Their heart rates were higher during feeding than before and after feeding; heart rate was not affected by age (Suiter & Ruark-McMurtrey, 2007). An older study found that oxygen levels drop *after* feeding in both bottle fed and breastfed babies (Hammerman & Kaplan, 1995).

Most studies on infant sucking and swallowing have focused on bottle feeding infants. Qureshi and colleagues (2002) found that infant suck rates in bottle feeding increase from 55 sucks per minute in the immediate postnatal period to 70 sucks per minute by the end of the first month. Swallow rates increase from about 46 to 50 swallows per minute over the same span. Feeding efficiency almost doubles over the first month. During the first month of life, an infant progresses from a 1:1:1 suck–swallow–breathe rhythm to a 2:1:1 or 3:1:1 rhythm. This development corresponds to the infant's increased ability to hold a larger bolus that is swallowed at one time.

Babies who exhibit short sucking bursts and shorter overall sucking times have more feeding difficulties at 6 weeks of age compared to babies who have longer, continuous sucking bursts and longer sucking times (Ramsay & Gisel, 1996). For this reason, it is important that you, as a lactation consultant, thoroughly assess the baby's early sucking pattern, if you have the opportunity. Work with the mother to help her baby continue with feedings rather than stop after short efforts, unless the baby is an ineffective feeder (e.g., preterm, oral anomaly, medicated). In particular, be aware that drugs administered during the mother's labor can affect nutritive sucking (NS) in the newborn (Torvaldsen et al., 2006; Jordan, 2006; Jordan et al., 2005; Baumgarder et al., 2003; Riordan et al., 2000). Letting the baby cry can compromise the infant's innate sucking behavior and result in a disorganized suck (as discussed in Chapter 13).

Sucking Rate

A breastfeeding baby sucks in a rhythm corresponding inversely to the amount of milk available. Thus high rates of milk flow result in slower sucking rates of about 1 suck per second, described as nutritive sucking. High-resolution ultrasound shows a wide variability in infant sucking patterns (Geddes, 2009b). Notably, the rate of nonnutritive sucking (NNS) is faster than nutritive sucking, averaging 2 sucks per second (Wolf & Glass, 1992). Nonnutritive sucking describes how a baby sucks on its hands and fingers, a parent's finger, a pacifier, or on the breast when milk volume is low.

The changes in sucking rate that occur during breastfeeding take place gradually. The baby sucks rapidly at the beginning of a feeding to initiate milk flow. Once letdown occurs and the infant swallows, the sucking pace slows. The sucking pattern will continue to alternate between nutritive and nonnutritive sucking throughout the feeding as the baby returns to more rapid sucking to stimulate further milk flow and then slower sucking to collect and swallow milk. When the baby switches to the other breast, the same pattern resumes.

Full-term neonates younger than 24 hours old exhibit less rhythmic sucking than older term infants. During the first 2 or 3 days, the baby sucks with several short, rapid bursts per swallow, indicating that the volume of colostrum is relatively small. Around the 3rd or 4th day, a regular feeding rhythm becomes established. This indicates that the mother is producing transitional milk with increased volume. At around 4 to 5 days, the full-term infant may or may not swallow with every suck, after the mother's letdown.

Physiology of Sucking

The earliest internal pictures showing how a baby sucks were published in 1958 using cineradiographic filming (Ardran et al., 1958a, 1958b). Considered cutting-edge technology at the time, these films were limited by their inability to image soft tissues. Later, ultrasound studies in the 1980s suggested that the baby's tongue moves in a peristaltic motion from the front of the mouth toward the back. In these images, it appeared that the nipple was drawn back completely to the juncture of the hard and soft palates (Bosma et al., 1990; Weber et al., 1986; Woolridge, 1986). Smith and colleagues (1988) described this action as more of a piston-like movement.

What appeared in earlier ultrasound technology to be stripping of the breast by the tongue may, instead, be the tongue modulating pressure changes that create suction

(Genna, 2008). High-resolution studies performed since the mid-2000s have combined ultrasound, video, and intra-oral pressure measurement in an attempt to refine our understanding of sucking dynamics (Geddes et al., 2008; Ramsay & Hartmann, 2005; Ramsay, 2004; Ramsay et al., 2004). These studies suggest that vacuum increases during the downward motion of the posterior tongue, and that peak vacuum occurs when the tongue is in the lowest position. Researchers have observed that lowering of the tongue coincides with milk flow in the nipple, which suggests that milk flow from the nipple into the infant's oral cavity coincides with the lowering of the infant's tongue and peak vacuum.

During sucking, the baby's tongue draws the nipple and areola into the mouth to form a cone-shaped extension of the breast that conforms to the shape of the baby's mouth, as shown in Figure 15.1. It is important to recognize that when the baby draws in sufficient breast tissue, the tongue is free from frictional movement against the breast. In other words, no in-and-out movement should occur. If the baby appears to slide back and forth on the nipple during feeding, chances are the mother will report discomfort.

When the baby sucks, the areola and nipple press upward against the upper gum and the hard palate. However, the nipple does not appear to reach completely to the juncture of the hard and soft palates. Ultimately the negative pressure of the baby's suck transfers milk with much greater milk flow when the tongue is down than when the tongue is up. The negative pressure, along with the alternate compression and release of the gums, moves the milk through the milk ducts and out the nipple. When the baby's jaw drops, the increased negative pressure allows the milk to move from the nipple to the baby's mouth.

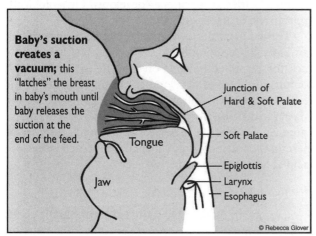

FIGURE 15.1 Sucking action. In breastfeeding, the tongue moves forward over the lower gum to grasp the breast tissue. The lips are flanged around the areola, and the tongue compresses the areola. The tongue, in combination with the cheek muscles and dropping of the jaw, help create negative pressure for suction.

Source: Printed with permission of Rebecca Glover, IBCLC.

Sucking Related to Milk Ejection

Multiple milk ejections are common during breastfeeding and facilitate milk transfer. The number of milk ejections is related to the amount of milk ingested by the baby (Geddes, 2009; Ramsay et al., 2004). Mothers may have 1 to 9 milk ejections per feeding, with an average of 2.5 being reported (Ramsay et al., 2006). Mothers typically notice only the first one, and many mothers do not feel their letdown at all.

Sucking increases the mother's prolactin level and releases oxytocin in a pulsatile manner (Yokoyama et al., 1994). The length of milk ejection (letdown) ranges from 45 seconds to 3.5 minutes (Geddes, 2009a) and occurs, on average, 2.5 times in a feeding (with a wide range from 0 to 9). Letdown is essential to the baby receiving sufficient milk (see Chapter 16). In one study, amounts of milk ranging from 0 to 13 mL were removed prior to milk ejection (Ramsay et al., 2004). The newborn is capable of adjusting his or her sucking rate, suggesting an ability to cope with variations in letdown (Geddes, 2009a).

~ Sucking at the Breast Versus a Bottle

Sucking action in breastfeeding involves the baby's entire mouth—lips, gums, tongue, cheeks, and hard and soft palates. The soft breast molds to the baby's mouth, and the baby actively suckles the breast to receive milk. This is quite different from the sucking motion used for extracting milk from a bottle, as shown in Figure 15.2. In bottle feeding, the baby draws the nipple into his or her mouth and must alter the mouth to accommodate the shape of the artificial nipple. The infant must also compress the nipple so that milk flows freely from the bottle. Ultrasound studies show that the baby's tongue pushes against the nipple, with compression of the nipple and a hook-like lift of the posterior tongue (Ramsay, 2004).

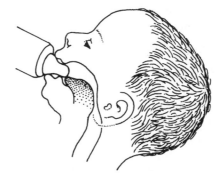

FIGURE 15.2 Bottle feeding action. In bottle feeding, the tongue thrusts upward and forward to control milk flow, gums and lips cannot create compression. There is an increased amount of air flow. Facial muscles are relaxed.

Source: Illustration by Marcia Smith.

What may appear to be dysfunctional sucking on a bottle—that is, wide jaw excursions—is not dysfunctional in breastfeeding. Wide jaw excursions are indicative of nutritive sucking in a breastfeeding baby. The Neonatal Oral–Motor Assessment Scale (NOMAS) is a tool designed to measure sucking effectiveness in full-term and preterm infants. An important distinction is made with this tool when evaluating breastfeeding infants for competency: sucking rhythm in breastfeeding depends on milk flow. Therefore, more than 1 suck per burst (e.g., suck–suck–swallow–breath) is not abnormal and should not be diagnosed as "disorganization" (da Costa & van der Schans, 2008).

Nyqvist (2008) found that preterm infants demonstrate rooting, efficient areolar grasp, and repeated short sucking bursts from 29 weeks gestation, as well as occasional long sucking bursts and repeated swallowing from 31 weeks gestation. The maximum number of consecutive sucks ranged between 5 and 24 sucks, with a median of 17. Full breastfeeding was attained at a median of 35 weeks gestation (specifically, between 32 and 38 weeks). The infants had adequate weight gain when fully breastfed. Nyqvist (2008) concluded that "very preterm infants have the capacity for early development of oral motor competence that is sufficient for establishment of full breastfeeding at a low postmenstrual age."

This finding belies the argument that preterm infants must "prove" themselves on a bottle before they are allowed to breastfeed. High flow rates from artificial nipples cause preterm infants to swallow continuously, thereby limiting their chances to breathe. Preterm infants can coordinate the suck–swallow–breathing pattern as early when breastfeeding as when bottle feeding. Moreover, a baby is better able to maintain stable body temperature and higher oxygen saturation while feeding at the breast (Morton, 2003). Nonetheless, the reality in the United States is that most babies cared for in a neonatal intensive care unit (NICU) will be bottle fed before initiating breastfeeding. See Chapter 23 for an exploration of NICU feeding issues, and ability-sensitive protocols that help establish breastfeeding in this population.

Alternating Breast and Bottle

Because of the very different ways in which babies suck on a bottle and on the breast, alternating between the two may potentially create problems for some babies. This situation is especially likely to occur in the early weeks when the baby is mastering his or her feeding technique. Artificial teats—both bottle nipples and pacifiers—may cause the baby to develop a preference for the teat over the breast. Milk flows immediately and faster from a bottle nipple. In contrast, when the baby nurses at the breast, he must suck actively to receive milk.

Healthy, full-term breastfed babies should not routinely be given an artificial nipple in the hospital. Multiple studies have found that the strongest risk factors for early breastfeeding termination are late breastfeeding initiation and supplementing the infant (Asole et al., 2009; Declercq et al., 2009; Pincombe et al., 2008; Chaves et al., 2007; Merten et al., 2005; Chezem et al., 2003). Compared with mothers experiencing baby-friendly practices, mothers experiencing no baby-friendly practices have been found to be approximately 8 times more likely to stop breastfeeding early.

Some parents consider other alternative feeding methods too stressful, time-consuming, or impractical. Those who feed supplements to their infants with a bottle will benefit from being taught paced bottle feeding (Wilson-Clay & Hoover, 2008; Law-Morstatt, 2003; Kassing, 2002), as described in Chapter 21. Feeding specialists have long noted that babies who cannot breastfeed well usually cannot bottle feed well either. When you encounter a baby who cannot breastfeed, carefully observing a bottle feeding can be an important part of your evaluation. For an infant who cannot breastfeed, bottle feeding can be a helpful tool when used therapeutically (Wilson-Clay & Hoover, 2008).

Consequences of Extended Bottle or Pacifier Use

Breastfeeding stimulates physiologically appropriate development of the muscular and skeletal components of the infant's orofacial complex (Viggiano et al., 2004). A study in the 1930s evaluated the teeth, facial contours, and mouths of thousands of people in non-industrialized cultures and skulls from burial sites. Nearly all had ideal occlusions and dental arches, and minimal decay (Price, 2008). This population—which lacked access to artificial formula, bottles, or pacifiers—developed physiologically appropriate orofacial structure.

The use of bottles and artificial nipples during infancy can have far-reaching health consequences. Babies who suck for extended periods on a bottle or pacifier may compromise proper development of the oral cavity and swallowing pattern. The greatest development of the craniofacial structure takes place during the first 4 years of life. Extended use of artificial devices in the child's mouth can, therefore, contribute to abnormal craniofacial development at a very sensitive period.

Orofacial Muscles

A vacuum builds up in a standard bottle as the baby withdraws milk. As the feeding continues, the negative pressure increases, opposing the suction exerted by the infant until the nipple seal is broken to allow equilibration inside and outside the bottle. This can lead to difficulty in generating suction or decreased suction strength for the baby (Fucile et al., 2009). A weakened suck, in turn, reduces the strength of the masseter muscle and increases the strength of the orbicularis oris muscles. Facial muscles subsequently develop in the exact opposite pattern from which nature intended. In contrast, breastfeeding requires the baby to use all the muscles of the mouth and jaw, thereby involving all the perioral musculature and leading to its proper development (Palmer, 2004).

Swallowing

Bottle feeding has the potential to alter proper development of swallowing as well—a problem that can extend into adulthood (Palmer, 1999, 2002). A proper adult swallowing pattern mirrors that of a breastfeeding baby. The tongue should not exert pressure on any teeth and should rest against the hard palate until the next swallow. In bottle feeding, the baby's tongue is placed at the back of the throat in a protective posture to prevent too much liquid from being swallowed. To limit the flow, the baby's tongue may exhibit a thrusting motion against the bottle nipple. This tongue thrusting can continue into adulthood, causing an adult to push against the teeth and create spaces. Tongue thrusting may be the greatest contributor to the development of a malocclusion (improper alignment of the teeth).

Malocclusion

Nonnutritive sucking and bottle feeding involve orofacial muscles different from those used in breastfeeding, and affect the palate differently as well. This behavior contributes to poor alignment of teeth and anomalous transversal growth of the palate—conditions that lead to posterior cross-bite (malocclusion). In this way, bottle feeding and nonnutritive sucking activity (pacifier use) increase the risk of posterior cross-bite (Vázquez-Nava, 2006). Breastfed children are less prone to develop a nonnutritive sucking habit compared to bottle fed children (Ngom et al., 2008).

Malocclusion in primary teeth has been shown to be directly related to the duration of pacifier sucking after 2 years of age and breathing through the mouth (Góis et al., 2008). In addition, research indicates that the incidence of malocclusion is higher among children who are not breastfed (Moimaz et al., 2008; Leite-Cavalcanti et al., 2007; Ovsenik et al., 2007; Peres et al., 2007; López Del Valle et al., 2006).

Oral Cavity

The greater the sucking action needed within the mouth, the greater the potential for collapse of the oral cavity. This process can narrow the dental arch to a V-shape rather than the normally wide U-shape. It also contributes to a high palate, which can infringe on the nasal cavity and increase resistance to air flow. Over time, these changes may lead to increased risk for obstructive sleep apnea in adulthood (Palmer, 2004).

∼ Latching the Baby

The moment of contact of the baby's mouth on the mother's breast is referred to as latching or attachment. A good latch enables the baby to take a large amount of breast tissue into his or her mouth. The baby needs to take in as much of the areola as possible, with a latch well behind the nipple. This enables the baby to generate a strong enough vacuum to elicit letdown. The baby is then able to suck and obtain milk. Removal of milk, in turn, relieves pressure in the breast and maintains milk production.

When a baby latches well, the mother will see long, drawing, nutritive, high-flow sucks. After copious milk production begins, she will also see and hear her baby swallow. In the first 24 to 48 hours after birth, the swallows often sound like small puffs of air after 3 to 4 high-flow, nutritive sucks. Although the mother may report a tugging or pulling sensation with a good latch, she should be free of pain, both during and after the feeding. If she experiences pain, she needs to adjust her baby's position or latch. Figures 15.3 and 15.4 show the differences between a baby who has a good latch and one who needs to be repositioned, respectively.

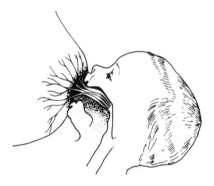

FIGURE 15.3   A baby well positioned at the breast.
Source: King FS. Helping mothers to breastfeed. Revised ed. Nairobi, Kenya: AMREF; 1992:14. Reprinted with permission.

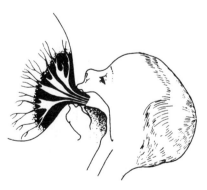

FIGURE 15.4   A baby poorly positioned at the breast.
Source: King FS. Helping mothers to breastfeed. Revised ed. Nairobi, Kenya: AMREF; 1992:14. Reprinted with permission.

Principles of an Effective Latch

An effective latch helps ensure adequate drawing in of the breast. In the position for optimal sucking, the breast is slightly above the center of the baby's open mouth. The baby's lips should flange out and open wide at an angle of approximately 140 degrees. The bottom lip will cover most of the areola, and the top lip will cover somewhat less of the areola in an asymmetrical, or off-center, latch.

An asymmetrical, or slightly off-center, latch seems to aid in achieving a deep latch. Positioning presents a problem when the baby's head and body are not in alignment or when the baby's head is not facing the breast. Suggesting to mothers that they position their baby "nipple to nose" will help them achieve optimal alignment. With the baby's nose and mother's nipple aligned, the mother can brush the upper lip with her nipple, causing the baby to aim up and not down (see Figure 15.5).

With a proper latch, the mother's breast tissue completely fills the baby's oral cavity, as depicted in Figure 15.1. The baby needs to be close to and facing the mother's breast so as to take in a large enough amount of breast tissue. Failing to take in enough breast tissue could cause the baby to have difficulty extracting milk and result in failure to gain weight. The infant might attempt to compensate for this problem by increasing suction and compressing the lips to hold the nipple securely, which could result in nipple soreness. A change in positioning can improve the baby's sucking.

When the baby is latched well, the tongue will be under the breast and will extend outward far enough to cover the alveolar ridge (bottom gum line). With a wide open mouth and flanged lips, the baby will take in a large mouthful of breast tissue. At this point, the baby's tongue forms a trough through which the milk will flow. The baby will then draw the nipple into the center of the mouth or tongue. The jaws will be well behind the nipple and compress the areola rhythmically. The baby's latch will continue while establishing a pattern of repeated bursts of suck–swallow–pause. A good latch usually means that the mother feels minimal discomfort, although transient soreness with the initial latch is common during the first few days postpartum.

The Baby's Latch in the First Few Days

A baby often experiences some difficulty with latch in the early days of breastfeeding, especially if the mother's labor and birth involved interventions and medications (see Chapter 12). If the baby misses the initial latch attempt, the mother can wait a few seconds and see if proximity to the breast triggers the baby's search response. If the baby seems disorganized, she can stroke the upper lip or philtrum with her nipple. If the rooting reflex appears to be weak, expressing milk onto the baby's lips will help the baby locate the breast.

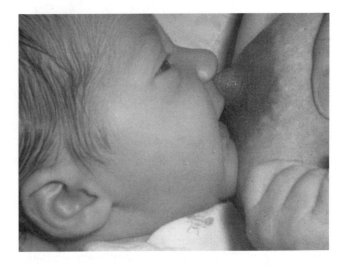

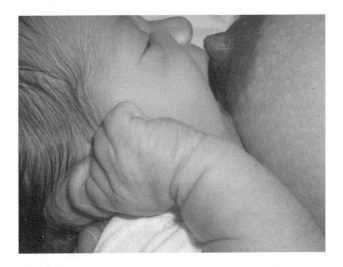

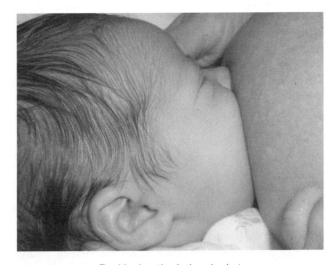

FIGURE 15.5   Positioning the baby nipple to nose.

Source: Printed with permission of Catherine Watson Genna, BS, IBCLC.

If the baby still does not latch, the mother can withdraw her breast, relax, reposition the baby, and repeat the rooting reflex stimulus. Establishing this routine will help the baby develop a pattern for getting onto the breast. Encourage the mother to think of the early days as a learning period and to not become discouraged if she and her baby have difficulty getting started. If the baby continues to be disorganized or becomes frantic, the mother can try to stimulate the sucking reflex with her finger, with expressed colostrum on it. This action may calm the infant, encourage rooting, and eventually achieve a good latch.

Milk Transfer

Before addressing possible problems with sucking and attachment, it is first helpful to understand two facets of the transfer process: (1) how the baby receives milk and (2) how interaction between the baby and the breast can affect milk transfer. Two essential elements for efficient milk transfer are a functioning letdown for the mother and appropriate sucking by the infant. It is important that everyone involved in the mother's and baby's care understand that milk transfer is an interaction between the mother and her baby. During this process, each exerts influence over the other. The manner in which the baby's mouth physically meets and then stimulates the breast is crucial to effective milk transfer.

The Transfer Process

Milk transfer occurs when the baby's sucking delivers a bolus of food to the nasopharynx and is swallowed. The mother's nipple, areola, and breast tissue form a teat within the baby's mouth. The baby's tongue cups along the sides of the teat and forms a trough. Milk reaching the back of the baby's mouth stimulates swallowing. Negative pressure retains the breast in the baby's mouth and may help milk move down the ducts. Thus the amount of breast tissue the baby takes in plays a role in how easily milk is extracted.

The baby alternately compresses the nipple and swallows when the back of the mouth fills with milk. Sucking typically occurs in a continuous cycle of suck–swallow–breathe (Arvedson, 2006). Throughout the sucking cycle, the baby's tongue continually covers the alveolar ridge. As the baby draws the end of the nipple back to within a few centimeters of the soft palate, the lower jaw and tongue rise to compress the breast. Milk enters the teat as a result of positive pressure in the alveoli created by the letdown reflex and suction caused by the jaw lowering. Although some milk is released when the breast is compressed, more is released when compression ends and the baby's jaw opens (Geddes et al., 2008).

Signs of Effective Milk Transfer

Evaluating the transfer of milk is a key element of a breastfeeding assessment. The vast majority of babies accomplish milk transfer remarkably well when the mother uses sound breastfeeding practices. Some babies, however, may have difficulty and require assistance. Watching the baby's sucking action and jaw movement in relation to the frequency of swallowing can offer clues about the effectiveness of milk transfer. Measuring pre-feed and post-feed weights on a sensitive, calibrated digital scale can identify this amount quite precisely if necessary, as in the case of a low-weight-gain or preterm baby.

Effective milk transfer is identified by the following signs:

- The baby moves from short rapid sucks to slow deep sucks early in the feeding.
- The mother notices her milk letting down.
- No dimpling or puckering of the baby's cheeks is noted.
- Breast tissue does not slide in and out of the baby's mouth when the baby sucks or pauses.
- No smacking or clicking sounds are evident with sucking.
- Swallowing is apparent after every 1 to 2 sucks.
- The baby is able to maintain a latch throughout the feeding.
- The mother's breast softens as the feeding progresses (noted after Stage II lactogenesis).
- The baby spontaneously unlatches and is satiated.
- The mother's nipple does not appear blanched or compressed when the baby unlatches.
- The baby is content between most feedings.
- The baby's voiding and stooling are appropriate for age.

Problems with Latch

It can sometimes take several feedings before a mother and baby achieve an effective latch. Helping mothers approach the early feedings in a calm manner and with a sense of humor decreases potential frustration in both the mother and the baby. If difficulties arise, encourage mothers to keep the attempts to breastfeed very short. Depending on the baby's tolerance, the mother may continue her attempts to establish a good latch for as long as 10 minutes. As soon as the baby cries, pushes away, or demonstrates other withdrawal or avoidance behaviors such as hiccoughing, coughing, gagging, or sneezing, she should stop the current attempt, calm the baby, and try again later.

The mother may also try feeding on the other breast or try holding her baby in a different position (see Chapter 14 for a discussion of positioning). If the baby rejects the breast after a few such attempts, urge that she stop all efforts for that feeding. She can snuggle skin to skin with her baby on her chest and watch for the return of approach behaviors such as tongue extension, mouthing movements, or rooting. If the baby fails to latch at that point, the mother can continue skin-to-skin contact at the breast and watch for hunger cues.

The mother will need to express milk from her breasts to maintain milk production if the difficulty with latching persists. She can feed her expressed milk to her baby with an alternative feeding method. The information in Table 15.1 will help you explore the possible causes for problems with latch so that you can determine the appropriate measures for a particular mother–infant dyad.

Assessing a Shallow Latch

A variety of factors can be observed during a feeding to assess whether the baby has achieved an effective latch. A baby that is latched well, with an ample amount of breast tissue taken into the mouth, will settle into a sucking rhythm and continue to nurse until satiated. A baby with a shallow latch will be unable to stay latched for more than several sucks, and may develop a pattern of the breast sliding in and out of the mouth throughout sucking. Dimpling or puckering of the baby's cheeks when sucking is another sign of a shallow latch. Clicking or smacking noises during suckling can also indicate a need to improve the latch, although some babies who are latched well also

seem to make these noises. Observing little or no swallowing during a feeding indicates low milk transfer and, therefore, a poor latch.

A shallow latch can result in the mother's nipple appearing flattened, creased, or blanched after the baby unlatches. Because a shallow latch is the primary cause of nipple soreness, it is important to assess the baby's latch any time a mother complains of pain during or after feedings. Latch should also be assessed if the baby is fussy during or after feedings, behavior that could indicate low milk transfer. Inadequate voiding or stooling is another sign of poor milk transfer that requires latch assessment. Little or no change in breast fullness from the beginning to the end of a feeding is another sign of poor milk transfer; this outcome would arise only after Stage II lactogenesis when the mother has copious milk.

Feeding Adjustments to Improve Latch

When a baby continues to have difficulty with latch, the mother needs to learn her options for alternative ways to manage feedings. Suggest that she provide lots of skin-to-skin contact without attempting to put the baby to breast. She can recline or lie on her back with the baby between her breasts, just as she would immediately after birth. If this initiates rooting, she can help guide her baby to the breast, making sure not to exert pressure. (See the discussion of biological nurturing in Chapter 14.)

The mother may have more success getting her baby latched using a position where her dominant hand is in control. A right-handed mother could use the side-sitting (also football or clutch) hold on the right breast or the

TABLE 15.1   Helping a Baby Who Cannot Get Attached

Cause	Suggestions for Management
The baby is being held in a position that requires him to twist his neck in order to breastfeed.	Help the mother hold her baby close, directly facing and slightly lower than the center of the breast.
The baby does not open his mouth wide enough.	Tease the baby with the nipple, by gently touching his upper lip, until he opens his mouth wide before attaching.
The baby has been given an artificial nipple and has a sucking preference. He may thrust or hump his tongue when he tries to attach and suckle	Give no artificial nipples to the baby; allow him only to suckle at the breast. If supplementation is necessary, use a small spoon, cup, or a tube at the breast.
The mother's nipples are flat because of engorgement.	Be sure the mother's breasts do not become too full because of limited feedings. If the breasts are engorged, express milk to help the nipple protrude and soften the areola. Try reverse pressure softening.
The mother's nipples are inverted to the point that the baby cannot get attached.	Draw out an inverted nipple with mild suction before the feeding, using an everter, inverted syringe or pump. Note that inverted nipples do not necessarily interfere with breastfeeding. Babies attach to the breast, not to the nipple.

cross-cradle hold with the left hand supporting the left breast (the positions would be reversed for a left-handed mother). Such positions will give the mother control over head movement and help her hug her baby to the breast as soon as the mouth is opened wide enough.

If her baby tends to approach the breast without a wide open mouth, the parents can encourage a wider opening. When the baby is content, awake, and happy, they can tickle the upper lip with a finger, talking to the infant all the time, saying slowly, "o..p..e..n.. w..i..d..e" while opening their mouth wide so that the baby will mirror the action. When the infant responds, they can gently put a finger into the mouth, pad side up, to suck on as a reward. Dipping the finger into the mother's expressed colostrum or milk serves as an added incentive. In addition, babies often imitate facial expressions.

One way to help a baby improve the latch is to make the nipple easier to grasp. The mother's nipple may be flat or inverted or might be poorly defined because of a full and rounded breast. Chapter 21 describes a number of techniques and devices that help to define the nipple better for the baby, thereby improving the ability to latch. A flexible approach that limits suggestions to only what a particular mother can tolerate may require providing more alternatives in some cases than in others.

The Baby Who Cannot Stay Attached

Some babies initially may achieve a good latch and then form a pattern of popping on and off the breast during a feeding. In such a case, the baby latches and begins to nurse, but after a short time falls away from the breast and cries or chokes. This might happen several times during a feeding. Table 15.2 presents the possible causes for this behavior and measures to address each cause. Failure to stay attached sometimes happens before the mother's milk has come in, although it could occur after as well. In particular, a strong milk ejection reflex can result in overactive milk production and overwhelm the baby.

Some situations can cause the baby to have trouble latching and generating enough sucking pressure to hold onto the breast. For example, a mother with very large breasts whose baby is born late preterm or small for gestational age (SGA) may experience this difficulty. The mother can help her baby stay latched by supporting her breast using the analogy of a "breast taco" or a "breast sandwich" (Wiessinger, 1998). In this analogy, the mother learns to hold her breast as she would a taco or sandwich horizontally—not vertically—to eat it. Likewise, she can help her baby take in a substantial part of her breast by flattening her breast so that it "fits" the plane of the infant's mouth. Mothers usually need this type of assistance only

TABLE 15.2 Helping a Baby Who Cannot Stay Attached

Cause	Suggestions for Management
The baby must reach or twist his neck to keep the breast in his mouth.	Be sure the mother is holding her baby close, directly facing and slightly lower than the breast, with his nose and chin touching the breast and the baby's ear, shoulder, and hip in alignment.
The baby is unable to breathe when he is at the breast.	Avoid flexing the baby's head forward in such a way that his nose is pushed against the breast. His head needs to be slightly extended so that his chin and nose are just touching the breast. Pull his bottom in more, and his head will angle out.
The mother is moving either her breast or her baby, or not supporting the baby enough so that the breast falls away.	Hold the baby in a side-sitting position with his head cradled in the mother's hand for greater head control (avoiding pushing at the back of his head). Help the mother identify a good attachment and focus on what it feels like so she can recognize the baby's gradual slipping off the breast. Put pillows or blankets under her arm so a fatigued arm muscle will not let the baby slip. Help her check during the feeding for good attachment and learn trauma-free unlatching and relatching so that both she and the baby develop the habits of a wide-open, mouth-full attachment. If you can see the problem and the mother cannot, she will continue doing the wrong thing.
The mother's milk is flowing too forcefully.	Be sure the mother's breasts do not become too full because of limited feedings. If the breasts are engorged, expressing milk will help the nipple to protrude. Suggest that the mother express milk before a feeding so that the flow is less forceful. Allow the baby to feed on only one breast per feeding, with no time limitations, until the initial oversupply has diminished. The mother may need to express milk from the other breast for comfort. If she has an overabundance of milk, she may want to nurse the baby on the same side two or three times before changing to the other breast.

in the early days after birth or until the preterm or late-preterm baby reaches the normal due date. You can reassure the mother that very soon her baby will be able to latch easily without extra help.

Figure 15.6 shows a mother using the taco hold. In this figure, the mother cups her breast in the C-hold and flattens the breast with her thumb and index finger so her baby can take in a mouthful of breast tissue. Her thumb is on the outer part of her areola. Mothers are usually advised to put their fingers behind the areola. For a mother with a large areola, however, this placement might be too far back to provide the necessary compression. Her breasts and areola might be so large that her breast would round back out, allowing the baby to slide down on her nipple. This is an example of the uniqueness of each mother and baby pair. When focusing on each dyad, flexibility and creativity are two of your most important tools!

Consequences of a Shallow Latch

As mentioned earlier, a shallow latch is the primary cause of nipple soreness. In turn, the pain—or anticipation of pain—when the baby latches can inhibit the mother's milk ejection reflex and prevent sufficient milk from reaching her baby. Because a poorly latched baby is unable to remove milk from the mother's breasts adequately, the mother is at risk for engorgement, plugged ducts, and mastitis. Milk production will diminish, and lactation failure is likely to result in the absence of any intervention. It is important that the mother pump or express her milk if the baby is not latching and breastfeeding effectively.

Consequences of a shallow latch are inevitable for the baby as well. Because of the mother's decreased milk ejection reflex, the breastfeeding infant receives primarily foremilk, which results in increased hunger, fussiness, and perhaps colic-like symptoms. The infant's urine and

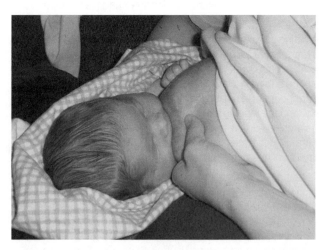

FIGURE 15.6 Assisting the baby with the taco or sandwich hold.

Source: Printed with permission of Anna Swisher.

stool output may be low, and jaundice may occur. If the baby is unable to obtain enough high-fat hindmilk, failure to gain adequate weight or even weight loss may occur. To preserve the baby's health, if human milk in not available, formula supplements may become necessary. This supplementation could mark the end to breastfeeding, unless the plan of care includes suggestions on ways to increase the mother's milk production. Making adjustments in the baby's latch can prevent the situation from progressing to this point.

Physical Issues That Can Affect Latch

In some cases, difficulty with latch may result from physical issues related to the mother, such as breast or nipple abnormalities. It could also result from her acute or chronic physical conditions such as low back pain, carpal tunnel syndrome, or pain related to delivery, particularly perineal or cesarean incision pain. Physical issues related to the infant that could affect latch include a cleft lip or palate, neurological or orthopedic problems, Down syndrome, a fractured clavicle, ankyloglossia (tight frenulum), or a high palate. If comfort measures do not produce improvement, these factors need to be explored as possible causes for the baby's difficulty with latch.

Some babies engage in rapid side-to-side head movements, making it difficult to achieve a good latch. When the baby's head movement stops, placing a couple of drops of milk or water on the baby's tongue as the mother attempts a latch may encourage the baby's mouth to open. The same technique can be done with tubing and a syringe at the breast.

∼ Problems with Sucking

Most feeding difficulties result from poor attachment or faulty positioning of the baby at the breast. In many cases, patience, practice, and repositioning of the baby's body and mouth on the breast will alleviate these sucking difficulties. Early sucking problems are associated with early cessation of breastfeeding (Mozingo et al., 2000). Suggesting that the baby will figure it out when the milk comes in does not provide the new mother with adequate help. Instead, she needs specific strategies and postdischarge support to help her develop good practices. If a problem with a baby's suck does not respond to adjustments in positioning and latching, a full assessment is needed.

Most attachment or sucking difficulties are short-lived. They usually resolve with the passage of time, as long as the baby receives sufficient calories. In some cases, a baby may have a weak or ineffective suck because of weakness from insufficient nourishment. Many times, a baby's sucking can be improved simply by consuming more calories. Intubation and other respiratory therapy are other factors to consider when evaluating an infant's suck, especially with preterm infants. It can take longer for these babies to develop normal nutritive and nonnutritive sucking skills (Estep et al., 2008; Poore et al., 2008; Stumm et al., 2008). A thorough assessment of both the mother and baby will help determine whether a baby has a truly dysfunctional suck.

Absence of Nutritive Sucking

Many times a baby may appear to achieve a good latch and then suck ineffectively or not at all. To assess such a child, first determine whether the infant is simply sleepy and not hungry at the moment. Sucking can be affected if a baby is being supplemented or is spending energy on nonnutritive sucking on a pacifier. Therefore, explore whether the baby is receiving any artificial feedings of water or formula, and if so, the amount per feeding and per day. Also learn if the baby is spending nonnutritive sucking on a pacifier, and if so, when and for how long. A key part of your assessment will be to find out *why* the baby is being supplemented, and *why* the parents are giving a pacifier. These factors can be corrected simply by elimination of the problematic practices. Clarification of the parents' motives and education about early bottle and pacifier use can help a baby return to exclusive breastfeeding easily, if that is the parents' goal.

Disorganized Sucking

Some babies have initial difficulty in mastering sucking. Disorganized sucking can result from a variety of causes—a delay in the first breastfeeding at birth, late-preterm birth, prematurity, maternal or infant medications, or illness. Neuromotor dysfunction, variations in oral anatomy, and artificial nipple use can affect sucking ability as well. Table 15.3 identifies causes of latch or sucking problems, and suggests measures to rectify them. As a lactation consultant, your careful assessment is an integral part of determining the appropriate course of action. Most breastfeeding problems relate to poor latch rather than dysfunctional sucking, although over time you may see

TABLE 15.3   *Causes of Latch or Sucking Problems*

Medication received by the mother during labor	Encourage childbirth educators to focus on labor support issues and to educate couples about the effects of epidurals and cesareans.
Forceps delivery or vacuum extraction	Watch positioning of the baby to avoid pressure on his head.
Post-birth interventions such as deep laryngeal suctioning or circumcision	Avoid putting the baby to breast immediately following deep suctioning or other oral insult until the baby demonstrates readiness. Avoid circumcision until the baby has fed well at the breast at least three times.
Prolonged crying, especially due to interventions	Prevent prolonged crying by helping the mother with her baby. Comfort the baby before putting him to breast. Teach the mother and staff the importance of feeding on cue rather than when the baby cries. Keep the mother and baby together rather than having the baby in the nursery.
Baby has a fractured clavicle or cephalhematoma	Position the baby in a manner that prevents pressure on the affected area.
Mother has tight, taut breast tissue with flat or inverted nipples	Massage breasts before the feeding. Use a hold that enables the mother to maintain control over her baby's head movement (side-sitting hold or cross-cradle hold). Use an inverted syringe to form the nipple (see Chapter 21). The mother may need to use a nipple shield (see Chapter 21).
Incorrect positioning at the breast	Correct any positioning problems. Make sure both mother and baby are comfortable.
Mother's lack of confidence in handling baby and putting baby to breast	Give encouragement to the mother and help her see that she and her baby will become more comfortable with one another with practice and time. Show the mother how to handle her baby and put him to breast. Avoid doing it for her.
High-arched or bubble palate	Use the side-sitting hold. Take the baby off the breast after 30–60 seconds and reattach. The second latch helps draw more tissue farther back into the baby's mouth.
Short or tight frenulum	Contact the pediatrician, dentist, oral surgeon, or ear-nose-throat specialist for evaluation and possible clipping of the frenulum.
Cleft lip	The lip usually molds around the breast to form suction. If this is not the case, the mother can cover the cleft area with her breast or finger. Massage the breasts before and during the feeding.

(Continued)

TABLE 15.3   Causes of Latch or Sucking Problems (*Continued*)

Cause	Suggestions for Management
Cleft palate	Nurse in a semiupright position. Hold the breast in the baby's mouth during feedings. Interrupt feeding as necessary to allow the baby to burp or breathe. Supplement with the best device for the individual baby. An obturator (a feeding plate placed over the cleft) may be helpful. The mother will need a referral to a cleft palate team.
Hypoglycemia in the baby	Feed the baby expressed colostrum via cup, spoon, or syringe. Use an artificial baby milk if expressed mother's milk is not sufficient for the baby's needs. Make sure that the baby is fed at regular intervals. Wake him to feed if necessary.
Hypotonia or hypertonia in the baby	Positioning is the key. Some hypertonic babies may need to find their own position of comfort. A hypotonic baby will need to be supported well. The mother may need to supplement if the baby does not feed well. These babies respond well to tube-feeding at the breast. Decrease external stimulation for the hypertonic baby. Use rousing techniques for the hypotonic baby, starting with infant massage. Use gentle massage to calm the hypertonic baby. Short, very frequent feeding (every 1½ to 2 hours) will be more effective than longer feedings at longer intervals. Condition the baby by establishing a routine for getting on the breast, especially if the baby's rooting reflex is not well developed. Supplement with expressed milk in a cup or bottle after nursing if the baby is unable to obtain enough through use of a tube-feeding device at the breast. Express milk and supplement the baby until the condition improves.
Baby engages in tongue sucking or tongue thrust	A baby who consistently sucks his tongue may have been doing so in utero for months. Have the baby learn to suck progressively on the mother's small finger, middle finger, and then thumb to gradually increase the baby's comfort level with larger sizes of objects in his mouth. Use finger feeding until the baby can latch on.
Baby has received bottles and prefers an artificial nipple	Because babies suck differently on an artificial nipple than they do on the breast, it is important to avoid using a rubber/silicone nipple as much as possible. The long, firm object stimulates his palate and initiates a suck almost immediately. He does not have to draw it into his mouth. Any kind of sucking stimulus on the bottle nipple will cause fluid to flow into his mouth; hence, he will be unable to suck nonnutritively on the bottle as he can on the breast. He will have to hump his tongue at the front of the nipple to control milk flow. When the breast is drawn into the baby's mouth, it conforms to the shape of his mouth, whereas the bottle nipple not only does not fill the baby's mouth, but he must alter his mouth shape to work with the artificial nipple. Discontinue the bottle and supplement with a cup, spoon, syringe, or medicine dropper.
Baby has a stuffy nose due to a cold or allergies	Nurse the baby in an upright position. Saline nose drops or a drop of the mother's milk in the baby's nostrils helps clear a stuffy nose. Using a bulb syringe to clear the nose may irritate the delicate mucous membranes and cause swelling.
Mother is taking medication that affects the baby through her milk	Ask the physician about switching to a drug that will have less effect on the baby. Alter feeding times and drug administration so that the baby nurses when the amount of drug in the mother's milk is lowest. If possible, delay drug use until the baby is older. If reactions are serious (i.e., extreme colic-like behavior or lethargy) and the drug cannot be discontinued, do not breastfeed. Pump and dump to maintain lactation.

many difficult and complex cases if you practice in the community.

Note that there is a difference between a *disorganized* suck and a *dysfunctional* suck. Babies may exhibit an uncoordinated suck in the first few days of life because of sucking habits in utero, birth interventions, or early artificial nipple feedings. Many times, uncoordinated or disorganized sucking resolves soon after birth, with practice and protected caloric intake. The initiation of any intervention in the hospital for a healthy term infant can result in poor or ineffective feeding behaviors. In addition, some babies may develop oral aversion owing to unpleasant experiences. Sometimes these interventions are necessary, as with intubating a preterm baby or suctioning after meconium aspiration. Given these possibilities, be sensitive to how you examine the baby, including the way you touch the infant's mouth and oral structure.

Management of Sucking Problems

Management of sucking problems involves assessment and peeling away the layers of the symptoms to find the root cause. For example, poor weight gain is a symptom of an underlying problem, not a problem in itself. In this example, ascertaining why the baby has poor weight gain and treating the cause offer true resolution of the underlying problem. Feeding the baby formula, in contrast, simply treats the symptom and fails to address the cause so that it can be resolved.

Sensitivity to the mother's emotional state and life situation will help relieve the stress parents feel when they experience a feeding problem with their baby. Collaborate with the mother on a feeding plan, being cautious not to overwhelm her with too many things to do. You can quickly see how you might develop two very different feeding plans for similar problems, depending on the parents' desires, tenacity, maturity, coping skills, and feeding goals.

Consider any long-term consequences of your feeding plan such as a bottle causing nipple preference or use of a nipple shield being stressful for a mother. It is possible that a bottle or nipple shield may be a useful tool that saves breastfeeding for a particular mother. For other mothers, use of these devices may make feeding a chore for the mother and a difficult procedure for the baby. Developing a practical plan that is workable given each family's unique needs will encourage the parents to actually use the plan.

Barger (2009) describes five levels of intervention for babies who exhibit sucking difficulty:

1. Non-interventive
2. Minimal
3. Low level
4. Moderate level
5. High level

When there is a true need for assistance, start with the least complex and intrusive method. Progress from the least invasive to the next level only when you determine it is clearly indicated. Use a technique that places the baby in control of the feeding whenever possible. Refer to Chapter 21 for further details on the techniques described in the remainder of this section.

Non-interventive Techniques

The least invasive approach to resolving a sucking difficulty is to first determine the probable cause and then consider whether the situation is one that will improve on its own, given a little time. If poor positioning is the cause, help the mother correct the positioning. Then wait for the "golden moment," the time when the baby is hungry and rooting with a wide open mouth. The mother can express colostrum onto her nipple to entice the baby to latch onto the breast and suck. If she cannot easily express her colostrum, she can drip some glucose water on the nipple to stimulate sucking. The sweeter the solution, the more vigorously the baby may suck. Make sure mothers

do not use honey, as contaminants in this food can cause botulism in infants.

Minimal Level of Intervention

If enticing the baby has been unsuccessful, you or the parent can place an index finger in the baby's mouth to initiate rhythmic sucking. This also works as a pacifying technique if the baby is fussy and unable to settle at the breast. Another technique is use of a supplemental feeding device at the breast, which gives the baby calories and stimulates sucking at the same time. Depending on availability of the mother's milk, the baby can receive, in order of preference, the mother's expressed milk, donor milk, or formula through the device. If the baby cannot latch and maintain a seal on the breast, a feeding tube at the breast will not be helpful. Conversely, a feeding tube may be useful for a baby who attaches and maintains a seal, but does not suck adequately.

Low-Level Intervention

Many times you will be able to assess the baby's oral structure visually. For some babies, you can easily identify a bubble palate, short tongue, or tight lingual frenulum. You can also observe whether the baby's tongue elevates to the roof of the mouth. Sometimes, however, frenulum tightness is more subtle and requires more than an assessment of its appearance. Therefore, the next level of intervention is to sweep your little finger under the tongue from side-to-side. If you encounter resistance, chances are the baby has a tight or wide frenulum that may need intervention (West & Marasco, 2008). Another low-level intervention is to insert your index finger into the baby's mouth to evaluate the oral structure and suck.

Moderate-Level Intervention

If less intrusive measures have been unsuccessful, you can place your index finger in the baby's mouth, with the pad side up, to organize the infant's sucking. This technique involves placing light pressure on the midline of the baby's tongue, and then pulling the finger out slowly to encourage the baby to suck it back in. The baby should receive verbal reinforcement when sucking correctly. Note that the baby is in control in both a minimal-level and low-level intervention. With this higher level of intervention, the caregiver exerts more control through manipulation of the finger in the baby's mouth. Its use is appropriate only after other measures have failed to elicit effective sucking.

A baby who is not breastfeeding effectively will need to receive nourishment by an alternative feeding method until the issue is resolved. Some babies respond well to finger-feeding with a supplemental nursing system. Parents can use this tool to help a baby who is having trouble sucking. The feel of a parent's finger may resemble the mother's breast more closely than a silicone or latex nipple. See Chapter 21 for a discussion on finger-feeding. A nipple shield may be a successful bridge to direct breastfeeding if the mother has flat or inverted nipples or edema that does not respond to reverse pressure softening or if the baby has a high bubble palate, tongue-tie, or thin buccal pads (Chertok, 2009; Chertok et al., 2006; Powers & Tapia, 2004; Meier et al., 2000; Bodley et al., 1996; Wilson-Clay, 1996).

High-Level Intervention

Suck training is the highest degree of sucking intervention. It involves stimulating specific parts of the baby's tongue, mouth, and lips to train the infant to suck. Usually, this type of training is handled by a speech language pathologist or an occupational therapist. If there is a need for suck training, other neurological problems, such as cerebral palsy, may be present. In such cases, the suck may be the first area in which the problem presents.

If you work in a hospital, speech language therapists and occupational therapists will be available to work with rehabilitating inpatients. If your hospital has a NICU or pediatric intensive care unit (PICU), your facility should have therapists trained to work with infants. Partner with them to assess babies with sucking and swallowing problems. If you work in private practice or in a community clinic, familiarize yourself with the practitioners in your area.

Some parents find that their babies' feeding ability improves with chiropractic care, massage therapy, or craniosacral therapy (see Figure 15.7). Developing a list of

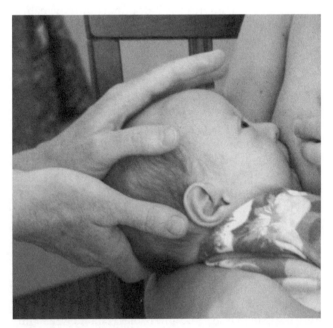

FIGURE 15.7   Referral to a craniosacral therapist may help resolve a sucking problem.

Source: Printed with permission of Anna Swisher.

reliable allied health professionals will enable you to refer parents appropriately. You will need to work in concert with the baby's caregiver and other specialists as a part of the healthcare team. Referral to an organization that assists the neurologically impaired child and family may be necessary as well. Refer to Appendix H for a list of national organizations that may be helpful for intervention referrals.

⮴ *Summary*

Although some babies need assistance in initiating effective suckling, the majority need no help. Caregivers need to trust in the innate abilities, reflexes, and instincts of both the mother and the baby to find a feeding method that works best for them. A sound understanding of infant sucking is essential for assessment and help, when necessary. Begin with the least invasive method when you need to intervene with the baby's suck. Partner with therapists trained in suck and swallow disorders to help parents resolve significant feeding problems. Many initial sucking difficulties resolve with a little time, as long as all parties take care to protect the mother's milk production and feed the baby sufficient calories.

⮴ *Chapter 15—At a Glance*

Facts you learned—

Sucking:

- Sucking stimulates saliva, gastrointestinal secretions, hormones, motility, milk production, and maternal yearning.
- Cholecystokinin (CCK) promotes satiety and sleepiness.
- Sucking rhythm corresponds inversely to the amount of milk available.
- Nutritive sucking is affected by CNS depressants.
- Suckling at the breast is very different from sucking on a bottle.
- Ineffective suckling places the mother at risk for engorgement, plugged ducts, mastitis, and compromised milk production.
- Ineffective suckling places the baby at risk for increased hunger, fussiness, colic-like symptoms, low urine and stool output, jaundice, and inadequate weight gain or weight loss.
- Latch difficulties may result from breast or nipple abnormalities, pain, cleft lip or palate, neurological or orthopedic problems, ankyloglossia, or high palate.

- Sucking can be disorganized due to illness, prematurity, medications given to the infant or mother, delay in the first breastfeeding at birth, neuromotor dysfunction, variations in oral anatomy, and nipple preference due to artificial nipples.
- Babies can develop oral aversion when they are subjected to intrusive interventions.
- When possible, the feeding should be controlled by the baby rather than by special devices or techniques.
- A baby who cannot suck or who has swallowing difficulties may have neurological deficits and should be referred to a speech language pathologist or occupational therapist.

Applying what you learned—

Teach mothers that:

- Wide jaw excursions indicate nutritive suckling.
- Alternating between breast and bottle can compromise breastfeeding if baby is not a robust nurser.
- Extended bottle or pacifier use may cause malocclusion and sleep apnea in adulthood.
- Audible swallows or long, drawing, nutritive, high-flow sucks indicate a good latch.
- The early days of breastfeeding are a learning period for both mother and baby.
- With a good latch, the breast is slightly above the center of the baby's open mouth, the lips are flanged, the bottom lip covers most of the areola off-center, and the tongue is under the breast and over the alveolar ridge, forming a trough.
- Efficient milk transfer requires a functioning letdown and appropriate suckling.
- A nipple shield may help a baby latch at the beginning of a feeding.
- Most feeding difficulties are caused by a shallow latch or faulty positioning.
- Most uncoordinated sucking is resolved with the passage of time and with increasing the baby's caloric intake.
- A baby who is sleepy or not hungry may not suck nutritively.

Teach the mother how to:

- Observe her baby for signs of a good latch and good milk transfer.
- Handle problems with the baby's latch and assist a baby who cannot stay attached.
- Maintain milk production when her baby is unable to nurse effectively.
- Preserve her baby's health with supplements when necessary.

∾ References

Ardran G, et al. A cineradiographic study of bottle feeding. *Br J Radiol.* 1958a;31(361):11-22.

Ardran G, et al. A cineradiographic study of breast feeding. *Br J Radiol.* 1958b;31(363):156-162.

Arvedson J. Part 1: Oral cavity, pharynx and esophagus. Swallowing and feeding in infants and young children. *GI Motility Online.* May 16, 2006. www.nature.com/gimo/contents/pt1/full/gimo17.html. Accessed May 22, 2009.

Asole S, et al. Effect of hospital practices on breastfeeding: a survey in the Italian region of Lazio. *J Hum Lact.* 2009;25(3):333-340.

Barger J. *Certified Lactation Specialist Course.* Wheaton, IL: Lactation Education Consultants; 2009.

Baumgarder D et al. Effect of labor epidural anesthesia on breast-feeding of healthy full-term newborns delivered vaginally. *J Am Board Fam Pract.* 2003;16(1):7-13.

Bodley V, Powers D. Long-term nipple shield use: a positive perspective. *J Hum Lact.* 1996;12(4):301-304.

Bosma J, et al. Ultrasound demonstration of tongue motions during suckle feeding. *Dev Med Child Neurol.* 1990;32(3):223-229.

Chaves R, et al. Factors associated with duration of breastfeeding. *J Pediatr (Rio J).* 2007;83(3):241-246.

Chertok IR. Reexamination of ultra-thin nipple shield use, infant growth and maternal satisfaction. *J Clin Nurs.* 2009;18(21):2949-2955.

Chertok I, et al. A pilot study of maternal and term infant outcomes associated with ultrathin nipple shield use. *JOGNN.* 2006;35(2):265-272.

Chezem J, et al. Breastfeeding knowledge, breastfeeding confidence, and infant feeding plans: effects on actual feeding practices. *JOGNN.* 2003;32(1):40-47.

da Costa S, van der Schans C. The reliability of the Neonatal Oral–Motor Assessment Scale. *Acta Paediatr.* 2008;97(1):21-26.

Declercq E, et al. Hospital practices and women's likelihood of fulfilling their intention to exclusively breastfeed. *Am J Public Health.* 2009;99(5):929-935.

Delaney A, Arvedson J. Development of swallowing and feeding: prenatal through first year of life. *Dev Disabil Res Rev.* 2008;14(2):105-117.

Estep M, et al. Non-nutritive suck parameter in preterm infants with RDS. *J Neonatal Nurs.* 2008;14(1):28-34.

Fucile S, et al. A controlled-flow vacuum-free bottle system enhances preterm infants' nutritive sucking skills. *Dysphagia.* 2009;24(2):145-151.

Geddes D. The use of ultrasound to identify milk ejection in women: tips and pitfalls. *Int Breastfeed J.* 2009a;4:5.

Geddes D. Ultrasound imaging of the lactating breast: methodology and application. *Int Breastfeed J.* 2009b;4:4.

Geddes D, et al. Patterns of respiration in infants during breast-feeding. Abstracts of Presentations at the 13th International Conference of the International Society for Research in Human Milk and Lactation (ISRHML). *J Hum Lact.* 2007;23:72.

Geddes D, et al. Tongue movement and intra-oral vacuum in breastfeeding infants. *Early Hum Dev.* 2008;84(7):471-477.

Genna W. *Supporting Sucking Skills in Infants.* Sudbury, MA: Jones and Bartlett Publishers; 2008.

Góis E, et al. Influence of nonnutritive sucking habits, breathing pattern and adenoid size on the development of malocclusion. *Angle Orthod.* 2008;78(4):647-654.

Hammerman C, Kaplan M. Oxygen saturation during and after feeding in healthy term infants. *Biol Neonate.* 1995;67(2):94-99.

International Lactation Consultant Association (ILCA); Mannel R, Martens P, Walker M, eds. *Core Curriculum for Lactation Consultant Practice*, 2nd ed. Sudbury, MA: Jones and Bartlett; 2007.

Jordan S. Infant feeding and analgesia in labour: the evidence is accumulating. *Int Breastfeed J.* 2006;1:25.

Jordan S, et al. The impact of intrapartum analgesia on infant feeding. *BJOG.* 2005;112(7):927-934.

Kassing D. Bottle feeding as a tool to reinforce breastfeeding. *J Hum Lact.* 2002;18(1):56-60.

Law-Morstatt L, et al. Pacing as a treatment technique for transitional sucking patterns. *J Perinatol.* 2003;23(6):483-488.

Leite-Cavalcanti A, et al. Breast-feeding, bottle-feeding, sucking habits and malocclusion in Brazilian preschool children. *Rev Salud Publica (Bogota).* 2007;9(2):194-204.

López Del Valle L, et al. Associations between a history of breast feeding, malocclusion and parafunctional habits in Puerto Rican children. *P R Health Sci J.* 2006;25(1):31-34.

Meier P, et al. Nipple shields for preterm infants: effect on milk transfer and duration of breastfeeding. *J Hum Lact.* 2000;16(2):106-114.

Merten S, et al. Do baby-friendly hospitals influence breastfeeding duration on a national level? *Pediatrics.* 2005;116(5):e702-e708.

Moimaz S, et al. Association between breast-feeding practices and sucking habits: a cross-sectional study of children in their first year of life. *J Indian Soc Pedod Prev Dent.* 2008;26(3):102-106.

Morton J. The role of the pediatrician in extended breastfeeding of the preterm infant. *Pediatric Ann.* 2003;32(5):308-316.

Mozingo JN, et al. "It wasn't working": women's experiences with short-term breastfeeding. *J Mat Child Nurs.* 2000;25(3):120-126.

Ngom P, et al. Prevalence and factors associated with non-nutritive sucking behavior: cross sectional study among 5- to 6-year-old Senegalese children. *Orthod Fr.* 2008;79(2):99-106.

Nyqvist K. Early attainment of breastfeeding competence in very preterm infants. *Acta Paediatr.* 2008;97(6):776-781.

Ovsenik M, et al. Follow-up study of functional and morphological malocclusion trait changes from 3 to 12 years of age. *Eur J Orthod.* 2007;29(5):523-529.

Palmer B. Breastfeeding: reducing the risk for obstructive sleep apnea. *Breastfeed Abstr.* 1999;18(3):19-20.

Palmer B. The importance of breastfeeding as it relates to total health. Kansas City, MO; January 2002. www.brianpalmerdds.com. Accessed May 21, 2009.

Palmer B. Sleep apnea from an anatomical, anthropologic and developmental perspective. Paper presented at: Academy of Dental Sleep Medicine; June 4, 2004. www.brianpalmerdds.com. Accessed May 21, 2009.

Peres K, et al. Effects of breastfeeding and sucking habits on malocclusion in a birth cohort study. *Rev Saude Publica.* 2007;41(3):343-350.

Pincombe J, et al. Baby friendly hospital initiative practices and breast feeding duration in a cohort of first-time mothers in Adelaide, Australia. *Midwifery.* 2008;24(1):55-61.

Poore M, et al. Patterned orocutaneous therapy improves sucking and oral feeding in preterm infants. *Acta Paediatr.* 2008;97(7):920-927.

Powers D, Tapia V. Women's experiences using a nipple shield. *J Hum Lact.* 2004;20(3):327-334.

Price WA. *Nutrition and Physical Degeneration*, 8th ed. Lemon Grove, CA: Price Pottenger Nutrition; 2008.

Qureshi M, et al. Changes in rhythmic suckle feeding patterns in term infants in the first month of life. *Dev Med Child Neurol.* 2002;44(1):34-39.

Ramsay D. Ultrasound imaging of the sucking mechanics of the term infant. Paper presented at: Human Lactation: Current Research and Clinical Implications; October 22, 2004; Amarillo, TX.

Ramsay D, et al. Ultrasound imaging of milk ejection in the breast of lactating women. *Pediatrics.* 2004;113(2):361-367.

Ramsay D, et al. Milk flow rates can be used to identify and investigate milk ejection in women expressing breast milk using an electric breast pump. *Breastfeeding Med.* 2006;1(1):14-23.

Ramsay D, Hartmann P. Milk removal from the breast. *Breastfeed Rev.* 2005;13(1):5-7.

Ramsay M, Gisel E. Neonatal sucking and maternal feeding practices. *Dev Med Child Neurol.* 1996;38:34-47.

Riordan J, et al. The effect of labor pain relief medication on neonatal suckling and breastfeeding duration. *J Hum Lact.* 2000;16(1):7-12.

Smith W, et al. Imaging evaluation of the human nipple during breast-feeding. *Am J Dis Child.* 1988;142(1):76-78.

Stumm S, et al. Respiratory distress syndrome degrades the fine structure of the non-nutritive suck in preterm infants. *J Neonatal Nurs.* 2008;14(1):9-16.

Suiter D, Ruark-McMurtrey J. Oxygen saturation and heart rate during feeding in breast-fed infants at 1 week and 2 months of age. *Arch Phys Med Rehabil.* 2007;88(12):1681-1685.

Torvaldsen S, et al. Intrapartum epidural analgesia and breastfeeding: a prospective cohort study. *Int Breastfeed J.* 2006;1:24. Comment in: *Int Breastfeed J.* 2006;1:25.

Vázquez-Nava F. Association between allergic rhinitis, bottle feeding, non-nutritive sucking habits, and malocclusion in the primary dentition. *Arch Dis Child*. 2006;91:836-840.

Viggiano D, et al. Breast feeding, bottle feeding, and non-nutritive sucking: effects on occlusion in deciduous dentition. *Arch Dist Child*. 2004;89(2):1121-1123.

Weber F, et al. An ultrasonographic study of the organization of sucking and swallowing by newborn infants. *Dev Med Child Neurol*. 1986;28:19-24.

West D, Marasco L. *The Breastfeeding Mother's Guide to Making More Milk*. New York: McGraw Hill Professional; 2008.

Wiessinger D. A breastfeeding tool using a sandwich analogy for latch-on. *J Hum Lact*. 1998;14(1):51-56.

Wilson-Clay B. Clinical use of silicone nipple shields. *J Hum Lact*. 1996;12(4):279-285.

Wilson-Clay B, Hoover K. *The Breastfeeding Atlas*, 4th ed. Manchaca, TX: Lactnews Press; 2008.

Wolf L, Glass R. *Feeding and Swallowing Disorders in Infancy*. San Antonio, TX: Therapy Skill Builders; 1992.

Woolridge M. Anatomy of infant suckling. *Midwifery*. 1986; 2:164-171.

Yokoyama U, et al. Releases of oxytocin and prolactin during breast massage and suckling in puerperal women. *Eur J Obstet Gynecol Reprod Biol*. 1994;53:17-20.

CHAPTER

16

Breastfeeding in the Early Weeks

The early weeks with a new baby are a time of great adjustment for families. Some parents sail through this time with little difficulty. Others encounter situations that require extra assistance. Anticipatory guidance at key times will help parents manage challenges more confidently. During the early weeks of breastfeeding, the mother establishes milk production and refines her breastfeeding technique. Your assistance during this critical time can help mothers avoid problems with sore nipples, engorgement, plugged ducts, and mastitis. Parents will benefit from your guidance and support as they learn how to respond to their babies' needs.

～ Key Terms

Alternate massage
Ankyloglossia
Autocrine control
Breast abscess
Breast compression
Candida albicans
Candidiasis
Cholecystokinin (CCK)
Colostrum
Edema
Engorgement
Feedback inhibitor of
    lactation (FIL)
Galactorrhea
Hyperprolactinemia
Labial frenum
Lingual frenulum
Mastitis
Methicillin-resistant
    Staphylococcus aureus
    (MRSA)

Milk bleb
Milk blister
Milk stasis
Palliative care
Phytoestrogens
Plugged duct
Post-term
Raynaud's phenomenon
Recurrent mastitis
Spontaneous lactation
Subclinical mastitis (SCM)
Sublingual
Suppressor peptides
Thrush
Transient nipple soreness
Vancomycin-resistant
    Enterococcus (VRE)
Vancomycin-resistant
    Staphylococcus aureus
    (VRSA)
Vasospasm

～ Commitment to Breastfeed

Why do some women breastfeed for months and years, and others wean after a few days or weeks? There is a perception in the industrialized world that, although breastfeeding is best, alternative methods of feeding an infant are acceptable. Generally, in developed countries, mothers who breastfeed do so out of choice, and against cultural norms, not because of tradition or a perceived necessity. This outlook has significant implications for the duration of breastfeeding. When a seemingly acceptable alternative exists, confidence and commitment can easily wane in the absence of support and encouragement.

Breastfeeding has been described as a fundamental gender right that needs reclaiming, so that women can "find power in honoring and validating their own experiences as breastfeeding mothers" (Smith, 2008). Hausman (2008) has examined breastfeeding in view of cultural gender roles, and describes how the formula companies shortchange women by framing artificial feeding as a "choice," couched in emotional terms. Poor women, young women, women of color, and women with less education find it most difficult to overcome constraints on breastfeeding. Social, cultural, and economic forces structure most people's daily lives and intimate decisions, including infant feeding choice. Recognizing the constraints that reveal the "choice" to be more a class privilege will help both lactation consultants and parents identify ways to challenge the status quo.

Reasons Women Continue Breastfeeding

A woman who says, "I will *try* to breastfeed," is quite different from one who says, "I *will* breastfeed." A woman who commits herself to breastfeeding is able to persevere despite any challenges that arise. Breastfeeding is a journey into the unknown and the unpredictable, one that involves ongoing learning. Part of a mother's persistence derives from her ability to recognize the need for help and then find it. In fact, a woman's perception of her ability to actively engage in decision making influences the likelihood of breastfeeding duration at 12 weeks after birth (Hauck et al., 2007). Thus encouraging women's involvement in decision making about breastfeeding helps promote breastfeeding.

Women who are confident in their commitment to breastfeed are better able to withstand both a lack of support from external sources and common challenges. Those who lack confidence are more likely to abandon breastfeeding when obstacles arise (Avery et al., 2009). Among women having breastfeeding problems, those who persevere tend to display an array of coping strategies and an ability to overcome difficulties (Hegney et al., 2008). They are more likely to rely on health professionals they can trust for support, and to have peers with whom they can share their experiences. In contrast, mothers who wean often express feelings of guilt and inadequacy and are more likely to be isolated.

A study of women in Hong Kong who breastfed for more than 6 months revealed that feeding difficulties were overcome despite family opposition and lack of societal acceptance of breastfeeding (Tarrant et al., 2004). Early contact and early breastfeeding are both key factors that influence how long a woman breastfeeds. Mothers benefit most from encouragement and guidance tailored to their individual needs that support their self-efficacy and their feelings of being capable and empowered (Hannula et al., 2008). Factors associated with breastfeeding for 6 months among mothers in an Australian group included the mother possessing a very strong desire to breastfeed, having been breastfed, having been born in an Asian country, and being an older age (Forster et al., 2006).

Mothers who see their babies grow, gain weight, rarely become ill, settle into nursing, and fall asleep during or after nursing are likely to view breastfeeding as successful. Satisfaction is higher when breastfeeding is comfortable and when any painful phases are short-lived. Conversely, mothers' reasons for quitting within the first year reveal a lack of self-confidence in regard to the nursing process. The belief that the baby was not satisfied by her milk alone was cited repeatedly as one of the top three reasons for ceasing breastfeeding. This belief was even more widespread among Hispanic and lower income mothers (Li et al., 2008). It takes time for mothers to find ways to work with the individual characteristics of their babies and to recognize that the baby's satisfaction is not totally the mother's responsibility. The infant's sucking competence, alertness, stamina, and abilities to self-regulate and to respond to soothing also influence the child's satisfaction with breastfeeding.

Increasing Women's Commitment

No single approach consistently increases all women's commitment to continue breastfeeding, though training

under the Baby-Friendly Hospital Initiative (BFHI) might have some potential for influence (Spiby et al., 2009). Continuity of care may also play a role. In one study, mothers who received process-oriented counseling and continuous care believed at day 3 after birth they understood their baby better than the control group, perceived stronger attachment, and enjoyed more breastfeeding and resting with the infant. At 3 months' postpartum, they talked more to their baby, perceived their baby to be more beautiful than other infants, and perceived more strongly that the infant was their own. In addition, they felt significantly more confident and closer with their baby (Ekström & Nissen, 2006).

Researchers have found that self-efficacy and confidence improve when parents are taught to respond to their baby's cues and states (Tedder, 2008). Tedder devised a program called HUG for parent educators; HUG is an acronym for "help, understanding, and guidance." Educational offerings abound online, and similar programs may be available in your community. The key is to help parents learn to understand their baby's behaviors as competent and communicative rather than to perceive them as helpless and manipulative.

Boosting a mother's confidence empowers her to continue breastfeeding. You can help the mother prioritize her baby's needs and reinforce her confidence with comments such as "He is growing so fast," or "She looks so healthy." Point out her abilities as well: "You're such a good mother" or "You pick up on your baby's cues really well." Help the mother recognize and respond to her baby's language and cues. Emphasize that she knows her baby better than anyone else. Validate her concerns and her wide range of emotions as a normal part of mothering.

Misconceptions That Interfere with Breastfeeding

Numerous unfounded beliefs about breastfeeding sometimes confuse parents and interfere with the delivery of sound medical advice. Parents and caregivers alike are vulnerable to these beliefs. You can assist both parents and caregivers to understand these misconceptions and recognize factors in sound breastfeeding practices. Some of the more common misconceptions are cited in this section.

Breastmilk

Misconception: The best way to tell that a baby is getting enough milk is that the infant sleeps for several hours after each feeding.

Sleeping is not an indication of the baby receiving enough milk. The more calorically deprived a baby is, the more the baby will sleep. Gastric emptying time varies greatly from baby to baby (Geddes, 2009). Mothers need to watch for the number of wet diapers and bowel movements, the baby's disposition during and between feedings, and other growth indicators (see Chapter 13).

Misconception: It is important to wait at least 2 to 3 hours between feedings so the breast can refill and the baby does not use the mother as a pacifier.

The breast is never empty. As the baby removes milk, the breast produces more milk. The shorter the period between feedings, the higher the fat content of the milk (Kent et al., 2006). Waiting a specified period between feedings can decrease milk production and lessen the amount of fat the baby receives (see Chapter 7). Additionally, sucking is soothing to the baby. Babies should be pacified at the breast, rather than on a rubber nipple—the breast is for nurture in addition to nutrition.

Misconception: A mother cannot make enough milk for more than one baby.

Most women can make far more milk than their baby requires and, in fact, can regulate production to their singleton's needs. Wet nurses once nursed as many as five babies simultaneously and produced as much as 2230 mL of milk per day (see Chapter 1). Exclusive breastfeeding of twins is common; exclusive breastfeeding of triplets or higher-order multiples, while posing a time and energy management challenge, is biologically feasible (see Chapter 15).

Misconception: Weaning is recommended when mothers are taking medication.

The American Academy of Pediatrics (AAP) advises that most maternal use of medications does not require weaning (see Chapter 10). Refer to the latest edition of *Medications and Mothers' Milk* (Hale, 2010) for information about specific drugs. You can also join the Medications Forum at www.ibreastfeeding.com to learn more.

Feedings

Misconception: Breastfeeding mothers and babies require more of the caregiver's time than do those who bottle feed.

Mothers who room-in with their babies in the hospital assume more care of their babies, thereby freeing up hospital staff to perform other tasks (see Chapter 12). Mothers who receive anticipatory guidance and appropriate teaching make fewer phone calls and visits to the pediatrician (see Chapter 2).

Misconception: Time at the breast needs to be limited in the early days to prevent nipple soreness.

Poor positioning is the major cause of sore nipples, not the amount of time a baby nurses. Babies need unlimited access to the breast. Early, frequent feedings increase the mother's milk production and avoid complications (see the discussion later in this chapter). Time limits increase the incidence of jaundice and inadequate weight gain in the baby as well as the incidence of engorgement and low milk production in the mother.

Misconception: Even with time limits, most breastfeeding women will experience nipple soreness.

The vast majority of sore nipples are a result of poor positioning of the baby at the breast. Women typically experience brief moments of latch tenderness or initial transient nipple soreness that disappears within a few days to a week after beginning breastfeeding. This transient pain does not interfere with breastfeeding. Breastfeeding should be pain free throughout the feeding after the first minutes of the baby beginning to feed, and between feedings.

Misconception: Mothers don't need to start breastfeeding until their milk "comes in."

Colostrum is present from approximately the 4th month of pregnancy onward. Delaying the start of breastfeeding can lead to engorgement, a delay or decrease in milk production, and interference with the mother's instincts (see Chapter 12). Mothers should be given the opportunity to breastfeed within 1 hour of birth, followed by unrestricted feedings.

Misconception: Newborn babies typically need to eat every 4 hours.

Breastfeeding babies may want to nurse as frequently as every 1 to 2 hours in the early days. Enforced scheduling of feedings ignores hunger cues and interferes with mothering. By learning how to read hunger cues, mothers can trust their babies to determine the timing of feedings. See Chapter 13 regarding infant hunger cues, and see the discussion of feeding frequency later in this chapter.

Misconception: After the mother's milk production is established, the baby will usually take most of the milk in the first 5 to 7 minutes.

Each baby's breastfeeding pattern is different, and the baby should determine the end of the feeding rather than having arbitrary time limits imposed (see Chapter 14). Healthy babies know when they are full and will detach from the breast, satiated. As babies become older, they are able to remove milk more quickly. A mother has multiple letdowns throughout a feeding, so the baby should be in charge of determining when the feeding ends.

Misconception: Mothers need to nurse from both breasts at every feeding; therefore, the mother should limit sucking time on the first breast so the baby will take the second breast.

The amount of time it takes a baby to remove both foremilk and hindmilk from a breast is unique to each baby. If the mother removes her baby from the breast before he or she receives hindmilk, the infant may ingest large amounts of foremilk, depending on the fullness of the breast. This could result in colic-like behavior or poor weight gain. Some babies nurse from only one breast at a feeding and will follow this pattern for all feedings, whereas others may nurse from one breast until late afternoon or evening and then nurse from both. Others will always nurse from both breasts. Initially, encouraging the baby to take the second breast after he or she comes off the first independently stimulates milk production in both breasts.

Formula

Misconception: Artificial baby milk is just as healthy as human milk.

Cow's milk is healthiest for cows, just as human milk is healthiest for humans. Artificial baby milk is inherently inferior to human milk for human babies, because there are profound differences between artificial baby milk and human milk. See Chapter 9 for a detailed discussion of the properties of human milk and the health risks associated with use of infant formula.

Misconception: Breastfeeding is essentially an alternative to formula feeding.

Breastfeeding is much more than delivery of human milk. It is a dynamic bonding process, which reinforces the biological relationship between a mother and her baby. Breastfeeding involves people, not simply infant food (see Chapter 3). This point is an especially important reminder to give to adoptive mothers and mothers with low milk production.

Supplementation

Misconception: Bottles given to breastfeeding babies do not interfere with breastfeeding.

Any artificial nipple given to an infant in the early weeks of establishing breastfeeding has the potential to create a preference for the artificial nipple (see Chapter 21). It is not necessary to feed breastfeeding babies with a bottle in the early days postpartum to train them to accept a bottle later.

Misconception: Water supplementation will help prevent or reduce jaundice in breastfeeding infants.

A jaundiced baby needs the increased stooling facilitated by the child's consumption of colostrum. The correct response to jaundice is to increase the number and effectiveness of feedings. Water supplementation can decrease the amount of human milk a baby consumes, which can increase bilirubin levels and result in weight loss (see Chapter 22). Water does not coat the gut as human milk does and does not have the laxative effect of colostrum, which helps with the excretion of meconium. Giving water to the baby can reduce effective sucking at the breast, increase the incidence of engorgement, and cause nipple preference when given by bottle. It also reduces the baby's calorie consumption and ability to self-regulate intake.

Misconception: Formula supplementation is necessary when the mother has low milk production.

Most times the solution to perceived low milk production is to increase the frequency of feedings and ensure correct positioning and attachment (see Chapter 18). The mother and baby need a full assessment to determine if the mother truly has low milk production or if the baby is failing to transfer milk. Alternate massage (breast compression) during a feeding will help increase the volume of milk transferred. If the mother has a delayed onset of milk production or true insufficient milk production, use of donor milk is preferable over artificial milk. See Chapter 25 for a discussion of problems with milk production.

Supplementing with artificial baby milk by bottle may potentially result in nipple preference, difficulty with attachment, less time at the breast, and inadequate milk removal. Additionally, formula exposes the infant to a greater risk of disease and sensitizes the child to cow's milk protein (see Chapter 9). It can also cause the mother to doubt her competence or ability to breastfeed. Breastfeeding babies should receive no artificial baby milk unless medically indicated. If the problem lies with the baby and not with the mother's milk production, the first choice for supplementation is the mother's pumped milk. If formula supplementation is medically necessary, as in the rare case of phenylketonuria (PKU), or if donated human milk is unavailable, formula should be given by the method that will interfere least with breastfeeding (see Chapter 21). As a lactation consultant, you should be sensitive to the parents' ability to handle the supplementation without feeling overwhelmed, given the stress of caring for a baby with feeding problems.

∾ *Establishing Milk Production*

Milk, in the form of colostrum, is present in the human breast from approximately the 4th month of pregnancy onward. At birth, the delivery of the placenta triggers a reduction in the woman's progesterone levels, which are very high during pregnancy. Progesterone inhibits prolactin, which is also elevated during pregnancy. As progesterone levels fall precipitously after birth, prolactin release becomes effective, leading to lactogenesis II.

In addition, the increased amounts of blood and lymph fluid present in the breast provide the nutrients needed for milk production. These fluids cause the breasts to become fuller, heavier, and sometimes tender. This normal fullness diminishes as regular, frequent nursing progresses. By about 2 weeks postpartum, when lactation is well established, the breasts become comfortably soft and pliable, even when they are full with milk. Regular, frequent feedings will maintain this condition.

A woman's production of milk requires a functioning letdown response and adequate milk removal on a regular basis. The process of milk production is believed to occur through local autocrine control after the initial postpartum period (Ben-Jonathan et al., 2006, 2008; Brennan et al., 2007). Removal of milk is just as important as nipple stimulation and letdown in ensuring ongoing milk production. When a baby nurses frequently, there is greater nipple stimulation and greater removal of milk and, consequently, increased milk production. Thus, to ensure ample milk production, the mother will want to avoid missed feedings, especially in the early days when she is still establishing milk production.

During the first month of life, the baby establishes patterns of milk intake that will continue through the next 12 months (Kent et al., 2006; Mitoulas et al., 2002). Parents need to avoid strict schedules for feeding, instead allowing the baby to lead the feedings. This flexibility supports the individual nature of infant needs and each mother's rate of milk synthesis and storage capacity. Each baby's feeding pattern reflects the infant's own internal rhythm.

One Breast or Two?

In the first few days of life, feedings may last only 10 to 15 minutes. In early feedings, it is common for the baby to nurse on only one breast at each feeding and then drift off to sleep. When put to the other breast, the infant may be too drowsy or too full to nurse. This drowsiness is due in part to the release of cholecystokinin (CCK) in the infant's system during sucking. A gastrointestinal hormone, CCK enhances digestion and sedation and induces a feeling of satiation and well-being. The baby's sucking releases CCK in both the baby and the mother. The baby's CCK level peaks immediately after a feeding and again 30 to 60 min-

utes later (Uvnas-Moberg et al., 1993). If the mother puts the baby to breast on the side that has not yet been nursed during the time between the two peaks, the infant may arouse enough to nurse.

As the days pass, copious milk production begins and the baby becomes more alert. Feeding times will lengthen and the baby will be more likely to feed at both breasts at the same session. Encourage mothers to remain flexible, especially in the early days while the mother and her baby are both establishing themselves as partners in this new venture. Let the baby be the guide. If milk production is plentiful and the baby is gaining weight, a mother need not be concerned about her baby's refusal of the second breast. This pattern is common in the early days and may persist for many weeks.

One-breast feedings can be adequate (Kent et al., 2006). Indeed, some babies never nurse on both breasts at a feeding. If the mother experiences uncomfortable fullness of the second breast, she can encourage her baby to nurse on that side to relieve the fullness and prevent engorgement. She can then begin the next feeding on the side that is fuller. Mothers returning to work, school, or for another separation may pump the full breast and store the milk.

Duration of Feedings

In general, babies' needs should determine feeding length. When the flow of milk diminishes from one breast, sucking rate will move from long, drawing nutritive sucks to a faster, gentler suck. Their eyes will close, their fists will relax, and their hands will fall away from their face. Many times, the baby releases the breast; when this occurs at the end of a long period of nutritive sucking it usually signals that the baby is finished with that breast. Allowing babies to end the feeding on their own helps ensure that they have received the high-fat hindmilk needed for optimal growth. Mothers can then offer the other breast until babies end the feeding, either by detaching, or drifting off to sleep.

If the baby tends to "linger" at the breast, the mother can watch for a change from nutritive to nonnutritive sucking. Nonnutritive sucking after a lengthy feeding is a sign that the baby has drained the breast. Continuing to suck at this point does not provide the stimulation necessary for increasing milk production, so the mother can remove her baby from the breast without significantly affect milk quantity. Even so, mothers should be encouraged to gauge their baby's needs. Some babies need to spend more time sucking at the breast for comfort than others.

Place No Time Limits

Hospital procedures and other practices that restrict feeding frequency and duration are detrimental to the initiation of breastfeeding. Limiting the time spent on a breast can result in the baby's receiving foremilk from both breasts and becoming too full to obtain a significant amount of hindmilk from either breast. This type of high-volume, low-fat feeding can result in poor weight gain and colic-like symptoms. As babies mature, they become more efficient at extracting milk, and the time spent at the breast will usually decrease. Flexibility on the mother's part will allow for variations in her baby's nursing style, hunger, and daily temperament.

Unlimited sucking time beginning directly after birth improves breastfeeding duration (DiGirolamo et al., 2008; Abolyan, 2006; Hofvander, 2005; Merten et al., 2005). Until breast tissue becomes accustomed to sucking, mothers may experience some initial nipple discomfort that usually peaks between the 3rd and 6th days postpartum. Decreasing the time or frequency of feedings does not prevent this tenderness. Although nipple soreness results primarily from improper positioning of the baby at the breast, it may also be due to the change in hormones after birth—akin to the breast tenderness felt by many women during the menstrual cycle. The best insurance against soreness is using a nursing position that places the baby's body facing the mother and ensuring a deep latch. Using these techniques, the mother can be comfortable nursing for as long as her baby requires.

Frequency of Feedings

During the first month after birth, feeding frequency for a healthy, fully developed baby may range from 8 to 14 or more feedings daily. Most babies require at least 8 to 10 feedings each day. A baby who nurses more frequently may nurse as often as every 1 to 2 hours, with nighttime feedings spaced further apart. The AAP (2005) recommends that non-demanding babies be aroused to feed if 4 hours have elapsed since the beginning of the previous feeding. When it is clear that the baby is gaining weight well and is breastfeeding more than 8 times during a 24-hour period, the mother need not wake her baby at night.

It is common for a baby to feed as often as every hour or hour and a half during the day or several times during the night. Considering the baby's feeding pattern over the course of a day will help a mother determine if she is meeting her baby's requirements. For example, a mother whose baby has gained well; has breastfed 10 times during the daytime; had 6 clear, heavy wet diapers; and 3 to 5 ample stools can relax if the infant sleeps longer that night and can enjoy her extra rest! This situation is very different, for example, from that of a lethargic baby who must be awakened to nurse, who has only breastfed fitfully 4 times in 24 hours, and who has only had 1 small stool or no stool and 3 very yellow, strong voids. Such a baby is in trouble and needs immediate medical help. Help moth-

ers learn to watch their babies rather than clocks, while being cognizant of feeding effectiveness.

By 8 to 12 weeks of age, a baby has usually developed a pattern of feeding every 2 to 3 hours, sometimes less often during the night. The longer nighttime stretch may alternate with a period of almost constant wakefulness and sucking at some other time of the day, generally the early evening. These patterns are referred to as clustered or bunched feedings. As babies mature and become more efficient breastfeeders, they will obtain more milk in a shorter period and may begin to space feedings further apart.

When providing anticipatory guidance to mothers, let them know that babies seem to nurse more frequently when they are teething, getting sick, or about to achieve a new developmental milestone (e.g., rolling over, sitting up, or crawling). The wider and shorter intervals for feeding with older babies are just general observations, not rules or requirements. The baby's needs and reasons for nursing change as the infant develops.

Increases in Frequency

A mother may notice that periodically her baby wants to nurse more frequently. All babies experience periods of sudden growth during their early months—and they react to these growth spurts by feeding more frequently. Such periods of increased feedings usually last only a few days. Mothers who nurse in response to their babies' cues may not even notice growth spurts. Often, however, mothers are aware of fussiness in a previously contented baby, a baby who wants to nurse more frequently than usual, or a baby who has suddenly begun to nurse more vigorously. You can prepare the mother for these events before they occur, so that such incidents do not undermine her confidence or cause her to consider early weaning. Reassurance, support, and a listening ear can be pivotal to a mother who finds herself with a fussy baby requiring a lot of attention. Encourage her to respond to her baby's needs during this growing time.

Growth spurts can occur at any time, although some take place at predictable ages. Specifically, these events typically occur when the baby is between 10 days and 2 weeks old, around 6 weeks old, around 12 weeks old, and around 6 months old. The 6-month growth spurt may also coincide with the baby's readiness to start solid foods. Mothers who have established robust milk production through frequent breastfeeding in the early postpartum days can carry through during these times until the growth spurt has passed. It is important to educate families about growth spurts, so that the mother doesn't perceive the first occurrence as indicating a bout of insufficient milk production and begin supplementation in response.

First Days at Home A baby whose feedings were restricted during the hospital stay may nurse more frequently when allowed to establish his or her routine. At home, the infant may feel overstimulated by eager parents or siblings and turn to nursing for comfort. He or she may react to the dramatic difference between the hospital environment (the first extrauterine experience) and the home, particularly at night. Although home births have better health and breastfeeding outcomes for infants, babies can still feel overstimulated by excited family members. Conversely, some babies may cope with overstimulation by sleeping, thereby missing feedings. Lowering excessive "noise" associated with today's frantic, high-tech lifestyles provides a soothing environment for the newborn.

Ten to Fourteen Days   The baby experiences a growth spurt approximately 10 to 14 days after birth and will want to nurse more often during this period. It is around this time that the mother may lose the initial fullness in her breasts. She may worry that increased feedings and smaller breasts indicate that her milk production is dwindling. Anticipatory guidance can help mitigate these concerns, which might otherwise cause the mother to question her ability to nourish her baby. Teaching parents to expect increased frequency in the baby's hunger around this time helps forestall worries about low milk production.

In the United States, samples of artificial baby milk will predictably arrive on parents' doorsteps during this span of time. Formula manufacturers obtain expectant- and new-parent information from direct marketing firms and mailing lists sold to them by retail stores, Internet orders or browsing, parenting magazines, and other sources (International Baby Food Action Network [IBFAN], 2007; Walker, 2007). This practice coincides with the 2-week growth spurt and exploits mothers' concerns at this stage. Chapter 28 discusses the sometimes unethical practices of the formula industry in more detail.

Three to Six Weeks   In addition to feeding more often in conjunction with a second growth spurt that occurs at around 3 to 6 weeks after birth, the baby may nurse more often in response to an increase in the mother's activity level at this time. By 6 weeks, mothers often resume many or all of their prepregnancy activities, including a return to work or school. The increase in activity may result in fewer feedings and reduced milk production. The baby's response is to nurse more frequently to rebuild milk production. The infant also may go to the breast more frequently for reassurance that his mother is still available for comfort.

Three and Six Months   As the baby continues to grow, feeding frequency will increase periodically to meet caloric needs. These growth spurts typically occur at about 3 and 6 months. The mother may incorrectly interpret these increased feedings as a sign of her baby's readiness to begin solid foods. Again, anticipatory guidance will prevent mothers from misinterpreting the increase in feeding frequency around 3 months as a need for other foods. Nevertheless, many babies are ready to begin solid foods at around 6 months of age; parents need to watch their infants for signs of readiness (see Chapter 17).

Other Increases in Feedings   Illness, overstimulation, emotional upset, or physical discomfort may cause a baby to turn to the breast for security and comfort. As a lactation consultant, you can help the mother through these times by reminding her that babies nurse for comfort as well as for nutrition. Remind her that when a baby is sick, she produces antibodies to the virus and passes these antibodies back to her baby. Breastfeeding is the only time in a mother's life when she will be able to protect her baby in this unique way. Being able to comfort her baby at the breast is one of the marvelous benefits of breastfeeding.

Studies have shown that breastfeeding relieves pain in infants (Shah et al., 2007; Gray et al., 2006), including the pain associated with medical procedures. Shah's review found that breastfeeding infants had smaller increases in heart rate, reduced crying time, and reduced duration of crying compared to neonates who were swaddled or who received pacifiers. Another study found breastfeeding to be analgesic to at least 6 months of age (Dilli et al., 2009).

Decreases in Frequency

A mother often becomes concerned when her baby begins dropping feedings, especially if she has not yet begun giving solid foods or other supplements. She may worry that the infant is not being nourished sufficiently if daily frequency suddenly drops from 8 or 9 to 6 or 7 feedings. This decrease in frequency is common when the baby reaches about 3 months of age. As babies grow, they obtain a greater amount of milk in a shorter period and sometimes go longer between feedings.

Encourage the mother to observe her baby's overall disposition and health. If the baby appears content, is voiding and stooling appropriately, gaining weight and height, and has good skin tone, she will know her child is well nourished and there is no cause for worry. If, however, decreased feedings occur when the baby is unhealthy or has inadequate growth, encourage the mother to contact her baby's healthcare provider immediately. A breastfeeding assessment is appropriate in these circumstances.

Signs of Sufficient Milk

There are a number of ways a mother can tell when her baby is receiving enough milk. Wet and soiled diapers are the best indication. Sufficient urine output to soak at least 6 or more regular diapers by the 4th day postpartum indicates adequate milk volume. The urine should be clear to pale yellow by this time, with no strong odor (as long as supplemental fluids are not given). If super-absorbent diapers are used, the number of diapers may be fewer. After day 4 or 5, stooling also indicates adequate milk transfer. In the first month, the baby should stool 3 or more times daily. Parents should call their baby's practitioner any time in the first month if their baby goes several days without producing at least 3 yellow, seedy stools larger than a quarter per day (see Color Plate 27). They should also call the provider immediately if the baby produces dark yellow voids, urea crystals (brick dust), or fewer than 6 wet diapers per day after the 4th or 5th day of life—these are all signs of dehydration.

As long as a baby is not typically placid or fussy, a pleasant disposition generally is a sign of adequate nourishment. A mother needs to understand that crying does not necessarily mean that her baby is hungry. Instead, she should be alert to other indications of adequate nourishment. Regular intervals of wakefulness, sleep, and feeding reassure a mother that she is providing her baby with enough milk. Healthy skin tone and color, alertness, engagement, and sustained eye contact are other signs of proper nourishment.

An infant's growth pattern shows whether he or she is thriving on the mother's milk. The most obvious signs are fat creases in the arms and legs, and outgrowing clothing. The mother should look for increases in length and head size, as well as regular weight gain. Weight loss of as much as 7 percent of birth weight during the first week of life is common. If feedings are restricted or ineffective in the early days, this weight loss can be as high as 10 or 12 percent. More frequent breastfeeding usually helps the baby regain the lost weight and return to birth weight by day 10. On the other hand, babies who nurse frequently from birth usually experience less initial weight loss and more rapid weight gain. Assure mothers that frequent and effective nursing creates the right amount of milk for the baby.

A mother whose baby has lost 10 percent of birth weight will likely be advised to supplement feedings. In such a case, the first choice as supplement should be the mother's own milk. She may find hand expression to be more effective in removing colostrum prior to Stage II lactogenesis. In addition, the baby's feeding ability needs to be assessed to identify the reason for the weight loss. Explore whether the mother received too many fluids during labor and delivery, whether feedings are too infrequent or ineffective, and whether the mother has impaired milk production or delayed onset of milk production. A complete feeding assessment will help determine the cause. Weight loss can also be sign of infection. If you encounter a baby whose mother has ample milk production and the baby transfers milk but is losing weight, an infection or other organic problem could be the root cause. Report this condition to the baby's doctor right away. Chapter 18 discusses problems and treatment of low milk production in more detail.

~ Leaking

It is common for women to experience milk leaking from their breasts during the first few weeks of breastfeeding. In most cases, leaking results from breast fullness or the mother's milk letting down. Leaking is a normal part of the process of breastfeeding. It can occur during a feeding from the opposite breast, directly before a feeding when the breasts are full, or if the mother misses a feeding entirely. The range of leaking is extremely variable from one woman to another.

For many women, milk leaking from the breast is an encouraging sign of plentiful milk production and indicates that their letdown reflex is functioning well. In most cases, leaking will subside as harmony develops between the baby's needs and the mother's milk production, usually by 6 weeks postpartum.

Failure to leak milk is not an indication that milk production is low. Indeed, many women never experience leaking. An absence of leaking may indicate that the sphincter muscles within the nipple function well to close off the nipple pores. It is possible that a mother whose breasts do not leak is feeding more frequently and, therefore, is less prone to leaking.

Causes of Leaking

Leaking can be caused by overly full breasts, stimulation during lovemaking, frequent milk expression, clothing that rubs against the nipples, overproduction of milk, or hormone imbalances. It may be a result of psychological conditioning of the mother's milk ejection reflex. A woman may leak in response to hearing a baby cry, picking up her baby to nurse, or simply thinking about breastfeeding or her baby. Oxytocin release also occurs during orgasm, which triggers the letdown reflex.

Controlling Leaking

Although women generally consider leaking to be a nuisance, they usually accept it as a part of breastfeeding and use appropriate measures to control it. Assure mothers that this phase of lactation passes quickly. The following techniques are suggested as ways to control leaking:

- Press the heel of the hand over the breast, or cross both arms and press them over the breasts.
- Wear absorbent breast pads and change them often.
- Feed the baby before sexual intercourse and use absorbent towels over bedding.
- Decrease pressure on the breast and elastic in the bra cup; loosen the bra or wear a larger size.
- Express or pump milk when it is necessary to miss or delay a feeding.

- Wear dark, patterned clothing or a sweater to conceal moist spots.
- Check for the use of medications or herbs that stimulate milk production, and discontinue their use if the mother's milk production is abundant.

Excessive or Inappropriate Leaking

Occasionally, a woman's leaking is excessive, or she may experience leaking past the early weeks of establishing breastfeeding. Excessive leaking can be a sign of an imbalance in other body functions. In some women, milk production greatly exceeds the baby's needs. In others, leaking continues after the baby weans or occurs at times unrelated to birth or breastfeeding. Such milk production post-weaning is termed galactorrhea, also referred to as spontaneous lactation.

Inappropriate milk production in a nonlactating breast may result from the use of medications such as thyrotropin-releasing hormones, theophyllines, amphetamines, opioids, or tranquilizers (Katz & Mazer, 2009; Racey et al., 2009). Chest or breast surgery, a fibrocystic breast, or herpes zoster may also stimulate nerves enough to induce milk production significantly. In some cases, a woman's body may be especially sensitive to normal levels of prolactin. If no underlying disorder is found through medical examination, the mother may find a decrease in breast stimulation to be helpful.

Galactorrhea is a symptom, not a disease. In particular, it may indicate an underlying health problem that causes elevated prolactin levels (hyperprolactinemia). Possible causes of hyperprolactinemia include hypothyroidism, hyperthyroidism, use of psychosis and anxiety medications, chronic renal failure, pituitary tumors, and uterine and ovarian tumors. Abnormal lactation may also occur in connection with surgery and stress related to such tumors.

Any unexplainable excessive milk flow during lactation, or milk production that continues beyond 3 to 6 months after the baby weans, is not normal. In such a case, the woman should be encouraged to have a complete physical examination. Infrequently, mothers may use medications to suppress lactation, but these medications are often only temporary measures. Generally, treatment of galactorrhea requires addressing the underlying cause (Lawrence & Lawrence, 2005).

～ Nipple Soreness

Although sore nipples occur with relative frequency, they are not an inevitable part of breastfeeding. Initial tenderness, or transient nipple soreness, is part of the typical postpartum course for the majority of mothers (Rebhan et al., 2008; Cadwell, 2007; de Oliveira et al., 2006).

Women often describe this condition as tenderness with the initial latch and first few sucks. The peak period of nipple tenderness occurs in the 1st week postpartum, particularly between the 3rd and 6th days after birth. It is possible that this period of tenderness is associated with the breast adjusting to the frequency of use in breastfeeding or to hormonal changes postpartum.

Pain is a sign that something is not right within the body—and this statement applies to nipple pain during breastfeeding as well. Nipple pain requires investigation if it occurs beyond the transient soreness of the first week or lasts after the first few sucks following attachment. Such pain can constitute a breastfeeding emergency because it is a common reason for early weaning. Nursing on a sore nipple is similar to painful friction on a scraped knee or knuckle. If left untreated, nipple pain can progress to the development of a crack. Such an open sore allows entry of bacteria and yeast that are present on the skin surface and may lead to infection. In addition, the increased severity of pain when untreated can decrease a woman's desire to put her baby to the breast. This, in turn, can lead to engorgement, reduced milk production, and premature weaning.

Causes and Prevention of Nipple Soreness

Numerous myths abound regarding the cause of nipple soreness, which the lactation consultant can help to dispel. One long-held belief states that a baby left too long on the breast will cause soreness; we now know this not to be true. Women were once encouraged to "toughen" their nipples prenatally with the hope of avoiding soreness—an unpleasant and unnecessary practice that damages nipple skin. There is also a belief that fair-skinned women are prone to nipple soreness. Atkinson's research (1979) corroborated this relationship, but Hewat and Ellis (1987) did not find a correlation.

Many cultural and commercial treatments for sore nipples exist, as discussed later in this section. Mothers need current, evidence-based information, especially when they receive questionable advice (often from older relatives or older healthcare providers). At the same time, you should remain sensitive to cultural beliefs and validate mothers' choices of long-held folk practices. When mothers receive suggestions that have been disproven or have limited validity, a tactful response may begin, "Yes, that is what practitioners have thought for years. New research now shows . . . ."

In an effort to not scare women, some breastfeeding advocates may downplay the possibility of nipple pain in the immediate postpartum period. It is important that mothers' complaints of nipple pain be neither minimized nor discounted. The truth is that perceptions of pain vary widely, and what might not be even noticeable to one mother may prove excruciating to another. Asking a mother to quantify her pain can help you determine if it is transient or symptomatic of true latch and sucking problems. The pain scale of 0 to 10, widely used by healthcare providers, is a helpful starting point, especially since mothers may have used it in labor and delivery.

Positioning and Attachment

The most common cause of nipple soreness is the manner in which the baby is latched to the breast. Prevention of nipple soreness requires correct positioning of the baby's body and attachment of the baby's mouth on the breast. Nursing is difficult when the baby does not face the breast and must swallow with his or her head turned to the side, flexed down to the chest, or tipped too far back. The mother's breast also experiences extra tension and negative pressure when poor positioning is used. In addition, bringing the baby to breast slightly off-center for an asymmetrical latch will help achieve a deep latch (see Figure 15.5 in Chapter 15). Prenatal education needs to emphasize these aspects of latch and postpartum caregivers need correct information regarding latch and positioning assessment.

Poor latch is frequently evident after the early introduction of an artificial nipple from a bottle or pacifier. Sucking on a bottle nipple is very different from sucking at the breast. With breastfeeding, the baby's sucking controls milk flow unless the mother's letdown is strong. With bottle feeding, the rate of flow is much faster, even with "slow-flow" nipples. In addition, milk flows from the bottle until the caregiver stops it. When mothers combine breastfeeding and bottle feeding during the time they are establishing breastfeeding, it may produce an unenthusiastic and incorrect suck when the baby returns to the breast. For all these reasons, artificial nipples should be avoided in the early days of breastfeeding unless used therapeutically (Wilson-Clay & Hoover, 2008; Kassing, 2002) or unless a bottle is the only alternative feeding device parents will accept.

Sucking Pressure

Sometimes nipple pain may result from anomalies in the infant's oral structure, such as ankyloglossia, a short tongue, or a high or bubble palate. Such anatomical differences can create difficulty with sucking (see Chapter 13). Clenching and compressing the nipple is common with late preterm, SGA, low-birth-weight (LBW), and post-term babies, due to their generally thin cheeks and sparse buccal fat pads. A very eager nurser combined with minimal milk flow in the first day or two may lead to pain, as can a mother pulling her baby off the breast without first breaking suction.

Strong pain due to sucking pressure beyond the first 4 or 5 days after birth, when mature milk should be established, might indicate the mother has low milk flow. In such circumstances, the baby increases sucking intensity in an effort to obtain milk. The center of the mother's nipple will often appear to have a bruise or "hickey" when this increased pressure occurs. Measurements of vacuum pressure in babies' mouths have revealed that infants of mothers who experienced continued pain with feeding had much higher baseline negative pressure and significantly lower milk intake (McClellan et al., 2008), despite professional help with positioning and latch. The reasons for the higher vacuum pressure are not clear.

Another infant response is to clamp down if the mother has a strong letdown. The baby may compress the nipple and areola to try to stop the overwhelming gush of milk. Sometimes the baby will slide down onto the nipple, or come off the breast choking or sputtering.

Other Factors

Nipple pain may also result from factors related to nipple shape, engorgement, or improper use of breast pumps or nipple shields. Breast and nipple skin can be tender from thrush (see Color Plate 38), impetigo, or eczema (International Lactation Consultant Association [ILCA], 2007). In addition, psoriasis (see Color Plate 39), herpes (see Color Plate 40), and poison ivy (see Color Plate 41) can damage the skin. Bacterial infection of the breast is common (Delgado et al., 2008, 2009; Kvist et al., 2008; Amir et al., 2006), and sensitivity to topical ointments can occur.

Assessment of Sore Nipples

Nipple soreness requires in-person assessment to determine the cause and suggest appropriate measures. It is important to note the age of the baby and when the soreness began. The mother's description of how the pain feels and at which times it feels a certain way can yield clues to the cause. Asking open-ended questions will help you elicit descriptive adjectives from the mother. "Burning" pain may indicate thrush; "throbbing" may indicate mastitis. Pain upon exposure to cold may indicate a vasospasm or even Raynaud's phenomenon. Note any chronic conditions of the mother, and identify medication usage. Ask about the use of soaps, creams, lotions, laundry products, and perfumes, especially recent product changes. Nipple soreness may also develop when the baby begins teething, or when the mother begins menstruating or becomes pregnant. Your assessment should address these milestones. Table 16.1 profiles a variety of breast conditions that can lead to nipple soreness.

Level of Soreness

Descriptors many lactation professionals use for nipple soreness include such terms as "cracked," "macerated," and "abraded." Mohrbacher (2008) developed a grading scale for identifying the severity of nipple trauma, similar

TABLE 16.1 A Comparison of Breast Conditions

Condition	Definition	Erythema	Skin Temperature	Edema of Skin	Description	Systemic Symptoms	Fever	Pain	Unilateral Versus Bilateral	Other
Breast fullness	The breast is full of milk but without obstruction of venous or lymphatic drainage, and the milk flows readily with suckling or pumping.	No	Occasionally increased	No	Firm, heavy	No	No	No	Usually bilateral	Occurs between postpartum days 3–5 when the "milk comes in"
Engorgement	The breast is "engorged" with milk and there is obstruction of venous and lymphatic drainage, which impedes the flow of milk with suckling or pumping.	Bilateral	Generalized warmth	Yes	Hard, enlarged, shiny	May have "milk fever"	< 38.4°C	Yes, generalized	Usually bilateral	Often confused with breast fullness
Blocked ducts (also termed "focal breast engorgement," "caked breast," or "plugged duct")	The breast has an area of localized milk stasis.	Often over a palpable lump	Little or no heat	No	Single lumpy area	Unlikely	Unlikely and if present < 38.4°C	Tender or pain is localized	Usually unilateral	May occur with a painful white bleb on the nipple (the bleb may be opened up with a sterile needle to relieve discomfort)

(Continued)

383

TABLE 16.1 A Comparison of Breast Conditions (*Continued*)

Condition	Definition	Erythema	Skin Temperature	Edema of Skin	Description	Systemic Symptoms	Fever	Pain	Unilateral Versus Bilateral	Other
Galactocele	A milk-retention cyst that is thought to result from a plugged duct.	No	No	No	Smooth rounded swelling	No	No	No	Usually unilateral	Compression of the cyst may cause milky fluid to exude from the nipple
Noninfectious mastitis (also termed "obstructive mastitis")	Secondary to ineffective and/or obstructed drainage of milk from the breast.	Yes	Warm to hot	Yes	Hard, usually wedge shaped	Yes in 50%-66% of women	Mild, < 37.5°C; acute, > 37.4°C– < 38.5°C; hyperacute: > 38°C	Yes, localized	Usually unilateral	See note*
Infectious mastitis	Results from untreated milk stasis and/or colonization with pathogenic bacteria.	Yes, usually but not always	Warm to hot	Yes	Hard, usually wedge shaped	No in 33%–50% of women	Mild, < 37.5°C; acute, > 37.4°C– < 38.5°C; hyperacute: > 38°C	Usually	Usually unilateral but may be bilateral	See note*
Breast abscess	A localized area of infection that has formed a barrier of granulation tissue.	Yes	Hot	Yes	Swollen lump, possibly fluctuant	May or may not be present	Severe	Often unilateral but may be bilateral	In neglected cases, the skin may be discolored with necrosis	

*The clinician cannot reliably differentiate non-infectious mastitis clinically from infectious mastitis. Treat with antibiotics if the mother is toxic/acutely ill, there are severe or bilateral symptoms, there are nipple fissures, or symptom resolution does not occur within 12 to 24 hours of improved milk removal.

Source: Betzold CM. Update on the recognition and management of lactational breast inflammation: differential diagnosis: infectious versus noninfectious mastitis. *J Midwifery Women's Health.* 2007;52(6):595–605. http://www.medscape.com/viewarticle/565616. Printed with permission of Elsevier Ltd.

to terms used in the medical field for other types of wounds. Table 16.2 outlines these four stages of nipple trauma, ranging from a superficial and intact nipple to one with deep damage throughout the dermis. These descriptors help lactation professionals quantify the severity of nipple damage in a consistent way with a common definition. They clarify whether the skin is broken and, if so, how deep the damage goes. Color Plates 42 through 45 illustrate each stage in this grading scale.

When assessing nipple soreness, note the appearance of the nipple before the feeding. If you observe signs of infection (angry, red streaks; swelling; pus), refer the mother to her caregiver right away. Have the mother attach the baby and nurse briefly. It is essential to see the baby's attachment and positioning during a feeding. You need to observe the baby's alignment and closeness to the breast, the mother's position, and the mouth–breast connection, as described in Chapter 14. After the feeding has progressed for a few minutes, ask the mother to remove the baby from the breast so you can examine the nipple. Blanching or flattening of the nipple indicates poor latch, as does the nipple appearing rounded at the top and flattened at the base.

If the mother reports that she ends feedings, rather than allowing the baby to self-detach, observe her technique. Pulling her baby off the breast without breaking suction can cause nipple pain and skin damage. Visually assess the baby's oral structure, paying close attention to the tongue, palate, labial frenum, and lingual frenulum. If no obvious cause can be found by observing the feeding, perform a digital exam of the baby's oral structure. Explain each step to the parents as you do it, both to educate and to reassure (see Chapter 21). Also explain the reasons for allowing the baby to end feedings.

Cracked Nipples

When soreness persists, a crack or fissure can develop, either crosswise or lengthwise along the nipple (see Color Plate 46). Infrequently a woman's nipple may fold over, causing a stress point at the fold. Bleeding may result during nursing when the baby stretches the nipple to twice its resting length. A significant amount of blood may cause vomiting or produce black stools. The baby's caregiver may want to interrupt breastfeeding for a short time to rule out internal bleeding. If the baby has black stools or vomits blood because of the cracked nipples, the symptoms will cease when the infant stops nursing.

When the integrity of the nipple skin has been compromised, the open wound serves as a pathway for bacteria into the mother's body and allows for the development of mastitis (breast inflammation or infection—discussed later in this chapter). It is important for the mother to cleanse her nipples. She may benefit from use of an antibacterial ointment such as mupirocin or polysporin, just as she would in case of a scraped knee or other open sore. If she applies the ointment after nursing, the ointment should be fully absorbed by the skin before the next feeding and not need to be wiped off. If the mother is concerned about the baby ingesting the ointment, she can gently wipe off any residue before nursing again. Encourage the mother to ask her caregiver for a recommended topical ointment.

Figure 16.1 presents the formula for a compounded ointment for treatment of cracked nipples that has found wide acceptance in Canada and the United States. Most compounding pharmacies have become proficient in preparing this ointment, which is available by prescription. The combination presented here gives a total volume

---

TABLE 16.2 Scale of Nipple Pain and Trauma

Stage I	Superficial intact	Color Plate 42	• Pain or irritation with no skin breakdown
Stage II	Superficial with tissue breakdown	Color Plate 43	• Could include redness (erythema), bruising (ecchymosis), red spots (petechiae), edema (swelling) • Pain reported • Could include abrasion, shallow crack or fissure, compression stripe, hematoma, shallow ulceration
Stage III	Partial thickness erosion	Color Plate 44	• Skin breakdown includes the destruction of the epidermis to the lower layers of the dermis • Could include deep fissure, blister, deep ulceration with more advanced erosion
Stage IV	Full thickness erosion	Color Plate 45	• Deeper damage through the dermis • Could include full erosion of some parts of the nipple

Source: Printed with permission of Ameda.

Mupirocin 2 percent ointment (not cream): 15 grams

Betamethasone 0.1 percent ointment (not cream): 15 grams

Add miconazole powder so that the final concentration is 2 percent miconazole

May also add ibuprofen powder, so that the final concentration of ibuprofen is 2 percent.

FIGURE 16.1 Dr. Jack Newman's all-purpose nipple ointment.

of approximately 30 g. clotrimazole powder to a final concentration of 2 percent may be substituted if miconazole powder is unavailable (Newman & Kernerman, 2009a).

If other healing methods prove ineffective, the mother may wish to interrupt breastfeeding for a day or two until her nipples heal. She can express her milk during that time. Table 16.3 summarizes the treatment options for cracked nipples.

Addressing the Cause

If positioning appears to be the cause of nipple soreness, help the mother make the necessary adjustments. The baby should be level with and facing the breast, with his or her body and head aligned. If the mother has been using only one position to nurse, using another position can provide relief to the sore area. The mother's body position is also important. If her arms tire during a feeding, the baby may not remain level with the breast and could slip down and exert more pressure on the nipple or slide to the nipple base.

Correcting Latch

The baby latch must consistently be latched effectively for milk transfer to occur as well as to ensure the mother's

comfort. The baby's mouth should open wide and optimally should be slightly off-center from the nipple. Because only the lower jaw moves, positioning the mouth so that the baby takes in more of the underside of the nipple will help compress the ducts most effectively. To encourage the baby to open wider, the mother can use a nursing position aided by gravity, such as the side-sitting (football or clutch) hold. Babies mimic facial expressions of others, so the mother can demonstrate a wide-open mouth and repeatedly say, "o . . . p . . . e . . . n," as the baby works to latch. This is useful for a baby who "chews" onto the nipple. The lips should flange outward, and the mouth should have a wide angle when the baby begins sucking. The mother needs to watch for correct lip placement and help her baby flange either or both lips when needed.

Babies who bite at the breast often respond well to prone positioning with the baby self-attaching, providing chin support or sublingual pressure (gentle pressure under the chin). Jaw clenching can cause nipple vasospasms (constriction of blood vessels within the nipple), identified by pain and blanching of the nipple. To avoid this problem, the mother can work with her baby to establish a good latch. Some helpful video clips demonstrating correct latch techniques can be found at various breastfeeding websites (see Appendix H).

Vasospasms

Vasospasms of the nipple during breastfeeding create a Raynaud-like phenomenon. Mothers have described this pain as stinging, tingling, burning, very painful, and persisting after the feeding. This phenomenon is characterized by a triphasic color change with the nipple turning white (blanches), then blue (cyanotic), and then red (rubor) (Page & McKenna, 2006; Anderson et al., 2004; Lawlor-Smith & Lawlor-Smith, 1997). Raynaud's phenomenon is a common condition that affects as many as 22 percent of women aged 21 to 50 (Olsen & Nielson,

TABLE 16.3 Causes and Treatment of Cracked Nipples

Causes	Actions for the Mother
All causes of sore nipples carried to extreme	• Consult physician about using ibuprofen, acetaminophen, or other painkiller. • Improve nutritional status, increasing protein, vitamin C, and zinc. • Refer to actions for sore nipples.
Nipple folds over (crack may appear at fold)	• Air dry breasts after feeding.
Local infection (baby with staph or other organism may have infected mother's nipples)	• Have physician check nipples, culture baby's throat and mother's nipples, and treat accordingly.
Baby overly eager at feedings	• Respond to feeding cues promptly. • Limit nursing times to 10 minutes per breast until nipple heals. • Pre-express milk to hasten letdown. • Nurse in a position that does not aggravate crack.

1978). Some mothers with nipple vasospasms report that this pain also occurs when they are exposed to cold, which is a marker for Raynaud's phenomenon. During breast-feeding, vasospasms may be caused by the baby compressing the breast so tightly as to interrupt blood flow to the nipple. Addressing the latch or cause for the compression may resolve the problem.

Treatment for vasospasm includes avoiding cold and applying heat to the nipples after a feeding. Caffeine and nicotine constrict blood vessels and have been shown to increase the severity of Raynaud's-related pain; thus removing caffeine from the mother's diet may bring relief. Increasing intake of vitamin B_6 has helped some mothers. Use caution when recommending supplementation with this vitamin, however, as high doses (e.g., 600 mg) can lower milk production. Additionally, vitamin B_6 passes readily into a mother's milk and too much can harm an infant's liver (Hale, 2010). Hale suggests not consuming more than 25 mg/day of vitamin B_6. Calcium-channel blockers, such as nifedipine, have been helpful for some mothers (Hale & Berens, 2002).

Many times, the lactation consultant's validation that a mother's nipple pain is abnormal and has a cause is a big relief to the new mother. See Chapter 25 for further discussion of Raynaud's phenomenon.

Ankyloglossia

Ankyloglossia, or tongue-tie, is a common cause of breast-feeding pain (see Color Plate 22). If the baby's lingual frenulum is too tight and the tongue is unable to extend over the lower lip, the frenulum may need to be clipped. A tight labial frenum on the upper lip (see Color Plate 23)

could also cause problems. See Chapter 13 for more information on oral anomalies. Refer the mother to a provider versed in assessment of this condition for evaluation and treatment of the infant, if appropriate.

Other Causes of Soreness

If dried milk sticks to the mother's bra or breast pads, she can avoid nipple damage by moistening the fabric before removing them. If the mother has been pulling her baby off the breast without releasing suction, she can learn to break suction with her finger between the baby's gums before removing the infant. When her soreness is relieved, she needs to understand the importance of allowing her baby to determine when to end the feeding. Pain connected to a retracted or inverted nipple may find relief from techniques that gently encourage eversion of the nipple, as described in Chapter 7.

Relieving Nipple Soreness

After identifying the cause of nipple pain, it is important to institute a plan for palliative care (care that provides pain relief) to address the mother's immediate physical comfort. The mother's care plan may combine alterations in her breastfeeding technique, pain relief, and applications to heal the skin. Use of a product that serves as a "quick fix" can be tempting. Some mothers may find an ointment or gel pad comforting, while others will prefer not to use them. Experience will help you become proficient at discerning the difference. Table 16.4 summarizes the treatment options for sore nipples.

TABLE 16.4 Causes and Treatment of Sore Nipples

Causes	Actions for the Mother
Soreness from newborn suckling	• Check to ensure that baby is put on and comes off breast properly. • Check to ensure that nipple is back far enough in baby's mouth. • Hold baby closely during nursing so nipple is not being pulled. • Use pure anhydrous lanolin or hydrogel pad as a temporary comfort measure.
Dried colostrum or milk causing nipple to stick to bra or breast pads	• Moisten bra or pads before taking off so as not to remove keratin.
Poor positioning	• Bring baby close to nurse, so he does not pull on breast. • Bring baby to breast so that he has a big mouthful of breast tissue.
Baby chewing or nuzzling onto nipple	• Form nipple for baby. • Set up pattern of getting baby onto breast, using rooting reflex.
Baby nursing on end of nipple	• Ensure that baby is positioned properly at breast. • Check for tight frenulum. • Check for inverted nipple. • Check for engorgement.

(Continued)

TABLE 16.4   Causes and Treatment of Sore Nipples (*Continued*)

Causes	Actions for the Mother
Baby chewing his way off nipple or nipple being pulled out of baby's mouth at end of feeding	• Remove baby from breast by placing a finger between baby's gums to ensure suction is broken. • End feeding when baby's sucking slows, before he begins to chew on nipple.
Baby overly eager to nurse	• Respond to feeding cues promptly. • Pre-express milk to hasten letdown and avoid vigorous sucking.
Inadequate letdown	• Use massage and relaxation before feedings. • Condition letdown by setting up routine for getting baby onto breast.
Nipples not allowed to dry	• Check for leaking milk. • Check that there are no plastic liners in breast pads. • Eliminate synthetic fabrics in bra and clothing; wear cotton or cotton blends. • Air dry breasts after feedings. • Change breast pads frequently.
Improper use of nipple shield	• Use shield only to draw nipple out, then have baby nurse on breast. • Avoid shields with inner ridges that irritate nipples.
Inadequate milk supply; baby tugging or sucking on empty breast	• Nurse more frequently (every 1 to 1½ hours). • Nurse long enough to facilitate good milk production.
Nipple skin not resistant to stress	• Improve diet, especially adding fresh fruits and vegetables and vitamin supplements. • Eliminate or decrease use of sugary foods, alcohol, caffeine, and cigarettes. • Check for use of cleansing or drying agents.
Natural oils being removed or keratin layers broken down by drying agents such as soap, alcohol, shampoo, or deodorant	• Eliminate irritants. • Wash breasts with water only. • Use lanolin or hydrogel pads after air drying.
Nipple irritated by going braless under rough clothing or by rubbing against bra during vigorous exercise	• Wear a bra or change to one with more support (sports bra). • Wear softer fabric blouse.
Residue of laundry products present on clothing	• Use less detergent, and rinse wash loads twice. • Try different laundry products.
Teething causes increased feedings, chomping down on nipple, irritation by a change in baby's saliva or medication used for baby's gums	• Wash breast after every feeding in plain warm water to remove baby's saliva or other irritants. • Breastfeed before giving solid foods rather than after. • Use soothing techniques instead of nursing to comfort baby. • Stop feeding after the first incident of biting and resume when baby is more hungry. • Keep finger ready to break suction and stop feeding when sucking pattern changes.
Baby falls asleep and clamps down on breast	• Remove baby before he falls asleep.
Teeth marks on breast (not usually cause for soreness but mother may say baby is biting)	• Alternate nursing positions.
Irritation from food particles in toddler's mouth	• Check toddler's mouth before feedings. • Offer toddler a sip of water or wipe his mouth with clean moist cloth before nursing. • Breastfeed before offering solid foods.
Mother menstruating or pregnant	• If menstruating, discomfort will last only a few days. • If pregnant, discuss plans for continued nursing or weaning.
Thrush (a yeastlike infection; see discussion thrush)	• Have physician check and prescribe medication for both of mother and baby. • Discard or boil any items that baby puts in his mouth.

There is no substitute for the lactation consultant's time, clinical judgment, and education of the mother on the basics of optimal latch and positioning for comfortable nursing. If pain persists, validate the mother's concerns and do not minimize her perceptions of pain (Morland-Schutz & Hill, 2005).

Alterations in Breastfeeding Technique

Starting a feeding with the least sore breast first will avoid the stronger sucking that occurs at the beginning of a feeding. Moreover, pumping for a couple of minutes before a feeding to initiate the milk ejection reflex will make milk readily available to the baby and reduce the stronger sucking. Eliminating prolonged nonnutritive (comfort) sucking at the breast will reduce the amount of irritation and allow longer periods between feedings for the nipples to rest.

If necessary, the mother can perform alternate massage to help sustain sucking and swallowing and relieve long periods of negative pressure. In alternate massage, the mother massages and compresses the breast each time the baby pauses during a feeding.

Use of a nipple shield can reduce the friction of a baby that slides back and forth on the nipple. Select the size closest to the mother's nipple, and teach her how to apply the shield correctly. Refer to Chapter 21 for more information on appropriate use of nipple shields.

Teaching the mother a variety of nursing positions can help her choose the options that alleviate nipple soreness. To avoid further irritation to a sore spot, she can keep the baby's chin, and thus the tongue, away from that area. Thinking of her breast as a clock can help the mother describe the location of the soreness. In turn, you can suggest nursing positions to minimize further irritation. Figure 16.2 illustrates the relationship between the most common nursing positions and the resulting sore spots. Other positions, such as with the mother and baby lying down with the baby's feet pointing above the mother's head, will also provide relief for the mother and distribute stress more evenly. See Chapter 15 for discussion of the various nursing positions.

Pain Relief

Some mothers find an anti-inflammatory such as ibuprofen helpful, if it is approved for use by the mother's caregiver. Mothers may obtain temporary relief by placing ice in a wet cloth and applying the cloth to their nipples prior to the baby latching. If this technique is used, the mother should make sure the ice is not placed directly on the skin.

Healing the Nipple Skin

Mothers should first consider whether they need to adjust their positioning and latch technique before using topical applications to treat sore nipples. Additionally, they should avoid any applications that need to be removed before a feeding, as unnecessarily removing topical agents can further aggravate any existing nipple damage. A mother sometimes may need to remove dead tissue from the skin, a process referred to as debriding (Wilson-Clay & Hoover, 2008).

A variety of topical agents have been used over the years to heal sore nipples. They include lanolin, vitamin E, tea bags, hydrogel pads, glycerin gel, antibiotic ointments, and compounded treatments. Research is mixed on the efficacy of these treatments.

For the lactation consultant, it is important to read research reports with a critical eye before recommending any clinical remedy. Some topical agents that are suggested for sore nipples actually delay healing time, and may cause irritation or an allergic reaction (ILCA, 2007). Some, such as regular lanolin, contain harmful substances such as pesticides. Oils, including vitamin E, do not facilitate moist wound healing. The oil stays on the surface of the skin and does not provide moisture for healing. In one

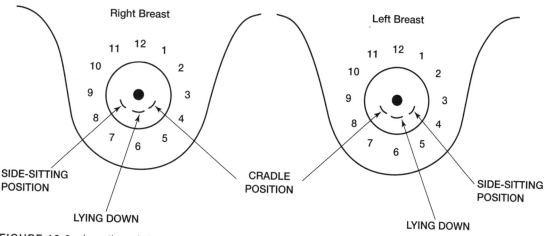

FIGURE 16.2 Location of nipple sore related to positioning.

study, increased serum concentrations of vitamin E were present in breastfed babies 6 days after ingesting milk from their mothers who were using topical vitamin E on their nipples (Marx et al., 1985). This finding is a cause for concern because high doses of vitamin E can cause liver damage (Hale, 2010).

Be sensitive to how a mother may perceive any negativity on your part about her using topical comfort measures. Many mothers bring their own ointments to the hospital, and commercial products are included in many breastfeeding gift bags. Discounting what the mother brought or is using may make her feel foolish or stupid, when she was actually planning ahead and using forethought. Barring the use of any harmful ingredients (such as the fat-soluble vitamins E and A, which are stored in the liver), there is no reason to criticize or discount the mother's choice. It is more constructive and empowering to praise her for thinking ahead and planning so well to deal with postpartum discomfort. If nothing else, the placebo effect may help her feel better and persevere through the transient soreness period.

Lanolin Use of hypoallergenic, medical-grade anhydrous, or modified, lanolin has been encouraged as a treatment for sore nipples for many years. Nevertheless, studies have produced mixed results regarding this product's efficacy. Many practitioners recommend that the mother apply her expressed milk to the sore area and allow for air-drying of the areola. Breastmilk was found to heal nipples faster than using lanolin (Mohammadzadeh et al., 2005). While modified lanolin may not be appropriate for routine use in all mothers, it may offer a perceived benefit to some mothers.

Hydrogel Dressing Hydrogel dressings have become popular as treatments for sore nipples. Gel dressings have been used in wound care for many years and help prevent scabbing and cracking. Any mother using gel pads needs to be taught how to use these products and instructed to discontinue using them if she sees signs of infection (redness, pus, bad odor). Some women with sore nipples report that cooled gel pads (stored in the refrigerator or an unopened packet in a cup of ice water) are very comforting. Other mothers do not like the sensation of cold on their breasts. Ask the mother first if cold is soothing to her before cooling the pads.

Be aware that the concept of "hot" and "cold" practices is very important in many non-Western cultures (including Latin America, Asia and Africa). This belief includes the necessity of maintaining a "hot–cold balance" within the body and with the environment after the birth of a baby (Kim-Godwin, 2003). Suggesting cold packs of any kind could be perceived as insensitive to mothers from these cultures. See Chapter 20 for a discussion of respectfully counseling families from different cultures than your own.

Peppermint Water Over the centuries, every culture has developed its own comfort measures for new mothers. Ask the families in your care which healing agents are typically used in their culture. For example, peppermint water is a cultural treatment for sore nipples in India. Studies show that women using peppermint water for sore nipples had a lower rate of nipple cracks compared to mothers using expressed breastmilk, lanolin, or a placebo (Sayyah Melli et al., 2007a, 2007b).

Interruption of Breastfeeding

When treatment fails to provide relief to sore nipples, some mothers prefer to stop breastfeeding for several feedings or even a few days in an attempt to preserve long-term breastfeeding. When a mother experiences an interruption in breastfeeding, she will need to pump to maintain milk production. The type of pump she needs to use depends on her stage of lactation. A hospital-grade pump is recommended during the early postpartum period to help establish milk production. By comparison, a mother who experiences sore nipples months after the birth can use her personal pump for this purpose. Many mothers also become proficient at hand expression.

If pumping exclusively, the mother can double pump for approximately 15 minutes, 8 to 12 times in 24 hours, or she can pump to match her baby's feeding frequency as closely as possible. Some mothers find that a small amount of olive oil dabbed on the flange before pumping lessens the pulling on the areola within the flange and makes pumping more comfortable (Wilson-Clay & Hoover, 2008). The pump should be set at the lowest suction level at the beginning of pumping to avoid pain. As her condition improves, the mother can increase the suction setting, although stronger suction does not necessarily produce better results. See Chapter 21 for further discussion of breast pumps.

When the mother is ready to resume breastfeeding, the baby can nurse at the breast when the mother feels ready. Depending on how quickly her nipples heal and how well the latch and suck have been improved, she can put the baby to breast for every second or third feeding. She can then increase the frequency of feedings at the breast as tolerated. Encourage the mother to maintain a lot of skin-to-skin contact during this time. Allowing the baby to self-attach may correct latch problems if they were the cause of the soreness. If not, skin-to-skin contact will still ensure that the baby continues to associate the mother's smell and skin with nurture and nourishment.

Candidiasis

A yeast infection usually develops from *Candida albicans*, a fungal organism commonly found in the mouth, gastrointestinal tract, and vagina of healthy persons. Under normal conditions, the body's flora keep *Candida* growth in check. Predisposing factors that may disturb the normal flora and lead to yeast infection include diabetes, illness, pregnancy, oral contraceptive use, poor diet, antibiotic therapy, steroid therapy, and immunosuppression. In addition, local factors such as obesity or excessive sweating provide consistently warm, moist areas in which *Candida* can thrive.

While *Candida* does not normally appear on skin such as the nipple, it may be present during lactation (Morrill et al., 2005). Yeast infection on the nipples has been associated with nipple damage early in lactation, mastitis, recent use of antibiotics in the postpartum period, long-term antibiotic use before pregnancy, and vaginal yeast infection. In one classic study, nearly two-thirds of mothers with vaginal yeast infections transmitted the infection to their infants (von Maillot et al., 1978). A baby may contract oral yeast while passing through the birth canal during delivery and, in turn, transfer the infection to the mother's nipple upon nursing. Preterm infants and infants in the NICU for other physical problems are especially prone to *Candida* infection (Kaufman, 2008; Vendettuoli et al., 2008; Manzoni et al., 2007, 2006). In these high-risk populations, *Candida* infection can be fatal.

Identifying a Candida Infection

A *Candida* infection that occurs in the baby's mouth is called thrush. Thrush presents as white patches that look like milk curds, as shown in Color Plate 24. The mother will not be able to wipe the patches off, which is how she can distinguish them from milk in her baby's mouth. In the diaper area, yeast may present as a raised, very red area with a sharply defined border. Babies with a yeast infection often seem to be gassy and fussy. Symptoms of vaginal yeast are usually difficult to miss. The vaginal area and vulva are tender and very red, with intense itching. There may also be a cheesy, white vaginal discharge.

A *Candida* infection affecting the nipple does not always present with visual symptoms. Although unusual, it is possible to see white patches or redness on the nipple (see Color Plate 38). The most obvious symptom is usually breast and nipple pain. When a mother presents with severely sore nipples after a period of pain-free breastfeeding, a yeast infection may be the cause. Mothers often describe the pain as intense and burning, radiating through the breast during or after feedings. Lawrence and Lawrence (2005) describe it as "feeling like hot cords burning in their chest wall."

Mothers with a yeast infection may not be able to tolerate either the feel of clothing on the nipple or the spray of water during a shower. They may feel a stinging sensation deep within the breast ducts and may experience pain between feedings. Sometimes the areola will have a very shiny, pinkish cast, which is easily detected with a small flashlight or other focused beam of light. Clinicians have observed a break in the skin similar to a positional compression stripe at the base of the nipple shank where the nipple joins the areola. There may also be some very slight edema noted in the areola (Berens, 2004).

Polymerase chain reaction/denaturing gradient gel electrophoresis (PCR-DGGE) is a newer technique for assaying bacteria and fungi, including *Candida*. This technique analyzes DNA and is considered highly reliable and sensitive in detecting both bacteria and fungi (Delgado et al., 2008; Woo et al., 2008). In one study, the bacterium *Staphylococcus epidermidis* was found in milk from mothers with nipple pain (Delgado et al., 2009). Mothers with mastitis had significantly higher rates of infection with strains that showed antibiotic resistance, including resistance to oxacillin, erythromycin, clindamycin and mupirocin. This increased resistance to common antibiotics may help explain chronic and/or recurring mastitis.

Candida and Breastfeeding

One study comparing yeast in breastfed and artificially fed infants found that *Candida* species were much less frequently encountered in infants who were predominantly breastfed than in those who were bottle fed. In contrast, yeast was observed much more frequently on the breasts of lactating women (Zöllner & Jorge, 2003). Another study found no yeast on 40 nonlactating women in the control group compared to positive *Candida* cultures in 23 percent of the lactating group. Twenty percent of these mothers had mammary candidiasis (Morrill et al., 2005).

Debate continues over whether yeast can reside within the breast ducts. Some mothers respond well to systemic treatments, suggesting possible internal yeast growth. A prospective study to detect *C. albicans* in the milk of women with severe nipple and deep breast pain found no significant difference between the control group and the mothers with pain (Hale et al., 2009). A *Candida* species was cultured in only one patient after the addition of iron to stimulate growth. The addition of pure *C. albicans* to milk samples suggested that milk does not inhibit *Candida* growth.

C. albicans does not appear to be present in milk ducts. Some researchers have conjectured that chronic breast pain may indicate subclinical mastitis, with no fever. Fluconazole—a medication often prescribed as a treatment for yeast infections—has mild antibiotic properties. Thus mothers who respond to systemic antifungal agents may be actually responding to these drugs' antibiotic properties (Wilson-Clay & Hoover, 2008).

Conversely, another study found that 30 percent of symptomatic women studied had positive breastmilk cultures for yeast, compared with 7.7 percent of controls. Among the 12 women from whom yeast was isolated, 11 grew *C. albicans*, suggesting that *Candida* species are found more often in breastfeeding mothers who report pain as compared with asymptomatic breastfeeding mothers (Andrews et al., 2007).

Treatment of a Candida *Infection*

When a mother has yeast on her nipples, her baby often has oral thrush; the reverse is also true. For this reason, it is imperative that both the mother and the baby receive treatment simultaneously, even if only one of them exhibits symptoms. In addition to the baby's mouth and mother's nipples, any other sites of infection need treatment. This includes the diaper area and vagina, as well as other family members who harbor the infection. It is important to follow the full course of treatment even after symptoms subside, as a yeast infection recurs very easily.

Treatment Options   The strain of yeast on the mother's nipples and the baby's mouth can be different from that found in a diaper rash. Unfortunately, many strains of yeast are resistant to the most commonly used medications. Various treatment regimens exist for both oral and nipple yeast infections. Antifungal topical agents used to treat yeast infections include nystatin, clotrimazole (1 percent), miconazole nitrate (2 percent), ketoconazole (2 percent), ciclopirox (1 percent), and naftifine hydrochloride. Although nystatin is often the first treatment suggested, the other topical agents are reportedly more effective (Lawrence & Lawrence, 2005). Clotrimazole and miconazole are available as over-the-counter products, whereas the other agents require a prescription.

The first-line treatment for oral yeast infection in the baby is usually nystatin, an oral antifungal agent. To administer this therapy, the mother rinses the baby's mouth with water after breastfeeding, shakes and pours nystatin into a cup, and then applies it to all surfaces of the baby's mouth with a cotton swab. The swab should never be dipped back into the original vial of nystatin. The mother can rinse her nipples with a solution made from 1 cup of plain, tepid water mixed with 1 tablespoon of vinegar, and air-dry them. She can then apply the antifungal cream sparingly so it soaks in by the time she is ready to feed again. The cream does not need to be washed off the nipple, though the mother should change breast pads at every feeding. Air drying and brief exposure of the breasts to sunlight or artificial light may be helpful, given that yeast thrives in dark, moist environments.

Gentian violet is a very effective treatment for both oral (Traboulsi et al., 2008) and nipple yeast infection. It is available as an over-the-counter product, and the mother should look for a 0.5 percent solution. To apply this treatment, she dips a cotton swab in the gentian violet and swabs the baby's mouth. When the baby latches onto the breast, the mother's nipple is treated by direct contact. Some clinicians advise that the mother swab both

of her breasts once a day as well. Newman and Kernerman (2009c) recommend applying gentian violet to the mother's breasts once daily for several days. The mother should discontinue use of gentian violet after the pain subsides. If her pain continues, she can use this treatment for up to a total of 7 days. Caution mothers that ulceration of the mucous membranes in the baby's mouth may result with excessive use or with use of gentian violet at strengths greater than 0.5 percent.

When discussing treatment options with a mother, it is important that a lactation consultant not prescribe medications without a license that includes prescriptive privileges. The explosion of media information and the increased sophistication of young parents have produced very informed consumers in recent years. These mothers may call you after having already researched yeast conditions and treatments exhaustively on the Internet. It is helpful to describe the treatments for yeast as a continuum. The lowest level of treatment includes home remedies such as rinsing the mother's nipples and exposing them to sunlight. The next level includes over-the-counter options such as topical antifungals and gentian violet. Further along on the continuum are the powerful, systemic antifungal treatments such as fluconazole and ketoconazole, which require prescriptions.

The mother should be encouraged to discuss treatment options with her own and her baby's caregivers, particularly in the event of persistent cases that do not respond to conventional topical medications. The protocol for treatment of breastfeeding candidiasis outlined in *Clinical Therapy in Breastfeeding Patients* (Hale & Berens, 2002) may prove helpful for the mother's healthcare provider in developing the plan of care. If the nipple soreness persists, referral to a dermatologist may be appropriate. Although culturing the breast for yeast has been difficult in the past, new techniques offer more precise measurement (Delgado et al., 2008; Andrews et al., 2007). Unfortunately, breast health problems such as yeast infection and mastitis continue to be ignored and under-researched in women (Amir & Ingram, 2008)—a phenomenon referred to as the "invisibility" of breastfeeding (Mulford, 2008).

Stopping the Spread of Yeast   Further considerations during the course of yeast treatment focus on family hygiene. Good hand washing before and after diapering, using the toilet, or breastfeeding will help stop the spread of yeast. Anything that comes in contact with the mother's breast needs to be boiled once a day for at least 20 minutes. Bras, breast shells and breast pump parts are vehicles for reinfection, and boiling kills the *Candida* bacterium. Moreover, the mother should discard items that go in the baby's mouth, such as bottle nipples, pacifiers, and teethers, after 1 week. Toys should be cleaned thoroughly with hot soapy water, and all of the family's clothing should be laundered in very hot water.

The mother's diet is believed by many care providers to be a factor in a persistent yeast infection (Gima, 2003). Other researchers have failed to confirm any statistical improvement in risk of infection with restricted diets (such as avoidance of sugars or yeast) compared to a well-rounded healthy diet (Hobday et al., 2008). The mother may try decreasing or omitting dairy products and sugars while increasing her intake of acidophilus, garlic, zinc, and B vitamins. If she is pumping, she can feed her fresh milk to her baby.

There is debate among lactation specialists as to whether giving previously frozen milk with *Candida* in it will reinfect a healthy baby. No studies have been conducted that definitively settle this question. Freezing does not kill *Candida*, and it is recommended that the frozen milk be pasteurized or discarded (Lawrence & Lawrence, 2005). To pasteurize it, the mother can heat the milk for approximately 20 minutes at a slow boil, in a double boiler or steamer to prevent direct contact with the water. In addition, the mother should label any milk she pumped during her infection so she will be sure to pasteurize it before feeding it to her baby.

∼ Engorgement

Engorgement describes the painful swelling that occurs when the breasts become overfull from failure to remove milk adequately or frequently enough. It is important to distinguish between this condition and the fullness that occurs as part of the normal physiological process as the mother's colostrum transitions to full milk production. Normal fullness is an expected part of lactation; engorgement is not.

Delivery of the placenta at birth triggers a reduction in a woman's progesterone levels. This precipitous drop in progesterone (from 55–200 ng/mL or more, down to 0 ng/mL) enables the mother's high prolactin levels to initiate mature milk production. Increased amounts of blood and lymph circulate in the breast and are the source of the nutrients needed for milk production. Enlarged blood vessels are often visible beneath the skin of the lactating breast. The fluids present in these veins cause the breasts to become fuller, heavier, and sometimes tender. Figure 16.3 shows a normally full breast. With unlimited, exclu-

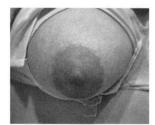

FIGURE 16.3   A normal full breast.
Source: Printed with permission of Linda Kutner.

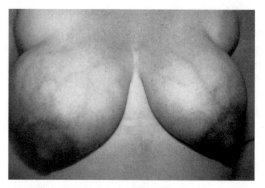

FIGURE 16.4   Engorged breasts.
Source: Printed with permission of Debi Bocar.

sive breastfeeding, this normal fullness diminishes. By about 10 days postpartum, when lactation is fully established, the breasts become comfortably soft and pliable, even when they are full of milk.

Engorgement occurs when the duct system is not cleared of colostrum or milk sufficiently, causing fluid to accumulate there. Increased pressure on the alveoli and milk ducts produces breasts that feel firm, hard, tender, and warm or hot to the touch. The skin may appear shiny and transparent, as shown in Figure 16.4. The nipples may flatten and, in extreme cases, may become indistinguishable from the rest of the breast. Table 16.5 characterizes four stages of breast fullness when describing engorgement (Kutner, 2009).

Causes of Engorgement

A mother can experience engorgement at any time during lactation whenever milk is not removed regularly. The most common time for engorgement to occur is in the early days postpartum, when breastfeeding is beginning and feeding patterns are irregular. Engorgement in the postpartum period can be iatrogenic, caused by medical interference with the natural process in the form of inappropriate regulations and schedules, and poor management of breastfeeding. Sometimes engorgement results from the mother having received IV fluids during labor,

TABLE 16.5   Four Stages of Breast Fullness

Stage	Definition
+1	Breasts are soft. Milk flows freely.
+2	Breasts are firm and nontender. Milk flows freely.
+3	Breasts are firm and tender. Milk release is slow and relief is obtained quickly.
+4	Breasts are hard and painful. Milk release is slow and relief is not obtained quickly.

which may lead to edema in her breasts as well as in her feet and ankles (see Figure 12.2 in Chapter 12).

Engorgement may also develop when the baby begins sleeping through the night and whenever the mother and baby miss feedings because of separation. It is a risk during the weaning process, especially if rapid weaning is necessary. Encourage mothers to remove milk from their breasts whenever they have a feeling of fullness, before they become uncomfortable. Figure 16.5 illustrates the causes and results of engorgement.

Consequences of Engorgement

Engorgement can compromise a mother's milk production. When milk remains in the breast for extended periods, the suppressor peptide—feedback inhibitor of lactation

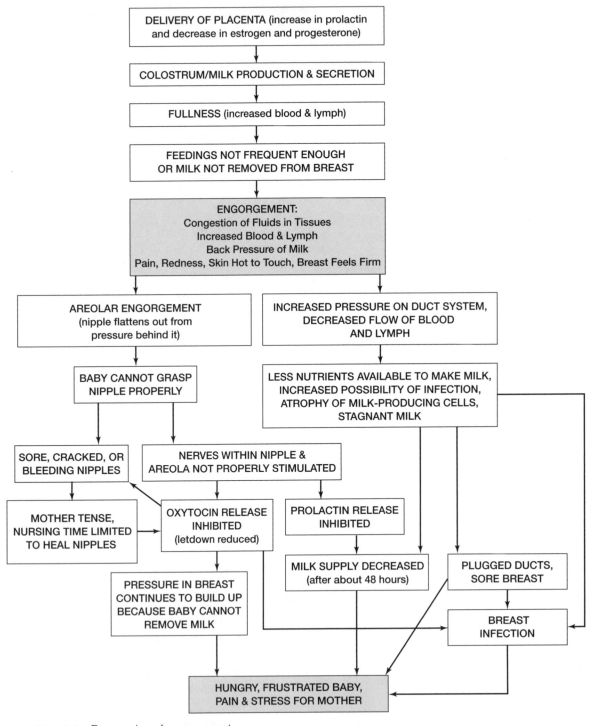

FIGURE 16.5   Progression of engorgement.

(FIL)—in human milk has a negative effect on milk production. Breast tissue elasticity allows milk storage for as long as 48 hours before the rate of milk production and secretion begins to decrease rapidly. Suppressor peptides are inhibitory peptides in human milk that bring about the cessation of milk secretion during milk stasis and engorgement (Grattan et al., 2008; Andrews, 2005; Buhimschi, 2004). Because unrelieved severe engorgement can result in lowered milk production, both mother and baby will need close follow-up.

Engorgement can adversely affect the mother's letdown mechanism as well. The flattened nipple of the engorged breast becomes difficult for the baby to grasp. The resulting shallow latch will fail to stimulate the nerves within the nipple and areola sufficiently, increasing the likelihood that letdown will not occur. Without letdown, the baby cannot remove milk from the breast efficiently and pressure in the ducts increases even more. Furthermore, when engorgement results in the baby grasping only the ends of the nipples, sore, cracked nipples can result and inhibit letdown even further.

With severe engorgement, the pressure on alveoli and ducts decreases the flow of blood and lymph to and from the breast. This slower flow increases the possibility of infection because the lymphatic system does not remove bacteria at a normal rate.

Engorgement also has the potential to harm breast tissue permanently. The increased milk pressure can cause some alveolar cells and myoepithelial cells to shrink and die off. This atrophy of milk-producing cells can permanently compromise the milk-producing ability of the breast for that particular breastfeeding experience.

Preventing Engorgement

Initiating breastfeeding within the first hour of life, as well as other breastfeeding-supportive practices identified in Chapter 12, helps prevent engorgement. When mothers and babies remain together 24 hours a day, the mother becomes familiar with her baby's hunger cues and learns to respond to them. Breastfeeding in response to baby cues for as long as the baby needs must be encouraged as the norm. Frequent feedings will help minimize engorgement—at least 8, and preferably more, in 24 hours, including night feedings. If breast fullness increases, the mother can be encouraged to wake her baby and nurse to remove milk.

For times when the baby is very sleepy and not nursing adequately, mothers need to know how to express their milk. In addition, each mother and baby must be assessed for correct latch and positioning if engorgement has occurred. If latch and positioning are not correct, it may lead to decreased milk removal (Mizuno et al., 2008). Parents should avoid the use of artificial nipples, which do not promote efficient sucking and may confuse the baby

upon returning to the breast. Education of maternity staff, midwives, and doulas must focus on these key areas for the postpartum period. Minimizing interference with breastfeeding is often the best preventive measure for engorgement.

Relieving Engorgement

Treatment of engorgement involves a combination of identifying and correcting the cause and offering palliative measures. Engorgement can be a frightening experience for a mother. It is helpful for her to know that this condition is temporary, and that engorgement usually resolves within 24 to 48 hours with proper treatment. If the mother has been limiting frequency or duration of feedings, encourage unrestricted feedings, at least every 2 hours or sooner if the baby desires and for as long as the infant needs. After the engorgement is resolved, suggest that the mother nurse at least 8 times in every 24-hour period. In addition, gentle breast compression during the feeding helps drain the breast more completely (Newman & Kernerman, 2009b). If breastfeeding alone does not reduce the engorgement, the mother may need to express milk between feedings. The Academy of Breastfeeding Medicine (ABM, 2009) protocol on engorgement calls for development of a uniform measurement system for rating engorgement, as well as more study for treatments and remedies.

If engorgement has progressed to the degree that the baby is unable to latch, the mother can express milk before a feeding to soften the areola. She may find expressing milk in the shower relaxing, with comfortably hot water spraying on her back and shoulders. Reverse-pressure softening, described in Chapter 21, has been helpful for many mothers in softening the areola and enabling the baby to latch (Cotterman, 2004).

Cold compresses applied between feedings will help decrease the mother's discomfort. A small bag of crushed ice or frozen pack of vegetables such as peas or corn conforms nicely to the shape of the breast. Refreezing the vegetables for reuse makes it an easy and affordable compress. The mother may also lie flat on her back to elevate the breasts and help reduce swelling. Cabbage leaves worn inside the bra provide a simple remedy that many mothers use. Table 16.6 summarizes the treatment options for engorgement.

Pumping for Engorgement

When appropriate guidelines are followed, pumping or hand expressing for engorgement will preserve the mother's milk production. Pumping for engorgement is usually necessary for only 24 to 48 hours to relieve the discomfort; continuing to pump beyond that time could maintain the mother's milk production at a level that is higher than needed. A double pump will remove milk

TABLE 16.6   Causes and Treatment of Engorgement

Causes	Actions for the Mother
Missed or infrequent feedings	• Room in with baby in the hospital. • Breastfeed baby 10 to 12 times each 24 hours, or more if he is willing, around the clock. • Watch baby for feeding cues, and respond to them. • Use rousing techniques for sleepy baby. • Increase skin-to-skin contact to encourage baby to nurse. The mother can remove her shirt and bra, and hold her baby with only a diaper on. • Pump breasts or hand express any time baby is unwilling or unable to nurse.
Milk removal not adequate at feedings	• Check that baby's latch and position are appropriate. • Stop the use of all artificial nipples. • Increase skin-to-skin contact during feedings. The mother can remove her shirt and bra and hold baby with only a diaper on. • Do breast compression during feedings to encourage baby to suckle. • Pump breasts or hand express *after* the feeding with a hospital-grade electric breast pump only to remove the milk that flows quickly and easily. • Pump breasts *between* feedings for comfort, if necessary, only as long as the milk flows quickly and easily.
Inadequate letdown due to edema and pain	• Relax in warm shower with water running over back, avoiding the breasts, and hand express to relieve fullness. • Breastfeed *after* the breast has softened enough to allow baby to latch on. • Use relaxation techniques and gentle breast massage during feedings. • Lie flat on back between feedings to elevate breasts. • Apply cool packs to the breasts and under arms. • Apply green cabbage leaves to breasts.

from both breasts at the same time. Some mothers prefer to single pump while they massage the affected breast. Briefly massaging and hand expressing milk before using the pump may increase flow significantly (Morton, 2009).

If engorgement occurs in only one breast, the mother does not need to pump the other one. Single pumping is appropriate when +2 or +3 engorgement is present and the baby is still able to nurse (see Table 16.5 for definitions of these levels). If the areola is firm or hard, the mother will need to pump before nursing. She should pump only long enough to soften the areola so that the baby can latch easily and not cause nipple trauma. The mother should then put her baby to breast to nurse. Following the feeding, she can pump her breast again if needed. If milk removal was easy and the mother heard her baby gulping, she can pump only until the milk stops flowing quickly. If swallowing was periodic and not sustained, she should pump for at least 10 minutes after the feeding. If the milk continues to flow quickly at the end of 10 minutes, she should continue to pump until the flow slows.

If the mother pumps only one breast at a time, she can use her other hand to massage the breast while she is pumping. She can apply cabbage leaves or ice packs to her breasts between feeding and pumping sessions as well. She will want to stop the pre-feed pumping as soon as possible, and pump after nursing only when necessary. Reassure the mother that she will be able to discontinue pumping very soon.

Cabbage for Engorgement

The use of fresh green cabbage leaves to treat engorgement was first described in *The Glory of Woman*, published in 1896. An article in 1988 was instrumental in reviving this traditional practice (Rosier, 1988). Research on the use of cabbage leaves is sparse, with no new studies of the topic having been undertaken in recent years. Roberts and colleagues (1995b) found that mothers reported significantly less pain with use of cabbage, either chilled or at room temperature, than before treatment. In addition, the mother who uses alternative treatments such as cabbage may derive some psychological value from this practice (Ayers, 2000).

A Cochrane Review found no difference between the use of cabbage and cabbage leaf extract in terms of the ability to relieve engorgement. Ultrasound treatment and placebo were equally effective. Use of Danzen (the trade name for serratiopeptidase, an anti-inflammatory agent used in Europe) significantly improved the total symptoms of engorgement when compared to placebo, as did bromelain/trypsin complex. Oxytocin and cold packs had no demonstrable effect on engorgement symptoms. The review concluded that prevention of engorgement should remain the key priority, rather than treatment after it occurs (Snowden et al., 2001).

Researchers have suggested that phytoestrogens present in cabbage contribute to reducing swelling in the tissues (Yildiz, 2006; Young et al., 2000). Cabbage is known to be effective on other parts of the body for reducing the swelling caused by sprains and strains. Many mothers have had positive results from the use of cabbage for reducing edema in breast engorgement and inflammation caused by plugged ducts and mastitis. Some mothers use prolonged applications of cabbage to wean or to suppress lactation. Folklore has it that farmers were careful to keep their cows out of the cabbage patch because consumption of cabbage decreased milk production.

Application of Cabbage to the Breast The procedure for applying cabbage is simple (see Color Plate 47). After discarding the outer leaves, pull off several leaves, wash them, pat them dry, and crush them slightly to break up the veins. Place the leaves on the engorged breasts and hold them in place with a bra. The remainder of the cabbage can be stored in the refrigerator and remain chilled for later use.

After application of cabbage for a short period, women report that their breast feels "different"—sometimes described as tingly and cool. The mother can remove the cabbage when she feels this sensation, when milk begins to leak, or when softening of breast tissue becomes apparent. She can then put her baby to breast, or pump if the baby still cannot latch. With severe engorgement, the cabbage will actually wilt from the heat of the breast. The mother can apply fresh leaves roughly every 2 hours for approximately 20 minutes in duration. As soon as the baby or pumping provides the needed relief, the mother should discontinue the use of cabbage. To dry up the milk completely, as in sudden weaning or suppressing lactation, the mother leaves cabbage on her breasts around the clock, changing it as needed until milk production ceases.

The amount of relief experienced by women from cabbage treatment varies. Some will find relief in as little as 20 to 30 minutes; others may need to apply the cabbage over a period of 24 hours. In some cases, the decrease of edema is so pronounced that the milk ducts will stand out in bold relief on the breast after the cabbage is removed.

Cabbage may help women with plugged ducts and mastitis as well, with the mother applying the cabbage to the plug or area where the mastitis inflammation is evident. She leaves it on the breast until she obtains relief. There are no reports of untoward effects from the cabbage (Roberts et al., 1995a, 1995b).

～ Plugged Ducts

Sometimes a plug forms in a duct, consisting of cells and other milk components shed within the ducts. A plugged duct causes localized soreness, swelling, lumpiness, or slight pain. The localized pain is not accompanied by a symptom in any other part of the body such as fever or flu-like symptoms, in which case a breast infection may be present.

Some plugs are absorbed quickly by the body and do not appear in the milk. A plug that is released and comes out with the milk may be brownish or greenish in color, and thick and stringy (see Color Plate 48). The mother can remove the mass manually with no ill effects. Although the baby may reject the milk with the plug due to the taste or texture, most babies easily return to nursing afterward. There is no known danger to the baby from such a plug.

Causes of Plugged Ducts

A plugged duct can result from incomplete milk removal or from outside pressure on specific areas of the breast. Any practice that inhibits the free flow of milk can create pressure. The source could be a tight or underwire bra, bunched-up clothing under the arm, or a baby sling. Plugged ducts may also result from consistently holding, carrying, or rocking the baby in the same position. Sleeping in a position that puts pressure on the breast or pressure from a breast pump flange can lead to a plugged duct as well.

In one study, a new mother experienced 7 episodes of blocked ducts during the first 19 weeks of lactation. Analysis found no detectable secretory immunoglobulin A (sIgA) present in her milk samples. Medical referral and further testing resulted in a diagnosis of selective IgA deficiency. Perhaps sIgA may be part of the mammary glands' defense system in addition to protecting the infant (Fetherston et al., 2008).

Treatment of Plugged Ducts

Plugs can be broken up and worked down the ducts by regular frequent feedings and hand massage in the direction of the plug toward the nipple. Applying moist heat over the area of the plug can help move it along the duct. Plugs can also be encouraged to move by using a nursing position in which the infant's tongue stimulates more milk flow in the area of the plug. Beginning a feeding on the breast with the plug will help with removal by taking advantage of the baby's more vigorous sucking early in the feeding. Another successful approach is massaging in front of the lump toward the nipple, and kneading close to and pushing toward the nipple (Campbell, 2006).

Consuming lecithin, a natural fat emulsifier, and reducing the amount of saturated fats in their diets helps women prevent recurring plugged ducts (Lawrence & Lawrence, 2005). Lecithin is most concentrated in organ meats, red meats, and eggs—foods whose consumption tends to be limited in modern diets. This reduction in lecithin intake may compromise the emulsification of fats in the mother's bloodstream and, therefore, the ability of the breast to clear the milk ducts (Scott, 2005). The recommended dosage of lecithin is 1 tablespoon 3 or 4 times daily or 1 to 2 capsules (1200 mg each) 3 or 4 times daily.

Table 16.7 identifies additional measures that can be taken to release a plug. Encourage the mother to make

TABLE 16.7   Causes and Treatments of Plugged Ducts

Causes	Actions for the Mother
Poor positioning	• Try a variety of positions for better milk removal.
Breasts overfull due to missed feedings, irregular nursing patterns, engorgement	• Nurse baby with his chin pointed toward the plugged duct. • If prone to plugged ducts, avoid missed feedings or pump to remove milk. • If baby does not adequately remove milk from the breasts, pump or express milk after feedings. • Nurse long enough on each breast for the baby to remove sufficient milk.
Incomplete removal of milk from the breast	• If baby does not remove milk, pump or express milk after feedings. • While nursing on affected side, use massage and heat to encourage drainage. • Nurse more frequently on affected breast. • Gently roll, pull, and rub plug down while in warm shower. • Use moisture to remove any dried secretions blocking nipple pores.
External pressure on the breast	• Avoid positions that put pressure on one spot for long periods, e.g., always sleeping on one side, always holding the baby one way, or baby sleeping on mother's chest. • Use larger nursing bra or a bra extender. • Avoid bunching up sweater or nightgown under arm during a feeding. • Use nursing bra instead of pulling up conventional bra to nurse in order to avoid pressure on ducts.

every effort to remove the plug quickly. A plugged duct can develop into a larger blocked-off area referred to as a "caked" breast and, left untreated, could develop into mastitis. Urge the mother to call her caregiver if a plug does not respond to treatment.

⤳ Milk Blister or Milk Bleb

Occasionally, milk will clog a nipple pore (see Color Plate 49). This site is referred to as a milk bleb or blocked nipple pore when it is open. When the skin closes over the pore and forms a blister, it is referred to as a nipple blister or milk blister. Many healthcare providers use all of these terms interchangeably.

Milk blisters and blebs are intensely painful, because milk cannot flow from the duct and stays in the breast. This type of blister or bleb is very different from the sucking blisters some mothers experience in the early days. Some specialists believe that nipple blisters lead to plugged ducts; others believe that plugged ducts actually cause the blisters (Newman & Kernerman, 2009a). Either way, these sores are terribly painful for most mothers who have them, and can lead to mastitis because of milk stasis.

One method for removing a blister is for the mother to soak her nipple with a warm wet compress or in a comfortably hot bowl of water. Sometimes very gentle rubbing with a soft cloth will remove the pore covering. The mother may even see the hardened plug of dried or crystallized milk come out. The mother can then nurse her baby, who may remove the plug through sucking. If this technique works, the mother usually feels instant relief as

the backed-up milk is removed (Genna, 2004). Soreness may remain for a few days.

The mother can use a topical antibiotic ointment to prevent infection of a blister. If the baby's sucking does not remove the plug, the mother may open a blister or bleb with a sterile needle (Newman & Kernerman, 2009a). The best time for doing so is immediately after breastfeeding the baby. When the blister is opened in this manner, the backed-up milk will often stream out and the mother usually feels immediate relief. Gentle breast compression will aid in draining the breast. If the mother does not wish to release the bleb herself, refer her to her healthcare provider. Encourage the mother to breastfeed her baby very frequently and thoroughly on the affected breast to prevent recurrence.

Ultrasound has also been used to treat plugged ducts. Newman and Kernerman (2009a) recommend a maximum of 2 treatments on 2 consecutive days, noting that ultrasound seems to prevent blocked ducts that always occur in the same part of the breast. The recommended dosage is 2 watts/cm^2, continuously, for 5 minutes to the affected area, once daily for up to 2 doses.

⤳ Mastitis

Mastitis is inflammation of the breast, usually (though not always) resulting from a bacterial infection. With this condition, the inflamed area of the breast becomes red, hot, and tender to the touch (see Color Plate 50). More than just a localized soreness, a breast infection usually produces fever and flu-like symptoms in the woman. Any time a breastfeeding mother feels flu-like symptoms, she needs to rule out the possibility of mastitis. If she has mastitis, she will want to begin treatment immediately to reduce the severity and to protect her milk production.

The occurrence of mastitis varies considerably, with estimates in the literature ranging from 3 to 20 percent depending on the definition (ABM, 2008). One large study on breast pain of all types found 11.8 percent of cases were due to lactational mastitis (Ohene-Yeboah, 2008). Foxman and colleagues (2002) found 9.5 percent of 946 U.S. women suffered from self-reported mastitis that was diagnosed by a healthcare provider within the first 3 months postpartum. Although most instances of mastitis occur in the first 6 weeks postpartum, a mother can get mastitis at any time. Nonlactational mastitis also occurs, and even mastitis during pregnancy. Rarely, infants can have mastitis.

Elevated cytokine levels in mother's milk have been reported during mastitis (Wöckel et al., 2008). Cytokines are regulatory proteins, such as interleukins and lymphokines that are released by immune system cells. They act as intercellular mediators in the generation of an immune response and serve as chemical messengers between cells. Cytokines can stimulate or inhibit the growth and activity of immune cells in response to the type of disease present.

Some mothers report their baby rejects the infected breast, possibly because of a salty taste resulting from increased sodium and chloride levels in the milk (Lawrence & Lawrence, 2005). If the baby will not nurse on that breast, the mother can pump the affected breast to prevent stasis. Many mothers may self-treat a breast infection and not seek medical treatment. A separate study, using the same cohort of 946 mothers described earlier, associated weaning with mastitis, breast or nipple pain, bottle use, and milk expression (pumping) in the first 3 weeks (Schwartz et al., 2002). A mother with symptoms of mastitis is at risk for weaning and needs immediate assistance.

Subclinical Mastitis

Many lactation consultants have encountered mothers who have chronic breast pain in the absence of fever (Wilson-Clay & Hoover, 2008). Such asymptomatic inflammation of mammary tissue is described as subclinical mastitis. It has been linked to lactation failure, suboptimal growth in early infancy, and increased risk of mother-to-child transmission of HIV via breastmilk (Aryeetey et al., 2008).

Research into milk enzymes carried out by the dairy industry shows promise as a way to detect subclinical mastitis. Levels of these enzymes can be assessed by measuring the concentration of sodium and milk immune factors in the affected mother's milk. Studies have confirmed a positive association between the sodium/potas-

sium ratio and breastmilk enzymes (Aryeetey et al., 2009; Rasmussen et al., 2008).

Subclinical mastitis is a special concern in mothers who are HIV positive (Lunney et al., 2010; Kasonka et al., 2006), as it could lead to poor maternal overall health and breast health. Improving health care for postpartum women, with an emphasis on managing maternal infections, is key to preventing this type of inflammation. More study into the consequences of subclinical mastitis is needed.

When a mother reports having had mastitis, or the symptoms of mastitis without accompanying fever, subclinical mastitis may be present. New assays for elevated enzyme and sodium/potassium levels may prove very helpful to these mothers and their healthcare providers in resolving chronic or recurring breast pain. For the lactation consultant, when you encounter a mother with breast pain, it is important that you ask open-ended questions to encourage the mother to describe and refine the kind of pain she is experiencing.

Figure 16.6 provides an example algorithm for identifying mastitis. As part of your problem-solving process, consider which clues might indicate subclinical mastitis. Think about what is happening in the mother's life: family stress, financial stress, fatigue from a new baby and older children. Perhaps she had one bout with mastitis and did not see her doctor. Maybe she took her medication for 5 days and failed to complete the entire prescription. Consider what other information you would try to obtain from her and what you would recommend to this mother.

Causes of Mastitis

Anticipatory guidance can alert mothers to times when breast infections are most likely to occur. In particular, mastitis commonly occurs during the newborn period, when the mother is more likely to be tired and when her immunity has been lowered by the burden of pregnancy. Research confirms that most inflammatory breast diseases associated with breastfeeding occur during the first 12 weeks postpartum—and that these conditions are the most common reason for early cessation of breastfeeding (Wöckel et al., 2008). Evidence suggests inflammatory mammary diseases are triggered or perpetuated in a large part by psychosocial stress. The underlying immunological processes remain largely unknown.

Mastitis is associated with milk stasis and engorgement. While a mother is working to establish breastfeeding, any interruption or change in nursing pattern can cause milk to remain in the ducts. An infection can also develop when the mother's time and energy become overextended, such as by a return to work or school, holidays, vacations, houseguests, family crises, or infant/other child illness.

This mother has come to see the lactation consultant (LC) as an outpatient in a pediatric practice, WIC clinic, or private practice. Her baby is 8 weeks old, and the mother is complaining of pain.

LC: How is nursing going for you and Chloe?
Mother: Not so good. It hurts.

LC: I'm sorry to hear that. What hurts?
Mother: My breast.

LC: Which part of your breast hurts?
Mother: Well, it hurts on the inside.

LC: It hurts on the inside of your breast. When does it hurt?
Mother: It hurts all the time, but especially after the baby nurses and at night.

LC: How would you describe your pain on a scale of 0 to 10, with 0 being no pain and 10 being the worst pain you've ever felt?
Mother: I would say it is a 1 all the time and a 2 or 3 at night.

LC: How do your nipples feel?
Mother: My nipples are fine. This is my third baby. I am sure Chloe is latching on right. She's gaining weight and pooping a lot.

LC: How can you best describe your pain—is it dull, aching, throbbing, burning, itching?
Mother: It's a dull ache most of the time, like the inside of my breasts are bruised. But there's no redness or hard lump. If my 3-year-old or 6-year-old hugs me, it hurts more. If Chloe bumps me while I'm holding her, it hurts, too.

LC: How is your stress level?
Mother: It's pretty high. My husband lost his job 2 weeks ago, and we're not sure if we'll have to move. And my mother was just diagnosed with cancer. She's only 55. I'm afraid I'll have to go back to work full-time.

LC: Wow, that's a lot to deal with. It sounds quite overwhelming. How are you taking care of yourself through all this?
Mother: I can barely take care of everyone else, much less myself.

LC: How is your postpartum health besides the breast pain?
Mother: Well, I had mastitis 3 weeks ago. My doctor called in an antibiotic, so I must be okay now. I haven't had any fever. And I don't have any redness or streaking.

LC: Which antibiotic was used, and for how long?
Mother: I think it was ampicillin. I took it for about 5 days and then I felt better. But this pain seems different.

FIGURE 16.6 Problem solving to identify mastitis.

Infection can develop when a crack in the nipple skin exposes a pathway into the breast for *Staphylococcus* and other invasive organisms. It can result from a plugged duct that went unnoticed or untreated, or that failed to respond to treatment. Infections often result from bacteria in the baby's mouth or in the home environment. Because the infection probably came from the baby's mouth or her home, the mother is likely to have produced antibodies to the infectious organism in her milk. Therefore, it is considered safe and desirable for the baby to continue to nurse through an infection. The mother needs to continue removing milk and the baby's sucking usually removes milk much more effectively than either a pump or hand expression does. Additionally, frequent feedings can prevent milk stasis from developing.

The Academy of Breastfeeding Medicine (2008) has identified the following events as predisposing factors for mastitis (although evidence for some remains inconclusive):

- Damaged nipple, especially if colonized with *Staphylococcus aureus*
- Infrequent feedings, scheduled feedings, or limited duration of feedings
- Missed feedings
- Poor attachment or weak or uncoordinated sucking leading to inefficient removal of milk
- Illness in mother or baby
- Overproduction of milk
- Rapid weaning
- Pressure on the breast (e.g., tight bra or car seatbelt)
- White spot on nipple or blocked nipple pore or duct: milk blister, granular material, *Candida* infection
- Maternal malnutrition (evidence of specific dietary risk factors in humans has not been identified)

Treatment of Mastitis

Treatments for mastitis include efficient milk removal, warm moist compresses to the site of inflammation, anti-inflammatory medication, and antibiotics. The mother needs total rest to help her body fight the infection. If she is employed, she will need to take sick leave or personal time off, if possible. Women can build a support system among relatives and friends for help with meals, grocery shopping, and caring for other children so they can rest and recuperate.

If it appears to you or the mother that she has a breast infection, recommend that she contact her primary healthcare provider immediately. If she is running a temperature higher than 100°F and her symptoms do not resolve within 24 hours, her caregiver will probably place her on antibiotic therapy for 10 to 14 days. In the absence of a fever, the caregiver may wait a few days to determine whether other measures are effective. The following basic measures are used to treat a breast infection:

- Heat: Apply warm, moist compresses to the inflamed area before and during the feeding.
- Rest: Get as much bed rest as possible.

- Remove milk from the breast: Nurse in a position that points the baby's chin toward the inflamed area.
- Breastfeed as often as possible: Use of breast compression and massage may help drain the breast more effectively.
- Call the caregiver for an antibiotic: Follow through on the entire regimen, even if the infection seems to clear quickly.

When mastitis develops, a feeding assessment will help ensure that the baby is latching and feeding effectively. Urge the mother to breastfeed as frequently as her baby desires and to express milk from the affected breast after every feeding if she feels it is not well drained. Soaking the affected breast in comfortably hot water for short periods facilitates blood flow and drainage. Having her baby begin a feeding on the affected breast will allow the baby's more vigorous sucking to drain the milk better.

Some clinicians have found relief from the application of cabbage leaves. Cabbage may work because it contains rapine, which some herbalists regard as an antifungal antibiotic (Yildiz, 2006; Lawrence & Lawrence, 2005). Anecdotal reports suggest that acupuncture and chiropractic care are effective for plugged ducts and mastitis. Table 16.8 lists treatment suggestions relative to specific causes of mastitis.

Recurrent Mastitis

Some mothers seem to be prone to recurring bouts of mastitis. For this reason, after a mother has recovered from a breast infection, she needs to be watchful for signs of recurring infection. She will want to be especially vigilant in removing milk regularly from her breasts. She needs to routinely express her milk whenever she must miss a feeding and should guard against becoming overly tired or overworked.

At the first sign of an infection or plugged duct, urge the mother to apply warm compresses, nurse more frequently, and get bed rest to shorten the length of the infection. If infection recurs within 2 months, the mother needs to see her caregiver. Some caregivers will prescribe medications over the telephone without ever seeing their patients with mastitis. This lack of care has resulted in chronic cases of subclinical mastitis, recurrent bouts, and even abscesses (Wilson-Clay & Hoover, 2008).

Maternal Factors

A mother who experiences recurrent mastitis should evaluate her hygiene, especially when handling her breast, as well as her diet, rest, and exercise. She may need to reduce her daily activities and commitments and prioritize them to achieve a more healthful and less stressed lifestyle while

TABLE 16.8 Treatment Options for Mastitis

Causes	Actions for the mother
Milk stasis: Poor milk removal from the breast	• Nurse as long as the baby desires. If breast is full after he is finished, express milk for relief.
Milk stasis: Breasts overfull due to missed feedings, irregular nursing pattern, or engorgement	• Avoid missed or delayed feedings. • When feedings are delayed, pump or hand express to remove milk from breasts.
Overwork	• Rearrange priorities and daily schedule. • Get help with tasks.
Low resistance to infection due to anemia, poor diet	• Improve diet. • Exercise. • Reduce stress.
Lack of adequate sleep; fatigue	• Take daytime naps or rest periods (sleep rebuilds the immune system). • Nurse lying down. • Take baby to bed at night.
Failure to clear a plugged duct	• Work plug down manually, if it is not too painful. • Have baby nurse with chin pointed toward plug.
Infection via cracked nipple	• Eliminate nonnutritive sucking. • Briefly soak breasts in saline solution (¼ tsp salt in 8 oz water) after feeding and air dry.
Infection passed from baby or other family member	• Treat primary infection in conjunction with mother's infection.

she is breastfeeding. Help from family and her other support network will be important. Many mothers raise their children without a father and without any extended family to whom they can turn for relief. In a mobile society where families move frequently, it is instructive to ask a mother how long she has lived in your area. Many mothers relocate during their pregnancy and have left behind their friends, family and caregivers.

Brainstorming to find social support sources is especially helpful to these mothers. Peer counselors, breastfeeding support groups, and church and other nonprofit groups can assist families in ways that go far beyond breastfeeding support. Many churches offer meals for postpartum mothers and support groups for new or single parents. Neighborhood preteens may be available to assist with simple household chores for less money than an older teen would charge. For the lactation consultant, it is essential to learn which private and government resources are available in your community so you can refer mothers who need help—lack of support is a risk factor for postpartum depression. As a caregiver, you can help form a safety net for the new mother by compiling a list of support avenues in your community and updating it often.

Anemia or other deficiencies predispose some women to recurrent mastitis. Recurring episodes also can occur when the mother fails to respond to a particular antibiotic or does not complete the entire course of treatment. Sometimes a woman will stop taking an antibiotic after several days because she no longer has symptoms of an infection. In reality, without the complete regimen of antibiotic, the infection may not fully clear and instead recur as soon as her resistance is lowered again. The bacteria also may be resistant to the antibiotic the mother takes, in which case a broader-spectrum antibiotic may be necessary.

Antibiotic-Resistant Bacteria

Antibiotic-resistant strains of *Staphylococcus aureus* have been increasingly found in mastitis and breast abscesses, and seem to be the main cause of lactational mastitis. A culture of the mother's milk and nipple and the baby's throat may help determine the appropriate antibiotic in such a case. Culturing milk to identify the specific pathogen may be problematic, however, as studies show mixed results. It is thought that the bactericidal action of human milk (especially lactoferrin) may reduce the bacterial cultures (Lacasse, 2008). The ability to use RNA sequencing holds great promise in this regard. Combining the use of culture with molecular techniques allows for better characterization of the bacterial diversity in milk from women suffering from infectious mastitis. Researchers have found that *Staphylococcus* strains seem to be the main cause of lactational mastitis (Delgado et al., 2008). This condition could be the result of some populations of bacterial species usually present in human milk growing (staphylococci) while others disappear (lactobacilli or lactococci).

Culturing is especially important, given the increase in antibiotic-resistant bacteria in today's world. Over the past 50 years, bacteria have become more resistant to antibiotics, especially those that are penicillin based. Methicillin-resistant *S. aureus* (MRSA) occurs more frequently now, and its eradication requires much stronger antibiotics than those usually used to treat *Staphylococcus* infection. MRSA occurs more commonly among people in hospitals and other healthcare facilities. It can also occur in the community and is associated with recent antibiotic use, sharing contaminated items, having active skin diseases, and living in crowded settings (Centers for Disease Control and Prevention [CDC], 2008).

Local resistance patterns for MRSA should be considered when choosing an antibiotic for such unresponsive cases while culture results are pending (ABM, 2008). Be aware that two of the antibiotics used to treat MRSA, vancomycin and teicoplanin, are expensive. They may be toxic and must be administered to the mother by intravenous infusion, typically while the patient is admitted to the hospital. Adding the oral antibiotic rifampin to vancomycin treatment increases its efficacy (Hale & Berens, 2002).

Vancomycin-resistant bacteria have also emerged over the past decade, including vancomycin-resistant *Enterococcus* (VRE). VRE is a nosocomial (hospital-acquired) infection. In 2004, it caused about 1 of every 3 infections in hospital intensive care units (MedicineNet.com, 2008). Given that most U.S. women deliver their children in hospitals, this is a worrisome trend. Another cause for concern is vancomycin-resistant *S. aureus* (VRSA) infection; in 2007, there were seven reported cases of VRSA in the United States. This development appears to be due to the transfer of a key antibiotic resistance gene from *Enterococcus* to *Staphylococcus* (Finks et al., 2009).

Research from the dairy industry shows that mastitis in dairy animals responds better to antibiotics infused with lactoferrin. Lactoferrin has a weak antibacterial effect when used alone, but appears much more effective when administered at a low concentration in combination with several antibiotics. The bacterial cure rate was greater for a bovine lactoferrin plus penicillin combination (33.3 percent) compared with penicillin alone (12.5 percent). The researchers concluded that lactoferrin added to penicillin is an effective combination for the treatment of stable *S. aureus* infections resistant to beta-lactam antibiotics (Lacasse et al., 2008). The application of this research into the field of human lactation merits further study.

Breast Abscess

An abscess is a localized collection of pus that forms from an infection that has no opening for drainage. Approximately 3 percent of mastitis cases progress to abscesses (Amir et al., 2004). An abscess in the breast usually forms from an untreated breast infection or one that did not respond to treatment. Indications of an abscess are the same as for mastitis—fever, flu-like symptoms, nausea, extreme fatigue, and aching muscles. However, symptoms may be less severe than with mastitis because the abscess is isolated from the rest of the breast. The infection site becomes red, swollen, and tender (see Color Plate 51). Occasionally, an abscess can occur in the absence of any systemic symptoms.

If treatment does not resolve what seems to be a plugged duct within 48 hours, the mother needs to see her physician to rule out an abscess. In one patient, an abscess improperly treated with hydrogen peroxide resulted in an oxygen embolism (Agostini, 2004). Abscesses have also been associated with development of arthritis (Dhulkotia et al., 2005; Demetriadi et al., 2004). Breast abscesses can occur in nonlactating women as well, including in a condition known as Zuska's disease (Guadagni & Nazzari, 2008). In Zuska's disease, keratinizing squamous epithelium replaces the lining of one or more ducts in the subareolar tissue (Lannin, 2004). An abscess can be a serious health hazard that requires the mother to see her physician immediately for treatment.

Treatment of an Abscess

A breast abscess usually is lanced and drained (see Color Plate 52) and the mother receives medication for the infection. A newer technique uses ultrasound to aspirate and irrigate the abscess. In one study, 10 cases of mastitis with 11 abscesses were treated with this technique and only one required surgical drainage (Ozseker et al., 2008). Abscesses are usually flushed with saline solution, though newer treatment may include the use of urokinase, a serine protein derived from human urine. Urokinase is used as a thrombolytic agent to treat severe deep vein thrombosis, pulmonary embolism, and myocardial infarction; it also helps drain complicated IV/dialysis/drainage lines. One study found that breast abscess drainage time was significantly less in a group of patients in whom urokinase was used compared to a group who received saline (Berná-Serna et al., 2009).

Breastfeeding with an Abscess

The mother may be able to continue to nurse on one or both breasts when she has an abscess. This decision will depend on the location of the abscess, the pain associated with it, and the medication prescribed by her physician. If the mother is unable to nurse, she will need to express milk from the affected breast, or she may choose to wean temporarily from that breast. Abscesses can be traumatic to mothers, and some will be adamant that they wish to wean. Be sensitive and respectful of the mother's feelings and engage in lots of reflective listening. Because the mother will need to continue to remove milk from the affected breast while it heals, she has time to consider or change her options about lactating on that breast.

If the mother wishes to continue breastfeeding on the affected breast, she can implement the suggestions in Table 16.8 for treating a breast infection. If she chooses to wean, give her the necessary information in a sensitive and tactful way. Many mothers practice one-sided nursing and produce sufficient milk for their baby. Whether she weans from the affected breast only or totally weans her baby, the mother will need to lower production slowly to avoid another infection. She can help prevent abscesses with appropriate, proactive breastfeeding management and immediate treatment of mastitis.

∽ Summary

The lactation consultant can provide much reassurance and assistance to breastfeeding women in the early weeks following delivery. Discussing common breastfeeding expectations can ease the mother through this time of great change. In addition, being available to her when difficulties arise and providing support and guidance will help her reach her breastfeeding goals. If you do not work in an outpatient setting, you can refer mothers to local and Internet resources for ongoing community support. The anticipatory guidance you provide for breastfeeding in the first days and weeks after birth, including sound breast care and breast health, will help to reduce unnecessary concerns. Educating mothers about prevention and treatment of nipple soreness, engorgement, thrush, plugged ducts, and mastitis may reduce their occurrence. If these problems do occur, giving mothers appropriate treatment options helps prevent prolonged occurrence or recurrence. You can help achieve consistency among caregivers in their approach to these events by educating them and being available as a resource.

∽ Chapter 16—At a Glance

Applying what you learned—

Counseling the mother:

- Help her prioritize her baby's needs.
- Boost her confidence.
- Point out positive things about her baby.

Teach mothers that:

- Limiting time at the breast does not prevent nipple soreness.

- Early use of artificial nipples may create nipple preference.
- Poor positioning is the major cause of sore nipples.
- Babies may breastfeed every 1–2 hours (8–14 feedings) in the early days.
- Water supplementation should not be given to breastfeeding infants.
- Formula supplementation is appropriate only if medically indicated, and only if human milk is not available or the baby has galactosemia (estimated rate: 1 case per 70,000 infants).
- Most medications are safe for breastfeeding, but check with the caregiver first before recommending any drug.
- The baby needs sufficient time at each breast to remove both foremilk and hindmilk.
- Regular frequent feedings will maintain milk production.
- The baby should determine when a feeding ends.
- A tight frenulum, tight frenum, short tongue, and palate shape may affect the infant's ability to latch and suck.

Teach mothers about:

- Risk factors of infant formula.
- Key times for increases and decreases in feeding frequency.
- Signs of sufficient milk transfer.
- Correct positioning and attachment.
- Importance of alternating breastfeeding positions.
- Causes and treatment of recurrent mastitis.

Teach mothers how to:

- Count wet and dirty diapers.
- Note the baby's disposition during and between feedings, and other growth indicators.
- Control leaking.
- Prevent and treat nipple soreness.
- Apply topical creams and ointments.
- Handle an interruption in breastfeeding due to soreness.
- Check for and treat thrush in the baby and yeast infection on the nipples.
- Stop the spread of yeast.
- Identify, avoid, and treat engorgement, plugged ducts, and mastitis.
- Use gentle breast compression to drain the breast.
- Prevent a breast abscess.

◠ References

Abolyan L. The breastfeeding support and promotion in baby-friendly maternity hospitals and not-as-yet baby-friendly hospitals in Russia. *Breastfeed Med.* 2006;1(2):71-78.

Academy of Breastfeeding Medicine (ABM). ABM clinical protocol #4: mastitis revision, May 2008. *Breastfeed Med.* 2008;3(3). www.bfmed.org, protocols tab. Accessed June 16, 2009.

Academy of Breastfeeding Medicine (ABM). ABM clinical protocol #20: engorgement. *Breastfeed Med.* 2009;4(2):111-113. www.bfmed.org, protocols tab. Accessed June 26, 2009.

Agostini A. Oxygen embolism after hydrogen peroxide irrigation of a breast abscess. *Gynecol Obstet Fertil.* 2004;32(5):414-415.

American Academy of Pediatrics (AAP). Policy statement on breastfeeding and the use of human milk. *Pediatrics.* 2005;115(2):496-506.

Amir L, et al. Incidence of breast abscess in lactating women: report from an Australian cohort. *BJOG.* 2004;111(12):1378-1381.

Amir L, et al. A case-control study of mastitis: nasal carriage of *Staphylococcus aureus. BMC Fam Pract.* 2006;7:57.

Amir L, Ingram J. Health professionals' advice for breastfeeding problems: not good enough! *Int Breastfeed J.* 2008;3:22.

Anderson J, et al. Raynaud's phenomenon of the nipple: a treatable cause of painful breastfeeding. *Pediatrics.* 2004;113(4):e360-e364.

Andrews J, et al. The yeast connection: is *Candida* linked to breastfeeding associated pain? *Am J Obstet Gynecol.* 2007;197(4):424.e1-424.e4.

Andrews Z. Neuroendocrine regulation of prolactin secretion during late pregnancy: easing the transition into lactation. *J Neuroendocrinol.* 2005;17(7):466-473.

Aryeetey R, et al. Subclinical mastitis is common among Ghanaian women lactating 3 to 4 months postpartum. *J Hum Lact.* 2008;24(3):263-267.

Aryeetey R, et al. Subclinical mastitis may not reduce breastmilk intake during established lactation. *Breastfeed Med.* 2009;4(3):161-166.

Atkinson L. Prenatal nipple conditioning for breastfeeding. *Nurs Res.* 1979;28(5):267-271.

Avery A, et al. Confident commitment is a key factor for sustained breastfeeding. *Birth.* 2009;36(2):141-148.

Ayers J. The use of alternative therapies in the support of breastfeeding. *J Hum Lact.* 2000;16(1):52-56.

Ben-Jonathan N, et al. Focus on prolactin as a metabolic hormone. *Trends Endocrinol Metab.* 2006;17(3):110-116.

Ben-Jonathan N, et al. What can we learn from rodents about prolactin in humans? *Endocr Rev.* 2008;29(1):1-41.

Berens P. Breast complications while breastfeeding. Presented at: La Leche League of Texas Area Conference; June 12, 2004; San Antonio, TX.

Berná-Serna J, et al. Use of urokinase in percutaneous drainage of large breast abscesses. *J Ultrasound Med.* 2009;28(4):449-454.

Brennan A, et al. The tammar wallaby and fur seal: models to examine local control of lactation. *J Dairy Sci.* 2007;90(1):E66-E75.

Buhimschi C. Endocrinology of lactation. *Obstet Gynecol Clin North Am.* 2004;31(4):963-979, xii.

Cadwell K. Latching-on and suckling of the healthy term neonate: breastfeeding assessment. *J Midwifery Women's Health.* 2007;52(6):638-642.

Campbell S. Recurrent plugged ducts. *J Hum Lact.* 2006;22(3): 340-343.

Centers for Disease Control and Prevention (CDC). Environmental management of staph and MRSA in community settings. July 2008. http://www.cdc.gov/ncidod/dhqp/ar_mrsa_Enviro_Manage.html. Accessed June 10, 2009.

Cotterman K. Reverse pressure softening: a simple tool to prepare areola for easier latching during engorgement. *J Hum Lact.* 2004;20(2):227-237.

de Oliveira L, et al. Effect of intervention to improve breastfeeding technique on the frequency of exclusive breastfeeding and lactation-related problems. *J Hum Lact.* 2006;22(3):315-321.

Delgado S, et al. PCR-DGGE assessment of the bacterial diversity of breast milk in women with lactational infectious mastitis. *BMC Infect Dis.* 2008;8:51.

Delgado S, et al. *Staphylococcus epidermidis* strains isolated from breast milk of women suffering infectious mastitis: potential virulence traits and resistance to antibiotics. *BMC Microbiol.* 2009;9:82.

Demetriadi F, et al. Post-partum polyarthritis associated with a staphylococcal breast abscess. *Rheumatology (Oxford).* 2004;43(6):810-811.

Dhulkotia A, et al. Breast abscess: a unique presentation as primary septic arthritis of the sternoclavicular joint. *Breast J.* 2005;11(6):525-526.

DiGirolamo A, et al. Effect of maternity-care practices on breastfeeding. *Pediatrics.* 2008;122:2:S43-S49.

Dilli D, et al. Interventions to reduce pain during vaccination in infancy. *J Pediatr.* 2009;154(3):385-390.

Ekström A, Nissen E. A mother's feelings for her infant are strengthened by excellent breastfeeding counseling and continuity of care. *Pediatrics.* 2006;118(2):e309-e314.

Fetherston C, et al. Recurrent blocked duct(s) in a mother with immunoglobulin A deficiency. *Breastfeed Med.* 2008; 3(4):261-265.

Finks J, et al. Vancomycin-resistant *Staphylococcus aureus,* Michigan, USA, 2007. *Emerg Infect Dis.* June 2009. www.cdc.gov/EID/content/15/6/943.htm. Accessed June 10, 2009.

Forster D, et al. Factors associated with breastfeeding at six months postpartum in a group of Australian women. *Int Breastfeed J.* 2006;12(1):18.

Foxman B, et al. Lactation mastitis: occurrence and medical management among 946 breastfeeding women in the United States. *Am J Epidemiol.* 2002;155(2):103-114.

Geddes D. Reflections on lactation: From outside to inside. Presented at: Hartmann & Hale Human Lactation Research Conference: The Next Frontier in Lactation Research: Outside Factors That Influence Breastfeeding Success; June 5, 2009; Amarillo, TX.

Genna CW. Nipple blebs/blisters. *Medela Breastfeeding Fact Sheet.* McHenry, IL: Medela; 2004.

Gima P. Yeast and thrush: Pat Gima's treatment plan. March 2003. www.breastfeedingonline.com/yeast.shtml. Accessed June 15, 2009.

Grattan D, et al. Pregnancy-induced adaptation in the neuroendocrine control of prolactin secretion. *J Neuroendocrinol.* 2008;20(4):497-507.

Gray P, et al. Pain relief for neonates in Australian hospitals: a need to improve evidence-based practice. *J Paediatr Child Health.* 2006;42(1-2):10-13.

Guadagni M, Nazzari G. Zuska's disease. *G Ital Dermatol Venereol.* 2008;143(2):157-160.

Hale T. *Medications and Mothers' Milk.* 14th ed. Amarillo, TX: Hale Publishing; 2010.

Hale T, Berens P. *Clinical Therapy in Breastfeeding Patients.* Amarillo, TX: Pharmasoft; 2002.

Hale T, et al. The absence of *Candida albicans* in milk samples of women with clinical symptoms of ductal candidiasis. *Breastfeed Med.* 2009;4(2):57-61.

Hannula L, et al. A systematic review of professional support interventions for breastfeeding. *J Clin Nurs.* 2008;17(9): 1132-1143.

Hauck Y, et al. Prevalence, self-efficacy and perceptions of conflicting advice and self-management: effects of a breastfeeding journal. *J Adv Nurs.* 2007;57(3):306-317.

Hausman B. Women's liberation and the rhetoric of "choice" in infant feeding debates. *Intl Breastfeed J.* 2008;3:10.

Hegney D, et al. Against all odds: a retrospective case-controlled study of women who experienced extraordinary breastfeeding problems. *J Clin Nurs.* 2008;17(9):1182-1192.

Hewat R, Ellis D. A comparison of the effectiveness of two methods of nipple care. *Birth.* 1987;14:41-45.

Hobday R, et al. Dietary intervention in chronic fatigue syndrome. *J Hum Nutr Diet.* 2008;21(2):141-149.

Hofvander Y. Breastfeeding and the Baby-Friendly Hospital Initiative (BFHI): organization, response and outcome in Sweden and other countries. *Acta Paediatr.* 2005;94(8): 1012-1016.

International Baby Food Action Network (IBFAN). *Breaking the Rules: Stretching the Rules 2007.* Penang, Malaysia: International Code Documentation Center; 2007.

International Lactation Consultant Association (ILCA); Mannel R, Martens P, Walker M, eds. *Core Curriculum for Lactation Consultant Practice,* 2nd ed. Sudbury, MA: Jones and Bartlett; 2007.

Kasonka L, et al. Risk factors for subclinical mastitis among HIV-infected and uninfected women in Lusaka, Zambia. *Paediatr Perinat Epidemiol.* 2006;20(5):379-391.

Kassing D. Bottle feeding as a tool to reinforce breastfeeding. *J Hum Lact.* 2002;18(1):56-60.

Katz N, Mazer N. The impact of opioids on the endocrine system. *Clin J Pain.* 2009;25(2):170-175.

Kaufman D. Fluconazole prophylaxis: can we eliminate invasive *Candida* infections in the neonatal ICU? *Curr Opin Pediatr.* 2008;20(3):332-340.

Kent J, et al. Volume and frequency of breastfeedings and fat content of breast milk throughout the day. *Pediatrics.* 2006;117(3):e387-e395.

Kim-Godwin Y. Postpartum beliefs and practices among non-Western cultures. *MCN.* 2003;28(2):74-78.

Kutner L. *Certified Lactation Specialist Course.* Wheaton, IL: Lactation Education Consultants; 2009.

Kvist L, et al. The role of bacteria in lactational mastitis and some considerations of the use of antibiotic treatment. *Int Breastfeed J.* 2008;3:6.

Lacasse P, et al. Utilization of lactoferrin to fight antibiotic-resistant mammary gland pathogens [published online ahead of print June 12, 2007]. *J Anim Sci.* 2008;86(13 suppl):66-71.

Lannin D. Twenty-two year experience with recurring subareolar abscess and lactiferous duct fistula treated by a single breast surgeon. *Am J Surg.* 2004;188(4):407-410.

Lawlor-Smith L, Lawlor-Smith C. Vasospasm of the nipple: a manifestation of Raynaud's phenomenon. *BMJ.* 1997; 314:644-645.

Lawrence R, Lawrence R. *Breastfeeding: A Guide for the Medical Profession*, 6th ed. Philadelphia, PA: Elsevier Mosby; 2005.

Li R, et al. Why mothers stop breastfeeding: mothers' self-reported reasons for stopping during the first year. *Pediatrics.* 2008;122:S69-S76.

Lunney K, et al. Associations between breast milk viral load, mastitis, exclusive breast-feeding, and postnatal transmission of HIV. *Clin Infect Dis.* 2010;50(5):762-769.

Manzoni P, et al. Risk factors for progression to invasive fungal infection in preterm neonates with fungal colonization. *Pediatrics.* 2006;118(6):2359-2364.

Manzoni P, et al. A multicenter, randomized trial of prophylactic fluconazole in preterm neonates. *N Engl J Med.* 2007;356(24):2483-2495.

Marx CM, et al. Vitamin E concentrations in serum of newborn infants after topical use of vitamin E in nursing mothers. *Am J Obstet Gynecol.* 1985;152:668-670.

McClellan H, et al. Infants of mothers with persistent nipple pain exert strong sucking vacuums. *Acta Paediatr.* 2008;97(9):1205-1209.

MedicineNet.com. Vancomycin-resistant enterococci (VRE). May 29, 2008. www.medicinenet.com/vancomycin-resistant_enterococci_vre/article.htm. Accessed June 3, 2009.

Merten S, et al. Do baby-friendly hospitals influence breastfeeding duration on a national level? *Pediatrics.* 2005; 116(5):e702-e708.

Mitoulas L, et al. Variation in fat, lactose and protein in human milk over 24 h and throughout the first year of lactation. *Br J Nutr.* 2002;88(1):29-37.

Mizuno K, et al. The important role of deep attachment in the uniform drainage of breast milk from mammary lobe. *Acta Paediatr.* 2008;97(9):1200-1204.

Mohammadzadeh A, et al. The effect of breast milk and lanolin on sore nipples. *Saudi Med J.* 2005;26(8):1231-1234.

Mohrbacher N. *Nipple Pain and Trauma Algorithm.* Piqua, OH: Evenflo; 2008.

Morland-Schultz K, Hill P. Prevention of and therapies for nipple pain: a systematic review. *JOGNN.* 2005;34(4):428-437.

Morrill J, et al. Risk factors for mammary candidosis among lactating women. *JOGNN.* 2005;34(1):37-45.

Morton J. Is use of breast pumps out of hand? Mothers who use "hands-on" technique see increase in milk production *AAP News.* 2009;30(6):14.

Mulford C. Is breastfeeding really invisible, or did the health care system just choose not to notice it? *Int Breastfeed J.* 2008;3:13.

Newman J. All Purpose Nipple Ointment (APNO). Revised 2009. www.nbcionline.org/index.php?option=com_content& view=article&id=76:all-purpose-nipple-ointment-apno&catid=5:information&Itemid=17. Accessed June 2, 2009.

Newman J, Kernerman E. Blocked ducts and mastitis. Revised February 2009a. www.nbcionline.org/index.php?option= com_content&view=article&id=7:blocked-ducts-a-mastitis&catid=5:information&Itemid=17. Accessed June 2, 2009.

Newman J, Kernerman E. Breast compression. Revised February 2009b. www.nbcionline.org/index.php?option=com_ content&view=article&id=7:blocked-ducts-a-mastitis&catid= 5:information&Itemid=17. Accessed June 2, 2009.

Newman J, Kernerman E. Using gentian violet. Revised 2009c. www.nbcionline.org/index.php?option=com_content&view= article&id=73:using-gentian-violet&catid=5:information&Itemid=17. Accessed June 2, 2009.

Ohene-Yeboah M. Breast pain in Ghanaian women: Clinical, ultrasonographic, mammographic and histological findings in 1612 consecutive patients. *West Afr J Med.* 2008;27(1):20-23.

Olsen N, Nielson S. Prevalence of primary Raynaud's phenomenon in young females. *Scand J Clin Lab Invest.* 1978; 37:761-776.

Ozseker B, et al. Treatment of breast abscesses with ultrasound-guided aspiration and irrigation in the emergency setting. *Emerg Radiol.* 2008;15(2):105-108.

Page S, McKenna D. Vasospasm of the nipple presenting as painful lactation. *Obstet Gynecol.* 2006;108(3 Pt 2):806-808.

Racey D, et al. Galactorrhoea is not lactation. *Trends Ecol Evol.* 2009;24(7):354-355.

Rasmussen L, et al. Milk enzyme activities and subclinical mastitis among women in Guinea-Bissau. *Breastfeed Med.* 2008;3(4):215-219.

Rebhan B, et al. Breast-feeding, frequency and problems: results of the Bavarian breast-feeding study. *Gesundheitswesen.* 2008;70(suppl 1):S8-S12.

Roberts K, et al. A comparison of chilled cabbage leaves and chilled gel paks in reducing breast engorgement. *J Hum Lact.* 1995a;11(1):17-20.

Roberts K, et al. A comparison of chilled and room temperature cabbage leaves in treating breast engorgement. *J Hum Lact.* 1995b;11(3):191-194.

Rosier W. Cool cabbage compresses. *Breastfeed Rev.* 1988; 1(12):28-31.

Sayyah Melli M, et al. A randomized trial of peppermint gel, lanolin ointment, and placebo gel to prevent nipple crack in primiparous breastfeeding women. *Med Sci Monitor.* 2007a;13(9):CR406-CR411.

Sayyah Melli M, et al. Effect of peppermint water on prevention of nipple cracks in lactating primiparous women: a randomized controlled trial. *Int Breastfeed J.* 2007b;2:7.

Schwartz K, et al. Factors associated with weaning in the first 3 months postpartum. *J Fam Pract.* 2002;51(5):439-444.

Scott C. Lecithin: it isn't just for plugged milk ducts and mastitis anymore. *Midwifery Today Int Midwife.* 2005;76:26-27.

Shah P, et al. Breastfeeding or breastmilk to alleviate procedural pain in neonates: a systematic review. *Breastfeed Med.* 2007;2(2):74-82.

Smith P. "Is it just so my right?" Women repossessing breastfeeding. *Intl Breastfeed J.* 2008;3:12.

Snowden H, et al. Treatments for breast engorgement during lactation. *Cochrane Database Syst Rev.* 2001;2:CD000046.

Spiby H, et al. A systematic review of education and evidence-based practice interventions with health professionals and breast feeding counselors on duration of breast feeding. *Midwifery.* 2009;25(1):50-61.

Tarrant M, et al. Becoming a role model: the breastfeeding trajectory of Hong Kong women breastfeeding longer than 6 months. *Int J Nurs Stud.* 2004;41(5):535-546.

Tedder JL. Give them the HUG: an innovative approach to helping parents understand the language of their newborn. *J Perinat Educ.* 2008;17(2):14-20.

Traboulsi R, et al. In vitro activity of inexpensive topical alternatives against *Candida* spp. isolated from the oral cavity of HIV-infected patients [published online ahead of print February 1, 2008]. *Int J Antimicrob Agents.* 2008;31(3):272-276.

Uvnäs-Moberg K, et al. Plasma cholecystokinin concentrations after breast feeding in healthy 4 day old infants. *Arch Dis Child.* 1993;68(1 spec no):46-48.

Vendettuoli V, et al. The role of *Candida* surveillance cultures for identification of a preterm subpopulation at highest risk for invasive fungal infection. *Pediatr Infect Dis J.* 2008;27(12):1114-1116.

von Maillot K, et al. *Candida* mycosis in pregnant women and related risks to the newborn. *Mykosen.* 1978;1:246-251.

Walker M. *Still Selling Out Mothers and Babies: Marketing Breastmilk Substitutes in the USA.* Weston, MA: NABA REAL; 2007.

Wilson-Clay B, Hoover K. *The Breastfeeding Atlas*, 4th ed. Austin, TX: Lactnews Press; 2008.

Wöckel A, et al. Inflammatory breast diseases during lactation: Health effects on the newborn-a literature review [published online ahead of print April 20, 2008]. *Mediators Inflamm.* 2008;298760. doi: 10.1155/2008/298760.

Woo P, et al. Then and now: use of 16S rDNA gene sequencing for bacterial identification and discovery of novel bacteria in clinical microbiology laboratories. *Clin Microbiol Infect.* 2008;14(10):908-934.

Yildiz F. *Phytoestrogens in Functional Foods.* Boca Raton, FL: CRC Press; 2006.

Young H, et al. Estrogenic effects of extracts from cabbage, fermented cabbage, and acidified Brussels sprouts on growth and gene expression of estrogen-dependent human breast cancer (MCF-7) cells. *J Agricult Food Chem.* 2000;48(10):4628-4634.

Zöllner M, Jorge A. *Candida* spp. occurrence in oral cavities of breastfeeding infants and in their mothers' mouths and breasts. *Pesqui Odontol Bras.* 2003;17(2):151-155.

Breastfeeding Beyond the First Month

As babies mature beyond their first month, breastfeeding will change in response to their increased age and development. Babies of this age are awake for longer periods, expanding their world in the direction of physical and social development. Parents learn to change childcare practices to accommodate new breastfeeding patterns. New challenges present themselves in the form of breastfeeding in public, traveling with a nursing baby, returning to work or school, and adjusting nursing routines as the baby grows.

Over time, parents learn to recognize their baby's unique means of communication. Waking and sleeping patterns, crying, cooing, smiling, and frowning all elicit parental responses and readjustments. The baby progresses from an awareness of the mother as a satisfier of his or her needs through the development of motor skills for self-amusement and an awareness of the surrounding environment. The infant experiences teething, crawling, standing, separation anxiety, experimenting with vocabulary sounds, self-feeding, and drinking from a cup. Mothers face the challenges of nursing a toddler and, ultimately, weaning. You can help parents appreciate these developmental milestones as they adjust their parenting role to accommodate and celebrate them.

∼ Key Terms

Allergens
Baby-led weaning
Bauer's response
Body length
Food intolerance
Gradual weaning
Head circumference
Minimal breastfeeding

Moro reflex
Mother-led weaning
Nursing strike
Palmer grasp
Pincer grasp
Prone position
Reflexes
REM sleep
Soporific
Tonic neck reflex

∼ Patterns of Growth in a Breastfed Baby

The World Health Organization Growth Charts, which use breastfed babies as the standard, validate the normal range of human infant growth. As observed by nursing mothers for millennia, breastfed babies gain weight quickly during the first 3 to 4 months of life. Their rate of growth then slows (WHO, 2006). Table 17.1 shows infant weight range from birth to 12 months for boys and girls.

Breastfed infants typically double their birth weight by 5 to 6 months of age, and triple it by 1 year. In the first few months after birth, breastfed infants generally grow at about the same rate as their formula fed counterparts. After this time, formula fed infants typically begin to exceed breastfeeding infants in weight, while breastfed infants tend to gain more length. Formula fed infants are less energy efficient, taking in more milk and using nutrients less effectively than infants who are breastfed (Dewey et al., 1992). Head circumference is similar for both breastfed and formula fed infants.

Body length and head circumference are indicators of appropriate growth. At 1 year of age, a baby's length is typically about 11/2 times the newborn's length at birth. In addition, brain growth is quite rapid in the first year of life. Head circumference should increase approximately 7.6 cm (3 inches) by 1 year of age. Body length and head circumference to are similar in breastfed and formula fed infants until after 4 months of age. Infants who are breastfed for 12 or more months are leaner than formula fed infants because of their lower energy intake (Dewey et al., 1993).

Like adults, babies come in all shapes and sizes, and there is great variance in the range of weight gain. If the parents of a petite, wiry infant are thin and small framed, chances are that their baby will be, too. Sometimes breastfed babies are chubby and parents wonder if they are overweight. Usually, they slim down in toddlerhood. Family practice researchers suggest monitoring the growth of exclusively breastfed babies by plotting routine weights and lengths on the WHO growth curve. Weight gain in

TABLE 17.1 Infant Weight Ranges

Girls (kg)	Boys (kg)	Month	Girls (lb/oz)	Boys (lb/oz)
2.3–4.4	2.3–4.6	Birth	5.1–9.11	5.1–10.1
3.0–5.7	3.2–6.0	1	6.9–12.9	7.1–13.3
3.8–6.9	4.1–7.4	2	8.6–15.3	9.0–16.4
4.4–7.8	4.8–8.3	3	9.11–17.3	10.9–18.4
4.8–8.6	5.4–9.1	4	10.9–19	11.14–20.1
5.2–9.2	5.8–9.7	5	11.8–20.4	12.12–21.6
5.5–9.7	6.1–10.2	6	12.1–21.6	13.8–22.8
5.8–10.2	6.4–10.7	7	12.12–22.8	14.1–23.9
6.0–10.6	6.7–11.1	8	13.3–23.6	14.12–24.8
6.2–11.0	6.9–11.4	9	13.11–24.4	15.3–25.1
6.4–11.3	7.1–11.8	10	14.1–24.14	15.11–26.0
6.6–11.7	7.3–12.1	11	14.9–25.12	16.1–26.11
6.8–12.0	7.5–12.4	12	15.0–26.8	16.5–27.3

Source: Data from World Health Organization. *The WHO Child Growth Standards*. Geneva, Switzerland: World Health Organization; 2006. http://www.who.int/childgrowth/standards/en. Printed with permission of the International Lactation Consultant Association.

breastfed infants can be higher than normal with no known adverse effects. Mothers with large volumes of milk that exceed what their infants need can avoid overfeeding with the help of a lactation consultant. Rarely, an infant who seems insatiable may need to be assessed for an overgrowth syndrome through an endocrinology and genetics consult (Osayande et al., 2009).

∾ Infant Development

In the first hours and days after birth, parents become acutely aware that their baby has a distinct personality. As they become familiar with the infant's waking and sleeping patterns, crying and cooing, and smiling and frowning, parents learn how to adapt their responses and parenting to meet their baby's specific needs. Despite each baby's individuality, there are many characteristics and patterns that all babies exhibit as they develop mentally, emotionally, and physically. Given this commonality, caregivers who have experience with a large number of infants are able to identify those who do not exhibit age-appropriate reflexes and developmental milestones. Babies develop as individuals within certain parameters. Parents need to be aware of developmental milestones and talk with their healthcare provider if their baby appears not to develop as expected.

Infant Development in the First Year

Normal infant development has a wide range of variation. Each baby progresses at his or her own rate. Humans develop progressively from head to foot and from the center of the body or torso out to the extremities. This progression aids us in attaining mobility. Parents usually look forward to new abilities as their baby develops. Parents who are aware of these developmental stages in advance can anticipate and respond appropriately to their baby's changes and growth. A mother specifically will learn to alter her nursing patterns and other caregiving to meet her baby's ever-changing needs.

Reflexes

Reflexes present at birth remain in place until the baby develops finer skills to replace them. These reflexes are necessary for survival. Reflexes such as rooting, sucking, grasping, and swallowing enable babies to obtain food. A gag reflex protects infants from choking while learning to take in food. Newborns exhibit the Moro reflex, startling in response to sudden noise. The Palmer grasp enables them to grasp their parents' fingers.

In addition, infants exhibit the tonic neck reflex—a normal body reflex, also referred to as the "fencer position"—until 3 or 4 months of age. When they lie on their backs, they extend the arm and leg on the side of the body opposite to the direction in which the head is turned. This prevents them from rolling over until adequate neurologic and motor development occurs. Pressure on the soles of a baby's feet will elicit Bauer's response, with the baby making movements similar to crawling or kicking. This reflex is exhibited when babies are given the opportunity to self-attach after birth (Colson et al., 2008).

Moro, Palmer grasp, and tonic neck reflexes disappear at about 4 months of age. Bauer's response and the

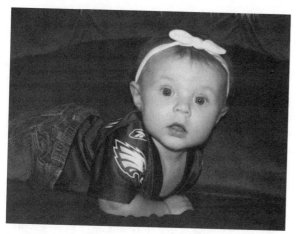

FIGURE 17.1   Baby at 3 months holding her head up.
Source: Printed with permission of Judith Lauwers.

rooting and sucking reflexes continue to about 9 months. Chapter 14 provides more information on the baby's innate feeding abilities.

Head and Body Control

Newborns are able to raise their heads purposefully from birth. These focused behaviors are often missed in Western hospitals, due to medicated births and rushed procedures (Smith, 2008). At about 3 months of age, babies can support their upper body with their arms when lying on the stomach and begin to raise their head from a prone position more consistently (see Figure 17.1).

By 4 to 5 months, as infants gain head and neck strength, they can raise the head higher and hold it for longer periods. They also become more alert and turn the head toward a voice or movement. During this same period, they begin to rest on the forearms as the torso becomes stronger.

By 6 months, large muscle motor development enables infants to roll over. The torso strengthens as they prepare for crawling. By 7 months, babies can roll over in either direction and can pull themselves to a standing position. Babies need to spend time on their tummies to achieve these developmental milestones.

Hand Movement

At 1 month, most babies will bring their hands near their face and keep their hands in tight fists. By 3 months, they will open and shut their hands and bring them to their mouth. They will start using their hands and eyes in coordination and will grab and shake toys.

At 4 to 5 months, infants are able to control hand movements and begin to play with their fingers. They wave and bat at objects, fascinated by movement.

By 6 months, infants master visually directed reaching so that they can grasp desired items and pull them toward their mouth. Tongue movement now allows them to take solid foods and begin to learn the social art of eating. Many babies at this age begin reaching for foods when they join the family for meals. Watching family members eat and grabbing for food are signs of developmental readiness to begin solids.

By 7 months, babies' hands and arms are more developed. They learn to wave goodbye and can transfer objects from hand to hand. They will struggle to get objects that are out of reach and will explore objects with their hands and mouth. They begin to use the thumb and forefinger to pick up objects, called the pincer grasp, at about 8 to 9 months of age.

Sitting

Sitting upright is one of the first developmental large motor milestones achieved by infants (Deffeyes et al., 2009). At 4 months, the baby's back is rounded and the head erect when held in a sitting position (see Figure 17.2). By 5 months, the body will be erect when supported. At 6 months, increased head and neck control make it possible to pull the infant to a sitting position. By this age, most babies can sit if they are propped. By 7 months, they can sit without being propped. By 9 months, they can sit well in a chair and pull themselves into a sitting position.

Crawling and Walking

Babies become very active by 7 months, a time when they expand their world through physical movements. Many babies begin the early stages of crawling at about 6 to 8 months, raising themselves onto their hands and knees and rocking back and forth (see Figure 17.3).

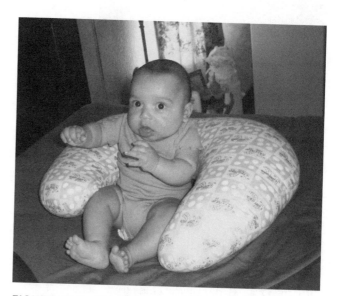

FIGURE 17.2   Baby at 4 months sitting with support.
Source: Printed with permission of Anna Swisher.

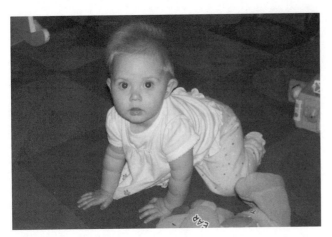

FIGURE 17.3   Baby at 6 months starting to crawl.
Source: Printed with permission of Judith Lauwers.

By 10 to 12 months, the beginning of locomotion has arrived. This is an expansive age for infants, as they vigorously and enthusiastically practice many new motor skills while avidly exploring the environment. They learn to cruise by using tables and chairs to balance as they begin to learn to walk (Figure 17.4). Babies progress from cruising to walking typically between 9 and 17 months of age. Because experience is a stronger predictor of skill improvement than age, babies need lots of opportunities and time for practice (Adolph et al., 2003). By 1 year, babies are interested in everything and show their pleasure and displeasure easily.

Mothers can help satisfy their babies' strong desire to explore by giving them freedom to move within safe lim-

its at home. Because babies are able to reach many items that can pose a danger to them, parents need to examine their house for potential hazards. As early as 10 months, babies can crawl up stairs but they cannot crawl down them. Children typically master stair ascent at about 11 months, several months after learning to crawl. They learn to descend stairs at 12 to 13 months (Berger et al., 2007). Parents in homes with stairs will want to spend time teaching their child to ascend and descend stairs. They may also want to place a baby gate at both ends of the stairs for safety, but should be cognizant that vigilance with mobile babies is crucial.

Many parents lived in one- or two-child households when they were young. They may not have been around babies or toddlers or know common-sense safety precautions. If you visit their home, be alert to potential hazards and gently point them out. Explain why something is dangerous so parents understand. A good idea for baby-proofing a home is for parents to get down and crawl around at the same level a baby would. New hazards that are easy to miss from a standing position become apparent at eye level. Objects such as cords, curtains, window blinds, and electrical outlets can all be dangerous to curious young explorers. For safety's sake, water should never be heated on the front burner of a stove in the home where a young child resides. Pot handles should be turned to the back so they cannot be reached and pulled down on the child.

Child safety information is available from many sources, including the Home Safety Council (www.home-safetycouncil.org). Many businesses provide child safety assessments and child-proofing services. Providing a list of those in your area may be helpful.

Sleep Pattern

Each baby's physical development determines when the infant will be able to sleep through the night. The ability to sleep for longer periods will increase as the baby's central nervous system develops. Differences in sleep organization and energy expenditure between breastfed and formula fed infants may indicate that breastfeeding enhances maturation of the central nervous system (Butte et al., 1992). Neuroimaging research can now probe the infant brain's intrinsic functional architecture. Such imaging shows that babies have synchronized spontaneous neuronal activity present even during natural sleep, in the form of resting-state networks in the brain, even in the absence of external stimuli (Fransson et al., 2009).

Newborns spend 50 percent of their time in REM (rapid eye movement) sleep, which is essential for brain growth and maturation. By 6 to 12 months of age, this proportion decreases to 30 percent. By comparison, adults spend only 20 percent of sleep time in REM sleep. Researchers have observed that among preterm infants,

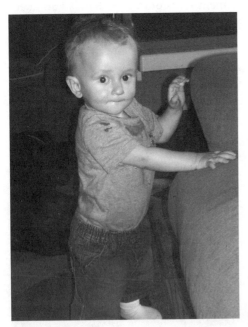

FIGURE 17.4   Baby at 1 year cruising with support of furniture.
Source: Printed with permission of Judith Lauwers.

those with low REM activity cry more and have more unfocused alert states in the neonatal period. In addition, they have lower mental development scores (Bayley II) at 6 months' corrected age compared to infants with high REM activity. This finding suggests that low REM activity may serve as an indicator of developmental risk, at least among preterm babies (Arditi-Babchuk, 2009).

As the baby approaches 3 months of age, the sleeping pattern usually shifts to at least one longer rest period and several naps each day. A baby's personality may determine during which part of the 24-hour cycle he or she sleeps for a longer period. The mother can adjust this cycle by initiating feedings more frequently during the day. When changes in the baby's sleep pattern occur, the mother may awaken with more fullness in her breasts than previously. Nursing her baby directly before she retires for the evening will promote the longest period at night and provide the mother with 5 or 6 hours of uninterrupted sleep.

At around 8 months of age, a baby may experience separation anxiety upon waking during the night and realizing that the mother is not nearby. Even after developing the ability to sleep for longer periods, a baby may experience disturbed sleep because of dreams. The need to nurse can also cause disturbed sleep. This sort of disruption is common during periods of rapid physical and mental growth, increased activity during the day, and teething. In the second year of age, the child may still need close physical contact to fall asleep.

Social Development

The baby's world broadens as he or she develops an awareness of the mother as the person who responds to the infant's needs. By 3 months, the infant regards the mother–baby dyad as a single entity, and the infant's need for her is absolute. The mother may have ambivalent feelings about such constant demands on her time and presence. She may enjoy the dependency because it helps her feel important and useful. At the same time, she may wish she had more time to herself for relaxation and recreation. She will continue to make adjustments as she defines her new role, enabling her to establish priorities in baby care while learning to postpone her own needs.

Interaction By 3 months, babies respond to stimuli and become very social. They begin to focus on objects around them and interact with both the parents and the environment (see Figure 17.5). Visual acuity becomes clearer, and infants will bat at objects in an attempt to touch and move them. They will respond more readily to high-pitched voices and may show interest in children while ignoring adults. This interest encourages siblings to entertain and interact with the infant.

At 3 months, the baby will be awake for more hours each day and will be much more alert and responsive.

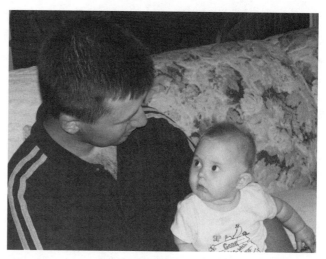

FIGURE 17.5 Baby at 3 months interacting with her father.
Source: Printed with permission of Judith Lauwers.

The mother will interact with the infant in ways other than breastfeeding, exposing him or her to everyday household sounds and providing bright, colorful toys and decorations. Varying positions and environment during the day will help provide the stimulation such a young child needs for physical and mental growth. Parents will enjoy playing with their baby. Encouraging tummy time promotes muscle development and prevents the baby's head from flattening because of lying supine the majority of the day.

Typical well-baby checks occur at 2 months and then at 4 months of age. Red flags for developmental delays by 3 months, as described by the Mayo Clinic (2008), include the following signs and symptoms:

- No improvement in head control
- No attempts to lift the head when lying in a face-down position
- Extreme floppiness
- Lack of response to sounds or visual cues, such as loud noises or bright lights
- Inability to focus on a caregiver's eyes
- Poor weight gain

At 10 to 12 months, the baby is eager to participate in family activities and will especially want to take part in mealtimes. Parents can offer finger foods that the baby can study, touch, turn over, and taste. Mealtime becomes a time of discovery and interaction. By participating in the feeding process, the infant experiences the independence he or she craves. As mobility increases, the child discriminates further between self and mother, freely moving away from the mother to explore the environment, while continually checking back for assurance that she will be there upon his or her return returns.

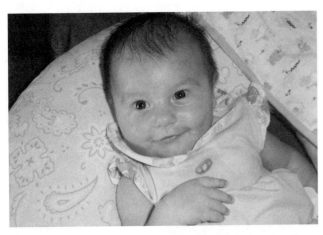

FIGURE 17.6 Baby at 2 months responding with a smile.
Source: Printed with permission of Judith Lauwers.

Disposition Smiles begin at around 2 months (see Figure 17.6). Big smiles are evident by 3 months, at which time babies recognize voices of their caregivers. They learn to express unhappiness, delight, and excitement during this time. Babies at this age may show a preference their parents, especially the mother, and may fuss when others provide care. At 3 months, infants are able to sense tension in a caregiver. They will respond with tension and fussiness, quieting down only when held in a calm and relaxed manner. Their eating and sleeping take on a more definite pattern, which may integrate easily into the family schedule.

By 4 months, babies have mastered the art of laughing aloud, to the delight of everyone around them. At this time, most parents have adapted their lives to the needs of their new baby and feel more confident in their parenting abilities. Their hours of patience, understanding, and love are rewarded by infants' responsiveness and development of elementary skills. Babies begin to gain independence through use of motor skills for self-amusement, and their demands on the parents decrease accordingly.

At about 9 months, babies' awareness of the mother's ability to be apart from them may bring on separation anxiety or dismay when a loved one leaves the room. As a result, they may cry in anticipation of the mother leaving or while she is away. They may wake during the night and cry out for reassurance that the parents are nearby. At this age, infants have learned that parents are important but do not have the awareness that they will return. Parents need to recognize this anxiety as a natural stage in their baby's development.

At 9 months, it is common for babies to prefer their mothers to their fathers. Their increased awareness of differences in people may cause them to react fearfully to strangers. Infants may continue their need for contact with the mother for reassurance. Parents do not need to protect infants from exposure to new people, however. Observing strangers will enhance babies' awareness of the

mother as a special person in their lives. Infants' fearful reactions to strangers are normal behavior at this age.

At 10 to 12 months, babies become so involved in physical achievements that they may feel overwhelmed by outside stresses such as contact with strangers, separation from the mother, and changes in schedule. They may react with shyness or fear, or begin clinging to the mother like a much younger baby. They may climb into the mother's lap to escape stresses as well as for emotional refueling. Although they may not appear tired, infants of this age need several periods of rest from active exploration each day to renew their energy.

Vocalization During the first year of life, researchers observe that early spontaneous facial movements undergo significant developmental change toward skill development for speech (Green & Wilson, 2006). By 4 to 5 months, babies begin to imitate sounds. By 6 months, babbling, cooing, and squealing mark the beginning of language. Babbling is the vocalization of vowel–consonant combinations. As they experiment with language, infants interact with those around them. Responding to infants' language efforts is essential for their development. This is a very active and social period for babies. At 10 to 12 months, their recognition vocabulary (words that the infant understands and responds to) increases noticeably, and children begin experimenting with vocabulary sounds. They expand their sociability, often seeming to interact with others in a negative manner by repeatedly saying, "No!"

Breastfeeding Behavior

Baby-friendly practices encourage a mother to nurse her baby immediately after birth. However, many babies do not actively feed at this time. They may be sleepy following delivery or simply need time to explore how to suck and grasp the breast. A baby who is allowed to self-attach is able to learn to breastfeed effectively, if the infant is not medicated and is full term, and if other problems are not present. Usually, breastfeeding patterns will settle in over the first several weeks after birth.

One Month By 1 month, infants are efficient at sucking and will actively nurse for 15 minutes or more at a feeding. They typically establish a pattern ranging between 8 and 16 feedings per day. Periods of increased appetite and growth can occur at any time. Babies typically experience appetite spurts at about 2 weeks, 6 weeks, 3 months, and 6 months of age. During this time, they nurse much more frequently, in spurts that last 2 to 3 days. Encourage mothers to respond with frequent feedings and lots of snuggling.

Anticipatory guidance about growth spurts will help prepare families for the possible arrival of "free" formula on their doorstep at about 7 to 10 days after birth. Formula companies obtain parents' personal information from a myriad of sources (e.g., Internet, drawings, retail stores, "baby fairs") to target times of vulnerability when the mother may question her milk production and begin the downward spiral of formula supplementation and eventual weaning (International Baby Food Action Network [IBFAN], 2007; Walker, 2007).

2 to 3 Months By 2 to 3 months, babies will typically spend less time at each feeding. Their sucking becomes more efficient as they mature, and they may use methods other than nursing for self-comforting. A mother may perceive this change as decreased interest in breastfeeding. Hormonal changes during this period may cause the mother's breasts to be less full. This may cause the mother to worry that she has lost her milk, which can increase her apprehension.

You can help mothers anticipate these changes as normal events in breastfeeding. Encourage the mother to focus on her baby's disposition, appearance, number of voids/stools, weight gain, interactions, and vigor. These signs will be reassuring to her and encourage her continuation of breastfeeding. Your open-ended questions, positive feedback, and descriptive statements may increase her security and confidence that she and her baby are competent and working in harmony. Their continued symbiotic relationship provides the infant with the precise amount of milk supporting optimal growth.

The mother may need to leave her baby regularly by 3 months. Many mothers must return to work—some as early as 6 weeks after birth. Make sure they know how to express milk to cover absences, as well as alternative feeding options other than a bottle. For example, breastfed babies often find the transition to a cup easier than a move to a bottle. Chapter 21 discusses expressing and feeding milk to the baby in more detail.

4 to 6 Months By 4 months, most babies become noticeably more efficient at nursing. Feedings shorten in length and may occur less frequently. Infants of this age become very interested in their surroundings and may shorten or miss some feedings because they are so curious about everything. When infants nurse at night, the nighttime intake may account for as much as 20 percent of the total 24-hour intake (Kent et al., 2006). Thus babies who are too busy to nurse often during the day may make up for it at night, given the opportunity.

Mothers need to watch their babies' output and weight gain during this time. Because the infant requires less time at the breast to satisfy hunger needs, the mother may consider feeding solid foods. You can remind her that a baby's swallowing mechanism and gastrointestinal tract are not mature enough to handle solid foods until 6 months of age or later. Assure her that her milk is still the ideal food to support her baby's growth. The American Academy of Pediatrics (AAP) recommends exclusive breastfeeding for the first 6 months of life.

At 4 months, babies continue to need their mothers' attention, yet expand their world beyond breastfeeding. Mothers can share in this growth by providing opportunities for their infants to develop to their full potential. Breastfeeding will continue to serve as a quiet, secure retreat from the stimulation of learning about the world apart from the mother.

By 4 to 5 months, babies may pat or stroke the breast and strain their body away from the mother to have a better look at her or to scan the environment. Mothers may regard this behavior as a sign of their babies' desire to separate themselves from exclusive breastfeeding or even as a rejection of them as mothers. Some babies may go through what is referred to by some as a "nursing strike." A nursing strike occurs when a baby who has previously been breastfeeding well becomes unhappy and fussy at the breast. Despite being hungry, the baby resists going to the breast, pulls off, and starts crying. In some instances, the baby may not cry but still pushes away. See Chapter 22 for further discussion of nursing strikes.

The apparent loss of interest or tendency toward distraction is actually a positive step forward in the baby's growth and development. It shows that infants are reaching out to learn more about the world around them. Breastfeeding continues easily during this expansive time as babies internalize their new knowledge and gain confidence.

By 6 months, the frequency of feedings usually will continue to diminish. The longest nursing usually will take place before being put to bed for the night. Solid foods will begin around this time, and the baby may wake more often during the night to nurse. Teething will begin soon, which can result in increased feedings for comfort and reassurance. The baby may drool, suck on his or her fingers, or chew on objects. Sucking can induce pain in the baby's tender gums and may cause the infant to pull off the breast abruptly.

These fluctuations in the nursing pattern, coupled with those caused by the baby's distractibility at this age, may result in less milk removal and the potential for engorgement, plugged ducts, and mastitis. Wiping the nipples with clear water after feedings will help prevent skin irritation. Regular milk removal will keep milk ducts open and prevent the development of plugs and infections.

Somewhere between 4 and 6 months, babies who have been sleeping through the night commonly begin waking at night to nurse. Developmentally, infants are doing more during the day. Nursing at night enables them to receive the calories they may have missed during the day. It also allows infants to reconnect with the mother. Cosleeping enables a baby to nurse frequently, maintains milk production, and provides the baby with a sense of security (Hicks, 2005).

7 to Twelve Months Most babies will have begun teething by 7 to 9 months of age. During this period, they will actively seek to nurse anytime and anywhere, pulling at the mother's clothing or attempting to unbutton her blouse. Babies may hold the breast with one or both hands while nursing. Over the next couple of months, they may become distracted easily, and mothers will need to find quiet locations for uninterrupted feedings.

By 10 to 12 months, newly found freedom can result in further changes in nursing patterns. Some babies increase the frequency and duration of their feedings as the many new events and experiences in their lives prompt a need for reassurance that there are safe and familiar aspects in the world. The constant need for reassurance and closeness, as well as increased feedings, may upset a mother who thought her baby was on the verge of weaning. She may feel discouraged by the infant's apparent lack of progress toward independence. You can assure her that satisfying the child's emotional needs now will lead to emotional growth and subsequent independence later.

By 10 to 12 months, babies mastered motor skills and established regular meal patterns. They may turn to the mother more frequently for comfort and reassurance, increasing the number of feedings. A mother may interpret this behavior as a sign that her baby is becoming overly dependent on her or on breastfeeding. The apparent dependence can be her baby's way of expressing a need for the reassurance of the safe, comfortable part of the world. It may indicate that an infant needs more time to adapt to his or her new experiences. You can let the mother know that her baby's current need for closeness will eventually lead to more independence. What may seem like a step away from independence may actually provide the security that will give the infant confidence to move toward self-reliance.

By 12 months, outside pressure may lead a mother to consider weaning. Her baby is now capable of obtaining nourishment away from the breast, and it may appear that the child is outgrowing breastfeeding. You can assure the mother that the infant still needs the security and comfort of nursing as a stabilizing factor in his or her life. Moreover, solid foods do not usually contain the special fatty acids present in human milk needed for continued brain growth. Only mother's milk contains the immune factors and antibodies specific to the baby's environment.

Remind mothers that the American Academy of Pediatrics recommends breastfeeding for the first year and beyond (AAP, 2005). The World Health Organization recommends breastfeeding for the first 2 years of life (WHO, 2002). The American Academy of Family Physicians recommends breastfeeding beyond infancy (AAFP, 2008). A large study by the Centers for Disease Control and Prevention (CDC: Infant Feeding Practices Study II) found that only 25.2 percent of babies were receiving any breastmilk at 12 months (USDHHS, 2009). Your encour-

agement can help mothers in your care to continue nursing at this stage of their babies' development.

There is a prevalent belief in U.S. culture that a mother's milk is no longer beneficial after the first year of an infant's life. You can educate parents about the continuing nutrition and protection afforded by human milk in the second year of life. If a mother chooses to wean at this time, your role is to support her decision. Help her replace her usual nursing periods with other types of close interaction. A mother who breastfeeds an older baby will benefit from support and encouragement, because it is difficult to breastfeed in a bottle feeding culture. Praise her for overcoming any obstacles, and validate the pride she feels in nourishing her child.

Overfeeding a Breastfed Baby Sometimes a mother may worry that her baby is nursing too frequently and for too long at a feeding. This worry could stem from a baby who seems to be overweight or who spits up milk. Babies are considered overweight if they are approximately two categories above the weight for height standard, as determined by standard height and weight charts. A normal weight gain is 1 to 2 pounds per month for the first 4 or 5 months of life. This rapid weight gain should not continue into the second half of the first year.

Some families have heavier babies who thin down in the second year, regardless of whether they are breastfed or bottle fed. If the baby is significantly heavier than other family members were, the child may be getting too much milk. An older baby who often spits up or vomits from an overly distended stomach may be overfed. In such a case, the mother's milk production may be overabundant. The mother can shorten or decrease feedings and substitute other activities for breastfeeding until the spitting up diminishes. Chapter 14 offers additional suggestions for dealing with overactive milk production.

Overfeeding may potentially occur when a baby nurses frequently for comfort or has a great sucking need. You can suggest to the mother alternative ways of comforting her baby so that she does not use feeding as a response to every cue. Encourage her to see the total picture of the developing mother–child relationship and to refine her parenting skills to meet her child's needs. As the months go by, the mother needs to interact with her baby through activities other than nursing in order to expand the infant's world in the direction of optimal physical and social development.

The following actions may assist the mother in avoiding overfeeding:

- Let the baby suck on his or her thumb or finger.
- Nurse at one breast per feeding and allow the baby to continue sucking on the less full breast.
- Learn other ways to interact with the baby—rock, carry, and keep the baby within view of the mother;

talk to the baby; change his or her position; play with and sing to the baby.

- Interest the baby in other activities—a stroll, toys, baby exercises, and so on.

Infant Development Beyond 1 Year

As a baby advances into toddlerhood, breastfeeding pattern reflects changes in the baby's social, emotional, and physical development. Many babies will continue to nurse far beyond 1 year. Others will wean themselves and never seem to miss breastfeeding. Providing anticipatory guidance to parents will relieve concerns and help them enjoy this exciting and entertaining stage of their children's lives.

Social and Emotional Development

Sometime between 12 and 15 months of age, the baby may again demonstrate a fear of strangers and a dislike for separation from the mother. The child may regress to earlier behaviors in an attempt to adjust to such incidents. A mother who works outside the home may be especially aware of these regressions. She will want to make certain that her baby's caretaker provides the attention and caring the child needs to develop emotional stability.

Overstimulation during the day or separation anxiety may cause a baby to wake at night. The child may especially appreciate the closeness of breastfeeding as a way to return to sleep. Love and reassurance freely given are likely to be the best cure for insecurity. Recognizing this fact may appease the mother of a baby who clings and nurses more frequently than she may wish. Many mothers separated from their babies during the day treasure their evenings and nights together. After all, the baby's outside interests soon will become more important than breastfeeding. The mother's love, patience, and understanding are rewarded when she sees her child as a secure and independent individual.

As the baby grows older, communication and play become increasingly important. The child's world extends to increase interaction with the father, who presents the novelty of another personality with different ideas and responses. A mother who returns home at the end of the day may offer this same type of diversion. When the baby begins to develop a close relationship with another person, the mother may worry that her role is diminishing. In reality, her baby needs her in new ways as he or she reaches out to others. This positive step in the child's development will eventually lead to the ability to identify and understand the separate interests of the parents. Eventually, the child will learn that absent parents will return, which minimizes emotional upset over temporary separations. Allowing the baby opportunities to become self-reliant and to proceed at a comfortable pace will encourage the child's growth and independence.

Breastfeeding Behavior

The expansion of the baby's world carries over to mealtimes. The mother can provide opportunities to breastfeed as she perceives her baby needs it. The infant will enjoy using a spoon for self-feeding and will practice picking up and drinking from a cup. As with all other tasks that the baby attempts, the mother will want to encourage exploration and practice. Accepting mistakes and spills as a part of learning is a helpful approach for parents to adopt concerning their child's eating habits.

In the second year of life, a child no longer requires as much food as in the first year, and becomes interested in other things. This shift in focus contributes to a decrease in appetite. The infant may have gained as much as 16 pounds in the first year and may double in weight after another 3 years. Food preferences become better defined, and a low-key approach to food selection may be the most effective method of ensuring an adequate diet. The mother can be satisfied if her 1-year-old eats one balanced meal a day plus two other partial meals and nutritious snacks.

The mother's milk will continue to provide significant calories, vitamins, and minerals and immunity to illness during this time. Breastfeeding is encouraged throughout the second year and beyond. The composition of milk changes as the baby's nursing pattern changes. The "weaning" milk of toddlers has a higher concentration of secretory immunoglobulin A (IgA), which helps protect young children who put their hands into their mouths as they explore an unsanitary world.

As their needs change during this expansive age, babies' breastfeeding patterns will fluctuate. They may nurse less frequently when they are busy experimenting with new skills, or more frequently because of an increased need for security or attention. They may also seek to nurse when they are getting ill. Testing other possibilities before putting the baby to breast helps the mother ensure that she does not initiate breastfeeding as the sole solution to her infant's bids for attention. This will ease the transition to a more comfortable pattern for the mother and child. Setting aside several special times during each day for total interaction with her baby will result in fewer interruptions at other times. These times will help a mother fulfill her baby's need for attention and social interaction in a positive manner.

~ Breastfeeding an Older Baby

As the baby grows and breastfeeding progresses, many events occur that require a mother to expand her childcare and parenting techniques. The lactation consultant can help her identify ways that breastfeeding fits into these events. The mother may need to make choices about how she will nurse in front of others or in public places. She may require suggestions for comforting her baby during teething or ways of coping with biting.

At some point, her baby may lose interest in nursing or develop a preference for one breast over the other. If a mother finds that she is still nursing her baby beyond the point at which she had planned to stop, you can help her reevaluate her goals. Anticipatory guidance will help the mother progress through breastfeeding in a rewarding and positive way. Knowing what to expect at each stage of breastfeeding may help the mother nurse as long as she originally planned, or even longer.

Breastfeeding in Public

Each individual mother makes her breastfeeding experience unique according to her attitudes and philosophies. Some mothers prefer to nurse only in the privacy of their homes. Others are comfortable breastfeeding in the homes of friends and family. Many women enjoy taking their babies along with them for shopping and dining out and are comfortable breastfeeding in public places. Some may be uncomfortable breastfeeding in the presence of other people, worrying that they are the center of attention and that others will disapprove.

Several U.S. states have passed legislation protecting a mother's and baby's right to breastfeed anywhere. Pointing this fact out may provide reassurance to mothers who question the acceptance of public breastfeeding. When a mother learns techniques that eliminate awkwardness and obscure her body from public view, she will often become more comfortable nursing in public.

A mother can gain confidence by watching other women nurse their babies, observing practical methods and other people's reactions. She may also feel more self-assured after she practices nursing in front of a mirror or another person. The baby's father is often a great "mirror" for the mother, as he may be more likely to give candid comments about what others might see. Another excellent place to try discreet nursing is within breastfeeding support groups, where other mothers can learn from one another.

If a mother knows she will be away from home during usual feeding times, she can prepare for discreet nursing by selecting appropriate clothing. Loose-fitting clothes allow easy access to the breast, and a sweater, jacket, or other such garment worn over her shoulders can conceal her breast from those who may view her from the side. A baby sling will provide support and extra cover, as well as ease in mobility. To avoid attracting attention, the mother can begin a feeding before her baby becomes overly hungry and starts to fuss. She will need to allow time for this feeding in her schedule.

A mother can also allow time to look for a comfortable place to nurse if she is unfamiliar with her location.

A spot that is out of the way of aisles and walkways will be more comfortable for the mother and less distracting for the baby. Such places include a corner table or booth in a restaurant, a bench next to a wall, sitting next to her partner or friends, a department store dressing room or lounge, or a parked car. Mothers should never breastfeed in a restroom or other highly unsanitary environment. A restroom is not an appropriate place for any type of eating!

With forethought and planning, a mother can choose a time and location for nursing in which she can be relaxed and comfortable. Most women grow in confidence as they learn they can breastfeed in public and that few people even notice. Breastfeeding in public has gained more acceptance as people recognize the importance of breastfeeding for lifelong health. To support this practice, many facilities now offer nursing lounges for mothers.

Traveling with a Breastfeeding Baby

The mother's physical recovery is nearly complete sometime after her baby is approximately 6 weeks old. At this point, she may be ready to leave home with her baby for extended periods. A baby between the ages of 6 weeks and 6 months is usually an ideal traveler. The child has a predictable routine, does not yet eat solid foods, and is not very mobile. Babies at this age often sleep through the monotony of an automobile, train, bus, or airplane ride, making the trip that much easier for parents. Traveling with a baby decreases the worry a mother might experience about being apart from her baby.

Planning for the Trip

Although traveling with a baby is more cumbersome than traveling alone, careful planning and preparation can help make it both convenient and enjoyable. So as not to become overburdened, parents can confine baby care items to those that are essential. Breastfeeding eliminates the need for supplemental foods or artificial baby milk, as well as the equipment necessary to prepare and transport them. It also eliminates the worry about the possibility of using contaminated water to reconstitute formula.

A lightweight diaper bag can double as a purse, and using disposable diapers will further decrease baggage. Parents can purchase diapers conveniently along the way, so only a few need to be packed. Several changes of baby clothing in the diaper bag, as well as plastic pants worn over diapers to contain potentially messy stools, will decrease the need to open suitcases in search of clothing while en route. For long trips, parents can take along a few items to keep the baby amused. Colorful pictures, rattles, and toys tied onto a string will all capture the baby's attention temporarily.

Traveling by Foot

A baby sling is convenient for walking with a baby. It is more versatile than a stroller, especially in crowded shops, on stairways, on hiking trails, and in the sand. Wearing the baby in a sling also helps prevent the baby from touching things in stores. Furthermore, the comfortable position and motion associated with a sling often lulls an infant to sleep. A lightweight cloth sling will fit easily into the mother's bag, ready to use at any time. For added protection in cold weather, parents can place the baby in the sling under their coat. Parents are cautioned to wear their baby safely, ensuring that the baby's face is visible and not pressed tightly against the wearer.

Traveling by Automobile

For safety, a baby should be strapped securely into an approved infant car seat when traveling by automobile. Infant car seats are also effective for other modes of travel and are more comfortable for the baby than adult seats. Parents should never hold their baby in a moving automobile, as a sudden stop could result in the parent losing hold and hurling the baby from the car or against the car's interior. Likewise, caution parents against carrying their baby in a sling or baby carrier while they are riding in the car: The force of the parent's body could cause serious injury to the baby in the event of a sudden stop.

A mother should be discouraged from breastfeeding during an automobile ride unless she is able to nurse with her baby remaining in the rear-facing car seat while she has her seat belt securely fastened. A bottle of expressed milk helps stretch out nursing times. In addition, parents can stop every 2 or 3 hours to allow for nursing and to permit the baby to move around freely. While repeated stops increase travel time, ultimately the journey will be more enjoyable when everyone arrives safely and comfortably at their destination. Allowing extra time for these accommodations is part of meeting everyone's needs.

At times, parents may need to endure the baby's crying if they cannot find a suitable distraction. This is probably the most difficult part of traveling with a child. It usually occurs near the end of the trip, when the parents are pushing to arrive at their destination. You can help parents understand that babies are not able to tolerate very long periods of travel. Encourage them to relax their schedule to accommodate their baby.

Traveling by Air

When planning a trip by air, a mother can request the roomier seat behind the bulkhead. Babies should be placed in their car seats strapped into a regular seat, if parents can afford a ticket for the baby. Otherwise, the baby will have to be held on a parent's lap. Strollers and other baby equipment can be well marked and checked with the luggage, leaving the mother free to carry her baby and only those items she will need during the flight. Airlines usually allow parents with small children to board the plane before other passengers so they can get settled and avoid waiting in line.

While on the airplane, mothers need to be aware that changes in cabin pressure may affect the baby's ears. Breastfeeding during takeoff and descent can help minimize this discomfort.

Teething and Biting

Babies typically cut their first tooth between 6 and 8 months of age, although teething can occur anywhere between 4 and 14 months. As a tooth erupts, it causes swelling and irritation in the gums. When the baby sucks, blood rushes to the gums, which adds to the swelling that is already present and causes immediate discomfort. Thus, when beginning to nurse, the baby may quickly pull away from the breast and cry out with pain. The mother may notice additional clues that her baby is teething, such as irritability, a slight fever, increased drooling, or unexplained spit up or loose stools. The baby may also begin waking during the night to seek comfort.

Overcoming Teething Pain

The baby soon discovers that chewing and rubbing the gums reduces teething pain. A teething baby may also rub the jaw or pull on an ear to relieve the discomfort—the same nerves to the teeth branch out to the face, cheek, and outer ear. A baby who cries out when the mother rubs the gums may be teething. Continued rubbing on the gums should be comforting and help the baby settle down. Providing the baby with a cooled teething ring or rubbing ice or a cold cloth on the gums before breastfeeding can relieve the soreness long enough to allow the baby to nurse comfortably. Providing suitable objects and hard foods such as toast for the baby to chew on helps relieve the pain and promote tooth eruption.

Parents may also soothe their baby's teething pain with over-the-counter pain relievers or locally acting over-the-counter preparations that temporarily numb gum tissue. The mother will want to consult her baby's caregiver before using such medications.

Discouraging Biting

Teething may cause the baby to clamp down on the breast during feeding. The mother can be especially observant at this time and watch for signs that the feeding is ending. When there is a slowing of the suck–swallow rhythm, she can remove the baby from her breast. If biting occurs in the middle of a feeding, the mother can remove her baby immediately; say, "No"; and wait a few minutes before resuming the feeding. If the baby bites again, she can end the feeding promptly and gently give another verbal reprimand.

Because of the sucking mechanics involved during breastfeeding, it is impossible for the baby to suck and bite at the same time. Clamping down tightly will interfere with the tongue compressing the nipple. A baby who bites probably is not hungry enough to nurse at that time. The mother can end the feeding and try again later when the baby's hunger returns. If she suspects teething pain to be the cause of biting, she can try some comfort measures and then resume nursing.

Biting may also occur at the end of a feeding as the baby falls asleep and closes the jaw. The mother can prevent such clamping down on her nipple by inserting her finger in the baby's mouth between the gums and removing her breast when she perceives that the child is nearly finished. Withdrawing her finger slowly will break suction and avoid discomfort. When a baby bites for the first time, the mother may react with an outcry and a startled jerk away from her baby. Let her know that this is a common reaction. She can be cautious not to respond so strongly in the future so that the baby does not interpret this reaction as a sign of rejection and discontinue nursing because of it. Assure her that she can overcome biting and that it need not be a reason to wean.

～ Sustaining Breastfeeding Beyond 1 Year

With loving patience from their parents, children outgrow their need to nurse in the 2nd, 3rd, or perhaps 4th year of life. Most often, cultural practices set the standards for weaning times in a society, without regard for the baby's biological needs. Within social groups where early weaning is common, a mother who chooses baby-led weaning is often pressured by lack of acceptance and misinformation about breastfeeding her older baby.

As a lactation consultant, you can suggest a number of techniques to help mothers continue breastfeeding for the recommended 2 years and beyond (WHO, 2002). As the baby becomes more alert and more easily distracted, breastfeeding in a quiet place will limit distractions and interruptions. When the mother adds supplemental foods to her baby's diet, she can breastfeed first and then offer the complementary food. A baby who has begun eating other foods may wish to breastfeed less frequently. The frequency and duration of nursing will continue to diminish as the child receives increased amounts of complementary foods. The mother can continue to respond to her baby's desire to nurse and allow her baby to lessen the number of feedings gradually while receiving sufficient complementary foods. Brochures and posters to encourage breastfeeding beyond 1 year are available from a promotion project in Australia (Queensland Government, 2009).

A landmark study compared siblings, one of whom was breastfed and one of whom was not, as well as siblings who were breastfed for different durations. Breastfed children were shown to have higher high school grade-point averages (GPA) and a higher probability of attending college (Rees & Sabia, 2009). Given that their sample contained a variety of adolescents, the researchers ruled out factors such as socioeconomic status in making the connection between breastfeeding and educational achievement. For every month a child was breastfed, the high school GPA increased about 1 percent and the probability of going to college increased about 2 percent. The researchers concluded that more than half of the estimated effect of being breastfed on high school grades can be linked to improvements in cognitive ability and health, and that one-fifth of the increased likelihood of going to college appears to be due to breastfeeding.

The role of self-regulation in appetite developed through breastfeeding may help prevent childhood obesity (Li et al., 2008; Grummer-Strawn & Mei, 2004). Leptin and ghrelin—two factors found in human milk—may also play a continued role as appetite regulators (Palou & Picó, 2009; Miralles et al., 2006). Antibody levels are higher in "weaning" milk, which benefits toddlers, who continually put objects in their mouths (Newman & Kernerman, 2009). Breastmilk continues to provide more than half of children's estimated zinc requirements after the introduction of complementary foods, even into the second year of life (Brown et al., 2009). Programs to promote and support breastfeeding can help change the erroneous belief that human milk has no value after the first year of a child's life.

Breastfeeding a Toddler

Some people believe that breastfeeding a baby beyond infancy will make the child more dependent on the mother. In fact, in cultures where mothers typically breastfeed beyond 12 months, babies walk and crawl earlier than children who are primarily bottle fed (Dewey, 2001). Many studies have shown that satisfying a baby's emotional needs encourages self-reliance. Normal sucking needs can last several years, and babies may require a substitute for sucking if weaning occurs before sucking needs subside. Some people believe that nighttime feedings cause the baby to continue waking at night. In reality, sleep patterns most often are the result of neurological development and environmental factors, rather than a reflection of the availability of breastfeeding.

Mothers who want to breastfeed into the toddler stage need reassurance that it is perfectly natural and normal to do so. The support of others within their social structure will validate their choice. They will be empowered further by informed professionals who can answer their questions. These mothers will benefit from the emotional support and practical suggestions of other mothers who understand their circumstances and are willing to listen to them.

Presenting the concept of breastfeeding a baby beyond infancy openly and with a sense of humor enables mothers to consider this parenting option objectively. Each society defines the term "older baby" differently when used in the context of breastfeeding. Many American women consider an older baby to be 18, 15, or even 9 months of age. Although most do not expect to continue breastfeeding their infants into the toddler years, they simply respond to their babies' breastfeeding needs on a daily basis as a natural part of mothering. Describing breastfeeding a toddler as an extension of the warm infant–mother relationship will help women view this practice positively. Breastfeeding toddlers fit very comfortably into family routines (see Figure 17.7).

Rewards of Breastfeeding a Toddler

Breastfeeding a toddler is rewarding and satisfying for the mother who recognizes that she is meeting her child's needs. It can be a source of great comfort and stability to the child, especially when the toddler feels stressed, is injured, has hurt feelings, is feeling shy, or is in a new and strange environment. Moreover, breastfeeding provides a comforting way for the active child to connect with the mother between explorations.

Particularly during the toddler period, breastfeeding offers the mother a reassuring way to communicate her love even though she and her child may be at odds over her child's behavior. A child who is able to communicate verbally can bring the mother great joy by expressing his or her feelings about breastfeeding. There can be love and humor in this relationship, with both mother and child being the giver and the receiver. These aspects of breast-

feeding serve as a transitional parenting technique from infancy to childhood.

Challenges to Breastfeeding a Toddler

Although breastfeeding a toddler can be very rewarding, it may also produce inconveniences and conflicts that rival those of the newborn period and cause mothers to consider weaning. The physical act of nursing a toddler can be quite different from the breastfeeding of an infant. The older baby may not wish to be held and will assume a position that allows the child to conveniently view the room, including standing or straddling. For a time, developing teeth may leave pressure marks on the areola until the toddler learns to hold the breast with the lips. Crumbs or food particles left in the child's mouth may also irritate the mother's nipples during feedings.

During this time, some women may consider weaning because they feel they have lost control of their bodies or that their babies are manipulating them. The child may insist on nursing at inconvenient or embarrassing moments, tugging at the mother's clothing, even partially disrobing her. The toddler may fondle her body, which embarrasses her when others notice. She may feel trapped and controlled by her child and resent that she did not expect this phase of breastfeeding.

The mother can prevent such potential negative feelings by guiding her child in breastfeeding, just as she guides other aspects of her child's life, such as eating, sleeping, and playing. She can limit breastfeeding to certain times and refuse to overindulge the child at inconvenient times. Feedings can be limited to coincide with the mother's needs so that breastfeeding continues to be a source of pleasure for both her and her child. If touching the other breast while breastfeeding is unpleasant, the mother can tell the toddler, "No." Help her adopt a balanced view of breastfeeding as an integral part of parenting so she can continue to enjoy this special relationship as her baby matures.

A mother can arrange some signals with her baby, as well as times for breastfeeding, that are reasonably acceptable to both. The family may adopt a special name for nursing to avoid embarrassment when the toddler asks to breastfeed while out in public. Rather than arguing with the child at every request, she can try to stretch the intervals between feedings. Her child may, for example, be satisfied with a drink or treat just before the usual time for nursing.

The mother may also suggest other activities to distract the toddler from wanting to nurse. Encourage her to remain flexible enough to adjust her approach if it causes stress in the child. The concept of time is often difficult for a child to comprehend, and nursing can be linked to a special location instead. For instance, the child will understand if the mother says, "Let's nurse when we get home

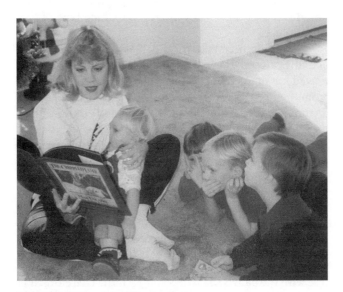

FIGURE 17.7 A toddler nursing.

Source: Printed with permission of Anna Swisher.

in Mommy's chair." Being consistent in restricting breast-feeding to a particular place is the key to making this prac-tice mutually satisfying for both mother and toddler.

Opposition from Others

Sometimes a baby's father will object to his older baby continuing to nurse. He may believe that the child appears too dependent while nursing. The father may also worry about the social and sexual implications of breastfeeding an older baby. If the mother complains about breastfeed-ing, the father may wonder why she continues. Help the mother learn what the father's precise objections are and develop a breastfeeding plan to resolve the issue. She can discuss with him the baby's physical and emotional needs at this stage of development, as well as her desire to con-tinue breastfeeding. If he continues to object, she can avoid nursing in his presence. The father may accept the situation better if he does not actually see the toddler nurse, or he may benefit from seeing other children con-tinue to nurse, as in a support group. He can also use websites and books about fathering as resources to learn more about this practice (Sears, 2006; Sears & Sears, 2006). The mother will benefit from your support if she continues breastfeeding despite the father's objection.

People other than the baby's father are often uncom-fortable seeing a woman breastfeed a toddler. Some moth-ers choose to breastfeed privately, while others are very comfortable nursing their child around others. Many mothers nursing past a year have formed Internet support groups and online forums—for example, www.007b.com provides support for normalizing breastfeeding of tod-dlers. Some mothers refrain from breastfeeding in front of people who are critical of their choice, so as to defray their negative reactions and avoid feeling intimidated by them. Mothers can benefit from other sources of emotional sup-port as they continue to do what is best for their children. Chapter 20 presents suggestions on helping mothers han-dle criticism about breastfeeding toddlers.

Siblings may resent the special attention the breast-feeding child receives from the mother. Reevaluating her children's needs and setting aside special time with each child may eliminate such reactions. The mother may inad-vertently be responsible for prolonging breastfeeding by nursing to prevent her toddler from disturbing her older children's toys or disrupting their play. Providing storage places and play areas that are inaccessible can prevent the baby from interfering with siblings, so that the mother does not resort to breastfeeding just to keep the toddler occupied.

You can listen to the mother's concerns with a sym-pathetic ear and help her work out solutions that fit her situation. Given that she may not know another person who will praise her for her efforts, it is incumbent on the lactation consultant to reassure her that she has chosen the right action for her child and family. Whether she chooses to wean or to continue breastfeeding, she needs an accepting listener who will support her in her decision. Attending a breastfeeding support group will also be help-ful to her, especially one with nursing toddlers.

~ Nourishment Away from the Breast

Mothers need to understand that any nourishment the baby receives away from the breast may alter the breast-feeding pattern. The greater the frequency and amount of other food, the greater the impact will be on breastfeed-ing. The lactation community distinguishes between sup-plementary feeding—food in place of the mother's milk—and complementary feeding—necessary nourish-ment that cannot be provided by the mother's milk.

Supplementary Feedings

The most common definition of a supplementary feeding is a food other than human milk fed to the infant follow-ing or in place of a breastfeeding. Some refer to it as "top-ping off" the breastfed infant with liquids other than mother's milk, such as water or infant formula.

Some consider the mother's expressed milk to be a supplementary feeding because the baby does not obtain it directly at the breast. The mother's milk is certainly preferred over water or formula. Encourage the mother to plan ahead and to express milk on a regular basis for these feedings. If she wishes to use formula for supplementary feeding, she needs to consider the WHO, UNICEF, and AAP recommendations, which call for a child to receive breastmilk exclusively to age 6 months. She also needs to check whether there is a history of allergies in the family and discuss with her baby's caregiver which type of for-mula to use.

Many mothers take their babies with them or plan activities around the baby's feeding times and never have a need for supplementary feedings. Others must be away from their babies for work or school. (See Chapter 24 for a complete discussion about working and continuing to breastfeed.) Mothers may also have doctor, dentist, or other professional appointments in which it is not con-ducive to take the baby. Planning for substitute feedings eliminates the worry of an unhappy and hungry baby at such times.

Feeding Method

Mothers need to introduce supplementary feedings in such a way that the amount of supplement does not inter-fere with the baby's breastfeeding pattern. Therefore, it is best to delay any supplementary feedings until the baby is at least 3 weeks old and has firmly established breastfeeding. Parents should initiate a supplementary feeding when the baby is not fussy or too hungry.

Because of the potential for nipple preference, parents may want to avoid bottles when other feeding methods are possible. Most babies will accept feeding by a cup, which avoids the nipple preference associated with a bottle. Learning to drink from a cup is often easier for breastfeeding babies than for those fed exclusively with a bottle. If a mother prefers to use a bottle, the baby's acceptance of this feeding method may require several attempts. A baby sometimes will accept a bottle, reject it the next few times, and then accept it again later. The mother can continue to offer the bottle until her baby accepts it. Encourage her to use paced feeding techniques to slow the feeding rate, as described in Chapter 21. Other babies happily take their milk any way they can get it, and switch between breast, cup, and bottle with ease.

Some mothers have found that their baby will not accept their expressed milk, which can be very worrisome for the parents. Some of these babies will drink only the bare minimum at daycare facilities or with the caregiver, and "reverse cycle" their feedings when reunited with their mothers. You can help mothers find creative ways to ensure their babies are fed. One mother reported that her husband was able to bring the baby to work when the baby needed to feed. Others have changed jobs (when possible) to a more mother-friendly environment in which they were able to either have the baby brought to them or to take nursing breaks. Some mothers arrange for child care near their work location so that they can nurse during the lunch hour.

If supplementary feeding results in a missed breastfeeding, the mother's breasts may become full. She can nurse or express milk just before she departs or she can express her milk while she is away. If she prefers that her baby nurse immediately when she returns, wearing a larger bra may help to avoid pressure on her full breasts that could cause blockage of her milk ducts. Mothers who work outside the home or return to school or an active social life soon learn how to manage such absences without experiencing discomfort from full breasts. Having prepared supplementary feedings ahead of time, they feel secure in their babies' willingness to accept substitute nourishment.

Complementary Feeding

Complementary feeding refers to the addition of new foods to the growing breastfed infant's diet that are intended to meet the energy and nutrient needs no longer met by the mother's milk alone. Some use this term interchangeably with "supplemental feeding" and interpret it as "topping off" the breastfed infant with liquids other than the mother's milk (i.e., water or infant formula). The most common definition of complementary foods refers to solid foods added to the maturing child's diet.

Mothers need to understand that the weaning process has begun when a baby receives the first complementary food. Early introduction of complementary foods is associated with unhealthful subsequent feeding behaviors such as early weaning and consumption of fatty or sugary foods (Grummer-Strawn et al., 2008). The introduction of solid foods begins to establish eating patterns that will last a lifetime. Thus parents recognize this event as a giant step in their baby's development that requires many decisions on their part. They wonder when to begin solid foods, which types of food are best, how to offer the food, and how to make sure their baby receives adequate nutrition. You can give parents the information necessary to help them make informed and responsible decisions about foods for their baby at this age.

Pressure to Begin Complementary Foods

New parents are deluged by messages from baby food manufacturers proclaiming the many advantages of commercially processed foods. Likewise, they often receive an overabundance of advice from family and friends regarding when and how to introduce these foods. Print and online media, as well as television programs, advocate various methods and times for starting solid foods. Parents must evaluate this assortment of facts and opinions in the context of their baby's needs. This process may represent one of the parents' first forays into advocating for their child as informed consumers, searching out and evaluating information available to them.

Counseling Implications

The lactation consultant can be a valuable source of information for parents about introducing solid foods to their baby. Provide them with clear, accurate, well-documented facts to eliminate their possible confusion resulting from contradictory advice. A mother needs encouragement and a high level of self-esteem to continue exclusive breastfeeding despite pressure to start solid foods. Reassure her that her baby looks and acts healthy and is well nourished from her milk alone. Assure her that she has adequate milk production and the capacity to increase milk production to meet her child's increased needs. You can be an active force in helping her delay solid foods until the child reaches an appropriate age by giving her the support that will build her confidence in her mothering skills.

Sometimes the baby's caregiver will suggest that a mother start her baby on solid foods when it does not seem appropriate or when the mother does not feel ready. Encourage her to ask the caregiver to clarify the reason for suggesting solid foods. Did the caregiver say that she may begin solid foods if she wishes or recommend solid foods for a specific reason? Perhaps the caregiver is not familiar with the AAP's recommendation that babies receive nothing but breastmilk before 6 months of age. In engaging with the caregiver, the mother can reinforce her breastfeeding goals and discuss such pertinent aspects of her baby's health as weight gain, family weight patterns, allergies, and anemia.

One of the counseling tips you can share with mothers is that their milk serves as "nutritional insurance" as their baby grows and begins other foods. Toddlers are notoriously picky eaters. One study found that 20.2 percent of mothers with 2-year-olds and 7.6 percent of mothers with 4-year-olds reported that their child was sometimes or often an irregular eater. Many of these children had exhibited feeding difficulties as early as 6 months (McDermott, 2008). Continuing to breastfeed lowers parents' stress by allowing them to introduce solid foods as a socialization measure, knowing that the mother's milk continues to provide the bulk of baby's nutritional needs from age 6 to 12 months.

Sleeping Through the Night

The suggestion for complementary feeding often occurs in relation to sleep issues, even though there is no conclusive evidence that a particular feeding method promotes longer nighttime sleep. Because human milk is digested more quickly than cow's milk, it seems reasonable that a breastfed baby would wake up hungry in the middle of the night. A baby who is exclusively breastfed at 5 months may sleep 8 hours at night. That same baby may have been awake every 3 or 4 hours during the night at 1 month old. It seems more likely, then, that the reason for longer sleep at 5 months is due to a more fully developed nervous system and is unrelated to nutritional factors.

Parents are sometimes told that a baby needs cereal just before going to bed to "fill the child up." In reality, sleeping through the night is a developmental event that parents may not be able to change by feeding the baby cereal. Adults with restless sleep often find a light snack such as warm milk helps before they retire; they do not choose a heavy meal that could cause indigestion and further encourage wakefulness. Warm milk contains a soporific (sleep-inducing) agent that helps people fall asleep. Given that fact, human milk is the ideal food for encouraging a baby to sleep.

Choosing the Appropriate Time

The introduction of solid foods expands a baby's dietary choices and serves to complement the mother's milk during weaning. Many factors must be considered in deciding when to add solid foods to a baby's diet. In general, the ideal time falls somewhere between the points at which the baby's system is mature enough to handle solid foods and at which the child needs more nutrients than can be obtained solely from the mother's milk. Beginning solid foods before 6 months or in response to growth spurts

seriously compromises milk production and may precipitate food allergies.

Babies of average birth weight with adequate fetal stores of fat and iron do well on mother's milk alone until about 6 months of age, which is why the AAP recommends exclusive breastfeeding as ideal nutrition that is sufficient to support optimal growth and development for the first 6 months after birth. Human milk provides all the calories, vitamins, and minerals in the proper proportions needed by the baby. In addition, its protective factors help prevent allergies and illness. Introducing other foods before the baby's body is ready for them can lead to frequent digestive upsets, increased upper respiratory infections, poor nutrient absorption, and excessive weight gain due to increased calorie consumption.

Researchers whose work has been sponsored by Nestlé suggest that rising rates of food allergies in early childhood reflect increasing failure of early immune tolerance mechanisms. They assert that the practice of delaying complementary foods until 6 months of age may, therefore, increase the risk of immune disorders. Their recommendation is that complementary foods be introduced when the child is approximately 4 months of age while maintaining breastfeeding for at least 6 months "if possible" (Prescott et al., 2008). However, the researchers' funding source suggests possible bias, underscoring the importance of critical discernment as you read and analyze research (see Chapter 27).

Lowered Risk of Allergy   Introducing complementary foods too early may increase the risk of food allergy in the infant. Some foods are more allergenic than others, and some food allergies are more persistent than others. A cautious approach would be to individualize the introduction of solids into the infants' diet. Complementary feeding can be introduced from the 6th month; egg, peanut, tree nuts, fish, and seafood introduction require caution (Fiocchi & Martelli, 2006). The optimal ages for introducing selected foods are dairy products at 12 months; hen's egg at 24 months; and peanut, tree nuts, fish, and seafood at about 36 months. Foods should be introduced one at a time, in small amounts. Parents should avoid mixed foods that may contain various food allergens unless tolerance to every ingredient has been assessed.

Longer breastfeeding duration is associated with a lower risk for eczema in infants whose mothers did not have allergies or asthma and a slightly lower risk for those infants of mothers with allergies but no asthma. Longer breastfeeding duration decreases the risk of recurrent wheeze, independent of maternal allergy or asthma status. The protective effect of breastfeeding on recurrent wheeze may also help protect infants against respiratory infections (Snijders et al., 2007).

A study in Qatar found that asthma, wheezing, allergic rhinitis, and eczema occurred less frequently in exclusively breastfed children, compared to infants nourished with partial breastfeeding and formula milk. The risk of allergic diseases, eczema, wheeze, and ear infection, in particular, were lower in children breastfed for more than 6 months, compared to those breastfed for less than 6 months (Bener et al., 2007).

Lowered Risk of Obesity Early introduction of solid foods correlates with higher weight at 8, 13, and 26 weeks of age. As research has shown, excessive weight gain in infancy can lead to lifelong obesity. It needs to be noted, however, that much of the research on infant and child nutrition is funded by formula manufacturers. Industry-funded studies frequently use negative semantics in describing the breastfed infant, with one study referring to the "relative undernutrition and slower growth" of breastfed babies" (Singhal, 2007). Another study noted that obesity risk at school age was reduced by 15 to 25 percent with early breastfeeding, rather than acknowledging that obesity risk is *increased* by 15 to 25 percent with artificial feeding (Koletzko et al., 2009). When reading research reports, especially when the work was funded by the artificial baby food industry, be mindful of how the studies "spin" the results to euphemize the pathology of artificial feeding results, and downplay the biological health resulting from normal human milk feeding.

Signs of the Baby's Readiness Babies display obvious outward signs that they are ready for solid foods when their internal functions have developed to the point where they can efficiently handle a more diverse diet. At approximately 6 months of age, neuromuscular development allows for chewing and swallowing nonliquid foods. Intestinal maturation promotes more complete digestion and absorption of a variety of foods. This enables a baby's body to handle the waste products from solid foods. The immunologic system has also begun to function, so that the infant no longer must depend on the protection provided by the mother's milk.

Other signs of a baby's readiness for additional foods include the eruption of teeth, the ability to sit up, the disappearance of the tongue extrusion reflex, improved eye–hand coordination, and the ability to grasp objects with the thumb and forefinger (Figure 17.8). The most obvious sign is the baby's behavior when others are eating. The infant may watch them intently, imitate their chewing, and reach for food while loudly vocalizing a desire for it. An intensified demand to nurse that is not satisfied after several days of increased breastfeedings may be an additional clue to the mother that it is time to begin solid foods.

Dewey (2007) has estimated the amount of energy provided by complementary foods at different ages, for infants in developing countries and in industrialized countries. At ages 6 to 8 months, these percentages are 33

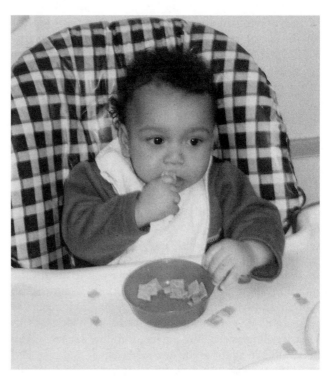

FIGURE 17.8 A 1-year-old feeding himself.
Source: Printed with permission of Anna Swisher.

percent and 21 percent, respectively. For ages 9 to 11 months, the percentage of energy provided by complementary foods is 45 percent for both groups. From 12 to 23 months, complementary foods provide 61 percent and 65 percent of energy needs, respectively. Dewey's findings are very helpful information to share, because they look at breastfeeding nutrition to 2 years of age.

Parents sometimes consider starting solid foods to solve an unrelated problem. Misconceptions about breastfeeding or about the baby's behavior patterns may cause parents to believe that some aspects of their relationship with their baby are feeding related. Such misconceptions may involve frequency of feedings, milk production, nutritional content of the mother's milk, sleep, crying, and infant development. By correcting these misconceptions, you can help parents avoid starting solid foods prematurely.

Supplementing to Provide Iron

Parents may consider starting solid foods to provide their baby with iron. In a healthy full-term baby, this step is not usually necessary. The mother's milk typically supplies sufficient iron until her baby's birth weight triples. Her milk contains lactoferrin, an iron-binding protein that increases the absorption of the normal amounts of iron that are available in the milk. Outside sources of iron disrupt this process. Specifically, adding iron too soon interferes with the disease-protection qualities of lacto-ferrin. Lactoferrin binds iron and increases its absorption, which robs some microorganisms of the iron they require to grow and multiply. Preterm infants and infants of anemic mothers will need iron supplementation whenever a hematocrit (hemoglobin blood test) determines that iron stores are low.

Introducing Complementary Foods

The introduction of solid foods should be a pleasant experience for both mother and baby. Slow and gradual introduction of foods will prevent the baby from feeling overwhelmed by this new way of eating. The infant's digestive system will also have a chance to get used to each new change in diet. Offering complementary foods to the baby after nursing is complete will maintain the mother's milk production. In addition, it allows the mother and baby to rely on breastfeeding as a means of relaxation and comfort during this time of change. With breastfeeding as a stabilizing factor in life, a baby will be better able to adapt to the new experience.

Infant food preferences may begin prenatally, as infants are exposed to different flavors in amniotic fluid (Mennella et al., 2004), and continue to evolve after birth, as they consume different flavors in their mothers' milk. This early flavor exposure may influence individual food preferences for life. Breastfeeding introduces the baby to the taste of a variety of foods. When solid foods are introduced, food preferences develop—due, it is thought, to the repeated exposures to a variety of foods (Nicklaus, 2009). Thus nutritional decisions during pregnancy and breastfeeding may influence a child's later nutritional choices through early flavor exposure (Beauchamp & Mennella, 2009).

Ideally, parents will begin at a slow pace, with 1 complementary feeding every 1 or 2 days. The best time to initiate this practice is when the baby is still hungry after a breastfeeding. Often, the afternoon and early evening hours are times when the baby may accept additional foods more readily. This period usually coincides with the time when the mother is most tired and busy with other tasks. Complementary feeding in this manner provides an opportunity for the father or other family member to interact with the child and offer the mother a break from baby care.

Age of the Baby

Breastfeeding should be allowed to diminish slowly as solid foods increase to the point that they become the primary source of nutrition for the child. The mother's milk can still meet three-fourths of her baby's nutrient needs during the second 6 months of life. Even during the baby's second year, her milk continues to be nutritionally valuable.

Not all babies will be able to wait until 6 months of age to start solid foods. Some babies who begin nursing constantly at 4 or 5 months and never seem to be satisfied may be biologically ready for additional nourishment from solid foods. Every baby will be ready for solid foods at a slightly different age. Parents can watch their baby for signs of readiness and discuss starting solids with their baby's primary healthcare provider.

By the age of 7 to 9 months, one or two complementary feedings a day with regular breastfeeding will satisfy the baby's nutritional needs. By 9 to 12 months, the infant becomes an active participant at family meals with three meals a day. The child will still require nutritious snacks several times a day, in addition to several separate nursing times. Breastfeeding will gradually decrease as the infant learns to eat balanced meals and drink from a cup.

Texture of Food

The foods initially offered during complementary feeding should be highly puréed and diluted with liquid. As the baby becomes accustomed to eating solid foods, liquid content can give way to a coarser texture. This will eventually transition to chunky foods, finger foods, and finally table foods. Delaying solid foods until 8 or 9 months avoids the need to prepare puréed foods. The baby can start with finger foods and chunky foods.

The texture of foods needs to be compatible with the baby's ability to chew and swallow. Table 17.2 presents guidelines for children's self-feeding ability as they develop and mature. As shown in the table, the average baby will begin eating small, chunky finger foods by 9 months. By 1 year of age, the child will be eating regular table food, cut into age-appropriate sizes, along with the rest of the family.

Type of Food

The type of food the baby receives depends on the child's age, the preferences of the parents or pediatrician, and the child's willingness to accept them. The baby will need to begin with nutrient-dense foods that are relatively high in protein (AAP, 2009), because the protein requirement in the baby's diet eventually begins to exceed what is received from the mother's milk. Single-grain infant cereals, such as rice or barley, provide additional energy and iron; thus these cereals are often the pediatrician's choice for the first complementary food. The mother can express some of her milk or use warm water to mix with the cereal. Cereal introduction is typically followed by vegetables, fruits, and meats, in that order. Babies do not require juice, and parents should limit its use. Babies also do not require desserts or sweeteners added to their foods. Sweet foods are a poor substitute for foods with greater nutritional value; they also cause tooth decay and promote poor eating habits.

La Leche League International (2004) recommends starting with banana, cooked sweet potato, or avocado chopped up so that infants can feed themselves safely. This would be followed by protein-rich meat or beans

TABLE 17.2 Child's Ability to Self-Feed

Age	Developmental Skills and Implications for Feeding
Birth to 6 months	Designed to suck, not chew
	Rooting reflex searches for food source
	Tongue-thrust reflex pushes out solid foods
	Sensitive gag reflex
6 months	Tongue-thrust and gag reflexes lessen; accepts strained, pureed solids
	Sits erect
	Begins teething
7 to 9 months	Holds bottle; may drink from cup
	Thumb-and-forefinger pickup (pincher grasp) begins
	Begins eating finger foods
	Begins mouthing chokable food and objects
	Bangs, drops, and flings
	Reaches for food and utensils
	Munches food
9 to 12 months	Self-feeding skills improve
	Holds bottle and cup longer
	Points, pokes, smears, and is messy
	Increased movement
	Masters finger foods
	Tries to use utensils; spills most food
12 to 18 months	Has prolonged attention span
	Participates in family meals
	Eats chopped or mashed family foods
	"Do it myself" desire intensifies
	Tilts cup and head while drinking; spills less
	Begins self-feeding with utensils
	Holds spoon better; still spills much
	Begins walking; doesn't want to sit still and eat
	Picks at others' plates
18 to 24 months	Molars appear; begins rotary chewing
	Spoon-feeds self without spilling much
	Learns food talk; signals for "more" and "all done"
	Wants to eat on the run
	Erratic feeding habits
	May become picky eater
	May wean
	Uses spoon and fork

Source: Adapted from *Feeding Infants and Toddlers: Feeding at a Glance: Birth to 24 Months.* 2006. http://www.askdrsears.com/html/3/t030500.asp. Accessed May 07, 2010.

cooked until tender and offered in small pieces, then whole-grain breads and cereals, and then fresh or cooked fruits (if canned, buy water-packed fruits). Yogurt, natural cheese, and cottage cheese can all be offered at 9 to 10 months of age, depending on the family history of dairy allergy. Whole milk and other dairy products, eggs, and citrus products can be offered after 1 year of age. Honey is not recommended until the child is at least 1 to 2 years old because of the risk of botulism spores.

Single-ingredient foods are the best choice, started one at a time at weekly intervals. This pacing provides an opportunity to identify potential food sensitivity and avert development of potential food intolerance or allergies. If the baby receives several foods together, the mother may be unable to identify which one causes a reaction. If food sensitivity occurs, the mother can discontinue the food and reintroduce it later. She may find that small amounts of a food can be tolerated, whereas larger amounts will cause reactions. Allergy considerations are discussed in more detail later in this chapter.

If the baby objects to a particular food, the mother can withhold it for several weeks before offering it again. The experience of trying new foods should be pleasant for the baby. Parents should not force the child to eat something that the infant finds unpleasant. They should also avoid starting new foods when the child is ill or has recently had an inoculation.

Giving the baby water with the solid food will meet the child's fluid needs without delivering extra calories. Additional water is often necessary to help rid the baby's body of the waste products in solid foods, especially those found in meats and egg yolks. Fruits, fruit juices, and vegetables pose less of a problem for the baby.

In the second year of life, a child no longer needs a special infant diet. At that time, he or she can begin sharing modified family meals, prepared without excessive salt or spices, cut into appropriate-sized pieces, and served at a moderate temperature.

Vegetarian Diet The American Dietetic Association's recently revised position on vegetarian diets states, "Well-planned vegetarian diets are appropriate for individuals during all stages of the life cycle, including pregnancy, lactation, infancy, childhood, and adolescence, and for athletes" (ADA, 2009). The key term here is "well-planned." Extremely restrictive vegetarian diets such as fruitarian and raw food diets are not appropriate for infants.

Most vegetarian families are well educated about their dietary choices, and know how to prevent nutritional deficiencies. The biggest concern with vegetarian diets is obtaining sufficient amounts of vitamin B_{12}. Severe vitamin B_{12} deficiency produces neurological symptoms in infants, including irritability, failure to thrive, apathy, anorexia, and developmental regression (Dror & Allen,

2008). Because vitamin B$_{12}$ is one of the vitamins in human milk whose quantity depends on maternal diet, it is imperative that vegetarian mothers consume vitamin B$_{12}$ supplements while breastfeeding (Chalouhi et al., 2008).

Infant growth is normal when infants of vegetarian mothers receive adequate breastmilk and the mothers' diets contain good sources of energy, iron, vitamin B$_{12}$, and vitamin D. Guidelines for the introduction of solid foods are the same as for other infants. Protein-rich foods include tofu, legumes, soy or dairy yogurt, cooked egg yolks, and cottage cheese. Foods rich in energy and nutrients such as legumes, tofu, and avocado should be used when the infant is being weaned.

Amount of Food Mothers often wonder how much complementary food they should feed to their babies. When first presenting a food, the mother will frequently prepare a small dishful, only to find that her baby scarcely tastes it. She can begin with a teaspoon or so of creamy-consistency food and then work up to a few tablespoons at a rate determined by the baby's appetite. Too often, babies are overfed because parents expect them to consume an entire jar of commercially prepared baby food in one sitting. Parents need to recognize when their baby has had enough.

At first, the mother can expect to see more food running down the sides of her baby's mouth than being swallowed. Such messiness, a normal and sometimes amusing part of this new experience, will decrease as the baby learns to use the newly developed swallowing mechanism. It will be evident again when the baby starts self-feeding. Some babies are not very interested in solid foods until they can handle the food themselves; others love to eat right from the start. Caution the mother not to overfeed an eager baby, as solid foods contain more calories per volume than milk. A young baby's mechanism for determining hunger is by volume of food. Overfeeding can manifest itself as constipation, spitting up, excessive weight gain, or a rapid decrease in breastfeeding frequency.

Allergy Considerations

When babies are breastfed exclusively, components in the mother's milk coat the intestinal tract to prevent foreign proteins from entering the baby's system and causing allergic reactions. Eventually the baby's body develops the ability to protect itself without the mother's milk. However, children of parents with a history of allergy appear to have a more prolonged dependence on the protective factors in human milk. These children have an increased susceptibility to ingested food proteins. The hereditary risk of food allergy seems to be lower when a baby is breastfed exclusively for several months (Venter, 2009). Avoidance of the most potent allergenic foods during the first year is effective in reducing allergic reactions in children.

The degree of response to foreign proteins varies widely from one baby to another. While some babies exhibit sudden and clear-cut allergic reactions, others may appear only slightly fussy or irritable. The signs of food reactions that may help a mother to recognize intolerance in her baby are highlighted in the following section. Food reactions may be mistaken for signs of illness or drug reactions, and vice versa. If symptoms persist, parents should contact the physician, as these symptoms may also indicate illness in the baby.

Signs of Food Intolerance

- Runny nose, stuffiness, and constant cold-type symptoms
- Skin rashes, eczema, hives, and sore bottom
- Asthma
- Ear infections
- Intestinal upset, gas, diarrhea, spitting up, and vomiting
- Fussiness, irritability, and colic-like behavior
- Poor weight gain due to malabsorption of food
- Red itchy eyes, swollen eyelids, dark circles under the eyes, constant tearing, and gelatin-like fluid in the eyes

Family History of Allergies

Parents with a family history of allergies should notify the physician whenever they suspect an allergic response in their baby. The physician can help them pinpoint the offending allergen and may provide medication to relieve the symptoms. To avoid potential sensitivity in her baby, the expectant mother should limit her consumption of milk and eggs, especially during the last month of pregnancy. She can substitute other foods to ensure a balanced, nutritious diet.

Excessive maternal consumption of a particular food may cause an allergic reaction in her baby. Mothers can avoid this sensitivity by eating a variety of foods in moderation. To eliminate a reaction entirely, a mother may need to exclude a food from her diet. By experimenting with known allergens, she can identify and eliminate the offending foods. If she eats a particular food and notices repeated symptoms with that food after she breastfeeds her baby, that food may be the cause.

If a mother eliminates a food from her diet, especially one such as cow's milk, which is high in protein and calcium, she will need to substitute another food or supplement to obtain the necessary nutrients to support lactation. Mothers do not need to eliminate foods from their diets unless they suspect that a particular food is causing problems. They can continue to consume in moderation any foods they have been accustomed to eating.

One study found that for women with food allergies, or with a previous allergic child, maternal omega-3 fatty acid supplementation from week 25 of pregnancy through 3 to 4 months' nursing resulted in lower incidence of allergic reactions (2 percent, compared to 15 percent in the placebo group). The incidence of immunoglobulin E (IgE)–associated eczema was also lower in the supplemented group (8 percent) than in the placebo group (24 percent). This simple dietary modification may be appropriate for a mother with a family history of allergic disease (Furuhjelm et al., 2009).

When the potentially allergy-prone baby begins consuming complementary foods, parents need to be especially cautious about introducing one food at a time and waiting at least 1 week for a possible reaction. Foods to avoid in the first year after birth include cow's milk and milk products, citrus fruits and fruit juices, eggs, tomatoes, chocolate, fish, pork, peanuts and other nuts, and wheat. A baby younger than 1 year of age should never receive honey because of its potential to cause infant botulism. The baby's skin should not be in contact with wool clothing and blankets or with lanolin products. There should be no smoking near the baby and preferably nowhere in the home.

⁓ Weaning

It is far too impersonal and arbitrary for a mother to allow cultural influences to dictate how long she will nurse her baby. The suitable time for weaning will define itself when the mother is knowledgeable about breastfeeding and weaning. Armed with the appropriate information, she will be confident that she is basing her decision on her baby's physical and emotional needs. She will then be less likely to allow misconceptions or pressure from others to cause her to initiate weaning before her baby is ready.

Baby-Led Weaning

The biologically normal and desired method for weaning is to allow the baby to self-wean. When a mother is relaxed about breastfeeding and has no pressures or problems that lead her to wean, she can allow her baby to establish his or her own nursing pattern and weaning time. Through baby-led weaning, the baby will drop feedings gradually and the mother will nurse only when the infant indicates a need for it. Normal biological weaning responds to the baby's developmental needs. It nurtures the child's eventual independence by allowing the baby to

determine the readiness to move to the next stage of development.

Signs a Baby Is Ready to Wean

When weaning takes place buffered from societal pressures, natural times for ending breastfeeding seem to fall between the periods of the baby's greatest developmental activity. Globally, the normal range for weaning is somewhere between 2 1/2 and 7 years of age (Stuart-MacAdam & Dettwyler, 1995), around when the first molars erupt. In Western cultures, the most common ages for weaning are 12 to 14 months, 18 months, 2 years, and 3 years.

The mother can follow her baby's hunger cues and subsequent pattern for weaning by neither denying nor initiating breastfeeding. The baby may become more self-reliant and go for long stretches without nursing, perhaps accepting a drink or snack as a substitute. The infant may show a disinterest in breastfeeding by being easily distracted at the breast, spending less time at feedings, frequently refusing the breast, and showing a greater interest in solid foods. These signs indicate to the mother that her baby may be ready to wean, and represent a natural step toward the baby's maturity.

A baby may start to wean when the mother does not want or expect it, and she may respond by trying to entice the infant to nurse more frequently. You can help her learn to appreciate the child's maturity by stressing the new achievements and showing her new ways to interact with the baby and continue their close relationship.

Sometimes a mother may overlook her baby's signs of readiness to wean and initiate feedings she could have eliminated. She may put her baby to breast as soon as the child awakens instead of preparing breakfast. She may nurse to keep the child quiet while she talks on the telephone or engages in other activities. If the mother wishes to change these patterns, she can read stories to her baby, offer a snack, or provide toys and activities to occupy the infant's time. Rocking, cuddling, singing, and holding can effectively replace the coziness and comfort of breastfeeding. Two resources that have been helpful to many mothers nursing beyond U.S. cultural norms are *Mothering Your Nursing Toddler* (Bumgarner, 2000) and *How Weaning Happens* (Bengson, 2000).

Mother-Led Weaning

Mother-led weaning describes a mother's attempt to end breastfeeding without having received cues from her baby. Your use of guiding skills will help the mother explore her goals and her baby's needs. Some mothers become impatient for their baby to wean. If a mother has begun to resent breastfeeding, it may be time for her to wean. She may be feeling pressure from others or may have received poor information or advice. She may be planning to return to work and believes that she must wean to do so. She may feel that her baby is no longer satisfied with breastfeeding.

Weaning is a transitional period that mothers need to manage with appreciation for the baby's needs. Many delay weaning so they can avoid bottles and progress directly to a cup. When a mother brings up the topic of weaning, she may actually be unsure whether she wishes to wean at that time. If she does want to wean, she may approach the subject with hesitation because she knows you advocate extended breastfeeding. Be sensitive to her cues and let her know that you will help her whether she chooses to wean or to continue breastfeeding. A non-judgmental approach will encourage her to express her concerns freely and to define her questions clearly, so that she can understand the nature of weaning.

Most mothers in the United States wean their infants before 9 months. Ending breastfeeding between 3 and 6 months is largely a matter of physical management. Mother-led weaning of a 3-year-old may involve a greater challenge, perhaps including bargaining with the child to establish acceptable substitute activities. Your role is to educate the mother about weaning, support her decision without judgment, and help her through the weaning process.

Gradual Weaning

If the mother wishes to initiate weaning, she can eliminate the least preferred feeding first, allowing at least 2 days for her baby and her breasts to adjust to the dropped feeding. In its place, the mother can substitute a drink, snack, cuddling, or a favorite activity. When she drops an early-morning feeding, for example, she can have breakfast ready when the baby awakens. When she drops a late-night feeding, she can consider alternative ways of getting the infant to sleep. As she and the baby adjust to each new substitution, she can proceed to drop another feeding, continuing in this manner for several weeks or months. The child may wish to continue one preferred feeding and may decrease the feeding frequency to once every few days until he or she stops breastfeeding entirely.

If weaning proceeds too quickly, the baby may react by demanding more attention, wanting to nurse more frequently, or exhibiting physical changes such as allergic reactions, stomach upsets, or constipation. Weaning too quickly may also cause the mother's breasts to become uncomfortable. She can express her milk to relieve this discomfort, while being careful not to express so much that she actually increases her milk production. She will want to watch for any symptoms of plugged ducts or mastitis, and can wear a supportive bra that is not binding to avoid these problems. She may want to consider comfort measures such as a pain reliever, ice packs, or cabbage leaves. The mother and baby both adjust better when weaning is gradual and tailored to their needs. By allow-

ing several months for weaning, any physical and emotional discomforts are minimal.

Miscues That Cause Mothers to Consider Weaning

Weaning ideally occurs when both the mother and the baby are ready for this step. If the baby no longer desires to nurse, encourage the mother to accept this sign of maturity and to discontinue putting the infant to breast. If the mother decides to end breastfeeding, she can find other ways of satisfying her baby's needs. In both of these situations, the mother usually learns to accept weaning without guilt or resentment.

Unfortunately, weaning sometimes results from misconceptions, outside pressure, or a change in personal circumstances. When this happens, the mother may react with anger, resentment, or guilt because she was unable to continue breastfeeding. Miscues that lead to untimely weaning are described in the following subsections.

Crying A mother may have a baby who cries a lot, which causes her to doubt that she is satisfying the child's hunger. This behavior may be stressful to the mother, causing her to consider weaning to avoid further stress. In such a case, you can help her explore the reason for the crying: Perhaps it is due to allergies, pain, distress, sensory integration issues, or hunger. Teach her comforting techniques and explain how she can increase milk production, if necessary. Teaching her about hunger cues and normal output may help to reassure her that her baby is getting enough milk. Feeling successful about her mothering skills will help her continue to breastfeed with confidence.

Teething, Biting, or Illness When teething, biting, or illness occurs, the mother may become frustrated and fatigued with trying to simultaneously manage breastfeeding and comforting her baby. She may decide to wean in an effort to decrease tension or so that someone else can feed the baby while she rests. You can help her understand that this stage is temporary. Further, bottle feeding is not likely to improve the situation if a baby is ill. Weaning at this time can produce the additional discomfort of engorgement and the inconvenience of trying to decrease milk production. In times of stress, a baby needs the closeness and reassurance of breastfeeding.

Nighttime Feedings Continued nighttime feedings may cause a mother to become so fatigued from lack of sleep that she does not function well during the day. If her baby is older, weaning may be the answer. Sometimes the solution is simply to drop night feedings. Help her explore the possible reasons for her baby's wakefulness—separation anxiety, habit, insufficient daytime feedings to satisfy hunger, or a need for attention. Perhaps she can respond to night feedings if she gets into the habit of napping during the day or cosleeping with her baby at night.

Changes in the Family Many times, a family's life becomes complicated with moving, job changes, illness, emotional upsets, or other stressful situations. It might appear that weaning would make life simpler for the mother at such a time. In reality, her baby's needs for security and continuity are even greater when significant changes occur in the child's life. Ending breastfeeding at this time could lead to fussiness, increased illness, and increased demands for attention. You can guide the mother in developing ways to integrate breastfeeding into her lifestyle so that she feels less stressed. If she does wean, she needs to do so gradually, so that her baby has time to adjust to the new environment.

The mother may consider weaning because she fears pregnancy and wants to start or resume taking oral contraceptives. You can give her some information about methods of contraception (see Chapter 19) that are compatible with breastfeeding and encourage her to discuss these options with her caregiver. Ideally, she will find a method that is acceptable to both her and her partner.

Sadly, breastfeeding babies have sometimes become emotional "footballs" between parents who are involved in divorce. Some mothers have felt pressured to wean to allow extended visitation between the father and child. In fact, visitation can take place in a way that accommodates breastfeeding. Information on breastfeeding in the context of family law and the best interests of the child is available at www.lalecheleague.org.

Societal Pressure Pressure or comments from family members or friends can prompt a mother to consider weaning. Suggestions that her baby is becoming too dependent because of breastfeeding may cause her to worry that this is actually the case. She can examine her breastfeeding pattern to determine whether she initiates nursing in response to all of her baby's bids for attention. In some instances, she may need to find other ways to respond. Self-reliance develops when the child can depend on the mother for comfort and security. She can continue to breastfeed knowing that it provides emotional benefits to her baby.

The baby's father may suggest weaning because he feels left out when he sees the mother and baby constantly together. Perhaps he misses evenings out together or simply would like more of his partner's attention. She can explore his reasons for wanting her to terminate breastfeeding and try to find a suitable compromise. Special times together for the couple or fewer feedings when he is home may satisfy the father. Ultimately, the mother may decide to wean to maintain harmony in the home; your role as lactation consultant is to support her in her decision.

A mother may be criticized for breastfeeding an older baby and begin to wonder if breastfeeding is still beneficial. Let mothers know that their milk has nutritional advantages for a toddler and that these effects are dose dependent. In other words, the more breastmilk received, the greater the nutritional benefits. Furthermore, the emotional security of breastfeeding can be a stabilizing factor in a child's life. To decrease criticism, the mother can avoid nursing in front of those who disapprove and keep a toy or snack ready as a distraction to postpone feedings. She can also avoid taking her child places when she anticipates the infant will become hungry or tired and wish to nurse.

If the mother senses others are receptive, she can attempt to educate them about the continuing benefits of breastfeeding. She may simply need to indicate her determination to continue nursing by standing firm and nursing discreetly. She will benefit from your encouragement and support to offset the negative influences around her. Contact with other women who are breastfeeding older babies will help build her confidence and maintain her perspective.

Untimely Weaning

Mothers must sometimes wean their babies abruptly, with no time for preparation or forethought. If emergency weaning is unavoidable, the mother must put aside her ideal vision of gradual, comfortable weaning. If she is able to take several days to wean, she can drop every other feeding the first day. In place of those feedings, she can express just enough milk to relieve discomfort but not so much that she stimulates further production. She can then eliminate the remainder of the feedings, making sure she includes extra nurturing and attention for her baby.

Emergency Weaning If a mother must wean immediately, she may experience 24 to 48 hours of painful engorgement, with the extent depending on how much milk she is producing and how often her baby has been nursing. Engorgement will subside gradually. If she likes, the mother can wrap her breasts in cabbage leaves to reduce swelling (see Chapter 16 for guidelines in applying cabbage to engorged breasts). Ibuprofen can relieve her pain and help reduce swelling. You may also want to refer the mother to her primary healthcare provider for prescription medications, as certain medications (e.g., antihistamines with pseudoephedrine, drugs in the ergot family, oral contraceptives with estrogen) are available that can lower milk production.

Placing ice wrapped in a towel on the breasts will help to reduce the swelling and pain associated with engorgement. The mother will want to avoid application of heat because it increases blood flow and swelling and can promote milk flow. Plugged ducts or mastitis might then occur because of the lack of milk flow through breastfeeding. Your attention and availability will be critical to the mother as she experiences this period of stress.

Some outdated medical literature and older relatives may recommend breast binding, a practice that can lead to plugged ducts and mastitis, and intensify the mother's pain or illness. Mothers should never bind their breasts!

Unintentional Weaning Sometimes a mother inadvertently weans her baby while actually wanting to continue nursing. Perhaps she started giving occasional bottles of formula and before she realized the consequences, her milk production had diminished. For some women, the hectic pace of the holidays can cause missed feedings and lead to reduced milk production, increased infant fussiness, and more supplementation. After the holidays are over, a mother may realize that her baby has begun weaning sooner than she had planned.

These mothers may feel breastfeeding has slipped away to the extent that they are unable or unwilling to turn back. They will especially need your acceptance and support at this time to help them through their disappointment. Should a mother express a desire to relactate, you can discuss the issues related to relactation as covered in Chapter 24.

Untimely weaning can shake a woman's confidence in her competence as a mother. Encourage her to continue giving her baby the same nurturing and attention she provided when she was breastfeeding, holding the infant close and providing eye contact during feedings.

Unavoidable Weaning Some circumstances outside the mother's control may lead to weaning. Perhaps the mother has developed a serious illness or requires medication that would pass through her milk and harm her baby. Perhaps she returns to work or school and finds it difficult to continue to breastfeed. Her baby may suddenly refuse to nurse and fail to resume breastfeeding. The mother may become pregnant, and her history of miscarriage or preterm birth may preclude breastfeeding. In other cases, the discomfort of sore nipples during pregnancy coupled with a decrease in milk production may suppress her desire to continue nursing.

After such forced weaning, the mother may grieve over the loss of breastfeeding. She may feel guilty or incompetent because she could not continue this part of her mothering role. Listening to and accepting her feelings will help her work through this personal loss. You can stress the benefits she provided her baby during the time she breastfed and emphasize her other mothering skills to substitute for the closeness of breastfeeding.

Minimal Breastfeeding

Many women find that minimal breastfeeding provides an attractive compromise to total weaning. Minimal breastfeeding describes a pattern of breastfeeding 1 to 3 times per day, with complementary foods providing the remaining nourishment for the baby. This practice may be an option when the mother and baby are separated for regular periods, as when the mother returns to work or school. Breastfeeding 2 to 3 times per day can help a mother continue to experience the special connection to her baby that accompanies breastfeeding. Many mothers use minimal breastfeeding (feeding 1 to 2 times per day) for an extended period as a comfortable transition to weaning.

After Weaning

It is common for mothers to feel some regret or sadness when breastfeeding ends, even if they had wanted to wean. Every woman benefits from support and understanding by those close to her so that she can resolve these feelings. You may be able to help the mother recognize that new skills for comforting her baby will replace breastfeeding, without minimizing her sadness at the loss of the breastfeeding relationship. Help her regard weaning as another step in her child's development, and encourage her to look forward to new stages. You can praise her for having met her child's need for both nutrition and nurturing. She will continue to nurture her child throughout his or her life, and she has set the stage for lifelong good nutrition.

If you sense that a mother's feelings are stronger than normal sadness, such as profound grief, she may benefit from counseling or therapy. You should also suggest that she see her primary healthcare giver to rule out clinical depression, as passage through life stages can be a trigger for dealing with other emotional issues. Keeping a current list of counselors or therapists who are sensitive to or who specialize in women's issues may prove helpful to mothers in your care over the years.

Physical Changes with Weaning

The mother may experience several physical adjustments after weaning, and your anticipatory guidance will prepare her for these changes. To avoid gaining weight, most women will need to adjust their diets to eliminate the excess calories they used during lactation. Some are pleased to find a sudden weight loss of a few pounds resulting from a loss of fluid and fat from the body's fat stores. If menstruation did not resume until after weaning, menstrual cycles may be somewhat irregular for a few months, with intermittent bleeding, light flow, or spotting.

For a few months after weaning, the breasts may become soft, flat, or droopy. Some women find that their breasts gradually return to their prepregnancy size, while other women's breasts remain larger than they were before they became pregnant. Some observe that their breasts never fully regain the fatty layer that was present before conception. The Montgomery glands recede, and the areola may remain darker than before pregnancy. Stretch marks may be apparent on the mother's breasts.

Continued Milk Secretion

Some mothers continue to secrete milk for several months after weaning. This flow will gradually diminish and turn to a colostrum-like consistency. If the mother is still spontaneously secreting milk 6 months after weaning, she should evaluate any circumstances that may be stimulating milk production. Perhaps she is holding her baby against her chest, wears clothing that rubs against her nipples, or is sensitive to sexual foreplay that involves her breasts.

The total cessation of milk secretion varies greatly from one woman to the next. It may last several weeks or as long as 1 year after weaning. Some hospital nurses and daycare workers report continuing to be able to express drops of milk years after weaning their own children. Perhaps it is the effect of working in an oxytocin-rich environment! After milk secretion has stopped completely, if the mother notices the appearance of a discharge, she will want to consult her caregiver to determine the cause. Sometimes old milk works its way out. Other times, fluid may result from an infection or growth. Review the discussion in Chapter 16 if it seems appropriate to investigate whether there is an underlying medical reason for the continued milk secretion.

∼ Summary

Anticipatory guidance helps parents recognize the normal events to expect as their babies develop throughout infancy and toddlerhood. Adjustments in routines and practices help accommodate breastfeeding to these developmental stages. Over time, the baby's world expands as he or she develops both physically and socially. The infant learns certain cues that elicit responses from the parents—cries, coos, smiles, or frowns, depending on the infant's needs. Although the baby's mother first represents the entire world to the infant, he or she soon expands awareness to others and the bigger world. Motor skills develop further as the infant begins to crawl and then walk. Teething, shorter feedings, separation anxiety, experimenting with vocabulary sounds, self-feeding, and drinking from a cup evolve gradually. Mothers find creative ways to nurse their toddler and eventually manage weaning.

This expansive time can be both exhilarating and challenging for parents. The lactation consultant's advice and support can increase parental confidence as mothers and fathers mature in their parenting role to meet their baby's needs.

∼ Chapter 17—At a Glance

Applying what you learned—

Teach mothers about:

- What to expect with each of the baby's developmental stages.
- The baby's innate reflexes of rooting, sucking, grasping, swallowing, and gagging.
- When the baby will be able to sleep through the night.
- Appetite spurts and decreased time at feedings because of efficiency in sucking.
- Adjusting breastfeeding when the baby begins teething.
- Typical weight gain.
- The fact that the breasts becoming less firm is unrelated to milk production.
- Delaying solid foods until 6 months or later.
- The value of breastmilk to the young child throughout the second year and beyond.
- Signs that the baby is ready for complementary foods.
- Resisting pressure to begin complementary foods too early.
- Cow's milk or other food allergy and signs of food intolerance.
- Role of family history in allergies.
- Signs a baby is ready to wean.
- Importance of baby-led weaning or gradual mother-led weaning.
- Miscues that cause mothers to consider weaning.
- Minimal breastfeeding as an alternative to weaning.
- Physical and emotional changes to expect after weaning.

Teach mothers how to:

- Adapt breastfeeding to each developmental stage.
- Adapt to changes in eating and sleeping patterns.
- Fit breastfeeding into resuming social activities.
- Help the baby overcome teething pain and discourage biting.
- Sustain breastfeeding beyond 1 year.
- Manage supplementary and complementary feedings.

∼ References

Adolph K, et al. What changes in infant walking and why. *Child Dev.* 2003;74(2):475-497.

American Academy of Family Physicians (AAFP). Family physicians supporting breastfeeding (position paper); 2008.

www.aafp.org/online/en/home/policy/policies/b/breastfeedingpositionpaper.html. Accessed June 30, 2009.

American Academy of Pediatrics (AAP). Policy statement on breastfeeding and the use of human milk. *Pediatrics*. 2005; 115(2):496-506. aappolicy.aappublications.org/cgi/content/abstract/pediatrics;115/2/496. Accessed June 30, 2009.

American Academy of Pediatrics (AAP); Kleinman R, ed. *Pediatric Nutrition Handbook*, 6th ed. Elk Grove Village, IL: AAP; 2009.

American Dietetic Association (ADA). Position of the American Dietetic Association: vegetarian diets. *J Am Diet Assoc*. 2009;109 (7):1266-1282.

Arditi-Babchuk H. Rapid eye movement (REM) in premature neonates and developmental outcome at 6 months. *Infant Behav Dev*. 2009;32(1):27-32.

Beauchamp G, Mennella J. Early flavor learning and its impact on later feeding behavior. *J Pediatr Gastroent Nutr*. 2009;48(suppl 1):S25-S30.

Bener A, et al. Role of breast feeding in primary prevention of asthma and allergic diseases in a traditional society. *Eur Ann Allergy Clin Immunol*. 2007;39(10):337-343.

Bengson D. *How Weaning Happens*. Schaumburg, IL: La Leche League International; 2000.

Berger S, et al. How and when infants learn to climb stairs. *Infant Behav Dev*. 2007;30(1):36-49.

Brown K, et al. Dietary intervention strategies to enhance zinc nutrition: promotion and support of breastfeeding for infants and young children. *Food Nutr Bull*. 2009;30(1 suppl):S144-S171.

Bumgarner N. *Mothering Your Nursing Toddler*. Schaumburg, IL: La Leche League International; 2000.

Butte N, et al. Sleep organization and energy expenditure of breast-fed and formula-fed infants. *Pediatr Res*. 1992;32: 514-519.

Chalouhi C, et al. Neurological consequences of vitamin B_{12} deficiency and its treatment. *Pediatr Emerg Care*. 2008; 24(8):538-541.

Colson S, et al. Optimal positions for the release of primitive neonatal reflexes stimulating breastfeeding. *Early Hum Dev*. 2008;84(7):441-449.

Deffeyes J, et al. Nonlinear analysis of sitting postural sway indicates developmental delay in infants. *Clin Biomech (Bristol, Avon)*. 2009;24(7):564-570.

Dewey K. Effects of exclusive breastfeeding for four versus six months on maternal nutritional status and infant motor development: results of two randomized trials in Honduras. *J Nutr*. 2001;131(2):262-267.

Dewey K. Nutrition, growth, and complementary feeding of the breastfed infant. In: Hale T, Hartmann P, eds. *Hale & Hartmann's Textbook of Human Lactation*. Amarillo, TX: Hale Publishing; 2007:415-423.

Dewey K, et al. Growth of breastfed and formula-fed infants from 0 to 18 months: the DARLING study. *Pediatrics*. 1992;89:1035-1041.

Dewey K, et al. Breast-fed infants are leaner than formula-fed infants at 1 year of age: the DARLING study. *Am J Clin Nutr*. 1993;57(2):140-145.

Dror D, Allen L. Effect of vitamin B_{12} deficiency on neurodevelopment in infants: current knowledge and possible mechanisms. *Nutr Rev*. 2008;66(5):250-255.

Fiocchi A, Martelli A. Dietary management of food allergy. *Pediatr Ann*. 2006;35(10):755-756, 758-763.

Fransson P, et al. Spontaneous brain activity in the newborn brain during natural sleep: an MRI study in infants born at full term. *Pediatr Res*. 2009;66(3):301-305.

Furuhjelm C, et al. Fish oil supplementation in pregnancy and lactation may decrease the risk of infant allergy. *Acta Paediatr*. 2009;98(9):1461-1467.

Green J, Wilson E. Spontaneous facial motility in infancy: a 3D kinematic analysis. *Dev Psychobiol*. 2006;48(1):16-28.

Grummer-Strawn LM, et al. Infant feeding and feeding transitions during the first year of life. *Pediatrics*. 2008;122(suppl 2):S36-S42.

Grummer-Strawn L, Mei Z; Centers for Disease Control and Prevention Pediatric Nutrition Surveillance System. Does breastfeeding protect against pediatric overweight? Analysis of longitudinal data from the Centers for Disease Control and Prevention Pediatric Nutrition Surveillance System. *Pediatrics*. 2004;113:e81-e86.

Hicks J, ed. *Hirkani's Daughters*. Schaumburg, IL: La Leche League International; 2005.

International Baby Food Action Network (IBFAN); Allain A, Kean Y. *Breaking the Rules: Stretching the Rules 2007*. Penang, Malaysia: International Code Documentation Center; 2007.

Kent J, et al. Volume and frequency of breastfeedings and fat content of breast milk throughout the day. *Pediatrics*. 2006;117(3):e387-e395.

Koletzko B, et al. Can infant feeding choices modulate later obesity risk? *Am J Clin Nutr*. 2009;89(5):1502S-1508S.

La Leche League International (LLLI). *The Womanly Art of Breastfeeding*, 7th ed. Schaumburg, IL: LLLI; 2004.

Li R, et al. Association of breastfeeding intensity and bottle-emptying behaviors at early infancy with infants' risk for excess weight at late infancy. *Pediatrics*. 2008;122(suppl 2):S77-S84.

Mayo Clinic. Infant and toddler health. January 5, 2008. www.mayoclinic.com/health/infant-development/PR00061/NSECTIONGROUP=2. Accessed June 18, 2009.

McDermott BM. Preschool children perceived by mothers as irregular eaters: Physical and psychosocial predictors from a birth cohort study. *J Dev Behav Pediatr*. 2008;29(3):197-205.

Mennella J, et al. Flavor programming during infancy. *Pediatrics*. 2004;113(4):840-845.

Miralles O, et al. A physiological role of breast milk leptin in body weight control in developing infants. *Obesity*. 2006; 14:1371-1377.

Newman J, Kernerman E. *Breastfeed a toddler: why on earth?* Rev. 2009. http://www.nbcionline.org/index.php?option=com_content&view=article&id=78:breastfeed-a-toddlerwhy-on-earth&catid=5:information&Itemid=17. Accessed April 17, 2010.

Nicklaus S. Development of food variety in children. *Appetite*. 2009;52(1):253-255.

Osayande A, et al. Clinical inquiries: How should you manage an overweight breastfed infant? *J Fam Prac*. 2009;58(6):E2.

Palou A, Picó C. Leptin intake during lactation prevents obesity and affects food intake and food preferences in later life. *Appetite*. 2009;52(1):249-252.

Prescott S, et al. The importance of early complementary feeding in the development of oral tolerance: concerns and controversies. *Pediatr Allergy Immunol.* 2008;19(5):375-380.

Queensland Government. Current breastfeeding campaign: 12+ months on the breast. Normal. Natural. Healthy. May 1, 2009. health.qld.gov.au/breastfeeding/bf_duration.asp. Accessed July 1, 2009.

Rees D, Sabia J. The effect of breast feeding on educational attainment: evidence from sibling data. *J Human Capital.* 2009;3:43-72.

Sears R, Sears J. *Father's First Steps: 25 Things Every New Dad Should Know.* Boston: Harvard Common Press; 2006.

Sears W. Fathering. 2006. www.askdrsears.com/html/10/t110100.asp. Accessed June 30, 2009.

Singhal A. Does breastfeeding protect from growth acceleration and later obesity? *Nestlé Nutr Workshop Ser Pediatr Program.* 2007;60:15-25; discussion 25-29.

Smith L. Why Johnny can't suck: impact of birth practices on infant suck. In: Genna CW, *Supporting Sucking Skills in Infants.* Sudbury, MA: Jones and Bartlett; 2008:57-78.

Snijders B, et al. Breast-feeding duration and infant atopic manifestations, by maternal allergic status, in the first 2 years of life (KOALA study). *Pediatrics.* 2007;151(4):347-351, 351.e1-351.e2.

Stuart-MacAdam P, Dettwyler K, eds. *Breastfeeding: Biocultural Perspectives (Foundations of Human Behavior).* New York: Aldine de Gruyter; 1995.

U.S. Dept. Health & Human Services, Centers for Disease Control and Prevention (USDHHS CDC). Division of Nutrition, Physical Activity and Obesity, National Center for Chronic Disease Prevention and Health Promotion. *Infant Feeding Practices Study II.* Atlanta, GA: USDHHS CDC; May 19, 2009. www.cdc.gov/ifps/index.htm. Accessed July 1, 2009.

Venter C. Factors associated with maternal dietary intake, feeding and weaning practices, and the development of food hypersensitivity in the infant. *Pediatr Allergy Immunol.* 2009;20(4):320-327.

Walker M. *Still Selling Out Mothers and Babies: Marketing Breastmilk Substitutes in the USA.* Weston, MA: NABA REAL; 2007.

World Health Organization (WHO). Infant and young child nutrition: global strategy on infant and young child feeding. Geneva, Switzerland: WHO; 2002. http://ftp.who.int/gb/archive/pdf_files/WHA55/ea5515.pdf. Accessed June 30, 2009.

World Health Organization (WHO). WHO Multicentre Growth Reference Study Group. *WHO Child Growth Standards.* Geneva: World Health Organization; 2006. www.who.int/childgrowth/standards/en/. Accessed May 10, 2009.

Problems with Milk Production and Transfer

Some mothers experience problems with establishing sufficient milk production to sustain their babies. Some babies may have difficulty transferring milk despite the mother having an ample supply. Still other mothers lack confidence in their ability to produce sufficient milk despite a healthy, thriving baby. The information presented in this chapter will assist you in helping a mother recognize when her milk production is truly low. You will learn to recognize when newborns are receiving sufficient amounts of milk as well as measures for increasing milk production and efficient transfer. With appropriate teaching and follow-up, you and the mother can maximize her chances of adequate milk production and a baby who thrives on mother's milk.

∽ Key Terms

Digital baby weight scale
Donor milk
Failure to thrive
Human Milk Banking
    Association of North
    America (HMBANA)
Insufficient milk
    production
Poor weight gain
Slow weight gain
World Health
    Organization (WHO)
    growth charts

∽ Perception of Insufficient Milk Production

A mother might perceive a problem with her milk for a number of reasons. She may believe it is not rich or satisfying enough. She may worry that her milk is causing an allergic response or excessive gas in her baby. By far the most common concern for mothers is that they have an inadequate amount of milk. One review found 35 percent of mothers who weaned early reported perceived insufficient milk as the primary reason (Gatti, 2008).

In fact, the most common reason women give for early weaning is the belief that they do not produce enough milk for their babies. Studies reveal that this is a universal belief, transcending nationalities and cultures. This is seen from studies including America (Hill & Aldag, 2007), Australia (Amir, 2006), Bosnia/Herzegovina (Simic et al., 2004), Brazil (Borges & Philippi, 2003), Cambodia (Straub et al., 2008), China (Xu et al., 2009), Hong Kong (Lee et al., 2006), India (Dhandapany et al., 2008), Israel (Shani & Shinwell, 2003), Japan (Otsuka et al., 2008), Mexico (Sacco et al., 2006), and Saudi Arabia (El Mouzan et al., 2009). This misperception often leads women to give their babies supplements, which in turn leads to insufficient milk production and often to untimely weaning.

When a mother says she does not have enough milk for her baby, you first need to determine why she believes this. Although it is possible that she has low milk production, the comment may actually result from a lack of confidence or a lack of knowledge about typical newborn behavior. Helping the mother identify whether she actually has a problem, and reassuring her when her production is fine, can have a tremendous influence on breastfeeding duration among your clients.

Reasons for Perceived Low Milk

There are differences between women who perceive they have insufficient milk and those who are confident in their ability to produce milk for their baby. Recognizing these differences will enable you to give these mothers the special help or information they need. Mothers who perceive their milk production to be insufficient worry that the baby does not seem satisfied and is fussy after feedings. They are also concerned about poor infant weight gain and what they consider too frequent feedings.

Some women lack confidence in their bodies' ability to function as nature intended. The medical profession's use of negative terminology in women's health could be a contributing factor. Such terms as lactation failure, failure to progress, and incompetent cervix can undermine a woman's self-confidence and self-esteem. Messages such as these can compromise a mother's confidence at a time when she is vulnerable to negativism.

Because many new parents do not live near their nuclear family, they may lack a strong support system and positive role models for birthing and parenting. Women who breastfeed in a culture saturated with bottle feeding messages face many societal challenges. Female friends and relatives may have bottle fed their babies. The expectations of society and the media are that babies are fed by bottles. Often, caregivers either have a lack of correct information regarding breastfeeding care (Chantry, 2009; Leavitt et al., 2009; Szucs et al., 2009; Brodribb et al., 2008) or are noncommittal to avoid causing mothers to "feel guilty" if they choose to bottle feed.

Parents want to know they are doing the best for their baby. The stress of becoming a new mother can feed into a woman's worries about competence. Most families in industrialized countries are small. Many parents have had little or no experience in caring for small infants. A mother's misconceptions about the realities of motherhood can cause her to question her choices and doubt her parenting abilities. Her preconceived notions of babies may not match the reality of her baby or her baby's needs. Misconceptions of normal behavior can create anxieties in inexperienced parents, who may incorrectly blame breastfeeding as the cause for fussiness, wakefulness, or other newborn behaviors.

High self-confidence and self-efficacy go hand-in-hand with a belief in sufficient milk production. In a Japanese study of 262 mothers, though most mothers intended to breastfeed exclusively, by 4 weeks postpartum fewer than 40 percent were doing so. Perceived insufficient milk was the primary reason for supplementation or weaning in 73 percent of these mothers. Mothers' perceptions were significantly related to their breastfeeding self-efficacy in the hospital after birth (Otsuka et al., 2008).

This corroborates an older study measuring parental self-efficacy, which also found a significant correlation between levels of maternal self-confidence and perceived insufficient milk (McCarter-Spaulding & Kearney, 2001). A qualitative study of Mexican mothers also found that they viewed crying as the primary symptom of insufficient milk production, and the most common coping strategy was to supplement with formula (Sacco et al., 2006).

Recognizing Sufficient Milk Production

It is important that the mother feels secure in her ability to breastfeed her baby and confident that she can produce the milk her baby needs. If she and her baby were discharged from the hospital at 48 hours or less after delivery, the baby's primary caregiver needs to see the infant within 2 to 4 days (American Academy of Pediatrics, 2004). The baby will typically have a second visit at around 2 weeks for a physical assessment and another weight check. It should be sooner if the baby's condition warrants it. These safeguards help to ensure a healthy baby and a confident mother.

Mothers have fewer worries about their milk production when they understand that milk removal triggers further milk production. Recognizing normal newborn behavior also assures them that they are meeting their babies' needs. Knowing how to tell that their baby is getting enough milk from nursing may prevent the unnecessary early weaning caused by a mother's perception that she does not have enough milk for her baby. The signs below indicate that breastfeeding is going well.

Signs That Breastfeeding Is Going Well

- By day 4 the baby has at least six wet diapers in each 24-hour period.
- The baby has pale, diluted urine.
- By day 4 the baby has three or more ample stools that are yellow or at least are turning yellow.
- The baby continues to have at least three stools in each 24-hour period until he or she is about 5 to 6 weeks old.
- The baby routinely breastfeeds at least 8 to 12 times in each 24-hour period.
- The mother's breasts feel softer after a feeding (although some women have no dramatic change).
- The mother's nipples are not painful during or after feedings.
- The baby regains birth weight by 10 to 14 days.
- The baby gains 4 to 8 ounces a week.
- During a feeding the baby's sucking rhythm changes and slows as he or she obtains milk; the mother may notice swallowing or gulping.
- The baby is alert and active.
- The baby is content between feedings, usually rests for 1 to 2 hours, wakes on his or her own, and signals to breastfeed again (although well-fed infants may be fussy for other reasons).

～ *Mothers at Risk for Low Milk Production*

Few mothers actually have insufficient milk production, although their numbers are increasing (West & Marasco, 2008; Marasco et al., 2000). Most cases of insufficient milk result from ineffective breastfeeding, which the mother can correct. Be careful not to confuse the maternal inability to produce adequate amounts of milk with the lack of opportunity to produce the milk.

Your role in the case of low milk production or transfer involves helping the mother explore the possible causes. Usually, multiple factors cause a baby to not gain adequate weight, some more significant than others. Factors may relate to the mother, to the baby, or to breastfeeding practices. When multiple factors exist at birth, it is important that the mother and baby receive follow-up. Figure 12.4 in Chapter 12 identifies potential problems for establishing either adequate milk production or effective milk transfer.

Poor breastfeeding technique may be the cause of slow or poor weight gain. Some feeding-related causes of low milk production are the baby's inability to suck well, improper positioning, or inadequate time at each breast. Mothers also find that their milk production diminishes after they begin supplemental or complementary feedings. Prolactin inhibitors and an inhibited or unstable letdown can cause problems with intake. A specific cause may not always be apparent. When the mother and baby are both more proficient at nursing, problems that cause low milk production often diminish. See Chapter 25 for a discussion of maternal factors for insufficient milk production.

Measures to Increase Milk Production

A need to increase milk production may occur at any time in the early days of lactation, at times of growth spurts, or whenever the baby nurses less often. A concern about milk production surfaces most often because of poor weight gain in the baby. Therefore while the mother takes measures to increase her milk production, she also needs to ensure that her baby receives sufficient nourishment. Paradoxically, the cause of the mother's reduced production may be the supplements she gives to her baby. Those supplements need to continue until her milk production increases sufficiently to provide total nourishment. You can work with a mother and baby while they increase milk production in a manner that is both safe for the baby and supportive of breastfeeding.

The degree to which a mother is able to increase her milk production depends on the baby's age, medical condition, and willingness or ability to nurse. The amount and length of time of any supplements the baby may have received are factors in the degree of any possible breast involution. The mother's condition can be a factor as well; see Chapter 25 for a more detailed discussion of maternal endocrine or surgical causes of insufficient milk. Success also depends on the degree of motivation the mother has for devoting the necessary time and energy to the task. Her baby needs to breastfeed at least 10 to 12 times in 24 hours for many days.

You can help the mother increase milk production by offering some of the suggestions presented in Table 18.1. Many mothers are able to increase milk production simply by altering their pattern of feedings and increasing the number of times they nurse daily. As with other aspects of breastfeeding, several measures can be considered when developing a plan with the mother to increase her milk production. Be careful not to overwhelm a mother with too many suggestions or with measures that do not appeal to her. Each mother's needs are different. The mother needs close contact and support from you, especially in the first few days when she is trying to sort out the methods that work most effectively for her.

Herbal Galactogogues

Some mothers respond well to galactogogues—foods, drinks, medications, or herbs believed to increase milk production. It is important to target any herb or medicine to the core reason behind true low milk production. Many varieties of herbs have been used as galactogogues, including fenugreek and blessed thistle. Some clinicians have found goat's rue and shatavari to be effective as well (West & Marasco, 2008b). *The Nursing Mother's Herbal* (Humphrey, 2003), *The Breastfeeding Mother's Guide to Making More Milk* (West & Marasco, 2008b) or the respective websites (www.lowmilksupply.org and www.makingmoremilk .org) may be helpful for mothers seeking an herbal approach.

Domperidone

Domperidone, a drug used to suppress nausea and vomiting, can increase milk production because of a side effect that increases prolactin levels. Before domperidone became available women used metoclopramide, which also raises prolactin levels. However, because of metoclopramide's other side effects of fatigue, irritability, and depression, domperidone is now preferred.

In 2004 the U.S. Food and Drug Administration (FDA) issued a warning against the use of domperidone by breastfeeding women (USFDA, 2004). Responses from breastfeeding experts underscored the long history of safe use of domperidone for increasing milk production in breastfeeding women. Domperidone is available in many countries, even as an over-the-counter medication. It is not available in the United States except by compounding, which is combining drugs to create a new substance.

TABLE 18.1   Measures to Increase Milk Production

Actions for the mother	• Rest as much as possible, and relax during breastfeedings to help the milk flow.
	• Spend 100 percent of her time with the baby for 48 hours, concentrating on increasing feedings and resting. Get help with all other tasks.
	• Take special precautions to prevent sore nipples.
	• Use local galactogogues (foods, drinks, or herbs believed to increase milk production).
	• Keep a record of feedings (both breastfeedings and any supplements). This can show how quickly the milk production is increasing and help the mother find a workable feeding pattern.
	• Use a hospital-grade electric breast pump to provide additional stimulation to the breasts.
	• Improve diet by eating more protein, fresh fruits and vegetables, and B vitamins.
Management of feedings	• Encourage letdown by relaxation techniques and following a daily feeding routine.
	• Prepare the baby so he is alert and ready to nurse by rousing or soothing him as needed.
	• Make sure the baby is attached for effective suckling.
	• Put the baby to both breasts at a feeding, several times each, to increase stimulation.
	• Encourage the baby to feed more frequently and longer, both day and night.
	• Nurse long enough for the baby to receive hindmilk. This will vary from one baby to another.
	• Nurse for comfort if the baby is fussy.
	• Get into bed with the baby for feedings to increase skin contact.
	• Resume night feedings if they had been dropped.

In addition to warning the public about use of domperidone, the FDA issued an Import Alert asking FDA personnel to be on the lookout for the drug being imported into the United States (USFDA, 2004). These warnings occurred at a time when the pharmaceutical industry was fighting against importation of drugs into the United States. The FDA issued the warning on the same day as the largest breastfeeding promotion campaign in U.S. history was launched by the Department of Health and Human Services.

Domperidone should not be the first approach to correcting breastfeeding difficulties. Its use is appropriate only after exploring all other factors that may result in insufficient milk production and responding appropriately. Problem solving should include correcting the baby's latch and sucking problems. Using breast compression during feedings and milk expression after feedings may also help to increase milk production (Newman & Kernerman, 2009b).

～ *Concerns About Infant Growth*

Several factors contribute to the total picture of a baby's adequate growth. Birth weight should double by 4 months and triple by 12 months (Lawrence & Lawrence, 2005). Body length is a significant indicator of growth. The baby should increase in length by 50 percent at 12 months.

Head circumference, which indicates brain growth, should increase by 3 inches (7.6 cm) at 1 year.

Other signs of healthy growth are sufficient voids and stools, which are frequent in the first month and less frequent thereafter. Bright eyes, an alert manner, and good muscle and skin tone also indicate a healthy baby. If there is a family history of small stature or slow weight gain, the parents' children will most likely exhibit a similar pattern. All these factors need to be considered before you determine that a problem may exist. Refer to the World Health Organization (WHO, 2006) growth charts in Appendix F to plot a slow-gaining baby's weight, height, and head circumference.

To ensure the health of every infant in your care, be alert to weight gain and to the factors that could contribute to low milk production. Understand each mother's and baby's feeding pattern to help you assess adequate growth. Consider all growth indicators and possible causes of poor growth as you and the mother develop a plan for improvement.

Newborn Dehydration

A baby can become dehydrated when he or she does not receive a sufficient amount of fluids. This can occur when a breastfed baby is not receiving an adequate amount of mother's milk. Many mothers and babies often leave the hospital before someone who is knowledgeable about breastfeeding has evaluated their breastfeeding technique. Consequently, some mothers may not have had a good breastfeeding before they go home. Because of short hospital stays, very few mothers have established milk production (lactogenesis II) before discharge. Recognizing the symptoms of dehydration will help you identify infants at risk.

Symptoms of Dehydration

- Few or no stools
- Scant urinary output
- Dark, strong smelling urine
- Infant sleeps at the breast
- Infrequent feedings
- Weight loss greater than 10 to 15 percent of birth weight
- Lethargy
- Weak cry
- Dry mucous membranes
- Lack of tearing
- Poor skin turgor
- Sunken fontanels

Preventing Dehydration

It is imperative that mothers and babies who go home early receive some form of follow-up shortly after discharge. There is never any reason for a healthy newborn to progress to the point of dehydration. Mothers need to know how to assess adequate breastfeeding. Hospital staff needs to teach the mother how to recognize when her baby achieves an effective latch. Just because a baby's jaw moves up and down does not mean he or she is taking in milk. Make sure mothers know the signs that breastfeeding is going well, in addition to the warning signs of potential problems (see Chapter 12).

It is often difficult to ascertain if a mother has established effective breastfeeding at the time of discharge if mature milk production has not begun. The mother and baby may need a follow-up visit to the physician's office, a lactation consultant, or health clinic within 1 to 2 days after discharge. Giving the mother a diary to document feedings, stools, and voids helps her to monitor her baby's intake and output. During the follow-up visit the office staff needs to understand and recognize the impact of the number of feedings, stools, and voids.

Weight Gain Issues

Concerns about the baby's weight usually surface during the first month. Poor intake, poor weight gain, or vomiting can be due to either organic or nonorganic causes. Behavioral causes can be tied to food refusal, food fixa-

tion, abnormal parental feeding practices, onset after a specific trigger, or the presence of anticipatory gagging. Organic causes include gastroesophageal reflux disease (GERD), milk allergy, idiopathic, or nutritional failure to thrive in which the child can respond to medication or nutritional therapy (Levy et al., 2009). Weight gain problems in breastfed infants that start after the first month are more likely to have organic causes (Lukefahr, 1990).

As discussed in Chapter 13, weight loss beyond 10 percent in the first week warrants an evaluation and assistance with breastfeeding. There should be no further weight loss after the third day for full-term infants. Weight gain should begin by day 4 when full milk production begins and the baby should regain back to birth weight by 10 to 14 days.

Breastfed and formula fed infants consume dramatically different amounts of calories. By 8 months a formula fed infant consumes about 30,000 more kcal than a breastfed infant (Garza et al., 1987). By 4 months of age gross energy intakes by exclusively breastfed infants are significantly less than current recommendations, which are based on artificial feeding. Breastfed infants have normal growth rates that differ from the growth rates of formula fed infants. They also have lower total daily energy expenditure, sleeping metabolic rates, rates of energy expenditure, rectal temperature, and heart rates (Garza & Butte, 1990).

In unfavorable environments babies may have higher than usual energy requirements. Rather than low milk production or intake, the baby's environment could explain the growth differences. This may be an issue for babies who live in high-poverty areas. Babies who lack restful sleep or who have multiple care providers may also have increased caloric needs (Butte et al., 1993). Although breastfed infants develop leaner body mass, the pattern does not continue into the second year (Butte et al., 2000). Because of the difference in growth in exclusively breastfed infants and those fed artificial baby milk, healthcare providers should replace outdated growth charts with the WHO growth charts based on breastfed children (WHO, 2006). See Chapter 13 for additional discussion about normal breastfed intake and growth rates.

Slow Weight Gain

Every child develops at his or her own rate. Some adolescents can experience a growth spurt and grow 6 inches in 1 year. Differences in growth rate are true for babies as well. Some babies naturally gain weight more slowly than others. It is important to distinguish between a baby who is not gaining weight adequately and one who is simply gaining weight slowly. A slow-gaining infant demonstrates slow and steady growth over time and grows proportionally for weight, length, and head circumference. Development will be age appropriate.

In the absence of other risk factors minimal intervention, if any, is required for this pattern of growth. You can observe breastfeeding to evaluate the mother's technique. Ask about her baby's feeding pattern and suggest any necessary changes if indicated. Some mothers believe they should nurse on only one breast at a feeding. Simply changing to two breasts can have a significant improvement in weight gain. Avoiding the use of pacifiers or bottles ensures adequate sucking time at the breast. Confirm that the mother is not trying to schedule or restrict feedings or limit her baby's time at the breast (see Chapter 19 for cautions about "baby training"). Review hunger cues with the mother to be sure she responds to her baby at appropriate times. If there are concerns, suggest that she have her baby weighed weekly and record weights to monitor growth. These measures may be all that is necessary for a slow-gaining infant.

Signs of Inadequate Weight Gain

You may not always have the opportunity to see mothers and babies who are at risk for low milk production or transfer before a problem develops. You need to recognize signs that alert you to problems. Babies who are not gaining adequately frequently sleep for long periods to conserve energy. They may fuss when removed from the breast and then go back to sleep as soon as they return to the breast. A mother may tell you she is nursing "all the time" because she cannot put her baby down with no fussing. Another mother may tell you she has a "good" baby who sleeps a lot and nurses infrequently. Poorly nourished infants usually sleep through the night and have few periods of quiet alert time.

A baby with poor weight gain often looks worried or anxious and holds his or her body in a flexed fetal position to help maintain temperature. A baby who has lost a large amount of weight will have hanging folds of skin on the thighs and buttocks. His or her cry may be high pitched like the "mew" of a cat. Urinary output may be decreased, or the baby may pass dark, concentrated urine. In an older baby urine may smell strongly of ammonia. A baby less than 5 to 6 weeks of age will pass few stools. A newborn infant without adequate intake may still be passing meconium after the 4th day of life.

Assessing Poor Weight Gain

If you question the adequacy of an infant's weight gain, evaluation of the mother's breastfeeding practices will help determine the cause. This applies to a newborn who has not regained birth weight by 14 days as well as an older baby who is not gaining or who is gaining less than 4 ounces per week in the first 3 to 4 months of life. Confirm whether the infant receives a minimum of 8 to 12 feedings per day around the clock and an appropriate number of complementary foods in the case of babies

6 months and older. The baby should be able to sustain sucking bursts without fatigue, with swallowing observed. The mother's breasts should feel softer after feeding. Be aware that some babies who seem to be swallowing are just swallowing their saliva, with little intake. On the other hand, many babies feed robustly and transfer milk well without audible swallowing. Caution against the use of pacifiers for a baby with poor weight gain. Emphasize to parents that all sucking needs to be nutritive (at the breast) to increase caloric intake.

If you are concerned that a baby may be an inefficient feeder, pre- and postfeeding weights will help assess milk transfer during the feeding. Use of a digital electronic scale ensures accuracy (Haase et al., 2009). When obtaining these measurements first weigh the baby naked. Then weigh the baby with a diaper on before nursing; this is your prefeed weight. Weigh the baby after the feeding to determine the milk transfer amount based on the difference in weight.

Ask the mother to pump after the feeding and measure the amount of residual milk that remained in the breast to help distinguish between ineffective milk transfer and low milk production. The pumped milk can be fed to the baby at the next feeding. If the parents use a bottle to feed the pumped milk, teach them paced feeding to slow the flow rate (Calgary Health Region, 2009; Wilson-Clay & Hoover, 2008; Kassing, 2002). See Chapter 21 for information about paced feeding.

Managing Poor Weight Gain

A baby with poor weight gain needs to be weighed at least twice a week to monitor weight. If the baby is an inefficient feeder, the mother needs to remove milk at the end of the feeding by hand expression or use of a breast pump. Pumping also provides nipple stimulation to maintain milk production. This is necessary until the baby is more effective at transferring milk.

The first goal in poor weight gain is for the baby to receive calories. Increasing his or her weight is essential. If the mother's milk production is low, the baby needs to receive supplemental donor milk or formula. If the baby is preterm or has other health problems, his or her physician can prescribe donor milk. Some insurance companies and Medicaid in some states may cover the use of donor milk for these babies. Compile a list of human milk banks, and become familiar with the Human Milk Banking Association of North America (HMBANA) guidelines, available at www.hmbana.org. Those who live outside Canada, the United States, or Mexico can check with their health ministry or department.

The second goal in poor weight gain is to increase the mother's milk production to the level that it can sustain her infant. Only then can the mother discontinue supplements. Supplementing the baby through a tube at the breast accomplishes both goals at the same time. The baby receives necessary nourishment and the mother's breasts receive the stimulation necessary for milk production. Pumping with a hospital-grade electric breast pump immediately after feedings further helps to increase milk production.

It is important that the baby's physician be updated on any feeding plan you and the mother develop. The mother's primary caregiver also needs to be involved if the mother has impaired milk production. Send a report of your consultation to both caregivers or call them with your evaluation and suggestions as appropriate. Encourage the mother to stay in close contact with you and her caregivers until the issue behind the baby's weight has been resolved. The mother can slowly decrease the amount the baby is supplemented when he or she begins to gain weight and when she is confident the baby is transferring more from the breast. Caregivers should become concerned when growth deviates downward by two major percentiles on the growth chart. When this occurs, the baby is diagnosed as failing to thrive.

Failure to Thrive

Failure to thrive (FTT) in an infant is defined as continuing to lose weight after 10 days of life, not regaining birth weight by 3 weeks of age, or having a weight gain below the 10th percentile beyond 1 month of age (Lawrence & Lawrence, 2005). In older infants a weight that is two standard deviations or more below where it should be on a standard growth chart is an indication of failure to thrive. A growth chart that shows normal weight for each age is a tool for determining whether growth is within established guidelines. Plotting the baby's predictable growth curve on a chart, using the WHO charts based on breastfed babies, helps assess his or her progress.

A baby who fails to thrive may be lethargic, hypertonic, irritable, and difficult to soothe (Figure 18.1). The infant may either sleep excessively or be continuously fussy, and his compromised status could relate to his physical condition or to that of his mother. Table 18.2 identifies causes related to the mother and infant. In many cases failure to thrive is a consequence of ineffective breastfeeding. It is important to realize that even a baby who appears to be satisfied can fail to thrive. An easy, placid baby is vulnerable to failure to thrive because he or she does not display appropriate hunger cues.

Failure to thrive can also result from an infection in the infant. For example, group B streptococcal ventriculitis can be manifested by progressive feeding difficulties and failure to thrive. This rare disease is not marked by fever, so often it is not diagnosed until the child develops intracranial hypertension (Collet et al., 2009; Miyairi et al., 2006). If you encounter a baby who is not gaining weight despite ample milk intake, an undetected infection may be present. The answer to a baby failing to thrive is

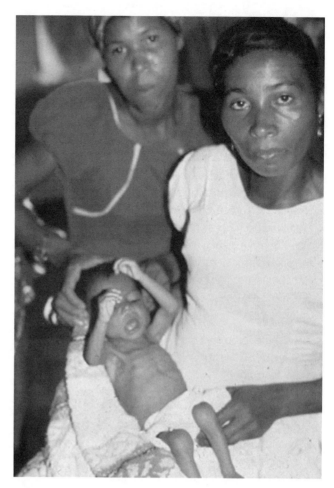

FIGURE 18.1 Infant who is failing to thrive.
Source: Printed with permission of Jan Riordan.

not to merely supplement with formula or to cease breastfeeding. The important action is to find the underlying *cause* of the failure to thrive and treat it.

What are the long-term effects of failing to thrive? One study of children at age 8 who had failed to thrive as babies concluded that early failure to thrive increased the incidence of short stature, poor arithmetic performance, and poor work habits (Black et al., 2007). Home visiting helped mitigate some of the negative effects of early failure to thrive, possibly by promoting maternal sensitivity and helping children build strong work habits that helped them in school.

Exploring the Cause of Failure to Thrive

The use of open-ended questions and a complete history of the mother and baby will help you identify the possible causes of failure to thrive. Explore issues related to the mother's pregnancy. Learning how much weight she gained may give you a clue to the possibility of an eating disorder or low fat in her milk. Asking what changes she noticed in her breasts during her pregnancy can help you determine if she has sufficient mammary tissue. Ask if

TABLE 18.2   Causes of Failure to Thrive

Maternal causes

- Previous breast surgery, either reduction or augmentation, or breast trauma
- Back or thoracic surgery
- Polycystic ovarian syndrome or history of infertility
- Hypoprolactinemia
- Anatomic position of the ducts
- Insufficient mammary tissue
- Hormonal disorders, including untreated hypothyroidism
- Sheehan's syndrome
- Disrupted neurohormonal pathways
- Inappropriate use of a nipple shield
- Retained placental fragments
- Poor breastfeeding practices, such as scheduling or restricting feedings

Infant causes

- Neuromotor problems
- Preterm or SGA infant
- Tight frenulum
- Systemic illness
- Sleepy infant
- Inability to compress breast adequately
- Mother's anatomy versus infant's oral cavity
- Disorganized suck
- "Good" baby who does not exhibit hunger cues

she has a history of infertility or miscarriage, because these can be markers for hormonal or thyroid disorders. Also ask what contraceptive method she is using to prevent another pregnancy. The use of birth control pills with estrogen, estrogen-emitting intrauterine devices, or estrogen patches can reduce milk production.

Ask about her labor and delivery to learn if there was excessive blood loss or if Pitocin or intravenous fluids were used. Hemorrhage or edema can delay the onset of milk production. Hemorrhage may be treated with methylergonovine (Methergine), which belongs to a class of drugs called ergot alkaloids. The ergot family includes bromocriptine and cabergoline, which can inhibit milk production.

Ask about the mother's general health. Although a mother's diet is rarely a factor in an infant's failure to thrive, learning about her overall eating pattern helps to paint a total picture. Ask whether she smokes cigarettes and how many per day. Smoking has been associated with low milk production (Hale, 2010), although studies are conflicting. Alcohol has been associated with a reduction

in milk let-down, infant intake, and infant sleep (Mennella & Pepino 2008; Mennella et al., 2005; Mennella, 2001). Learning about her alcohol consumption helps to rule this out as a cause. Learn whether she has had any breast procedure such as a biopsy, cyst removal, augmentation, or reduction. Ask specifically if she ever had a breast injury, because this may not occur to her when you inquire about breast procedures. Color Plate 53 shows a scar on the breast from a childhood injury.

Explore issues related to the mother's breastfeeding. Ask if she experienced any breast engorgement or mastitis, because pathological engorgement can lead to the loss of milk-producing cells. Obtain a clear picture of her breastfeeding routine, including how often her baby nurses, for how long, and whether on one or both breasts at a feeding. If she limits feeding length or restricts the number of feedings, she could down-regulate milk production. Ask how many voids and stools her baby had in the previous 24 hours, and their color and size. Scant or no stooling is a marker for inadequate intake. Green stools could indicate an imbalance in foremilk and hindmilk.

Explore issues related to parenting practices. Learn whether she uses a pacifier and how frequently. Some studies correlate pacifier use with fewer feedings and reduced breastfeeding duration (Karabulut et al., 2009; Kronborg & Vaeth, 2009; Parizoto et al., 2009). Others refute such a correlation (Jenik et al., 2009; O'Connor et al., 2009). Similarly, ask how much time her baby spends in a swing or other pacifying apparatus since use of devices to delay or avoid feedings can contribute to underfeeding. Ask if she uses a particular parenting program or feeding schedule. "Baby training" programs that place rigid restrictions on feedings are associated with low weight gain and reduced milk production (Aney, 1998; Marasco & Barger, 1998). See Chapter 19 for further discussion of such programs.

Managing Failure to Thrive

If failure to thrive is suspected, measures must begin immediately to reverse the pattern of weight loss. The actions taken depend on whether the issues affecting lactation lie with the baby, the mother, or both. Your assistance and support can be pivotal in helping a mother reverse her baby's weight pattern. Interventions may be required for a long time, so help her form realistic expectations. It is very common for the mother of an infant who is failing to thrive to feel highly stressed. As her baby's condition begins to improve, caution the mother to proceed slowly as she decreases the amount of supplement and frequency of milk expression. Sometimes interventions are required for the entire time the baby is breastfed.

Assess the baby's latch, sucking technique, and positioning at the breast. If oral anomalies are noted or if you cannot determine why the baby fails to transfer milk, the baby should be referred to an appropriate specialist. For example, babies with ankyloglossia are often referred to ear, nose, and throat specialists or to pediatric dentists for frenotomies (clipping the frenulum). Submucosal clefts and other subtle oral anomalies can easily be missed by care providers. Babies with ineffective sucking are often referred to an occupational therapist or a speech language pathologist.

Assess milk transfer with pre- and postfeeding weights on a digital baby scale. If the baby does not transfer at least 2 ounces or more and the mother is able to pump that amount, refer her to the baby's physician for assessment. If the baby is able to transfer 2 ounces, increasing frequency and duration of feedings may be appropriate.

It will be necessary to make adjustments in the mother's breastfeeding routine. Ask her to nurse her baby 10 to 12 times in 24 hours around the clock until he or she has three stools per 24 hours for 3 days in a row. Suggest she switch breasts when the baby's sucking pattern changes and swallowing ceases. In addition, use of alternate breast compression during the feeding increases milk flow (Newman & Kernerman, 2009a). Limiting feedings to 40 minutes per session—regardless of which combination of feeding methods are used—helps prevent fatigue and stress on both the part of the baby and the mother.

Address milk production by asking the mother to pump immediately after nursing. Massage and hand expression before pumping has been found to increase milk production significantly (Morton et al., 2009). Use of a hospital-grade electric breast pump and double pumping for 10 to 15 minutes or until milk stops flowing help stimulate milk production. She can then massage her breasts and pump a few minutes more.

Protecting the baby's health is a priority. It is essential to meet the baby's caloric needs with frequent feedings and supplements as recommended by the baby's physician. Follow the physician's guidelines for supplementation until the baby is gaining well and the baby's doctor states that supplementation can be discontinued. Keep the baby's doctor apprised of any increased ability to transfer milk by direct breastfeeding and/or any increase in the mother's milk production. Ensure that the baby visits his physician frequently and that any change in his weight is monitored closely. Urge the mother to stay in close contact with you and her baby's physician.

The mother may need help coping with her regimen for improving her baby's condition. As the situation improves you can help her identify any intervention that produces the most stress; she can then try to eliminate or decrease that aspect of the feeding plan. Mothers frequently ask to discontinue nighttime supplements when things improve. Continuing to breastfeed at least once during the night takes advantage of higher night-time prolactin levels.

Supplementing the Baby

It is crucial that a baby who is failing to thrive receive adequate nourishment while the mother is increasing her milk production. If milk production is too low to give sufficient calories, she will need to supplement her baby with donor milk or formula until her milk production increases. Avoiding pacifiers ensures that all sucking is nutritive.

Generally, encourage the mother to breastfeed first and follow with the supplement. However, if her baby is frantic to eat, he may nurse better if he receives a small amount of supplement first (15 mL or a half-ounce). Pumping after feedings provides further stimulation for milk production, and the pumped milk can be fed to her baby. As milk production improves supplements can decrease slowly along with continuing to increase the number of breastfeedings.

Amount to Supplement Mothers must regulate supplements and give them in measured amounts. This helps ensure that the baby does not receive too much supplement and consequently becomes disinterested in nursing. Suggest that the mother plan the number of ounces to feed her baby during a 24-hour period. A standard physician order of "nurse first and supplement afterward" may be misleading. Some babies nurse as few as 6 times a day, whereas others nurse as many as 12 or more times. A baby who nurses more frequently could consume so much formula that nursing may never resume.

The mother can ask her baby's caregiver how much supplement per day her baby must receive. The recommended number of milliliters or ounces can then be divided into two, three, or four feedings, depending on the amount. The baby can receive supplements at predetermined times through a tube at the breast. If the baby does not finish it at one feeding, he or she may not require as much supplement in per day. On the other hand, he or she may need the remaining amount sometime later within that 24-hour period. Urge the mother to watch her baby carefully for signs of hunger and to respond accordingly.

Feeding Assessment A feeding assessment helps to determine the amount of supplement the baby needs. Optimally, the baby will not have nursed for his or her normal interval before the assessment. However, you want to let the mother know not to hold the baby off just because you are going to do an assessment. A frantic, overly hungry baby can be difficult to calm to nurse. Additionally, crying stresses parents and care providers alike. The mother should delay expressing her milk until after the feeding assessment as well.

Weighing the baby on a sensitive digital scale before and after a feeding (ac/pc weight) establishes how much is consumed during the feeding (Figure 18.2). The mother

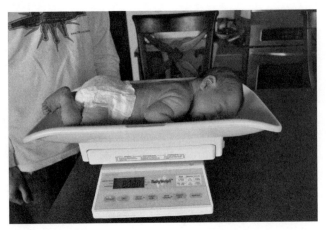

FIGURE 18.2   Baby being weighed on a digital scale.

Source: Printed with permission of Anna Swisher.

478 to 1356 mL (16–46 oz) during a 24-hour period (Kent et al., 2006). This wide range demonstrates quite a variation in "normal."

There are differing points of view among lactation and pediatric caregivers about the use of scales and test weights. Quantification of infant feeding damaged breastfeeding in the early 20th century, and some lactation advocates view test weights as further medicalizing breastfeeding (Sachs et al., 2006). However, clinical test weights are a core component of a comprehensive feeding assessment for lactation consultants. Accurate weight is especially crucial in abnormal feeding situations such as a preterm or compromised infant or for mothers with insufficient milk. Work with mothers of preterm infants reveals that mothers find test weights helpful (Calgary Health Region, 2009; Hurst et al., 2004).

can then pump her breasts to measure the amount of any residual milk left in the breast. The amount of milk the infant consumed, added to the amount of residual milk, gives a good indication of the mother's milk production over the preceding 2 or 3 hours. More than one ac/pc weight may be needed if you doubt whether the transfer amount was indicative of average intake and if you are dealing with failure to thrive or other serious weight loss. Additional test weights over a couple of day will provide a clearer picture of the baby's ability to transfer milk adequately.

Knowing what the baby consumed compared with what should have been consumed will give you and the mother an accurate measurement of the amount of supplement her baby requires. Table 18.3 provides calculations to determine a baby's total daily requirements. Divide the daily total by the number of feedings the infant takes or should take during a 24-hour period. A convenient reference list for determining feeding requirements appears in Appendix E.

Keep in mind that feeding charts are guidelines. Although charts can be helpful tools when a baby is not gaining, they are not ironclad rules. Babies differ in the amounts of milk they consume. Breastfed babies typically consume an average of 788 mL (26.65 oz) with a range of

Weaning From the Supplement   The process of eliminating formula and increasing milk production to replace it may take several weeks of concentrated effort. Watching for small daily successes aids the mother in reaching her goal of exclusive breastfeeding. Encourage her to keep a record of how much supplement her baby receives as well as the number of breastfeedings, wet diapers, and stools.

The baby needs enough supplements to provide nourishment for adequate growth. At the same time the mother's breasts need sufficient stimulation to increase milk production. Any reduction in supplement needs to be based on confidence that milk production has increased sufficiently to warrant it. Caution her to decrease the amount of supplement slowly, with frequent weight checks to make sure her baby continues to gain. A mother should never dilute formula in an attempt to cut back on supplements, because this can lead to insufficient caloric intake for the baby.

Counseling the Mother

A baby who fails to thrive plays into a mother's fears and insecurities about her parenting and her ability to breastfeed. It is important that you approach the mother with sensitivity, offering validation and reassurance. Your close contact with her, if desired by the mother, helps to give

TABLE 18.3   Determining the Number of Ounces an Infant Needs

Example for an infant weighing 4 pounds and 2 ounces	
Convert infant's weight to ounces.	4 lb + 2 oz = 66 oz
Divide total ounces by 6 to determine amount required for a 24-hour intake.	66 oz ÷ 6 = 11 oz
Divide the 24-hour requirements by the number of feedings per 24-hour period to determine how much is required per feeding.	11 oz ÷ 8 feedings = 1.37 oz per feeding
	11 oz ÷ 6 feedings = 1.83 oz per feeding

her the support and objectivity she needs. She may cry frequently and need to express her fears and feelings of guilt. Lack of familiarity with infant development and a lack of follow-up support from the healthcare system are factors in most cases of failure to thrive. See Chapter 25 for a discussion of biological insufficient milk and ways to counsel and help those mothers to optimize their breastfeeding. In a case of breast trauma, especially augmentation or reduction surgeries, the mother will need to come to terms with impaired milk production.

~ Summary

Healthcare providers have a responsibility to give mothers the breastfeeding information and support they need. This empowerment increases maternal confidence in their ability to provide sufficient milk to their baby. A mother who is physically unable to establish adequate milk production or an infant who is physically unable to achieve milk transfer is uncommon in the general population. However, these circumstances comprise a large part of lactation consultations beyond the postpartum period. Lactation consultants in private practice often receive referrals for such occurrences.

Inappropriate breastfeeding technique is the cause of many problems with milk production and transfer. Some problems may result from numerous complex issues on the part of the mother, the baby, or both. Identifying the cause and taking appropriate action is crucial to preventing serious consequences for the baby. No breastfed baby should reach the point of dehydration or failure to thrive. Be alert to significant barriers to milk production or effective milk transfer. Understanding the issues presented in this chapter will help you, as a practitioner, avoid such serious consequences.

~ Chapter 18—At a Glance

Applying what you learned—

Teach the mother about

- When to consult a healthcare practitioner
- Signs her baby's weight needs to be monitored with a baby weight scale
- Signs of a healthy slow weight gain
- Signs that a baby is not gaining adequate weight
- Causes of failure to thrive and the importance of supplementing the baby

Teach the mother how to

- Recognize sufficient milk production
- Avoid practices that compromise milk production
- Avoid newborn dehydration
- Increase milk production
- Recognize signs of adequate growth in her baby
- Recognize and manage failure to thrive

~ References

American Academy of Pediatrics. Committee on Fetus and Newborn. Hospital stay for healthy term newborns. *Pediatrics*. 2004;113:1434-1436.

Amir L. Breastfeeding—managing "supply" difficulties. *Austr Fam Physician*. 2006;35:686-689.

Aney M. Babywise advice linked to dehydration, failure to thrive. *AAP News*, April 1998. www.aapnews.aappublications.org/cgi/content/abstract/14/4/21. Accessed August 1, 2009.

Black M, et al. Early intervention and recovery among children with failure to thrive: follow-up at age 8. *Pediatrics*. 2007; 120:59-69.

Borges A, Philippi T. Opinion of women from a family health unit about the quantity of mother milk produced. *Rev Lat Am Enfermagem*. 2003;11:287-292.

Brodribb W, et al. Breastfeeding and Australian GP registrars: their knowledge and attitudes. *J Hum Lact*. 2008;24:422-430.

Butte N, et al. Higher energy expenditure contributes to growth faltering in breast-fed infants living in rural Mexico. *J Nutr*. 1993;123:1028-1035.

Butte N, et al. Infant feeding mode affects early growth and body composition. *Pediatrics*. 2000;106:1355-1366.

Calgary Health Region. Women's & infant health clinical practice guidelines. Oral feeding protocol: Neonatal. Updated February 14, 2009. www.calgaryhealthregion.ca/programs/neonatology/Protocols.htm. Accessed July 28, 2009.

Chantry C. Academy of Breastfeeding Medicine's primary goal is to educate physicians worldwide in breastfeeding and human lactation. *Breastfeed Med*. 2009;4(1):47-48.

Collet E, et al. A 6-week-old infant with failure to thrive: insidious presentation of group B streptococcal ventriculitis. *Arch Pediatr*. 2009;16:360-363.

Dhandapany G, et al. Antenatal counseling on breastfeeding—is it adequate? A descriptive study from Pondicherry, India. *Int Breastfeeding J*. 2008;3:5.

El Mouzan M, et al. Trends in infant nutrition in Saudi Arabia: compliance with WHO recommendations. *Ann Saudi Med*. 2009;29:20-23.

Garza C, Butte N. Energy intakes of human milk-fed infants during the first year. *J Pediatr*. 1990;117:S124-S131.

Garza C, et al. Growth of the breastfed infant. In: Goldman A, et al., eds. *Human Lactation*, vol. 3. New York: Plenum Press; 1987:109-121.

Gatti L. Maternal perceptions of insufficient milk supply in breastfeeding. *J Nurs Scholarsh*. 2008;40:355-363.

Haase B, et al. The development of an accurate test weighing technique for preterm and high-risk hospitalized infants. *Breastfeed Med*. 2009;4:151-156.

Hale T. *Medications and Mothers' Milk*. 14th ed. Amarillo, TX: Hale Publishing; 2010.

Hill P, Aldag J. Predictors of term infant feeding at week 12 postpartum. *J Perinat Neonatal Nurs.* 2007;21:250-255.

Humphrey S. *The Nursing Mother's Herbal.* Minneapolis: Fairview Press; 2003.

Hurst N, et al. Mothers performing in-home measurement of milk intake during breastfeeding of their preterm infants: maternal reactions and feeding outcomes. *J Hum Lact.* 2004;20:178-187.

Jenik A, et al. Does the recommendation to use a pacifier influence the prevalence of breastfeeding? *J Pediatr.* 2009; 155:350-354.

Karabulut E, et al. Effect of pacifier use on exclusive and any breastfeeding: a meta-analysis. *Turk J Pediatr.* 2009;51:35-43.

Kassing D. Bottle-feeding as a tool to reinforce breastfeeding. *J Hum Lact.* 2002;18:56-60.

Kent J, et al. Volume and frequency of breastfeedings and fat content of breast milk throughout the day. *Pediatrics.* 2006;117:e387-e395.

Kronborg H, Vaeth M. How are effective breastfeeding technique and pacifier use related to breastfeeding problems and breastfeeding duration? *Birth.* 2009;36:34-42.

Lawrence R, Lawrence R. *Breastfeeding: A Guide for the Medical Profession*, 6th ed. Philadelphia: Elsevier Mosby; 2005.

Leavitt G, et al. Knowledge about breastfeeding among a group of primary care physicians and residents in Puerto Rico. *J Commun Health.* 2009;34:1-5.

Lee W, et al. A population-based survey on infant feeding practice (0-2 years) in Hong Kong: breastfeeding rate and patterns among 3,161 infants below 6 months old. *Asia Pac J Clin Nutr.* 2006;15:377-387.

Levy Y, et al. Diagnostic clues for identification of nonorganic vs organic causes of food refusal and poor feeding. *J Pediatr Gastroenterol Nutr.* 2009;48:355-362.

Lukefahr JL. Underlying illness associated with FTT in breastfed infants. *Clin Perinatol.* 1990;29:468-470.

Marasco L, Barger J. Cue vs. scheduled feeding: revisiting the controversy. *Mother Baby J.* 1998;3:38-42.

Marasco L, et al. Polycystic ovary syndrome: a connection to insufficient milk supply? *J Hum Lact.* 2000;16:43-48.

McCarter-Spaulding D, Kearney M. Parenting self-efficacy and perception of insufficient breast milk. *JOGNN.* 2001; 30:515-522.

Mennella J. Alcohol's effect on lactation. Review. *Alcohol Res Health.* 2001;25:230-234.

Mennella J, et al. Acute alcohol consumption disrupts the hormonal milieu of lactating women. *J Clin Endocrinol Metab.* 2005;90:1979-1985.

Mennella J, Pepino M. Biphasic effects of moderate drinking on prolactin during lactation. *Alcohol Clin Exp Res.* 2008; 32:1899-1908.

Miyairi I, et al. Group B streptococcal ventriculitis: a report of three cases and literature review. *Pediatr Neurol.* 2006; 34:395-399.

Morton J, et al. Combining hand techniques with electric pumping increases milk production in mothers of preterm infants. *J Perinatol* 2009;29:757-764.

Newman J, Kernerman E. Breast compression. Revised February 2009a. www.nbci.ca/index.php?option=com_content&view=article&id=8:breast-compression&catid=5:information& Itemid=17. Accessed July 30, 2009.

Newman J, Kernerman E. Domperidone, getting started. Revised 2009b. www.nbci.ca/index.php?option=com_content&view=article&id=14:domperidone-getting-started-&catid=5:information&Itemid=17. Accessed July 30, 2009.

O'Connor N, et al. Pacifiers and breastfeeding: a systematic review. *Arch Pediatr Adolesc Med.* 2009;163:378-382.

Otsuka K, et al. The relationship between breastfeeding self-efficacy and perceived insufficient milk among Japanese mothers. *JOGNN.* 2008;37:546-555.

Parizoto G, et al. Trends and patterns of exclusive breastfeeding for under-6-month-old children. *J Pediatr.* 2009;85:201-208.

Sacco L, et al. The conceptualization of perceived insufficient milk among Mexican mothers. *J Hum Lact.* 2006;22:277-286.

Sachs M, et al. Feeding by numbers: an ethnographic study of how breastfeeding women understand their babies' weight charts. *Int Breastfeeding J.* 2006;1:29.

Shani M, Shinwell E. Breastfeeding characteristics and reasons to stop breastfeeding. *Harefuah.* 2003;142:426-428, 486.

Simic T, et al. Breastfeeding practices in Mostar, Bosnia and Herzegovina: cross-sectional self-report study. *Croat Med J.* 2004;45:38-43.

Straub B, et al. A descriptive study of Cambodian refugee infant feeding practices in the United States. *Int Breastfeed J.* 2008;3:2.

Szucs K, et al. Breastfeeding knowledge, attitudes, and practices among providers in a medical home. *Breastfeed Med.* 2009; 4:31-42.

U. S. Food Drug Administration (USFDA). FDA Talk Paper: FDA warns against women using unapproved drug, domperidone, to increase milk production; June 7, 2004. www.fda.gov/Drugs/DrugSafety/InformationbyDrugClass/ucm173886.htm. Accessed February 13, 2010.

West D, Marasco L. *The Breastfeeding Mother's Guide to Making More Milk.* New York: McGraw-Hill; 2008.

Wilson-Clay B, Hoover K. *The Breastfeeding Atlas*, 4th ed. Austin, TX: Lactnews Press; 2008.

World Health Organization (WHO). WHO Multicentre Growth Reference Study Group. WHO child growth standards. Geneva: World Health Organization; 2006. www.who.int/childgrowth/standards/en. Accessed May 10, 2009.

Xu F, et al. Breastfeeding in China: a review. *Int Breastfeed J.* 2009;4:6.

4

Special Care

Changes in the Family

Sleep and rest, sleep and rest,
Father will come to thee soon;
Rest, rest, on mother's breast,
Father will come to thee soon.

—*Alfred, Lord Tennyson (1809–1892)*
Lullaby, *from* The Princess

Family dynamics, roles, and relationships all take on new dimensions when a baby enters the picture. As a couple merge into new roles as parents, both the mother and father undergo adjustments with one another and with their baby. If other children are at home, their adjustments to the new baby present further challenges. You can provide assistance and support as the family settles into newly defined roles and relationships.

∼ Key Terms

Amenorrhea
Anovulatory
Anticipatory stage
Attachment
Baby blues
Baby training
Barrier methods
Contraception
Edinburgh Postnatal
    Depression Scale
Fertility
Formal stage
Implants
Informal stage
Injectables
Intrauterine device (IUD)
Kegel exercises
Lactational amenorrhea
    method (LAM)

Lochia
Menses
Natural family planning
Oral contraceptives
Patches
Perineum
Personal stage
Posttraumatic stress
    disorder
Postpartum depression
Postpartum psychosis
Sexual abuse
Sterilization
Tubal ligation
Urethra
Uterus
Vaginal ring

∼ Acquiring the Parental Role

One role common to most people is that of parent. Becoming a parent is a stressful experience (Randall & Bodenmann, 2009), even if a joyous one. Although young adults must receive special instruction to qualify for driving an automobile, for employment, and for other life skills, industrialized society does little to formally prepare couples for the important job of parenting. Fewer couples live near their extended families, and many have no family support system for everyday parenting. Many couples are on their own as they use trial and error to establish themselves as parents.

Babies are attuned to recognize and prefer their mothers. Bonding to the baby by both the mother and father in the first hours and days of life seems to encourage the acceptance of their roles as parents and ensure their attachment to the baby (Figure 19.1). Bowlby, well-known for his theories about parent–child attachment, maintains that good maternal care is essential for a mother's psychological health as well (Barett, 2006). The mother's physical recovery and the development of realistic expectations can help her maintain a positive perspective. This may help her transition more smoothly to the role of mother, just as her partner redefines his role as a new father. The couple can support one another through this transition by helping one another adjust to the changes occurring in their lives.

Studies show that parents experience greater declines in marital satisfaction compared with nonparents (Lawrence et al., 2008, 2007). Planning pregnancies and

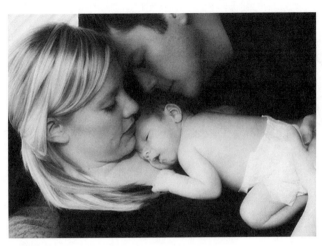

FIGURE 19.1 A mother and father enjoying their new baby.
Source: Printed with permission of Leila Farber.

the quality of the relationship before conception generally help protect marriages from these declines. Although these family transitions can strain couple relationships, they also provide opportunities to strengthen marriage (Schulz et al., 2006). Indeed, one study of new fathers found that change in the relationship was common "and often resulted in a more closely united relationship" (Fägerskiöld, 2008). Babies in industrialized nations are increasingly born to single mothers; the father may or may not be involved. See Chapter 20 for more discussion about counseling the single mother.

Learning About Parenting

Many of today's parents search for information and social support on the Internet. However, there are considerable differences based on gender, age and socioeconomic factors. First-time middle class mothers ages 30 to 35 are most active in looking up health and parent information on the Internet. At the same time several studies report diminishing class differences on parent Web sites. An important factor in the increasing number of parents who turn to the Internet for information and interaction is the weakened support many of today's parents experience from their own parents, relatives, and friends (Plantin & Daneback, 2009).

No amount of preparation can totally predict a couple's parenting style and interactions with their unique children. However, parents typically progress through predictable stages as they prepare for and care for their first child. The four classic stages of role acquisition are anticipatory, formal, informal, and personal (Bocar & Moore, 1987; Mercer, 1981). A study focusing on fathers coined stages as "To be overwhelmed," "To master the new situation," and "To get a new completeness in life" (Premberg et al., 2008).

Anticipatory Stage

The anticipatory stage is when parents begin to learn about their new roles. They may take classes, read books, and browse parenting blogs, forums, and other Internet media. They often begin asking questions of their own parents and other family or friends who already have children.

Formal Stage

After taking in and considering new information, parents move into the formal stage. During this time they begin to view their roles as parents more personally. They often strive for "parenting perfection" with a goal of doing it "just right." This includes getting breastfeeding "right" (Hall & Hauck, 2007).

Informal Stage

The frustration of trying to achieve perfection and the realization that "just right" is very individual leads parents into the informal stage. This stage is a time of modifying, blending, and individualizing their roles to fit their unique family.

Personal Stage

As parents become more comfortable in their parenting role, they move into the personal stage. Their style of parenting evolves to be consistent with their personalities—parenting that fits them like an old glove. The roles of the mother and father grow and change in response to the needs of their baby, their family backgrounds, and the couple's interactions. Both parents define their roles gradually through experience, which is enhanced and made more enjoyable through open communication between them. They become more relaxed with each child.

Parenting Programs

There are many effective parenting programs and books to help parents in their journey through these stages. Others cause concern within the healthcare profession. Some parenting programs and authors have been around for decades, including well credentialed professionals such as Barbara Coloroso (2009), Dr. William Sears (2009), Dr. Kevin Leman (2009), Drs. Cloud and Townsend (2009), and Drs. Cline and Fay (2009). Programs include Parent Effectiveness Training (PET, 2009), 1-2-3 Magic (2009), and Systematic Training for Effective Parenting (STEP, 2009). These authors and programs advocate consistency, treating children with respect, and teaching children logical and natural consequences. They typically do not stress specific infant regimes, such as restricted feedings, and tend to focus on children past the infancy stage.

A few programs based on a rigidly structured approach to child rearing are so worrisome that the American Academy of Pediatrics (AAP) passed a resolution in 1998 to investigate and monitor them. Parents who follow these rigid programs may find it difficult to move beyond the formal stage of parenting to develop a personal style. There are concerns both about the potential physical problems that can ensue from parents following such strict rules and about the psychological outcome of children left to "cry it out" (Francis, 1998; Hunter, 1998; Child Abuse Prevention Council of Orange County, 1996).

Baby Training Programs

Several books and parenting programs teach parents to schedule feedings with a key goal for the baby to sleep through the night as early as 8 weeks of age. These teachings contradict the AAP's guidelines on infant feeding and baby care. Such books and programs tend to promote their parenting method as the "right" way to raise a child, with no scientific or evidence-based medicine for any of their teachings. These books and programs fre-

quently become popular with young parents. Table 19.1 contrasts AAP infant feeding policy (AAP, 2005) and the AAP Media Alert on scheduled feedings (AAP, 1998) with the general approaches of books that promote scheduling.

Parents Drawn to These Programs

The generation of young people in Western cultures who are having babies today reached adulthood during a time of economic prosperity. Couples may begin their lives together as educated professionals establishing or maintaining demanding careers. The parenting approaches of baby training programs pander to couples in this lifestyle. The approach dovetails with the description of this age group by Twenge (2006) as "smart, brash, even arrogant, and endowed with a commanding sense of entitlement." This may easily include the belief that parents are entitled to full nights of uninterrupted sleep and that babies should not be "the center of the family universe" (Ezzo & Bucknam, 2006). Time for "me" is a key ingredient in this philosophy (Hogg & Blau, 2005), many times at the expense of the baby and breastfeeding. Lack of knowledge about infant physiology and the day-to-day care of

TABLE 19.1   Advice from American Academy of Pediatrics Versus Baby Training Books and Programs

Source	Feeding Frequency	Longest Interval Between Feedings	Who Should Design Feeding Schedule	How to Know if Baby Needs Feeding
American Academy of Pediatrics (AAP), www.aap.org	On demand: "8–12 feedings at the breast every 24 hours" (Breastfeeding Policy Statement, 2/05)	4 hours (Breastfeeding Policy Statement, 2/05)	Babies, because those "designed by parents may put babies at risk for poor weight gain and dehydration" (AAP Media Alert, 4/98)	An infant's feeding cues: "increased mouthing, or rooting. Crying is a late indicator of hunger." (AAP Media Alert, 4/98)
Baby Training or Scheduling Books and Programs	Watch for fewer than 8–12 feedings in 24 hours or lip service to feed 8 times, but contradictions of "every 4 to 6 hours," which would preclude 8 or more feedings. Watch for terms like "snacking," "using mother for a pacifier," or other derogatory terms for nursing often.	Watch for terms like: "never wake a sleeping baby," or "never wake the baby at night."	Parents. Watch for language stating that either the parents are in control or the baby is in control—language that describes an antagonistic, power-struggle relationship. Watch for books and programs with scant scholarly references to back up claims, especially if they contradict well-established evidence-based research.	Watch for a disregard of feeding cues or "yes, but" language that discounts the validity of cues compared with the clock or the parents' authority to dictate feeding times. Watch for any book advocating "crying it out" as desirable and normal in infants.

Source: Compiled by Patricia Donohue-Carey, BS, LCCE, CLE, Anh Gordon, MD, and Anna Swisher, MBA, IBCLC. Reprinted by permission of Patricia C. Donohue-Carey, FACCE, CLE, and Anh H. Gordon, MD.

a baby can set parents up for unrealistic expectations of what to expect with their new baby.

A baby's grandparents may give such books to their children. If they fed their children on a schedule and let them "cry it out," these books provide affirmation that the grandparents did the right thing. Parents who ascribe to such programs may be in a peer group with other first-time parents who are using them. Parents may be spiritually invested in religiously based parenting programs, such as Growing Families International. They teach parents to form a "like-minded . . . moral community" within a social sphere that can become a closed loop (Gordon, 1999; Terner & Miller, 1998). Because parents rely on the program for parenting details, it may be difficult for them to move beyond the formal stage of learning to mature in their parenting style. Of greater concern to medical and mental health professionals are the behaviors observed in some infants subjected to these teachings. Infants can demonstrate detachment, depression, eating issues, and self-stimulating and self-soothing behaviors (Webb, 2003; Williams, 1999, 1998).

Effect on Breastfeeding

Baby training programs blame "demand" feeding for sleep deprivation, maternal depression, low milk production or quitting breastfeeding, failure to thrive, and selfish children. Parents are encouraged to let their babies cry from 15 minutes to an hour at a time. Anticipatory guidance is especially important for these parents, preferably prenatally during childbirth or breastfeeding classes. Mothers who use baby training techniques frequently experience low milk production, low infant weight gain, or breast rejection by the baby. Infrequent feedings down-regulate milk production, and many of these mothers lose their milk entirely by 3 to 4 months postpartum (Moody, 2002; Aney, 1998).

Mothers who schedule feeding as part of a broader parenting philosophy are sometimes told that lactation consultants have a bias toward "attachment parenting" and don't understand the "new paradigm" in lactation. They are urged to never cosleep, never nurse the baby to sleep, and to not use a baby sling or feed frequently (Ezzo & Bucknam, 2006; Ezzo & Ezzo, 2002). You can try to help these parents understand the reasons behind your recommendations regarding breastfeeding practices. Staying up-to-date on lactation research enables you to discuss the scientific reasons behind the variance in each mother's milk storage capacity and synthesis rate (Cox et al., 2008; Kent, 2007; Kent et al., 2006; Mitoulas et al., 2002).

Baby training books and programs dismiss the idea that crying is harmful to babies. Teaching parents about the effects of stress and extended crying on infants may be helpful (Gordon & Hill, 2009; O'Connor & Spagnola,

2009; Moore et al., 2007; Gordon & Hill, 2006). Demonstrated effects of infant crying include "increased heart rate and blood pressure, reduced oxygen level, elevated cerebral blood pressure, initiation of the stress response, depleted energy reserves and oxygen, interrupted mother-infant interaction, brain injury, and cardiac dysfunction" (Ludington-Hoe et al., 2002). Most of the research on crying it out has been done on children older than 1 year (Gordon & Hill, 2006). Both animal and human research findings show that there can be long-term effects of early adversity, such as caregiving deprivation (O'Connor & Spagnola, 2009).

One important claim from these books to address with parents is that nonscheduled babies miss feedings. Although this is usually not the case with healthy, full-term babies, parents of a preterm, ill, jaundiced, or newborn baby who does not demonstrate hunger cues *will* need to temporarily "watch the clock." They often must rouse the baby to feed frequently enough, not allowing more than 4 hours without feeding (AAP, 2005). They need to make sure the baby eats at least 8 to 12 times in 24 hours. They also need to monitor diapers by counting voids and stools. However, this occurs after the initial postpartum sleepiness stage.

Parents who follow baby training for religious reasons may be responsive to theological reasoning. Respected Christian leaders reject the materials (MacArthur, 2000; Dobson, 1999; Hanegraaf, 1998–1999), and several articles argue against the teachings on theological grounds (Webb, 2003; Cox, 2001; Terner & Miller, 1998). Use of reflective listening will enable you to be accepting of these parents without implying endorsement of their practices. A nonjudgmental approach is important to creating a climate in which parents can question the information. Although you may have strong feelings about rigid parenting techniques, it is important that you share information objectively and give current and relevant resources. Conversely, if you have used these teachings and approaches with your own children, it is important to not project your personal biases into your work with families. Your credentialing as a healthcare provider requires you to practice evidence-based care.

You have a unique opportunity to empower parents who find it difficult to move beyond the formal stage of acquiring their parental role. After you address scheduled feedings and present information from reliable medical sources, you need to step back from the situation and the parents' practices. Document any concerns you have regarding the baby's health or mother's milk production. Stay in close communication with the parents' physicians or other caregivers. Be sure the baby's caregiver is aware if a mother is using scheduled feedings so the baby's weight gain and signs of infant depression can be monitored.

∼ *Becoming a Mother*

Although women respond to motherhood in their own ways, they generally have one characteristic in common: They have little or no idea of what to expect in their babies' behavior and development! They may have formed opinions on child care only to find that much of what they know does not work with their baby. They may have had preconceived ideas about types of babies and find that theirs is another type entirely. Mothers eventually realize they need to develop their own parenting skills. Their competence and confidence grow with practice, experimentation, observation, and self-education.

Every mother has some adjustments to make after her baby is born. This is a wonderful phase in a family's life. At the same time it can be frustrating. A mother may not feel prepared for the fact that caring for a baby is a 24/7 job. She cannot return to her life as she knew it. A pitfall of counseling an experienced mother is to assume she does not need your support. She is constantly making adjustments, and although her questions and concerns will be different from those of a first-time mother, they are just as significant. She often must help others in the family, such as siblings and grandparents, make their own adjustments. Having a supportive person with whom she can share her concerns can be especially important to her.

Emotional Adjustments

Emotions during the postpartum period rival those of the adolescent years. Hormonal shifts are dramatic within the first 24 hours after giving birth. Suddenly, the mother has a baby who is entirely dependent on her. At the same time she is coping with extraordinary body changes, and her emotions are subject to biochemical, psychological, and societal influences. Her birth experience may have been exhilarating, confusing, exhausting, or devastating. Her ideas about parenting and her expectations of herself, her baby, and her family may not reflect the reality of her situation.

Lactation Consultant's Role

Help mothers see that their reactions are normal and that the blissful image of a perfect mother is far from reality. Encourage each mother to develop realistic expectations about her baby and about motherhood. Help her see that not all problems with her baby are associated with breastfeeding. If she is considering weaning, help her understand that weaning may not solve her other problems. Her baby will still cry, and she will still feel tired and tied down at times. Bottle feeding mothers have these challenges, too!

Normal Postpartum Adjustments

There is a tendency to assume that even the most highly educated woman is comfortable with and adequately prepared for parenting. However, women often feel unprepared for their new role as mother. They may lack personal experience in caring for a baby and may not have family close by to support them in the early weeks. A mother's uncertainty may show up as a specific concern or worry, such as handling a fussy baby or insufficient milk production (Otsuka et al., 2008). A mother who has quit working will experience a loss of income. The dynamics in her relationship with the baby's father may change as well. Additionally, decreased contact with adults can create feelings of isolation and loneliness.

Motherhood is a new, constant job, and the stress of the new expectations may seem overwhelming at times. The mother may have a baby who is continually fussy, rarely sleeps and fails to live up to her expectations of a happy, responsive baby. She may have had a disappointing or unpleasant birth or may have experienced an unwanted pregnancy. Poor nutrition and lack of rest can also cause emotional distress in the new mother, especially when coupled with the many adjustments to a new baby.

Women's emotional adjustments to motherhood vary greatly during the postpartum period. Some women need do no more than make room for the new baby. Many women, however, have a few rough days balanced by high moments. This brief despondency, referred to as baby blues, frequently appears around the third day postpartum and could last for a couple of weeks. The mother may have bouts of tearfulness and sadness, mingled with happiness and excitement. These emotions are more common in women who have their first baby. A positive birth experience and an abundance of emotional support and practical help following the birth help to minimize baby blues.

Postpartum Depression

Postpartum depression affects at least 10 to 15 percent of postpartum women, including more than 600,000 American mothers in 2003 alone (Jolley et al., 2007). The rate is higher in women with preexisting depression (Misri, 2002). The hormonal response of women with postpartum depression was found to be similar to women with early life stresses (Jolley et al., 2007). Postpartum depression creates mood changes, loss of pleasure, poor concentration, low self-esteem, guilt at failing as a mother and wife, sleep disturbances, fatigue, and a flat affect in voice tone. Typically, the mother is depressed from 1 to 6 weeks postpartum. Some women become clinically depressed for weeks or months after giving birth. These women require professional help that is beyond your role as lactation consultant.

A woman suffering from postpartum depression generally feels unable to cope with life and worries that something is not "right." She may even entertain occasional thoughts of harming herself. This requires urgent evaluation by a psychiatrist (Kendall-Tackett, 2005), preferably one who has a special interest in antenatal and postpartum women. These psychiatrists are more likely to support breastfeeding and try to treat the mother without interfering with breastfeeding. Loss of control is a significant emotion experienced after the birth of a baby and is not an identifying symptom of postpartum depression.

Effective education helps the mother and other family members understand the difference between baby blues and postpartum depression. Postpartum depression is a common illness and is treatable, like any other biological illness. When the mother and her partner understand this, there is less likely to be obstacles around diagnosis and treatment, and the mother may get help more quickly.

Identifying Women at Risk It is very important during your intake that you ask about the mother's mental health history. You will want to know if she has had clinical depression, anxiety disorder, or any other mental ailment such as bipolar disorder or attention deficit disorder. Ask what medications she has taken in the past, and what therapy or support system she has used. Ask what medications she intends to take now that the pregnancy is over. Some medications are not recommended during pregnancy (e.g., lamotrigine or lithium) but may be resumed after the baby is born.

A mother in the throes of postpartum depression may lack confidence in her ability to breastfeed. Depressed women may also be less likely to initiate breastfeeding and to do so exclusively. They are at risk for decreased breastfeeding duration, a sudden dramatic drop in milk production, increased breastfeeding difficulties, and less breastfeeding self-efficacy (Dennis & McQueen, 2009). She may say she is lonely, has no visitors, and has no place to go. She may not answer her telephone, or she may stay away from home in an attempt to keep busy. She may demonstrate a lack of tolerance for other family members and feel detached from her baby, evidenced by a failure to refer to her baby by name. Premature weaning occurs more frequently among depressed women (Hasselmann, 2008).

Nurses play a crucial role in the early identification and treatment of these postpartum mood disorders (Doucet et al., 2009), as do other healthcare providers who may interact with these mothers. Advising a social service consultation is appropriate if you observe worrisome mother–baby interactions in the hospital. Lactation consultants should never attempt to counsel an emotionally distressed mother alone. Gently urge the mother to contact her caregiver for an evaluation and referral to a psychiatrist. In addition to counseling treatment may involve medications, most of which are compatible with breastfeeding. You can be a source of information for the mother by citing current medication information and providing her with resources.

Edinburgh Postnatal Depression Scale Depression makes it difficult, if not impossible, to experience real pleasure and joy. The Edinburgh Postnatal Depression Scale (EPDS, Figure 19.2) was developed to help primary care health professionals detect mothers suffering from postnatal depression. These mothers may cope with their baby and with household tasks, but their enjoyment of life is seriously affected, and it is possible that there are long-term effects on the family. The Edinburgh Scale (Cox et al., 1987) is an easy self-rating depression scale that indicates the normal range of postpartum emotions and degree of danger for depression.

Developed at health centers in Livingston and Edinburgh, the scale consists of 10 short statements. The mother underlines one of four possible responses that describe how she has been feeling during the past week. Mothers who score above the threshold of 92.3 percent are likely to be suffering from a depressive illness. The EPDS score should not override clinical judgment or careful clinical assessment to confirm diagnosis. The scale will not detect mothers with anxiety neuroses, phobias, or personality disorders. Another helpful screening tool is the Beck Depression Inventory (BDI). This tool measures the severity and depth of depression symptoms. It is available at no cost on the Internet at Real-Depression-Help.com.

Postpartum Psychosis An estimated 1.2 of 1000 postpartum women develop psychosis within 90 days of delivery (Valdimarsdóttir et al., 2009). This involves symptoms far more serious than those of baby blues or depression. The mother's symptoms may progress beyond insomnia, fatigue, and depression. Postpartum psychosis occurs on a much more intense level than postpartum depression. It can lead to a loss of control, rational thought, and social functioning. The mother experiences overwhelming delusions and hallucinations (Gale & Harlow, 2003).

Because of the severity of depression the mother may attempt suicide. This illness is a medical emergency. A British review found that suicide accounted for 12.5 percent of maternal deaths from 2003 to 2005. A significant minority died from substance misuse and other accidents that may have been associated with psychological distress (Centre for Maternal and Child Enquiries, 2007).

A mother experiencing postpartum psychosis may be at very high risk for harming her baby and other children. The priority is to keep the mother and her child safe and to get her into effective treatment immediately (Spinelli, 2009). The world was horrified in 2001 by the multiple murders by a mother with a history of severe

Instructions for users:

The mother is asked to underline the response that comes closest to how she has been feeling in the previous 7 days. All ten items must be completed. Care should be taken to avoid the possibility of the mother discussing her answers with others. The mother should complete the scale herself, unless she has limited English or has difficulty with reading. The EPDS may be used at 6–8 weeks to screen postnatal women. The child health clinic, postnatal check-up, or a home visit may provide suitable opportunities for its completion.

Name: _____ Baby's Age: _____
Address: _____

As you have recently had a baby, we would like to know how you are feeling. Please UNDERLINE the answer that comes closest to how you have felt IN THE PAST 7 DAYS, not just how you feel today.

1. I have been able to laugh and see the funny side of things.
   a. As much as I always could – 0
   b. Not quite so much now – 1
   c. Definitely not so much now – 2
   d. Not at all – 3

2. I have looked forward with enjoyment to things.
   a. As much as I ever did – 0
   b. Rather less than I used to – 1
   c. Definitely less than I used to – 2
   d. Hardly at all – 3

*3. I have blamed myself unnecessarily when things went wrong.
   a. Yes, most of the time – 3
   b. Yes, some of the time – 2
   c. Not very often – 1
   d. No, never – 0

4. I have been anxious or worried for no good reason.
   a. No, not at all – 0
   b. Hardly ever – 1
   c. Yes, sometimes – 2
   d. Yes, very often – 3

*5. I have felt scared or panicky for not very good reason.
   a. Yes, quite a lot – 3
   b. Yes, sometimes – 2
   c. No, not much – 1
   d. No, not at all – 0

*6. Things have been getting on top of me.
   a. Yes, most of the time I haven't been able to cope at all – 3
   b. Yes, sometimes I haven't been coping as well as usual – 2
   c. No, most of the time I have coped quite well – 1
   d. No, I have been coping as well as ever – 0

*7. I have been so unhappy that I have had difficulty sleeping.
   a. Yes, most of the time – 3
   b. Yes, sometimes – 2
   c. Not very often – 1
   d. No, not at all – 0

*8. I have felt sad or miserable.
   a. Yes, most of the time – 3
   b. Yes, quite often – 2
   c. Not very often – 1
   d. No, not at all – 0

*9. I have been so unhappy that I have been crying.
   a. Yes, most of the time – 3
   b. Yes, quite often – 2
   c. Only occasionally – 1
   d. No, never – 0

*10. The thought of harming myself has occurred to me.
   a. Yes, quite often – 3
   b. Sometimes – 2
   c. Hardly ever – 1
   d. Never – 0

Response categories are scored 0, 1, 2, and 3 according to increased severity of the symptoms. Items marked with an asterisk are reverse scored (i.e., 3, 2, 1, and 0). The total score is calculated by adding together the scores for each of the ten items. Users may reproduce the scale without further permission providing they respect copyright by quoting the names of the authors, the title and the source of the paper in all reproduced copies.

FIGURE 19.2 Edinburgh Postnatal Depression Scale (EPDS).

Source: Reprinted by permission from Cox LL, Holden JM, Sogovsky R. Detection of postnatal depression: development of the 10-item Edinburgh Postnatal Depression Scale. *Brit J Psych.* 1987;150:782-786. © 1987 The Royal College of Psychiatrists. The Edinburgh Postnatal Depression Scale may be photocopied by individual researchers or clinicians for their own use without seeking permission from the publishers. The scale must be copied in full and all copies must acknowledge the following source: Cox LL, Holden JM, Sogovsky R. Detection of postnatal depression: development of the 10-item Edinburgh Postnatal Depression Scale. *Brit J Psych.* 1987;150:782-786. Written permission must be obtained from the Royal College of Psychiatrists for copying and distribution to others or for republication (in print, online, or by any other medium). Translations of the scale, and guidance as to its use, may be found in Cox JL, Holden J. *Perinatal Mental Health: A Guide to the Edinburgh Postnatal Depression Scale.* London: Gaskell; 2003.

postpartum depression and two suicide attempts. She drowned her five children, including her baby, whom she had breastfed for 4 months (O'Malley, 2004).

Kauppi et al. (2008) examined 10 cases of filicide (murder of one's own child) and found that these mothers all had clear depressive symptoms, including an irrita-ble, severely depressed mood with crying spells, insomnia, fatigue, anxiety, and preoccupation with worries about the baby's well-being and the mother's ability to care for the baby. The mothers' conditions deteriorated rapidly to sui-cidal or psychotic thoughts. Each mother killed her baby when she and the baby were left alone against her will.

The babies were well tended before the murders. Most of the mothers reported emotionally troubled histories with their own parents, especially their mothers. All the mothers had experienced trauma in either childhood or adulthood. Another study found that 72 percent of 39 mothers studied had previous mental health treatment before murdering their children; 38 percent of these occurred in the postpartum period (Friedman et al., 2005). A Japanese analysis of 96 cases also found that mental disorders were frequent and postpartum depression was associated with infanticide (Taguchi, 2007).

Survivors of Sexual Abuse

There are three forms of sexual abuse. The one most commonly referenced is physical sexual abuse, which involves intercourse and other forms of touch. Psychological sexual abuse can be just as devastating, with the victim being forced to view something sexual, or the perpetrator taking inappropriate interest in the victim's sexual development. Verbal sexual abuse also occurs, with erotic talk or innuendo.

The World Health Organization (WHO) estimates the prevalence of forced sexual intercourse and other forms of sexual violence involving touch at 7 percent among boys and at 14 percent among girls under 18 (WHO, 2009). WHO reports that "violence against infants and younger children is a major risk factor for psychiatric disorders and suicide, and has lifelong sequelae including depression, anxiety disorders, smoking, alcohol and drug abuse, aggression and violence towards others, risky sexual behaviours and post traumatic stress disorders." There is also a greater likelihood of revictimization by the adult survivor's male partner (Rivera-Rivera et al., 2006; Arias, 2004).

Most sexual abuse survivors (84–98 percent) have never revealed their history to a physician (Kirkengen, 2001). Marriage, pregnancy, birth, and breastfeeding can all serve as reminders of the mother's own family upbringing. For women who have suppressed the memory of abuse, pregnancy and childbirth are common times for a sexual abuse survivor to remember her past abuse. Other triggers may be:

- A daughter or granddaughter reaches the age when she (the mother or grandmother herself) was abused
- The perpetrator dies or others disclose abuse by the same perpetrator
- Media coverage of others who were abused
- Times of stress such as surgery, death of a loved one, or quitting smoking

Because of the intimate nature of breastfeeding, past sexual abuse may cause a disruption or disturbance in breastfeeding. Memories, flashbacks, and feelings from the abuse may interfere with the mother's ability to have her baby at the breast. Flashbacks are a sign of posttraumatic stress disorder (PTSD) and require professional help. Memories may be triggered by the sounds or feelings of giving birth, the sensation of the baby at the breast, the loss of control felt in the early days of parenting, or even the sight of milk during letdown. Any of these events can trigger a flashback that causes the woman to feel uncomfortable with breastfeeding (Kendall-Tackett, 2009).

A history of sexual abuse or assault is common among new mothers (Kendall-Tackett, 2009). Women with histories of sexual abuse are still likely to breastfeed, and abuse survivors have breastfeeding rates similar to nonabused women. One study reported 53.6 percent of survivors intending to breastfeed, compared with 40.6 percent of nonabused women (Benedict et al., 1994). Another study found that sexually abused women are twice as likely to initiate breastfeeding as nonabused mothers (Prentice et al., 2002). Because of the high rate of sexual abuse, you will very likely work with mothers who have this background. Becoming familiar with and sensitive to this population's needs is an important part of your counseling skills.

Identifying a Sexual Abuse Survivor   In some instances a woman may feel comfortable telling you about her sexual abuse because you take the time to listen to her concerns. Assisting the mother with such an intimate topic draws on your ability to listen intently with warmth and caring and to regard the woman with openness and acceptance. You may first wonder about a history of abuse from the way the mother positions herself for feedings or from an apparent discomfort with holding her baby while discussing breastfeeding.

Some warning signs that may indicate a history of sexual abuse are late prenatal care, substance abuse, mental health concerns, eating disorders, poor compliance with self-care, or sexual dysfunction. Rates of teen pregnancy, prostitution, and promiscuity are higher among sexual abuse survivors. Other markers are being a high achiever, having dysfunctional relationships, fear of medical procedures, discomfort with touch, and morbid obesity. Mistrust of authority figures, fear of being out of control or dependent, and gender preference for baby and caregiver are also common. The mother may feed expressed milk to her baby with a bottle and not put him to breast (Kendall-Tackett, 1998). Although these signals do not necessarily indicate a history of sexual abuse, they are signs that can alert you to the possibility.

Breastfeeding Implications for the Survivor   The most stressful time in breastfeeding for a survivor is during the early postpartum period, when the new mother feels stressed, tired, and vulnerable. Although all new mothers experience fluctuations in their emotions at this time, abuse survivors may be more emotionally fragile due to memories of abuse or depression. Because sexual assault tends to occur at night or at bedtime, nighttime breastfeeding can be especially difficult. Having someone feed her milk to the baby for nighttime feedings may help this situation. When the baby gets older and becomes more playful, the mother may seem reluctant to continue breastfeeding. Reviewing normal infant behaviors may be reassuring to the mother and help her breastfeed longer.

Be prepared to meet the mother's needs and to support her decisions. Her choices in breastfeeding may include expressing her milk and feeding it to her baby by bottle. Each mother's reactions to a situation may vary widely, and you must meet the mother on her own terms. Some mothers find breastfeeding too uncomfortable to continue. Others find breastfeeding to be quite healing. Statistically, women who have overcome abusive backgrounds received emotional support from a nonabusive adult during childhood, received therapy, and have a nonabusive, stable, and emotionally supportive relationship with their mate (Kendall-Tackett, 2009). Be alert to the mother's feelings and provide support when possible, including support for weaning if that is her choice.

A lactation consultant is not qualified to treat or investigate sexual abuse situations. Unless you are a licensed counselor or therapist and have special training in this area, refer the mother to a licensed therapist or counselor who specializes in women's issues, preferably one who is familiar with breastfeeding mothers. You can network with counselors in your community to provide appropriate breastfeeding information. Helpful books for mothers dealing with depression or past abuse include *The Hidden Feelings of Motherhood: Coping with Stress, Depression and Burnout* (Kendall-Tackett, 2005) and *Survivor Moms: Women's Stories of Birthing, Mothering and Healing after Sexual Abuse* (Sperlich & Seng, 2008). See Appendix H for additional resources for abuse survivors and women in domestic violence situations.

Physical Recovery After Birth

After a woman gives birth many changes take place within her body to return it to its prepregnant state. Having just completed 9 months of pregnancy, she may feel disappointed that her abdomen still protrudes because of stretched muscles. Her walk may seem more of a waddle because of loosened pelvic ligaments and stitches or pads. The fullness in her breasts may be slightly uncomfortable, and she may have little energy left to cope with her appearance and the stresses of daily life. Assure mothers that these physical responses are normal. For the first 6 weeks new mothers need rest for physical recovery. A mother who receives insufficient rest can develop excessive bleeding, exhaustion, dizziness, or weak pelvic floor

muscles. Add breastfeeding to the mix, and she may experience sore nipples or a breast infection.

Encourage mothers to get as much bed rest as possible. Staying in her bathrobe for the first few weeks may discourage a new mother's visitors from staying too long. She can nap when her baby naps and nurse lying down to catch up on needed rest. A reminder of the need for moderation is especially helpful in the early weeks after delivery. By this time the mother will begin to feel energetic and restless at home and could be more apt to overexert herself. Caution her to minimize household tasks and to not resume strenuous activities too quickly. Her family can help by limiting visitors during that time. Many mothers today must return to work or school within 6 weeks, which can be overwhelming. You can strategize with the mother to identify as much support as possible, at home, at work, and at school.

Familiarize the mother with normal physical changes that occur during the weeks after delivery. In addition to the usual postpartum recovery involving the uterus and perineum, she may experience variations in body functions or minor physical irritations. The resumption of menstruation and the possibility of another pregnancy are a concern for many new mothers. Breastfeeding speeds uterine recovery, encourages the mother to rest while nursing, relieves breast fullness, and delays the return of fertility and menses.

Uterus

The uterus, which attained a weight of about 2.5 pounds by delivery, begins to diminish in size soon after the baby's birth. By 1 week postpartum it has decreased to about 1 pound, and at 6 weeks it is usually reduced to approximately 2 ounces. This time of involution is accompanied by a discharge of blood, mucus, and tissue called lochia, which is the gradual sloughing off of the extra tissue lining the uterus. Its color transforms from red to pink and then to white in about 3 to 4 weeks. A change in color from pink to white and back to red may indicate that the mother's level of physical exertion is too high. She needs to report this to her caregiver and cut back on her activity level.

There is often an increase in lochia flow during feedings because of uterine contractions caused by the release of oxytocin. The contractions may cause what is commonly referred to as afterpains, which usually last for only a few days to 1 week. Multiparous women may find these contractions more severe. The mother can reduce afterbirth pains by emptying her bladder before breastfeeding and by doing deep breathing. Ibuprofen can alleviate the discomfort, if approved for use by her caregiver, as well as any prescription pain reliever her caregiver prescribed, such as hydrocodone. Reassure the mother that the pains are nature's way of limiting blood loss and returning her body to its prepregnant state.

Perineum

A vaginal delivery causes swelling and tenderness in the perineum, the region between the vagina and rectum. An episiotomy, a surgical incision between these two points, enlarges the vaginal opening during delivery. The incision may increase postpartum swelling and cause a pulling sensation. Ice packs, sitz baths, sprays, cooling cotton pads, and medications can provide comfort for the mother.

Perineal floor exercises, known as Kegel exercises, help the mother regain muscle tone in the pelvic floor, where stretching is most pronounced during labor. If these muscles remain weak, the uterus may tip or sink down into the vagina and the mother may have difficulty controlling urination. To perform Kegel exercises the woman inhales and then tightens the muscles surrounding her vagina, urethra, and rectum as she exhales. You can help mothers visualize this by telling them these are the same muscles used to stop the flow of urine. Performing Kegel exercises regularly throughout the day helps return muscle tone and enables the mother to control urination.

Body Functions

In the first few days postpartum the mother may notice changes in her body functions. She may need to urinate frequently as she loses extra fluids accumulated during pregnancy. Some women have difficulty urinating, especially if they had a catheter inserted in the bladder to keep it empty during labor and delivery. A mother might not have a bowel movement until 2 or 3 days postpartum.

Initially, a woman who delivered vaginally may find it unsettling to assume a position that is similar to the position in which she had recently delivered her baby. She may fear expelling her uterus, rupturing her episiotomy, or increasing her pain. A mother who had a cesarean delivery may have difficulty with bowel movements until her intestines resume normal functioning. The manipulation of the intestines during cesarean delivery causes gas and temporary bowel dysfunction. The mother may find relief from deep breathing exercises, rocking back and forth in a rocking chair, and alternating between abdominal tightening and relaxing. Encourage her to drink plenty of fluids and to eat high fiber, high water fruits. She may require a stool softener if other methods fail. Medications used by many caregivers to reduce gas have not been shown to cause problems for breastfeeding babies.

Minor Irritations

Among other minor irritations, some women experience backaches in the early weeks because of the hormones that softened or loosened the sacroiliac ligaments and allowed more flexibility of the pelvic structure for birth. Backaches are also associated with the use of epidural anesthesia (Ruppen et al., 2006; Smith, 2009). Heat, massage, pelvic rocking exercises, and correct lifting and breastfeeding positions help provide relief. Heavy perspiration, particularly at night, results from the body removing surplus fluid from pregnancy. The mother can wear cool, loose clothing and take frequent showers to help her feel better. The extra-large sanitary pads used postnatally may be irritating. As the lochia discharge subsides, the mother may be more comfortable with a minipad.

Changing Priorities

Caution mothers that when they overexert physically, their baby may be fussy the next day. An overactive lifestyle can lead to a breast infection. Each mother makes her own decision about the importance of a task. She may need to relax her standards and priorities concerning household chores. Many mothers return to full- or part-time work, school, volunteer work, in addition to caring for older children. Perhaps she can make some compromises or trade-offs that will allow her the time she needs for herself and her baby. Encourage her to resume obligations slowly, to watch her baby and other family members for signs of distress, and to cut back when possible. Help her realize that the intense amount of time her baby now consumes will diminish rapidly. As the baby becomes efficient in expressing and meeting his or her needs, the mother's schedule will become more relaxed, and a new "normal" will develop.

The mother can be creative in meeting her previous obligations. She could explore telecommuting, working at home, employing a teenager, or trading favors with another mother. She might participate in only those activities where her baby is welcome, arrange to take her baby with her, or work out some other method to suit her needs. There are organizations of mothers who have made a variety of lifestyle decisions, such as the National Association of At Home Mothers. Searching the Internet may lead to connections with other mothers for adult conversation and a sense of community. Many online forums and blogs provide mother-to-mother support. La Leche League even has online meetings for breastfeeding women (www.lalecheleague.org).

The mother's ability to adapt her lifestyle to motherhood will depend on her emotional state, her physical recovery, her maturity, and the support she receives from family and friends. She can hasten her recovery and her return to a workable schedule by resting during the early weeks. Help her form realistic expectations, and point out options in household chores, child care, and career, work, or schooling.

∼ *Becoming a Father*

Men experience social, emotional, and behavioral adjustments as they redefine themselves as fathers. A new father will adapt to a changed relationship with his partner, now a mother. He will embrace changes brought about by a new family member—a newborn baby who poses a very serious responsibility. His role expands to one of supporter and helpmate to his wife and protector and provider for his newborn infant. This represents an awesome responsibility to many men, and each will adjust in his own way. It is important that the mother accept her partner's definition of his new role. Encourage couples to share their feelings with one another, both positive and negative, openly and honestly.

Men learn their paternal role through society's definitions, experience with their own fathers, and peer pressure from other men. Pressure or encouragement from within his family is also a factor in a man's growth as a father. Each father chooses his own level of involvement in the care and nurturing of his baby. Being actively involved in the pregnancy and the birth enhances his level of participation (Sears, 2006).

Fathers and Common Parenting Issues

Anticipatory guidance can help fathers ease into the parenting role. Even before the childbearing years, boys and girls alike deserve exposure to discussions of infant feeding and the importance of breastfeeding. Often, you have an opportunity to provide such education through school, hospital, and community outreach programs. Planting the seed for future generations empowers them to make knowledgeable choices regarding infant feeding. Early education results in breastfeeding becoming more acceptable and, therefore, the norm.

When a couple discovers they are expecting, they frequently seek out prenatal classes to prepare for parenting. Learning what to expect and how to cope helps both parents ease into their roles. Much focus in prenatal breastfeeding education is on the mother. However, educating fathers regarding the realities of breastfeeding strengthens their involvement and validates their reactions in the early postpartum period. Fathers often express concerns related to breastfeeding, such as limited initial opportunity to develop a relationship with their children, feeling inadequate, and feeling separated from their partners. Incorporating sensitivity to these concerns and appropriate guidance into breastfeeding classes helps fathers know what to anticipate.

Prenatal classes need to address issues related to the mother and father as a couple. Couples who perceived higher social support in pregnancy reported significantly lower levels of distress 6 weeks postnatally (Castle et al.,

2008). With the mother seemingly immersed in the care of their new baby, the father may feel as though he has lost his partner. Early parenting is both physically and emotionally intense, whether the baby is breastfed or not. Fortunately, breastfeeding simplifies some aspects of these early days. Nighttime feedings are easier for both the mother and father, because there is no special preparation required for feeding and the baby's food is always available.

Other aspects of life with a new baby benefit from anticipatory guidance, including physical recovery from childbirth and changes in roles of the couple as new parents. Although breastfeeding enhances a woman's physical recovery from childbirth, the mother still experiences fatigue, discomfort, and breast changes in the early days. Although parenting expands the couple's relationship to a wonderfully new dimension, the change is not without periods of stress and uncertainty. You can acknowledge these points when educating couples and emphasize that such reactions are normal. Encourage them to communicate with one another regarding their feelings and to keep a focus on their relationship as a couple through this time of great change.

Fathers' Reactions

Fathers experience a hormonal response to their babies' cries, with a rise in prolactin and testosterone levels (Delahunty et al., 2007). Not surprisingly, they are also more responsive to infant cues than are nonfathers (Fleming et al., 2002). The father can bond with his baby through infant care tasks like bathing, burping, and diapering. He can help the mother with positioning to breastfeed, carry the baby in a sling, and provide skin-to-skin contact. Fathers benefit from learning about infant cues and responsiveness to recognize what is normal and how to interact with their young infants.

Researchers interviewed couples during pregnancy and between 3 and 4 months postpartum about their needs in transitioning to parenthood. They found that the couples felt unprepared. Mothers turned to social networks, including parents, friends and colleagues, health professionals, and prenatal/postpartum groups for support. In comparison, men appeared to lack support networks and reported having no one to turn to other than their partner and work colleagues (Deave et al., 2008). Helping strategies include involving partners in breastfeeding sessions, rewriting educational materials to be more inclusive of fathers, increasing future parents' awareness of relationship changes, and promoting active discussion of potential changes.

In the early postpartum period, the baby initially may show a preference for the mother. The father needs time alone with the baby to develop his own parenting style and bond with his child. Although he may have different methods from the mother, his methods are no less important or effective. He needs encouragement in his new role. Fathers may be further encouraged by the fact that they are the first person in their baby's life who teaches him that food and love must not always come from the same person! Books that are helpful in assisting the father in his personal parenting journey include *Becoming a Father: How to Nurture and Enjoy Your Family* (Sears et al., 2003) and *Fathering Right from the Start: Straight Talk about Pregnancy, Birth and Beyond* (Heinowitz, 2001).

Paternal Postpartum Depression

Fathers can experience postpartum depression as well as mothers. Paternal depression, like maternal depression, adversely affects infant learning (Kaplan et al., 2007). The average rate of depression among new fathers is 10 percent, twice the rate in the general population of men (Paulson et al., 2006). The rate increases to 20 percent at 3 to 6 months. Postpartum depression in mothers and fathers is associated with less positive parent–infant interactions and poorer sleep regulation for the child. These affects do not continue at 2 years after maternal depression, whereas previous paternal depression continues to affect interaction with the child.

Depression tends to be higher among fathers in nontraditional family structures. Fathers are three times more likely to be depressed if the mother is mildly depressed and eight times more likely when the mother is moderately to severely depressed. Depression disrupts parental collaboration and affects the early family. Negotiating their role change to father and mother creates tension in the couple and contributes to depression. The child's temperament can contribute as well.

Support for the Mother

A breastfeeding mother benefits from an abundance of emotional support from those close to her. Ideally, a major portion of this support comes from the baby's father. Discussing plans for breastfeeding enables couples to share their opinions and concerns and arrive at mutual decisions. The breastfeeding experience is much more rewarding and fulfilling when shared by the entire family in a positive and accepting atmosphere.

Support by the father takes many forms. It can range from physical care of the baby to helping with household chores to a strong philosophical support. A lack of sharing of tasks often becomes a source of the mother's complaints. She may wish that her mate would take more initiative in helping or that he were more competent with baby care and household chores. You can help her understand that learning these tasks is like learning a new job. Her partner needs time and encouragement to develop confidence and competence. Because mothers typically spend more time with the baby than fathers do, they tend to learn quickly how to interact with and care for their baby. A mother needs to be patient and give her mate the same opportunity to learn what works for him and how he fits in. When the mother encourages the father in his new role, she often finds that he becomes her best supporter and an outspoken advocate of breastfeeding.

Learning about breastfeeding enables fathers to provide their partners with practical help. A father who attends prenatal classes may be better able to assist his partner in tangible ways, such as helping her get comfortable. He can fill in pieces of information the mother may have forgotten and provide encouragement when she is having a bad day. Prenatal classes expose fathers to the normalcy of breastfeeding and the reasons why breastfeeding is important for babies. They learn practicalities of breastfeeding, such as the economics, the ease of nighttime feedings, health issues, and overall convenience. These influences may further cement their support of their partner's decisions to breastfeed.

Interaction with the Baby

Each father chooses his own manner and level of involvement with his baby. Ideally, a father participates in the birth process and begins to bond with his baby immediately after birth. Such involvement increases the likelihood that the father will respond more openly and readily to the baby than one whose first interaction occurs after the baby comes home. Devoting the first hours and days to becoming acquainted with his newborn child enables the father to learn the skills necessary to care for him or her. Mothers and fathers both need to learn these parenting skills; they do not come naturally as some parents expect.

A father's help can be invaluable in the postpartum period and beyond. He can help soothe a fussy baby through walking, rocking, singing, and cooing. He can share in his baby's care and provide the mother some free time alone. He can bathe, burp, diaper, and play with his baby. Bringing the baby to the mother for nighttime feedings helps her get needed sleep.

Many mothers find that their mates' involvement increases as the baby gets older and responds to his attentions. Whatever type of interaction the father chooses, the mother should be careful not to discourage his efforts by criticizing the way he does things to the point that he limits his involvement. She can offer instructive guidance, particularly when a certain practice might be harmful to the baby (e.g., she can point out the need to support the baby's head when carrying or holding him). Encourage the mother to avoid unwarranted criticism. Although the father may do things differently from the mother, his way may be very satisfying for him and his baby.

Babies whose fathers interact with them continually and consistently show an eagerness for learning. They may have a more positive self-image and show more confidence in relating to males. These babies are more likely to have a sense of humor and a longer attention span. Fathers benefit as well from interacting with their babies. They can learn how to care for the baby, can read to him or her, and can be supportive in easing the intensity of motherhood.

∽ Changes in Family Relationships

The responsibility of being parents presents a major adjustment to many couples. At times, some new parents may feel resentment toward their baby for disrupting their lives and interfering with their freedom. Help them understand that such ambivalence is normal and often is balanced by deep feelings of affection and love for their infant. Parents do not need to feel guilty about their reactions. Encourage them to share their feelings honestly and openly with one another.

The need for open and honest communication is especially great during the first few months of parenthood. Both partners feel inadequacies and a need for support in establishing their new roles as father and mother. They may react strongly to the ways in which the other performs his or her role. They may resent the fact that the baby now receives a lot of the affection and intimacy previously monopolized by the other partner. Remaining sensitive to one another's needs helps them make compromises and adjustments.

Sexual Adjustments

Open communication between the couple and the passage of time are major factors in reestablishing enjoyable sexual relations. By reassuring the mother that the need for sexual adjustment is common to most new parents, you can make it easier for her to discuss her feelings with her partner. New babies consume a great deal of time and energy, and at the end of a tiring day lovemaking may seem like just one more chore. As the mother settles into her new role, she may be encouraged to look for ways to boost her energy level. She can nap when her baby naps, nurse lying down, and cosleep. You can help the mother look at her dietary practices and offer her suggestions for improvement through quick and healthy food choices (see Chapter 8). The mother can also explore ways to prioritize her household tasks and ask for help to maximize her efficiency.

Reducing the mother's workload both at home and at work or school may give her more time and energy to enjoy companionship, conversation, and lovemaking with her partner. New fathers, as well as new mothers, need to be reassured that they are good parents. Fatherhood is a part of manhood, and a confident man is more likely to inspire an enthusiastic sexual response from his partner. He needs to be understanding about the physical demands of motherhood.

Resuming Sexual Intercourse

The recovery period after birth may take several months. Many caregivers advise women that they may resume sexual intercourse after the 6-week checkup, whereas some suggest waiting until the mother's lochia discharge has completely stopped. The 6-week checkup indicates how the mother's recovery is progressing and whether any complications exist. Some couples resume sexual relations before this checkup. The mother should listen to her body before resuming intercourse.

Emotional Adjustments

In the early weeks or months after giving birth some women have little or no desire for lovemaking or other forms of intimacy. It may take several months for a new mother to regain her desire or for her responses to return to normal. Such a reaction may be due in part to the fact that her baby provides her with sufficient affection and emotional gratification, and she does not feel a need for further intimacy. You can assure the mother that this response is normal and that it usually subsides as she adjusts to her maternal role. Other women find motherhood exhilarating and that the hormones of mothering and nursing increase their libido. This is normal as well.

A woman's breasts may be overly sensitive during foreplay or, at the other extreme, she may experience no sensual response to her partner's touch. Her responses usually return to normal within several months after delivery, although for some women this change continues throughout lactation. Some women describe themselves as becoming sexually aroused or experience an increased sensuality when nursing the baby. The sensation is a result of the hormone oxytocin released during both lactation and sexual orgasm. Women need reassurance that nothing is wrong or inappropriate and that they can enjoy this aspect of breastfeeding.

Either partner may be reluctant to engage in foreplay that involves the woman's breasts for fear of passing on germs. If the breast skin is healthy and unbroken, chances of transmitting an infection are minimal. The mother produces antibodies to her partner's germs, which pass to her baby through her milk and protect him or her from infection. She can shower or wash her breasts before nursing the baby after sex.

Physical Adjustments

A new mother may experience some physical discomfort when she first resumes sexual intercourse. The hormones involved with lactation cause a decrease in vaginal lubrication, which may result in discomfort. The mother can relieve this discomfort with a water-based artificial lubricant. Birth interventions can interfere with her desire for intimacy in the postpartum period. Intercourse may be painful because of an episiotomy, abdominal incision, or internal injury from the use of forceps. If either partner lacks physical sensations during intercourse, it may be the result of stretched pelvic floor muscles. Kegel exercises help with general toning of the perineal area.

Overfull or leaking breasts may be a source of discomfort for the mother. Sexual orgasm releases the hormone oxytocin, which also facilitates the letdown of the mother's milk. Therefore leaking during intercourse is very common and indicates a positive hormonal response. If the couple is uncomfortable with the dampness that results, a towel can protect bed linens. In addition, an adjustment in positioning can alleviate pressure on the woman's breasts. Nursing the baby before intercourse decreases fullness as well as leakage.

Adjusting Sexual Routine

Adjustments in positioning can help alleviate physical discomfort caused by painful incisions or full breasts. A change in the couple's timing for lovemaking can also help. They may be tense if lovemaking begins at a time when the baby usually wishes to nurse or even if the baby is pleasantly awake. Nursing the baby immediately before bedtime and taking advantage of moments alone during nap time can provide parents an opportunity for intimacy. Spontaneity is a challenge with children. Many parents find scheduling a "date" or a set time for intimacy helps keep their relationship connected.

The stresses of discomfort and demands of the baby are easier to cope with when there is tenderness between partners. Often, it is effective for couples to have a period of rekindling their tenderness for each other by spending time just holding and cuddling. It is important for a couple to understand that the need for sexual adjustment is normal and common to new parents regardless of whether the mother is lactating. Variations in technique or routine can enhance lovemaking. If the mother experiences discomfort or lack of response in her breasts during foreplay, developing new patterns of foreplay can be an enjoyable solution. It is reassuring to both parents to learn that what they are experiencing is normal and that coping requires simply a little understanding and willingness to adapt.

Menstruation and Fertility

Menstruation and fertility are delayed for varying periods during lactation. The delay occurs as part of the mother's physiological response to her baby's sucking and other stimuli. This alters the release of brain hormones and reproductive hormones, thus disrupting the cycle of ovulation and menstruation. The single most important factor in suppressing ovulation during lactation is the early establishment of frequent and strong sucking (Academy of Breastfeeding Medicine [ABM], 2006; McNeilly, 2001). A variety of hormones is involved, with links between levels of gonadotropin-releasing hormone, luteinizing hormone, follicle-stimulating hormone, prolactin, and estrogen.

Return of Menses

In the initial postpartum period and for several months thereafter a breastfeeding mother experiences a phase of amenorrhea (lack of menstruation). The menstrual cycle can be delayed for several months, followed by a period of resumed menstrual cycles that may be anovulatory (producing an inadequate ovum). The length of amenorrhea and infertility is linked to breastfeeding frequency, short intervals between feedings, duration of feedings (ABM, 2006), the presence of nighttime feedings, and the absence of supplemental foods in the baby's diet.

Menstruation may resume at any time during lactation and greatly depends on overall breastfeeding patterns. In women who breastfeed exclusively, the rate of return of menses is between 19 and 53 percent by 6 months postpartum (Lawrence & Lawrence, 2005). Although a very small percentage of women resume menstruation as early as 6 to 12 weeks, others may not menstruate until breastfeeding has ceased totally. Some women produce a scanty show before their full menstrual cycles resume. The onset of menstruation should not be confused with any normal or abnormal postpartum bleeding. If the mother suspects abnormal bleeding, she should consult her caregiver.

Some women report they are bleeding at around days 42 to 56. This can signal an end to lochial discharge, or it may reflect a change in the mothers' activity level (Visness et al., 1997). If a mother experiences other bleeding, or bleeding with breastfeeding difficulties, encourage her to seek immediate healthcare advice. Menstruation causes no significant changes in the composition of the mother's milk, and mothers can continue nursing during menstrual cycling. Hormonal changes may alter the taste of her milk, however, which can prompt the baby to be fussy during a feeding or even refuse to nurse. The baby's reaction may also result from heightened tension in the mother or to swelling in the breast caused by menstrual edema and hormones. Any of these factors can affect letdown.

Contraception

Parents face important decisions about birth control during the postpartum period. They may gather information about various contraceptive devices through reading, talking with friends, and consulting their caregiver. Often, a woman may ask about birth control methods that are compatible with breastfeeding. Some women fear another close pregnancy and will not breastfeed if it precludes using a method that provides full protection. These women may not be receptive to a family planning method that relies on breastfeeding and their body's signals. You are not responsible for a mother's final choice; you are responsible only for ensuring that your guidance is based on scientific evidence and that it supports her goals.

Parents have many contraceptive options. There are advantages and disadvantages of each, especially when a mother is breastfeeding. The options they may consider include lactational amenorrhea, combined oral contraception, the progesterone-only pill, injectable methods, implants, intrauterine devices (IUDs) and systems, barrier methods, and sterilization (Hughes, 2009). Resources for education may help the mother find the solution that is best for her. Birth control options need to be considered in light of their effect on lactation (ABM, 2006). Refer to the Academy of Breastfeeding Medicine's Clinical Proto-

col #13, "Contraception and Breastfeeding," for the Academy's principles for contraception considerations during lactation, and a summary of the advantages, disadvantages, and impact of these methods on lactation. The protocol is available online at www.bfmed.org/Resources/Protocols.aspx.

Lactational Amenorrhea Method The absence of ovulation and menstruation during lactation is not merely a convenience to the mother. Research has demonstrated that lactation can delay the return of fertility during the postpartum period (Radwan et al., 2009; Subhani et al., 2008; Romero-Gutiérrez et al., 2007; Aryal, 2006). Women who breastfeed fully (that is, frequently, day and night) and who experience lactational amenorrhea are more than 98 percent protected from pregnancy for 6 months after birth (Kennedy et al., 1998; Hight-Laukaran, 1997; Labbok et al., 1997, 1994). This protection is called the lactational amenorrhea method (LAM) of contraception (Figure 19.3).

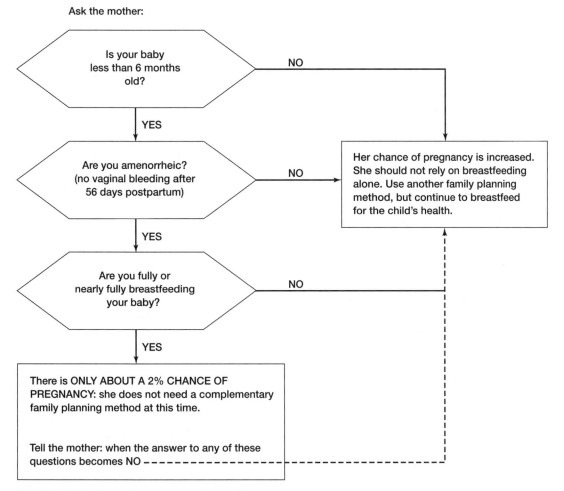

FIGURE 19.3 Lactational amenorrhea method.

Source: Institute for International Studies in Natural Family Planning. Labbok M, Koniz-Booher P, Cooney K, Shelton J, Krasovack K (eds). *Guidelines for Breastfeeding in Family Planning and Child Survival Programs.* Washington DC: Georgetown University; 1990. Reprinted with permission.

Three conditions are necessary for the mother to rely on the LAM to prevent pregnancy:

- First, the mother's menses must not have returned.
- Second, the mother must breastfeed around the clock, without significant amounts of other foods in her baby's diet.
- Third, the baby must be younger than 6 months of age.

If any one of these conditions is not met, the mother is at increased risk of pregnancy and should supplement with another contraceptive method to ensure adequate protection. Shaaban and Glasier (2008) found that only 1.5 percent of unintended pregnancies occur when all the prerequisites of LAM were present. For LAM to be most effective it is recommended that the baby breastfeed beginning soon after birth and continue to breastfeed exclusively, day and night, for 6 months. The use of artificial nipples such as a bottle or pacifier interferes with the frequency and duration of sucking at the breast, and the mother should avoid them.

LAM offers a method of protection from pregnancy at a vulnerable time in a mother's life—the first 6 months postpartum. It does so with no side effects to either the mother or child. Many mothers find this an excellent opportunity to be in tune with their bodies' natural rhythms. LAM requires only that the mother learn the three conditions and that she breastfeed her child in an optimal manner. Such a method, which allows a mother to meet both her needs and her baby's needs in a safe manner and which costs the family nothing, needs to be included in prenatal and postpartum education.

Emphasize to mothers, however, that as soon as there is a decline in breastfeeding, either because the baby begins solid foods or supplements or because he or she is nursing less often, contraceptive protection decreases. Over 61 percent of breastfeeding mothers with unintended pregnancies (the same cohort as above) failed to use contraception because they believed breastfeeding would prevent pregnancy (Tilley, 2009).

Natural Family Planning Periodic abstinence, or natural family planning, involves charting the basal body temperature (temperature taken on waking, at around the same time each day) or checking vaginal secretions. It requires keeping a careful calendar record of menstrual periods to predict fertile days. This method is more reliable than the rhythm method, which estimates the woman's fertile period from the calendar records of menstrual periods alone.

In total natural family planning, changes in cervical mucus before ovulation help signal the beginning of the fertile days. Women who are familiar with natural family planning probably have more success with it postpartum than new users, because the signs can be quite different during lactation. Cervical mucus patterns in the first few breastfeeding months postpartum may be less clearly defined than after regular cycles have resumed. Mucus changes from a scant semisolid white or yellowish matter to an abundant thin, clear, watery, and slippery fluid that allows the sperm to penetrate the canal of the cervix easily.

Fluctuations in the woman's basal body temperature aid the couple in determining fertile periods. During menses and up to ovulation, basal body temperature is at its lowest. After ovulation the temperature rises, leveling off until just before the onset of menses. Monitoring mucous and temperature changes identifies the 5 to 7 days per month when pregnancy may occur. Clients interested in using natural family planning can read *Breastfeeding and Natural Child Spacing: How Ecological Breastfeeding Spaces Babies* (Kippley, 2008a), *The Seven Standards of Ecological Breastfeeding: The Frequency Factor* (Kippley, 2008b), or visit the website for the Couple to Couple League at www.ccli.org.

Oral Contraceptive Combination oral contraceptives contain the hormones estrogen and progesterone. They appear to cause the most difficulty in lactating women, especially in the early postpartum period before lactation is well established. Estrogen can lower milk production (WHO, 2004; International Planned Parenthood Federation, 2002; Koetsawang, 1987; Tankeyoon et al., 1984). A Cochrane review of hormonal contraception during breastfeeding criticizes the WHO studies and calls for new randomized controlled trials (Truitt et al., 2003). The long-term effects of oral contraceptive use on babies are not known. Some research suggests an increased risk of infant acute leukemia with use of oral contraceptives (Schnyder et al., 2009). The effect of this hormonal exposure on the reproductive potential of these children needs consideration.

Generally, advice to breastfeeding women is that they use nonestrogen contraceptive methods. Progestin-only oral contraceptives (the mini-pill) do not appear to interfere with milk production and therefore are acceptable during lactation (Bjarnadottir et al., 2001; Kelsey, 1996). However, the long-term effects remain unknown. Slight adverse effects were noted in some mothers and children but the mini-pill appeared to be safe for lactating women. Generally, women should not use this method before 6 weeks postpartum. Practitioners have received numerous anecdotal reports of mothers experiencing drops in milk production after starting the progesterone-only pill. Milk production recovers when mothers discontinue taking the pill.

Intrauterine Device The IUD is a copper or hormonal device placed into the uterus. The copper affects the lining of the uterus and prevents a fertilized egg from implanting (Epigee Women's Health, 2009). The nonhormonal IUD does not seem to have any effect on lactation (Koetsawang, 1987). Hormonal IUDs prevent pregnancy by releasing the hormone progesterone. This causes a thickening in the cervical mucus and acts as a barrier to prevent sperm from entering the uterus, thereby preventing implantation of a fertilized egg. Hormonal IUDs need replacement within 1 year (Epigee Women's Health, 2009). Use of a progesterone-releasing IUD was associated with a slight decrease in milk volume, compared with use of a copper IUD (Kelsey, 1996), but this study has not been replicated.

Vaginal Ring The vaginal ring is a hormone-releasing ring a woman can self-insert. One study found similar effectiveness rates between the efficacy of a progesterone-releasing vaginal ring and a copper IUD in lactating mothers. Milk production and infant growth were within normal limits for women who used a vaginal ring and those who used an IUD (Sivin, 1997). At least one vaginal ring on the U.S. market contains both progesterone and estrogen. Although the company website says that it contains "half the estrogen of a commonly used oral contraceptive," a mother might be prudent to consider nonestrogen alternatives (NuvaRing, 2008).

Implants Levonorgestrel is a progestin implant made of a small plastic rod(s) inserted surgically under the skin of the upper arm. The rod(s) slowly releases progesterone into the body for up to 3 years. Levonorgestrel can also be implanted in the uterus for long-term use (up to 5 years). This type of contraception is used in women who have given birth.

A 3-year study compared levonorgestrel uterine implants with a copper IUD. No statistically significant differences were found between groups with regard to all infant physical growth parameters and various infant development tests (Shaamash et al., 2005). Another uterine implant emits etonogestrel. A similar 3-year study found no statistically significant growth or development differences (Taneepanichskul et al., 2006).

Injectables Injectables are progesterone injections given every 3 months. These include the trade names Depo-Provera and NET-EN. Infertility may last up to a year or longer after the depot subsides. Many lactation consultants have noted a connection between the administration of injectables immediately postpartum and impaired milk production. Clinical studies show no statistical impact on lactation; however, the participants did not receive the depot injection until after 6 weeks postpartum (Danli et al., 2000; Elfituri et al., 2006). The ABM (2006) recommends that mothers delay use of progesterone injectables until lactation is well established. This makes sense because it is the precipitous drop in progesterone postpartum that initiates stage II lactogenesis (Kennedy et al., 1997).

Be aware that there is a paternalistic attitude among some care providers that "many uninsured or underinsured women lose access to care shortly after their delivery, and are unable to readily access contraceptive services postpartum" (Allbusiness.com, 2009). The philosophy is that low-income women will not return for their traditional postpartum visit and thus should be given birth control injections in the hospital before discharge (Rodriguez & Kaunitz, 2009). Patients are often concerned about the side effects, including changes in menstrual cycle, body weight, and mood disturbances. Instead of respecting women's concerns about this drug and exploring nonhormonal alternatives, proponents advise caregivers to "redesign counseling strategies to improve contraceptive continuation and improve patient adherence" (Bakry et al., 2008).

Littlecrow-Russell (2000) described her experience of being pressured to receive the depot injection as a low-income, breastfeeding mother. As a lactation consultant you may work with adolescents, minorities, or low-income women who have received the progesterone depot shot without informed consent. You may need to ask additional open-ended questions to help the mother recall or determine when and what she was given, especially if she is encountering low milk production with no other risk factors. You can try to empower the mother to take charge of her own health care and fertility, including requesting her own medical records, if she does not know or understand what she was given.

Patches The "patch" is a birth control system that delivers hormones directly through the skin into the bloodstream via a thin patch. It is a combination contraceptive, containing both estrogen and progesterone with effectiveness rates similar to combination oral contraceptives. The U.S. Food and Drug Administration (2008) requires the U.S. manufacturer of this contraceptive to include warnings that users of the birth control patch are at higher risk of developing serious blood clots, also known as venous thromboembolism, than women using birth control pills. Venous thromboembolism can lead to pulmonary embolism.

Barrier Methods Barrier methods include condoms, diaphragms, cervical caps, and the use of a spermicide, with or without physical barriers. Spermicides prevent pregnancy by destroying sperm before they can reach and fertilize an egg. Studies of spermicides show variable failure rates averaging 21 to 26 percent for typical users. A male condom is a thin latex or silicone sheath that covers the penis. A female condom is a thin polyurethane sheath with two soft rings at each end. One ring, covered with the polyurethane, fits over the cervix and acts as an anchor. The larger, open ring stays outside the vagina, covering part of the perineum and labia during intercourse. Male condoms have about a 14 percent failure rate (Epigee Women's Health, 2009). Diaphragms and cervical caps have a higher failure rate among women who have had vaginal births (Epigee Women's Health, 2009).

Sterilization   Some mothers choose sterilization through bilateral tubal ligation, a procedure that ties the mother's fallopian tubes to prevent conception. Most mothers in the United States who choose tubal ligation have the procedure almost immediately postpartum. Although there is no evidence that tubal ligation hampers milk production, the operation immediately postpartum can potentially affect the mother's pain level. The intravenous (IV) fluids she receives can increase edema and make it difficult for her baby to latch in the early days.

Some fathers choose sterilization by vasectomy, in which the vas deferens (the main duct through which sperm travel during ejaculation) is snipped. Sterilization is a permanent decision (Hatcher et al., 2008). Parents considering this option may want to let time lapse before deciding to end their family size.

Points for Parents to Consider   Most caregivers' offices provide information on family planning, sex education, parenting, and sterilization. Literature and Internet information on each of the individual birth control methods are readily available. Prenatal classes can encourage couples to discuss contraception with their providers during pregnancy so they have time to research what will work best as a breastfeeding family. The obstetric provider knows the woman's general medical history, family history, and other needs that may influence her options.

The choice of contraceptive method is the couple's responsibility. Restrict your help to that of suggesting options that are compatible with breastfeeding rather than giving advice. The following considerations may be helpful to parents in selecting a form of contraceptive:

- Religious and ethical feelings about birth control and the types that are acceptable
- Concerns regarding contraceptive effectiveness and the possibility of another pregnancy
- Choice of who will take responsibility for contraception
- Convenience in terms of remembering to use it and wishing to use it every time
- Association between the method and intercourse
- Long-term health risks of hormonal contraception
- Expense, inconvenience, use of foreign objects, messiness, and loss of spontaneity

⁓ Sibling Reactions and Adjustments

Homecoming for parents and their new baby can range from a very smooth adjustment to a distant or demanding attitude by siblings. Reactions depend on many factors, including the age of the child and the length of his or her separation from the mother. Prepare the mother for possible changes in her older children, and let her know that these reactions are common. She may be engrossed with the baby and feel less close to her other children for a while. This can cause the children to display jealousy and perhaps develop a closer relationship with their father or other relative in the early weeks, while appearing distant with the mother. Relationships will mend as all family members learn to bond with the baby in their own way (Figure 19.4).

Preparing for the New Baby

Parents can begin preparing their children for the baby's arrival by sharing the events of pregnancy with them. They can explain how a baby develops, visits their mother will make to her caregiver, and what she will do in the hospital. They can read books to their children that show a

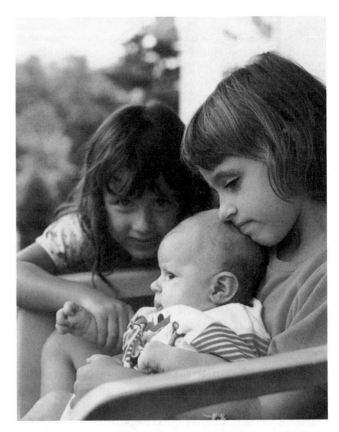

FIGURE 19.4   Siblings enjoying time with their new brother.
Source: Printed with permission of Debbie Shinskie.

new baby in the family. Children can participate in preparing for the baby by helping with baby clothes and equipment and packing the mother's suitcase. If the child's sleeping arrangements will change, it should be done early and in a way that the older child does not feel crowded out by the new baby.

The mother can make a construction paper booklet with pictures about what it is like in the hospital (physicians, nurses, nursery pictures), coming home, at home with the baby (bathing, sleeping, nursing, crying), and the new family. Looking at their family's current baby pictures can be fun, too. She can prepare the child for what new babies do, such as nursing, sleeping, and crying, and the fact that they are not yet able to play. There are many children's books that show breastfeeding as a normal, routine part of infant care and family life. You can find up-to-date lists by a quick Internet search.

Parents can explain any changes that will take place in usual family activities and the reasons for the changes. The mother can involve her child in caring for the new baby, enlisting help with such things as bringing diapers and clothes to her and holding, talking, and getting the baby to smile. Siblings can visit a family with a new baby to see what a baby looks and sounds like and how it has changed their family.

Preparing for a Home Birth

Many families prefer the option of home birthing as the natural, low-intervention way to welcome their new baby into the world. It is the parents' decision whether their other children attend the labor and birth. Some parents are concerned that the intensity of labor could frighten a young child. The level of participation parents are comfortable with probably depends on the age, maturity, and personality of the children.

Regardless of whether the child is present for the labor and birth, the continuous presence of the mother in the home eliminates the concern about the child's reaction to her absence. Other siblings are able to see the baby during or immediately after birth. They can welcome the new baby to their home, free from hospital interventions and interruptions. A caregiver for the children can tend to their needs during and after labor.

Preparing for the Mother's Absence

If the mother plans to give birth in a hospital, it is important that the older child be prepared for her absence during her hospital stay. The child will want to understand where the mother is going, why, for how long, and what she will do while she is there. Visiting the hospital during the pregnancy helps the older child understand what will take place. Many hospitals offer sibling classes and tours,

and sibling visitation during the mother's postpartum stay can be worked out at that time. The mother can plan to maintain contact with her family through telephone calls and visits. Because of the brevity of U.S. hospital stays, the mother is usually away only one or two nights.

Choosing to have siblings present at the baby's birth requires preparation about what birth is like and how the mother will act. When siblings are present, a caregiver needs to be present to meet the needs of the children during the experience. The sibling can decide whether he or she is comfortable being present at the actual time of delivery. This may be easier to arrange in a free-standing birth center than in a U.S. hospital.

Adjusting to the New Baby

Whenever a new baby joins a family, the role of each family member is redefined and expanded. An older child who previously had been the "baby of the family" loses the position as the center of attention. Older children may need to assume responsibility for tasks previously performed by their parents. Parents may expect them to dress themselves, help with household chores, and generally fend for themselves instead of always relying on someone to help them. The ease with which they can do this depends on their age at the time of the sibling's birth, their personality, and their sense of security.

Each child needs time and understanding in assuming a new role in the family. The parents can help with this adjustment by making the child feel special in new ways. The mother can begin fostering her older child's emotional growth by giving her undivided attention the first time they are together after the birth of the baby. She can have another adult hold the baby while she renews contact with her older child and expresses her love. After the family is settled the parents can create situations where each child can look at, touch, or hold the baby. Setting aside special moments each day for the other children individually lets each one know how she appreciates their unique qualities.

Sibling's Behavior During Feedings

During feedings a sibling may want to be included in the closeness and interaction between mother and the new baby. The mother can accommodate this by nursing her baby where there is ample room for all family members, such as the bed, couch, or floor. She can plan activities to share with her toddler during nursing times, such as reading books, playing simple games ("I spy something red"), and activities (paper and crayons, tea party, puzzles, or playing music).

If a toddler who had weaned asks to nurse again the mother's awareness of his needs and her willingness to respond favorably are reassuring to him. He may want only to taste the milk, in which case the mother can put some of her milk in a cup to satisfy his curiosity. This renewed interest in breastfeeding is usually temporary. Occasionally a toddler resumes nursing on a regular basis, and the mother may need your support in tandem nursing (see Chapter 14).

Adjustment Challenges

Despite parents' efforts toward a smooth transition, some toddlers and young children exhibit regressive behaviors when a new baby arrives. Reactions can include whining, baby talk, bed-wetting or accidents from a previously toilet-trained child, waking during the night, clinging to the mother, or hitting the baby. Such behavior may be the child's way of seeking attention. A child often develops mixed feelings. The child may enjoy cuddling and talking to the baby but at the same time may find it difficult to share the mother's attention with the baby.

The mother can reassure her child that she understands and accepts these feelings. She can read to him about new babies and emphasize his importance as an older child in protecting and amusing their baby. She can help him find his new position in the family by giving him special opportunities to demonstrate his capabilities in caring for the baby. She can point out the many benefits and privileges of being more independent and self-reliant. Spending focused time with each parent—especially the mother—can help alleviate the older child's feelings of displacement and help the adjustment to being the new older brother or sister.

〜 Summary

Your availability and support to couples will encourage them as they mature into the parental role. Understanding typical postpartum adjustments and aspects of physical recovery may help mothers avoid needless worry. Prenatal education about the differences between baby blues, postpartum depression, and postpartum psychosis is crucial. Fathers have their own unique adjustments as they provide support to the mother and learn how to interact with their new baby. The mother and father will experience changes in their sexual relationship. You can educate them on contraceptive options that are compatible with breastfeeding. Siblings benefit from preparation for the birth, as well as extra patience, love, and understanding as they adjust to the new baby. This is an exciting time for the family as they welcome a new baby into their home and learn to respond to one another in new ways.

〜 Chapter 19—At a Glance

Applying what you learned—

Counseling the mother:

- Encourage mothers to express their feelings.
- Encourage women to develop friendships with other new mothers.
- Encourage realistic expectations about the baby and parenthood.
- Help mothers see that not all problems with the baby are related to breastfeeding.
- Help mothers cope with baby blues.
- Recognize when baby blues progresses to depression or psychosis.
- Recognize your limitations and when to refer.
- Recognize characteristics of survivors of sexual abuse.

Teach parents about

- Dangers of baby training programs
- Physical recovery and emotional adjustments after birth
- Changes in priorities with a new baby
- Importance of the father's support to the mother
- Importance of the father's role and bonding with the baby
- Changes in the family's relationship
- Sexual adjustments and physical discomfort
- Lactational amenorrhea method and other contraceptives
- How to respond to their baby's needs
- Helping siblings prepare for and adjust to the new baby

〜 References

1-2-3 Magic. www.parentmagic.com. Accessed September 20, 2009.

Academy of Breastfeeding Medicine (ABM) Protocol Committee. ABM clinical protocol #13: contraception during breastfeeding. *Breastfeed Med.* 2006;1:43-51.

AllBusiness.com. ED Legal Letter. Start postpartum contraception early. September 1, 2009. www.allbusiness.com/medicine-health/health-health-care-by-target/12709372-1.html. Accessed September 24, 2009.

American Academy of Pediatrics (AAP). Media Alert: AAP addresses scheduled feedings vs. demand feedings. April 20, 1998. www.ezzo.info/Aney/mediaalert.pdf. Accessed September 21, 2009.

American Academy of Pediatrics (AAP). Policy statement on breastfeeding and the use of human milk. *Pediatrics.* 2005;115:496-506.

Aney M. *Babywise* linked to dehydration, failure to thrive. *AAP News*; April 1998.

Arias I. The legacy of child maltreatment: long-term health consequences for women. *J Womens Health*. 2004;13:468-473.

Aryal TR. Retrospective reporting of the duration of post-partum amenorrhea: a survival analysis. *Kathmandu Univ Med J*. 2006;4:211-217.

Bakry S, et al. Depot-medroxyprogesterone acetate: an update. *Arch Gynecol Obstet*. 2008;278:1-12.

Barett H. Parents and children: facts and fallacies about attachment theory. *J Fam Health Care*. 2006;16:3-4.

Benedict M, et al. *Long-term effects of child sexual abuse on functioning in pregnancy and pregnancy outcome* (Final report). Washington, DC: National Center on Child Abuse and Neglect; 1994.

Bjarnadottir R, et al. Comparative study of the effects of a progestogen-only pill containing desogestrel and an intrauterine contraceptive device in lactating women. *Br J Obstet Gynaecol*. 2001;108:1174-1180.

Bocar D, Moore K. *Acquiring the Parental Role. Lactation Consultant Series #16*. New York: Avery Publishing Group; 1987.

Castle H, et al. Attitudes to emotional expression, social support and postnatal adjustment in new parents. *J Reprod Infant Psych*. 2008;26:180-194.

Centre for Maternal and Child Enquiries. Saving mothers' lives 2003–2005 (Full report) Reviewing maternal deaths to make motherhood safer 2003–2005. London: CMACE; December 2007. http://www.cmace.org.uk. Accessed September 19, 2009.

Child Abuse Prevention Council of Orange County. Religious parenting programs: their relationship to child abuse prevention. Parenting Program Review Committee, May 14, 1996. www.ezzo.info/Aney/childabusepreventioncouncil.pdf. Accessed September 19, 2009.

Cline F, Fay J. 2009. www.loveandlogic.com. Accessed September 20, 2009.

Cloud J, Townsend H. 2009. www.cloudtownsend.com. Accessed September, 20, 2009.

Coloroso B. 2009. www.kidsareworthit.com. Accessed September 20, 2009.

Cox D, et al. Studies on human lactation: the development of the computerized breast measurement system; 1998. Updated 2008. www.biochem.biomedchem.uwa.edu.au/page/69859. Accessed March 1, 2009.

Cox J. Utah chapter, American Academy of Pediatrics. Got time? *The Growing Times; Salt Lake City, UT*: September/October 2001.

Cox L, et al. Edinburgh postnatal depression scale (EPDS). *Br J Psych*. 1987;150:782-786.

Danli S, et al. A multicentered clinical trial of the long-acting injectable contraceptive Depo Provera in Chinese women. *Contraception*. 2000;62:15-18.

Deave T, et al. Transition to parenthood: the needs of parents in pregnancy and early parenthood. *BMC Pregnancy Childbirth*. 2008;8:30.

Delahunty K, et al. Prolactin responses to infant cues in men and women: effects of parental experience and recent infant contact. *Horm Behav*. 2007;51:213-220.

Dennis C, McQueen K. The relationship between infant-feeding outcomes and postpartum depression: a qualitative systematic review. *Pediatrics*. 2009;123:e736-e751.

Dobson J. Focus on the family. Radio broadcast August 25, 1999: in response to on-air question. www.ezzo.info/Focus/dobsontranscript.htm. Accessed September 22, 2009.

Doucet S, et al. Differentiation and clinical implications of postpartum depression and postpartum psychosis. *JOGNN* 38:269-79; 2009.

Elfituri A, et al. 18-month progestogen: only contraception during breast-feeding in Libyan women. *PAN Arab Med J*. 2006;5:28-32.

Epigee Women's Health. Types of birth control; 2009. www.epigee.org. Accessed September 25, 2009.

Ezzo G, Bucknam R. *On Becoming Baby Wise: Giving Your Infant the Gift of Nighttime Sleep*, 4th ed. Simi Valley, CA: Parent-Wise Solutions; 2006.

Ezzo G, Ezzo A. *Let the Children Come Along the Infant Way*. Louisiana, MD: Growing Families International; 2002.

Fägerskiöld A. A change in life as experienced by first-time fathers. *Scand J Caring Sci*. 2008;22:64-71.

Fleming A, et al. Testosterone and prolactin are associated with emotional responses to infant cries in new fathers. *Horm Behav*. 2002;42:399-413.

Francis B. Growing Families International: an extreme response to attachment parenting. *Christian Assoc Psych Studies West Newsl*. 1998;25:2, 7.

Friedman S, et al. Child murder committed by severely mentally ill mothers: an examination of mothers found not guilty by reason of insanity. 2005 Honorable Mention/Richard Rosner Award for the best paper by a fellow in forensic psychiatry or forensic psychology. *J Forensic Sci*. 2005;50:1466-1471.

Gale S, Harlow B. Postpartum mood disorders: a review of clinical and epidemiological factors. *J Psychosom Obstet Gynaecol*. 2003;24:257-266.

Gordon A. Differing parenting philosophies. Presented at the La Leche League International Texas Area Conference, Dallas, Texas, June 1999.

Gordon M, Hill S. Is "crying it out" appropriate for infants? A review of the literature on the use of extinction in the first year. Poster presented at the World Infant Mental Health Conference, Paris, France, July 2006. www.infantsleep.org. Accessed September 21, 2009.

Gordon M, Hill S. Parenting advice about sleep: where have we been? Where are we going? Paper presented at: the Society for Research in Development Biennial Conference, April 1-4, 2009; Denver, CO. www.infantsleep.org. Accessed September 21, 2009.

Hall W, Hauck Y. Getting it right: Australian primiparas' views about breastfeeding: a quasi-experimental study. *Int J Nurs Stud*. 2007;44:786-795.

Hanegraaf H. Christian Research Institute: commentary on radio broadcast of The Bible Answer Man, July 28, 1998, October 6, 1998, October 8–9, 1998, October 26, 1998, October 27, 1998, March 25–26, 1999. www.ezzo.info/Rein/prominent.htm. Accessed February 14, 2010.

Hasselmann M. Symptoms of postpartum depression and early interruption of exclusive breastfeeding in the first two months of life. *Cad Saude Publ.* 2008;24(Suppl 2):S341-S352.

Hatcher R, et al. *Contraceptive Technology*, 19th ed. New York: Thomas Reuters; 2008.

Heinowitz J. *Fathering Right from the Start: Straight Talk about Pregnancy, Birth and Beyond.* Novato, CA: New World Library; 2001.

Hight-Laukaran V, et al. Multicenter study of the lactational amenorrhea method (LAM) II: acceptability, utility, and policy implications. *Contraception.* 1997;55:337–346.

Hogg T, Blau M. *Secrets of the Baby Whisperer*, 2nd ed. New York: Ballantine Books; 2005.

Hughes H. Postpartum contraception. *J Fam Health Care.* 2009; 19:9-10, 12.

Hunter B. *The Power of Mother Love.* New York: Waterbrook Press; 1998.

International Planned Parenthood Federation. IMAP statement on hormonal methods of contraception. *IPPF Med Bull.* 2002;36:1-8.

Jolley S, et al. Dysregulation of the hypothalamic-pituitary-adrenal axis in postpartum depression. *Biol Res Nurs.* 2007;8:210-222.

Kaplan P, et al. Infant-directed speech produced by fathers with symptoms of depression: effects on infant associative learning in a conditioned-attention paradigm. *Infant Behav Dev.* 2007;30:535-545.

Kauppi A, et al. Maternal depression and filicide-case study of ten mothers. *Arch Womens Ment Health.* 2008;11:201-206.

Kelsey J. Hormonal contraception and lactation. *J Hum Lact.* 1996;12:315-318.

Kendall-Tackett K. Breastfeeding and the sexual abuse survivor. *J Hum Lact.* 1998;14:125-130.

Kendall-Tackett K. Trauma in the lives of postpartum women: sexual abuse/assault in the lives of childbearing women. Presented at the Hale & Hartmann Lactation Research Conference, Amarillo, Texas, June 5, 2009.

Kendall-Tackett K. *The Hidden Feelings of Motherhood: Coping with Stress, Depression and Burnout*, 2nd ed. Amarillo, TX: Pharmasoft Publishing; 2005.

Kennedy K, et al. Premature introduction of progestin-only contraceptive methods during lactation. *Contraception.* 1997;55:347-350.

Kennedy K, et al. Users' understanding of the lactational amenorrhea method and the occurrence of pregnancy. *J Hum Lact.* 1998;14:209-218.

Kent J. How breastfeeding works. *J Midwifery Women's Health.* 2007;52:564-570.

Kent J, et al. Volume and frequency of breastfeedings and fat content of breast milk throughout the day. *Pediatrics.* 2006;117:e387-e395.

Kippley S. *Breastfeeding and Natural Child Spacing: How Ecological Breastfeeding Spaces Babies.* Raleigh, NC: Lulu.com; 2008a.

Kippley S. *The Seven Standards of Ecological Breastfeeding: The Frequency Factor.* Raleigh, NC: Lulu.com; 2008b.

Kirkengen AL. *Inscribed Bodies: Health Impact of Childhood Sexual Abuse.* Dordrecht, The Netherlands: Kluwer; 2001.

Koetsawang S. The effects of contraceptive methods on the quality and quantity of breast milk. *Int J Gynaecol Obstet.* 1987;25(Suppl):115-127.

Labbok M, et al. Multicenter study of the lactational amenorrhea method (LAM) I: efficacy, duration, and implications for clinical application. *Contraception* 1997;55:327-336.

Labbok M, et al. The lactational amenorrhea method (LAM): a postpartum introductory family planning method with policy and program implications. *Adv Contracept.* 1994; 10:93-109.

Lawrence E, et al. Marital satisfaction across the transition to parenthood. *J Fam Psychol.* 2008;22:41-50.

Lawrence E, et al. Prenatal expectations and marital satisfaction over the transition to parenthood. *J Fam Psychol.* 2007; 21:155-164.

Lawrence R, Lawrence R. *Breastfeeding: A Guide for the Medical Profession,* 6th ed. St. Louis, MO: Elsevier-Mosby; 2005.

Leman K. www.drleman.com. Accessed September 20, 2009.

Littlecrow-Russell S. Time to take a critical look at Depo-Provera. A publication of the population and development program at Hampshire College, July 5, 2000. www.cwpe .org/files/criticallook.pdf. Accessed September 20, 2009.

Ludington-Hoe S, et al. Infant crying: nature, physiologic consequences, and select interventions. *Neonat Netw.* 2002; 21:29-36.

MacArthur J. Grace Community Church: public statement, July 25, 2000. www.ezzo.info/GCC/macarthur.htm. Accessed September 20, 2009.

McNeilly A. Neuroendocrine changes and fertility in breastfeeding women. *Prog Brain Res.* 2001;133:207-214.

Mercer R. A theoretical framework for studying factors that impact on the maternal role. *Nurs Res.* 1981;30:73-77.

Misri S. *Shouldn't I Be Happy? Emotional Problems of Pregnant and Postpartum Women.* New York: Free Press; 2002.

Mitoulas L, et al. Variation in fat, lactose and protein in human milk over 24 h and throughout the first year of lactation. *Br J Nutr.* 2002;88:29-37.

Moody L. Case studies of moms who had problems using Babywise or Preparation for Parenting, 2002. www.angelfire .com/md2/moodyfamily/casestudies.html. Accessed September 20, 2009.

Moore E, et al. Early skin-to-skin contact for mothers and their healthy newborn infants. *Cochrane Database Syst Rev.* CD003519; 2007.

NuvaRing. Consumer information. 2008. www.nuvaring.com. Accessed September 22, 2009.

O'Connor T, Spagnola M. Early stress exposure: concepts, findings, and implications, with particular emphasis on attachment disturbances. *Child Adolescent Psych Mental Health.* 2009;3:24.

O'Malley S. *Are You There Alone? The Unspeakable Crime of Andrea Yates.* New York: Simon & Schuster; 2004.

Otsuka K, et al. The relationship between breastfeeding self-efficacy and perceived insufficient milk among Japanese mothers. *JOGNN.* 2008;37:546-555.

Parent Effectiveness Training. 2009. www.gordontraining.com. Accessed September 20, 2009.

Paulson JF, et al. Individual and combined effects of postpartum depression in mothers and fathers on parenting behavior. *Pediatrics.* 2006;118:659-668.

Plantin L, Daneback K. Parenthood, information and support on the internet. A literature review of research on parents and professionals online. *BMC Fam Pract.* 2009;10:34.

Premberg A, et al. Experiences of the first year as father. *Scand J Caring Sci.* 2008;22:56-63.

Prentice J, et al. The association between reported childhood sexual abuse and breastfeeding initiation. *J Hum Lact.* 2002;18:219-226.

Radwan H, et al. Breast-feeding and lactational amenorrhea in the United Arab Emirates. *J Pediatr Nurs.* 2009;24:62-68.

Randall A, Bodenmann G. The role of stress on close relationships and marital satisfaction. *Clin Psychol Rev.* 2009; 29:105-115.

Rivera-Rivera L, et al. Physical and sexual abuse during childhood and revictimization during adulthood in Mexican women. *Salud Publica Mex.* 2006;48(Suppl 2):S268-S278.

Rodriguez M, Kaunitz A. An evidence-based approach to postpartum use of depot medroxyprogesterone acetate in breastfeeding women. *Contraception.* 2009;80:4-6.

Romero-Gutiérrez G, et al. Actual use of the lactational amenorrhoea method. *Eur J Contracept Reprod Health Care.* 2007;12:340-344.

Ruppen W, et al. Incidence of epidural hematoma, infection, and neurologic injury in obstetric patients with epidural analgesia/anesthesia. *Anesthesiology.* 2006;105:394-399.

Schnyder S, et al. Estrogen treatment induces MLL aberrations in human lymphoblastoid cells. *Leuk Res.* 2009;33:1400-1404.

Schulz M, et al. Promoting healthy beginnings: a randomized controlled trial of a preventive intervention to preserve marital quality during the transition to parenthood. *J Consult Clin Psychol.* 2006;74:20-31.

Sears W. Fathering. 2006. www.askdrsears.com. Accessed September 21, 2009.

Sears W. www.askdrsears.com. Accessed September 21, 2009.

Sears W, et al. *Becoming a Father: How to Nurture and Enjoy Your Family,* 2nd ed. Schaumburg, IL: La Leche League International; 2003.

Shaaban O, Glasier A. Pregnancy during breastfeeding in rural Egypt. *Contraception.* 2008;77:350-354.

Shaamash A, et al. A comparative study of the levonorgestrel-releasing intrauterine system Mirena versus the Copper T380A intrauterine device during lactation: breast-feeding performance, infant growth and infant development. *Contraception.* 2005;72:346-351.

Sivin I, et al. Contraceptives for lactating women: a comparative trial of a progesterone-releasing vaginal ring and the copper T 380A IUD. *Contraception.* 1997;55:225-232.

Smith L. *Impact of Birthing Practices on Breastfeeding,* 2nd ed. Sudbury, MA: Jones and Bartlett; 2009.

Sperlich M, Seng J. *Survivor Moms: Women's Stories of Birthing, Mothering and Healing after Sexual Abuse.* Eugene, OR: Motherbaby Press; 2008.

Spinelli M. Postpartum psychosis: detection of risk and management. *Am J Psychiatry.* 2009;166:405-408.

Subhani A, et al. Duration of lactational amenorrhoea: a hospital based survey in district Abbottabad. *J Ayub Med Coll Abbottabad.* 2008;20:122-124.

Systematic Training for Effective Parenting (STEP). Step into parenting. 2009. www.steppublishers.com. Accessed September 20, 2009.

Taguchi H. Maternal filicide in Japan: analyses of 96 cases and future directions for prevention. *Seishin Shinkeigaku Zasshi.* 2007;109:110-127.

Taneepanichskul S, et al. Effects of the etonogestrel-releasing implant Implanon and a nonmedicated intrauterine device on the growth of breast-fed infants. *Contraception.* 2006; 73:368-371.

Tankeyoon M, et al. Effects of hormonal contraceptives on milk volume and infant growth. WHO Special Programme of Research, Development and Research Training in Human Reproduction. Task Force on Oral Contraceptives. *Contraception.* 1984;30:505-522.

Terner K, Miller E. More than a parenting ministry: the cultic characteristics of Growing Families International. *Christ Res J.* 1998;20. www.equip.org/articles/the-cultic-characteristics-of-growing-families-international. Accessed September 20, 2009.

Tilley I, et al. Breastfeeding and contraception use among women with unplanned pregnancies less than 2 years after delivery. *Int J Gynaecol Obstet.* 2009;105:127-130.

Truitt S, et al. Combined hormonal versus nonhormonal versus progestin-only contraception in lactation. *Cochrane Database Syst Rev.* 2003:CD003988.

Twenge J. *Generation Me.* New York: Free Press (Simon & Schuster); 2006.

U.S. Food and Drug Administration. FDA approves update to label on birth control patch. January 18, 2008. www.fda.gov/NewsEvents/Newsroom/PressAnnouncements/2008/ucm116842.htm. Accessed September 21, 2009.

Valdimarsdóttir U, et al. Psychotic illness in first-time mothers with no previous psychiatric hospitalizations: a population-based study. *PLoS Med.* 2009;6:e13.

Visness C, et al. The duration and character of postpartum bleeding among breastfeeding women. *Obstet Gynecol.* 1997;89:159-163.

Webb C. Is the Babywise method right for you? What you should know about Babywise and Growing Kids God's Way. *Tulsa Kids;* Tulsa, OK: TK Publishing, Inc.; July 2003.

Williams N. Counseling challenges: helping mothers handle conflicting information. *Leaven.* 1998;34:19-20.

Williams N. Dancing with differences: helping mothers handle conflicting information, including scheduled feeding and sleep training. Presented at the La Leche League International Conference, Orlando, Florida, July 5, 1999.

World Health Organization (WHO). *Medical Eligibility Criteria for Contraceptive Use,* 3rd ed. Geneva: World Health Organization; 2004.

World Health Organization (WHO). Violence and injury prevention and disability. Prevention of child maltreatment; 2009. www.who.int/violence_injury_prevention/violence/activities/child_maltreatment/en/index.html. Accessed September 25, 2009.

Special Counseling Circumstances

Lactation consultants meet women from many walks of life and with many different lifestyles. Clients range from low income, minority, and non-native speaking to wealthy, highly educated professionals. Each woman has commonalities in wanting to breastfeed and benefiting from sensitive support. Tailoring your approach and counseling style to women's circumstances helps support them in their specific options, decisions, and challenges. Breastfeeding is difficult when a woman encounters negative reactions from significant people in her life, including employers. Single, adolescent, and low-income mothers face special challenges. Meeting the needs of women from other cultures and countries requires awareness of and respect for their traditions and beliefs. These issues are all explored in this chapter, as well as the important role of support groups for breastfeeding women.

～ Key Terms

Acculturated
Anticipatory guidance
Culturally competent care
Lifestyle
Mother-to-mother
  support group
Opposition to
  breastfeeding
Outreach counseling

～ Mother's Lifestyle

Some women have factors in their lives that detract from breastfeeding and interfere with building understanding and rapport with caregivers. Mothers who live in the city differ in their frame of reference from those who live in suburbia or a more rural setting. Low-income families and those from other cultures may have values and health practices that differ from your own. It is important that you not make unfounded assumptions about others' lifestyle choices. You cannot presume that a mother is married or that the baby's father is living with the mother and baby, or even that there is enough food for the family to eat. Single-parent households are common, and a breastfeeding woman who is solely responsible for her baby's care may have many challenges in her life.

Women with unwanted or unplanned pregnancies are less likely to breastfeed. Analyses of 18 countries found a significant association between unintended pregnancies and less likelihood of prolonged breastfeeding (Hromi-Fiedler & Pérez-Escamilla, 2006). Domestic abuse, or intimate partner violence, is much more common than caregivers might believe. Violence toward pregnant women significantly increases risk for low-birth-weight infants, preterm delivery, and neonatal death; it also affects breastfeeding initiation and duration (Sarkar, 2008). Intimate partner violence continues into the postpartum period, and adolescents may be at even higher risk than their adult counterparts for domestic violence (Chambliss, 2008). A teenage mother usually is coping with single parenthood as well as normal adolescent changes. All these circumstances present special counseling challenges. Your approach and availability to the mother can greatly influence her mastery of the situation.

Having realistic expectations for each mother and her goals for breastfeeding is important. Beliefs and practices vary widely among cultural groups. Breastfeeding, especially exclusive breastfeeding, may be more than some mothers can handle or even desire. Learn about cultural differences and trends in your community so that you can respond to the individual needs of each mother. Remaining flexible and objective in your approach helps mothers fit breastfeeding into their lifestyles. By working in partnership with the mother, you can develop innovative approaches for providing accurate information and support to all women.

∿ Opposition to Breastfeeding

Despite the strong endorsement of breastfeeding by governments, the American Academy of Pediatrics (2005), the World Health Organization (1989), and other major health organizations, mothers often receive questions and comments that prompt them to explain and defend their decision to breastfeed. Such remarks can undermine a mother's confidence and cause her to doubt her decision or her capability to breastfeed. Most of those who comment do not truly oppose breastfeeding; they simply do not understand it. When the mother is confident in her decision to breastfeed, she may be able to educate some of these people and familiarize them with the feeding patterns of a breastfed baby.

Opposition to breastfeeding often manifests itself as subtle undermining of a mother's efforts rather than blatant remarks. Healthcare professionals and lay persons alike, quick to state that breastfeeding is "the best" infant food, often point to breastfeeding as the cause when the baby cries or the mother expresses a concern. The mother is encouraged to "rest" and feed her baby with a bottle, implying that breastfeeding and bottle feeding are interchangeable and that breastfeeding is exhausting. Mothers benefit from your education and support to get them through challenging times when doubts surface that undermine their confidence.

A mother may receive opposition from strangers, friends, her employer, colleagues, coworkers, her caregiver, the baby's grandparents and other relatives, and even the baby's father. It is more difficult for the mother to cope with objections from people close to her. It is no surprise that mothers who have a strong support system for breastfeeding have better outcomes (Souza et al., 2009; Britton, 2007). You can help a mother identify the various breastfeeding supporters within her network of friends and family. Their support helps her through the challenges she may face when others oppose or question her choice to breastfeed. You can also provide positive support, suggest ways for her to manage the opposition, and make an extra effort to boost her morale and self-confidence.

Strangers

When a mother is confident and knowledgeable about her decision to breastfeed, she is less likely to yield to the opinions or rude remarks of a stranger. To minimize the potential for such comments, she can ensure that she is discreet when she breastfeeds in public. She can wear clothing that allows easy access to her breast while still providing coverage. Practicing discreet breastfeeding in front of a mirror will help her become confident with techniques that work for her. Discreet breastfeeding does not mean disguising the fact that the mother is breastfeeding. Breastfeeding in public normalizes breastfeeding and helps increase cultural acceptance.

Friends

Opposition from friends may prove more difficult for the mother to handle. Depending on the nature of the friendship, a mother may attempt to educate a friend who opposes breastfeeding. She needs to find a comfort level with such a friend to maintain both their relationship and her breastfeeding. Developing friendships and relationships with people who are supportive of breastfeeding or who are breastfeeding mothers themselves can help her become more confident with breastfeeding (Rossman, 2007; Ekström & Nissen, 2006).

Employer

Maternal employment, the most common reason for milk expression, is also a major barrier to continued breastfeeding (Labiner-Wolfe et al., 2008). Early return to work is a key barrier to both breastfeeding initiation and duration (Chuang et al., 2010). When mothers work full-time, employers play a critical role in their breastfeeding success (Mills, 2009). Lack of support for breastfeeding employees is common. Many women who return to work while they are breastfeeding experience negative reactions from their employers. A Cochrane review found no trials that evaluated the effectiveness of workplace interventions in promoting breastfeeding among women returning to paid work after the birth of their child. The impact of such intervention on process outcomes is also unknown (Abdulwadud & Snow, 2007).

A mother's ability to negotiate with her employer for time to pump her milk may vary. A low-income hourly employee has less power and voice in the workplace than a senior partner in a law firm who has a private office and positional power. However, high education and income are no guarantees, either. One anesthesiologist reported weaning her baby by 5 months for the same reason many unskilled, hourly workers wean: no private place to pump, coworker criticism, and few breaks for doing so.

A mother may reduce the stress and tension of an unsupportive work environment by speaking frankly with her employer about her plans to breastfeed. She can discuss any special needs she has, such as breastfeeding her baby at work or expressing milk for her baby, as well as her desire to accommodate breastfeeding after returning to work.

The mother may need to convince her employer that any needs related to breastfeeding will not interfere with her job performance. She can point out that the health benefits of breastfeeding result in less time off and less use of health benefits (U.S. Department of Health and Human Services [USDHHS], 2008a). Employers who have had previous experience with breastfeeding employees often react more positively to combining employment with breastfeeding (Dunn et al., 2004). Employer support has risen to about 26 percent of employers offering some sort of lactation support program, up from 19 percent in 2005 (Shellenbarger, 2007). You can work to increase employer support by educating your community about breastfeeding's importance to infant and maternal health.

You will want to stress the implications and benefits for the organizations (Mills, 2009). Employers are more responsive when they recognize breastfeeding's importance and the cost savings to the company (National Business Group on Health, 2009; USDHHS, 2008b). The monograph *Advancing Women's Health: Health Plans' Innovative Programs in Breastfeeding Promotion* describes model programs and promotion within the insurance industry. It explores eight organizations that promote breastfeeding coverage and provide benefits to breastfeeding employees (American Association of Health Plans, 2001).

Many women are uncomfortable approaching their employer, especially if they work in a male-dominated profession or have little job security. They may worry that they are jeopardizing their position with such a "feminine" request. These mothers need to consider which aspects of the job are compatible with breastfeeding. They may find websites, forums, books and other media for employed breastfeeding mothers helpful. You can encourage them to learn their legal rights and how to approach their employer before the baby arrives. Be sure to address employment issues in prenatal education classes as part of your anticipatory guidance.

In some cases a woman may be unable to resolve her employer's lack of support. If the situation undermines her breastfeeding, she may need to reevaluate her priorities and motives regarding working and breastfeeding. She can refer unreasonable and unfair treatment by an employer to her human resources department, local labor relations board, or, in the United States, the Equal Employment Opportunity Commission. Some work environments are not compatible with breastfeeding. You can assist the mother in developing a plan within the parameters of her employment. See Chapter 24 for further discussion of combining breastfeeding with employment.

Physician

It is often difficult for a mother when her physician does not support breastfeeding. Women value their physicians' opinions and trust their judgments about their family's health care. A physician who does not seem committed to breastfeeding may be unsupportive and unintentionally give misinformation. If the mother has good rapport with her physician, she may be able to resolve differences about breastfeeding. If she finds it difficult to work with her physician, she may need to consider whether this relationship is in the best interests of her and her baby.

Well-meaning physicians may not realize that their remarks to a woman can undermine her confidence. A mother with an unsupportive physician needs a lot of extra contact and confidence building. Anticipatory guidance will help this mother through times of change and uncertainty. A perceived lack of support by a physician may actually stem from lack of knowledge and experience with breastfeeding. Giving her research articles to share with her physician can reinforce her efforts and raise the physician's level of appreciation for the importance of breastfeeding and understanding of breastfeeding care. See Chapter 2 for further discussion of the relationship between physicians and mothers with respect to breastfeeding.

Grandparents and Other Relatives

Throughout the world the baby's grandmother has a pivotal role in a mother's breastfeeding experience. This role has been studied from South Asia (Ingram, 2003) to Brazil (Giugliani et al., 2008) to China (Raven et al., 2007) and points in between. A new mother often turns to her own mother for encouragement and wisdom as she assumes her parenting role. Breastfeeding is a part of feminine identity. Women from the 1940s on were discouraged from breastfeeding for a variety of poor reasons, which remain part of many grandmothers' understanding of the childbearing continuum. It is often difficult for their daughters to disregard these beliefs without feeling guilty.

Turnbull-Plaza et al. (2006) found in Mexico that the maternal grandmother, the physician, and the paternal grandmother had the greatest positive influence on a mother's exclusive breastfeeding. Ironically, these are the same people who also most influence breastfeeding's interruption. The paternal grandmother also plays a powerful role in many traditional cultures, such as Malawi (Bezner et al., 2008).

A grandmother may see the choice to breastfeed by her daughter as a reflection on her own parenting decisions. Grandparents often sympathize with the strains of early parenting, such as lack of sleep, coping with crying, and physical recovery from birth. They may perceive that breastfeeding increases these strains and may therefore encourage the mother to reduce stress by supplementing breastfeeding or weaning. A mother who receives negative comments from her mother or mother-in-law needs to understand the grandmother's concern for both the mother and baby. She may not want her daughter to experience the same disappointment and failure that she did. On the other hand, she may be envious that her daughter can do something she was not able to do.

New mothers have described a need for their own mothers to value breastfeeding and to provide loving encouragement. The researchers term this "grandmother breastfeeding advocacy" (Grassley & Eschiti, 2008). Mothers also needed their own mothers to acknowledge the barriers to breastfeeding, to confront myths they might believe, and to learn and accept current breastfeeding knowledge, especially if the grandmothers did not breastfeed.

You can help a mother recognize that her own mother did the best she could with the information and support that was available to her at the time. She can gently explain that she understands that her mother did her best and that she is now doing the same today for her child with current information. The grandmother may not understand the typical feeding pattern of a breastfed baby. She may worry that her grandchild's frequent feedings indicate inadequate nourishment. She may not know that loose stools are normal for breastfeeding babies and may believe it indicates diarrhea. Remarking about her concerns can undermine the new mother's confidence and come through as lack of support.

You can encourage the mother to be patient and understanding of any relative, especially a grandparent, whose opposition stems from a genuine concern for her and her baby. She can attempt to educate the grandparents and enlist their support by giving them literature. She might ask the grandmother to accompany her to a breastfeeding support group meeting. At times a mother may simply need to accept the grandmother's point of view and not allow it to affect her breastfeeding. She can stay firm in her resolve while remaining kind and considerate.

Health, breastfeeding, and grandparenting organizations have information geared directly to grandparents (Texas Dept. State Health Services, 2008). There are many Internet and media resources, including grandparenting blogs (Olds, 2008). You can direct mothers to media and print resources with current recommendations. They may also address past beliefs or practices in a respectful way. Recommendations may include:

- Babies should be breastfed for at least 1 year or longer.
- Putting a baby to bed with a bottle is unsafe and causes tooth decay.
- Feeding cereal through the bottle can cause the baby to choke.
- Feeding solid foods to babies before they are 4 to 6 months old can cause health problems.
- Placing the baby on his or her back to sleep helps reduce the risk of sudden infant death syndrome.
- Babies should not be exposed to secondhand smoke.

Occasionally, a grandmother may be overly helpful or overly controlling. She may pressure a mother to breastfeed who may not actually want to do so. If you encounter an overbearing grandmother in the hospital, you can encourage nurses to limit visitors. If you are visiting the mother in her home and the grandmother is dominating the conversation, you might ask her to help with the baby or with other children. You may need to simply state that you and the mother need to meet privately. The Health Insurance Portability and Accountability Act (HIPAA) does not permit you to discuss the mother's situation with her in front of others unless she gives verbal permission.

When the grandmother is not present, you can ask the mother how she feels and what her breastfeeding goals are. If the mother tells you that she does not want to breastfeed or that she would rather bottle feed, your role is to support the mother, not add to any coercion in her life. You can teach her about using "I feel...when" messages to communicate her feelings. Sometimes by empowering the mother to stand up for herself, you can empower her to choose freely to breastfeed, pump, combine breastfeeding and bottle feeding, or to formula feed, if that is her desire. Having the skills to help a mother learn to express her desires (even if those are not the choices you would like to see her make) is an important part of being a healthcare giver in general and a lactation consultant specifically.

Baby's Father

It is especially difficult for a mother to encounter opposition from the baby's father. A father's preference typically is significant in the mother's choice for infant feeding. Demographics show that low socioeconomic status of the father is associated with bottle feeding rather than breastfeeding (Glenn & Quillin, 2007). Thus his opposition weighs greatly on her decision to initiate or continue breastfeeding (Kong & Lee, 2004; Rose et al., 2004; Chang & Chan, 2003). A father may seem unsupportive of breastfeeding because he wants his child to be independent and worries that breastfeeding will make the baby too dependent on the mother. It can be helpful for him to learn that meeting a child's present needs actually leads to greater independence in the future. Sharing information with the baby's father about the importance of breastfeeding provides a springboard for discussing the mother's need for his support and their mutual need for support from each other.

Open communication between the father and mother about parenting may improve the couple's long-term relationship. Men who feel supported by their partners in their role as father are more sensitive and playful with their children than are fathers who are involved in less satisfying relationships (Shannon et al., 2006). If the father believes breastfeeding interferes with the couple's sex life, you can communicate to the parents that having a baby changes all parents' sex lives, no matter how they feed their baby.

The father's opposition may stem from the same concerns as those of grandparents and other relatives—the health and well-being of his partner and baby. You can point out the positive aspects of this concern and suggest ways for the mother to reassure and educate the father that breastfeeding is beneficial to the entire family and that *not* breastfeeding increases health risks for both the mother and baby (Ip et al., 2009). Financial costs of artificial feeding are also a consideration, both the product purchase and the increased healthcare costs.

Since the 1970s there has been a growing expectation that the father be involved in the day-to-day care of his children (McKellar et al., 2008). However, many fathers feel unsure of how to embrace parenthood. The father–infant relationship is influenced by the parents' relationship as well as the father's psychological well-being (Condon, 2006). Involving fathers in breastfeeding support is a part of changing attitudes toward breastfeeding in communities where formula feeding is seen as the normal way to feed a baby (Ingram & Johnson, 2009; Ingram, 2008). If the father feels left out of his baby's care because he is not able to participate in feeding, the mother can suggest ways for him to be involved other than with feedings. She can remind him that most babies start solid foods at 6 months and he can enjoy feeding the baby then. See Chapter 19 for more discussion of the father's interactions.

Western culture promotes women's breasts in a sexual manner in all forms of media (Palmer, 2009). As a man's role changes from mate to father, it may be difficult for him to regard his partner's breasts as having a nonsexual role. The father may subconsciously believe that the baby is invading his territory. The biological purpose of the female breast has always been to nurture babies. You can encourage the couple to discuss these issues with sensitivity and understanding. Some couples respond well to humor. Others might be offended by levity.

As the baby grows older a previously supportive father may question the need or appropriateness of continuing to breastfeed. He may worry about a son's loss of masculinity due to an overdependence on the mother. The mother can remind the father about the health benefits of breastfeeding for their baby at any age, both nutritionally and developmentally. Breastfeeding is dose dependent, with longer duration providing greater pro-

tection against diseases (Brugman et al., 2009; Khan et al., 2009). The mother can help her partner understand their baby's needs and her desire to continue breastfeeding. Networking with families of older nursing babies and children enables the father to meet breastfeeding families and find it more acceptable. See Chapter 19 for further discussion of the father's role in supporting breastfeeding.

A mother who cannot resolve the father's opposition to breastfeeding needs a great deal of support and will benefit from a breastfeeding support group and continued contact with a lactation consultant when possible. If she decides to wean her baby because of the father's opposition, your role is to accept this decision and to help her wean gradually and with love. Help the father understand the need for her to wean slowly to avoid mastitis. Avoid placing yourself in the middle of a conflict between a mother and an unsupportive partner. You can listen, suggest educational resources for the father, and offer extra support and encouragement. It is important that you help the mother cope with her situation without judging or becoming enmeshed in any conflicts.

If a father seems jealous, be aware that although some women interpret jealousy as a sign of love, jealousy is a marker for intimate partner violence (Power et al., 2006). The issues in this relationship may be far more problematic than the breastfeeding education or problem you may be helping with on the surface. Print and Internet resources provide avenues to improve the health of the parents' relationship. You need to be discreet, tactful, and sensitive to how and if you present these resources. Moe (2007) found that unconditional and empathetic institutional and/or social support helped women to continue resisting the coercive control tactics of their partners. You can be a part of that unconditional and empathetic support.

Because of the intimate nature of your role with mothers, you are in a unique position to witness a couple's interaction. If you see bruises or unexplained injuries, suspect domestic violence, or witness the father verbally ridiculing or abusing the mother, you can mention this privately to the mother. Provide her with hotline numbers and local community resources, such as battered women's shelters or safe houses (see the resources in Appendix H). If she denies the situation or makes excuses, you can gently reflect what you see to her and encourage her to talk with her caregiver or a counselor about what is occurring. If you suspect the baby or other children are being abused, you are legally required to report it to the appropriate authorities in most countries.

Mother's Confidence

Maternal confidence is a significant predictor of the duration and level of breastfeeding (Britton & Britton, 2008; Kang et al., 2008; Ystrom, 2008; Noel-Weiss, 2006). A mother who is confident in herself and in her commitment to breastfeed will continue despite setbacks or problems. Likewise, there is a correlation between low parental confidence and a high perception of milk insufficiency (Gatti, 2008; Otsuka et al., 2008). Enhancing a mother's feelings of self-efficacy and increasing her confidence in her ability to breastfeed help her persevere if she encounters difficulties (Hegney et al., 2008; Memmott & Bonuck, 2006).

A positive breastfeeding experience is very empowering to women. Prenatal and postnatal care needs to go beyond education to encompass enhancing the mother's confidence regarding breastfeeding (Elliott & Gunaratnam, 2009). You can help build the mother's confidence by pointing out positive aspects of her relationship with her baby and praising her for how well her baby is growing. Positive, sincere feedback helps the mother recognize that she is doing well at mothering and validates her choice to breastfeed.

∼ Low-Income Mothers

The income level of many mothers in your care may be near or below the poverty level. This is especially the case if you work in a public health clinic or hospital or a Women, Infants, and Children (WIC) office. Poverty is often associated with lower self-esteem, limited expectations, and lower educational and occupational levels. Low-income women may live in an area in which many unfavorable conditions exist. They may face the challenge of overcrowding, run-down housing, crime, and inadequate community services. They may experience physical and mental health problems, broken families, relocation, isolation, alienation, or language differences.

Low-income women may not attend childbirth classes because of cost, availability, or lack of interest. In one study attendance at childbirth classes was associated with a 75 percent increase in the odds that a child would be breastfed. It also cited significant sociodemographic disparities in attendance at childbirth classes (Lu et al., 2003).

The mother may have received prenatal care in one place and delivered her baby in another. She may seek attention for her sick children from a clinic or emergency room. Her well children may receive no preventive health care. You can inform her of local health services and suggest that she take advantage of programs that assist low-income populations with health services and supplemental foods. For example, Healthy Start participants' rates of ever breastfeeding (72 percent) and putting infants to sleep on their backs (70 percent) were significantly higher than nonparticipants (Rosenbach et al., 2009). In the United States the WIC program provides these services. See Chapter 2 for further discussion about

the U.S. WIC program and the Canada Prenatal Nutrition Program.

Breastfeeding rates in 1999 through 2006 were significantly higher among women with higher income (74 percent) compared with those who had lower income (57 percent) (National Center for Health Statistics [NCHS], 2008). Lower income is associated with a shorter duration of breastfeeding as well (Wallby, 2009).

Psychosocial Issues

Other barriers can impede a low-income mother's commitment to initiate or continue breastfeeding. She may lack support and accurate information, and may even face challenges related to survival (England et al., 2003). Low-income mothers often hold two jobs and have little discretionary time or money. Life can be a series of crises. Statistically, substance abuse and alcoholism are high among this population. One study showed that 25 percent of at-risk women did not breastfeed or quit breastfeeding because of the fear of passing "dangerous things" to their infants through their milk (England et al., 2003). In a survey of low-income formula feeders, 84 percent knew that breastmilk was better for their babies but chose not to breastfeed due to concerns about pain, smoking, and work (Noble et al., 2003).

Family and community support for breastfeeding can be lacking in a low-income community. Low-income mothers often believe they cannot control their lives and surrounding, and may feel detached from society. A sense of despair or stress can prevail. Inadequacies prevail in income, child care, education, preventive health services, and lifespan. Their lives are often saturated with violence, which places them as unsafe even in their own homes (Chin & Solomonik, 2009). The mother may believe that her immediate circle of relationships is not comfortable or supportive. She might distrust you because her life is insecure and you represent the "system" that has been unkind to her. She may consider breastfeeding to be one more stress in her life and may worry that breastfeeding will be one more failure in her life. She also may be unaware of the many community resources available to low-income women.

Decision to Breastfeed

Research has shown that a low-income woman is more likely to choose breastfeeding if she has a higher level of education (Singh et al., 2007), is married (Khoury et al., 2005), or has greater self-efficacy (McCarter-Spaulding & Gore, 2009). The greatest motivator seems to be a support person she respects who had a positive breastfeeding experience. Access to support and accurate information play vital roles in her breastfeeding experience. Her perception of family and peer support is another factor, particularly from another woman with whom she is close.

Medical personnel, respected for their expertise, can be instrumental in encouraging low-income women to continue breastfeeding. You can help these women recognize that babies are healthier, and therefore happier, when their mothers breastfeed. Let the mother know that more women breastfeed now, so she will not feel that she is different. Praise her for making an intelligent decision based on sound medical fact rather than fads or advertising claims.

Introduction of artificial baby milk, particularly through the hospital, undermines a mother's confidence in her ability to breastfeed. A low-income woman may be especially susceptible to bottle feeding messages. She may believe that a substitute is equally good or perhaps better because it is more "scientific." There may be little family or community support for breastfeeding compared with bottle feeding. The use of infant formula is implicitly advocated when it is given by postpartum hospital staff in gift packs. Receiving 'free' formula negatively affects breastfeeding rates (Kaplan & Graff, 2008; Rosenberg et al., 2008).

Your support during the mother's hospital stay and the first week postpartum can be critical to her breastfeeding. More than in other populations, a low-income woman may find that breastfeeding builds her self-confidence and self-esteem. Realizing that breastfeeding contributes to her child's well-being and that she accomplished it through her own resources enhances her self-image. This can improve her parenting skills and encourage her to share her success with others. Some women report that child rearing was the experience that enabled them to become active learners, as they became advocates for their children's health. Self-esteem is associated with higher rates of exclusive breastfeeding (Britton & Britton, 2008).

Peer Support

Breastfeeding rates among low-income women increase when their local healthcare clinics expand breastfeeding support to include classes, one-on-one instruction, and peer counselors. Mothers have significantly higher breastfeeding initiation rates when they receive a combination of peer counseling support through prenatal home visits, daily perinatal visits, postpartum home visits, and telephone counseling as needed. They reportedly breastfeed exclusively longer, remain amenorrheic longer, and their infants have fewer diarrheal episodes (Anderson et al., 2005). Breastfeeding interventions with a component of lay support (such as peer support or peer counseling) are more effective than usual care in increasing the short-term breastfeeding rate (Chung et al., 2008).

Peer counselor support has a positive effect on breastfeeding initiation and duration, as does the mother's choice to breastfeed exclusively. A successful example is the Rush Mothers' Milk Club, a neonatal intensive care unit support group for mothers of preterm infants. This club has had outstanding success at helping primarily low-income women pump for their preterm babies. Many have gone on to breastfeed directly (Meier et al., 2004). A study of peer support for African American women indicated that women who attended support groups were more than twice as likely to intend to breastfeed compared with women who did not (Mickens, 2009).

Although breastfeeding discussion groups can serve as an effective teaching arena, attendance may be minimal for low-income women. Many women are overwhelmed with work, child care, and obtaining the necessities of life. Adding a class to the mother's load may be more than she can handle. Those who are receptive are more likely to attend meetings in surroundings they find comfortable such as a private residence, church, or community center. When participants have a major role in planning and organizing such meetings, they feel part of the process. They can also determine the day, time, and topics that are most relevant to them.

A low-income woman may be very isolated, with no support system and no acquaintances who breastfed. Discussion groups with other mothers who face the same challenges can provide the peer support she needs to succeed and help build trust in your services. To make the meetings enjoyable, keep presentations short and focused. Address issues that are relevant to the mother's needs, using a casual, informal approach that encourages discussion.

Teaching and Support Strategies

When a mother is in crisis, you need to put aside theoretical and background information for the moment and first concentrate on the problem at hand. Adopt an approach that accounts for unchangeable factors such as personality or the limitations of her lifestyle. Suggestions need to be practical rather than general. Simply advising that she nurse her baby more often will not be as useful as helping her figure out times and ways she can do it. Help her with practical solutions to improve nutrition for herself and her family. Refer her to a local WIC clinic or food bank for nutritious foods to supplement her diet.

A low-income mother's literacy level could impede her ability to absorb information. Offer attractive, simply written brochures with illustrations that cover only the essential points she needs to know. Make sure the reading level of the material is appropriate, being sensitive to visual images and the amount of words on each page. If too many words make a brochure overwhelming, she may not read or absorb the information.

When teaching the mother about breastfeeding techniques, reinforce verbal explanations with visual aids.

Provide her with a checklist of the suggestions you discussed as a reminder. If you are assisting her over the phone, reinforce the basic points of your conversation. Try to get some feedback from the mother to indicate that she has understood your message and will act on your suggestions. Make sure she understands the consequences of her practices, and be patient and persevering in areas of importance. The mother and baby will both benefit from your sincerity and concern.

Make sure women know when you are available and how to contact you. Reach out to them in their neighborhoods through community bulletin boards, clinics, and other public places. If you provide home visits, it is important that you be conscious of safety issues. Low-income homes are often in high-risk areas. Plan visits during daylight hours. Leave behind information with a colleague or family member that includes where you will visit, times you expect to arrive and leave, and the route you will take. A map or GPS and a cell phone are essential when visiting a client's home. Recognize that circumstances may make it unsafe for you to visit a mother's home alone. In this case arrange to have someone accompany you on the visit or meet with the mother in a different location. Be sensitive and tactful when you discuss these arrangements with the mother to avoid offending her.

∿ Single Mothers

A mother may have sole responsibility for her baby because of divorce, separation, death of her partner, a choice to remain unmarried, or a situation that requires the baby's father to be away from home for extended periods. The number of single mothers has increased dramatically over the past several decades. All measures of childbearing by unmarried women increased in the United States to historic levels in 2007, with 39.7 percent (over 1.7 million) of all births (over 4.3 million) to unmarried women—a 26 percent increase over the previous 5 years. Among women aged 20 to 24 years, 60 percent of births were to unmarried women (NCHS, 2009b).

In 2007 nearly one-third of children in the United States (22 million children) were living with one parent, usually their mother (Kids Count Data Center, 2009). The share of children in one-parent families has nearly tripled since 1970, when the rate was 11 percent (Amato, 2008). Low-income children and children of color are most affected. In 2007, 65 percent of non-Hispanic black children, 49 percent of Native American children, and 37 percent of Hispanic children lived in one-parent households (Kids Count Data Center, 2009).

A single mother may live alone or may reside with her parents or a friend. Each situation presents unique challenges. There are over 10.4 million single-mother families in the United States alone (U.S. Census Bureau, 2007).

These women juggle one or more jobs, schooling or training, household responsibilities, and parenting. In 2007, 32 percent of single-parent families with related children had incomes below the poverty line, compared with 6 percent of married families (Kids Count Data Center, 2009). When economic hardship and stressful living conditions are present, children are at greater risk of poor achievement as well as behavioral, psychological, and health problems (Amato & Maynard, 2006).

A mother who lives with her parents can benefit from their support and security. At the same time she may struggle to maintain her identity as an adult and a mother and to preserve an identity as a family unit for herself and her baby. It can be difficult for two family units to live harmoniously in the same home. The mother may receive criticism about her parenting, and other family members may discipline her child. Lack of privacy can interfere with her breastfeeding. Many mothers view their return home as a temporary situation until they secure other living arrangements.

When a mother's single status has resulted from divorce or the death of a spouse, emotional stress and other demands of the aftermath can result in missed feedings and lowered milk production. Her baby may tune in to her emotional state and want to nurse more frequently. Breastfeeding can provide comfort to both the mother and baby in such times of stress. Any increase in frequency helps maintain milk production as well.

A single mother will benefit from your support since she may have little or no support system among friends and family and no one with whom she can share concerns or parenting responsibilities. She may attempt to be a "supermom" as she tries to meet her baby's needs along with those of everyday life. This leaves little time for herself. She can compromise by doing simple things, such as taking a walk with her baby in a backpack or stroller or exercising with other mothers and babies. Her nutritional status may be affected because of a lack of desire or time to prepare well-balanced meals. Single mothers are likely to appreciate your care and concern. They can also contact a local Parents Without Partners or other support group. Many churches have single-parent ministries that offer food assistance, free automobile care, parenting classes, and childcare services.

∿ Teen Mothers

The United States continues to have the highest rate of teen pregnancy in the world, though teen birth rates have declined globally. The U.S. teenage pregnancy rate dropped 40 percent from 1990 to 2005, reaching an historic low of 7 percent of women aged 15 to 19 years before creeping up again in 2006 and 2007 (NCHS, 2009a). Twenty-three percent of unmarried births (over 394,368) in 2007 were to teenagers (NCHS, 2009b). Rates fell much more for younger than for older teenagers (NCHS, 2009b). Some teens breastfeed, although rates are lower for teen mothers than for adults, partly because of lack of knowledge.

It is important to recognize that many young people becoming parents today lack active guidance from parents and other adults (Parker & Williams, 2000). Figure 20.1 identifies common reasons teens become pregnant. Most pregnant teens do not marry the father of their baby, because they do not feel pressured socially to have a mate or a father for their babies. The overwhelming majority of births to teenagers are to unmarried women (NCHS, 2009b). They may not complete high school because of the demands on their time. They may be unable to care for their babies because they lack the skill or income. They often have no job skills and are dependent financially on their families and society. Young mothers wish to be treated as adults and do not respond well to lecturing, advice, or a patronizing manner that suggests an adult–child relationship. They need you to listen to their concerns and respond as you would with an older mother.

A Brazilian multidisciplinary group demonstrated the value of interventions for teen mothers (Oliva et al., 2008). They provided integral support during pregnancy and medical follow-up for the mother and child after birth. The teens had a good social network, which included support from both family and fathers of the infants. They considered themselves good mothers and felt happier after their maternity experience. They demonstrated responsibility in family planning and correct contraceptive use, with low levels of repeat pregnancy. Almost half of the mothers were employed, and 24 percent returned to their education. The children of mothers receiving this approach to care were breastfed longer and had greater vaccination coverage than the average for the area (Oliva et al., 2008).

Approaching a teen mother sensitively and respectfully enables you to be a positive influence in her life. You can empower her to form her own individuality, take ownership of her life, acquire her maternal role, and learn to advocate for her baby. Because she is in the process of learning to think abstractly, it is normal for her adolescent focus to be self-centered. Talking to a teen mother about the benefits of breastfeeding for her (or the risks of not breastfeeding) may carry more weight than a litany of information about the baby's health.

Prenatal Issues

There is a frequent pattern of inadequate prenatal care and poor nutrition among pregnant teens. Some young mothers attempt to hide or deny their pregnancy in the early months. Consequently, they begin prenatal care much later than usual, many times as late as the end of the second trimester. Teens, therefore, have a higher incidence of prematurity, low-birth-weight infants, stillbirths, and neonatal death than do adult mothers (March of Dimes, 2009).

A pregnant teenager may be fearful and unhappy about the physical changes that occur with her body during pregnancy. She may feel apprehensive about the impending labor and delivery. She may be concerned about the reactions of family, friends, teachers, and her baby's father. Depending on the degree of her emotional adjustment to pregnancy, she could doubt her self-worth and have a poor self-image.

Many teenagers have poor eating habits. Pregnant teenagers need to understand the importance of good nutrition to the developing fetus and to the mother's body. Pregnancy compromises the health of a young mother, whose own growth needs compete with the growth needs of her baby. She may be reluctant to gain weight and can be encouraged and praised for the weight she gains and its benefit to her baby. She may need to consume more food than older mothers and benefits from ongoing individualized advice regarding her diet. The adolescent who recently experienced puberty may require even more calories to support the rapid growth that follows. If she lives with her parents, she may have limited influence on meal planning. Nutrition education is a primary achievement for all pregnant teenagers. Figure 20.2 shows how a teen mother's health can affect her baby.

After the Baby Is Born

Adolescent mothers often feel threatened and overwhelmed by the hospital environment and may be reluctant to ask for anything from the nursing staff. Consequently, they may be less likely to arrange for immediate or prolonged contact with their babies after birth. Teens may not understand the importance of early contact for bonding and may consider the social aspect of visitors to be more important. Hospital personnel can be

---

- It will never happen to me. (denial and invulnerability)
- Everyone else has a baby. (power, social status, peer pressure)
- I thought he'd marry me. (seeking permanence)
- I didn't mean to. (date-rape, substance abuse, impulsivity)
- I wanted out of the house. (physical, emotional, sexual, substance abuse)
- It's not fair—I used birth control. (ignorance, inconsistent or improper use)

FIGURE 20.1   Reasons teens become pregnant.

Source: Printed with permission of Denise Parker and Nancy Williams, 2000.

- Some teens may need to change their lifestyle to improve their chances of having a healthy baby. Unhealthy foods, smoking, alcohol, and drugs can increase the risk that a baby will be born with health problems, such as low birth weight (less than 5 1/2 pounds).
- Teens are more likely than women over age 25 to smoke during pregnancy. Babies of women who smoke during pregnancy are at increased risk for premature birth, low birth weight, and sudden infant death syndrome, or SIDS. Women who smoke during pregnancy also have an increased risk for pregnancy complications, including placental problems.
- Teens are least likely of all maternal age groups to get early and regular prenatal care. From 2000 to 2002 an average 7.1 percent of mothers under age 20 received late or no prenatal care, compared with 3.7 percent for all ages.
- A teenage mother is at greater risk than women over age 20 for pregnancy complications, such as premature labor, anemia, and high blood pressure. These risks are even greater for teens younger than 15 years.
- Of 19 million new cases of sexually transmitted infections (STIs) reported each year, more than 9 million affect young people ages 15 to 24. These STIs include:
  - Chlamydia, which can cause sterility in the affected individual and eye infections and pneumonia in the newborn.
  - Syphilis, which can cause blindness, maternal death, and infant death.
  - HIV, the virus that causes AIDS. Treatment during pregnancy greatly reduces the risk of an infected mother passing HIV to her baby

FIGURE 20.2 The effect of a teen mother's health on her baby.

Source: March of Dimes National Foundation. Facts you should know about teen pregnancy. White Plains, NY: March of Dimes; 2009. www.marchofdimes.com/printableArticles/14332_1159.asp. Accessed October 2, 2009. Used with permission.

sensitive to this and invite interaction between the mother and her baby rather than relying on the mother to ask that someone bring her baby to her. Childbirth is a time of vulnerability for all new mothers. For a teen mother, whose confidence is very fragile, it may be the first realization of the responsibility ahead of her.

After she is at home with her baby, a young mother may question her adequacy as a parent and have difficulty coping with the daily responsibilities of parenthood. In some cases her own mother raises the baby, with the mother having little to do with her baby's care. The mother's maturity and attitude are determining factors in how she copes with parenthood and breastfeeding. The less-mature teenager may have difficulty devoting love and attention to her baby at a time when her own needs for such nurturing are so great. However, other young mothers are ready to accept the responsibilities of motherhood and respond in much the same way as an older mother.

Teen mothers often lose their closest friends when the baby arrives. Their friends may find it difficult and uncomfortable to relate to the new mother or may simply be pursuing typical adolescent activities and no longer have shared interests. Inviting a close friend to accompany her to a support group for parenting or breastfeeding may help the friend feel engaged and increase the likelihood that the friend remains part of the young mother's life (Bonyata, 2005).

Breastfeeding Decision

Not surprisingly, breastfeeding rates among teenage mothers are much lower than among adult mothers, 43 percent compared to 65 percent for mothers aged 20 to 29 years. Mexican-American infants born to mothers under 20 years of age have a significantly higher breastfeeding rate (66 percent) compared with non-Hispanic white (40 percent) and non-Hispanic black infants (30 percent) (NCHS, 2008).

Breastfeeding is especially important to the teen population. Babies of teens are in most need to receive the health benefits of breastfeeding. Teens tend to deliver earlier, have lower-birth-weight babies, and have more delivery complications. They typically live in less healthful environments, and their children face significant risks. According to the Centers for Disease Control and Prevention (2009) children of teens are more likely to:

- Have lower cognitive attainment and proficiency scores at kindergarten entry
- Exhibit behavior problems
- Have chronic medical conditions
- Rely more heavily on publicly provided health care
- Be incarcerated at some time during adolescence until their early 30s
- Drop out of high school
- Give birth as a teenager
- Be unemployed or underemployed as a young adult

As with adult mothers who choose not to breastfeed, teens are less likely to be married and more likely to have low educational and income levels. Knowledge, positive beliefs, and supportive cultural norms also predict future intentions to breastfeed. Parental norms are more important than peer norms on teen breastfeeding beliefs (Swanson et al., 2006). Younger, single teens who are enrolled in school and have little exposure to breastfeeding need the most outreach and encouragement. Studies show these factors consistently across countries and cultures, including Scottish (Swanson et al., 2006), Canadian (Walsh et al., 2008), Native Canadian (Martens, 2001), Native American (Walkup et al., 2009), Brazilian (Fujimori et al., 2008; Nakamura et al., 2003), and British (McMillan, 2009).

A qualitative, descriptive study found that teens chose breastfeeding mainly for infant health reasons, closeness, and bonding (Wambach & Cohen, 2009). Those who weaned cited perceptions of insufficient milk production, nipple/breast pain, school or work time demands, problems with pumping, and feelings of being overwhelmed and frustrated. Adolescents may be less likely to speak out or advocate for their needs. Many who wean have not used available help and may regret weaning earlier than intended. Teens that breastfed beyond 6 weeks received significant support (emotional, informational, and instrumental) from their family, friends, school, and their babies. This confirms an earlier study on the effects of self-esteem and social support on breastfeeding in adolescents. The study found that teen mothers who breastfeed are likely to have a higher self-esteem and that social support was related to breastfeeding at 6 weeks postpartum (Gaff-Smith, 2004).

Back in 1988, Dr. Marianne Neifert found that, similar to the adult population, the majority of teens decide whether to breastfeed before the third trimester of pregnancy. This demonstrates the need to reach teens in early pregnancy regarding infant feeding and to capitalize on opportunities to incorporate breastfeeding into school curricula for all students. Neifert et al. (1988) found that most teens choose to breastfeed because it is "good for the baby"; they identify the "closeness" of the nursing relationship as what they enjoy most with breastfeeding. They also cite concern about modesty and the need to return to school within 2 months postpartum as obstacles. These obstacles still exist today.

Some teens breastfeed to establish control, seeing breastfeeding as the one thing that only they can do for their baby. They may breastfeed to limit the biological father's involvement in the baby's care for as long as possible. Some teens find themselves in a power struggle with their mothers over the care of the baby. The teen may want to assert herself as a parent, but her mother may believe she is too young to care for a baby. Providing the teen mother with accurate information on baby care may help the teen allay her mother's misgivings. The teen's mother may feel threatened by her daughter's desire to breastfeed. Perhaps she did not breastfeed her daughter and may worry that her grandchild will not receive proper nutrition. She may worry that her daughter's choice to breastfeed reflects negatively on her own child-rearing techniques (see the discussion on grandparents earlier in this chapter).

Support from grandparents helps to empower the teen as a parent. Feelings of parental competence in turn helps to increase the teen's self-esteem (Feldman-Winter & Shaikh, 2007). Breastfeeding is an investment in the new grandchild's lifelong health. Sometimes this involves listening to the grandmother's story of failed breastfeeding. Lactation consultants are seeing increased numbers of young mothers whose mothers breastfed and who are very supportive and encouraging of their daughters nursing. These breastfeeding grandmothers are passing the gift on to another generation, reclaiming the culture for the normalcy of nursing one's baby.

Breastfeeding Management

Teens have the same potential for milk production as do older women, because the greatest proliferation of mammary ducts occurs during pregnancy (Stout, 1992). It was common for girls to marry and have children in their teens before industrialization, and girls still marry young in traditional societies. It may be that adolescents in developed countries do not breastfeed often enough for robust milk production. Those who encounter difficulties are less likely than adults to overcome them and continue breastfeeding. Asking open-ended questions helps a teen learn to quantify her breastfeeding pattern and clarify her needs:

- How many times did your baby breastfeed over the past 24 hours?
- How many minutes did your baby nurse on each side?
- How many times does your baby pee and poop each day?
- How many bottles of formula do you give your baby each day?
- How much formula is in each bottle?

Teens are inclined toward exaggeration, so when a teen tells you that her baby cries "all day long," help her measure what that means. Help her learn that she can reduce her baby's crying by using a sling or snuggly carrier. Teach her infant hunger cues so she can learn to begin a feeding before her baby starts crying. If she says her baby "never sleeps," suggest that she keep a notepad handy to record naps. If she complains that her baby "is always hungry," suggest that she count the number of feedings in a 24-hour period. She may find her baby is eating in a perfectly normal pattern. Whereas this might be tedious for a more mature mother with a better grasp of time, it may help a young mother learn to modulate, analyze, and describe her baby's behaviors more observantly.

Teens may feel overwhelmed by parenting responsibilities. They especially need support for breastfeeding from family and friends. They may lack futuristic thinking, failing to anticipate the consequences of their actions and not understanding that a problem can be resolved "in the moment." Don't immediately discount the strengths of many teen parents, however. Some teens have an excellent support system and breastfeed for the same amount of time as the average adult breastfeeding mother.

Interactions with Teenage Mothers

A teenage mother usually has a great need for a one-to-one relationship with someone who cares about her and understands her needs. She wants consistency and personal involvement in this relationship. It is important to get to know her as an individual and not just as the baby's mother. An adolescent mother needs a trusting relationship with her mother, grandmother, partner, or pregnancy coordinator (Dykes et al., 2003). Ask her about herself—how she is adjusting, how the birth went, how she feels, and what her needs are. Demonstrating interest in her as a person builds rapport and develops trust in the relationship. Help her see how she benefits from breastfeeding her baby. Lactation consultants who work with teen mothers have seen the growth, maturation, and increased self-confidence with subsequent babies.

Teaching

Interaction with teens often takes place in a class or other educational setting, such as a public health clinic or a maternity home. To meet their needs effectively, find out what the teens already know about breastfeeding and what they would like to learn. This can be a challenge, because teen mothers often do not volunteer information and may not ask questions, fearing peer ridicule. Asking teens to write out their questions or concerns anonymously encourages them to think about the situation and protects their privacy.

Because teens may not attend every educational offering or appointment, you need to cover breastfeeding basics whenever possible. New information needs to be given in simple, clear terms that do not overwhelm them. After 15 minutes of new information teens typically lose interest, so you need to make the time together both humorous and informative. Allow for nonthreatening participation, and plan meaningful interaction. To demonstrate the importance of positioning the baby, for example, teens can be asked to swallow some water looking straight ahead and then to repeat it, turning their head to the side. This demonstrates how difficult it is for babies to swallow with their head turned. A doll will help you demonstrate how to hold their baby. A golf ball can illustrate the size of a newborn's stomach. Use audiovisual aids and handouts that depict other teens, rather than adults, in breastfeeding and parenting situations. When teaching teens in a group setting, be available to talk with them individually.

Encourage teens to bring family or friends with them to classes to help build a support system. Giving information about breastfeeding to friends and family can help them learn how to support the mother. Recognize that the teen may not have help or support for breastfeeding at home. Her mother may not have breastfed, and her peers are much less likely to have breastfed. Interactions between the teen and her mother may or may not be positive. She may be in disfavor with her family because of her pregnancy. Her mother also may have unresolved issues about her own breastfeeding experience or lack of it. Convey your support to the teen and be accepting of her situation.

Teens want to learn but don't want to be told what to do (Nelson, 2009). Nelson also suggests addressing myths such as pain during breastfeeding with teens. Active learning strategies such as Internet searches may be helpful as guided discovery. Although teens are egocentric, teens in this study believed that "the baby comes first." The author also suggested that a sensitive, "hands-off" approach might be more well accepted than touching the teen mother. Become familiar with organizations that assist teen mothers. Agencies that reach out to teenage mothers in the United States include WIC, the March of Dimes, and the USDHHS. See Appendix H for source information for these organizations.

∽ Cultural Competence in Helping Mothers

Countries are becoming increasingly diverse, as globalization has increased work opportunities and decreased barriers to travel and emigration. Table 20.1 details the increasing population diversity within the United States. As a healthcare provider it is important that you provide families with culturally competent care. This means treating families from cultures other than your own with sensitivity and respect for their beliefs and traditions. Noble and Noble (2009) reported that 77 percent of healthcare professionals caring for breastfeeding mothers in urban areas did not achieve a score of cultural competence. Healthcare professionals "have a moral, ethical and legal responsibility to provide medical care that transcends cultural and linguistic boundaries" (Feldman-Winter et al., 2007).

The National Center for Cultural Competence (2003) considers the critical components of culturally competent healthcare services as an understanding of

- Beliefs, values, traditions, and practices of a culture
- Culturally defined, health-related needs of individuals, families, and communities
- Culturally based belief systems of the etiology of illness and disease and those related to health and healing
- Attitudes toward seeking help from healthcare providers

Familiarity with customs, beliefs and healing traditions that shape a person's approach to health and illness is important in treatment and interventions. Healthcare services must be received and accepted to be successful.

TABLE 20.1   Increasing Diversity in the U.S. Population

- African Americans compose 13.1% of the population and 15% of children are black/African American.

- Hispanics compose 14.7% of the population and 21% of children are Hispanic.

- The number of Asian and Pacific Islanders from many different countries and cultures grew 72% from 1990 to 2000.

- The Native American and Alaska Native population grew 26% since 1990.

- By 2030 approximately 25% of the U.S. population will self-identify as Hispanic and 14.5% as black.

- Over 54 million people speak a language other than English.

- 11.9 million people live in linguistically isolated households where no one over the age of 14 speaks English "very well."

- There are over 300 languages spoken in the United States.

Source: National Center for Cultural Competence, Georgetown University Center for Child and Human Development. Goode T, Dunne C, rev eds. *Policy Brief 1: Rationale for Cultural Competence in Primary Care.* Washington, DC: NCCC; 2003. Reprinted by permission..

The National Center for Cultural Competence (2003) identified seven compelling reasons why it is important to provide culturally competent care:

1. To respond to current and projected demographic changes

2. To eliminate long-standing disparities in the health status of people of diverse racial, ethnic, and cultural backgrounds

3. To eliminate disparities in the mental health status of people of diverse racial, ethnic, and cultural groups

4. To improve the quality of services and health outcomes

5. To meet legislative, regulatory, and accreditation mandates

6. To gain a competitive edge in the marketplace

7. To decrease the likelihood of liability/malpractice claims

Families who leave their native country have several characteristics in common when they work toward becoming part of a new culture. They share a sense of loss of their own culture, an environment in which they developed a set of beliefs and attitudes that are central to their lives. A person's degree of acculturation (integration into a new culture) depends on how firmly they cling to traditional values. Members of succeeding generations replace old values with new ones as cultural differences become more diffuse.

Other factors that influence behavior are age, educational and social exposure, the intent to return to their country of origin, economic status, contact with older relatives, and the part of the country in which they reside. The lower classes tend to hold onto traditional values, whereas the middle and upper classes generally incorporate new practices into their value system. Practically speaking, this means that women from other cultures exhibit a wide range of value systems, family support, and interest in breastfeeding.

Family Dynamics

In many Western cultures the individual is the basic social entity and the building block of all social relations and institutions. In other cultures the family is the dominant unit, and decision making is the responsibility of the family rather than the individual member. Decisions may be the responsibility of the eldest male or other male figure in the family group. Extended family often provides a support system for raising children. To counsel effectively you must take care not to interfere with family dynamics. Instead, you can strengthen family support by providing clear, accurate information in a climate of acceptance.

Because cultural beliefs form our view of reality, a woman's cultural convictions may be more important to her than science-based practices. Working within the mother's framework helps her achieve her personal breastfeeding goals. A Hispanic woman may, for instance, insist that she not breastfeed in the early days after delivery because her colostrum is insufficient. Although you may educate her otherwise, trying to convince her to accept your information may be nonproductive. Rather, you might suggest that she let her baby "practice" breastfeeding 8 to 12 times a day for when the mature milk is established.

Health and Illness Behaviors

Cultural beliefs may create health and illness behaviors that vary significantly from your own. Understanding these differences will avoid alienating a mother with recommendations that are irrelevant or ignored. A mother's culture affects the way she regards health and the measures she takes to prevent or treat illness. She may place considerable reliance on cultural patterns as a method of coping. Cultural and religious practices can be therapeutic and foster social support from her community. To counsel a woman from another culture effectively, you need to understand her values and cultural practices and learn how they can influence her breastfeeding.

Cultural Beliefs Regarding Breastfeeding

Approaching women with cultural sensitivity requires flexibility. Learn about their beliefs and adapt your suggestions to meet their needs. There are many Internet resources such as EthnoMed (2009) for culturally competent care to educate you on specific groups' beliefs and needs. EthnoMed contains information about cultural beliefs, medical issues, and related topics about health care for immigrants to the United States, many of whom are refugees fleeing war-torn parts of the world. Inappropriate advice can upset or confuse a mother and cause friction with other family members. You risk your credibility and rapport with the mother if you discredit beliefs she has held her entire life. Do not try to change culturally based practices unless they are detrimental to the mother's or baby's health. It is the mother's responsibility to accept or reject the information you give her.

Each mother's cultural heritage and economic standing have a direct bearing on how long she breastfeeds and her ability to deal with reactions from her partner, family, or friends. Values and priorities vary greatly among women of different cultural backgrounds. Some regard healthcare providers and the scientific community with great respect. Others place more faith in self-care or folk medicine. Some cultures regard colostrum as valueless or undesirable and do not encourage breastfeeding until the second or third postpartum day. You can inform these mothers about the medical value of colostrum, realizing at the same time that their cultural beliefs may predominate, as in the example above.

You can seek ways to work around culturally based practices so they benefit rather than harm breastfeeding. For example, some women of Mexican heritage who work outside in the heat believe their milk will spoil in their breasts during the day, and so they wean before returning to work. One caregiver used this belief as a motivating factor to continue to breastfeed by instructing the women to express out the "bad" milk and throw it away, and then to nurse their babies when they returned home. The mothers were able to continue breastfeeding, with formula supplements given to the babies during the daytime, similar to the way some other working mothers manage breastfeeding.

In an intervention where postpartum Cambodian mothers were given culturally important foods, breastfeeding initiation rates increased from 16.6 percent in the hospital to 66.6 percent 3 months after the intervention (Feldman-Winter et al., 2007). The concept of "hot" and "cold" forces being "good" and "bad" for mothers is common in Asian culture. Some traditions discourage new mothers from consuming cold foods and beverages for several weeks or months (Raven et al., 2007). Hot teas and soups help these mothers meet their fluid requirements. Some cultural beliefs place limitations on activity for the postpartum mother that an uninformed caregiver may interpret as a lack of compliance. By recognizing this you can encourage the involvement of extended family in the mother's care. Cultural restrictions may carry over to how others relate to the baby as well. Certain ways of touching the baby or referring to the baby may be taboo. Always ask permission when you wish to touch the baby. Gentle, honest inquiries about the mother's customs help you learn appropriate responses. Most families are delighted when caregivers express an open, honest interest in their culture.

Language and Communication

Cultural barriers may seem greater when accompanied by a language difference. A sensitive understanding of the woman's culture and language is essential to establishing effective communication. Speak slowly and clearly, and provide simple explanations. Maximizing communication is especially important if the mother has a breastfeeding problem she needs to discuss. A woman with limited English proficiency (LEP) may be able to speak and understand English well enough about breastfeeding in general. When she has a specific problem, however, she may need to converse in her native language to be understood and to comprehend your advice.

The ability to communicate in a non-native language influences how patients feel about the quality of their care. Compared with English-speaking patients, those with limited proficiency report less satisfaction with medical encounters, have different rates of diagnostic testing, and receive less explanation and follow-up (Ramirez et al., 2008). An interpreter can facilitate the transmission of health education. However, having an interpreter does not substitute for the provider speaking the same language in patients' ratings of their providers and the quality of interpersonal care (Ngo-Metzger et al., 2007).

Bilingual Aids

If you are not bilingual, you can make the effort to learn common phrases used in breastfeeding in the languages used by mothers in your community (see the Spanish glossary in Appendix G). Many communities offer classes in conversational medical terminology, called "meducation." It would be helpful to have the services of a colleague who can speak comfortably in a second language. If you practice in a hospital, a translator should be on staff or a language translation service should be available. Effective communication including interpreter and translation services is an important aspect of patient safety (Joint Commission, 2009).

If there is no one available in your practice who speaks the language of a particular mother, you can ask her if she has a bilingual friend or relative who can assist. Optimally, the interpreter will be another woman, because the mother may be reluctant to share intimate information with a male other than her partner. Try to ensure that the interpreter is communicating accurately and not adding opinions or values that differ from what you are attempting to convey to the mother.

Women who have difficulty reading English probably will not benefit from lengthy print articles or books on breastfeeding. Brief pamphlets with simple themes and illustrations written at an appropriate reading level can help these mothers. You might want to have literature specific to your practice translated so that the mothers can best understand your services. Demonstrations with visual aids and the use of flash cards with translations are helpful. Teaching aids and breastfeeding information in many different languages are available through La Leche League International and other sources (see Appendix H). Local social services may be helpful as well.

Body Language and Customs

Because body language is an important communication tool, personal contact is preferable to phone contact to enable you to be alert to differences in body language. In some cultures nodding and smiling do not denote understanding as they do in Western society. You cannot assume that a mother comprehends what you are saying because of these gestures. Watch for nonverbal cues and messages through the mother's facial and body expressions. For example, a nod of the head accompanied by a bland or puzzled look can imply confusion. To ensure that a woman understands your instructions, you can ask her to repeat them or to demonstrate what you have shown her. You can also demonstrate a technique and summarize the important points at the end of your conversation. Use of listening skills is critical in determining motivation to breastfeed and cultural factors that may be involved.

Visiting a woman in her home helps you obtain a more complete picture of her physical and emotional environment. Some families might be reluctant to invite strangers into their homes or may feel embarrassed by their living arrangements. At the same time they may respond to a friendly and sincere interest in their welfare. Learn cultural customs of greeting and inclusion of others before you make this visit. Become familiar with the cultural practices of the ethnic groups in your community. For example, it is customary to remove one's shoes upon entering the home in many Asian countries. Americans tend to be very businesslike and customarily do not accept offers of tea and food on a home visit, considering it a professional call and inappropriate to mix "business" with socializing. However, offers of tea or food are important rituals in some cultures, and it can be considered rude to refuse.

Taking cues from your clients helps you respond appropriately and show your interest and respect for the woman and her culture. If you are unsure about proper etiquette in a particular situation, ask your client what the correct practice is. Most immigrants are pleased to share their customs. Remember that the Western way is not the best or only way. Most other countries and cultures have higher breastfeeding rates than the United States and Western culture has much to learn. Remain open to the ideas and choices that work in other places.

Promoting Breastfeeding to Women of Other Cultures

In addition to learning to function within a woman's culture, you may face the challenge of promoting breastfeeding among an ethnic group that favors formula feeding. A woman from that culture who breastfed her own baby can help your promotion efforts. She can help you learn beliefs and child-rearing practices that dominate her culture. She can also help you understand effective measures for supporting and educating mothers.

Many Hispanic women initiate breastfeeding at high rates but do not breastfeed exclusively, especially before their mature milk comes in. "No tengo leche" ("I don't have milk") is a common postpartum refrain. Prenatal intervention can help alter this belief. Thirty-two percent of mothers exposed to Healthy Families America education reported exclusive breastfeeding during the first week postpartum compared with 20 percent who did not receive the intervention (Sandy et al., 2009). However, both Hopkinson and Konefal Gallagher (2009) and Petrova et al. (2007) reported limited success with interventions aimed at increasing exclusive breastfeeding among predominantly Hispanic mothers.

Immigrant women in a large study had higher breastfeeding initiation and longer duration rates than native women, even after controlling for socioeconomic and demographic differences (Singh et al., 2007). This study examined a large nationally representative sample to explore breastfeeding patterns among 12 ethnic groups with varying levels of acculturation. Breastfeeding rates and duration decrease for immigrant children who are born in the United States (Mistry et al., 2008). It is important to reverse this trend, because breastfeeding is associated with improved health outcomes for infants of immigrant mothers. This is especially pertinent for children at greater risk for food insecurity (Neault et al., 2007).

Lack of knowledge and misinformation are reported to be major barriers to breastfeeding for Vietnamese immigrants in Canada (Sutton et al., 2007). Inability to communicate in English and a lack of effective transportation were key obstacles to women's ability to access mainstream prenatal and postpartum health programs and services. Another study suggested that mothers chose bottle feeding because of conflicts between Vietnamese cultural practices and the Canadian norms. Family members were unable to conduct important postpartum rituals considered important to the mothers' health and milk quality (Groleau et al., 2006). Breastfeeding education for immigrant families also needs to address the feasibility and practicality of breastfeeding when the mother works or attends school.

McLachlan and Forster (2006) examined the breastfeeding attitudes and practices of mothers from Vietnam, Turkey, and Australia who gave birth in Australia at a Baby-Friendly Hospital. Vietnamese women had the lowest rate of breastfeeding initiation (75 percent) compared with Turkish women (98 percent) and Australian women (84 percent). They believed their partners were more negative about breastfeeding and did not value the properties of colostrum as much as the other two groups. Forty percent of the breastfeeding Vietnamese mothers gave their baby formula while in the hospital.

Receiving free formula samples in the hospital undermines a mother's confidence in her ability to produce milk. It sends a message that her caregivers do not take her decision to breastfeed seriously and implies that formula feeding is the accepted cultural method of feeding (Rosenberg et al., 2008). Castrucci et al. (2008) studied breastfeeding initiation rates on both sides of the border between a county in Texas and a state in Mexico. Attempted breastfeeding before hospital discharge was 81.9 percent in Mexico compared with 63.7 percent in Texas. This underscores the importance of connecting mothers to strong community resources.

Exclusive breastfeeding rates were 15.6 percent at 2 months postpartum among a group of Chinese immigrant mothers in Canada. After implementation of a feeding hotline, 20 percent of new Chinese mothers in Vancouver indicated that they had used the hotline. Among these women, the rate of exclusive breastfeeding was 44.1 percent (Janssen et al., 2009). In a study of ethnic minority groups in the United Kingdom, first- and second-generation immigrant mothers were less likely to initiate breastfeeding and to breastfeed for at least 4 months. For every additional 5 years spent in the United Kingdom, immigrant mothers were 5 percent less likely to breastfeed for at least 4 months (Hawkins et al., 2008).

As is true for all babies, the children of immigrant mothers have worse health if they are not breastfed. In a study of immigrants, 83 percent of mothers initiated breastfeeding while 36 percent of immigrant households reported food insecurity. The non-breastfed infants were more likely to be in fair or poor health and to have more hospitalizations. Breastfeeding especially protects children of immigrants who are at greater risk for not having enough food to eat in their homes (Kaplan & Graff, 2008). A mother who wishes to acculturate in her new home country may believe that formula feeding is one way to achieve it. Family support for breastfeeding is an integral part of breastfeeding education. In the absence of an extended family, a mother tends to rely heavily on the father's infant feeding preference. Prenatal education should actively seek to include the father and members of the extended family.

Historically, immigrant mothers of African descent breastfeed at higher rates than U.S.-born African American mothers (Singh et al., 2007). One study found the most common reason for not breastfeeding among WIC mothers was fear of difficulty or pain during breastfeeding (35.6 percent), particularly among African American and white mothers. Hispanic mothers were more likely to report perceived infant breast rejection. Not having enough milk was the most common reason reported (23.4 percent) for quitting breastfeeding. Hispanic mothers were more likely to cite perceived insufficient milk and infant breast refusal as reasons for quitting. African American mothers were more likely than white mothers to report quitting because of a return to work. The researchers concluded that there are racial and ethnic differences in why women quit breastfeeding. They suggest that culturally sensitive breastfeeding interventions are necessary (Hurley et al, 2008).

A breastfeeding pamphlet for African American families is available from the National Women's Health Information Center website. It appears the group is no longer active. Low-income African American mothers may be encouraged to breastfeed by supportive messages from healthcare providers in the perinatal period. The role breastfeeding can play in preventing childhood illnesses should be emphasized (Sharps et al., 2003).

Women generally wish to do what is best for their babies and are more likely to follow your suggestions when they fully understand the reasons behind your advice. While learning about a woman's culture and her unique beliefs, you can clarify your own beliefs. You need to be aware of how your own convictions, customs, and prejudices may affect your ability to counsel women from cultures different from your own. Accept the mother where she is and work to put your beliefs aside while providing care. Intercultural experiences provide an opportunity for personal growth by enabling you to view yourself and others more objectively.

∾ Mother-to-Mother Support Groups

As breastfeeding rates continue to rise in the Western world, most babies leave the hospital being breastfed, either partially or exclusively. However, many of these mothers fail to continue because they lack the necessary support and information. Midwifery care and the home-birth model support breastfeeding initiation in countries where traditional birthing is the norm. Mother-to-mother support groups help create the community of breastfeeding, especially in societies where it has been lost for generations. Breastfeeding support groups such as La Leche League and breastfeeding cafés provide help through Internet websites, forums, podcasts, and blogs (such as Mocha Milk, a blog specifically for breastfeeding mothers of color). They also provide written materials, counseling services, regular meeting groups, and special programs (Figure 20.3). It is important to become aware of and involved in the lactation services and support available within your community.

Support groups reinforce women's traditional patterns of seeking and receiving advice from relatives and friends. A mother can seek help at any time, day or night, and help usually is available in her own community. Experienced mothers lead discussion groups and offer support to new mothers, helping them gain a feeling of self-reliance and reassurance. Starting a mother-to-mother support group can provide a needed service to women in your community and further the promotion of breastfeeding. See the discussion in Chapter 2 regarding a lactation consultant's relationship to mother-to-mother support groups.

The goal of a mother-to-mother support group is to educate women about options, to help them make informed choices, and to support them in reaching their goals. The group should accommodate the style and needs of the women and the community it serves. Contact between a counselor and mother is encouraged from the baby's birth through weaning. These groups usually emphasize exclusive breastfeeding for at least 6 months, baby-led weaning, and limited separation of mother and baby. Helping mothers manage breastfeeding and working, supporting early weaning, and other variations in breastfeeding styles that require compromises reflect the group's flexibility and acceptance.

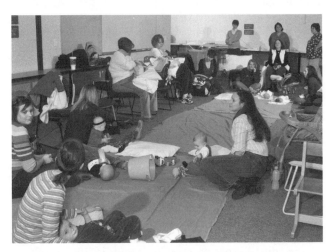

FIGURE 20.3   Mothers and their babies in a support group.
Source: Courtesy of St. John's Hospital, Springfield, Illinois..

The positive working relationship you develop with peer counselors, the mothers they counsel, and their caregivers are essential to meeting women's needs. Be careful not to place yourself, counselors, or mothers in opposition to other members of the medical community. This discourages healthcare providers from referring mothers to you and diminishes your credibility in the community. Open communication and cooperation between the medical community and other breastfeeding counselors is essential, with the mother making decisions based on information from both.

Outreach Counseling

A mother-to-mother support group provides anticipatory guidance to help mothers learn what to expect, avoid potential problems, and resolve issues before they become obstacles. Inviting women to group meetings and contacting them by phone or e-mail are effective forms of outreach. Other ways to actively reach out to women include speaking at childbirth classes and clinics, sharing information with professionals, and speaking to high school health classes.

Regular meetings for breastfeeding mothers in the community provide a valuable counseling opportunity. Meeting formats should encourage friendly and informal discussion and provide a supportive environment for a mother who lacks contact with other breastfeeding women. The primary factors influencing meetings should be the needs of the women who attend. The goal should be to involve mothers as much as possible and help them feel comfortable in taking part with questions, demonstrations, small group discussions, and book reviews.

If a support group is not available in your community, you can provide ongoing support and appropriate written materials. In the absence of community support, it is especially important that you provide follow-up to mothers after hospital discharge and after they have experienced a difficulty. You might also help develop a mother-to-mother support group, train group leaders, or be available as a resource to the group.

⁓ *Summary*

You can provide valuable support and guidance to mothers navigating through special circumstances. When a mother experiences opposition to her breastfeeding, you can offer a listening ear, praise, and practical suggestions, especially when the opposition is from someone close to her. You can also be a valuable resource to a mother who is experiencing challenges such as low income, single parenthood, or teen parenthood. Such mothers often bear burdens that go well beyond the scope of breastfeeding.

They benefit from thoughtful suggestions and referrals tailored to their special needs. Cultural competence in an increasingly global world is crucial for client safety and satisfaction. A mother whose culture or nationality differs from your own needs your openness and flexibility. Mother-to-mother support groups provide valuable technical and emotional help to mothers. These groups benefit from your support as well.

∼ Chapter 20—At a Glance

Applying what you learned—

Counseling the mother:

- Help her cope with opposition to breastfeeding.
- Educate an unsupportive father about health risks associated with not breastfeeding.
- Avoid placing yourself in the middle of conflicts with an unsupportive family member.
- Build the mother's confidence with positive feedback.
- Adapt your counseling to each woman's income level, educational level, lifestyle, and support system.
- Give practical suggestions rather than general advice.
- Use visual aids to reinforce verbal explanations.
- Provide reading materials at an appropriate literacy level.
- Reach out to mothers in their own neighborhoods.
- Help mothers access supplemental food programs.
- Recognize the needs of single mothers.
- Refer women to a breastfeeding support group.

Recognize special needs of a teenage mother:

- Need for sound prenatal care and nutrition
- Ability to feel adequate as a parent
- May be engaged in a power struggle with her mother
- Tendency not to breastfeed often enough for robust milk production
- Need for a one-to-one relationship
- Need to be treated as an adult
- Need for concrete suggestions and simple, clear information

Tailor counseling and expectations to cultural differences:

- Accept health and illness behaviors that do not compromise breastfeeding.
- Ask permission before touching the mother or baby.
- Learn customs and body language to help you respond appropriately.
- Learn phrases in common languages within your community.
- Teach with visual aids and return demonstrations.
- Enlist help from other women in the culture to promote breastfeeding.

∼ References

Abdulwadud O, Snow M. Interventions in the workplace to support breastfeeding for women in employment. *Cochrane Database Syst Rev.* 2007;(3):CD006177.

Amato P. Recent changes in family structure: implications for children, adults, and society. National Healthy Marriage Resource Center; 2008. www.healthymarriageinfo.org/docs/May08changefamstructure.pdf. Accessed October 2, 2009.

Amato P, Maynard R. Decreasing nonmarital births and strengthening marriage to reduce poverty. *Future of Children.* 2006;17:117-141.

American Academy of Pediatrics (AAP). Policy statement on breastfeeding and the use of human milk. *Pediatrics.* 2005;115:496-506.

American Association of Health Plans. Health plans' innovative programs in breastfeeding promotion. August 2001. www.aahp.org. Accessed September 25, 2009.

Anderson A, et al. A randomized trial assessing the efficacy of peer counseling on exclusive breastfeeding in a predominantly Latina low-income community. *Arch Pediatr Adolesc Med.* 2005;159:836-841.

Bezner Kerr R, et al. "We grandmothers know plenty": breastfeeding, complementary feeding and the multifaceted role of grandmothers in Malawi. *Soc Sci Med.* 2008;66:1095-1105.

Bonyata K. Encouraging teen moms to breastfeed. October 10, 2005. www.kellymom.com/bf/start/prepare/teenbf.html. Accessed October 2, 2009.

Britton C, et al. Support for breastfeeding mothers. *Cochrane Database Syst Rev.* 2007;(1):CD001141.

Britton J, Britton H. Maternal self-concept and breastfeeding. *J Hum Lact.* 2008;24:431-438.

Brugman S, et al. Prolonged exclusive breastfeeding reduces autoimmune diabetes incidence and increases regulatory T-cell frequency in bio-breeding diabetes-prone rats. *Diabetes Metab Res Rev.* 2009;25:380-387.

Castrucci B, et al. Attempted breastfeeding before hospital discharge on both sides of the US-Mexico border, 2005: the Brownsville-Matamoros Sister City Project for Women's Health. *Prev Chronic Dis.* 2008;5:A117.

Centers for Disease Control and Prevention (CDC). Adolescent reproductive health: about teen pregnancy. 2009. www.cdc.gov/reproductivehealth/AdolescentReproHealth/AboutTP.htm. Accessed October 2, 2009.

Chambliss L. Intimate partner violence and its implication for pregnancy. *Clin Obstet Gynecol.* 2008;51:385-397.

Chang J, Chan W. Analysis of factors associated with initiation and duration of breast-feeding: a study in Taitung Taiwan. *Acta Paediatr Taiwan.* 2003;44:29-34.

Chin NP, Solomonik A. Inadequate: a metaphor for the lives of low-income women? *Breastfeed Med.* 2009;4:S41-S43.

Chuang C, et al. Maternal return to work and breastfeeding: a population-based cohort study. *Int J Nurs Stud.* 2010; 47(4):461-474.

Chung M, et al. Interventions in primary care to promote breastfeeding: an evidence review for the U.S. Preventive Services Task Force. *Ann Intern Med.* 2008;149:565-582.

Condon J. What about dad? Psychosocial and mental health issues for new fathers. *Aust Fam Physician.* 2006;35:690-692.

Dunn B, et al. Breastfeeding practices in Colorado businesses. *J Hum Lact.* 2004;20:170-177.

Dykes F, et al. Adolescent mothers and breastfeeding: experiences and support needs. An exploratory study. *J Hum Lact.* 2003;19:391-401.

Ekström A, Nissen E. A mother's feelings for her infant are strengthened by excellent breastfeeding counseling and continuity of care. *Pediatrics.* 2006;118:e309-e314.

Elliott H, Gunaratnam Y. Talking about breastfeeding: emotion, context and "good" mothering. *Pract Midwife.* 2009; 12:40-46.

England L, et al. Breastfeeding practices in a cohort of inner-city women: the role of contraindications. *BMC Public Health.* 2003;3:28.

EthnoMed. Integrating cultural information into clinical practice; 2009. www.ethnomed.org. Accessed October 3, 2009.

Feldman-Winter L, et al. Breastfeeding promotion tailored to meet the needs of a diverse society. Breastfeeding Promotion in Physicians' Office Practices (BPPOP III). Teleconference presentation. March 22, 2007. www.aap.org/ breastfeeding/files/PPT/Teleconference2(1).pps. Accessed October 2, 2009.

Feldman-Winter L, Shaikh U. Optimizing breastfeeding promotion and support in adolescent mothers. *J Hum Lact.* 2007;23:362-367.

Fujimori M, et al. The attitudes of primary school children to breastfeeding and the effect of health education lectures. *J Pediatr.* 2008;84:224-231.

Gaff-Smith M. Psychosocial profile of adolescent breastfeeding mothers. *Birth Issues.* 2004;13:98-104.

Gatti L. Maternal perceptions of insufficient milk supply in breastfeeding. *J Nurs Scholarsh.* 2008;40:355-363.

Giugliani E, et al. Intake of water, herbal teas and non-breast milks during the first month of life: associated factors and impact on breastfeeding duration. *Early Hum Dev.* 2008; 84:305-310.

Glenn L, Quillin S. Opposing effects of maternal and paternal socioeconomic status on neonatal feeding method, place of sleep, and maternal sleep time. *J Perinat Neonatal Nurs.* 2007;21:165-172.

Grassley J, Eschiti V. Grandmother breastfeeding support: what do mothers need and want? *Birth.* 2008;35:329-335.

Groleau D, et al. Breastfeeding and the cultural configuration of social space among Vietnamese immigrant woman. *Health Place.* 2006;12:516-526.

Hawkins S, et al. Influence of moving to the UK on maternal health behaviours: prospective cohort study. *BMJ.* 2008; 336:1052-1055.

Hegney D, et al. Against all odds: a retrospective case-controlled study of women who experienced extraordinary breastfeeding problems. *J Clin Nurs.* 2008;17:1182-1192.

Hopkinson J, Konefal Gallagher M. Assignment to a hospital-based breastfeeding clinic and exclusive breastfeeding among immigrant Hispanic mothers: a randomized, controlled trial. *J Hum Lact.* 2009;25:287-296.

Hromi-Fiedler AJ, Pérez-Escamilla R. Unintended pregnancies are associated with less likelihood of prolonged breast-feeding: an analysis of 18 Demographic and Health Surveys. *Public Health Nutr.* 2006;9:306-312.

Hurley K, et al. Variation in breastfeeding behaviours, perceptions, and experiences by race/ethnicity among a low-income statewide sample of Special Supplemental Nutrition Program for Women, Infants, and Children (WIC) participants in the United States. *Matern Child Nutr.* 2008;4:95-105.

Ingram J. The father factor: men can make the difference. *Pract Midwife.* 2008;11:15-16.

Ingram J, Johnson D. Using community maternity care assistants to facilitate family-focused breastfeeding support. *Matern Child Nutr.* 2009;5:276-281.

Ingram J, et al. South Asian grandmothers' influence on breast feeding in Bristol. *Midwifery.* 2003;19(4):318-27.

Ip S, et al. A summary of the agency for healthcare research and quality's evidence report on breastfeeding in developed countries. *Breastfeed Med.* 2009;4:S17-S30.

Janssen P, et al. Development and evaluation of a Chinese-language newborn feeding hotline: a prospective cohort study. *BMC Pregn Childb.* 2009;9:3.

Joint Commission. Patient safety. Hospitals, language, and culture. Standards in support of language and culture. The Joint Commission 2009 Requirements Related to the Provision of Culturally Competent Patient-Centered Care Hospital Accreditation Program (HAP). May 18, 2009. www.jointcommission.org/PatientSafety/HLC/HLC_Joint_Commission_Standards.htm. Accessed October 3, 2009.

Kang J, et al. Effects of a breastfeeding empowerment programme on Korean breastfeeding mothers: a quasi-experimental study. *Int J Nurs Stud.* 2008;45:14-23.

Kaplan D, Graff K. Marketing breastfeeding: reversing corporate influence on infant feeding practices. *J Urban Health.* 2008;85:486-504.

Khan F, et al. The beneficial effects of breastfeeding on microvascular function in 11- to 14-year-old children. *Vasc Med.* 2009;14:137-142.

Khoury A, et al. Breast-feeding initiation in low-income women: role of attitudes, support, and perceived control. *Womens Health Issues.* 2005;15:64-72.

Kids Count Data Center. Annie E. Casey Foundation, Baltimore, MD; 2009. http://datacenter.kidscount.org/. Accessed October 1, 2009.

Kong S, Lee D. Factors influencing decision to breastfeed. *J Adv Nurs.* 2004;46:369-379.

Labiner-Wolfe J, et al. Prevalence of breast milk expression and associated factors. *Pediatrics.* 2008;122(Suppl 2):S63-S68.

Lu M, et al. Childbirth education classes: sociodemographic disparities in attendance and the association of attendance with breastfeeding initiation. *Matern Child Health J.* 2003;7:87-93.

March of Dimes National Foundation. Facts you should know about teen pregnancy. White Plains, NY: March of Dimes;

2009. www.marchofdimes.com/printableArticles/14332_1159.asp. Accessed October 2, 2009.

Martens P. The effect of breastfeeding education on adolescent beliefs and attitudes: a randomized school intervention in the Canadian Ojibwa community of Sagkeeng. *J Hum Lact.* 2001;17:245-255.

McCarter-Spaulding D, Gore R. Breastfeeding self-efficacy in women of African descent. *JOGNN.* 2009;38:230-243.

McKellar L, et al. Enhancing fathers' educational experiences during the early postnatal period. *J Perinat Educ.* 2008;17:12-20.

McLachlan H, Forster D. Initial breastfeeding attitudes and practices of women born in Turkey, Vietnam and Australia after giving birth in Australia. *Int Breastfeed J.* 2006;1:7.

McMillan B, et al. Studying the infant feeding intentions of pregnant women experiencing material deprivation: methodology of the Looking at Infant Feeding Today (LIFT) study. *Soc Sci Med.* 2009;68(5):845-849.

Meier P, et al. The Rush Mothers' Milk Club: breastfeeding interventions for mothers with very-low-birth-weight infants. *JOGNN.* 2004;33:164-174.

Memmott M, Bonuck K. Mother's reactions to a skills-based breastfeeding promotion intervention. *Matern Child Nutr.* 2006;2:40-50.

Mickens A, et al. Peer support and breastfeeding intentions among black WIC participants. *J Hum Lact.* 2009;25(2):157-162.

Mills S. Workplace lactation programs: a critical element for breastfeeding mothers' success. *AAOHN J.* 2009;57:227-231.

Mistry Y, et al. Infant-feeding practices of low-income Vietnamese American women. *J Hum Lact.* 2008;24:406-414.

Moe A. Silenced voices and structured survival: battered women's help seeking. *Violence Against Women.* 2007;13:676-699.

Nakamura S, et al. School girls' perception and knowledge about breastfeeding (Portuguese). *J Pediatr.* 2003;79:181-188.

National Business Group on Health. Investing in workplace breastfeeding programs and policies: an employer's toolkit; June 2009. www.businessgrouphealth.org. Accessed October 2, 2009.

National Center for Cultural Competence, Georgetown University Center for Child and Human Development. Goode T, Dunne C, rev eds. *Policy Brief 1: Rationale for Cultural Competence in Primary Care.* Washington, DC: NCCC; 2003.

National Center for Health Statistics (NCHS). Breastfeeding in the United States: findings from the National Health and Nutrition Examination Surveys 1999–2006. (McDowell M, et al). NCHS data briefs, no. 5. Hyattsville, MD: NCHS; 2008.

National Center for Health Statistics (NCHS). Births: preliminary data for 2007. (Hamilton B, et al). National Vital Statistics Reports, 57(12); 2009. Hyattsville, MD: NCHS; 2009a.

National Center for Health Statistics (NCHS). Changing patterns of nonmarital childbearing in the United States. (Ventura S). NCHS data brief, #18. Hyattsville, MD: NCHS; 2009b.

Neault N, et al. Breastfeeding and health outcomes among citizen infants of immigrant mothers. *J Am Diet Assoc.* 2007;107:2077-2086.

Neifert M, et al. Factors influencing breastfeeding among adolescents. *J Adolesc Health Care.* 1988;9:470–473.

Nelson A. Adolescent attitudes, beliefs, and concerns regarding breastfeeding. *MCN Am J Matern Child Nurs.* 2009;34:249-255.

Ngo-Metzger Q, et al. Providing high-quality care for limited English proficient patients: the importance of language concordance and interpreter use. *J Gen Intern Med.* 2007;22(Suppl 2):324-330.

Noble L, et al. Factors influencing initiation of breast-feeding among urban women. *Am J Perinatol.* 2003;20:477-483.

Noble L, Noble A, Hand I. Cultural competence of healthcare professionals caring for breastfeeding mothers in urban areas. *Breastfeed Med.* 2009;4(4):221-224.

Noel-Weiss J, et al. Randomized controlled trial to determine effects of prenatal breastfeeding workshop on maternal breastfeeding self-efficacy and breastfeeding duration. *JOGNN.* 2006;35:616-624.

Olds S. Grandmothers and breastfeeding. Super granny: how today's grandmothers have fun with, relate to, and communicate with our grandchildren. Sunday, May 25, 2008. http://omasally.blogspot.com/2008/05/grandmothers-and-breastfeeding.html. Accessed October 1, 2009.

Oliva G, et al. Integral care for pregnant adolescents: impact on offspring. *Int J Adolesc Med Health.* 2008;20:537-546.

Otsuka K, et al. The relationship between breastfeeding self-efficacy and perceived insufficient milk among Japanese mothers. *JOGNN.* 2008;37:546-555.

Palmer G. *The Politics of Breastfeeding: When Breasts are Bad for Business,* 3rd ed. London: Pinter & Martin, Ltd.; 2009.

Parker D, Williams N. *Lactation Consultant Series Two: Teens and Breastfeeding.* Schaumburg, IL: La Leche League International; 2000.

Petrova A, et al. Maternal race/ethnicity and one-month exclusive breastfeeding in association with the in-hospital feeding modality. *Breastfeed Med.* 2007;2:92-98.

Power C, et al. Lovestruck: women, romantic love and intimate partner violence. *Contemp Nurse.* 2006;21:174-185.

Ramirez D, et al. Language interpreter utilization in the emergency department setting: a clinical review. *J Health Care Poor Underserved.* 2008;19:352-362.

Raven J, et al. Traditional beliefs and practices in the postpartum period in Fujian Province, China: a qualitative study. *BMC Pregn Childb* 2007;7:8.

Rose V, et al. Factors influencing infant feeding method in an urban community. *J Natl Med Assoc.* 2004;96:325-331.

Rosenbach M, et al. Characteristics, access, utilization, satisfaction, and outcomes of healthy start participants in eight sites. *Matern Child Health J* DOI 10.1007/s10995-009-0474-1; July 10;2009.

Rosenberg K, et al. Marketing infant formula through hospitals: the impact of commercial hospital discharge packs on breastfeeding. *Am J Public Health.* 2008;98:290-295.

Rossman B. Breastfeeding peer counselors in the United States: helping to build a culture and tradition of breastfeeding. *J Midwifery Womens Health.* 2007;52:631-637.

Sandy J, et al. Effects of a prenatal intervention on breastfeeding initiation rates in a latina immigrant sample. *J Hum Lact.* 2009;25(4):404-411; quiz 458-459.

Sarkar N. The impact of intimate partner violence on women's reproductive health and pregnancy outcome. *J Obstet Gynaecol.* 2008;28:266-271.

Shannon J, et al. Fathering in infancy: mutuality and stability between 8 and 16 months. *Parent Sci Pract* 2006;6:167-188.

Sharps P, et al. Health beliefs and parenting attitudes influence breastfeeding patterns among low-income African-American women. *J Perinatol.* 2003;23:414-419.

Shellenbarger S. Work & family mailbox. *Wall Street Journal,* September 27, 2007. Available at http://online.wsj.com/article/SB119084364634840467.html. Accessed October 3, 2009.

Singh G, et al. Nativity/immigrant status, race/ethnicity, and socioeconomic determinants of breastfeeding initiation and duration in the United States, 2003. *Pediatrics.* 2007; 119 Suppl 1:S38-S46.

Souza M, et al. The use of social network methodological framework in nursing care to breastfeeding women. *Rev Lat Am Enfermagem.* 2009;17:354-360.

Stout R. Composition of milk in adolescents. *J Adolesc Health.* 1992;13:261.

Sutton J, et al. Barriers to breastfeeding in a Vietnamese community: a qualitative exploration. *Can J Diet Pract Res.* 2007;68:195-200.

Swanson V, et al. The impact of knowledge and social influences on adolescents' breast-feeding beliefs and intentions. *Public Health Nutr.* 2006;9:297-305.

Texas Dept. State Health Services. Nutrition services section. Just for grandparents. #13-06-11288; September 2008.

Turnbull-Plaza B, et al. The role of social networks in exclusive breastfeeding. *Rev Med Inst Mex Seguro Soc.* 2006;44:97-104.

U.S. Census Bureau news. Single-parent households showed little variation since 1994, Census bureau reports; March 27, 2007. www.census.gov/Press-Release/www/releases/archives/families_households/009842.html. Accessed October 2, 2009.

U.S. Department of Health and Human Services (USDHHS). Health Resources and Services Administration (HRSA), Maternal and Child Health Bureau. Employees' guide to breastfeeding and working; 2008a. www.womenshealth.gov/breastfeeding/programs/business-case/employees-guide.pdf. Accessed October 1, 2009.

U.S. Department of Health and Human Services (USDHHS). Health Resources and Services Administration (HRSA), Maternal and Child Health Bureau. The business case for breastfeeding; 2008b. www.womenshealth.gov/breastfeeding/programs/business-case/breastfeeding-businesscase-for-managers.pdf. Accessed October 1, 2009.

U.S. Department of Health & Human Services (USDHHS). Office on Women's Health. National Women's Health Information Center. An easy guide to breastfeeding for African American women; Washington, DC: USDHHS; 2006. www.womenshealth.gov/Pub/BF.AA.pdf. Accessed February 14, 2010.

Walkup J, et al. Randomized controlled trial of a paraprofessional-delivered in-home intervention for young reservation-based American Indian mothers. *J Am Acad Child Adolesc Psych.* 2009;48:591-601.

Wallby T, Hjern A. Region of birth, income and breastfeeding in a Swedish county. *Acta Paediatr.* 2009;98:1799-1804.

Walsh A, Moseley J, Jackson W. The effects of an infant-feeding classroom activity on the breast-feeding knowledge and intentions of adolescents. *J Sch Nurs.* 2008;24(3):164-169.

Wambach K, Cohen S. Breastfeeding experiences of urban adolescent mothers. *J Pediatr Nurs.* 2009;24:244-254.

World Health Organization. *Protecting, Promoting, and Supporting Breastfeeding: A Joint WHO/UNICEF Statement.* Geneva: WHO; 1989.

Ystrom E, et al. The impact of maternal negative affectivity and general self-efficacy on breastfeeding: the Norwegian Mother and Child Cohort Study. *J Pediatr.* 2008;152:68-72.

Breastfeeding Techniques
and Devices

The United States and other developed countries are fascinated with technology. Breastfeeding is no exception, with a variety of devices marketed to facilitate feedings. In such a climate, it is important for caregivers and parents alike to ask themselves what a woman truly needs in order to breastfeed. Moreover, what do parents truly need in order to care for an infant? Advertisements for baby-care items often focus on separation of the mother and baby, implying that separation is the desired norm. This trend is evident in breastfeeding devices as well, with use of a breast pump often reflecting an assumption that the mother and baby will be apart. Appropriate and conservative use of breastfeeding devices increases your effectiveness with mothers. Overuse of devices can overwhelm a new mother and make breastfeeding seem like a lot of work—many times, *too* much work. Teaching mothers techniques to assist with feedings helps them to become self-sufficient and to reach their breastfeeding goals.

∼ Key Terms

Alternate feeding method
Breast massage
Breast pump
Breast shells
C-hold
Cup feeding
Dancer hand position
Digital techniques
Disorganized suck
Drip milk
Dysfunctional suck
Flat nipple
Human Milk Banking
    Association of North
    America (HMBANA)
Holder pasteurization
Human milk bank
Hydrogel dressing

Inverted nipple
Inverted syringe
Manual expression
Nipple shield
Nursing supplementer
Olfactory senses
Oral aversion
Paced feeding
Pacifiers
Paladai
Pinch test
Pooled milk
Reverse pressure softening
Spoon feeding
Suck reorganization
Tube feeding
Uncoordinated suck

∼ Breastfeeding Techniques

Some simple techniques to assist breastfeeding are helpful to women prenatally and in the early weeks postpartum. Performing a pinch test, for instance, helps the mother determine whether her nipple will evert for feedings. Learning how to massage her breasts helps her with early feedings and facilitates removing milk from her breasts through pumping or hand expression. Supporting her breast during feedings can help the baby maintain a good latch during the early days of nursing.

Pinch Test

The pinch test can be used prenatally to assess a mother's nipples for protrusion. When a mother learns she has retracted or inverted nipples near the end of her pregnancy, she can begin manipulating her nipples to help increase protraction. Figure 21.1 shows a mother's breast before performing the pinch test. To test the protractility of the nipple, the mother grasps the base of the nipple with her forefinger and thumb, as in Figure 21.2. She then presses the thumb and forefinger together several times around the base.

If the nipple moves forward it is a normal, protracting nipple and needs no special intervention. A retracting nipple moves inward rather than outward, as depicted in Figure 21.2. It may benefit from the use of a nipple eversion device or a breast pump after the baby is born. A nipple may appear to be inverted on visual inspection and then evert when pinched. Although this type of nipple may need shaping before latching the baby, it will most likely not interfere with breastfeeding. A completely inverted nipple appears inverted on visual inspection and does not respond to stimulation. This type of nipple may improve with manipulation. See Chapter 7 for a discussion on differences in nipples.

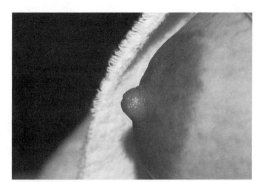

FIGURE 21.1   Pinch test: nipple at rest before compression.

Source: Printed with permission of Kay Hoover.

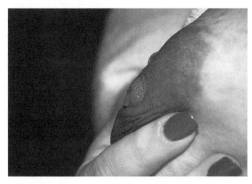

FIGURE 21.2   Pinch test: nipple retracts after compression.

Source: Printed with permission of Kay Hoover.

Breast Massage and Compression

Breast massage, or breast compression, can be helpful for breastfeeding mothers at various times and for a variety of reasons. Any form of massage encourages the mother to relax. Because touch causes myoepithelial cells to contract, breast massage helps stimulate letdown. During breast massage oxytocin levels increase and remain high throughout the massage (Yokoyama et al., 1994). Massage works in combination with oxytocin and the myoepithelial cells to help "push" the milk down the ducts where it is available for the baby to remove or for the mother to express. Squeezing increases positive pressure inside the breast, facilitating the movement of milk from an area of high pressure to an area of low pressure (the baby's mouth).

A mother often instinctively shapes her breast, provides support, and massages her breast while nursing her baby. You can point out these behaviors and praise her for naturally knowing what to do. Affirming her intuitive behavior helps build her confidence in herself and in her body. Breast massage can be especially useful to mothers attempting to relactate or to initiate lactation to nurse an adopted baby. The mother can massage her breasts just before a feeding, hand expression, or pumping to stimulate letdown. She can combine it with relaxation techniques such as deep breathing and visualization.

For a baby who seems impatient for milk to flow, the mother can massage to enhance letdown before putting her baby to breast. Performing massage before manual expression or pumping helps initiate letdown in these instances. Edema of the nipple and areola can cause the nipple to retract with a pinch test, thereby confusing mothers who had no nipple retraction prenatally. This is especially the case when a mother's labor is induced or when she has a long labor followed by a cesarean delivery, because of the massive fluid infusion.

Massage stimulates milk flow to alleviate engorgement, a plugged duct, or mastitis—all situations in which milk stasis increases difficulty. When the baby pauses during a feeding, alternate massage encourages sustained sucking in a sleepy baby or inefficient feeder. Alternate massage also increases the volume of fat content per feeding (Morton, 2004). Online sample clips of videos and demonstrations of hand expression are available at the Stanford School of Medicine Newborn Nursery (2009b).

Breast Compression

Breast compression is similar to massage focuses more on squeezing milk into the baby's mouth. To use this technique the mother holds her breast with one hand, with her thumb on the top of the breast and her other fingers on the bottom, well behind the areola. When her baby begins flutter sucking instead of sucking nutritively ("drinking"), she compresses the breast by squeezing gently. The compression simulates a letdown, often triggering another sucking burst (Newman & Kernerman, 2009). The mother can repeat this throughout the feeding whenever she notices the baby is not sucking effectively. This technique is helpful in the early days, especially with ineffective feeders, but is not necessary when the baby needs no help.

Breast Massage Technique

The techniques for breast massage are useful to teach mothers and easy for mothers to learn (Figure 21.3). Beginning at her chest wall the mother uses the palm of her hand to exert gentle pressure on the breast, massaging in a circular motion from the chest wall toward the nipple. Make sure she uses the palm of her hand and not her fingers. She continues in this manner, rotating her hand around the breast. Encourage her to focus on the areas of greatest milk duct development, which are under the breast and along the side under the arm. A mother with large breasts can support her breast with the other hand while she massages it. Women from a culture other than

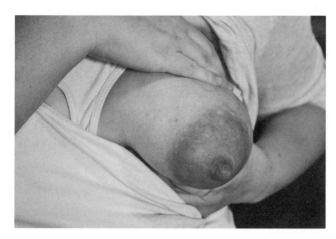

FIGURE 21.3 Breast massage.

Source: Printed with permission of Anna Swisher.

your own may have variations in breast massage that accomplish the same purpose.

Oketani Breast Massage

The Oketani method, named after a Japanese midwife, is a form of breast massage popular in Japan and other Asian countries as a way to stimulate milk production. The massager, typically a midwife, moves her fingers in motions to simulate the baby's sucking. One study found that the method significantly increased fat in the milk in the late lactating period but not in the early postpartum period. Casein (protein) amounts were increased by massage in the early postpartum period. The researchers found that lactose was not significantly changed (Foda et al., 2004). It makes intuitive sense that fats and other solids can be increased by massage, because these tend to adhere to the alveoli; the increased pressure from massage helps move them through the ducts.

Reverse Pressure Softening

Practitioners have observed that many mothers who receive intravenous fluids in a hospital delivery have edema in their breasts and extremities. This often results in flattening of the areola, similar to engorgement. A reverse pressure softening technique helps move the fluid away from the areola so the baby can latch. Table 21.1 shows this procedure, with instructions for the mother. The procedure has also proven helpful in relieving engorgement and triggering the mother's letdown reflex (Cotterman, 2004).

C-Hold

A mother often finds it helpful to support her breast for feedings in the early days when she and her baby are learn-

ing to latch. Some women are uncomfortable touching and handling their breasts and may need verbal encouragement and "hands-on" assistance. Cupping the breast with one hand similar to the shape of the letter "C"—referred to as the C-hold—forms the breast and nipple to help the baby latch. Continuing this throughout the feeding supports the weight of the breast and keeps the nipple from slipping out of the baby's mouth. The mother cups the breast in her hand, placing her thumb on top and her fingers below (see Figure 14.2 in Chapter 14). Make sure the mother places her hand well behind the areola so that her fingers do not interfere with her baby's latch. If the baby's chin, jaw, or lips touch the mother's hand, she needs to move her hand back toward the chest wall. The fingers and thumb can slightly compress the breast to help form it for the baby. Guide the mother to compress the breast so that it matches the plane of the baby's mouth, like a "breast taco" or "breast sandwich" (Wiessinger, 1998). When the mother senses that her baby no longer needs assistance, she can discontinue holding her breast at feedings.

Dancer Hand Position

A slight variation of the C-hold is useful with premature infants and other babies who have weak muscle development and find it difficult to hold their jaw steady while they suck. This position, the Dancer hand position, begins in the C-hold position. The mother then brings her hand forward to support her breast with the first three fingers. She supports the baby's chin in the crook of her hand between her thumb and index finger (see Figure 14.3 in Chapter 14). The mother can bend her index finger slightly so that it gently holds the baby's cheek on one side, with the thumb holding the other cheek. This hold helps decrease the available space in the baby's mouth and increases negative pressure. The use of steady, equal pressure while holding her baby's cheeks avoids interfering with the rooting reflex. As the baby's muscle tone begins to improve, the mother can move her thumb back on top of the breast, with her index finger supporting the baby's chin.

⁓ Breastfeeding Devices

Sometimes a mother may have a special need for a breastfeeding device to assist her with feedings or the care of her breasts. After careful assessment, you can make appropriate suggestions to facilitate breastfeeding. Starting with the least invasive methods for approaching a problem leads to fewer complications and later difficulties. Mothers who use breastfeeding aids often need special counseling suggestions and close follow-up during their use.

TABLE 21.1   Reverse Pressure Softening Technique

You (or your helper, from in front, or behind you) choose one of the patterns pictured. To see your areola better, try using a hand mirror. Place the fingers/thumbs on the circle touching the nipple. If swelling is very firm, lie down on your back, and/or ask someone to help by pressing his or her fingers on top of your fingers. Push gently but firmly straight inward toward your ribs. Hold the pressure steady for a period of 1 to 3 full minutes.

Relax, breathe easy, sing a lullaby, listen to a favorite song or have someone else watch a clock or set a timer. It is okay to repeat the inward pressure again as often as you need. Deep "dimples" may form, lasting long enough for easy latching. Keep testing how soft your areola feels. You may also press with a soft ring made by cutting off half of an artificial nipple. Offer your baby your breast promptly while the circle is soft.

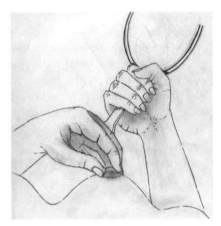

One handed "flower hold." Fingernails short, fingertips curved, placed where baby's tongue will go.

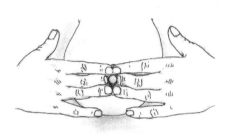

Two handed, one-step method. Fingernails short, fingertips curved, each one touching the side of nipple.

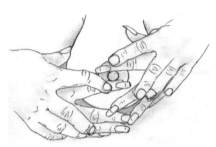

You may ask someone to help press by placing fingers or thumbs on top of yours.

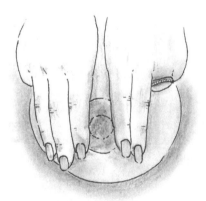

Two step method, two hands, using 2 or 3 straight fingers each side, first knuckles touching nipple. Move ¼ turn, repeat above and below nipple.

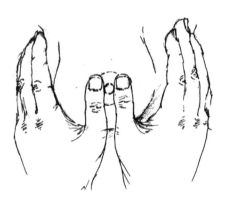

Two step method, two hands, using straight thumbs, base of thumbnail even with side of nipple. Move ¼ turn, repeat, thumbs above and below nipple.

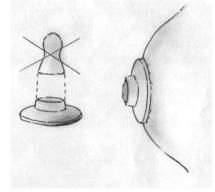

Soft ring method. Cut off bottom half of an artificial nipple to place on areola to press with fingers.

Source: Printed by permission of Lactation Education Consultants, © 2010. May be reproduced for noncommercial purposes. K. Jean Cotterman, RNC, IBCLC. Illustrations by Kyle Cotterman.

Lubricants on the Breast and Nipple

Glands within the areolar skin normally keep the nipple area soft and pliable. An artificial lubricant is necessary only if this natural lubrication has been disturbed and needs to be replaced. A lubricant may be necessary prenatally when a mother has excessively dry skin, eczema, or other dermatological condition. It can also replace moisture when the improper use of drying agents or other practices have removed the natural lubrication. After breastfeeding begins mothers can apply a lubricant if their nipples become sore or cracked. Research varies on the effect of breast lubricants (see the discussion on sore nipples below and in Chapter 16), however many mothers believe that topical treatments reduce soreness. You can guide them in making appropriate decisions.

Lubricants to Avoid

The choice of breast lubricant must take into consideration its potential effects on the health of both the mother's breast skin and her baby. Mothers should avoid any lubricant that contains petroleum, because it inhibits skin respiration and can actually prolong nipple soreness. Petroleum-based products include baby oil, petroleum jelly, cocoa butter, A and D ointment, and dimethicone. Additionally, mothers should avoid products that contain alcohol, which are drying to the skin. They also should not use vitamin E oil due to the potential for elevated levels in the baby (Marx et al., 1985) and sealing of an open wound with a crack.

If the baby's mother or father has a family history of allergies, the mother should avoid exposing the baby to a potential allergen such as peanut oil or massé cream. Women with a family history of wool allergy should avoid lubricants that contain wool derivatives. Any product the mother must wash off can further irritate sore nipples from rubbing the nipple with a washcloth. Mothers receive a variety of breast creams in the hospital that also are available in most pharmacies. Generally, although these products do no harm, they are ineffective in the prevention of sore nipples and may delay a mother from seeking early help.

Acceptable Applications

Many lactation experts suggest application of the mother's colostrum or milk for the treatment of sore nipples. The prophylactic benefit of human milk to infants is well established, and it may help in the treatment of nipple soreness as well. One study found that although expressing milk did not help prevent cracked nipples, fewer mothers had nipple pain in the group that applied their expressed milk (Akkuzu & Taskin, 2000).

Hypoallergenic, medical-grade, anhydrous lanolin may help severely dry or sore nipples. This form of lanolin does not contain the concerning levels of pesticides or alcohols that contribute to allergic response and are therefore less of a risk in allergic patients. A small amount massaged gently into the nipple and areola after a feeding is sufficient. When applied correctly after a feeding, the skin absorbs the lubricant before the next feeding.

Some practitioners recommend hydrogel dressings in the form of gel pads. The pads are worn between feedings to soothe sore nipples. Those designed for breast use are circular and flat, with two sides of film that the mother peels off before use. They can be stored in the refrigerator to provide the additional comfort of coolness. Some gel pads can be washed and reused. Mothers should discontinue the use of gel pads if they experience further soreness or irritation. One study found a higher infection rate with gel pads than with lanolin (Brent et al., 1998). Another study found the opposite, with infection in some

of the lanolin users and none in the hydrogel group (Dodd & Chalmers, 2003). Gel pads are water based and keep the skin moist. If using gel pads some lactation consultants recommend air drying the nipple before feeding.

There is no substitute for clinical judgment and experience when you work with mothers. You should first address the root cause of soreness and determine if correcting latch and positioning will remedy the problem. If soreness persists and you perceive that the mother wants "something" to fix the problem, the use of lanolin or gel pads can help her through a period of transient soreness and extend breastfeeding duration. Instruct the mother to discontinue gel pad use and contact her physician if she sees any sign of infection.

Inverted Syringe for Flat or Inverted Nipples

Some clinicians suggest the use of an inverted syringe to help mothers evert a flat or inverted nipple. This technique has been used prenatally as well as before a feeding. In the prenatal period the mother should first check with her primary caregiver to determine whether such nipple stimulation is safe during her pregnancy. For certain women nipple stimulation prenatally can lead to preterm labor.

When using an inverted syringe to evert the nipple, the mother needs a syringe with a barrel slightly larger than her nipple. Usually a 10- to 20-mL syringe works well. After cutting off the tapered end of the syringe, she reverses the plunger direction to provide a smooth surface against the breast. Caution the mother not to place the cut end against her breast, because the sharp edges could damage her breast tissue. With the smooth end of the syringe placed over her nipple, the mother then pulls gently on the plunger (Figure 21.4). There are commercial eversion products, such as the Evert-It nipple enhancer, a syringe with a soft, flexible tip made of silicone. The mother can use either end to provide suction to help her

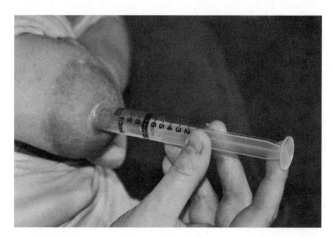

FIGURE 21.4 Inverted syringe used to pull out the nipple.

Source: Printed with permission of Anna Swisher.

nipples protrude for easier latch. Another, the Latch Assist, resembles a miniature bicycle horn pump and is used in the same manner.

It is important that the mother do the pulling on the syringe and not you or another caregiver, because only she can assess her comfort level. Instruct her to gentle pressure and to hold the pressure for about 30 seconds and then release. If she experiences pain, she should stop the procedure. and she should never pull hard enough to cause pain or color changes in the nipple. After each use the syringe should be washed in hot, soapy water and then rinsed and air-dried for the next use (Kesaree et al., 1993).

Women can use this technique prenatally two or three times a day until the baby is born, holding the plunger out for 30 seconds two or three times in each session. After birth, use of the syringe helps evert the nipple for babies that have difficulty latching. There has been debate among lactation professionals about the use of syringes for nipple eversion as a "use for which the device is not intended." If you practice in a hospital, ask for guidance from your administration. If you are in private practice, use your judgment to determine if this use is appropriate or if a commercial device specifically for nipple eversion would be more prudent.

Breast Shells

Plastic breast shells are worn against the breast inside the bra. The bra should be a cup size larger than the shell to avoid pressing the shell too tightly against the breast. The shells should have several openings for air circulation to keep the skin from becoming softened and susceptible to chapping. Mothers can sometimes achieve a similar effect to that produced by the shell by cutting a small hole in the bra that allows the nipple to protrude.

Women have used breast shells prenatally to improve nipple protractility from the gentle pressure placed on the areola which stretches and pushes the nipple forward (Figure 21.5). There is no clear research to support the premise that wearing breast shells prenatally everts nipples. Anecdotally, women have reported good results. Mothers wear breast shells in the early days postpartum to protect their clothes from milk that leaks between feedings. Make sure mothers know they cannot save milk that accumulates in a breast shell worn between feedings because of possible bacterial growth. However, a mother can collect milk in a breast shell worn on the opposite breast during a feeding. If she plans to save the drip milk, she must be sure the shell is clean and placed on the breast immediately before the feeding.

Some mothers use breast shells to relieve engorgement, wearing them for about 20 minutes before feedings. Wearing them between, or for short periods before, feedings can help shape a flat or inverted nipple to improve latch. Shells can protect a sore nipple between feedings

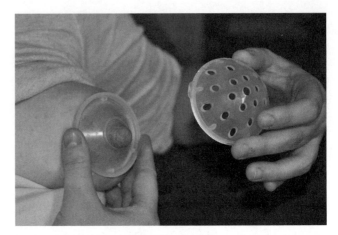

FIGURE 21.5 Breast shell on the breast.
Source: Printed with permission of Anna Swisher.

and prevent rubbing against clothing that could irritate the skin further. Caution mothers not to wear breast shells while they sleep and not to use them excessively.

Researchers measured the recommendation to use shells and found that it was associated with a shortened duration of breastfeeding (Alexander et al., 1992). The researchers did not measure whether women actually used the shells or for how many hours per day or how many weeks before giving birth. It may be that women associated the recommendations for devices with breastfeeding being too difficult.

Nipple Shield

A nipple shield is an artificial nipple placed over the mother's nipple during a feeding so the baby latches on to the nipple shield to nurse (Figure 21.6). Used throughout time, nipple shields have been made out of glass, metal, and even lead (Gordon & Whitehead, 1949). Older studies with rubber and latex shields reported significant decreases in the volume of milk transfer (Amatayakul et al., 1987; Jackson et al., 1987). Today's nipple shields are made of thin silicone. Some have cutouts to allow the baby's nose and chin to remain in contact with the breast (Figure 21.7).

Considerations when using nipple shields include selection of correct size and material (silicone, never rubber or latex), infant preference, possible breast tissue damage, adequate sucking stimulation, correct shield placement during feeding, and adequate milk transfer. Never use a baby bottle nipple as a nipple shield. Whenever you use alternative feeding methods, the mother's preference for the method is an important consideration. Your clinical expertise will help you gauge the best intervention for each mother and baby.

Optimally, nipple shields should be used under the care of a lactation consultant to ensure appropriate use. However, nipple shields are widely available in many

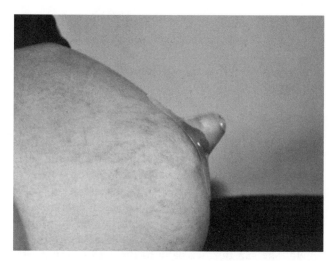

FIGURE 21.6 Nipple shield on the breast to help the baby latch.

Source: Printed with permission of Anna Swisher.

retail stores, and online. Many mothers buy them without input from a lactation consultant, based on recommendations from friends or relatives. It is common for mothers to bring nipple shields to the hospital before birth.

Appropriate Use of a Nipple Shield

A nipple shield should not be the first intervention for latching difficulties or sucking concerns. Other techniques need to be tried first, such as a change in positioning, forming the nipple, reducing breast fullness, nipple eversion techniques, and active sucking. As with any breastfeeding device, a nipple shield can be a useful transitional tool for breastfeeding when used wisely (Chertok, 2009; Wilson-Clay & Hoover, 2008; Chertok et al., 2006; Meier et al., 2000; Wilson-Clay, 1996).

Meier et al. (2000) found a significant increase in milk transfer when preterm babies used a nipple shield. The mean transfer was 18.4 mL with the nipple shield versus 3.9 mL without. The outcome was so significant that researchers halted the control group not using the nipple

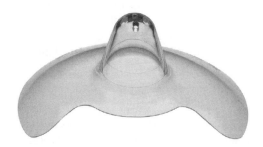

FIGURE 21.7 Contact nipple shield with cutout to allow contact with the breast.

Source: © Medela, Inc., 2010.

shield (Meier et al., 2000). It appears that a nipple shield helps babies with low tone (including preterm and small for gestational age) sustain suction within the oral cavity by holding the nipple in the mouth. The nipple shield may compensate for the lack of fat buccal pads and weak suck common in these babies (Wilson-Clay & Hoover, 2008).

A nipple shield has also been used for babies with a short tongue, tight frenulum, or high palate. It can help a mother who has flat or inverted nipples that have not responded to other attempts to improve latch. A shield can also aid the transition to direct breastfeeding when a baby has been bottle fed and refuses the breast. If a mother is considering weaning because of breastfeeding difficulties, a shield can buy the mother and baby time to work through the difficulty and preserve breastfeeding (Wilson-Clay & Hoover, 2008; Wilson-Clay, 1996).

Chertok (2009) reported no statistically significant differences in infant weight gain for 54 dyads using nipple shields for 2 months. A large majority of the women (89.8 percent) reported a positive experience with nipple shield use, and 67.3 percent reported that the nipple shield helped prevent breastfeeding termination. An earlier pilot study of 32 mothers measuring maternal prolactin and cortisol levels as well as infant weight gain also reported no significant differences in weight gain or milk production while using nipple shields (Chertok et al., 2006).

Method for Using a Nipple Shield

The baby's sucking draws the mother's nipple into the shield and it is best to begin with the smallest shield possible that accommodates both the baby's mouth and the mother's nipple. This enables the baby to obtain a deeper latch. Never try to force a large, prominent nipple into a small shield. Nipple shields are typically available in 16-, 20-, 21-, 24-, 25-, and 26-mm sizes.

With the appropriately sized shield, make sure the mother understands how to apply it for the best fit:

- Moisten the edges of the shield.
- Fold it back so that it is almost inside out.
- Place it snugly over the nipple with the mother's nipple centered in the shield.
- Smooth the shield over the nipple.
- If the baby needs encouragement to suck, insert expressed milk into the shield with a syringe (Figure 21.8).

When used appropriately, a nipple shield optimally is in place for only a few minutes at the beginning of the feeding. Sometimes, smoothing the shield over the nipple draws the nipple into the shield. The mother can nurse for several minutes with the shield in place until her baby's sucking draws the nipple into the shield. After a few more minutes she can remove the shield and then quickly put

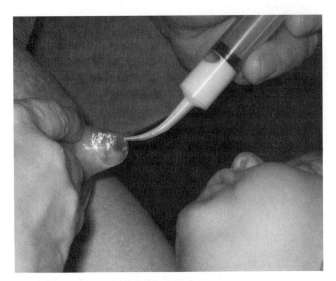

FIGURE 21.8 Filling nipple shield with milk to entice baby to suck.

Source: Printed with permission of Catherine Watson Genna, BS, IBCLC.

her baby back to breast to suck without the shield. A preterm or low-birth-weight infant may need the shield in place for the entire feeding to transfer milk.

Monitoring and Follow-up

The need for a nipple shield is a symptom of an underlying problem and mothers should follow up with a lactation consultant and/or their infants' healthcare provider. The mother needs to monitor her baby's intake and output carefully during the shield's use, with a daily record of feedings, voids, and stools. She should check her baby's weight periodically; prefeeding and postfeeding weight checks determine if the nipple shield allows the baby to transfer milk adequately.

Some mothers may need to pump when they are using a nipple shield in order to maintain sufficient milk production. However, if a baby is transferring milk well with the nipple shield, excessive pumping in the early days could result in overactive milk production. On the other hand, a mother with a late preterm baby who feeds ineffectively with a nipple shield needs to pump to establish and maintain her production. Every mother and baby's case is unique and requires a feeding plan tailored to their individual needs.

Encourage mothers to consider the shield as a bridge to work through a breastfeeding difficulty, and to wean from the shield as soon as is practical. Most infants who need to mature and fatten up transition from a nipple shield easily once they can milk the breast as effectively without it as with it. In the instances of severely inverted nipples that will not evert or uncommon infant anomalies such as a submucosal cleft, the mother may need to use a

shield for the entire time she breastfeeds. Give her lots of praise and affirmation for persevering, and help her feel positive about her experience. Mothers have nursed with a nipple shield for their entire duration of breastfeeding with no adverse effects.

Weaning the Baby From the Shield

When you and the mother decide that the time is right to work toward weaning from the shield, the mother may benefit from practical suggestions. A past recommendation of trimming the shield gradually is not advisable because the trimmed edges of silicone could lacerate the baby's mouth or the mother's nipple. Rather, the mother can watch for cues that her baby might nurse without the shield. She can put her baby to the breast periodically without the shield when it "feels right" to see whether he or she will nurse without it. Often, a sleepy baby is less likely to resist the transfer from shield to breast. Some babies are more receptive after the initial fullness at the beginning of a feeding has decreased. Increased skin-to-skin contact with the mother aids in the transition from shield to breast. The mother can try slipping the shield out when the baby has nursed well and is in a satiated sleeping state; often, the baby will continue to suck. Some babies can be encouraged to nurse directly when cobathing with the mother.

Pacifiers

Pacifiers can help meet the sucking needs of a bottle fed baby but they are often a source of difficulty for a breastfeeding baby. The debate about pacifier use for breastfeeding babies intensified when the American Academy of Pediatrics (AAP) recommended use of a pacifier to reduce sudden infant death syndrome, as discussed in Chapter 13 (AAP, 2005b).

Pacifiers offer no nutritional benefit to an infant. They expend calories and, in some instances, can contribute to slowed growth. Studies suggest that pacifiers also increase the incidence of candida and ear infections (Mattos-Graner et al., 2001; Warren et al., 2001). The AAP and the American Academy of Family Physicians (AAFP) recommend weaning children from pacifiers in the second 6 months of life to prevent otitis media (Sexton & Natale, 2009). Pacifiers can also cause malocclusion (Charchut et al., 2003; Larson, 2001; Palmer, 2004; Zardetto et al., 2002).

Appropriate Use of a Pacifier

Because pacifiers are so prevalent, mothers need to receive instructions on safe pacifier use. Figure 21.9 shows two types of pacifier designs. The first type, with an "orthodontic" shape, elicits a different sucking pattern from all other nipples (Nowak et al., 1994; Wolf & Glass, 1992).

Additionally, the multiple parts have the potential to harbor bacteria, thrush, and mold. The second type is a solid piece of molded silicone with no separate parts and may be a safer choice for the baby. The pacifier's material also may be a safety issue. Because of a growing concern about latex allergies, mothers may want to avoid latex pacifiers. A 1998 recall occurred because one brand contained phthalates, which can be harmful in large doses; phthalates are no longer used in pacifiers. Parents should never connect a pacifier to a cord around the baby's neck because of the potential for strangulation. If their baby has a medical or therapeutic need for a pacifier, parents can work with their occupational therapist to select one that is best for their baby's particular needs (Wolf & Glass, 1992).

Preterm Babies Preterm infants benefit from sucking on pacifiers during gavage feeding (Barlow et al., 2008; Poore et al., 2008). A Cochrane review found that nonnutritive sucking decreased the length of hospital stay significantly in preterm infants (Pinelli & Symington, 2005). Accelerated maturation of the sucking reflex, decreased intestinal transit time, and increased rates of weight gain are all positive effects of pacifier use in these infants. Electrical stimulating pacifiers appear to help mature the preterm infants' sucking rhythm.

Alleviating Pain A pacifier helps calm infants who must undergo painful procedures and may be an especially effective way to reduce testing stress for severely ill babies (Elserafy et al., 2009; Kapellou, 2009). Fussy, term babies in neonatal intensive care units (NICU) may benefit from a pacifier if feedings are restricted or for times when they are NPO (Latin term, *nil por os*, meaning "nothing by mouth") for medical reasons. Pacifier use for these babies avoids excessive crying which increases blood pressure, heart rate, and calorie expenditure.

Gastroesophageal Reflux Disease (GERD) Some occupational therapists recommend pacifiers for babies with gastroesophageal reflux disease (GERD). A pacifier allows the baby to suck for comfort and to salivate, which coats the esophagus and reduces pain. Constant sucking at the breast can cause the baby to consume excess amounts of milk, overfilling the baby's stomach and aggravating the disease (Boekel, 2000). See the discussion on gastroesophageal reflux disease in Chapter 13.

Concerns with Breastfeeding

Mothers need to ensure that her baby's time spent sucking on a pacifier does not compromise time needed at the breast. Excessive pacifier use interferes with the symbiotic relationship of the baby increasing the mother's milk production through sucking. Therefore pacifiers can negatively affect a mother's milk production in relation to her baby's needs. A baby who uses a pacifier frequently may show poor weight gain from having inadequate time at the breast. Less time at the breast can also cause insufficient milk drainage, which, in turn, can result in engorgement or mastitis for the mother.

Missed Hunger Cues When a baby uses a pacifier, it is easy for parents to miss hunger cues. The baby may suck on the pacifier, grow hungrier, spit out the pacifier, and start crying—a late indicator of hunger (AAP, 2005a). A baby who is frantic and hungry is difficult to soothe enough to latch and nurse. Sucking on a pacifier can also tire some babies—especially late preterm babies (35–37 weeks)—causing the baby to fall asleep and miss a feeding. Because the baby was sucking on a pacifier, the parents were unable to see hunger cues their baby would have demonstrated. Rather than using a pacifier in response to crying, encourage parents to respond to early hunger cues and help them learn other ways to comfort their baby (see the discussion of crying in Chapter 13).

Lower Breastfeeding Rates Pacifier use in the neonatal period is detrimental to exclusive and overall breastfeeding and should be avoided (Howard et al., 2003). Pacifier use has been shown to result in a shorter duration of breastfeeding and fewer feedings (Karabulut et al., 2009; Kronborg & Vaeth, 2009). One study reported a strong relationship between daily pacifier use and weaning by 3 months (25 percent use vs. 12.9 percent nonuse). Other studies suggest that although pacifier use does not necessarily cause early weaning, it may be a marker for breastfeeding difficulties or decreased maternal motivation to breastfeed (Benis, 2002; O'Connor et al., 2009). The AAP recommends that, "For breastfed infants, delay pacifier introduction until 1 month of age to ensure that breastfeeding is firmly established" (AAP, 2005b).

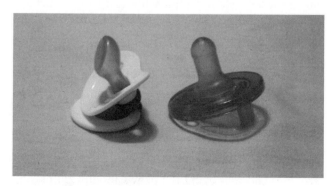

FIGURE 21.9 Two types of pacifiers.
Source: Printed with permission of Anna Swisher.

Guidelines with Breastfeeding A pacifier should not replace sufficient breastfeeding, interaction, or skin contact with the mother. It should be used only after the baby's needs for food, comfort, and human contact are fully met. Encourage mothers to tune into their baby's cues. A baby that settles when being held may simply have needed comfort. A baby that remains unsettled and roots should be put to breast before being given a pacifier. If the baby does not want to nurse and continues to demonstrate a need to suck, a pacifier may be appropriate.

～ Digital Techniques

The baby's oral cavity is extremely sensitive and contains many nerve fibers and impulses. Too much inappropriate stimulation can result in an aversion to anything going into the mouth, including the breast. Inserting your finger into a baby's mouth should be done only when necessary and within your scope of practice. The use of digital techniques ranges from calming a baby to assessing the oral cavity to improving the baby's suck. At the most advanced level a clinician may use digital manipulation to alter a dysfunctional suck.

Barger (2009) identified four levels of digital intervention for infants who have difficulty sucking. When a mother needs assistance, the caregiver should start with the least intrusive method and progress to a higher degree of intervention only when other less intrusive methods have failed. Refer to Chapter 15 for further discussion on the four levels of digital intervention.

Minimal Level: Pacifying the Baby

The least invasive digital technique involves the evaluator or parent touching the baby's lips with an index finger, pad side up. The caregiver waits for the baby to latch onto the finger and draw it into his or her mouth (Figure 21.10). Parents may use this to pacify their baby or to initiate sucking at the beginning of a feeding. They can also use it in conjunction with a tube feeding system at the breast to increase the baby's calorie intake, described later in this chapter under finger feeding. Passively presenting your finger in this way is a minimal level of intervention, with the baby in total control when sucking on your finger.

Low Level: Evaluating the Oral Cavity

Digitally evaluating the infant's oral cavity is a low-level intervention used by many clinicians when assessing an infant's suck. With the baby relaxed, placing your fingertip on the upper lip should trigger the rooting reflex. When the baby's mouth opens, place your finger pad side up. When the baby draws your finger into his or her mouth, subtly move your finger to feel the inside of the oral cav-

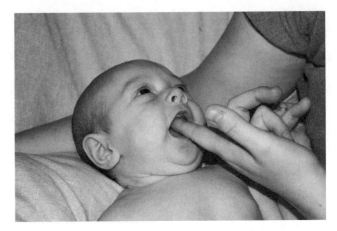

FIGURE 21.10 Index finger inserted pad side up to pacify baby.

Source: Printed with permission of Kori Martin.

ity and the palate. Assess whether the palate is normal, flat, or excessively high. As the baby sucks notice whether the tongue covers the alveolar ridge and cups around the bottom of your finger to form a trough. Detect whether the tongue moves rhythmically from front to back. Assessing these elements helps determine if a problem exists. Evaluating the oral cavity, although a bit more invasive, still places the baby in control of sucking on the finger.

Moderate Level: Suck Reorganization

It is common for a baby to exhibit an uncoordinated or disorganized suck, especially a baby who is preterm or late preterm. Uncoordinated sucking often resolves with the passage of time as the baby's system and reflexes become more mature. Increasing the baby's caloric intake can also help resolve a disorganized suck. Use of a nursing supplementer can provide fluids at the breast while the baby sucks; the flow of fluid regulates suck and therefore improves sucking for some babies. It should first be determined if these methods achieve the desired result before attempting any digital manipulation.

Digitally manipulating a baby's suck should be done only if the baby alone cannot achieve organized sucking. As the baby draws in your finger, pad side up, place slight downward pressure on the midline of the tongue and pull your finger out slowly to encourage the baby to suck it back in. Verbal praise reinforces appropriate movement. This may be all the baby needs to organize sucking into an effective rhythm and movement.

High Level: Suck Training

The technique known as suck training involves tapping, stroking, and massaging the baby's tongue, gums, and palate. A baby who needs suck training should be referred to a professional who is trained and skilled in this field, such as a physical therapist (PT), occupational therapist (OT), or speech therapist (SLP or SLT) with specialization in infant disorders. A need for suck training may indicate other neurological deficits, with the suck being one of the first areas where the problem manifests. Do not attempt to handle this situation alone, and do not cavalierly manipulate a baby's sucking.

Suck training is beyond the scope of practice for most nurses and lactation consultants, unless you have obtained special training in this area or are also an occupational therapist or speech therapist. In suck training the therapist places an index finger in the baby's mouth, pad side up, and stimulates certain portions of the oral anatomy to train the baby to suck. There are different types of stimulation, including the therapist's finger "walking" back on the tongue. Different tools and textures are also used.

Close coordination of care and communication between the therapist, the lactation consultant, and the baby's primary physician helps to ensure that the family obtains the appropriate level of help, while protecting the potential to breastfeed. If the baby is definitively diagnosed with neurological or other physical problems, community support and parent education groups are recommended.

∼ Milk Expression

There are times in most women's breastfeeding when they need to remove milk from their breasts. Mothers need to understand that no matter what method of milk expression they use, they cannot remove milk from their breasts as effectively as the sucking of a robust baby. The baby combines suction, negative pressure, and rhythmic compression of the areola with his or her gums. Just as a mother and baby need time to learn how to nurse, a mother may express several times before she becomes proficient and is able to obtain the desired amount of milk. Gentle breast massage may help relax and soothe the mother so she can express more milk.

Manual Expression

Knowing how to hand express their milk enables women to be self-reliant, no matter what circumstances arise in the course of breastfeeding. They can extract milk during a brief separation and despite a broken pump, power failure, natural disaster, or low battery. Learning to be independent and to function without a need for devices can instill further self-confidence. The mother is able to express anytime and anywhere without waiting. Hand expression is free and quiet, and the mother is in charge of the pressure. Milk collection by hand expression has been shown to have lower contamination rates compared with milk collection using a breast pump (Boo, 2001).

Mothers of preterm babies are encouraged to hand express their milk, in addition to using a breast pump. In a study where mothers combined hand expression and pumping with an electric breast pump in the first 3 days, milk output increased by 48 percent (Morton et al., 2009). One mother reportedly increased her milk production by hand expression and tube feeding the baby the pumped milk at the breast (Lopes de Melo & Murta, 2009).

Technique for Manual Expression

In preparing to express by hand the mother should first wash her hands well. If she wishes she can gently massage her breast and apply a warm, moist cloth for several minutes before expressing her milk. Both techniques help promote milk flow. Massaging her breast throughout her expressing session will continue to promote the flow of milk.

To begin expressing she can lean slightly forward with her nipple aimed at the collection container, as shown in Figure 21.11. Steps in milk expression include the following:

- Grasp the breast as when using the C-hold.
- Place the thumb behind the areola above the nipple.
- Place the index finger behind the areola below the nipple.
- Press the thumb and index finger inward gently toward the chest wall.
- Firmly press on the ducts beneath the areola between the finger and thumb.
- Continue the cycle of pressing and releasing the thumb and forefinger.
- Move the thumb and forefinger placement to compress ducts around the areola.

Initially, it may take several attempts until milk begins to drip. Milk will spray out with greater force after the milk lets down. Caution the mother not to squeeze the nipple itself and not to move her fingers along her skin. Such actions have little or no benefit to expressing milk and can irritate the breast tissue. A demonstration of hand expression is available online at the Stanford School of Medicine (2009a).

Many mothers find a variation of this method of hand expression that works equally well or better. Some women, for example, express by cupping the breast with the C-hold, gently massaging and applying pressure on the ducts. Encourage mothers to experiment with various hand positions until they find what works best for them. There is no one correct way for this or many other techniques. Honor individual choices by not commenting

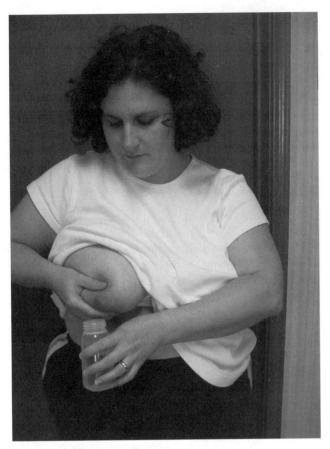

FIGURE 21.11   Mother hand expressing her milk.

Source: Printed with permission of Anna Swisher.

negatively or insisting on the mother's conforming to a certain technique. Practice and adaptation are keys to hand expression working for the mother. When she masters hand expression, it can be as fast and efficient as a breast pump. Teaching hand expression to mothers increases their self-confidence. The more comfortable a woman becomes with massage and hand expression, the more comfortable she becomes in all areas of her mothering experience.

Use of a Breast Pump

Breast pump use has soared within the past 20 years, in part because of the Western world's enthusiasm for technology and fixation on gadgets to "fix" things. Breast pumps have become a standard baby shower gift and many women who plan to breastfeed own one before they give birth.

Appropriate Use of Pumps

Lactation consultants struggle with the complex issue of pump use. A qualitative study interviewed 12 long-term lactation consultants about the impact of pumps on breastfeeding practices (Buckley, 2009). The respondents reported that "technological birth" has led to "technological breastfeeding." The dangerous trend toward normalizing technology as a part of childbirth has translated to the use of technology in breastfeeding. The overuse of high-tech obstetrical interventions increases breastfeeding problems that must then be managed with breast pumps. Breast pumps seem to satisfy women's desire for control over a process they did not trust to unfold easily, similar to the perception that labor interventions offer greater control over the unpredictable process of birth.

Pumping enables working women to continue to lactate and provides an efficient means for mothers to express milk for preterm, sick, or impaired infants. However, the wide availability of pumps, and the perception that they are a requirement for breastfeeding, is distressing to those who worry that pumps contribute to the medicalization (Avishai, 2007) and objectification (Sweet, 2006) of breastfeeding. Breast pumping may be seen to create a dichotomy in breastfeeding, posing the question of whether it is the mother or the mother's milk that is most important to the baby (Lepore, 2009). Lactation consultants need to be careful not to promote pumping and other gadgets to the detriment of breastfeeding.

Ethical Considerations Some consider breast pump sales and rentals as a part of a lactation consultant's or hospital's income to be controversial. Hospital-grade pumps are expensive and represent a significant capital expense when purchased or a high overhead expense when leased. A lactation consultant who rents or sells breast pumps to clients needs to ensure that the service is conducted within the professional Code of Ethics. Many lactation consultants choose not to lease or sell pumps to avoid this dilemma. Others consider that if a mother is going to use a pump, it is important that she receive expert help in selecting and using one.

Need for Support and Follow-up When a mother is using a breast pump, no matter the reason, close contact with a lactation consultant helps identify any difficulties with pumping or with maintaining milk production. Her needs are especially great when she is using a mechanical device to empty her breasts and maintain milk production without the emotional gratification of her baby nuzzling at her breast. Her reactions to using a breast pump may range from fear of possible pain, to embarrassment, to irritation, to passive acceptance, or to gratitude and relief. It is common for mothers who are pumping for preterm babies to vacillate between these feelings.

If the need for a pump has resulted from a health problem, the mother may be anxious about the outcome and want to share her concerns with someone. If she will be pumping for an extended time she may experience periods of discouragement and will benefit from your reassurance and support. A mother who is preoccupied with the situation requiring that she pump may not pay close attention to the information you provide her. Make a special effort to offer clear instructions and explanations. In a NICU setting, where you work with mothers over weeks or months, understand that you may need to repeat instructions multiple times before the mother can take the information in.

Although her present circumstances may be stressful, you can help a mother view pumping as a positive tool in the resolution of her need for the device. Encourage her to regard pumping as more than a means of obtaining milk—it is her lifeline to breastfeeding her baby and by pumping regularly she can maintain the potential to breastfeed. It is something that only she can do for her baby and in a situation in which she can do little else, pumping can help a mother to feel involved and essential.

Selecting a Breast Pump

In selecting a breast pump the mother should consider her baby's age and condition and how long she needs to pump. If she will pump at work, she can consider the amount of time she has available for pumping, facilities for pumping and storage, affordability, and personal preference. If she is pumping in the absence of direct breastfeeding, she needs an efficient electric pump to ensure sufficient milk production.

Familiarize yourself with the many types of available breast pumps, as well as the ease with which mothers can obtain them. Provide practical information such as descriptions and prices of various pumps, how they are used, and their advantages and disadvantages. Breast pumps manufactured by companies that sell artificial baby milk or feeding products may not be the best choice. Advise mothers to select a pump manufactured by a company with a good performance record. Some mothers like the automatic cycling provided by leading pump manufacturers. Others prefer being able to release the suction themselves. Mothers must avoid long periods of uninterrupted vacuum that could damage breast tissue. Your guidance will help mothers select the appropriate pump for her specific needs.

Flange Size

The mother needs a flange size that fits her breast and nipple and does not cause friction against the nipple. Her nipple should move freely inside the tunnel without contacting the sides of the tunnel during suction. One manufacturer provides a nipple template for sizing; be aware that the nipple expands by a few millimeters during pumping (Wilson-Clay & Hoover, 2008). For mothers whose nipples are too large for the standard sized flanges (24-, 25-, or 26-mm), flanges ranging from 27 to 40 mm are available depending on the manufacturer. The 40-mm flanges are glass and very expensive. Mothers who have small nipples and areolas benefit from special inserts that rest inside the flange to achieve the proper fit. How-

ever, the inserts can cause sore breasts or nipples in some women.

Criteria for Selecting a Breast Pump

- Does it cycle quickly, similar to the rhythm of the baby's suck? Or is the mother able to self-cycle, at a rate that is comfortable for her?
- Is the flange shape comfortable and an appropriate size for the mother's breast?
- Are smaller and larger flanges available?
- Are inserts available for the flanges for very small areolas and nipples?
- Can standard-size bottles be used for collecting milk?
- Are the pump parts dishwasher safe?
- Is the pump easy to assemble, with few parts?
- Is the pump easy and comfortable to use with the type of hand or arm motion required?
- If the pump is electric, is the power source adequate (i.e., type of outlet—two or three prongs—and amount of voltage)?
- Is the pump quiet?
- Is the pump easy to transport?
- Is the pump affordable for the length of time it is required?
- Are quick service and overnight replacement available?
- What period and what parts does the warranty cover?
- Are written instructions provided that are easy to understand?
- Is there someone at the company who is knowledgeable in breastfeeding to answer questions and resolve problems?
- Is there a toll-free number to call with questions?
- Is there an up-to-date website?

Hand-Held Breast Pump

Many mothers use a hand-held breast pump as an occasional supplement to breastfeeding or to relieve engorgement in the early postpartum period. A hand-held pump consists of a collecting bottle and flange that fits over the breast. A piston, trigger, or motor provides the suction. Hand-held pumps may be either manual (Figure 21.12), battery operated (Figure 21.13), or a combination of battery and electric. A wide variety of styles and prices is available.

A manual pump that uses natural movements will be the most comfortable for the mother. Motorized hand pumps provide suction either with a control button so the mother can regulate pressure or with an autocycling motor that controls the suction. Foot pedal models are also available. An early hand-held breast pump, still found in some stores today, was the "bicycle horn" pump. The name derives from its resemblance to the horn on a

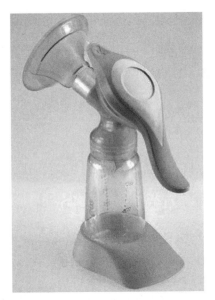

FIGURE 21.12   Hand-held manual breast pump.
Source: © Medela, Inc., 2010.

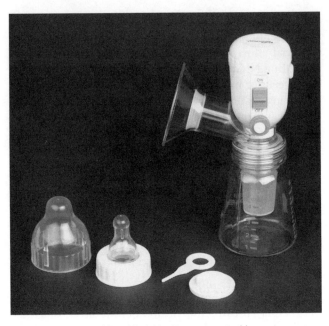

FIGURE 21.13   Hand-held battery-operated breast pump.
Source: Printed with permission of Lumiscope, a Graham-Field Brand.

bicycle. This pump can damage a mother's nipple and harbors bacteria that could be dangerous to the baby. Mothers should not use hand pumps that use a bulb to generate suction.

A few battery-operated double pumps on the market are designed for hands-free operation (Figure 21.13). Performance of these pumps is questionable. There are also bras available designed to provide hands-free operation of electric breast pumps. Mothers can make their own hands-free bras by cutting vertical slits in a cheap sports bra and avoid the expense of a special bra.

Electric Breast Pump   Electric breast pumps are useful in the regular absence of nursing when the mother and baby cannot be together (Figure 21.14). Electric pumps most closely mimic the baby's sucking rhythm and provide the stimulation that is necessary to maintain milk production. They offer the option of pumping both breasts at the same time, as shown in Figure 21.14, thus saving time and increasing breast stimulation. A recent Cochrane review found no significant differences in prolactin levels or quantity from double pumping, although simultaneous pumping is obviously faster (Becker et al., 2008). Heavy-duty double electric breast pumps are produced for both hospital and consumer use.

Hospital-Grade Pump   Hospital-grade electric breast pumps are the best option for mothers who need the most efficient pumping. Mothers with an ill baby, a preterm or late-preterm baby, or multiples (who are usually preterm) typically use this pump. Hospital-grade pumps are very expensive to purchase, so most mothers rent them from

an authorized rental station for use at home. Hospital-grade pumps are approved by the U.S. Food and Drug Administration for multiuse. This designation requires that the pump provider disinfect and clean the pump between rentals to prevent cross-contamination. Each user purchases a personal pump kit, which should not be resold. Many women who use pumps for lengthy or regular separation, such as full-time employment, invest in a quality consumer version of the double electric pump.

Consumer Pump   The U.S. Food and Drug Administration approves consumer pumps for single use only. Multiuse of consumer pumps can theoretically cause cross-contamination and is therefore not recommended. The

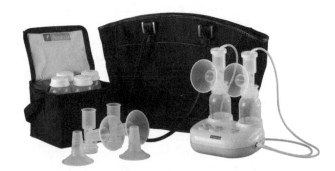

FIGURE 21.14   Electric double breast pump.
Source: Printed with permission of Ameda.

reality is, however, that many women trade, borrow, or purchase previously used pumps. The motor and diaphragm parts on the consumer pumps are not conducive to multiple use, and the pressure may be lower than needed. You can encourage mothers to research the risks of used pumps. If a mother insists on using a previously owned pump, suggest that she obtain a new pump kit and that she have the pressure checked.

Pumping Guidelines

Because the use of breast pumps accompanies an interruption in breastfeeding, the mother may need specialized counseling. For this reason many lactation consultants have pumps and accompanying equipment readily available for demonstration and hands-on teaching. Mothers need complete written instructions as well as a demonstration of proper equipment use. Trying different pumps helps a mother find one that works best for her. She can use a sterilized, autoclaved kit solely for test pumping.

Conditioning Letdown for Pumping When a baby sucks at the breast, the stimulation on the mother's nipple triggers letdown her milk to let down. A breast pump or manual expression does not provide the same degree of stimulation as that of the baby. Massaging her breasts briefly and expressing a few drops of milk by hand helps the milk let down and encourages the mother with faster results.

The mother's emotional state may be a factor in her ability to establish letdown. She can prepare mentally for pumping and arrange to pump at times when she feels rested and unhurried. An atmosphere that is conducive to pumping includes privacy, a comfortable chair, a picture of her baby, and perhaps a recording of her baby's sounds to listen to while pumping. Other techniques for establishing letdown appear in Chapter 7.

When a mother finds it difficult to let down while pumping, she may become tense, agitated, and upset, which may inhibit her letdown even further. After first confirming that she is using a quality pump with correct pressure and using good technique, you can encourage her to continue pumping to obtain the readily available milk. Often, the regular routine of pumping helps the mother relax and patiently work toward increasing her milk production. Correctly fitting breast flanges helps provide the stimulation needed for her milk to let down.

Pumping Technique The mother needs to wash her hands and get comfortable before she begins pumping. Moistening the flange of the pump with her milk or olive oil can help obtain a good seal and decrease skin friction. Large-breasted women may find it helpful to place a rolled towel under their breasts for support during pumping.

Centering the nipple in the flange ensures that breast tissue touches the sides. The mother should use only as much suction as is needed to maintain milk flow throughout her pumping session. Advise that she begin with the suction on the lowest setting and gradually increase suction strength as necessary.

If the mother is double pumping with an electric pump or two battery pumps, 10 to 20 minutes total pumping time may be sufficient. You can suggest that she pump for 10 to 20 minutes, or a minute or 2 after the milk stops flowing. Mothers who pump long term have found that massaging their breasts after the milk stops flowing, and then pumping again for a few minutes, yields more milk and better drainage of the breast (Morton, 2004).

A mother who is single pumping may find it helpful to alternate between breasts several times throughout her pumping session to capitalize on the multiple letdowns that occur simultaneously. She can pump 5 to 7 minutes on one breast and then switch to the other breast for another 5 to 7 minutes. She can then return to the first breast for 3 to 5 minutes of pumping and repeat that time on the second breast (massaging her breasts if necessary to promote flow). She can finish on the first breast with 2 to 3 minutes of pumping and then the second breast for another 2 to 3 minutes.

Encourage mothers to tailor pumping times to their specific needs and circumstances. Mothers can expect to pump varying amounts of milk on different days and at different times of the day. If her baby breastfeeds some or most of the time, pumping can be adapted to the baby's breastfeeding schedule. A mother may pump in place of a missed feeding, between feedings, or on one breast while feeding the baby on the other breast. Experimenting will help her find which arrangement best suits her and her baby's needs.

Pumping for a Hospitalized Baby When a baby is hospitalized and unable to nurse, the mother initially needs to pump at least 8 to 12 times every 24 hours, regardless of the amount of milk she obtains. Regular milk removal helps the mother build and maintain milk production so she has sufficient milk when her baby is able to nurse. It is easier to down-regulate than to try to increase milk production. There is quite a range in normal infant intake, so pumping within that range is desirable, with a range of 478 to 1,356 mL (16.17–45.86 oz) (Kent et al., 2006).

Initiating copious milk production helps establish long-term lactation. This is especially important in times of stress. If the mother needs to collect large amounts of milk for her baby, she can pump more frequently and try to reduce stress and get sufficient rest. A mother may find that one breast produces more milk and lets down more easily than the other. This is normal and is common in most women (Engstrom et al., 2007; Hill et al., 2007). Both breasts need regular milk removal to establish milk production and avoid complications.

Pumping during the night may produce larger quantities of milk because prolactin levels are highest at that time. The mother may benefit from a 4- or 5-hour stretch of sleep to maintain her health and energy. She can pump during the night whenever she wakes naturally and can drink extra fluids just before bedtime to facilitate waking. As the time grows closer for her baby to come home, she can begin to pump more regularly at night.

A mother who uses a breast pump to protect lactation can ask her healthcare practitioner to write a prescription for insurance reimbursement. Progressive insurance companies support breastfeeding, recognizing that families have fewer health claims with breastfed children (American Association of Health Plans, 2001). Medicaid reimburses for electric pump rentals for preterm and ill babies. In the United States, Women, Infants, and Children clinics provide hospital-grade electric pumps for mothers of preterm and ill babies. If a mother has financial problems, encourage her to explore these avenues. Hospital NICUs have hospital-grade electric pumps for use in the hospital; the mother needs a pump for home use as well. Some hospitals have loaner hospital-grade pumps available through grants and donations.

Collecting and Storing Human Milk

Mothers collect milk for a variety of reasons. They may store it in the freezer for emergencies and for regular separation, such as working or attending school. They may store it for a short-term separation such as a shopping trip, wedding, or other social outing. Preterm, physically disabled, or ill infants may need expressed milk for an extended period of time. Many mothers donate their milk to human milk banks to be given to other babies, children, or sick adults.

If a mother expresses her milk to relieve breast fullness or collects drip milk during a feeding, she can save it for later use. She should not save milk that accumulates in a breast shell worn between feedings. It has been against her skin for a lengthy time and could have increased bacterial growth. When the mother is taking a medication proven to be harmful to her baby, she should not give her milk to her baby. Data are conflicting about whether or not milk pumped during a yeast infection harbors enough *Candida* to reinfect the baby. No *Candida* was found in milk cultured from women with breast pain, although the milk did not seem to inhibit the growth of *Candida* in samples (Hale et al., 2009). Some sources suggest that mothers who wish to reuse milk pumped during thrush heat treat the milk (Mohrbacher & Stock, 2003; Amir & Hoover, 2002). A multiple child-care setting may require varying guidelines for milk storage. The mother can review safety issues with the care provider. You can assist them by providing up-to-date guidelines and educating the child-care staff.

Storage Container

Milk must be stored in a manner that preserves its quality and keeps it from spoiling. The mother should clean collection containers and any pump parts that have contact with the milk after every use. She can wash them in hot, soapy water and then thoroughly rinse and air-dry them, or simply cycle them through a dishwasher. Some mothers like to use microwave-safe steam bags that allow the parts to be steam cleaned in the microwave. Although expensive they are convenient for some mothers.

Glass containers are the best choice for milk storage. Glass does not absorb the milk's antibodies or other proteins. It is easy to clean and offers protection against contamination of the milk during storage. A hard plastic (polypropylene) container is the next best choice for storage. A drawback to this container is that the interior surface can scratch and make cleaning difficult. Soft plastic (polyethylene) baby bottle liners are not recommended for storing milk. When milk is stored in soft plastic containers such as bottle liners, certain antibodies in the milk reduce in concentration. Additionally, such soft plastics are difficult to seal and may puncture easily. As discussed in Chapter 10, many plastic bottles are made with bisphenol A, a chemical correlated with health hazards. Thus mothers should be sure any old bottles given to them or bought at a resale shop do not contain bisphenol A.

The amount of milk stored in each container varies as the mother determines how much her baby consumes in her absence. To minimize waste, she initially should store her milk in small amounts, usually 1 to 2 ounces. As the baby starts consuming more at a feeding, small amounts are useful for topping off when the baby is still hungry after a full bottle. If the milk will be frozen, she needs to leave space for expansion during freezing.

Labeling the container with a waterproof marker assists the mother and other caregivers. The label should include the date and time the milk was expressed and possibly the amount of milk contained. If the milk is to be given to the baby by another caregiver with multiple children, the mother's and baby's full names should be written on the label. The baby's last name is important because some babies and mothers do not have the same last name. The mother can transport the milk in a container that is ready for feeding to reduce the possibility of the caregiver contaminating the milk while pouring.

Storage Time

Storage times vary, depending on how soon the baby will receive the expressed milk. A protocol for storing milk for healthy full-term infants is available from the Academy of Breastfeeding Medicine (ABM, 2004). The Centers for Disease Control and Prevention (CDC, 2007) have published milk storage guidelines for full-term infants. Mothers do not always have immediate access to refrigeration.

The CDC guidelines account for variables inherent in milk collection such as amount of contamination and definition of room temperature. If a mother is not sure that she will use her milk within 3 to 5 days, she should freeze it as soon as possible (CDC, 2007). She can place her expressed milk directly in the freezer after collecting it.

A mother can store her milk in a freezer for up to 1 year, depending on the type of freezer. In a freezer that is part of a refrigerator unit with a separate door, the milk will keep for up to 6 months. A deep freezer will keep the milk for up to 1 year, depending on the temperature. To avoid extremes of temperature, milk should not be stored on the refrigerator or freezer door or near the freezer's defrosting unit. Also caution mothers not to store their milk near an automatic ice maker, which has a variance in temperature that can affect the milk. The optimal temperature in the freezer is 0°F, or minus 18–20°C.

A mother may complain that her milk smells bad after it has been frozen for a short while. The odor seems related to the level of lipase in the milk. Gently warming the milk before freezing, never to the point of boiling, avoids this odor. Although warming the milk lowers some of the immunoglobulins, it prevents the mother from discarding her milk because of the odor. Her milk is always a better option for her baby than artificial milk.

Special Guidelines for the NICU Infant

Milk collection and storage guidelines vary depending on the reason the mother is collecting her milk. Guidelines often focus on mothers with healthy babies who are collecting milk for convenience or employment. Such guidelines are not appropriate in all situations. A mother who is collecting milk for her baby in the NICU requires more strict guidelines to ensure her baby's safety. Each NICU will provide specific protocols for collection and storage.

Whenever possible, the mother should express her milk just before feeding the baby. If the milk will not be used within 1 hour, it should be refrigerated immediately. If the baby is ill or preterm and will not receive the fresh milk within 24 hours, the mother should freeze it. Mothers who collect milk for a preterm infant need to place milk from each pumping session in a separate storage container to minimize handling and contamination of the milk (Human Milk Banking Association of North America [HMBANA], 2006).

When a baby goes to the NICU, staff will give the mother specific instructions on how to collect and store her milk. Mothers should be assisted to begin expressing their milk within the first 6 hours after delivery to provide the stimulation necessary for establishing adequate production. A mother may assume that because she and her baby are separated due to prematurity or illness, breastfeeding is no longer an option for her. Encourage NICU staff to educate mothers about early pumping to help maximize their milk production potential. Guidelines may vary from one hospital to another. If your hospital does not offer neonatal intensive care, parents will need guidelines for milk collection and storage from the NICU that cares for their baby. Make sure parents receive this information before the mother leaves the hospital.

Combining Containers of Milk

Mothers often have questions about the procedure for storing milk from more than one pumping session or from both breasts at the same pumping session. When a mother pumps both breasts at the same time for a well baby, she can combine both containers of milk for storage. She can also combine milk from different pumping sessions, with the label stating the date and time of the earliest pumping. She can add newly pumped milk to refrigerated milk after the newly pumped milk cools. The CDC does not recommend adding fresh milk to already frozen milk within a storage container. It suggests keeping the two separate.

Defrosting and Warming Human Milk

Appropriate labeling makes it easy for the mother to use milk based on when she expressed it, using her oldest milk first. If she has a large stock of milk in her freezer, she can arrange the milk with the oldest containers toward the front.

Milk can be thawed by placing it in the refrigerator overnight (ABM, 2004; CDC, 2007) or by warming it rapidly in a pan of warm water or under a stream of warm tap water. A microwave oven should not be used for warming milk. Microwaved liquid may contain hot spots that could burn the baby's mouth. Additionally, microwaving substantially decreases activity of anti-infective properties in human milk (Quan et al., 1992).

When the mother's milk sits in the refrigerator or freezer, the fat rises to the top of the milk. Gently swirling the milk throughout the warming process mixes the fat. After stored milk has been warmed, it needs to be used immediately. Milk should be used or discarded within 24 hours of thawing. To ensure the safety of the milk, the mother should not refreeze thawed milk. Both the CDC and the ABM state that milk remaining at the end of a feed should be discarded and not reused. However, there are no current studies showing the bacterial growth in bottles of human milk after feeding.

Human Milk Banking

A mother's expressed milk is more appropriate for her baby than any other alternative feeding choice. Her antibodies reflect the family environment, and her milk production is tailored to her baby's needs. However, sometimes a mother may be unable to provide enough milk through either breastfeeding or expression, especially in the case of preterm infants (Henderson, 2008; Hartmann, 2003; Cregan et al., 2002). In such cases the baby can receive donor milk from other women, in preference to infant formula.

Today, there is a growing trend among parents to purchase human milk through the Internet or obtain milk from a relative or friend (Thorley, 2008). The contaminated formula scandals have also increased this trend (Fowler, 2008). Greater awareness of the importance of human milk increases the likelihood of encountering parents who consider these alternatives. Giving mothers information nonjudgmentally about the viruses that can be transmitted and suggesting the donor be screened are appropriate. Be aware that in some countries screened fresh donor milk is used in NICUs (Grøvslien & Grønn, 2009). Home pasteurization is also used.

Human milk banks offer a safe alternative to mothers who cannot breastfeed or who cannot produce enough milk for a compromised baby. The first human milk bank was established in 1909 in Vienna, with the first one in the United States opening in 1911 in Boston. A milk bank is a collection point where healthy nursing mothers donate their milk (Figure 21.15). In the early 1980s there were 23 milk banks in Canada and 30 in the United States. These numbers declined rapidly with the isolation of human immunodeficiency virus (HIV) in human milk and an increase in preterm formulas (Balmer & Wharton, 1992). Research has demonstrated improved outcomes for infants given human milk, and the risks of artificial formula now are more widely recognized by the public and the medical community. Thus the demand for banked human milk is skyrocketing.

Human Milk Banking Association of North America (HMBANA)

Human Milk Banking Association of North America (HMBANA), a not-for-profit organization established in 1985, provides uniform standards for human milk banking. In 2008 member banks processed more than 1.4 million ounces of milk (Geraghty et al., 2010). Improved laboratory testing and pasteurization techniques have eradicated concerns about disease transmission. The safety of human milk banking is becoming better known, as more NICUs use it and witness the positive outcomes. At least one milk bank in North America is able to label the milk with nutritional content analysis (protein and lipid percentages and calorie content). This enables neonatologists to provide the most fragile babies with the best nutritional match possible. Milk banks are also able to provide human milk from mothers on dairy-free diets and fat-free human milk for babies suffering with chylothorax (Updegrove, 2009).

As of 2009 there were 12 operating milk banks in North America, with more scheduled to open. Information about the milk banks is available at www.hmbana .org. Donor milk can be shipped overnight anywhere in the United States and Canada. Regional donation is becoming more convenient for mothers as new depots open (Geraghty et al., 2009). Some milk banks receive support from an associated hospital. Mothers who are interested in additional information can contact HMBANA or an area milk bank directly.

Recipients of Donor Milk

Milk banks prioritize the dispensing of milk based on the greatest need, for example, hospitalized and the most medically fragile infants (HMBANA, 2008). Recipient hospitals cover processing fees and shipping costs for babies receiving donor milk as inpatients. Nonprofit milk banks also depend on donations or grants. Recipient families pay a processing fee, but the milk bank does not deny any recipients who have a medical need. Medicaid programs in the United States provide coverage on a state-by-state basis, so reimbursement is variable.

Donated milk is processed, pasteurized, and dispensed by prescription to infants, children, and, rarely, adults with a medical need. Babies may need donor human milk because they are temporarily unable to breastfeed, are intolerant of human milk substitutes, or suffer from digestive disorders or severe diarrhea. Some preterm or very ill infants need donor milk until their mother increases her milk production to meet their needs.

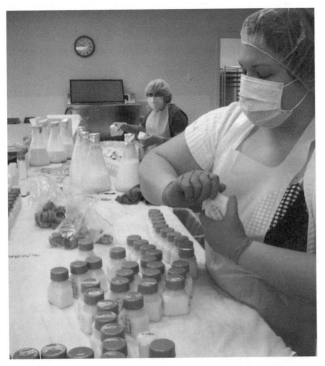

FIGURE 21.15 Human milk being processed at a milk bank.
Source: Printed with permission of Mothers' Milk Bank at Austin.

Infants with autoimmune disorders, inborn errors of metabolism, or conditions such as cystic fibrosis benefit from human milk. The condition may not show up until several weeks or months after birth. The mother may be unable to relactate and therefore turns to a milk bank to help her baby survive.

Procedure for Donating Milk

Mothers who express and save milk for another person's baby find great emotional gratification and reward in knowing they are helping a baby in need. Some donors are bereaved mothers whose babies have died (see the discussion on counseling grieving parents in Chapter 23). You can facilitate the use of milk banks for donors and recipients by providing information to mothers in your care who have plentiful supplies.

Learn the location of milk banks as well as their policies regarding milk collection and distribution. HMBANA provides such information for health professionals. When a mother expresses a desire to become a donor, you can provide her with general information and refer her to the nearest milk bank. Because each milk bank has slightly different procedures, it is best for the mother to communicate directly with the milk bank.

Some potential donors may be disqualified from donating milk, such as mothers who are ill or who are taking certain medications. Mothers can check with the specific milk bank for exclusions. Donors learn hygienic techniques for milk expression, with appropriate hand washing, washing and disinfecting of pump parts, and handling of disinfecting equipment. They learn how to label their milk, proper milk storage, and proper technique for transporting their milk to the bank. Milk banks provide containers for mothers to pump and store their milk for shipping.

Milk banks require that mothers freeze their milk and attach the label to the jar before placing it in the freezer to ensure that it adheres. Mothers must insulate the milk well to prevent thawing, so it stays frozen until it arrives at the milk bank. The mother should collect milk in a sterile container and mark it with her name, collection date, number of ounces, and the name and dosage of any drugs she is taking. Milk banks accept excess stockpiled milk if the mother meets the donor requirements. The individual milk bank provides its specific collection and storage guidelines.

Screening and Processing of Donated Milk

Milk banks thoroughly screen potential donors for lifestyle and medical history risks before the donors are accepted. The mothers also have blood tests and provide a written agreement from the mother's doctor and the baby's doctor that she is a viable donor and her donating poses no detriment to her baby. Most mothers commit to donating a certain amount of milk (e.g., 100 oz), though one-time donations are also accepted.

Frozen donor milk is thawed in a refrigerator at the milk bank and pooled under clean conditions. The milk then undergoes heat treatment at 62.5°C (Holder pasteurization) for 30 minutes to kill HIV and other viruses and bacteria that may be present. Fortunately, heat-treated milk retains most of its immunological and nutritional properties, although vitamin C is destroyed by heating. The pasteurized milk is rapidly cooled and refrozen. Each batch is cultured for bacteria, and any batch containing bacterial growth is discarded or saved for research purposes. The milk bank also conducts routine antigen testing similar to that of blood banks to further rule out the presence of HIV, hepatitis B, cytomegalovirus, human T-cell lymphotropic virus, and syphilis.

Presently, only one milk bank in North America provides raw human milk (San Jose, CA). The milk bank screens the pool of raw milk for bacteria, which must have an acceptably low level of bacteria colonies of normal skin flora. When colonies are unacceptably high, or if any bacteria other than normal skin flora are present, the milk is excluded from raw use.

For-Profit Milk Banking

Breastfeeding advocates have been troubled by for-profit milk banking attaching an economic value to human milk, which further objectifies the milk as "product" (Palmer, 2009). One for-profit entity, Prolacta Bioscience, receives milk donations from unpaid mothers and sells its processed, patented milk and human milk fortifiers to hospitals (Prolacta Bioscience, 2009a; Austin, 2006; Ensor, 2006). Prolacta has also entered into a "co-promotion" marketing agreement with Abbott Nutrition, the formula manufacturer, for Abbott to sell Prolacta's products, along with its artificial baby milks (Prolacta Bioscience, 2009b).

The MilkShare website provides networking for private donors, stating that it prohibits selling or buying of milk. By August 2008 about 16,000 families reportedly engaged in private milk donation (MilkShare, 2008). As the long-term health implications of artificial feeding become better known in Western culture and as formula scandals continue to unfold, such activity may become more frequent.

∾ Alternate Feeding Methods

The need for an alternate feeding method means a mother's idealized view of breastfeeding has not materialized. Approach the issue of alternate feeding methods gently and with a lot of support. The mother needs an opportunity to verbalize her concerns and fears about her situation and her baby. She needs to know her options and their risks and benefits to breastfeeding. Enabling the mother to make the choice about what fits best in her life gives her some control over an otherwise tenuous situation.

The options available for a breast alternative include a cup, a spoon, a syringe, a tube-feeding device used at the breast, a tube device used for finger feeding, and an artificial nipple and bottle. The mother needs to understand the appropriateness of a method to her baby's situation. She also needs to know the cost and the care and cleaning of the device she will use. She needs thorough instructions, both verbal and written, with demonstration and close follow-up until the baby is breastfeeding without the supplemental method.

Spoon Feeding

Occasionally, all babies need is an infusion of calories to get them started with breastfeeding. If the baby is unable to latch or sustain a suck, the mother can express colostrum onto a spoon. To feed the baby by spoon, she places the tip of the spoon gently at the tip of the baby's tongue and ladles the colostrum onto the tongue a few drops at a time (Figure 21.16). Most babies love the taste of colostrum and will extend their tongues to lap it. This small feeding may rouse the baby enough for feeding. The range of intake for a 7.5-pound baby in the first day of life ranges from 10.2 to 108.8 mL (0.3–3.6 oz) so even a small amount is important to the baby (Casey et al., 1986).

Cup Feeding

Cup feeding offers a baby-led alternative for a baby who is unable to breastfeed (Figure 21.17). The cup provides an initial sensory stimulus to the baby's lips, olfactory senses, and tongue. A younger baby will lap the milk, which promotes appropriate tongue movement used during breastfeeding. He can pace his intake, and because he is in control, respiration is easier, and swallowing occurs

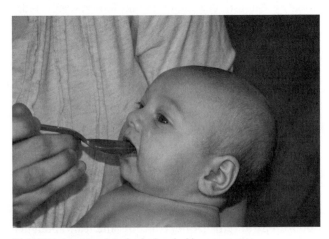

FIGURE 21.16   A baby being fed by a spoon.
Source: Printed with permission of Anna Swisher.

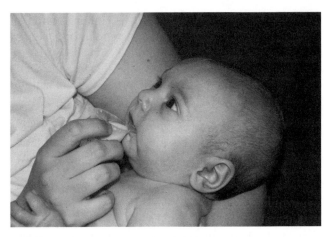

FIGURE 21.17   A baby being fed by a cup.
Source: Printed with permission of Kori Martin.

when he is ready. Babies as young as 30 weeks' gestation are capable of maintaining heart rate, respiration, and oxygenation while cup feeding (Lang et al., 1994). At 30 to 34 weeks, babies lap by protruding their tongues into the cup to obtain small boluses of milk. They often hold the milk in their mouth for some time before swallowing. As the baby matures, a sipping action begins to develop.

Procedure for Cup Feeding

Cup feeding is easy for a mother and baby to learn. It may take the baby only four or five feedings to catch on to the technique. A small cup with rounded edges works best, such as a shot glass, a medicine cup, or a hollow-handed medicine spoon. The small plastic cups used by fast-food restaurants for catsup are a convenient choice, as are disposable small paper cups.

The mother needs to allow the baby to lead this activity and to rest between swallows. Pouring milk directly into the baby's mouth increases the risk of aspiration. Slow pacing also is important for avoiding aspiration. If the baby resists the cup, it is best to pause and try again later.

Paladai Mothers in India have used a small cup-like device called a paladai for centuries. One study compared the use of a bottle, cup, and paladai in 100 newborn infants. Infants took the maximum volume in the least time and stayed calmest with the paladai. Spilling was higher with the cup, especially with preterm infants. Infants could accept feedings with the paladai or cup before the bottle, with the youngest baby at 30 weeks gestational age (Narayanan & Bambroo, 2002). A newer pilot study comparing the paladai with bottle feeding in preterm infants found increased spillage, increased feeding times, and more stress cues (Aloysius & Hickson, 2007). If parents want to use a cup, they should avoid using "sippy" cups because the spout does not allow the baby's tongue to trough. The spout also makes it hard for the caregiver to gauge the amount given.

Steps in Cup Feeding

- Fill the cup about halfway or less, with about 10 to 15 mL ($\frac{1}{3}$ to $\frac{1}{2}$ oz) of milk.
- Tuck a cloth under the baby's chin to catch any spills.
- Hold the baby in a semisitting position.
- Bring the cup to the baby's lips and rest the rim of the cup on his lower lip so that it touches the corners of his mouth.
- Tip the cup until the milk touches the baby's lips.
- The baby will begin to lap the milk from the cup. His tongue will form a trough to bring the milk to the back of his throat so that he can swallow it.

Choice to Cup Feed

Cup feeding provides a low level of intervention that is much less invasive than finger feeding or the use of an artificial nipple. One key limitation with cup feeding, however, is that the baby does not get any practice sucking. Spillage is also greater, with one study reporting that 38.5 percent of milk taken from the cup spilled onto the baby's bib (Dowling et al., 2002). That aside, cup feeding is helpful in assisting babies in learning to extend their tongues over the alveolar ridge. It also results in fewer oxygen desaturations than with other methods.

A Cochrane review (Collins et al., 2008) found that cup feeding significantly decreased "no breastfeeding or only partial breast feeding" on discharge home. However, cup feeding also significantly increased the length of hospital stay by up to 10 days. The review found a high degree of noncompliance in the largest study of cup feeding, indicating dissatisfaction with this method by staff and/or parents. The expense of NICU stays, especially in the United States, is significant enough to prevent adoption of cup feeding as the norm in NICU settings.

One study found that twice as many mothers who had cup fed their babies were still breastfeeding at 3 months compared with those who bottle fed (Rocha et al., 2002). Cup-fed infants demonstrate significantly more mature breastfeeding behaviors when compared with bottle fed infants over 6 weeks (Abouelfettoh, 2008). Although neither group breastfed in the hospital, the cup-fed group had a significantly higher proportion of breast-feedings 1 week after discharge.

A hospital study found that supplemental feedings, whether by cup or bottle, had a detrimental effect on breastfeeding duration among mothers who delivered vaginally. There were no differences between cup-fed versus bottle fed groups for breastfeeding duration in this study. Interestingly, among infants delivered by cesarean, cup feeding significantly prolonged exclusive, full, and overall breastfeeding duration. Perhaps supplementation with two or more cup feedings provided calories to sustain the babies until their mothers' mature milk production, which may have been delayed due to the cesareans (Howard et al., 2003).

Tube Feeding

A tube-feeding device can be used during breastfeeding to provide supplemental nutrition while the baby sucks at the breast. A commercial nursing supplementer consists of a plastic bag or bottle designed to hold fluid. The mother suspends the supplementer by a cord around her neck or clips it to her clothing at shoulder level so that it rests between her breasts. Thin, flexible tubing leads from the container to the end of the mother's nipple (Figure 21.18). Manufacturers make "starter" supplementers that attach directly to a bottle. A less expensive noncommercial supplementer can be constructed with the use of a number 5, 6, or 8 French oral gastric tube on the end of a syringe or placed in a bottle (Figure 21.19). Video clips demonstrating the use of supplementers can be found on breastfeeding websites and on YouTube. If a syringe and feeding tube are used, exercise caution and demonstrate paced feeding to parents so the baby receives a comfortable flow.

Procedure for Tube Feeding

The substance used in tube feeding can be either expressed human milk or artificial baby milk. Some infant formulas are thick and do not flow well through the narrow tubing. If the mother uses powdered formula, she needs to shake it well to avoid clogging the tubing. Some sources suggest avoiding the use of powdered formulas in a tube-feeding device because of the potential for clogging and the infant thus receiving insufficient supplementation. Human milk

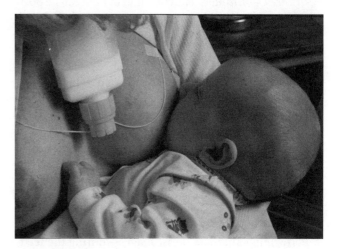

FIGURE 21.18 Baby breastfeeding with a commercial nursing supplementer.

Source: © Medela, Inc., 2010.

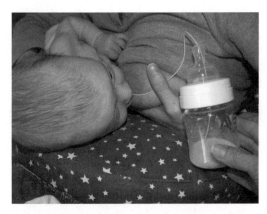

FIGURE 21.19   Baby breastfeeding with a homemade supplementer using a bottle and tubing.

Source: Printed with permission of Anna Swisher.

fortifiers can also clog tubing. Potential for clogging may be a factor in parents' decision because of the increased cost of ready-to-feed formula.

Placement of Tubing   The feeding tube should extend a few centimeters beyond the end of the nipple. Taping it to the breast keeps it in place. The tape needs to be long enough to prevent it from coming loose in the baby's mouth. Paper tape is the least irritating to the mother's skin. Many mothers have found it more comfortable to use an adhesive bandage. The mother threads the tube through the pad part of the bandage and can leave the bandage on all day without having to remove it. She should check her baby's mouth daily to make sure that the tube is not irritating the roof of his or her mouth. After every use the tubing needs to be flushed with cold water, washed with hot soapy water, and then rinsed with clear water.

Position of Container   The container of milk can be positioned level with, above, or below the baby's head, depending on the desired rate of flow. The level of the container initially should be adjusted so the baby has about one suck per swallow. As the baby's suck becomes stronger and milk flow increases, the container can be lowered. Some commercial supplementers have a flow-control valve that responds to the baby's sucking, and some have various sizes of tubing to adjust flow rate. It is unnecessary to compress the tube manually to control milk flow. In fact, doing so can damage the device or result in the baby expending energy on nonnutritive sucking.

Assisting the Baby   Some babies may initially object to having the tube in their mouths and require time to accept it. Performing alternate breast massage during the feeding increases milk flow and encourages the baby to suck. If the baby is not at risk, the mother can start a feeding without the supplementer and use it only when her baby

needs additional nourishment. Some babies become so accustomed to nursing with the tubing that they refuse to nurse without it. Others seem to figure out that the milk is coming from the tubing, slide off the mother's breast, and suck on the tube like a straw. Taping the tubing farther back on the mother's nipple, either flush with her at-rest nipple or a few centimeters behind it, encourages the baby to grab more of the mother's breast tissue to obtain the milk. Some mothers tape the tubing below the nipple to keep the baby from sliding down the tubing.

Amount of Supplement   When it is evident that the baby is receiving increasing amounts of milk from the breast, the mother can reduce the amount of supplement at each feeding. Such clues will be softer, emptier-feeling breasts after a feeding or increased amounts of milk left in the supplementer accompanied by good weight gain. Test weights measure the intake of the mother's milk and supplement to monitor the mother's production. For example, the mother puts 30 mL (1 oz) of expressed milk or formula into the supplementer. She weighs the baby, nurses, and then weighs the baby again. If the baby gains 60 mL (2 oz) and there is nothing left in the supplementer, then 30 mL (1 oz) was received from direct breastfeeding and 30 mL (1 oz) from the supplementer during the feeding.

Daily milk production usually seems highest in the morning, and the mother can reduce the amount of supplement accordingly. Encourage her to watch for changes in sucking rhythm and supplement flow during feedings and to switch breasts for optimal stimulation of milk production. She can observe signs of sufficient nourishment, such as wet diapers, ample stooling, good skin turgor, weight gain, and a consistent pattern of eating and sleeping. When she and her baby's caregiver are confident that milk production is adequate, based on clinical evidence such as the baby's output and the mother's milk production, supplements can be decreased slowly and finally discontinued.

Choice to Tube Feed

A tube-feeding device encourages nutritive sucking at the breast. The mother can adjust it to deliver more fluid when her milk production is low and less fluid as her production increases. A mother who has been expressing milk for an ill baby may need to use a supplementer during the transition from milk expression to nursing. If the baby has been receiving the mother's milk from a bottle, the mother can replace use of the bottle with tube feeding. A mother who is relactating or inducing lactation may find this device helpful for supplementing her baby's intake while she increases production. A baby who has difficulty nursing at the breast can be encouraged by the flow of milk from the supplementer.

For a baby who will latch, a tube-feeding device is the least invasive supplemental method. It avoids the possibility of nipple preference from a bottle nipple and provides the mother with the breast stimulation she needs (Borucki, 2005). The baby sucks at the breast and the tip of the tube simultaneously, and the flow of supplement from the container encourages continued sucking. In this way the baby receives nourishment at the same time as oral stimulation. Additionally, the mother receives natural stimulation of her breasts to encourage milk production.

Some mothers use a tube-feeding device for the entire course of breastfeeding. These usually are either adoptive mothers or mothers with impaired milk production because of true insufficient milk production, breast reduction, or breast augmentation. They benefit from encouragement while they persevere in nurturing their baby at the breast (West & Marasco, 2008). The adoptive breastfeeding website, www.fourfriends.com/abrw, contains many practical hints for mothers who use nursing supplementers.

Finger Feeding

Finger feeding is another means of getting nourishment to the baby (Figure 21.20). Whereas in tube feeding the tubing is placed on the end of the mother's nipple, in finger feeding the tubing is placed on the end of the caregiver or parent's finger. Finger feeding is more invasive than tube feeding. As with any alternative feeding method, if the mother uses finger feeding too long, the baby may come to prefer it to the breast. Finger feeding can be beneficial for a baby who has low muscle tone, who has a disorganized suck, or who needs stimulation to elicit sucking. This is common in babies from heavily medicated births whose central nervous systems are depressed. Although caregivers need to use a glove when demonstrating finger feeding, parents can generally finger feed without gloves. Because of the potential for allergy, latex gloves should not be used.

Procedure for Finger Feeding

As with tube feeding, you may use either a commercial nursing supplementer or number 5, 6, or 8 French oral gastric tubing on the end of a syringe that has the plunger removed. Removing the plunger allows the baby greater control over feeding. Another alternative, placing tubing in a bottle, gives the baby total control over milk flow. Place the appropriate amount of expressed milk or substitute in the container attached to the tubing. Prime the tubing with the milk and crimp it to stop the flow until it is positioned. Hold the baby in an upright or semi-upright position. Place the container of milk level with, above, or below the baby's head, depending on the desired rate of flow. You can raise or lower the syringe or supplementer to achieve the appropriate flow.

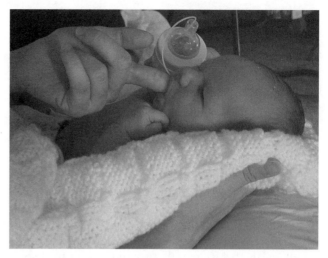

FIGURE 21.20   Baby being fed with tubing attached to the mother's finger.

Source: Printed with permission of Anna Swisher.

Ensure that the nail of the index finger is short and smooth. If the mother has long nails, she can wear a non-latex glove to prevent scratching and protect the baby from possible bacteria under her nails. Because the finger does not elongate as the nipple would in the baby's mouth, place the end of the tube flush with the finger or a few centimeters behind it to prevent the tubing from poking the baby. If you wish, you can tape the tubing to your finger. Gently tickle the baby's lips so she opens her mouth for your finger. Never push your finger into her mouth. Wait until the baby invites you to insert your finger, and then place the fat pad of your finger with the tube on it into the baby's mouth against the hard palate (the fingernail will be against the baby's tongue).

The baby's condition and the indication for finger feeding determine the number of times this technique is used and the amount of milk the baby receives. Holding the baby against the breast as for breastfeeding, at a 45-degree angle, avoids milk getting into the baby's ears. The goal is to elicit one suck per swallow, as with breastfeeding. More than four sucks per swallow may be tiring to the baby.

Evaluating the baby's actions during finger feeding can be a helpful diagnostic tool. Finger feeding is not a useful feeding method for a baby that does not respond to the finger by sucking, cannot sustain sucking bursts, or take three or four sucks to form a bolus big enough to swallow. A baby that does not suck may need to be syringe fed, with the parent pacing the feedings, or possibly gavage fed. Increased calories through gavage or syringe feeding may lead to more effective sucking.

Encourage the mother to check her baby's mouth several times each day to make sure the tubing is not irritating the roof of the mouth. After every use, she needs to flush out the tubing with cold water, wash with hot soapy water, and rinse with clear water. Water can be siphoned through the tube by sucking on the other end if necessary.

Syringe Feeding

Some clinicians use a standard or periodontal syringe either with finger feeding or at the breast (Figure 21.21). As with all alternate feeding methods, be cautious when using a syringe. Feeding a baby with a syringe places the caregiver in control, not the baby. Teach parents to deliver the milk bolus just a little bit at a time and not to squirt the milk into the baby's mouth. Squirting the milk could cause aspiration, especially when done by someone who is inexperienced with the use of a syringe.

Teach parents to keep the syringe forward and in the middle of the baby's mouth, to avoid poking the baby's tongue, gums, or palate. If using a syringe with a finger, place the syringe in the corner of the baby's mouth. Placing a small amount of milk toward the front third of the tongue encourages the baby to extend it outward. Some babies quickly become proficient at sucking on a syringe and learn to pace themselves. When sucking begins, the mother can move her baby to the breast to begin a feeding.

Bottle Feeding

Baby bottles carry the powerful influence of cultural acceptance and encouragement, often to the point of excluding breastfeeding. Some mothers may lack support for the use of any alternative feeding device other than a bottle. A mother may decide she is only comfortable with the use of the bottle, or she may try another alternative feeding method for some time and decide to switch to a bottle.

Long-term use of artificial nipples can weaken a baby's suck and contribute to malocclusion. There is a

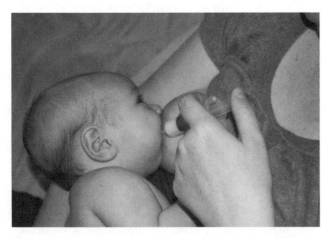

FIGURE 21.21   Baby breastfeeding being fed by syringe.
Source: Printed with permission of Kori Martin.

marked difference between the breast and an artificial nipple within the baby's oral cavity during feeding. In breastfeeding the baby's entire oral cavity fills with breast tissue, not just with the nipple. No artificial nipple on the market can conform to the individual shape of the baby's mouth as the breast does.

Another consideration is the difference in the baby's mouth action on the breast and with a bottle (Geddes et al., 2009, 2008; Ramsay et al., 2004; Smith, 1988). On the breast, the baby is in charge. The breast responds to the baby's sucking action with varying degrees of milk flow, with milk flow stopping when the baby stops sucking. A bottle provides a continuous flow of fluid, and the baby must clamp the nipple to stop the flow. The action changes to one of protecting the airway when a baby sucks on a bottle. No bottle and nipple is able to mimic baby-led feeding at the breast.

Appropriate Use of Bottles

Bottle supplementation is associated with breastfeeding problems. Preterm infants often receive a bottle before breastfeeding, even though studies have shown that oxygenation rates are more stable with breastfeeding (Chen et al., 2000; Meier, 1988). Cost pressures of managed care in the United States result in the shortest stays possible. Therefore getting the baby to nipple feed tends to be a key goal rather than full direct breastfeeding.

Used appropriately, a bottle can be a therapeutic tool to help a baby learn to breastfeed (Wilson-Clay & Hoover, 2008; Kassing, 2002). The mechanics of suck–swallow–breathe that feeding specialists observe in healthy babies can form a basis for appropriate bottle feeding (Wolf & Glass, 1992). Some lactation consultants have observed that it may not be so much the nipple that causes problems as it is the rate of flow. Even "slow-flow" nipples continue to drip when the bottle is turned upside down and squirt when barely compressed.

Selecting a Bottle Nipple

Mothers who combine breastfeeding and bottle feeding usually want to avoid a bottle nipple that has a small base (Figure 21.22). Babies that suck on this type of nipple, tend to purse their lips, an action they may repeat when put to breast. A nipple with a large base forces the baby's mouth to open wide as with breastfeeding (Figure 21.23). The wide base can help minimize latch difficulties when switching back and forth between breast and bottle.

Some babies have difficulty pulling a nipple with a large base back far enough into the mouth to flange their lips on the wide part of the base. Instead, they slide down and purse their lips around the narrow part of the nipple. A few bottles on the market have a shorter teat, illustrated by the nipple on the left in Figure 21.23. If the mother

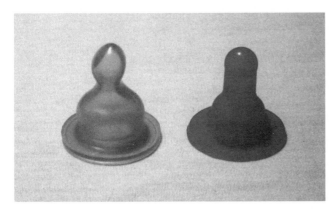

FIGURE 21.22 "Orthodontic" shaped nipple on left and premie nipple on right.

Source: Printed with permission of Anna Swisher.

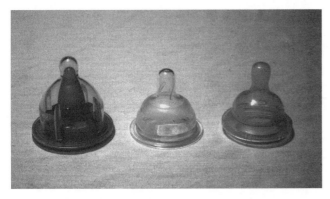

FIGURE 21.23 Three different types of nipples for a baby or infant bottle feeding.

Source: Printed with permission of Anna Swisher.

hears smacking or clicking when the baby drinks from a bottle, she can try a different nipple, avoiding one that causes the baby's lips to purse.

Another issue related to artificial nipples is the choice between latex and silicone. Latex nipples are cheaper and are available in more shapes than those made of silicone. They do not last as long, however, and can become rather gummy, particularly after boiling. There is also concern that boiling latex can release nitrates, which are potentially carcinogenic. Many people are latex allergic and using latex products could precipitate an allergic reaction in a susceptible infant. Although silicone nipples are firmer and more expensive, they withstand boiling better than the latex ones and thus last considerably longer. Silicone nipples are a potential source of silicone ingestion, however.

Selecting a Feeding Bottle

It probably does not much matter what type of bottle a mother uses. The use of bisphenol A–free materials in plastic bottles has become a consideration (see Chapter 10) and has increased popularity of glass bottles, which previously had almost disappeared from store shelves in the United States. It is important that the mother clean the bottle thoroughly with a bottle brush that can reach into every crevice. Elongated "0" shaped bottles designed for easy holding by the baby cannot be cleaned as easily as a plain bottle. Another consideration is choosing a bottle that is easiest for the feeder to hold comfortably, especially as feedings may take a long time (Wolf & Glass, 1992). Using an angled bottle may give the baby more control, especially when feeding in an upright or semi-upright position.

Baby bottles come in many themes and colors, including brand soft drinks. This cuteness factor perpetuates the bottle as an icon of babyhood (Palmer, 2009). The use of soft drink symbols can set the stage for early consumption of unhealthy beverages as normal and desirable.

Responding to the Baby's Hunger Cues

A bottle delivers milk without much effort on the baby's part. Parents need to watch for cues that their baby is responding favorably to the feeding and is able to suck on the nipple appropriately. Table 21.2 presents the signs of stability, disorganization, and dysfunction in nipple feeding. In addition to watching the baby's responses, parents can optimize their method of bottle feeding in the following ways:

- Touching the corner of the baby's mouth to stimulate sucking
- Allowing the baby to root for the nipple
- Inserting the nipple into the baby's mouth and over the tongue
- Positioning the baby in a flexed position so his head is above the stomach and midline.
- Holding the bottle at a horizontal angle to prevent a rapid rate of flow (it is okay for baby to take in some air)
- Pacing the feeding by removing the bottle after every two or three sucks, so the baby can order his suck-swallow-breathing, slow the feeding, and better emulate breastfeeding.
- Avoiding a rocking motion while feeding to avoid overstimulation.
- Avoiding constantly moving the nipple in the baby's mouth, which may cause stress.
- Observing the baby for signs of stress.

TABLE 21.2   Infant Cues During Nipple Feeding

Signs of Stability in Nipple Feeding	Signs of Disorganized Nipple Feeding	Signs of Dysfunctional Nipple Feeding
• Smooth, regular respirations • Hand activity near face with good consistent postural control • Organized and calm with optimal color and oxygen saturation • Focused and alert • Good coordination of suck, swallow, breathe • Sustained awake behavior	• Sucking bursts vary in length consisting of usually 5–10 sucks each • Flaring of nose; uncoordinated suck, swallow, breathing • Worried look • Extraneous movement of upper extremities • Head turning • Irregular jerky jaw excursions • Lack of response to nipple insertion • Rapid deterioration of normal sucking pattern denotes potential aversion to the nipple • Difficulty latching or initiating sucking	• Lack of role change between nonnutritive and nutritive suck; nonnutritive is usually faster • Excessively wide jaw excursions • Restricted range of motion at temporal mandible joint with jaw clenching • Flaccid or retracted tongue with absence of tongue groove • Hyperactive gag

Source: Reprinted with permission from Seton Healthcare Network.

Stress Cues During Bottle Feeding

Teach parents to observe their baby during bottle feeding and to watch for stress cues. Stress cues are avoidance behaviors that tell the parent something is bothering the baby. They include frowning, wrinkling the brow, squinting, or closed eyes as if in pain. The baby may appear tense and may flail or have clenched fists. Milk may spill out of the baby's mouth. The baby may stop sucking and gag, choke, or sputter or may become stiff and arch his or her back. Signs of stress during bottle feeding include

- Color change
- Tachypnea, or nasal flaring
- Shallow breathing
- High-pitched crowing noise
- Drooling
- Gulping
- Coughing
- Choking
- Changes in oxygen needs
- Squirming
- Arching
- Yawning
- Hiccuping
- Finger splaying
- Increased fussiness
- Saluting sign
- Covering face with hands
- Looking away from caretaker
- Tongue extension
- Falling asleep

- Changes in vital signs
- Hypertonicity or motor flaccidity

Inexperienced parents tend to ascribe cognitive behaviors to newborns that are not age appropriate. These behaviors do not mean the baby is "mad" or "stubborn." Help parents see that their baby is trying to convey stress or discomfort and that something about the feeding is not working. Paced feeding can calm the baby and help make feedings a pleasant learning experience.

Paced Feeding to Mimic Breastfeeding

Many babies feel overwhelmed by the amount of fluid and the rate of delivery with bottle feeding. You can help parents mimic breastfeeding by teaching them paced feeding, a very simple technique that parents can do easily. The goal of paced feeding is for the baby to suck, swallow, and breathe as in breastfeeding. Although babies can suck and breathe at the same time, when they attempt to swallow and breathe at the same time they can aspirate milk into their lungs and nasal cavity (Wolf & Glass, 1992). Paced feeding slows bottle feeding to better mimic what the baby would do at the breast.

When they use paced feeding, parents often observe their frantic, worried baby become calm with relaxed hands, a smooth brow, and open eyes. Point out this composure and alertness to parents, and teach them what to look for. The baby learns that feeding does not have to be an aversive experience. A baby who gulps down a full bottle quickly is doing so in an attempt to breathe. Paced feeding helps the baby coordinate sucking with breathing.

A few minutes of slow paced feeding can raise the trust level of a baby who is unenthusiastic about feeding at the breast. It can calm the baby enough to be put to the breast. A baby who cannot sustain a suck on the bottle, whose mouth leaks milk, or who elicits no "pop" sound when the bottle is pulled out needs to be referred to a physician. If the baby exhibits such low tone when feeding, a physical or neurological problem may be present. Babies are born to breastfeed. When something does not work, parents need to investigate it, not ignore it, or sacrifice breastfeeding "on the altar of ignorance" (Newman & Pitman, 2000). Paced feeding is a helpful diagnostic and therapeutic tool. It is also a gentler and healthier way to bottle feed any baby.

Instructions for Paced Feeding

- Hold the baby at a 45-degree angle or greater. Provide postural support to the neck, shoulders, back, and torso. Some babies calm better if they are swaddled. This may be helpful in preventing the baby's arms from flailing. Other babies transition better to breastfeeding by being held on the mother's bare chest, with the bottle near her breast.
- Tickle the baby's upper lip, just as the mother would with her nipple. When the mouth opens, let the baby pull the bottle nipple in; do not force the bottle into the baby's mouth.
- Hold the bottle at an angle that is as close as possible to the angle of the breast, so the baby's neck angles slightly up at its most open position, providing a clear airway.
- Allow the baby three or four sucks and remove the bottle, resting the nipple on the baby's upper lip. Observe what the baby does. Most babies swallow, then breathe, and then open their mouths and root for the nipple.
- Put the bottle back to the baby's mouth for three or four sucks and remove the bottle again. Continue in this pattern for the rest of the feeding.

Another method of paced feeding is to hold the bottle horizontally in the baby's mouth so that a limited amount of milk enters the nipple. The baby takes in more air, but the delivery rate is greatly slowed, allowing the baby to breathe between swallows (Wilson-Clay & Hoover, 2008). Swallowing fluids too rapidly, which can lead to apnea, bradycardia, and fatigue aspiration, is a greater concern than swallowing air.

Bottle Feeding the "Breastfeeding Way"

The advantages of breastfeeding for the mother and baby extend far beyond nutritional and immunological benefits. When a mother chooses to breastfeed, she is making a health choice. She is choosing a method of communicating with her infant that is unique to breastfeeding. This lifestyle and relationship is the natural and normal one for new mothers. A mother who bottle feeds exclusively can make certain adaptations so she and her baby receive some of the benefits of a breastfeeding relationship.

Mothers hold their babies in several different positions for breastfeeding. Babies breastfeed from both the right and left sides of the mother's body and receive a different visual perspective when they change breasts. Bottle fed babies can receive the same advantage by being cuddled in the right arm for one feeding and in the left arm for the next feeding. Likewise, breastfeeding involves skin-to-skin contact between the mother and baby that is continuous throughout a feeding. Bottle feeding mothers can make a point to provide frequent skin-to-skin contact with their babies.

There may be a temptation with bottle feeding to prop the bottle rather than hold the baby. This practice is dangerous for the baby and is strongly discouraged as the baby can easily choke on or aspirate the milk. Breastfeeding mothers instinctively "groom" their babies while they nurse by stroking, patting, and otherwise touching their babies with their free hand. This is a bit more difficult to do while bottle feeding. Bottle feeding mothers can be encouraged to snuggle and hold the baby for at least 15 to 20 minutes after a feeding so the baby can benefit from this mothering. They can also be encouraged to carry their baby in a sling or baby carrier.

Breastfed babies enjoy periods of nonnutritive sucking at the breast, usually at the end of a feeding. A bottle fed baby is unable to suck nonnutritively on a bottle because any mouth movement results in milk flow. A bottle feeding mother could give her baby a pacifier at this time. If she is bottle feeding because of low milk production or ineffective nursing on the baby's part, encourage her to pacify the baby at her breast.

Breastfed babies often have the opportunity to cuddle in bed with the mother during feedings, with both of them napping while the baby nurses. A bottle fed infant does not generally have this opportunity. Lying down with her baby after eating provides this special time.

When parents choose to use artificial baby milk and bottles for feeding, it is the role of the healthcare professional to provide them with appropriate feeding guidelines to minimize the risk to their baby. This information assists women prenatally as they make their infant feeding choice. Maternity staff who teach postpartum patients need to include complete and correct information for those who choose to bottle feed (Redmond, 2009), including the potential hazards in preparation and cleaning. Often, much information regarding proper bottle feeding and use of an artificial baby milk is glossed over or not discussed at all. This does a disservice to parents and to their babies and does not provide true informed consent for their decisions.

A comprehensive review found that mothers who bottle fed their babies failed to receive sufficient information on bottle feeding to make informed decisions.

They reported negative emotions such as guilt, anger, worry, uncertainty, and a sense of failure. Reported mistakes in preparation of bottle feeds were common (Lakshman et al., 2009). Parents need complete and accurate information to make responsible decisions. Chapter 9 discusses the information parents need to bottle feed as safely as possible.

∾ Summary

There are specific uses for the various breastfeeding devices and techniques available to mothers. Practitioners should recommend them only when there is a clear need. If used inappropriately, some breastfeeding aids can have a negative impact on breastfeeding. Begin with the least invasive methods for dealing with a problem to minimize interference. Provide guidance, support, and follow-up to ensure that the mother has a clear understanding of the proper use of any device. When mothers must be away from their babies during feedings, help them select a method of milk expression that best suits their needs. Learning hand expression may be all the mother requires. Make sure mothers know the proper collection and storage techniques for preserving the nutritional quality of their milk. Human milk banks provide donated milk for preterm and ill infants. Help parents learn alternate feeding methods that work best for them. Above all, serve as an advocate for the mother and baby remaining together with minimal interventions. Incorporate special aids into care plans only when necessary.

∾ Chapter 21—At a Glance

Applying what you learned—

Counseling precautions:

- Begin pumping immediately when initiation of breastfeeding is delayed.
- Use digital techniques appropriately.
- Use suck training only if you have appropriate training.

Teach mothers how to

- Do the pinch test to determine nipple eversion.
- Do breast massage to help early feedings.
- Use reverse pressure softening.
- Use the C-hold support.
- Use the Dancer hand position for preterm infants and those with weak muscle development.
- Apply lubricants to the breast appropriately.

- Use an inverted syringe or everter for flat or inverted nipples.
- Wear breast shells appropriately.
- Use drip milk safely.
- Use a nipple shield appropriately and wean their baby from it as soon as is appropriate.
- Select and use a pacifier appropriately.
- Manually remove milk from their breasts.
- Select and use a breast pump.
- Condition letdown for pumping.
- Pump for a hospitalized baby.
- Collect and store their milk for healthy infants and NICU infants.
- Combine, defrost, and warm their milk.
- Donate milk to a milk bank.
- Cup feed and spoon feed as baby-led feeding alternatives.
- Tube feed with a supplementer.
- Select and use bottles and nipples appropriately.
- Pace bottle feedings according to hunger cues, and watch for stress cues.

∾ References

Abouelfettoh A. Cup versus bottle feeding for hospitalized late preterm infants in Egypt: a quasi-experimental study. *Intl Breastfeed J.* 2008;3:27.

Academy of Breastfeeding Medicine (ABM). Clinical protocol number #8: human milk storage information for home use for healthy full term infants; 2004. www.bfmed.org/Resources/Protocols.aspx. Accessed October 1, 2009.

Akkuzu G, Taskin L. Impacts of breast-care techniques on prevention of possible postpartum nipple problems. *Prof Care Mother Child.* 2000;10:38-41.

Alexander J, et al. Randomised controlled trial of breast shells and Hoffman's exercises for inverted and non-protractile nipples. *Br Med J.* 1992;304:1030-1032.

Aloysius A, Hickson M. Evaluation of paladai cup feeding in breast-fed preterm infants compared with bottle feeding. *Early Hum Dev.* 2007;83:619-621.

Amatayakul K, et al. Serum prolactin and cortisol levels after suckling for varying periods of time and the effect of a nipple shield. *Acta Obstet Gynecol Scand.* 1987;66:47-51.

American Academy of Pediatrics (AAP). Policy statement on breastfeeding and the use of human milk. *Pediatrics.* 2005a115:496-506.

American Academy of Pediatrics (AAP). Policy statement. Task Force on Sudden Infant Death Syndrome. The changing concept of sudden infant death syndrome: diagnostic coding shifts, controversies regarding the sleeping environment, and new variables to consider in reducing risk. *Pediatrics.* 2005b;116:1245-1255.

American Association of Health Plans. Health Plans' innovative programs in breastfeeding promotion. August 2001. www.aahp.org. Accessed September 15, 2009.

Amir L, Hoover K. *Candidiasis and Breastfeeding*. Lactation Consultant Series Two, Unit 6. Schaumburg, IL: La Leche League International; 2002.

Austin M. Got breast milk? Buyers are willing to pay but booming trade raises safety, ethical questions. *The Denver Post*. Sunday, March 26, 2006. www.starnewsonline.com/article/20060326/NEWS/203260331?Title=Got-breast-milk-Buyers-are-willing-to-pay. Accessed October 1, 2009.

Avishai O. Managing the lactating body: the breast-feeding project and privileged motherhood. *Qual Soc*. 2007;30:135-152.

Balmer S, Wharton B. Human milk banking at Sorrento Maternity Hospital, Birmingham. *Arch Dis Child*. 1992;67:556-559.

Barger J. *Certified Lactation Specialist Course*. Wheaton, IL: Lactation Education Consultants; 2009.

Barlow S, et al. Synthetic orocutaneous stimulation entrains preterm infants with feeding difficulties to suck. *J Perinatol*. 2008;28:541-548.

Becker G, et al. Methods of milk expression for lactating women. *Cochrane Database Syst Rev*. 2008;CD006170.

Benis M. Are pacifiers associated with early weaning from breastfeeding? *Adv Neonatal Care*. 2002;2:259-266.

Boekel S. Gastroesophageal reflux: the breastfeeding family's nightmare. Presentation at ILCA Conference, Washington, DC, July 27, 2000. www.repeatperformance.com/product.asp?ProductCode=%27ILCA00S3%27 for order. Accessed February 15, 2010.

Boo N, et al. Contamination of breast milk obtained by manual expression and breast pumps in mothers of very low birth-weight infants. *J Hosp Infect*. 2001;49(4):274-281.

Borucki L. Breastfeeding mothers' experiences using a supplemental feeding tube device: finding an alternative. *J Hum Lact*. 2005;21:429-438.

Brent N, et al. Sore nipples in breast-feeding women: a clinical trial of wound dressings vs. conventional care. *Arch Pediatr Adolesc Med*. 1998;152:1077-1082.

Buckley K. A double-edged sword: lactation consultants' perceptions of the impact of breast pumps on the practice of breastfeeding. *J Perinatal Educ*. 2009;18:13-22.

Casey C, et al. Nutrient intake by breast-fed infants during the first five days after birth. *Am J Dis Child*. 1986;140:933-936.

Centers for Disease Control and Prevention (CDC). Proper handling and storage of human milk. May 22, 2007. www.cdc.gov/breastfeeding/recommendations/handling_breastmilk.htm. Accessed September 27, 2009.

Charchut S, et al. The effects of infant feeding patterns on the occlusion of the primary dentition. *J Dent Child*. 2003;70:197-203.

Chen C, et al. The effect of breast- and bottle feeding on oxygen saturation and body temperature in preterm infants. *J Hum Lact*. 2000;16:21-27.

Chertok I. Reexamination of ultra-thin nipple shield use, infant growth and maternal satisfaction. *J Clin Nurs*. 2009;18:2949-2955.

Chertok I, et al. A pilot study of maternal and term infant outcomes associated with ultrathin nipple shield use. *JOGNN*. 2006;35:265-272.

Collins C, et al. Avoidance of bottles during the establishment of breast feeds in preterm infants. *Cochrane Database Syst Rev*. 2008;CD005252.

Cotterman K. Reverse pressure softening: a simple tool to prepare areola for easier latching during engorgement. *J Hum Lact*. 2004;20:227-237.

Cregan M, et al. Initiation of lactation in women after preterm delivery. *Acta Obstet Gynecol Scand*. 2002;81:870-877.

Dodd V, Chalmers C. Comparing the use of hydrogel dressings to lanolin ointment with lactating mothers. *JOGNN*. 2003;32:486-494.

Dowling D, et al. Cup-feeding for preterm infants: mechanics and safety. *J Hum Lact*. 2002;18:13-20.

Elserafy F, et al. Oral sucrose and a pacifier for pain relief during simple procedures in preterm infants: a randomized controlled trial. *Ann Saudi Med*. 2009;29:184-188.

Engstrom J, et al. Comparison of milk output from the right and left breasts during simultaneous pumping in mothers of very low birthweight infants. *Breastfeed Med*. 2007;2:83-91.

Ensor D. Breast-milk enterprise raises concerns among those who view collection and distribution as a philanthropic endeavor. *San Diego Union-Tribune*, February 12, 2006.

Foda M, et al. Composition of milk obtained from unmassaged versus massaged breasts of lactating mothers. *J Pediatr Gastroenterol Nutr*. 2004;38:484-487.

Fowler G, Ye J. Got milk? Chinese crisis creates a market for human alternatives. *Wall Street Journal*, September 24, 2008.

Geddes D, et al. Tongue movement and intra-oral vacuum in breastfeeding infants. *Early Hum Dev*. 2008;84:471-477.

Geddes D, et al. Ultrasound imaging of infant swallowing during breast-feeding. *Dysphagia*. DOI 10.1007/s00455-009-9241-0; July 22, 2009.

Geraghty S, et al. Guidelines for establishing a donor human milk depot. *J Hum Lact*. 2010;26(1):49-52.

Gordon I, Whitehead T. Lead poisoning in an infant from lead nipple-shields: association with rickets. *Lancet*. 1949;2:647-650.

Grøvslien A, Grønn M. Donor milk banking and breastfeeding in Norway. *J Hum Lact*. 2009;25(2):206-210.

Hale T, et al. The absence of *Candida albicans* in milk samples of women with clinical symptoms of ductal candidiasis. *Breastfeed Med*. 2009;4:57-61.

Hartmann P, et al. Physiology of lactation in preterm mothers: initiation and maintenance. *Pediatr Ann*. 2003;32:351-355.

Henderson J, et al. Effect of preterm birth and antenatal corticosteroid treatment on lactogenesis II in women. *Pediatrics*. 2008;121:e92-e100.

Hill P, et al. Comparison of milk output between breasts in pump-dependent mothers. *J Hum Lact*. 2007;23:333-337.

Howard C, et al. Randomized clinical trial of pacifier use and bottle feeding or cupfeeding and their effect on breastfeeding. *Pediatrics*. 2003;111:511-518.

Human Milk Banking Association of North America (HMBANA). *2006 Best Practice For Pumping, Storing and Handling of Mother's Own Milk in Hospital and at Home*, 2nd ed. Raleigh, NC: HMBANA; 2006.

Human Milk Banking Association of North America (HMBANA). *Guidelines for the Establishment and Operation of a Donor Human Milk Bank*. Raleigh, NC: HMBANA; 2008.

Jackson D, et al. The automatic sampling shield: a device for sampling suckled breast milk. *Early Hum Dev.* 1987;15:295-306.

Kapellou O. Blood sampling in infants (reducing pain and morbidity). *Clin Evid (Online)* pii: 0313; Jan 7, 2009. http://clinicalevidence.bmj.com. Accessed February 15, 2010.

Karabulut E, et al. Effect of pacifier use on exclusive and any breastfeeding: a meta-analysis. *Turk J Pediatr.* 2009;51:35-43.

Kassing D. Bottle feeding as a tool to reinforce breastfeeding. *J Hum Lact.* 2002;18:56-60.

Kent J, et al. Volume and frequency of breastfeedings and fat content of breast milk throughout the day. *Pediatrics.* 2006;117:e387-e395.

Kesaree N, et al. Treatment of inverted nipples using a disposable syringe. *J Hum Lact.* 1993;9:27-29.

Kronborg H, Vaeth M. How are effective breastfeeding technique and pacifier use related to breastfeeding problems and breastfeeding duration? *Birth.* 2009;36:34-42.

Lakshman R, et al. Mothers' experiences of bottle-feeding: a systematic review of qualitative and quantitative studies. *Arch Dis Child.* 2009;94:596-601.

Lang S, et al. Cup feeding: an alternative method of infant feeding. *Arch Dis Child.* 1994;71:365-369.

Larson E. Sucking, chewing, and feeding habits and the development of crossbite: a longitudinal study of girls from birth to 3 years of age. *Angle Orthod.* 2001;71:116-119.

Lepore J. Baby food: If breast is best, why are women bottling their milk? *The New Yorker,* January 19, 2009.

Lopes de Melo S, Murta E. Hypogalactia treated with hand expression and translactation without the use of galactogogues *J Hum Lact.* 2009;25(4):444-447.

Marx CM, et al. Vitamin E concentrations in serum of newborn infants after topical use of vitamin E in nursing mothers. *Am J Obstet Gynecol.* 1985;152:668-670.

Mattos-Graner R, et al. Relation of oral yeast infection in Brazilian infants and use of a pacifier. *ASDC J Dent Child.* 2001; 68:33-36.

Meier P. Bottle- and breast-feeding: effects on transcutaneous oxygen pressure and temperature in preterm infants. *Nurs Res.* 1988;37:36-41.

Meier P, et al. Nipple shields for preterm infants: effect on milk transfer and duration of breastfeeding. *J Hum Lact.* 2000; 16:106-114.

MilkShare; 2008. http://milkshare.birthingforlife.com. Accessed September 28, 2009.

Mohrbacher N, Stock J. *The Breastfeeding Answer Book,* 3rd ed. Schaumburg, IL: La Leche League International; 2003.

Morton J. Breastfeeding the preterm infant, lessons for all. Presented at the Amarillo Conference on Human Lactation: Current Research and Clinical Implications, Breastmilk for Pre-term Babies, Amarillo, Texas, October 21, 2004.

Morton J, et al. Combining hand techniques with electric pumping increases milk production in mothers of preterm infants. *J Perinatol.* 2009;30:14.

Narayanan I, Bambroo A. Alternative methods of feeding low birthweight infants: an additional support to kangaroo mother care. Presented at the 4th International Workshop on Kangaroo Mother Care, Cape Town, South Africa, November 27, 2002.

Newman J, Kernerman E. Breast compression; February 2009. http://www.nbci.ca/index.php?option=comcontent&view=article&id=8:breast-compression&catid=5:information&Item id=17. Accessed September 28, 2009.

Newman J, Pitman T. *The Ultimate Breastfeeding Book of Answers.* Roseville, CA: Prima; 2000.

Nowak A, et al. Imaging evaluation of artificial nipples during bottle feeding. *Arch Pediatr Adolesc Med.* 1994;148:40-42.

O'Connor N, et al. Pacifiers and breastfeeding: a systematic review. *Arch Pediatr Adolesc Med.* 2009;163:378-382.

Palmer B. Sleep apnea from an anatomical, anthropologic and developmental perspective. Presentation at the Academy of Dental Sleep Medicine, Philadelphia, June 4, 2004.

Palmer G. *The Politics of Breastfeeding: When Breasts are Bad for Business,* 3rd ed. London: Pinter & Martin, Ltd; 2009.

Pinelli J, Symington A. Non-nutritive sucking for promoting physiologic stability and nutrition in preterm infants. *Cochrane Database Syst Rev.* 2005;CD001071.

Poore M, et al. Patterned orocutaneous therapy improves sucking and oral feeding in preterm infants. *Acta Paediatr.* 2008;97:920-927.

Prolacta Bioscience. www.prolacta.com; 2009a. Accessed September 28, 2009.

Prolacta Bioscience. Abbott co-promotion agreement frequently asked questions; October 4, 2009b. http://www.prolacta.com/faq_abbott.php. Accessed February 15, 2010.

Quan R, et al. Effects of microwave radiation on anti-infective factors in human milk. *Pediatrics.* 1992;89:667-669.

Ramsay D. Ultrasound imaging of the sucking mechanics of the term infant. Presented at the Amarillo Conference on Human Lactation: Current Research and Clinical Implications, Amarillo, Texas, October 22, 2004.

Redmond E, et al. Contamination of bottles used for feeding reconstituted powdered infant formula and implications for public health. *Perspect Public Health.* 2009;129:85-94.

Rocha N, Martinez F, Jorge S. Cup or bottle for preterm infants: effects on oxygen saturation, weight gain, and breastfeeding. *J Hum Lact.* 2002;18:132-138.

Sexton S, Natale R. Risks and benefits of pacifiers. *Am Fam Physician.* 2009;79:681-685.

Smith WL, Erenbert A, Nowak A. Imaging evaluation of the human nipple during breast-feeding. *Am J Dis Child.* 1988;142:76-78.

Stanford School of Medicine. Newborn Nursery at LPCH. Hand expression of breastmilk. http://newborns.stanford.edu/Breastfeeding/HandExpression.html. Accessed September 27, 2009a.

Stanford School of Medicine. Newborn Nursery at LPCH. Maximizing milk production with hands on pumping. 2009b. http://newborns.stanford.edu/Breastfeeding/MaxProduction.html. Accessed September 27, 2009b.

Sweet L. Breastfeeding a preterm infant and the objectification of breastmilk. *Breastfeed Rev.* 2006;14:5113.

Thorley V. Sharing breastmilk: wet nursing, cross feeding, and milk donations. *Breastfeed Rev.* 2008;16:25-29.

Updegrove K. Personal interview. Mothers' Milk Bank at Austin; September 29, 2009.

Warren J, et al. Pacifier use and the occurrence of otitis media in the first year of life. *Ped Dentist.* 2001;23:103-107.

West D, Marasco L. *The Breastfeeding Mother's Guide to Making More Milk*. New York: McGraw-Hill; 2008.

Wiessinger D. A breastfeeding tool using a sandwich analogy for latch-on. *J Hum Lact*. 1998;14:51-56.

Wilson-Clay B. Clinical use of silicon nipple shields. *J Hum Lact*. 1996;12:279-285.

Wilson-Clay B, Hoover K. *The Breastfeeding Atlas*, 4th ed. Austin, TX: Lactnews Press; 2008.

Wolf L, Glass R. *Feeding and Swallowing Disorders in Infancy*. San Antonio, TX: Therapy Skill Builders; 1992.

Yokoyama Y, et al. Release of oxytocin and prolactin during breast massage and suckling in puerperal women. *Eur J Obstet Gynaecol Reprod Biol*. 1994;53:17-20.

Zardetto C, et al. Effects of different pacifiers on the primary dentition and oral myofunctional structures of preschool children. *Pediatr Dent*. 2002;24:552-560.

Temporary Breastfeeding Situations

At times a new mother may face an interruption or a temporary obstacle with breastfeeding that requires extra encouragement and suggestions. Jaundice, for example, is common in the early days, and understanding its relationship to breastfeeding practices helps parents reduce its incidence and severity. Later in the breastfeeding journey, some babies seem to lose interest in breastfeeding or to prefer one breast to another. Mothers who experience a delay in the initiation of breastfeeding, wish to nurse an adopted baby, or decide to relactate will also benefit from advice and support. You can help these mothers recognize that breastfeeding is a means of nurturing their babies as well as feeding them.

∼ Key Terms

Acute bilirubin
   encephalopathy (ABE)
Albumin
Alternate massage
Apnea
Bili-bed
Bili-blanket
Bili-light
Blood incompatibility
Breast compression
Breastfeeding-associated
   jaundice
Breastfeeding jaundice
Breastmilk jaundice
Conjugation
Coombs' test
Edema
Exchange transfusion
Fiberoptic blanket
Gestational age
Hemoglobin
Hemolysis
Hospital-grade electric
   breast pump

Hyperbilirubinemia
Inducing lactation
Involution
Jaundice
Kernicterus
Lactogenesis
Late-onset jaundice
Late preterm infant
Normal newborn jaundice
Nursing supplementer
Pathologic jaundice
Phototherapy
Physiologic jaundice
Prolactin receptor cells
Rebirthing
Relactation
Remedial cobathing
Respiratory distress
   syndrome
Ruptured membranes
Switch nursing
Transcutaneous bilimeter
Wallaby wrap

∼ Hyperbilirubinemia (Jaundice)

Clinically, hyperbilirubinemia (jaundice) is the most commonly treated medical condition in the healthy newborn. It is apparent in up to 60 percent of full-term infants in their first week of life and in nearly all preterm infants (Watson, 2009). Visually, jaundice is identified by a progressive yellow coloring of the skin and the whites of the eyes. In some cases weakness and loss of appetite occur. Most jaundice is physiologic and clears up spontaneously within a few days with no intervention and no ill effects. However, jaundice can be dangerous if levels rise too high or when other risk factors are present (Watchko, 2009). Figure 22.1 describes the various levels of risk factors for jaundice.

All jaundice warrants investigation and follow-up. It can be challenging for clinicians to differentiate between normal and abnormal jaundice patterns (Gartner & Herschel, 2001). Jaundice becomes clinically significant when it develops within the first 24 hours of the baby's life, when bilirubin rates increase rapidly, when levels become exaggerated, or when the condition is prolonged beyond 2 weeks in term babies and beyond 3 weeks in preterm babies. High bilirubin levels appear to occur more often among Asians, Native Americans, and Eskimos. Jaundice rates are also higher in babies who live at higher altitudes, perhaps because the decrease in oxygen levels at high altitudes leads to an increase in hemoglobin and number of red blood cells (Maisels & Watchko, 2000).

Types of Jaundice

At birth, a healthy newborn's bilirubin level has historically been measured as 1.5 mg/dL or less. Over the next 3 to 4 days, it has been observed to rise to a peak of approximately 6.5 mg/dL. Bilirubin then returns to a normal level of less than 1.5 mg/dL by around the 10th day of life (American Academy of Pediatrics [AAP], 2004). This natural rise and fall of the newborn's bilirubin is referred to as physiologic jaundice.

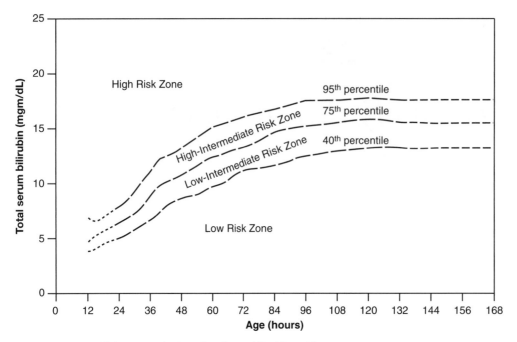

FIGURE 22.1   Risk factors for jaundice (hyperbilirubinemia).

Source: Bhutani VK et al. Predictive ability of a predischarge hour-specific serum bilirubin for subsequent significant hyperbiliruinemia in healthy term and near-term newborns. *Pediatrics.* 1999;103:6-14. Reprinted with permission of the American Academy of Pediatrics.

It is normal for jaundice to last longer in healthy, breastfed babies (Gartner, 2007). In infants with mild jaundice, the yellow coloring may be difficult to detect visually under artificial light. Physiologic jaundice is distinguished from high bilirubin levels resulting from poor breastfeeding, later onset of jaundice, or pathology. Jaundice is considered nonphysiologic when the bilirubin level reaches above 12 mg/dL and the jaundice has no identifiable cause. The term pathologic jaundice applies when a disease process causes elevated bilirubin.

Bilirubin levels change hourly in a newborn. Whereas a full-term newborn may be considered healthy with commonly considered "high" levels, a very preterm baby may be able to sustain kernicterus at seemingly "low" levels. Maisels (2006) suggests that the terms "newborn jaundice" or "neonatal bilirubinemia" better describe this phenomenon rather than current terminology of physiologic and pathologic jaundice. However, until researchers and policymakers refine and standardize these definitions, the present standard definitions used by the AAP serve as the best guide.

Physiologic Jaundice (Normal Newborn Jaundice)

In utero, the fetus produces large amounts of red blood cells, necessary for transporting oxygen to the fetus from the mother's blood via the placenta. This is the baby's only source of oxygen until leaving the mother's womb and drawing in oxygen through the lungs. The hemoglobin (a protein) portion of the body's red blood cells transports oxygen. Newborn infants have more hemoglobin than adults do, and healthy full-term infants are born with both fetal and adult hemoglobin. Although fetal hemoglobin is efficient in handling oxygen in utero, only adult hemoglobin is efficient after birth. Because the infant does not need fetal hemoglobin after birth, the infant's body breaks it down, separates it, and reuses the globin portion. The heme portion undergoes many changes, the final byproduct of which is bilirubin.

Conjugated Bilirubin   Although every infant is born with an increased concentration of bilirubin, not all infants have the high concentrations that result in the visible yellow coloring associated with jaundice. Under normal conditions the bilirubin becomes bound chemically to proteins, such as albumin, which transport it to the liver. Many infants are able to dispose of bilirubin through this physiologic process. The liver converts the bilirubin through a process of conjugation into a form that can pass through the bile to the intestine. In the intestine it undergoes further changes that enable the baby's stools and, to a much lesser extent, urine to excrete it. Bilirubin that is conjugated, or bound (attached to albumin), is not in itself harmful to the baby, because it remains in the bloodstream.

Unconjugated, Unbound Bilirubin   Frequently, a newborn's red blood cells break down more quickly than the immature body can process, resulting in a temporary buildup of bilirubin. Physiologic jaundice occurs when bilirubin production exceeds the liver's ability to process it. Bilirubin levels will gradually decline as the excess hemoglobin breaks down, bacteria colonize the intestines, and the transition from fetal to adult hemoglobin occurs. The decreased rate of bilirubin conjugation in physiologic jaundice, allows unbound, unconjugated bilirubin to circulate freely in the bloodstream. This unbound bilirubin can migrate to other parts of the body with high fat content, such as the brain, skin, muscle tissue, and mucous membranes, where it deposits (Figure 22.2).

Kernicterus In extreme cases elevated bilirubin can place the infant at risk for bilirubin encephalopathy, leading to long-term neurological damage. Under certain conditions that disrupt the blood–brain barrier—such as prematurity, asphyxia, starvation, and hemolytic disease—bilirubin can pass the blood–brain barrier and deposit in nerve cells in the brain. Bilirubin has a toxic effect on brain and nerve cells and can result in neurological damage known as kernicterus, or acute bilirubin encephalopathy (ABE). In the extreme, ABE can cause death. The AAP (2004) suggests that the term ABE best describes this high elevation of bilirubin and that the term "kernicterus" be used for the chronic, long-term sequelae associated with brain damage from ABE.

The bilirubin level at which ABE occurs varies with the gestational and postnatal age of the infant. Birth weight, the presence of other disease, and the availability of albumin-binding sites are also factors. Generally, a healthy, full-term infant will not develop ABE when the bilirubin level is below 20 mg/dL (Stevenson et al., 2004).

In a review of 125 kernicterus cases reporting serum bilirubin levels ranging from 20.7 to 59.9 mg/100 mL, no specific bilirubin level threshold coincided with the onset of ABE (Johnson et al., 2009). However, a preterm infant can progress quickly to bilirubin encephalopathy and to the chronic stage of kernicterus. A disproportionate number of the 125 cases were late preterm infants, 34.9 percent of whom were large for gestational age and not treated as preterm. Statistically, infants most at risk for kernicterus are those born at 35 to 38 weeks' gestation, male, and Asian. Other risk factors are infants that have bruising, that develop jaundice within 24 hours of birth, that remain visibly jaundiced at discharge, or that have a previous sibling who had jaundice (AAP, 2001).

Special Health Conditions Conditions such as hepatitis, galactosemia, biliary atresia, or sepsis cause an abnormality of excretion or reabsorption of bilirubin. Bruising, blood incompatibility, lack of enzymes, or antibodies against the baby's own red blood cells can create a rapid rise in bilirubin level. Many diseases and drugs can lead to the production of autoantibodies, which destroy red blood cells and may cause anemia (Dugdale & Chen, 2008). The direct Coombs' test is used to detect the presence of these autoantibodies and to help diagnose the cause of anemia, jaundice, or red blood cell abnormalities. Glucose-6-phosphate dehydrogenase (G6PD) deficiency, the most prevalent enzyme deficiency, is estimated to affect 400 million people worldwide (Nkhoma et al., 2009). This deficiency is a hereditary genetic defect that causes newborn hyperbilirubinemia and chronic hemolytic (red cell destruction) anemia. Although most people with G6PD deficiency have no symptoms, certain drugs or infections can cause acute hemolysis (Cappellini & Fiorelli, 2008).

Breastfeeding-Associated Jaundice

Breastfeeding-associated jaundice is a term used to describe jaundice that results from such iatrogenic causes as scheduled feedings, routine mother–infant separation, unnecessary formula supplements, and pacifier use. A new mother unfamiliar with what to expect with breastfeeding may fail to nurse her newborn frequently enough for adequate nourishment. Likewise, the use of labor medications may result in sleepy babies who then have difficulty nursing (Jordan et al., 2009) resulting in inadequate intake of the mother's milk.

Elevated bilirubin levels in breastfeeding-associated jaundice result not from dehydration but from caloric deprivation and the resultant decreased stooling. This inadequate intake of milk could be considered "starvation jaundice of the newborn" (Gartner, 2007) or "breast-nonfeeding jaundice" (Gartner, 2001). Frequent cases of exaggerated jaundice in a hospital or community of breastfed babies may indicate a need to improve breastfeeding policies and support.

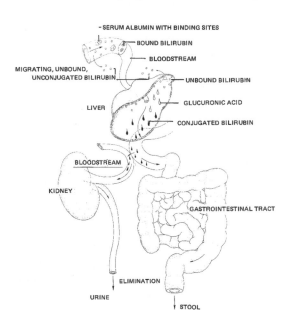

FIGURE 22.2 How the body handles bilirubin.

Breastfeeding-associated jaundice is usually preventable through appropriate breastfeeding practices. Establishing policies of obstetrical care based on the Ten Steps to Successful Breastfeeding (available at www.unicef.org) helps eliminate practices that lead to this type of jaundice. When jaundice occurs, treatment includes increasing the number and quality of breastfeedings, observing the baby's attachment and positioning, listening for swallowing, and using pre- and post-feed test weights. Rooming-in and frequent skin-to-skin contact facilitate an increase in the number of feeding opportunities. A study of 358 exclusively breastfed newborns found significant positive correlations between the frequency of feedings and meconium stooling in the first 24 hours of life. Babies that nursed more than 13 times in 24 hours had lower bilirubin level on days 3 and 7 (Okechukwu & Okolo, 2006).

Breast compression (alternate massage) can help increase the flow of milk for a baby with a weak and ineffective suck (Newman & Kernerman, 2009a). The mother can also hand express her colostrum and spoon or syringe feed it to her baby (see Chapter 21 for alternative feeding options). A baby who is an effective feeder can be given unlimited access to the breast, with no restrictions on frequency or duration. However, unlimited sucking is not productive for a baby with an ineffective suck, which is common in babies born late preterm.

Although optimal breastfeeding does not entirely eliminate neonatal jaundice, it can lead to a pattern that may actually be beneficial to infants (Gartner & Herschel, 2001). Research shows that bilirubin acts as a powerful antioxidant and may provide protection against free radical cellular damage after birth (Kapitulnik & Maines, 2009; Sedlak et al., 2009). The question to ask may be whether artificially fed infants that do *not* exhibit normal newborn jaundice levels lack this protection (Newman & Kernerman, 2009b).

Prolonged Physiologic Jaundice (Breastmilk Jaundice)

Prolonged physiologic jaundice—also called late-onset or breastmilk jaundice—becomes apparent later than physiologic newborn jaundice. It typically occurs between the 4th and 7th days of life, when mature milk begins to replace colostrum. In this type of jaundice, bilirubin reaches a maximum concentration by the 2nd or 3rd week and may persist through the 6th week of life, even up to 15 weeks. A baby with breastmilk jaundice is lively and does not appear to be sick. Some research suggests that the enzyme β-glucuronidase in human milk increases intestinal absorption of bilirubin and contributes to this type of jaundice. However, this may not be the case since high concentrations of this enzyme already exist in the baby's gut (La Torre, 1999).

Continuation of jaundice into the third and later weeks of life in a healthy breastfed newborn is actually a normal extension of physiologic jaundice. Frequent and effective breastfeeding started soon after delivery minimizes weight loss and helps the baby gain weight quickly. Such optimal breastfeeding practices are associated with reducing the incidence and intensity of breastfeeding jaundice.

Prolonged physiologic jaundice is usually a self-limiting and benign condition, with most cases requiring no interruption in breastfeeding. Just as with newborn physiologic jaundice, it can be treated with increased feedings and exposure to sunlight (although the AAP does not recommend sun exposure; see the discussion on vitamin D in Chapter 8). Despite bilirubin levels in this type of jaundice rarely rising to dangerous levels, these infants still need to be monitored because of the potential for toxicity (Gartner, 2007).

Because there is an association between urinary tract infections and late-onset jaundice (Xinias et al., 2009; Ghaemi et al., 2007), culturing urine for infection is recommended when a baby has prolonged jaundice. As with any occurrence of jaundice, parents need the reassurance that nothing is wrong with the mother's milk. Prepare them for a long period of resolution if the baby's skin is still yellow after the second week. If a mother's previous baby experienced late-onset jaundice, you can offer her anticipatory guidance that this baby may have it as well.

Pathologic Jaundice

Pathologic jaundice can result from conditions such as infections in the blood or liver, diseases of the liver, obstructions in the gastrointestinal system, and interference with the binding of bilirubin in the bloodstream. Many of these circumstances are also associated with jaundice in an adult. Clinical evaluations and various tests are performed to pinpoint specific diseases. Treatment of the disease, as well as treatment of the jaundice, is necessary in these situations. Because of its diverse nature, it is possible for pathologic jaundice to appear any time after birth thus making diagnosis of the type of jaundice relatively difficult.

Blood incompatibility and certain drugs can also result in pathologic jaundice. A breastfeeding mother and baby should discontinue any drugs that contribute to the buildup of bilirubin. Blood incompatibility occurs when a mother with blood type O becomes pregnant with a baby having blood type A, B, or AB. The mother's blood contains naturally occurring antibodies to type A and B; these antibodies can cross the placenta and destroy (hemolyze) the baby's red blood cells (National Center for Biotechnology Information, 2005). In addition to the G6PD enzyme deficiency noted earlier, there are more than 50 known red cell enzyme deficiencies associated with newborn jaundice (Gartner, 2007).

Detection of Jaundice

Jaundice is visible when the bilirubin level reaches 5 to 7 mg/dL. Among babies with visible jaundice, 15 percent have a bilirubin level of 10 mg/dL or higher. Approximately 3 percent of these babies have exaggerated or sustained bilirubin levels because of a normal development process in their ability to conjugate and excrete bilirubin. If the infant is ill or preterm, the safe level for bilirubin is lower, and the resulting jaundice requires quicker treatment and close monitoring.

Progression of Yellowing

As jaundice levels increase, the body's yellowing progresses from the head down to the chest, to the knees, lower legs and arms, and finally to the hands and feet. Bilirubin levels correspond to the visual jaundicing of the baby's body (Kramer, 1969):

- Shoulder: 5 to 7 mg/dL
- Umbilicus: 7 to 10 mg/dL
- Below the umbilicus: 10 to 12 mg/dL
- Below the knees: greater than 15 mg/dL

Testing Bilirubin Levels

Clinicians who suspect jaundice or detect it visually perform either a transcutaneous light meter test or a blood test to determine the bilirubin level. Many hospitals routinely check bilirubin levels of all newborns after 24 hours of life, at the same time when they rule out disease and infection. Blood types of both mother and baby are evaluated as well, to rule out blood incompatibility. Assessment of the Coombs' test performed at birth is coordinated with these other tests to check for antiglobulins in the baby's blood.

A baby with a high bilirubin count typically receives multiple heel sticks throughout the course of treatment. Breastfeeding during painful procedures effectively reduces pain responses (Dilli et al., 2009; Saitua et al., 2009; Shah et al., 2009; Osinaike et al., 2007; Uga et al., 2008). In fact, breastfeeding has been found to be analgesic up to 6 months of age (Dilli et al., 2009). Mothers can request breastfeeding during heel sticks to reduce their babies' pain level.

Parents can request a less invasive initial jaundice assessment procedure as well. Transcutaneous bilirubin (TcB) measurement systems are noninvasive handheld devices similar to a small handheld calculator or flashlight. When held over the baby's skin, usually the torso, a number appears on the screen to indicate bilirubin level. TcB systems have been used for years as a quick, noninvasive way to screen babies. Depending on the bilirubin level indicated by the meter, the baby then has a serum bilirubin drawn (heel stick).

Newer TcB devices are reliable substitutes for serum bilirubin measurements (Maisels et al., 2004). Measuring bilirubin levels on the sternum yields better results than on the forehead, which can be affected by race (Holland & Blick, 2009). Although another study found that the TcB test underestimated serum bilirubin levels, especially in patients with high levels, TcB is considered useful as a screening tool (Marco Lozano et al., 2009). Parents concerned about repeated heel sticks might ask for an initial bili-flash, as these devices are called, followed by serum testing as needed. The hospital may or may not have bilimeters.

Treatment of Jaundice

When a bilirubin level is significant, several types of treatment are appropriate, depending on the baby's condition. For less severe jaundice regular visual observation and periodic testing of bilirubin levels may be sufficient. Physiologic jaundice is usually very mild and causes no known lasting effects in a healthy full-term infant. In most cases bilirubin values rise slowly (less than a 5-mg/dL increase in 24 hours). Bilirubin reaches a noticeable level by the third day of life and remains slightly elevated for several days, falling by the end of the first week. Active treatment is rarely required as long as levels remain within a safe range. Figure 22.3 provides an AAP graph for evaluating bilirubin risk level.

The incidence of dangerous bilirubin levels is associated with disjointed care during the first week after the baby's birth. A study of kernicterus events found multiple providers at multiple sites, an inability to identify the at-risk infant, and an inability to manage severe hyperbilirubinemia in a timely manner (Johnson et al., 2009). Families need to have a newborn medical weight and color check within 3 to 5 days of birth. Unfortunately, in the United States infants often are not seen until 2 weeks for the traditional wellness check.

In one large provider network, newborn follow-up was inconsistent and commonly delayed (Profit et al., 2009). Only 37 percent of all infants (and 41 percent of exclusively breastfed infants) were seen before 6 days of age. Steps can be taken in the early postpartum period to reduce the incidence and severity of jaundice by increasing effective feedings. Phototherapy and, when severe, blood exchange transfusions are also treatments.

Increased Feeding

Increasing the frequency and effectiveness of feedings in the early days helps to reduce bilirubin levels in the infant. Increased feedings stimulate stooling, thereby reducing intestinal reabsorption of bilirubin (MacDonald et al., 2005). The incidence of jaundice is decreased when meconium, which is laden with bilirubin, is passed quickly.

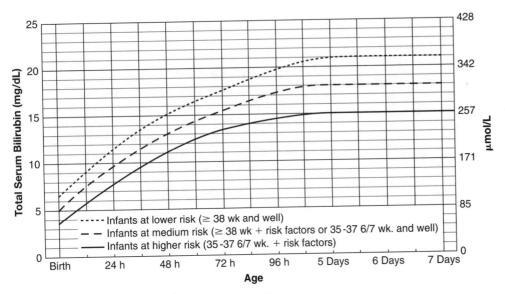

- Use total bilirubin. Do not subtract direct reacting or conjugated bilirubin.
- Risk factors = isoimmune hemolytic disease, G6PD deficiency, asphyxia, significant lethargy, temperature instability, sepsis, acidosis, or albumin < 3.0g/dL (if measured)
- For well infants 35-37 6/7 wk can adjust TSB levels for intervention around the medium risk line. It is an option to intervene at lower TSB levels for infants closer to 35 wks and at higher TSB levels for those closer to 37 6/7 wk.
- It is an option to provide conventional phototherapy in hospital or at home at TSB levels 2-3 mg/dL (35-50 μmol/L) below those shown but home phototherapy should not be used in any infant with risk factors.

FIGURE 22.3   Identifying bilirubin risk level.

Source: American Academy of Pediatrics (AAP) Subcommittee on Hyperbilirubinemia. Clinical practice guideline: management of hyperbilirubinemia in the newborn infant > 35 weeks of gestation. *Pediatrics.* 2004;114:297-316. Reprinted with permission of the American Academy of Pediatrics.

Because colostrum has a laxative effect on the baby, early and frequent breastfeeding helps prevent jaundice by elimination of bilirubin from the gut. Additionally, frequent feedings help the mother establish milk production, thus increasing the baby's fluid intake and weight gain in the early weeks.

Water supplementation causes a baby to void, not stool, and therefore is not shown to reduce serum bilirubin levels (MacDonald et al., 2005). If the baby is not breastfeeding well or if the mother has a delayed onset of mature milk, she can pump and supplement with her expressed milk. If she is initially unable to obtain adequate amounts from milk expression, she needs to supplement with donor milk or artificial baby milk.

Phototherapy

When bilirubin approaches a level that requires more aggressive treatment, the baby may be placed under a special fluorescent light, called a bili-light, for phototherapy. A bili-light works in the same way as sunlight to break down bilirubin, forming products that are colorless and able to be excreted without conjugation. A full-term newborn with bilirubin levels reaching 20 mg/dL is a candidate for phototherapy; treatment often is begun when the level exceeds 15 mg/dL. The bilirubin levels at which the

AAP (2004) recommends phototherapy based on the baby's age are:

- 25 to 48 hours of life: 15 mg/dL or above
- 49 to 72 hours of life: 18 mg/dL or above
- Greater than 72 hours of life: 20 mg/dL or above

Keeping informed of current recommendations enables you to help mothers persevere in breastfeeding through the temporary challenges jaundice presents. In the past parents and caregivers frequently placed babies near a sunny window, because bilirubin breaks down when exposed to sunlight or its equivalent. The AAP (2004) does not recommend the use of sunlight as a reliable therapeutic tool because of concerns about sun exposure for a newborn. If parents state they plan to use sunlight exposure, encourage them to ask their care provider for guidelines.

Types of Phototherapy   Maximum skin exposure is desirable for traditional phototherapy conducted in the hospital. The infant, with eyes covered to protect them from the light, is placed in an isolette to maintain body heat and usually remains under the bili-light continuously except for brief feeding periods (Figure 22.4). Some hospitals

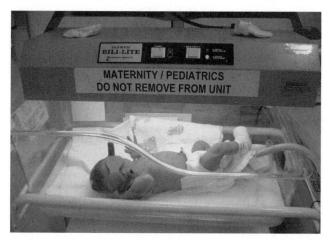

FIGURE 22.4   Baby receiving treatment under a bili-light.
Source: Printed with permission of Jeremy Kemp.

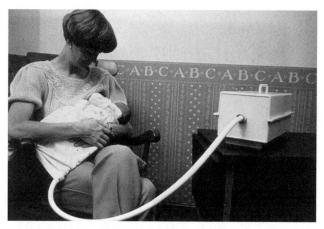

FIGURE 22.6   Fiber optic blanket for treating jaundice.
Source: © Medela, Inc., 2010.

encourage parents to touch their babies while they are under the lights to provide skin contact and additional opportunities for bonding.

Phototherapy can cause the baby to have sluggish responses and a noticeably weak sucking reflex. More frequent and shorter feedings, as well as supplemental expressed breastmilk, can improve the baby's feeding behavior. However, because these symptoms may also be a sign of something more serious, encourage the mother to observe her baby's feeding behavior during treatment, at the breast and with supplementation, so that she can report any changes to the healthcare team.

Traditional phototherapy using overhead bili-lights increases separation of mothers and infants and thus may have a negative impact on breastfeeding. Newer phototherapy options include the use of a bili-bed (Figure 22.5) and a bili-blanket or fiberoptic blanket (Figure 22.6), both of which can be placed in the mother's room. A bili-bed provides light underneath the baby, so he is able to lie in an open bed. No eye patches are needed, and parents can hold their baby's hand, stroke his body, and gaze into his eyes.

Home phototherapy using a fiberoptic blanket provides similar advantages to the bili-bed for the treatment

of jaundice in the full-term newborn. Parents can hold their baby, and the mother can even nurse him during treatment. A receiving blanket placed over the bili-blanket keeps the baby warm. Eye patches are unnecessary, and treatment can take place at home with the family's support system around them. Compliance with home phototherapy may be a problem for some families, as is ongoing follow-up after discharge.

While home phototherapy is an option for some parents with private insurance or the ability to self-pay, it may not be possible for low-income families. Medicaid in the United States, for example, does not provide home health coverage for this type of medical equipment. Home phototherapy options vary in Canada as well (Goulet et al., 2007). When counseling parents who face a possible extended hospital stay for their newborn due to normal physiologic jaundice, you can suggest they explore the option of home phototherapy with the baby's caregiver, if appropriate. Familiarize yourself with the availability of home phototherapy in your community and confirm which equipment is available in your area before suggesting it to families. It is helpful to point out the options of these therapies to parents, who may be overwhelmed by their baby having jaundice and by the thought of their baby needing an extended hospital stay. Talk with your hospital's case manager about the types of community resources for home health care.

Exchange Transfusion

A baby whose bilirubin levels fail to drop after phototherapy may require a blood exchange transfusion. The AAP (2004) recommends this serious step for babies whose bilirubin counts reach the levels indicated in Figure 22.3. Babies with dangerously high levels receive a combination of exchange transfusion and intensive phototherapy. Fortunately, babies rarely need blood exchange

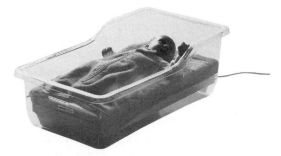

FIGURE 22.5   Bili-bed for treating jaundice.
Source: © Medela, Inc., 2010.

transfusions. They were done more commonly in the 1940s and 1950s before the advent of RhoGAM, an immunoglobulin preparation that prevents Rh-negative mothers from making antibodies to their baby's Rh-positive blood.

Treatment of Jaundice in a Preterm Infant

Jaundice that is not truly physiologic occurs more frequently in preterm infants and may last for up to 3 or 4 weeks. The preterm infant's digestive system takes longer to mature to the point at which it can detoxify and eliminate bilirubin. In addition, the infant's brain is especially sensitive to bilirubin, and levels that are permissible in the preterm infant relate inversely to the degree of prematurity.

Experience with preterm infants demonstrates that neurological impairment can occur with physiologic jaundice, even at lower levels of bilirubin. Because other factors may be causing the rise in bilirubin levels, these babies may be put on intravenous (IV) fluids and receive nothing by mouth while tests are run. If direct breastfeeding is suspended temporarily, the mother should pump to protect her milk production. Staff in the neonatal intensive care unit (NICU) can help her with collection and storage guidelines. As discussed in Chapter 23 about late preterm infants, the mother may need to express milk in addition to direct breastfeeding.

There is a strong correlation between lower gestational age and risk for hyperbilirubinemia. The AAP (2004) recognizes that even though newborns of 37 weeks' gestation and above are considered to be at term, they may not nurse as well as more mature infants. Babies born at 37 weeks' gestation are much more likely to develop a serum bilirubin level of 13 mg/dl or higher than are those born at 40 weeks' gestation. Practitioners are urged not to treat late preterm newborns as term newborns in the management of hyperbilirubinemia. Infants of 35 to 37 weeks' gestation have significantly lower birth weights, significantly higher serum total bilirubin levels on days 5 and 7, and are 2.4 times more likely to develop significant hyperbilirubinemia than are those of 38 to 42 weeks' gestation (Sarici et al., 2004).

Parental Concerns About Jaundice

A lactation consultant involved in prenatal education is in a key position to educate parents about birthing practices that have an impact on breastfeeding. Because newborn jaundice occurs so frequently, it is helpful for all expectant parents to learn about this condition. Anticipatory teaching during pregnancy helps their understanding if their baby develops jaundice. Let parents know that jaundice is a common newborn condition that can be evaluated and treated with great success. Reinforce information for parents after their baby is born to help them integrate the facts. Encourage them to focus on ways they can ensure contin-

ued close contact with their baby in the event their baby experiences significant jaundice and requires treatment.

Optimal Birth Practices

When parents learn about the factors associated with jaundice, they can take action to minimize its occurrence. This includes avoiding unnecessary drugs during pregnancy and choosing a birthing environment that promotes early, uninterrupted breastfeeding. Delivering their baby at home or in a birthing center reduces unnecessary interventions. If the mother chooses a hospital birth, she can seek her doctor's support to nurse her baby immediately after birth and very frequently in the early days postpartum.

A woman who goes into labor on her own reduces the amount of IV fluids she receives. Women have the right to refuse an elective induction performed solely for convenience and without medical need. Choosing a care provider who does not require routine IV administration helps avoid the edema associated with a delay in stage II lactogenesis that can also affect a baby's ability to latch (Nommsen-Rivers et al., 2009). Refusal of elective induction for nonmedical need may also lower her risk for a cesarean section, which is implicated in delayed onset of milk production and even more IV fluids (Smith, 2010). Minimizing the types and amounts of medications taken during labor and delivery (which pass through to the baby), reduces the incidence of depressing the baby's central nervous system and ability to suck effectively (Smith, 2008).

Concerns About Their Baby

Parents can reduce emotional stress by arranging to be with their jaundiced baby whenever possible. They can request treatment at the mother's bedside with intervals of interaction for holding, gazing, and breastfeeding. If the baby must remain hospitalized after the mother's discharge, the mother can request to stay with her baby in the room. If the baby is readmitted to the hospital, parents can ask whether rooming-in is available; this may be dictated by the size of the hospital and the type of facility. Family-centered care may be more possible at a children's hospital. Insurance coverage may determine where the baby is treated which could limit the parents' options.

To eliminate separation from their infant, parents can explore home phototherapy rather than an extended hospital stay if it is appropriate and economically feasible. Encourage them to stay well informed of their baby's condition and treatment and to discuss concerns with their baby's caregiver. You can reassure parents that the long-range outcome for babies who experience jaundice is excellent. Breastfeeding is the most important thing they can do for their baby during treatment. If breastfeeding is interrupted, you can assist the mother with pumping and help her return to exclusive breastfeeding after treatment has ended (see Chapter 21 for more information on pumping).

Vulnerable Child Syndrome

Researchers have found a high incidence of vulnerable child syndrome after treatment for newborn jaundice (Kemper et al., 1989). Vulnerable child syndrome is a psychological condition parents experience—identified by Green and Solnit (1964)—usually following their child's serious illness, hospitalization (including for prematurity), or survival of a life-threatening event (Nelson, 2007). The parent sees the affected child as being vulnerable to illness and becomes hypervigilant. Despite no differences in infant health problems, parents of babies that experienced jaundice requiring treatment were more likely to judge the health problems as serious and to take the baby to the emergency room (Kemper et al., 1990).

Anticipatory guidance given prenatally can empower parents to be proactive, prudent, and effective advocates in caring for their baby. Maternal anxiety level at discharge predicts later incidence of vulnerability perception (Allen et al., 2004). Asking for the parents' input and providing reassurance through the treatment period will help the mother maintain lactation and encourage her to look ahead to resolution. Treatment for nonpathologic jaundice is typically brief—only a day or two. Attentive, collaborative care may reduce the parents' feelings of powerlessness or victimization. This in turn may help to reduce the incidence of perceiving their child as unusually vulnerable or fragile (Kokotos & Adam, 2009).

Working with the Baby's Doctor

Parents of a jaundiced baby can work with their baby's doctor to develop a care plan that allows them easy access for frequent feedings. Understanding the cause and treatment of their baby's jaundice will help them recognize that it will most likely resolve within a few days or weeks. They can remain in close communication with the doctor to learn which screening tool will be used for detecting bilirubin levels, the results of the tests, and any further testing that will be needed.

Parents can ask when the jaundice is expected to clear and the type of treatment their baby will receive. They can discuss options and criteria for home phototherapy and express their desire for a treatment plan that allows their baby to breastfeed during the procedure (e.g., a bili-blanket or wallaby wrap). If the baby will receive treatment under a bili-light, they can clarify how often the mother may breastfeed and how frequently the parents can hold their baby. If breastfeeding is interrupted, they can ask the rationale for the decision and the criteria for when breastfeeding can resume. Table 22.1 provides further suggestions for counseling parents of a jaundiced baby.

TABLE 22.1   Counseling the Parents of a Jaundiced Baby

Parents' Concern	Suggestions
Parents feel bewildered by procedures and other aspects of baby care	• Discuss questions with the baby's physician and other caregivers. Research available information.
Separation of mother and baby	• Arrange for bedside treatment of baby, if possible, using portable bili-blanket or bili-bed. • Arrange for regular intervals of interaction for eye and skin contact.
Treatment is interfering with breastfeeding	• Arrange for fiberoptic blanket or bili-bed phototherapy. • Arrange for regular contact with baby and frequent feedings. • Use relaxation techniques to promote letdown. • Arrange for uninterrupted feedings.
Baby has sluggish responses and a weak sucking reflex	• Begin more frequent feedings. Use breast compression while nursing to encourage sucking. • Use a tube-feeding device. • Use cup, spoon, or syringe feedings if latch is poor.
Physician is considering interruption in breastfeeding	• Ask for recheck of bilirubin level after baby is breastfed or supplemented with mother's milk. • Ask for frequent checks of the baby's bilirubin level.
Breastfeeding must be interrupted	• Begin expressing milk as soon as possible to establish and maintain milk production.
Prevention of jaundice	• Avoid exposure to chemicals during pregnancy. • Avoid jaundice-producing drugs during labor and delivery. • Nurse within 1 hour after birth and frequently thereafter.

~ Delayed Onset of Breastfeeding

At times, circumstances do not permit a new mother to begin breastfeeding immediately after her baby's birth. A short-term delay can occur lasting from a few hours to a couple of days if the baby is born with a low body temperature, aspirates meconium at birth, receives low Apgar scores, or exhibits symptoms of infection. Such conditions may necessitate that the baby and mother be separated until the condition is stabilized.

In the case of possible infection, some hospitals isolate the mother and baby together to avoid a separation. Prematurity, respiratory distress syndrome, and other birth complications can require several weeks or months of hospitalization. Although breastfeeding can most likely begin at some point during the hospitalization, it may not be possible in the early days.

Babies who are born with health problems need their mother's milk to aid in their recovery. The importance of receiving human milk has led healthcare providers around the world to encourage mothers to express milk for their compromised babies or to nurse them (Dougherty & Luther, 2008; Nye, 2008; Isaacson, 2006). Some women who intend to breastfeed give up their plan when they are separated from their infant or when breastfeeding is delayed for another reason. Caregivers involved with these mothers and babies can reassure them that a temporary delay does not preclude breastfeeding. Women who understand that breastfeeding is still possible need a great deal of encouragement, support, and information on how to establish and maintain milk production until they can breastfeed.

Expressing Milk to Maintain Lactation

When a delay occurs in breastfeeding, it is important that the mother begin milk expression as soon as possible and that she continue to express milk on a regular basis to establish and maintain milk production. Even if the baby's prognosis is poor, the mother can be comforted knowing that she is providing milk for her baby. If the baby is not yet able to receive breastmilk, expressing her milk provides the mother the opportunity to be involved in a parenting role.

Suggest to the mother that she express her milk at least 8 to 10 times every 24 hours, including at least once at night when prolactin levels are highest. If she drinks fluids before bedtime, she is likely to wake during the night to urinate and can take advantage of this night waking by expressing milk. If her baby remains hospitalized after her discharge and she is unable to room-in or stay nearby, she will need to travel to and from the hospital to visit her baby. A routine of expressing milk and trying to recover physically from childbirth can add to the mother's anxiety and exhaustion. Sleep and rest will be at a premium for her during this time. She may have other children at home who need her and, depending on the length of her baby's hospitalization, she may be required to return to work or school before her baby is discharged.

Establishing letdown may be difficult for a mother who is worried about her sick baby and must turn to a breast pump in place of her baby for establishing and maintaining milk production. She can tape a picture of her baby to the breast pump and play a recording of her baby's sounds while she is expressing. She may also find that expressing her milk is more successful when she is at the hospital near her baby.

The type of breast pump the mother uses will influence her milk production. High quality, hospital-grade, electric double pumps usually provide the best yield. Some mothers find that their milk production decreases over time (de Aquino & Osório, 2009), while others produce more milk than their baby needs. Mothers may find that their milk production corresponds to the baby's condition, decreasing when the baby's condition worsens. You can reassure a mother that stimulating the production of prolactin receptor cells in the breasts will help her milk production rebound after the baby begins nursing.

It may be useful to combine the use of an electric pump, hand pump and manual expression. An electric pump, which requires less effort on the mother's part and is convenient for maintaining milk production on a long-term basis, can be rented one for use at home. Public assistance programs such as Women, Infants, and Children (WIC) in the United States may provide hospital-grade pumps for mothers in these situations. Some hospitals also have grant programs that loan hospital-grade pumps for a small deposit. A hand pump is useful when the mother's electric pump is inaccessible. Many women express milk manually or with a hand pump and do not use an electric pump. Knowing how to hand express ensures that the mother is not reliant on a pump in case one is not available at a particular time. Hand expression several times a day before pumping has been shown to increase milk production significantly (Morton et al., 2009). See Chapter 21 for guidelines on storing and transporting expressed milk for a hospitalized baby.

Transition to Breastfeeding

When her baby is ready to begin nursing, the mother may need help in making a smooth transition from milk expression to breastfeeding. Ideally, the first breastfeeding takes place in the hospital as the baby's condition improves. If the mother returns to the hospital for feedings, NICU staff can provide her with a place to nurse her baby and assist her with feedings. For some babies, the first feeding may not occur until after the baby is home.

The mother may find her baby's first feeding at the breast to be stressful, feeling unsure of how to breastfeed and doubting the adequacy of her milk production. Her baby may be confused about how to suck at the breast and may have a poor sucking reflex, or may initially appear to be disinterested in breastfeeding. The mother may need to increase her milk production and adjust to the difference between the pump and her baby's sucking pattern. These are all issues she can work through with varying degrees of success, depending on her baby's condition. If prematurity caused the delay in breastfeeding, the outcome for transitioning to direct breastfeeding as her baby matures can be very positive. She will benefit from your support and advice until the transition is complete.

A mother who is unable to nurse every 2 or 3 hours will need to continue expressing milk to maintain production. If she is nursing frequently and her baby is not transferring milk adequately, she may need to supplement with her expressed milk or infant formula until milk transfer improves. It may take several days or even months to reach the goal of exclusive breastfeeding. Encourage the mother to concentrate on enjoying her baby and to take things one day at a time. The following guidelines may help the mother make the transition from expressing to breastfeeding.

Conditioning the Baby to Breastfeed

- Express milk onto a breast pad and place it near the baby.
- Place a picture of the mother in the baby's view.
- Provide frequent skin-to-skin contact.
- Conduct practice sessions at the breast.
- Shape and hold the breast for the baby with the Dancer hand position.
- Express milk into the baby's mouth.
- Consider use of a nipple shield, especially for babies who have been bottle feeding.
- Use a tube-feeding device for feedings.

Mothers Who Return to Bottle Feeding

Because of the health importance of human milk, caregivers strongly urge mothers to breastfeed their ill or preterm babies (Groh-Wargo & Sapsford, 2009; Sisk et al., 2006; Sweet, 2008). Some of these mothers may not have planned to breastfeed and prefer to provide their milk through expressing or nursing only as long as it is medically necessary. When the baby is out of danger, these women typically switch to formula. Even short-term breastfeeding can foster an intimate bond between a mother and baby. Remember that your role is to support the mother in her choices, which includes guiding her through weaning when it is her wish.

∼ Relactation

Relactation is defined as reestablishing milk production in a mother who has greatly reduced milk production (de Aquino & Osório, 2009) or who has stopped breastfeeding (Ogunlesi, 2008). It may follow untimely weaning or separation of the mother and baby, as with a low-birthweight infant or hospitalization of the mother or baby.

Healthcare practitioners are urged to consider recommending relactation when mothers wean prematurely and are willing to reconsider nursing their baby. Because of the emotional and physical demands of relactation, approach the topic sensitively and tactfully. The mother may not know that it is possible to relactate. If her baby is in the NICU or readmitted to the hospital for illness, you can make her aware of this option and give her more information if she seems interested.

Banapurmath et al. (2003) evaluated whether mothers with babies less than 6 weeks old can initiate or establish lactation. Mothers who had either stopped breastfeeding or were not able to initiate breastfeeding received help with establishing lactation at an outpatient clinic. Within 10 days 91.6 percent of mothers established lactation, with 83.4 percent achieving complete lactation. The study concluded that it is possible to help most mothers with lactation difficulties when the baby is less than 6 weeks old.

Reason for Relactating

When discussing relactation with a mother, it is important to explore the reasons she did not initially begin or continue with breastfeeding. A baby's allergic reaction to artificial baby milk is one of the most common motives for relactation. The mother may have weaned due to misinformation and regrets the decision. She may be in the bargaining stage of grief over forced weaning. Her milk production may have down-regulated or was never established. Her baby may have rejected the breast or sucked poorly and she was unable to establish breastfeeding. Her interest in relactation may result from family pressure or guilt. Perhaps she wants to use breastfeeding as a factor in her favor for a divorce or custody dispute. Understanding her motivation without judgment will enable you to find the best counseling approach.

One study on relactation reported that healthy babies were weaned due to time demands or mothers' perceptions of health problems. The primary reason for relactating was the child's negative reaction to weaning (e.g., incessant crying or refusal to eat). Nineteen mothers were able to relactate between less than 1 day and 3 months postpartum (Marquis et al., 1998).

Relactating to feed abandoned and orphaned infants or when a mother is too sick to nurse is an age-old tradition in most cultures, especially in African countries, and is usually done by grandmothers (Ogunlesi, 2008). Promoting relactation by healthy, non-HIV/AIDS grandmothers could help provide a partial solution to the overwhelmingly difficult feeding options for babies whose mothers are HIV/AIDS positive. A study in Burkina Faso found that 74 percent of women would accept breastfeeding by a wet nurse if they themselves were HIV/AIDS positive. In addition, 70 percent would be willing to be a wet nurse for an infant born to an HIV-infected woman (Nacro et al., 2009).

Realistic Expectations

Understanding the reason for a mother discontinuing or failing to initiate breastfeeding, as well as her reason for wanting to relactate, will help you assist her in achieving her goals. A mother who is highly motivated and enthusiastic about relactation is likely to have a higher degree of success. On the other hand, a woman whose decision to relactate is at another person's urging may lack the motivation to persevere.

The mother's motivation to relactate needs to be tempered by realistic expectations. Explore how the mother defines successful relactation and how she will react if her milk production does not meet the full needs of her baby or if she is unable to relactate at all. You can help her assess her expectations honestly and provide a realistic and supportive picture that invites her thoughtfulness and aids in her decision.

A mother who wishes to relactate needs a clear understanding of the steps required for achieving her goal. Encourage her to determine her sources of support and how those in her immediate household feel about the process. A mother who experiences opposition to her plans to relactate will need to consider how to proceed despite the lack of support. You can help her identify people in her life who support her efforts, such as a peer counselor, WIC nutritionist, or even a friend. After you determine that the mother is motivated to carry through with relactation, you can address issues of milk production and ways to help the baby breastfeed directly.

Process of Relactation

Estrogen concentrations fall rapidly immediately after birth, and prolactin levels drop to normal by about 3 weeks in a woman who is not breastfeeding (Lawrence & Lawrence, 2005). The degree of postpartum breast involution is a factor in successful relactation. The amount of time that elapsed since weaning or since the baby's birth is also a factor, with the least time being best. Effective breast emptying within the first few weeks postpartum is associated with the proliferation of prolactin receptors in the mammary cells (Hill et al., 2009). The window of opportunity for prolactin receptor proliferation is narrow (Peaker & Wilde, 1996; Wilde & Hurley, 1996). Therefore, a mother may not have triggered enough receptor cells before involution set in if she did not breastfeed beginning at birth. On the other hand, if she initiated breastfeeding well and had lactation interrupted by poor advice or a temporary medical condition, she may have a sufficient number of prolactin receptors.

Another factor in relactation success is the amount of breast stimulation the mother receives, which depends on the baby's willingness to suck at the breast. The baby's frequent sucking is by far the most efficient way to increase milk production. If the baby will take the breast, sucking along with the use of a tube-feeding device at the breast provides stimulation for the mother's breasts and nourishment for the baby simultaneously. During a breastfeeding, switch nursing and breast massage help increase milk flow. With switch nursing the mother alternates between both breasts several times during a feeding.

Frequent and continuous skin-to-skin contact in a relaxed, unpressured atmosphere may entice the baby to latch. A baby that is drowsy or in a light sleep state may be encouraged to latch with skin-to-skin contact and some expressed milk or formula on the end of the mother's nipple. If the baby is unable to suck, the mother can initiate pumping using a double electric breast pump, matching the frequency to her baby's feeding pattern. The baby may become more interested in sucking when milk is available, so breast massage can also help. Expressing milk between feedings provides further stimulation to increase milk production.

Adjusting her lifestyle will help the mother accommodate the relactation process, and practical ways to simplify her life can optimize her efforts. Encourage her to rest as much as possible, to eat nutritiously and to accept offers from family and friends to perform errands, care for other children, and prepare meals. A young teen or retired neighbor may be willing to help her for part of the day. Her faith community such as her church or synagogue may have volunteers to help new mothers as well. If she can afford it, and it is available, a doula service can help with household routines. The mother may also want to examine possible milk-reducing substances in her life, such as oral contraceptives, nicotine, or herbs like peppermint and sage (Humphrey, 2003). Make sure the mother knows that alcohol is *not* a galactogogue and can inhibit milk yield (Mennella & Pepino, 2008; Mennella et al., 2005). See the discussion of galactogogues in Chapter 18.

The mother needs to supplement with donor milk or infant formula until she is confident that her milk production is established at a level that will serve as her baby's sole form of nourishment. As milk production increases, the amount of supplement her baby receives can be reduced accordingly. The mother must work closely with her baby's caregiver to make sure that she decreases the supplement in relation to her milk production and that she monitors her baby's weight closely as the supplement decreases.

Increasing the Mother's Success

A mother's feeling of success with relactation depends in large part on her expectations. Encourage her to view breastfeeding as a means of nurturing her baby and not just a feeding method. Help her measure success in terms of bonding with her baby rather than the amount of milk she produces or the length of time she nurses. Many mothers who relactate benefit from the support provided by groups such as breastfeeding after breast surgery (www.bfar.org) and adoptive breastfeeding groups.

The mother's success with relactation is influenced by the amount of time that has passed since the baby was at the breast, as well as the feeding method used since that time. It is also important to explore the mother's previous breastfeeding routine to identify the need for possible adjustments. Confirm that she understands basic breastfeeding practices and biologically normal infant behaviors, especially in the areas of touch, feeding, and sleep.

Re-creating the birth experience has helped some mothers with relactation (Shinskie, 1998; Harris, 1994). Rebirthing, or remedial cobathing, simulates the birth experience with the baby and mother spending gentle, calming time together in warm bath water. After some time the mother reclines, places the baby on her abdomen, and allows her baby to crawl unassisted to the breast, root, and latch. Cobathing is calming for both mother and baby and may help the baby latch and breastfeed directly. This technique is similar to the self-attachment process used in biological nurturing (Colson et al., 2008). See Chapters 15 and 16 for more suggestions on encouraging the baby to nurse and increasing milk production.

∾ *Nursing an Adopted Baby*

Nursing an adopted baby can provide emotional satisfaction for both mother and infant as long as the mother has realistic motives and expectations. A woman who had a previous pregnancy is technically considered to be relactating for the adopted baby, even if she never gave birth or breastfed a biological child. A woman who has never been pregnant and is attempting to produce milk is considered to be inducing lactation. Induced lactation differs from relactation because the woman has experienced none of the mammary changes associated with pregnancy.

Healthcare providers, adoptive case workers, and social services managers have become much more aware of and supportive of adoptive nursing in recent years (Adoption.com, 2009; Bryant, 2006; AAP, 2005; American Academy of Family Physicians, 2001). You can respond to a receptive mother well before her baby arrives with timely resources such as the adoptive breastfeeding website (www.fourfriends.com/abrw), blogs, and books about nursing adopted babies.

This mother requires unique and personalized care (Wittig & Spatz, 2008). It is time consuming to induce lactation in the absence of a pregnancy. Without the estrogen concentrations of pregnancy that prepare a woman's breasts for lactation, prolactin may not have a sufficiently potent stimulative effect on milk secretion. If the mother's inability to conceive resulted from a hormonal imbalance, that same imbalance could affect her chances of inducing lactation (West & Marasco, 2008).

It is common for adopted children to seemingly reject breastfeeding and their mothers initially (Gribble, 2006). Such rejection can be devastating to the mother, especially if she struggled with infertility in trying to become pregnant. Understandably, some women may take the rejection personally to the extent that they withdraw nurturing. You can assist mothers in locating networks to support them in sensitive parenting and breastfeeding. The baby's willingness to nurse may improve over time.

A mother may or may not be able to nourish her adopted baby entirely on her milk alone. If she begins breastfeeding with this goal in mind, she may believe that her attempts are unsuccessful and disappointing. If her motive is to have an emotionally gratifying experience for herself and her baby and an opportunity to develop a warm and loving bond with her baby, she will find greater satisfaction in her nursing experience.

Supplements to Assist Induced Lactation

Some adoptive mothers initiate hormonal regimens to mimic the hormones of pregnancy. The Newman-Goldfarb protocols use combination oral contraceptives for a period of time, followed by medications such as domperidone to raise prolactin levels (Hormann, 2007). Pumping is also initiated (Newman & Goldfarb, 2002). Although no peer-reviewed journal study has been published, over 2,000 women reportedly have used the protocols to induce lactation (Newman & Goldfarb, 2008).

Over the years different medications have been used to initiate lactation. Some of these, including antipsychotic medications, are no longer commonly used. In one study of women who received estrogen and either metoclopramide or chlorpromazine to begin milk production, along with frequent sucking (Kramer, 1995), those who had breastfed previously did not require estrogen. A mother in another study initiated full milk production by the time her adopted baby was 4 months old (Cheales-Siebenaler, 1999). Older studies report varying degrees of success in inducing lactation (Auerbach & Sutherland, 1985; Auerbach & Avery, 1981; Kleinman et al., 1980).

Process of Inducing Lactation

The relactation techniques discussed earlier also apply to the process of inducing lactation for adoptive mothers. An adoptive mother can use all the same measures as biological mothers for nipple preparation. These measures include avoiding drying agents such as harsh soaps and checking for inverted nipples. Breast massage and back rubs help increase blood circulation to and within the breast, as nerves in the breast radiate from the area between the shoulder blades. The mother will benefit from massaging her breasts from 5 to 8 times daily over a period of 3 to 6 months.

An adoptive mother may benefit from attending a support group for breastfeeding or adoptive nursing women while she waits for her baby's placement. Often, parents receive only a few days' warning before they receive their baby, with little time for preparation. On the other hand, if the mother knows when the baby's birth is expected, she can begin pumping to stimulate milk production up to 1 month before placement, pumping several times a day for 10-minute sessions. By the time placement occurs, she should be pumping every 2 to 3 hours throughout the day. A hospital-grade electric breast pump with a double setup provides the most effective nipple stimulation. It may be some time before she sees any results from her pumping, and she can be encouraged by even the smallest amount of milk she produces.

Many adoption agencies cooperate with the adoptive parents' plans to breastfeed and may arrange to have the baby fed with an alternate feeding method to minimize nipple preference. They may also provide for breastfeeding sessions if placement does not occur soon after birth.

The length of time it takes for a woman's milk to appear and the amount of milk produced vary with each mother and baby. Regular milk removal is necessary for continued milk production (Czank et al., 2007; Hill et al., 2009). The baby's sucking provides the best stimulation for establishing lactation, so the amount of milk produced will increase more rapidly after the baby begins sucking at the breast. The baby's age is also a factor, with babies younger than 3 months being more likely to suck when placed at the breast. Hand expression before pumping or directly breastfeeding may help increase milk production (Morton et al., 2009). In fact, one Australian study showed that milk output nearly doubled when the mother massaged and expressed milk before and after feedings (Nursing Mothers' Association of Australia, 1985). Having the baby sleep in bed with the mother to suck sleepily for comfort throughout the night may also enhance milk production.

Feeding the Baby

The mother's milk production may not be copious enough to sustain her baby's growth, and the quantity may increase much more slowly than that of a biological mother. In fact, in most cases adoptive mother's milk supply is not adequate for totally nourishing her baby. Anecdotally, adoptive mothers typically produce one-third to one-half of their infants' needs. The mother most likely will need to supplement her baby with donor human milk or an appropriate infant formula to ensure optimal nourishment. You can encourage her to focus on bonding, oral and jaw development, and visual coordination that come with breastfeeding rather than on the quantity of milk. She can provide the supplement through a tube-feeding device to reduce the amount of time she needs to spend feeding her baby. She also can save time and reduce anxiety by preparing an entire day's feeding equipment and donor milk or formula at one time.

When inducing lactation, the baby's health and well-being must always take priority. Caution the mother to proceed slowly with any decrease in supplement, ensuring that the decrease corresponds with the amount of milk her baby receives directly from the breast. Make sure she understands that she must decrease the supplement rather than diluting it. As a general guide, it is best to limit the decrease to no more than 25 mL per feeding, and to monitor the baby's growth and output for 4 to 7 days before decreasing it further.

A diary of supplemental feedings and nursing sessions—with attention to frequency, duration, and the baby's disposition—will help the mother monitor her baby's intake. Encourage frequent visits to the baby's caregiver for weight checks and the monitoring of other signs of growth. Sample pre- and post-feeding weights on an accurate digital scale, coupled with a daily weight check at the same time every day, helps the mother determine how much supplement, if any, her baby requires.

An adopted baby's nursing schedule is similar in frequency and duration to that of the baby of a biological mother. The age at which the baby begins solid foods and initiates weaning is also similar to biological babies. Because the adoptive mother usually does not produce enough milk for her baby's total nourishment, she will need extra support and encouragement. Adoptive breastfeeding support websites provide helpful suggestions, support, and e-mail lists (see www.fourfriends.com/abrw). You can help the mother educate caseworkers and other caregivers who are responsible for her baby's welfare, emphasizing the beneficial nature of the nurturing

TABLE 22.2 Counseling a Mother Who Is Relactating or Inducing Lactation

Mother's Concern	Suggestions for Mother
Inadequate letdown	• Use relaxation techniques.
Establishing milk production	• Begin nursing as early as possible. • Use regular supplements and decrease the amount as milk production increases. • Use breast massage. • Breastfeed frequently. • Get sufficient rest. • Eat a nutritious diet. • Keep a diary of breastfeedings and formula feedings.
Baby is reluctant to nurse	• Use soothing techniques and increase skin-to-skin contact. • Apply the mother's milk or a sweet substance to the nipple (not honey). • Slowly drop the mother's milk into the side of the baby's mouth before placing the baby on the breast. • Use a nursing supplementer.
Preparation for breastfeeding	• Massage the mother's back and breasts. • Stimulate the nipples manually. • Stimulate milk production by using a breast pump. • Avoid soap and other drying agents on the breasts.
Low milk supply	• Supplement the baby with formula; do not dilute. • View breastfeeding primarily as a means of nurturing the baby's emotional health. • Have the baby checked frequently for weight gain. • Monitor the baby's weight while replacing formula with breastfeeding.
Nipple preference in the baby	• Use a nursing supplementer, cup, spoon, or dropper.
Mother is frustrated with partial breastfeeding	• Simplify bottle preparation techniques or use a nursing supplementer. • Learn to appreciate breastfeeding as a nurturing relationship with the baby.

relationship between her and her baby. Table 22.2 provides suggestions for counseling a mother who is attempting to relactate or induce lactation.

~ Breastfeeding During Disasters

Disasters focus global attention on feeding babies as safely as possible when emergencies strike. From the 2004 Indonesian tsunami, to the 2005 Hurricane Katrina in the United States, and the 2010 earthquake in Haiti, the plight of society's most vulnerable population—infants and young children—captured worldwide interest. As described in the 2009 World Breastfeeding Week theme, breastfeeding plays a vital role in emergency response worldwide (Figure 22.7). World Breastfeeding Week is cel-

ebrated by over 120 countries to encourage breastfeeding and improve the health of babies around the world (UNICEF, 2009). The 2009 initiative urged communities to inform mothers, breastfeeding advocates, communities, health professionals, governments, aid agencies, donors, and the media about how they can actively support breastfeeding before and during an emergency.

Many organizations and governments have put emergency feeding guidelines into place to help mothers continue breastfeeding and to relactate. Because the use of artificial infant milk carries a much higher risk for illness and death, cross-nursing by non–HIV-positive women is also appropriate in emergency situations. Infant feeding recommendations in emergencies are shown in Table 22.3.

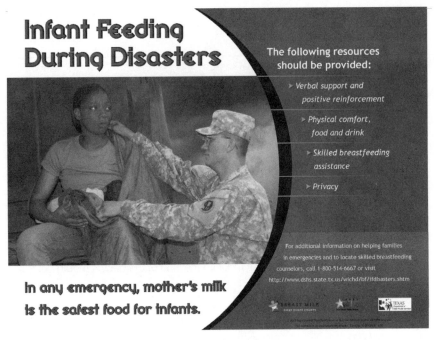

FIGURE 22.7 Breastfeeding support during a disaster.

Source: © Texas Department of State Health Services.

TABLE 22.3 Guide for Action on Infant and Young Child Feeding in Emergencies (IFE)

	Emergency Preparedness	On the Ground	Support from Afar
Government/national policy makers	• Develop/strengthen national infant and young child feeding policy and emergency preparedness plans/policies to include IFE. • Enact strong national *Code* legislation. • Translate key resources. • Orient and train key staff on IFE. • Coordinate/link to networks of expertise. Make plans to prevent and handle donations of BMS, bottles, and teats in emergencies. • Give the media clear guidelines on IFE. • Include breastfeeding promotion, protection, and support in emergencies for the general public.	• Ensure that basic support for breast-feeding mothers is integrated across all sectors of emergency response. • Prevent/handle donations of BMS, bottles, and teats. • Monitor and report *Code* violations.	• Watch out for appeals for donations of BMS, bottles, and teats, and act to stop them.
National breastfeeding advocates/counselors/trainers	• Undertake orientation and further training on infant feeding in emergencies. • Identify and network with agencies, local emergency committees, and communities, involved in emergency response. • Organize a seminar on 'helping mothers and babies in emergencies' for emergency workers. • Create a network of experienced staff available for training and/or deployment in emergencies. • Organize, with government and NGO allies, a press conference or media event on IFE. • Update your website with key links to resources.	• Get involved in early protection and support of breastfeeding. For example: training community counselors and emergency relief staff, individual counseling, mother to mother support, phone line support. • Adapt materials and key messages to the context of the emergency.	• Identify agencies that support breastfeeding in emergencies and offer them your help. • Respond to negative stories and/or appeals for donations in the media.

(Continued)

TABLE 22.3 Guide for Action on Infant and Young Child Feeding in Emergencies (IFE) (*Continued*)

	Emergency Preparedness	On the Ground	Support from Afar
Aid agencies/NGO and UN staff	• Integrate Operational Guidance on IFE into agency guidance and policies. • Orientate all emergency response staff on IFE. • Identify networks of expertise, e.g. breastfeeding counseling, in countries/regions of operation. • Enroll health/nutrition staff in IFE training. • Communicate a clear plan to all staff on preventing/handling donations of BMS, bottles and teats. • Lobby the government and donors to include breastfeeding support in emergency action plans.	• Integrate IFE into minimum response across sectors—nutrition, health, shelter, protection, etc. • Implement skilled programs to protect support and promote breastfeeding. • Act to prevent/handle donations of BMS, bottles and teats.	• Support "on the ground" staff by not soliciting or accepting donations of BMS. • Support fund raising and send money instead of BMS.
Health professionals	• Increase your breastfeeding support skills and follow a breastfeeding counseling training course, or at minimum, an IFE training course for health/nutrition workers in emergencies. • Implement the BFI (in hospitals and in community health services). • Advocate for updated training on Breastfeeding Counseling and HIV and Infant Feeding Counseling at national /local level. • Gather information on what support is available for breastfeeding at national /local level (lactation consultants, peer counselors, mother to mother support groups). • Organize training/a seminar for colleagues on IFE.	• Ensure that mothers and their children are kept together. • Implement the 10 Steps to Successful Breastfeeding in appropriate reproductive, maternal newborn and child health programs in emergencies. • Ensure that skilled breastfeeding and infant feeding support is available for mothers antenatally, at delivery, and postnatally for 2 years. • Ensure that skilled childbirth attendance is available for pregnant women. • Ensure that breastfeeding is fully supported for HIV-infected mothers unless AFASS conditions for replacement feeding are all in place.	• Be vigilant for local appeals of donations of infant formula, other BMS, and bottles/teats to emergencies, and act to stop them.
Mothers/caregivers	• Exclusively breastfeed your baby until s/he is 6 months of age. • Continue to breastfeed your baby to 2 years or beyond. • Encourage your local mother support group(s) to discuss emergency preparedness. For example, plan ways that the group could staff a safe place for mothers and provide mother-to-mother support to breastfeeding if large numbers of people are made homeless. • Make contact with local emergency authorities and community groups and tell them about IFE.	• Offer support to other mothers who are having difficulties or to mothers of newborns in an emergency. • Consider wet nursing if needs are identified, e.g. orphans, very ill mothers. • Help organise safe places for mothers with mother-to-mother support for breastfeeding.	• Identify agencies that support breastfeeding in emergencies and fundraise for them.

Note: AFASS: Acceptable, feasible, affordable, sustainable and safe. BMS: Breastmilk substitute. NGO: Non-governmental organization.

Source: World Alliance for Breastfeeding Action (WABA). Breastfeeding–a vital emergency response: are you ready? 2009. http://worldbreastfeedingweek.org/images/english_2009actionfolder.pdf. Accessed December 3, 2009. Reprinted by permission.

You can work with your local community's emergency responders and healthcare facilities to raise awareness that in a disaster, formula donations do more harm than good. After the 2004 Indian Ocean tsunami, formula donations resulted in immediate decreased rates of breastfeeding and higher rates of diarrhea and death among young children (UNICEF, 2009). During the Balkan civil war crisis in 1999, relief agencies were inundated with massive quantities of unsolicited infant feeding products, with 40 percent of 3,500 metric tons being infant food (Borrel et al., 2001). Any donated formula needs to be ready-to-feed, not powdered, and should be reserved for infants whose mothers are not present to lactate. Protecting and promoting breastfeeding equates to lives saved. Some countries experiencing disasters have shown the largest increases in breastfeeding rates (over 20 percent increase), including Madagascar, Sri Lanka, and Pakistan. Breastfeeding rates have also increased in Zambia, Mali, Ghana, and Benin (UNICEF, 2009).

ᨱ Baby Losing Interest in Breastfeeding

Some babies seem to appear disinterested in nursing as early as 3 or 4 months and most commonly around 7 months of age. The baby may appear happy to go to the breast and mouth the nipple but then acts disinterested or cries. This could happen suddenly, or the baby may gradually decrease the number of feedings. Most often, such disinterest in breastfeeding lasts only a few days to a week. However, some periods of nursing abstinence may continue for 3 or 4 weeks. The mother might become uncomfortable from overfull breasts or feel emotionally drained from trying to satisfy her baby. Encourage her to relax and be patient as she learns to manage the change in her breastfeeding pattern. She can maintain milk production by expressing her milk regularly and putting her baby to breast frequently without pressure to nurse.

This temporary phase of apparent disinterest in nursing is not a sign of weaning. Few infants self-wean before 1 year of age. In addition, toddlers are not fussy when they wean (Bengson, 2000; Bumgarner, 2000); they are simply ready to move on to their next stage of development. A baby in the throes of a nursing strike is unhappy, hungry and unable to settle to breastfeed. Reassure the mother that this phase will pass and that her baby will probably return to a regular nursing pattern within several days.

If a nursing strike persists for more than a few days, encourage the mother to contact her baby's caregiver. Babies sometimes refuse to nurse because they are in pain. Thrush, for example, is painful in adults (Clarkson et al., 2007), and it makes sense that it causes discomfort in babies as well. A baby who appears healthy could have an ear infection or other illness, even in the absence of a fever. During the time the baby is not breastfeeding, the mother will need to protect her milk production by pumping as frequently as her baby was nursing. She also needs to feed her baby by an alternate method until breastfeeding resumes.

Possible Causes of a Baby's Disinterest

It is sometimes difficult to pinpoint the cause of a baby discontinuing breastfeeding and you can help the mother understand her growing baby's changing needs. Many times disinterest in breastfeeding occurs during a particular developmental stage and subsides as the baby matures. The baby may simply be more efficient at nursing and obtains more milk in a shorter period. It may be that the baby is easily distracted by new objects and people, in which case the mother can either move away from the distraction or end the feeding and resume when the baby seems more interested. She can shift her position so the baby faces the activity while nursing and can let the baby play and nurse intermittently at the breast.

Extra evening or late night feedings may make up for missed daytime feedings. A baby who needs the mother's undivided attention while nursing may nurse better late at night when the house is quiet and the baby is too sleepy to be distracted. Retiring to a quiet darkened room for these brief periods of breastfeeding can help. The mother can make a point to not talk, read, work on her laptop, or watch television during feedings. Some babies may seem disinterested in breastfeeding if their parents manipulate their schedules in an attempt to encourage them to sleep through the night. These babies have difficulty knowing when they may breastfeed.

A baby who has an ear infection or a head cold with a stuffy nose will have difficulty nursing. Nursing in an upright position or with the side-sitting hold takes pressure off the baby's ears and facilitates nasal drainage. The mother can assist the baby by massaging her breasts and expressing milk before nursing to promote letdown. Performing breast compression during the feeding also helps her baby obtain milk more easily. Encourage the mother to consult her baby's caregiver about medications for decreasing her baby's mucus production or mechanical methods for removing mucus before nursing.

Teething pain can make sucking uncomfortable and cause the baby to nurse sporadically, fuss, and pull away from the breast. Comfort measures to ease gum pain, such as rubbing the gums with a cool washcloth or allowing the baby to bite on a cooled teether, usually renews an interest in nursing. If pain causes the baby to bite the mother when at the breast, the mother may unintentionally rebuff her baby with an overwhelming reaction and cause her baby to feel rejected. This could result in the baby associating nursing with the mother becoming upset because of the biting, thereby not wanting to risk trying it again.

Skin-to-skin contact between the mother and baby helps to reestablish trust. The mother can undress and take the baby to bed or into the bath with her, holding the baby close to her body with her breasts exposed and gently latching for a feeding if the baby seems receptive. Use of a baby sling also provides increased intimacy to build the baby's trust with the mother.

A baby may reject nursing because sucking needs are satisfied in another way, such as sucking on a thumb or other object. The mother can put her baby to breast whenever she observes this behavior. Sometimes receiving solid foods or supplemental bottles causes the baby to become less interested in breastfeeding. If the mother is giving her baby supplemental foods, she can review the quantity and frequency with her baby's caregiver to be sure she is not overfeeding him.

What the Mother Can Do

The mother can examine events in her life to determine if her own overexertion, tension, poor eating habits, or fatigue led to her baby's decreased feedings. She can pay close attention to caring for herself with adequate rest, nutrition, exercise, and stress reduction. During menstruation the taste of her milk and the scent of the secretions on her skin may change slightly, making feedings seem less familiar and therefore less desirable to the baby. In this situation the baby's interest in nursing will be renewed after the end of the menstrual cycle. The mother can discontinue any medication she might be taking that reduced milk production, such as pseudoephedrine or birth control pills. There may be the possibility that the mother is pregnant and the taste of her milk has changed or milk production is reduced.

The mother can express her milk regularly to maintain milk production and prevent engorgement until her baby nurses again. She also needs to work out an alternate method of feeding her baby, recognizing that use of a bottle and artificial nipple has the potential for nipple preference because of the difference between sucking at the breast and on a bottle nipple. Choosing an alternate feeding method such as cup feeding avoids this obstacle. Your objectivity can help the mother establish priorities and work toward resuming breastfeeding with her baby. Table 22.4 provides measures to encourage the baby to breastfeed.

TABLE 22.4 Encouraging a Baby to Breastfeed

Issue	Advice for the Mother
Baby	• Check for illness or teething pain and contact his caregiver if necessary. • Discontinue any use of pacifiers. • Take a warm bath with the baby, with dim lighting, such as candles. The tranquility will relax the mother, and often, the baby as well. Co-bathing works well for newborns that cannot latch, and it often is effective for older babies who resist nursing.
Mother	• Cleanse the breasts with clear water before feedings to remove deodorant, lotions, or other substances. • Discontinue the use of any new brand of deodorant or lotion. • Get plenty of rest, consume adequate protein and fresh vegetables, and drink sufficient fluids to promote a feeling of well-being. • Hand express or pump between feedings to maintain milk production. • Determine if she is pregnant or taking any new medications.
Managing feedings	• Nurse in a quiet, dark room without distractions. • When ready to go to bed for the night, take the baby to bed with her to nurse. • Attempt to nurse when the baby is almost asleep, or put him to breast when he first falls asleep. • Express a little milk onto the nipple or the baby's lips to encourage him to feed. • Feed the baby by an alternative method for a few minutes, and then put him to breast. • Feed the baby in the presence of other breastfeeding babies. • Hold the baby in an upright position for easier breathing during feedings. • If the baby prefers one breast, transfer him to the other breast by gently sliding him over rather than turning him around. • Use breast compression while the baby is at the breast to increase milk flow. • If the baby's gums are sore, rub them with ice or a finger before the feeding. • Increase skin contact with the baby before feedings. • Use relaxation techniques and breast massage before feedings. • Increase evening and nighttime feedings. • Nurse before offering any dietary supplements. • Reduce the amount of supplements being given to the baby. • Supplement liquids with a cup or other method that avoids an artificial nipple. • Put the baby to breast when he begins sucking on his thumb or other object.

⌒ *Baby Prefers One Breast*

It is common for a baby to display a preference for one breast over another. Although it is often difficult to determine a cause, one factor may be the mother's hand preference. If a woman is right-handed, her baby may seem to prefer her left breast when held in a cross-cradle position. She may also tend to put the baby to breast on the left side more often while she uses her right hand for other tasks, unconsciously promoting a preference. Or she may simply feel more comfortable holding the baby with her dominant hand. By evaluating her breastfeeding patterns, she can adjust positions so her baby nurses comfortably on both breasts.

It is also common for one breast to produce more milk than the other. One study found the right breast produced more milk (Engström et al., 2007), another found the left breast produced more (Hill, 2007), and still another found that both breasts had similar storage capacities with output statistically similar between breasts (Prime et al., 2009). There is wide variance in normal milk production between breasts and in most cases the greater producing breast would be sufficient to meet the needs of one baby. Marked breast asymmetry or a marked difference in production could alert you to possible hypoplasia, surgery, or injury. A feeding assessment provides you and the mother with appropriate information.

A baby may dislike the appearance or feel of one of the mother's breasts, perhaps owing to a mole, hair, or other difference. If the baby seems to dislike the smell of the skin on one side due to deodorant or perfume, the mother could eliminate these products and wash with clear water before nursing. In rare cases a baby may seem to dislike the taste of the milk in one breast; feeding the milk to the baby with a cup can help rule this out. Refusal may result from a plug of thick milk that has broken loose and is traveling through the ducts and out of the nipple. As soon as the plug clears, usually after one pumping session, regular nursing typically resumes.

The mother may have engorgement on one breast and firmer tissue in the areolar area, which does not allow for a comfortable and productive suck. When this occurs, hand expressing or pumping to soften the breast tissue may encourage the baby to nurse on that breast. The baby's birth experience may have involved trauma to one side of the face, chin, neck, or shoulder, causing pain when the baby is held in certain positions. Careful attention to positioning may entice the baby to nurse equally well on both breasts. After the discomfort is relieved, the baby usually returns to the refused breast.

Historically, breast rejection has been reported to be a marker for breast tumors (Saber et al., 1996; Hadary et al., 1995; Goldsmith, 1974). You can share this information with a mother as appropriate without being alarmist. Other case studies report no rejection by the baby of the affected breast (Petok, 1995). If you work with a mother whose baby continues to reject one side, without a logical reason, recommend that she see a physician experienced with the lactating breast to rule out all possibilities (Molckovsky et al., 2009; Mason & Johnson, 2008).

Encouraging the Baby to Feed at Both Breasts

The mother can try various methods to get her baby back on both breasts. She can begin feedings on the preferred breast to promote letdown and express some milk from the other breast to start the baby on it. Alternatively, she could begin with the less preferred breast, after first having obtained letdown by preexpressing her milk. She could do this at times when the baby is sleepy and unaware of being on the less preferred breast. She can also entice the baby with expressed milk on her nipple. Using the side-sitting (also clutch or football) hold sometimes fools the baby into thinking he is on the preferred breast, especially if he has an earache or other sensitive ear condition. Sometimes simply putting the baby to breast in any new position may do the trick.

The mother can express milk from the less preferred breast regularly to relieve any discomfort and maintain milk production. Some women decide to nurse primarily or totally on one breast. One breast can produce a sufficient amount of milk for the baby. Although the breast may be slightly larger for a time, the mother can conceal this size difference with loose-fitting clothing.

⌒ *Summary*

Temporary breastfeeding challenges can be overwhelming to parents regardless of the duration. Preserving breastfeeding may involve altering the baby's feeding routine or supplementing while the mother increases her milk production. It may mean promoting milk production for relactation or adoptive nursing. It may require maintaining lactation with the use of a breast pump for a nursing strike. Your support and suggestions will help mothers navigate these challenges more smoothly. Anticipatory guidance and timely education help achieve satisfying outcomes for mothers and babies.

⌒ *Chapter 22—At a Glance*

Applying what you learned—

Counseling the parents:

- Assure parents that a temporary setback does not preclude breastfeeding.
- Empower parents to be proactive, prudent, and effective advocates.

- Encourage parents to keep themselves well informed of their baby's condition and treatment plans.
- Support mothers in their choices, including weaning when it is their wish.
- Assure adoptive mothers that breastfeeding involves nurturing and not simply feeding.

Teach mothers about:

- Discontinuing drugs that contribute to the buildup of bilirubin.
- Requesting treatment at the mother's bedside and time for eye and skin contact.
- Requesting home phototherapy with a bili-bed or bili-blanket if appropriate and available.
- Expectations and management for relactating and nursing an adopted baby.
- Frequent and continuous skin-to-skin contact.
- Pumping frequency to match her baby's feeding patterns.
- Cobathing to encourage self-attachment.

Teach mothers how to:

- Feed frequently (10–14 times a day) in the early days to reduce bilirubin levels.
- Use a tube-feeding device at the breast to encourage the baby to nurse.
- Establish letdown and express milk to maintain lactation.
- Transition the baby to breastfeeding and reestablish milk production.
- Proceed slowly with any decrease in supplement.
- Encourage a baby who seems disinterested in breastfeeding.
- Persevere through a nursing strike.
- Encourage a baby to feed at both breasts.

~ References

Adoption.com. Breastfeeding the adopted child; 2009. www.adoption.com. Accessed October 5, 2009.

Allen E, et al. Perception of child vulnerability among mothers of former premature infants. *Pediatrics.* 2004;113:267-273.

American Academy of Family Physicians. Breastfeeding: position paper; 2001. http://www.aafp.org/x6633.xml. Accessed October 5, 2009.

American Academy of Pediatrics (AAP), Subcommittee on Neonatal Hyperbilirubinemia. Neonatal jaundice and kernicterus. *Pediatrics.* 2001;108:763-765.

American Academy of Pediatrics (AAP), Work Group on Breastfeeding. Breastfeeding and the use of human milk. *Pediatrics.* 2005;115(2):496-506.

American Academy of Pediatrics. (AAP), Subcommittee on Hyperbilirubinemia. Clinical practice guideline. Management of hyperbilirubinemia in the newborn infant 35 or more weeks of gestation. *Pediatrics.* 2004;114:297-316.

Auerbach KG, Avery J. Induced lactation. A study of adoptive nursing by 240 women. *Am J Dis Child.* 1981;135:340-343.

Auerbach KG, Sutherland A. *Relactation and Induced Lactation.* Garden City Park, NY: Avery Publishing; 1985.

Banapurmath S, et al. Initiation of lactation and establishing relactation in outpatients. *Indian Pediatr.* 2003;40:343-347.

Bengson D. *How Weaning Happens.* Schaumburg, IL: La Leche League International; 2000.

Borrel A, et al. From policy to practice: challenges in infant feeding in emergencies during the Balkan crisis. *Disaster.* 2001;25:149-163.

Bryant C. Nursing the adopted infant. *J Am Board Fam Med.* 2006;19:374-379.

Bumgarner N. *Mothering Your Nursing Toddler,* rev ed. Schaumburg, IL: La Leche League International; 2000.

Cappellini MD, Fiorelli G. Glucose-6-phosphate dehydrogenase deficiency. *Lancet.* 2008;371:64-74.

Cheales-Siebenaler NJ. Induced lactation in an adoptive mother. *J Hum Lact.* 1999;15:41-43.

Clarkson J, et al. Interventions for preventing oral candidiasis for patients with cancer receiving treatment. *Cochrane Database Syst Rev.* 2007;CD003807.

Colson S, et al. Optimal positions triggering primitive neonatal reflexes stimulating breastfeeding. *Early Hum Dev.* 2008;84:441-449.

Czank C, et al. Hormonal control of the lactation cycle. In: Hale T, Hartmann P. *Hale & Hartmann's Textbook of Human Lactation.* Amarillo, TX: Hale Publishing; 2007.

de Aquino R, Osório M. Relactation, translactation, and breastorogastric tube as transition methods in feeding preterm babies. *J Hum Lact.* 2009;25(4):420-426.

Dilli D, et al. Interventions to reduce pain during vaccination in infancy. *J Pediatr.* 2009;154:385-390.

Dougherty D, Luther M. Birth to breast—a feeding care map for the NICU: helping the extremely low birth weight infant navigate the course. *Neonat Netw.* 2008;27:371-377.

Dugdale D, Chen Y. Coomb's test. Medline Plus. November 23, 2008. www.nlm.nih.gov/medlineplus/ency/article/003344.htm. Accessed October 10, 2009.

Engström J, et al. Comparison of milk output from the right and left breasts during simultaneous pumping in mothers of very low birthweight infants. *Breastfeed Med.* 2007;2:83-91.

Gartner L. Breastfeeding and jaundice. *J Perinatol.* 2001;21(Suppl. 1):S25-S29; discussion S35-S39.

Gartner L. Hyperbilirubinemia and breastfeeding. In: Hale T, Hartmann P. *Hale & Hartmann's Textbook of Human Lactation.* Amarillo, TX: Hale Publishing; 2007.

Gartner L, Herschel M. Jaundice and breastfeeding. *Pediatr Clin North Am.* 2001;48:389-399.

Ghaemi S, et al. Late onset jaundice and urinary tract infection in neonates. *Indian J Pediatr.* 2007;74:139-141.

Goldsmith HS. Milk-rejection sign of breast cancer. *Am J Surg.* 1974;127:280-281.

Goulet L, et al. Preparation for discharge, maternal satisfaction, and newborn readmission for jaundice: comparing postpartum models of care. *Birth.* 2007;34:131-139.

Green M, Solnit A. Reactions to the threatened loss of a child: a vulnerable child syndrome. *Pediatrics*. 1964;34:58-66.

Gribble K. Mental health, attachment and breastfeeding: implications for adopted children and their mothers. *Int Breastfeed J*. 2006;1:5.

Groh-Wargo S, Sapsford A. Enteral nutrition support of the preterm infant in the neonatal intensive care unit. *Nutr Clin Pract*. 2009;24:363-376.

Hadary A, et al. The milk-rejection sign and earlier detection of breast cancer. *Harefuah*. 1995;128(11):680-681, 744.

Harris H. Remedial co-bathing for breastfeeding difficulties. *Breastfeed Rev*. 1994;11:465-468.

Hill P. Comparison of milk output between breasts in pump-dependent mothers. *J Hum Lact*. 2007;23:333-337.

Hill P, et al. Association of serum prolactin and oxytocin with milk production in mothers of preterm and term infants. *Biol Res Nurs*. 2009;10:340-349.

Holland L, Blick K. Implementing and validating transcutaneous bilirubinometry for neonates. *Am J Clin Pathol*. 2009;132(4):555-561.

Hormann K. *Breastfeeding an Adopted Baby and Relactation*. Schaumburg, IL: La Leche League, International; 2007.

Humphrey S. *The Nursing Mother's Herbal*. Minneapolis, MN: Fairview Press; 2003.

Isaacson L. Steps to successfully breastfeed the premature infant. *Neonat Netw*. 2006;25:77-86.

Johnson L, et al. Clinical report from the pilot USA Kernicterus Registry (1992 to 2004). *J Perinatol*. 2009;29(Suppl. 1):S25-S45.

Jordan S, et al. Associations of drugs routinely given in labour with breastfeeding at 48 hours: analysis of the Cardiff Births Survey. *Br J Obstet Gynaecol*. 2009;116:1622-1629, discussion 1630-1632.

Kapitulnik J, Maines M. Pleiotropic functions of biliverdin reductase: cellular signaling and generation of cytoprotective and cytotoxic bilirubin. *Trends Pharmacol Sci*. 2009;30:129-137.

Kemper K, et al. Jaundice, terminating breast-feeding, and the vulnerable child. *Pediatrics*. 1989;84:773-778.

Kemper K, et al. Persistent perceptions of vulnerability following neonatal jaundice. *Am J Dis Child* 1990;144:238-241.

Kleinman R, et al. Protein values of milk samples from mothers without biologic pregnancies. *Pediatrics*. 1980;97:612-615.

Kokotos F, Adam H. The vulnerable child syndrome. *Pediatr Rev*. 2009;30:193-194.

Kramer L. Advancement of dermal icterus in the jaundiced newborn. *Am J Dis Child*. 1969;118:454-458.

Kramer P. Breast feeding of adopted infants. *Br Med J*. 1995;311:188-189.

La Torre A, Targioni G, Rubaltelli F. Beta-glucuronidase and hyperbilirubinemia in breast-fed babies. *Biol Neonate*. 1999;75(2):82-84.

Lawrence R, Lawrence R. *Breastfeeding: A Guide for the Medical Profession*, 6th ed. St. Louis, MO: Elsevier Mosby; 2005.

MacDonald M, et al., eds. *Avery's Neonatology: Pathophysiology and Management of the Newborn*, 6th ed. Philadelphia: Lippincott Williams & Wilkins; 2005.

Maisels M. What's in a name? Physiologic and pathologic jaundice: the conundrum of defining normal bilirubin levels in the newborn. *Pediatrics*. 2006;118(2):805-807.

Maisels M, et al. Evaluation of a new transcutaneous bilirubinometer. *Pediatrics*. 2004;113:1628-1635.

Maisels M, Watchko J, eds. *Neonatal Jaundice. Monographs in Clinical Pediatrics*. Amsterdam: Harwood Academic Publishers; 2000.

Marco Lozano N, et al. Neonatal jaundice: clinical evaluation of a transcutaneous bilirubinometer. *An Pediatr (Barc)*. 2009;71(2):157-160.

Marquis G, et al. Recognizing the reversible nature of child-feeding decisions: breastfeeding, weaning, and relactation patterns in a shanty town community of Lima, Peru. *Soc Sci Med*. 1998;47:645-656.

Mason G, Johnson O. Inflammatory breast cancer: patient advocate view. *Semin Oncol*. 2008;35:87-91.

Mennella J, et al. Acute alcohol consumption disrupts the hormonal milieu of lactating women. *J Clin Endocrinol Metab*. 2005;90:1979-1985.

Mennella J, Pepino M. Biphasic effects of moderate drinking on prolactin during lactation. *Alcohol Clin Exp Res*. 2008;32:1899-1908.

Molckovsky A, et al. Approach to inflammatory breast cancer. *Can Fam Physician* 2009;55:25-31.

Morton J, et al. Combining hand techniques with electric pumping increases milk production in mothers of preterm infants. *J Perinatol*. 2009;29:757-764.

Nacro B, et al. Prevention of mother to child transmission of HIV in Burkina Faso: breastfeeding and wet nursing. *J Trop Pediatr*. Oct 2009 [Epub ahead of print].

National Center for Biotechnology Information. Hemolytic disease of the newborn (Dean L); 2005. www.ncbi.nlm.nih.gov/bookshelf/br.fcgi?book=rbcantigen&part=ch4. Accessed October 6, 2009.

Nelson R. How to spot and treat vulnerable child syndrome. *Pediatr News*. 2007;41:28.

Newman J, Goldfarb L. Newman-Goldfarb protocols for induced lactation decision tool. ILCA Abstracts. *J Hum Lact*. 2008;24:102.

Newman J, Goldfarb L. Newman-Goldfarb protocols; November 2002. www.asklenore.com. Accessed October 13, 2009.

Newman J, Kernerman E. Breast compression; February 2009a. www.nbci.ca/index.php?option=com_content&view=article&id=8:breast-compression&catid=5:information&Itemid=17. Accessed October 6, 2009.

Newman J, Kernerman E. Breastfeeding and jaundice; 2009b. www.nbci.ca/index.php?option=com_content&view=article&id=79:breastfeeding-and-jaundice&catid=5:information&Itemid=17. Accessed October 6, 2009.

Newman T, et al. Outcomes among newborns with total serum bilirubin levels of 25 mg per deciliter or more. *N Engl J Med*. 2006;354:1889-1900.

Nkhoma E, et al. The global prevalence of glucose-6-phosphate dehydrogenase deficiency: a systematic review and meta-analysis. *Blood Cells Mol Dis*. 2009;42:267-278.

Nommsen-Rivers L, et al. Delayed onset of lactogenesis is common in a cohort of California primiparae. *FASEB J*. 2009;23:344-348.

Nursing Mothers' Association of Australia. Adoptive breastfeeding and relactation. Nunawading, Victoria: Nursing Mothers' Association of Australia; 1985.

Nye C. Transitioning premature infants from gavage to breast. *Neonat Netw.* 2008;27:7-13.

Ogunlesi T, et al. Non-puerperal induced lactation: an infant feeding option in paediatric HIV/AIDS in tropical Africa. *J Child Health Care.* 2008;12(3):241-248.

Okechukwu A, Okolo A. Exclusive breastfeeding frequency during the first seven days of life in term neonates. *Niger Postgrad Med J.* 2006;13:309-312.

Osinaike B, et al. Effect of breastfeeding during venepuncture in neonates. *Ann Trop Paediatr.* 2007;27:201-205.

Peaker M, Wilde C. Feedback control of milk secretion from milk. *J Mammary Gland Biol Neoplasia.* 1996;1:307-315.

Petok ES. Breast cancer and breastfeeding: five cases. *J Hum Lact.* 1995;11(3):205-209.

Prime D, et al. Using milk flow rate to investigate milk ejection in the left and right breasts during simultaneous breast expression in women. *Int Breastfeed J.* 2009;4:10.

Profit J, et al. Delayed pediatric office follow-up of newborns after birth hospitalization. *Pediatrics.* 2009;124:548-554.

Saber A, et al. The milk rejection sign: a natural tumor marker. *Am Surg.* 1996;62:998-999.

Saitua I, et al. Analgesic effect of breastfeeding when taking blood by heel-prick in newborns. *An Pediatr.* 2009;71:310-313.

Sarici S, et al. Incidence, course, and prediction of hyperbilirubinemia in near-term and term newborns. *Pediatrics.* 2004;113:775-780.

Sedlak T, et al. Bilirubin and glutathione have complementary antioxidant and cytoprotective roles. *Proc Natl Acad Sci USA* 2009;106:5171-5176.

Shah V, et al. Effectiveness and tolerability of pharmacologic and combined interventions for reducing injection pain during routine childhood immunizations: systematic review and meta-analyses. *Clin Ther.* 2009;31(Suppl. 2):S104-S151.

Shinskie D. Use of rebirthing to facilitate latch in neurologically impaired baby. *Clin Issues.* 1998;3:4-5.

Sisk P, et al. Lactation counseling for mothers of very low birth weight infants: effect on maternal anxiety and infant intake of human milk. *Pediatrics.* 2006;117:e67-e75.

Smith L. *Impact of Birthing Practices on Breastfeeding*, 2nd ed. Sudbury, MA: Jones and Bartlett; 2010.

Smith L. Why Johnny can't suck: impact of birth practices on infant suck. In: Genna C, ed. *Supporting Sucking Skills in Infants.* Sudbury, MA: Jones and Bartlett; 2008.

Stevenson D, et al. NICHD Conference on Kernicterus: research on prevention of bilirubin-induced brain injury and kernicterus: bench-to-bedside-diagnostic methods and prevention and treatment strategies. *J Perinatol.* 2004;24:521-525.

Sweet L. Expressed breast milk as "connection" and its influence on the construction of "motherhood" for mothers of preterm infants: a qualitative study. *Int Breastfeed J.* 2008;3:30.

Uga E, et al. Heel lance in newborn during breastfeeding: an evaluation of analgesic effect of this procedure. *Riv Ital Pediatr.* 2008;34:3.

UNICEF. UNICEF in emergencies. Breastfeeding a crucial priority for child survival in emergencies; 2009. www.unicef.org/emerg/index_50471.html. Accessed October 12, 2009.

Watchko J. Identification of neonates at risk for hazardous hyperbilirubinemia: emerging clinical insights. *Pediatr Clin North Am.* 2009;56:671-687.

Watson R. Hyperbilirubinemia. *Crit Care Nurs Clin North Am.* 2009;21:97-120, vii.

West D, Marasco L. *The Breastfeeding Mother's Guide to Making More Milk.* New York: McGraw-Hill; 2008.

Wilde C, Hurley W. Animal models for the study of milk secretion. *J Mammary Gland Biol Neoplasia.* 1996;1:123-134.

Wittig S, Spatz D. Induced lactation: gaining a better understanding. *MCN Am J Mat Child Nurs.* 2008;33:76.

Xinias I, et al. Bilirubin levels predict renal cortical changes in jaundiced neonates with urinary tract infection. *World J Pediatr.* 2009;5:42-45.

High-Risk Infants

Expectant parents anxiously anticipate giving birth, bringing their baby home, and settling in as a family. Unfortunately, some parents must return home alone and leave their baby in the special care of medical personnel. Hospitalization of a high-risk infant creates trauma, anxiety, stress, and uncertainty for parents. All parents respond in their own way to such an untimely separation and their need for support is just as individual. The transition from hospital to home presents another stressful and challenging time. Familiarizing parents with normal reactions and ways of coping helps them learn how to interact with their baby and plan for the homecoming. Understanding what these families experience helps you tailor counseling to meet their unique needs.

～ Key Terms

Adipose tissue
Apnea
Appropriate for gestational age
Blood sugar levels
Bradycardia
Cyanosis
Enteral
Extremely low birth weight (ELBW)
Gastrostomy
Gavage tube
Glucuronic acid
Grief process
High-risk infant
Human milk fortifier
Hyperalimentation
Hypercapnia
Hypoxemia
Hypoxia
Intrauterine growth retardation (IUGR)

Kangaroo care
Lactoengineering
Low birth weight (LBW)
Nasogastric (NG)
Late preterm
Neonatal intensive care unit (NICU)
Orogastric (OG)
Parenteral
Percutaneous endoscopic gastrostomy (PEG) tube
Postterm infant
Preterm infant
Renal solute load
Small for gestational age (SGA)
Small-for-date
Tertiary
Very low birth weight (VLBW)

～ Prolonged Hospitalization of the High-Risk Infant

Beyond a brief glimpse of their baby at birth, parents of a high-risk infant may have little opportunity for interaction in the first hours. Depending on the baby's condition, it may be several days or weeks before they can hold or even touch their baby. Likewise, it may be several weeks or months before the mother is able to breastfeed her baby directly. In the absence of breastfeeding, she will need to learn how to initiate and maintain milk production by expressing her milk. The family must also cope emotionally with the trauma of a high-risk infant. More information on delayed and interrupted breastfeeding appears in Chapter 24.

Parents' Reactions

Care of high-risk infants in a neonatal intensive care unit (NICU) is delivered in the safest and gentlest way possible to achieve the best outcomes medically, nutritionally, and developmentally for the infant. Parents' first experience with the NICU will most likely be seeing their infant lying unclothed in an open radiant warmer or an isolette, connected to machinery with tubing (Figure 23.1). The equipment and its correlation to their baby's chances for survival can be overwhelming. The NICU environment can be a frightening scene, even when parents are prepared to expect it and have been given an explanation for all the life-sustaining devices.

Parents sometimes find it difficult to focus on their high-risk baby as an individual. Even with a favorable prognosis, they may worry about their baby's survival. They will want to know what can be done to help him, how soon he will be out of danger, how soon he will be disconnected from tubes and monitors, and when he can go home. They may feel helpless, wanting to do something for their baby and not knowing what or how. Parents who plan to breastfeed may wonder how soon their baby can go to breast. Mothers who plan to bottle feed may be asked to pump and provide their colostrum and, later, their milk

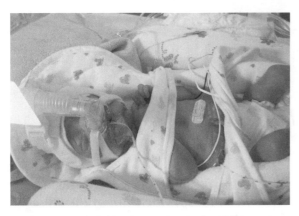

FIGURE 23.1   Seeing their infant in the NICU can be unsettling to parents.

Source: Printed with permission of Leslie and Brad Jackson.

for the baby while he is in the NICU. In this setting your care ranges from assurance for the parents who prepared extensively for their baby's arrival to giving very basic information to mothers who never planned to breastfeed and who know nothing about it.

The experience in the NICU can resemble arriving in another country where a foreign language is spoken. Learning common NICU acronyms (Table 23.1) enables you to discuss the baby's care with the parents and health-care providers. You can help parents formulate questions for their baby's caregivers. Stress the importance of asking for explanations and clarification of anything they do not fully understand. They may find it difficult to absorb and process all the information they receive from you and other caregivers. Consequently, you may find that you need to continually repeat, review, and clarify important points for the mother about breastfeeding her high-risk infant. Be patient, and recognize that her inability to remember does not reflect disinterest.

TABLE 23.1   Common NICU Abbreviations

A & B: Apnea and bradycardia

Bili: Bilirubin

BP: Blood pressure (see low blood pressure)

BPD: Bronchopulmonary dysplasia

cc or mL: Metric measures of liquid; 30 cc (or mL) is 1 ounce; 5 cc is ~1 teaspoon

CNS: Central nervous system (brain and spinal cord) or clinical nurse specialist

CPAP: Continuous positive airway pressure (air or oxygen delivered under a small amount of pressure)

CPR: Cardiopulmonary resuscitation

CPT or Chest PT: Chest physiotherapy (vibrating or tapping on the chest)

ET: Endotracheal (refers to a tube placed through the mouth or nose to the windpipe)

Gms or grams: Metric weight; 450 grams = 1 pound; 1 kilogram (kg) = 1,000 grams

HMD: Hyaline membrane disease (another name for respiratory distress syndrome)

HI-FI: High-frequency ventilator

ID: Infectious disease or identification

IMV: Intermittent mandatory ventilation (i.e., no. of breaths per minute by the ventilator)

IV: Intravenous (by vein)

IVH: Intraventricular hemorrhage

LP: Lumbar puncture (getting sample of spinal fluid using a needle)

NEC: Necrotizing enterocolitis

NG: Nasogastric (tube going from nose to stomach)

NICU: Neonatal intensive care unit

NPO: Nothing by mouth

O_2: Oxygen

OG: Orogastric (tube going from mouth to stomach)

OT: Occupational therapist

PDA: Patent ductus arteriosus

PIC or PCVL: a tiny catheter or tube placed into a vein to give fluids or nutrition

PT: Physical therapist

PVL: Periventricular leukomalacia

ROP: Retinopathy of prematurity

RDS: Respiratory distress syndrome

SIDS: Sudden infant death syndrome

SIMV: Synchronized intermittent mandatory ventilation (machine breaths timed to baby's)

TPR: Temperature, pulse, and respiration

TTNB: Transient tachypnea of the newborn

TPN or TNA: Total parenteral nutrition (nutrition by vein)

UAC: Umbilical artery catheter

UTI: Urinary tract (kidney or bladder) infection

UVC: Umbilical venous catheter

VS: Vital signs (temperature, pulse, respiration, blood pressure)

Source: Meriter Health Services. Preemie health, introduction to the neonatal intensive care unit (NICU); 2009. Reprinted by permission of Brad and Leslie Jackson.

Feelings of Detachment and Grief

Hospitalization of a newborn is highly stressful and overwhelming, especially when the baby is born preterm or in a compromised condition. The experience is likely to be one of the greatest life challenges that parents face (Dyer, 2005a, 2005b). Many parents of high-risk infants experience feelings of guilt, loneliness, and anxiety. They may avoid contact with parents who have healthy babies. While in the hospital, mothers may detach themselves from other mothers and babies. Parents may try to avoid involvement with their own baby in an instinctive effort to protect themselves from becoming attached to a baby they may lose. This is a very common and natural reaction. Such feelings usually subside when the parents are able to accept their baby's condition.

Parents sometimes disconnect so much that they may abandon the baby emotionally, mentally, and even physically; though most parents work through their loss and do not progress to this extreme. Regardless of the baby's prognosis, parents typically move through stages of grief, similar to those shown in Figure 23.2, as they mourn the loss of their healthy "dream" baby. After parents have grieved for and mourned the healthy baby they expected, they can begin to accept the baby they have.

It is common for high-risk infants to be transferred to a different facility that can provide a higher level of care. The very fact that transfer to a special care facility is necessary underscores the seriousness of their baby's condition. Parents go through a very real grief experience when it is necessary to transfer their infant to another facility. The new medical personnel caring for their infant, although very competent, are complete strangers to them. Furthermore, the parents may be separated from their baby by a distance that makes visitation difficult.

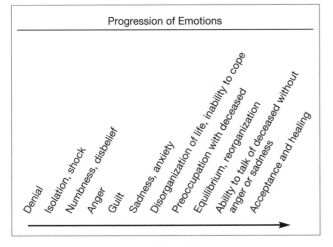

FIGURE 23.2 Sequence of the grief process.

Need for Support

A critically ill or preterm infant adds one more stressor to a life already filled with stress (Chin & Solomonik, 2009). Parents of a high-risk infant are tired and anxious, which can put a strain on their relationship. Many times crisis brings out unresolved conflicts in a couple's relationship, with the baby's condition serving as a catalyst for problems rising to the surface (Howland, 2007). Thus disagreements or arguments you observe in the parents' interactions may be unrelated to the baby's condition. Encourage parents to seek out sources of support, both in the hospital and within their community. Most hospitals assign case managers to help families through this type of crisis. Social service consultations are available, and most hospitals have chaplains trained in grief and crisis counseling. Talking with other parents who have experienced similar situations can help them realize that their reactions are typical and may give them techniques for coping.

Hospitals with level III NICUs often have support groups for families that are facilitated by trained staff. Support groups are also available in many communities for parents of high-risk infants, as well as online. Participating in group discussions provides parents the opportunity to share their feelings and concerns and to learn to put their reactions into perspective. The hospital's social caseworkers should also have local resources available. It may be helpful for you to compile a resource list specifically for feeding issues. You can also refer parents to resources in their communities of faith, such as a pastor, priest, or rabbi.

Mothers of high-risk infants who have sources of support are more likely to continue breastfeeding (Meier et al., 2004). Breastfeeding promotion and staff training in the NICU increase exclusive breastfeeding rates early after discharge, especially among infants born at very low birth weight (VLBW) (Renfrew et al., 2010; Dall'Oglio, 2007). Familiarize yourself with available support and make appropriate referrals. Because of modern mobility, many people do not live near their own parents and need to establish a circle of support. Therefore, inquire about the mother's family and friends as support systems. In addition, many NICU parents are low-income or minorities with a history of drug use. Consequently, they may have many other social needs as well.

A high-risk infant requires a great deal of attention and care, and parents' needs often go unrecognized or unmet. Your sincere interest in the mother can encourage her to talk about her labor and delivery experience. A mother who perceives that her needs are validated is more likely to share her anxieties about her birth, her baby, and her coping abilities. Asking the mother about her sleep, her appetite, and her postpartum pain shows concern about her as a person. Additionally, she will receive information and advice from many sources and may need you to listen to her in an accepting, objective, and interested manner. Sincere and honest concern is natural; let her know that you care and that you are there to support her.

Neonatal Intensive Care Unit

The NICU is an overwhelming environment for both the parents and their baby. The mother's voice and rhythmic body sounds comfort her baby in the womb. The surroundings are dark and comforting, with only subtle variance in diffused light. The baby is continuously bathed in warm amniotic fluid, constantly fed, and rocked by the mother's movements.

In contrast, the NICU can be a noisy environment with continuous white noise and harsh mechanical sounds occurring at varying times. Voices often are indistinct, and the constant bright lighting lacks any daily rhythm. Sound levels at three NICUs were found to exceed recommended levels of < 45 dB, including at night, when they should not exceed 35 dB (Darcy, 2008). Overstimulation of a preterm infant's auditory system can trigger responses of apnea, heart rate fluctuations, blood pressure fluctuations, and oxygen saturation changes. Preterm infants exposed to prolonged excessive noise are also at increased risk for hearing loss, abnormal brain and sensory development, and speech and language problems (Brown, 2009).

As evidenced by the care available to infants in special care facilities, tremendous medical advances have improved the morbidity and mortality rates of high-risk infants. There are three levels of NICUs. Level I NICUs provide routine newborn care. Level II NICUs care for newborns that may require monitoring and care beyond routine newborn care (typically, babies over 33 weeks who are "growers and feeders"). Level III NICUs (tertiary care) are high-risk facilities equipped to care for the smallest and sickest babies. These include very preterm infants (micro-preemies) and full-term infants with severe or potentially life-threatening conditions.

Regional level III NICUs care for babies transported from the surrounding geographical area. Many times babies can be cared for at the hospital where they were born. This can be a comfort to the parents when the hospital is near their home. In some instances a high-risk pregnancy is detected early enough so the woman can deliver in a tertiary care facility that has the means to care for both her and her baby.

Often, the mother of a high-risk infant has had a cesarean and will not leave the birth facility for 3 or 4 days, requiring that she be separated from her new baby. NICU case managers can assist families with information on extended-stay resources, such as Ronald McDonald Houses and Family Rooms. Information is available at www.rmhc .com. These corporate-sponsored facilities offer free accommodations for parents visiting sick children.

Care of a High-Risk Infant

Most touching that takes place with a high-risk infant in the NICU is either technical or medical in nature. The baby thus may learn to associate touch with unpleasant events. There is debate among healthcare professionals regarding how much stimulation is appropriate for a high-risk infant (see the discussion on kangaroo care later in this chapter). Being aware of current research in NICU care helps you advocate for a breastfeeding-friendly environment that encompasses the best of high-tech developmental care. You can share with the mother ways she can nurture her infant through gentle, warm, and loving touch.

Massage Gentle massage therapy for NICU infants is associated with improved motor development and earlier hospital discharge (Ho et al., 2009). Clinically stable preterm infants have shown faster weight gain and earlier discharge with various types of massage (Gonzalez et al., 2009). Massage that incorporates kinesthetic stimulation (Massaro et al., 2009) combined with massage oil, for example, has been found to promote greater infant weight gain than with massage oil alone (Arora et al., 2005). A 2004 Cochrane review found similar results but questioned the methodological quality and selective reporting of outcomes in the included studies (Vickers et al., 2004).

Nonnutritive Sucking Nonnutritive sucking is an important skill for the NICU infant, especially before beginning oral feeds. Nonnutritive sucking on a pacifier can improve the baby's state regulation and is a comfort measure during lengthy separation from the mother, gavage feeding, and painful procedures (Dougherty & Luther, 2008). For babies who cannot yet receive breastmilk, nonnutritive sucking on the mother's drained breast can help elicit breastfeeding behaviors. This allows the baby to practice coordinating the pattern of suck–swallow–breathe without the theoretical risk of aspiration. The baby begins to associate the mother's breast with the smell of her milk and learns that her breast is a cozy, pleasant place to be. The review by Pinelli and Symington (2005) noted a significant decrease in length of stay in preterm infants receiving nonnutritive sucking intervention.

Nourishment A high-risk infant may receive nourishment initially through hyperalimentation, intravenously receiving a solution of amino acids, glucose, electrolytes, and vitamins. The baby then progresses to gavage feedings via nasogastric (NG) tubing or orogastric (OG) tubing. Both NG tubing (passed through the nasal passage down to the stomach) and OG tubing (passed through the mouth and down the throat) can be used for either continuous or intermittent feeding. OG feeding is also used for a baby with structural nasal anomalies or for a baby receiving continuous positive airway pressure (CPAP) (Birnbaum & Limperopoulos, 2009). Because imprinting affects babies' feeding abilities, preterm or ill babies may develop oral aversions (McNeil, 2008; Pinelli & Symington, 2005; Wolf & Glass, 1992). Occasionally, the baby may have a percutaneous endoscopic gastrostomy (PEG) tube placed through the skin directly into the stomach. After achieving the ability to tolerate enteral feedings and growing more clinically stable, the infant can progress to oral feedings, including feeding at the breast. In the mother's absence the baby can be fed via an alternative feeding method such as cup, spoon, bottle, or dropper (Kumar, 2010).

Bottle Feeding Bottle feeding is deeply entrenched in the culture of NICU care. Most babies in the United States are fed by bottle due to staff time constraints and familiarity with bottle feeding. The ability to suck—referred to as "nippling"—is a key developmental goal for the infant before hospital discharge. Historically, this goal was achieved on a bottle teat (Shaker & Woida, 2007). One of the regrets that parents report is when medical staff, and not the parents, give the first bottle to their baby. Parents can ask to be present if possible, to observe and to par-

ticipate in their baby's feedings and care as soon as possible.

High-risk infants optimally would not receive feedings with artificial nipples and bottles. Bottle feeding is associated with physiological and biochemical changes in the infant such as hypoxemia, hypoxia, hypercapnia (high carbon dioxide levels), apnea, bradycardia (slow heart rate), and cyanosis (Thoyre & Carlson, 2003; Chen et al., 2000; Blaymore-Bier et al., 1997; Meier, 1988). If bottles are used, therefore, the staff needs to assess the baby for complications, including apnea and bradycardia.

You can advocate for evidence-based practices that protect breastfeeding, such as limiting pacifiers to appropriate use and not requiring successful bottle "nippling" before direct breastfeeding. Table 23.2 describes preterm feeding behaviors and their progression in both breastfeeding and bottle feeding. An innovative NICU oral feeding protocol has been instituted in some NICUs. It is based on the Calgary Health Region model, which describes stages of the infant's readiness to feed, not just weight and gestational age (Table 23.3).

TABLE 23.2 Development of Preterm Infant Feeding Behavior

	Breastfeeding	Bottle Feeding
Immature	• Licking predominates • Little rooting evident • Shallow latch or difficulty maintaining latch • Occasional short sucking bursts of ~ 3-5 sucks • Pattern of bursts is ~1-5 sucks, pause and breathe • ≤ 5 minutes of nutritive suckling	• Predominantly expression/compression rather than suction usually ~ 2-3 seconds • If suction is present it is of low amplitude • Pattern is irregular or arrhythmic • Expression/suction is not paired with swallow • < 50% of expressions/sucks are organized into bursts • ≤ 10 sucks per burst when burst present • Breathing not consistently integrated into expression and swallow
Mixed	• Some rooting • Repeated short sucking bursts of ~ 6-15 sucks • Swallowing beginning to be integrated into sucking bursts • ~ 6-10 minutes of nutritive suckling	• Predominantly expression/compression • Expression/compression pattern rhythmic usually ~ 1/second (55/minute) • Alteration of suction/expression emerging but arrhythmic • Expression/suction inconsistently paired with swallow • 50-90% of expressions/sucks organized into bursts • Pauses irregular and generally long • 10-20 sucks per burst
Mature	• Obvious consistent rooting • Deep latch maintained • Repeated long sucking bursts of ~ 15-30 sucks • Swallows audible • Pattern of bursts: suck/swallow/breathe or suck/suck / swallow/breathe • 11 minutes of sucking	• Rhythmic alteration of suction and expression/compression • Rate increases ~ 65/minutes • Suck of consistently high amplitude • Swallows consistently paired with suck • > 90% of sucks organized into bursts • Pauses more regular and short • 10-40 sucks/burst

Source: St. David's Round Rock Medical Center, 2400 Round Rock Ave., Round Rock, Texas; July, 2009. Developed by Kathy Amell, LVN, IBCLC, RLC, and Heather Anderson, MS, CCCSP. Adapted from Calgary Regional Health Center.

TABLE 23.3 Neonatal Oral Feeding Guidelines

PRE-ORAL

Infant Characteristics
- Handling intolerance
- Weak physiologic, motor and state regulation
- None to very weak oral reflexes
- None to very weak NNS skills

Goals
- Minimize negative stimulation
- Promote behavioural organization
- Establish and maintain mother's EBM supply
- 0% oral intake

Interventions
- Developmental care
- Skin to skin care (Kangaroo care?)
- Positive experiences to facial area
- Support mother lactation
- Tube feeding only

NON-NUTRITIVE

Infant Characteristics
- Stable with handling
- Able to maintain physiologic, motor and state stability with NNS practice
- Oral reflexes emerging
- Demonstrates licking and rooting
- Learning to latch
- Ready to practice NNS bursts

Goals
- Positive oral stimulation and NNS
- Support mother's EBM supply
- 0% oral intake

Interventions
- Skin to skin care
- Facilitate hand to mouth contact
- Allow infant to nuzzle at pumped breast
- Use soother
- Place warm drops of milk on infant's lip when tube feeding to promote licking
- Once infant attains NNS stability, offer NNS during tube feedings

NUTRITIVE SUCKING STAGE I

Infant Characteristics
- Emerging readiness cues, e.g., manages secretions and maintains quiet alert state
- Good NNS; emergent but not sustained SSB coordination
- Oral intake <10% daily volume

Goals
- Oral practice only
- Infant able to take small amounts orally in a controlled setting
- Focus on quality of feeding more than quantity taken
- Experience is positive for infant and caregiver

Interventions
- Minimize distracting stimuli
- Intervene to prevent distress
- Do not push feedings
- **Therapeutic tasting** – drip milk onto soother from 1 ml syringe 1 drop at a time
- **External pace** before infant becomes distressed. Remove nipple to lip, allow infant to take several swallows and breathe. Wait for baby to open mouth to cue you to place nipple back in mouth.
  - **Breastfeeding**
    - Breastfeeding practice at pumped breast
    - Pair tube feeding with BF practice
    - If disorganized, try NNS first
  - **Bottlefeeding**
    - Swaddle, side lying elevated on pillow
    - Start with NNS x 1–2 minutes
    - Slow flow nipple; Check for excessive milk flow

Heed infant disengagement cues, Slow down oral feeding progression, May need to move back one stage

Abbreviations:
B – bottle   BF – breast feed
GA – gestational age
NNS – non-nutritive sucking
NS – nutritive sucking
OG/NG – orogastric/nasogastric
SSB – suck-swallow-breathe
TFI – total fluid intake
WOB – work of breathing

Alberta Health Services

I03367A ©Alberta Health Services, (2009/11)

NUTRITIVE SUCKING STAGE II

Infant Characteristics
- Inconsistent but identifiable readiness cues, e.g., hand to mouth, increased activity
- Functional to good SSB coordination
- Improved endurance but not enough for full feeding
- Oral intake 10% to <80% of daily volume

Goals
- To ease the transition to full oral feeding by supporting endurance, skills and physiologic stability

Interventions
- Watch for disengagement/distress cues and assess infant's readiness to continue
- If oxygen saturation drops, consider smaller OG/NG tube
- Facilitate breastfeeding opportunities
- Side lying, swaddle, lie on pillow, offer soother first to organize SSB coordination
- Slow flow nipple. Check for excessive milk flow
- Externally pace to prevent distress. Wait for baby to open mouth to cue you to place nipple back in mouth.
- Do not jiggle or rotate nipple during recovery phases. If infant is too sleepy, wake infant by sitting up rather than using mouth stimulation.
- Focus on quality of feeding experience rather than quantity of feed taken.
- Track daily % oral intake vs tube feeding:

  Stage IIA: 10% to <25%
  - Maximum 5–10 minute oral feeding time (BF or B)
  - Oral practice only when cueing; likely 1–2 times/day
  - Assess whether infant needs nonpumped vs pumped breast
  - Indwelling NG/OG; NNS and/or therapeutic tasting with tube feeds

  Stage IIB: 25% to <50%
  - Typically >10 minute oral feeding time
  - BF/B opportunities dependent on infant cues; aid to awake state a.c.
  - NNS and/or therapeutic tasting with tube feeds
  - Occasional full bottle taken

  Stage IIC: 50% to <80%
  - Maximum 30 minutes oral feeding time
  - Offer BF/B opportunities every time infant cues
  - May or may not need supplementation after BF/B; determine TFI range to allow flexibility in amount of tube feeding top-up needed.
  - Consider removing OG/NG for BF/B

Disengagement/Distress Cues: Physiologically unstable (↓in HR, RR, O₂), ↑WOB, color Δ, motor stress cues (squirming, finger splaying), loss of bolus, gulping, coughing, disorganized SSB, fatigue, shutting down (eyes glaze over), feedings >30 minutes

NUTRITIVE SUCKING STAGE III

Infant Characteristics
- Sustains SSB throughout feeding
- Infant has endurance to maintain nutritional intake and support growth
- Demonstrates clear hunger cues, e.g., hand to mouth, wakes to feed
- Demonstrated satiation cues, e.g., falls asleep at end of feeding
- ≥80% oral feedings

Goals
- Full oral feeding that supports growth
- Feeding experience positive for infant and caregiver

Interventions
- Continue sidelying positioning and external pacing as required
- Transition to cue-based feeding before discharge
- If infant demonstrates disengagement cues, delay feeding till infant cues again
- Consider no top-up if infant consumes ≥80% of feed
- Encourage breastfeeding mothers to spend long blocks of time in nursery to facilitate cue-based feeding
- Parents should bring in the nipple and feeding regime that they want to use at home
- Ideally infant should spend >3 days in stage III pre-discharge

Readiness Cues: Manages secretions, improving state regulation, physiologic stability and endurance, NNS skills, hunger cues (licking, rooting), effective latch, functional SSB coordination with or without external pacing, satiation cues

Advance feeding interventions as per infant cues

Source: Alberta Health Services; September, 2009. http://www.calgaryhealthregion.ca/programs/neonatology/Protocols.htm. Printed with permission.

Cup Feeding An Egyptian study found that cup-fed late preterm infants exhibited more mature breastfeeding behaviors when compared with bottle fed infants over 6 weeks of age. These infants had a mean gestational age of 35.13 weeks and a mean birth weight of 2,150 g. They also received a significantly higher percentage of feedings at the breast 1 week after NICU discharge (Abouelfettoh et al., 2008).

Full-term infants have been observed to use their oral musculature (buccinator, masseter, and temporalis) more in breastfeeding and cup feeding than in bottle feeding (Gomes et al., 2006). This suggests that cup feeding might be more desirable than bottle feeding to promote the infant's oral structural growth and development.

Maternal presence and NICU staff workload are key constraints to cup feeding. Many mothers are limited to one visit a day, especially when they must return to work, are single parents, or have other children. Additionally, staff time to provide cup feeding is problematic in a cost-conscious healthcare environment. Thus although cup feeding is associated with higher rates of breastfeeding at discharge (see Chapter 21), the longer hospital stay (up to 10 days) may be prohibitive (Collins et al., 2008).

Breastfeeding High-risk infants can transition from gavage to direct breastfeeding without the use of bottles. Classic research has shown that it is physiologically less stressful for a preterm infant to suck on the human breast than on an artificial nipple (Anderson, 1993, 1989; Meier, 1988). Direct breastfeeding is possible for babies as young as 30 weeks' gestation and as small as 1,100 g (Nyqvist, 2008).

Every baby is different in his or her capabilities and should be assessed on an individual basis. Although many preterm babies are ineffective feeders, each should be given a chance to breastfeed directly once they are physiologically stable. In one study 57 of 71 preterm babies established full breastfeeding at an average of 36 weeks' gestational age, with a range of 33.4 to 40.0 weeks (Nyqvist et al., 1999).

An individual feeding plan helps the baby progress predictably from parenteral feeding through each stage until reaching the ability to breastfeed directly, as described in Table 23.3. Websites and other media resources abound for parents of babies in the NICU, including blogs and parent forums. *Best Medicine: Human Milk in the NICU* (Wight et al., 2008) and *Breastfeeding Special Care Babies* (Lang, 2002) provide easy-to-read in-depth references.

The mother's hospital stay provides an opportunity for caregivers to dispel myths and provide anticipatory guidance on initiating lactation. Unsupportive healthcare practices have been cited as reasons for breastfeeding failure among many groups of mothers. Chief among them are inconsistency, inaccurate information, and lack of support. Identified barriers to breastfeeding a preterm infant include (Wight & Morton, 2007):

- The intimidating physical environment of the NICU
- Individual infant medical factors
- Ill, stressed, or medicated mothers
- Family environment and experience with breastfeeding
- Financial constraints
- Well-meaning but misinformed healthcare providers

Parenting in the NICU

Family-centered care is an approach that develops a partnership between staff and families. A family-centered NICU allows unrestricted parental presence and involvement in infant caregiving. This environment maintains open communication between parents and staff (Griffin, 2006). It is challenging for parents to embrace the parental role when their baby is in the NICU. Initiating as much meaningful interaction as possible can help parents minimize the impact of early separation from their high-risk infant. The overwhelming nature of the experience can cause parents to feel hesitant or fearful about interacting with their baby. You can help bridge this gap by inquiring about and addressing their concerns. Encourage their participation and provide explanations in simple and concrete terms.

Supporting Parents Cleveland (2008) identified six key needs for parents of NICU infants. These needs can be met in a welcoming environment with supportive policies and practices that provide emotional support and parent empowerment. Parent education should provide opportunities to practice new skills through guided participation. The six key needs are as follows:

1. Accurate information and inclusion in the infant's care
2. Vigilant watching-over and protecting the infant
3. Contact with the infant
4. Being positively perceived by the nursery staff
5. Individualized care
6. Therapeutic relationship with the nursing staff

One study found that family satisfaction with communication in the NICU improved to 95 percent with a few simple interventions. Interventions included educating providers about family communication, distributing contact cards to families, and putting up a poster of providers in the unit (Weiss et al., 2009). Another educational-behavioral intervention program for parents was associated with improved parent mental health outcomes, enhanced parent–infant interaction, and reduced hospital length of stay (3.8 fewer days in NICU) (Melnyk et al., 2006). A follow-up analysis of this program found cost savings of at least $4,864 per infant (Melnyk & Feinstein,

2009). The authors estimate that implementing this program in NICUs across the United States could save the healthcare system more than $2 billion per year.

Needs of Fathers Fathers, who often experience a sense of lack of control in the NICU experience, benefit from individual attention. Care and communication, especially with a male physician, was reported as positive and useful according to one study (Arockiasamy et al., 2008). Specific activities help a father regain a sense of control and help him fulfill his various roles of protector, father, partner, and breadwinner. Engaging fathers in the NICU is a much more difficult task than with mothers, primarily because the mother is the most frequent visitor (after the initial postpartum period). Optimally, family care needs should be identified and incorporated into the developmental plan of care (Johnson, 2008).

Fathers return to work quickly after their infant's birth, and work continues to be a primary focus. This is partly to provide financially for the family as well as for the comfort of their work expertise to compensate for their feelings of inadequacy or novice in the NICU. Not surprisingly, the most stressful part of the NICU experience for fathers is juggling their time between work and family needs. These stressors are often invisible to healthcare providers (Pohlman, 2005).

Needs of Teen Parents Educating teen parents of high-risk infants is a special challenge. Boss et al. (2010) found most teens could name their infant's diagnosis and treatment but often underestimated the seriousness of the baby's condition. Teens were hesitant to ask for clarification of technical language, and reported that speaking with a physician was confusing to them. Parental knowledge was better when physicians make explicit efforts to communicate with parents. It helps to ask teen parents many open-ended questions, to use simple terminology, and to demonstrate understanding of teaching such as milk expression, pumping, applying a nipple shield, positioning, and latch. Don't assume a teen mother understands what you are saying just because she agrees verbally.

Interaction with Their Baby Parents often are not aware of what is normal and expected for their baby in the NICU. It is helpful to point out what to expect based on their baby's condition and gestational age. Parents express less anxiety and more realistic expectations when they recognize their baby's behavioral capabilities. They can visit, touch and fondle their baby as much as the baby's condition allows (Figure 23.3). Babies have better weight gains and quicker recoveries when their mothers hold and care for them during hospitalization.

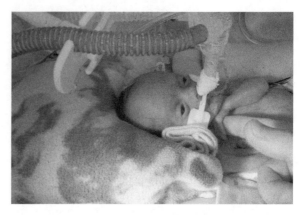

FIGURE 23.3 A parent interacting with her infant in the NICU.

Source: Printed with permission of Leslie and Brad Jackson.

Eye-to-eye contact between the parents and their baby is important as well. If eye patches are used, parents can ask that they be removed during their visit. When the baby is stable enough, they can request time alone with their baby to interact as a family without the presence of hospital staff. Encourage them to take part in caring for their baby as well with feeding, bathing, and diapering.

As parents transition to becoming their infants' primary caregivers, nurses can move to roles of educators and supporters (Nyqvist & Engvall, 2009). This transition is especially important in the days preceding the baby's discharge. Privacy screens and rooming-in when the baby is able gives parents the chance to bond with their baby and embrace their parental role. Encourage mothers to arrange private time whenever the baby's condition permits.

Pressure of Other Demands Be mindful that logistical constraints such as caring for siblings and transportation to and from the hospital may interfere with parents' ability to interact with their baby. Time commitments present challenges for the mother in terms of rest, expressing her milk, and caring for other children or family members. The father, feeling overwhelmed by rising medical bills, may focus on his job because he fears losing the income and insurance on which his family depends. Many employed mothers must also return to work before the baby comes home, robbing them of rest and bonding time.

Although committed parents want to spend as much time as possible with their baby, parents feel pressured by all these demands. They should not be made to feel guilty or negligent if they cannot visit their baby as often as you or others consider appropriate. Assume parents are doing the best they can in a difficult situation, unless you observe behaviors that suggest otherwise.

Although discussion in this chapter involves two parents, 39.7 percent of births in 2007 in the United States were to single mothers, and 23 percent of these were to teens. Teens are at the highest risk for problem pregnancies and low-birth-weight (LBW) babies. They may have little or no support from family and may be living on their own, with friends, or in a shelter. In such cases social services become even more vital for the well-being of the mother and baby. See Chapter 20 for more discussion on teen mothers.

Taking the Baby Home

Parents' emotions can be a mixture of elation, anxiety, caution, and insecurity in their roles as full-time caretakers. Many parents of hospitalized infants perceive their baby as needing ongoing special care, which may be true in some cases. The parents are often anxious at the time of discharge and overwhelmed at the thought of caring for their baby full time. While some have advance notice that their baby will go home, discharge may occur relatively quickly for other parents.

Baby's Health Status

The physical stability a high-risk baby must demonstrate before discharge includes normal breathing, oxygenation, voiding, stooling, and body temperature. In addition to tolerating feedings by mouth, sucking, swallowing, and breathing must be coordinated—at either the breast or bottle. The baby will have a "sleep study" to determine if sleep apnea is a risk. Small infants are discharged today much earlier than in the past, and babies are no longer required to reach a "magic" weight. Today, it is common for an infant to go home when she is able to maintain her temperature in an open crib, gains weight appropriately on full oral feedings, and is in stable medical condition.

Discharge Planning

The mother can prepare for her baby's homecoming by arranging for household help when possible, freezing meals for later use, stocking up on grocery items, and any other preparations that will maximize her time with her infant. Before discharge, the baby's caregiver will schedule a postdischarge visit and discuss the baby's feeding plans, as well as any special care procedures or restrictions that are needed. If supplements are required, the mother needs to clarify how much and how often she must feed them to her baby. The NICU also coordinates community care with the baby's primary care physician, including sharing medical records.

The Academy of Breastfeeding Medicine (2004) has a protocol for the preterm infant's transition from the NICU to home. If you work in a NICU or with NICU graduates, you may want to compare these guidelines with your facility's existing policies and see if any of the protocols can be adapted for your use.

Home Environment

After arriving home with their baby, parents have many additional concerns unrelated to feedings. Because auditory pathways continue to develop during the neonatal period, they need to plan for quiet in the home environment (Goines, 2008). This can be a challenge in the chaotic environments of many NICU families. Other health problems may require that the infant go home with a heart monitor or sleep apnea monitor. He may have an NG tube or PEG tube in place for feedings. It is easy to see why breastfeeding can fall by the wayside quickly when a baby has multiple health issues and care is so intensive.

A study of breastfeeding experiences among NICU families found that at 6 weeks after discharge 71 percent of infants continued to receive at least some mother's milk (Wheeler, 2009). Reasons for discontinuing pumping or breastfeeding included the mothers' own physical and emotional problems, infant health concerns, and lack of time and support.

Today, 66 percent of U.S. mothers with children aged 17 years or younger are employed. Among employed mothers, 74 percent work full time (Parker, 2009). Women in countries with ample family leave or where fewer mothers are employed outside the home may be able to spend more time with their baby in the NICU. In the United States, however, many women have exhausted their maternity leave or personal leave options by the time their high-risk baby comes home and must arrange for special caregivers. This exerts an additional emotional and financial toll on the parents.

Some mothers split their maternity leave, taking off a brief time after the birth, returning to work while the baby is in the NICU, and then taking the remainder of their leave after the baby is home. In the United States, maternity leave can be as brief as 6 weeks. Resources such as home health services, specialized daycare providers, and respite caregivers may be helpful for these mothers. If the mother loses her job, case management can help the family check into benefits such as Women, Infants, and Children (WIC), Medicaid, and other social services.

Many parents experience an initial phase of excitement, followed by exhaustion, until the transition is completed and enjoyment and self-confidence return (Klaus et al., 2000). After the baby is home, the parents most likely will feel drained, both physically and emotionally, and their baby will still be recovering physically. Encourage parents to limit visitors to allow quiet time with other family members as they reestablish relationships and integrate the baby into the family.

Baby Care and Feeding at Home

You can assist the mother through the transition home by increasing your contact with her before her baby's discharge. Inquire about her most pressing concerns, and refer her to appropriate assistance as necessary. Mothers of high-risk infants are concerned about crying, breathing noises, spitting up, and infant behavior, all of which relate to feeding. It is important to address these issues with parents.

Preterm or sick infants often do not demonstrate overt hunger cues. Therefore mothers may be unaware of the cues given by their babies in the early days. It is helpful to point out any subtle cues such as rooting that indicate the baby's readiness to feed. Also, teach typical infant responses that show a sign of overstimulation, such as the baby's breathing changes, frowning, back arching, arm waving, hiccoughing, and avoidance of eye contact. See the discussion about these cues in Chapter 13. One helpful video resource is "A Premie Needs His Mother" (2002), by Jane Morton, MD.

Crying behavior of a preterm high-risk infant varies according to gestational age. Infant cries may be more high pitched and uneven than those of a full-term baby, and more frequent as well. A preterm baby may have a greater incidence of reflux as well (Birch & Newell, 2009; Di Fiore et al., 2009; Boekel, 2000). These behaviors can be very trying for parents as they learn how to console their child. Anticipatory guidance helps them learn what to expect and how to cope with crying.

Mothers who lack necessary information regarding their babies' care and expected behavior may be more anxious and less confident in caring for their babies. Your assistance and support can help ease this anxiety and build maternal confidence. Ongoing support through postdischarge follow-up can assist these mothers in their baby's transition to home.

～ Preterm Infant

Preterm birth is a serious health problem that costs the United States alone more than $26 billion annually. It is the leading cause of newborn death (March of Dimes, 2009). Babies who survive an early birth often face the risk of lifetime health challenges, including breathing problems and mental retardation. Babies born even a few weeks early have higher rates of death and disability than full-term babies.

The preterm birth rate in the United States has increased by 36 percent since the 1980s. Despite a modest decline in the 2007 preterm birth rate, the number of babies born too soon continues to top more than 540,000 each year. The preterm birth rate declined for babies born at 34 to 36 weeks' gestation (late preterm) and among babies born to African American and white women. The March of Dimes attributes the slight decrease to the multiorganizational attention to the problems of late preterm babies.

Most preterm infants weigh less than 5.5 pounds (2500 g). If the rate of intrauterine growth is normal the infant is deemed appropriate for gestational age (AGA). If intrauterine growth was slowed, referred to as intrauterine growth retardation (IUGR), the baby is considered small for gestational age (SGA). Full-term babies can also be small for gestational age or large for gestational age (LGA). Preterm babies are classified by birth weight as follows:

- Low birth weight (LBW): under 5 lb, 8 oz (2500 g)
- Very low birth weight (VLBW): under 3 lb, 5 oz (1500 g)
- Extremely low birth weight (ELBW): under 2 lb, 3 oz (1000 g)

According to the March of Dimes (2009) LBW is a factor in 65 percent of all neonatal deaths. In 2006, 8.3 percent of live births in the United States were LBW, 1.5 percent were VLBW, and 0.5 percent were ELBW. ELBW babies born at 27 weeks' gestational age or younger are highly susceptible to all the possible complications of preterm birth. Up to 50 percent of these infants die before hospital discharge (Jones & Carter, 2008). Because health problems increase with lower birth weights, it is important to learn a baby's gestational age and birth weight, even if it is months later and the baby appears to be healthy.

Baby's Appearance and Health Status

A preterm infant's skin is loose and wrinkled, with a gelatinous appearance. Blood vessels and bony structures are visible owing to very little subcutaneous fat. Fine downy hairs may be present on the sides of the face and on the forehead, back, and extremities. Hair on the baby's head is scanty, and there are usually no visible eyebrows. The baby's eyelids may still be fused (Figure 23.4). The ears may fold in many positions, lacking full development of the cartilage needed to support them. Because skull growth is complete before other body growth, the baby's head appears large in proportion to the rest of his body.

Despite the fact that the preterm infant's heart is usually well developed, the lungs and rib cage may not function efficiently at birth due to muscular weakness. Heat regulation is poorly developed, requiring that caregivers stabilize and carefully monitor the baby's body temperature. Due to immature liver and digestive systems and low levels of glucuronic acid, preterm infants tend to have a higher rate of physiological jaundice than do full-term

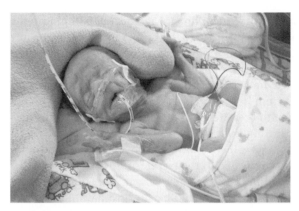

FIGURE 23.4   Infant born at 25 3/7 weeks, with eyes fused.
Source: Printed with permission of Leslie and Brad Jackson.

infants. (See Chapter 22 for an in-depth discussion on jaundice.) Because iron stores deposit during the last 6 weeks of pregnancy, babies who are born before that time probably require iron supplements. It is important to evaluate each baby for iron status, as all preterm infants do not automatically require iron supplements. Preterm infants also have higher risk for other health conditions (AAP, 2007), including:

- Respiratory distress syndrome (RDS)
- Chronic lung disease/bronchopulmonary dysplasia (BPD)
- Respiratory syncytial virus (RSV)
- Retinopathy of prematurity (ROP)
- Apnea and bradycardia
- Anemia of prematurity (low blood cell count)
- Heart murmurs

Feeding Effectiveness

It is important to evaluate each dyad for feeding effectiveness. Because of limited amounts of adipose tissue, small for gestational age or preterm infants often have problems regulating their blood sugar and body temperature. They frequently exhibit early feeding problems, and may require supplementation with their mother's expressed milk, donor milk, or with an artificial baby milk until their condition has stabilized and they begin to gain weight. Even after their condition stabilizes, these infants often require very frequent feedings, as if they are trying to gain the weight they should have gained in utero. These babies typically spend a lot of time at the breast, nursing frequently and for long periods.

Bottle feeding research reveals that sucking maturity and coordination peak at different times and different rates among preterm infants from 26 to 29 weeks' gestational age, with independent oral feeding from 34 to 38 weeks' gestational age (Amaizu et al., 2008). These findings may help explain a similar variance among 34- to 37-week preterm breastfeeders. Nyqvist (2008) observed that babies at 29 weeks' gestational age demonstrated obvious rooting and efficient areolar grasp. They repeated short sucking bursts from 29 weeks and occasional long sucking bursts and repeated swallowing from 31 weeks. These infants achieved full breastfeeding with adequate weight gain between 32 and 38 weeks (median, 35 weeks). Another study of bottle feeding measuring sucking strength suggests that significant neurobehavioral maturation occurs between 35 and 40 weeks' postconceptual age. Birth weight may also be a marker for feeding strength in the most preterm infants (Wrotniak et al., 2009).

Ability to Breastfeed

Practices differ for determining a preterm infant's physical ability to breastfeed. Readiness to breastfeed begins when the baby becomes stable, and each preterm infant needs an individual assessment irrespective of size or ability to suck on a bottle. Preterm infants are ready to breastfeed when they are able to coordinate sucking and swallowing (Nyqvist, 2008). They will put their fists to their mouths and feed with only occasional disruptions in breathing and heart rate.

Requirements for Readiness

Requiring a preterm infant to reach a certain weight before beginning to breastfeed is a questionable practice. Size does not necessarily correlate with an infant's ability to coordinate sucking, swallowing, and breathing—evidenced by the fact that sucking motions and swallowing of amniotic fluid occur early in gestation. For more on gestational development of newborn reflexes, refer to Table 13.2.

Many caregivers continue to withhold breastfeeding until the infant first "proves" the ability to bottle feed well. This practice, based on the premise that breastfeeding is more "stressful" for the preterm infant, has no basis in fact. Preterm infants who bottle feed actually have more oxygen desaturations during a feeding than breastfeeding infants and, as mentioned earlier, exhibit more episodes of apnea and bradycardia. Despite this, preterm babies in the United States typically may have breastfed only one to four times per day before discharge or may only achieve token breastfeeding. They rarely progress to complete direct breastfeeding before they go home.

Promoting Breastfeeding of the Preterm Infant

By keeping current on breastfeeding recommendations for preterm infants you can update NICU staff to ensure that they base their care on correct, evidence-based information. Presenting factual information to mothers does not allow for a "neutral" position regarding infant feeding.

Artificial feeding is clearly the suboptimal way to feed a baby. Withholding facts to avoid "making the mother feel guilty" keeps valuable information from parents and it is paternalistic and disempowering. Parents deserve to learn all the facts to make decisions based on current, evidence-based information.

Sisk et al. (2006) found anxiety and maternal stress levels of mothers of VLBW infants who initially planned to formula feed to be similar to those of mothers who intended to breastfeed. Of those who intended to formula feed, 85 percent initiated pumping. They provided at least 50 percent of their infants' enteral intake for the first 3 weeks and 32.8 percent did so for the entire stay. They all expressed appreciation that the staff helped them with milk expression.

Caregivers encountered by the mother while her baby is in the NICU can be very influential in promoting breastfeeding for her baby. Having a specific protocol that covers education, skin-to-skin time at the breast, non-nutritive sucking, and the transition to breastfeeding can make a difference (Table 23.3).

An evidence-based breastfeeding program (Meier et al., 2004) was initiated to provide education and support to mothers and their VLBW infants. Two years later, breastfeeding initiation was 72.9 percent. Outcomes for low-income African American women were the highest reported in the literature to that point. The outcomes approach the national health objective despite the mothers having had significant risk factors for initiating and sustaining lactation. These findings have important implications for clinicians, researchers, administrators, and policymakers.

Breastfeeding education about prematurity often focuses on the significant advantages that a mother's milk offers to her baby. It is helpful to point out these benefits to the mother. Only her milk is the same age as her baby, and it changes to meet her baby's changing needs. At a time when she can do little else for her baby, expressing her milk is something she can do to provide a valuable contribution to her baby's health and development.

Expressing Milk

A mother may feel overwhelmed by the birth of her preterm baby and need hands-on lessons in establishing lactation, supported by written instructions. Nursing staff on the postpartum unit can help her develop a plan for milk expression that meets her and her baby's needs until her baby can breastfeed directly. A mother who cannot breastfeed her preterm infant should begin to express milk within 6 hours of delivery (see Chapter 21 for a discussion on pumping for a hospitalized baby).

Because most NICUs encourage the use of human milk for babies, mothers may feel pressured to provide milk for their babies in the NICU. The family is overwhelmed and reeling from the shock of their baby's birth;

be careful not to focus on management of pumping to the exclusion of sensitivity to their other needs. It is probably the first time this mother has had to face pumping for a child. If she was planning to breastfeed, she anticipated settling comfortably into nursing after the birth, not separated from her baby and facing a crisis. Those who did not plan to breastfeed may need time to process the idea of expressing their milk. Mothers report that providing their milk gave them a way to be physiologically and emotionally connected to their preterm infant in the NICU. Expressed milk was "highly valued," but the separation placed pressure on the mother to "produce milk as integral to her sense of motherhood" (Sweet, 2008).

Initially, the mother may be able to express only a few drops of colostrum, and hand expression may work best for this small quantity. You can assure the mother that this is the normal progression for lactation, that the amount increases gradually, and that the initial small quantities provide essential health benefits to her baby. The mother's colostrum can be spoon-fed to her baby, if oral feedings are tolerated, or added to the NG or OG tube. The mother can also drip some colostrum onto a breast pad and place it in the isolette to familiarize her baby with her scent.

Frequent pumping in the early weeks determines the amount of milk the mother is able to produce long term (Groh-Wargo, 2009). It is, therefore, very important that the mother pump as often as she can in the first few days after birth. Research suggests that mothers with smaller storage capacities may need to pump more frequently (Kent et al., 2009, 1999; Mitoulas, 2004). A pumping diary can help a mother keep track of her efforts. An easy-to-read, full color primer is available from Lactnews.com.

To establish lactation the mother needs to express at least 8 to 10 times every 24 hours, with one session during the late evening or early morning hours. Recommend that she allow at least 10 to 15 minutes of expressing time for each breast, using a hospital-grade electric breast pump (Morton et al., 2009; Wight et al., 2009; Morton, 2004). If she pumps both breasts at the same time, she can pump for 10 to 15 minutes total time. Longer pumping sessions do not increase milk yield, though the mother can increase volume by pumping more frequently throughout the 24 hours. Adding hand expression before five of the daily pumpings and breast massage during pumping sessions has shown to lead to faster expression of milk and may produce increased amounts, especially after the mother's full milk production is established (Morton et al., 2009; Morton, 2004).

Mothers delivering extremely preterm infants appear sometimes to have delays initiating lactation and establishing adequate milk production (Wight & Morton, 2007; Hartmann, 2004; Cregan et al., 2002). Betamethasone, the corticosteroid administered to hasten preterm lung development, may have a negative impact on lactation. The effect appears to depend on how soon before birth the medication is administered (Henderson et al., 2009, 2008; Hartmann, 2004). Because this medication is vital to the preterm infant's lung maturity, withholding it is not an option. Be aware of this connection and follow these mothers closely.

Stimulating Letdown

Stimulating the milk-ejection reflex helps the mother obtain the greatest amount of milk in the least time. Sensory stimulation through a picture or piece of the baby's clothing can help. The use of auditory and visual relaxation is another method. Massaging the mother's back while she is pumping can promote milk ejection as well (Lang, 2002).

Some mothers have used galactogogues such as fenugreek or blessed thistle, or prescription medications such as metoclopramide or domperidone (Hale, 2010; Gabay, 2002). However, herbs or medicines that present no problem with full-term infants could be harmful to a very preterm or sick infant. They could also interact with medications the baby is receiving. For this reason, many neonatologists do not want mothers using herbal galactogogues. It is *crucial* that the mother discuss any planned galactogogue use with the neonatologist before use.

Fluctuations in Milk Production

The mother's milk production may fluctuate in response to her baby's condition, dropping in volume if the baby experiences a setback. Although her baby may be doing well medically, seeing other babies nearby who have debilitating, terminal conditions can be disheartening and overwhelming for mothers. Encourage mothers to take frequent breaks for fluids, nutrition, pumping, and walking outside the unit if possible.

Changes in a mother's lifestyle may also affect her milk production, especially for a mother who returns to work while her baby remains in the NICU. Over time, she may notice an unexplained decrease in volume or that it takes longer for her milk to let down. Sometimes the opposite is true, and the mother produces much more milk than her baby is able to use. Any excess milk can be stored for later use or donated to a milk bank to help other preterm and ill infants. Many mothers of preterm infants encounter problems with milk production and following up with these mothers is a high priority to support them through fluctuations in volume.

Significance of Human Milk for the Preterm Infant

Human milk can be vital to the progress of a high-risk infant, who is at risk for developing a variety of infections. Chapter 9 discusses the increased risk for infection in babies that do not receive human milk. Immunologi-cal properties in human milk can help protect preterm infants. Healthcare providers in the NICU setting need to emphasize the importance of the mother's milk for her high-risk infant and encourage the mother to provide her milk to her baby.

Many caregivers recommend that a preterm infant receive his mother's milk regardless of whether the mother planned to breastfeed. The World Health Organization's (1980) second choice for infant nutrition, after mother's own milk, is donor milk. The AAP (2005) also recommends donor milk if the mother is "unable or unwilling" to provide her milk for her baby. Like their full-term counterparts, artificially fed preterm infants have lower neurodevelopment than preterm infants fed human milk, including mature donor milk (Vohr et al., 2007, 2006; Lucas et al., 1998; 1994; Lucas et al., 1996). Artificial baby milk is associated with lower intelligence scores during childhood as well (Kramer et al., 2008; Smith, 2003). See Chapter 9 for more information on the specificity of human milk for human babies, and Chapter 21 for a discussion of human milk banking.

Health Importance to the Preterm Infant

Human milk helps establish enteral (through the digestive system) tolerance and allows for an earlier discontinuation of parenteral (intravenous) nutrition. Its laxative effect helps clear meconium, especially with the early milk, colostrum. The neurological outcomes from receiving human milk compared with artificial milk are especially important for babies born too early. Human milk has a higher antioxidant capacity than formula, and the oxidative stress associated with prematurity has been shown to be reduced by exclusive human milk feedings (Ledo et al., 2009). Although breastfeeding a preterm infant poses challenges in the early days and weeks, the challenges seem less imposing in light of the wealth of benefits provided by human milk and the avoidance of increased risks of artificial feeding.

In light of the health concerns that accompany prematurity, the mother's milk becomes all the more important to the baby. Human milk offers preterm infants the advantages of receiving physiological amino acids and fat. It provides greater bioavailability of nutrients, a lower renal solute load, enzymes to aid digestion, and anti-infective protection. Artificial milk greatly increases the incidence of necrotizing enterocolitis (NEC). As discussed in Chapter 9, human milk has the ideal protein balance for babies weighing 1500 g or more. Babies below that weight may need increased calories, carbohydrates, minerals, and proteins (Wight et al., 2008).

Human Milk Fortifiers

VLBW and ELBW infants present unique nutritional challenges. There is reasoned concern that human milk may not provide sufficient nutrition for preterm infants, especially VLBW under 1,500 g (Wight et al., 2008; Schanler, 2007; Wight & Morton, 2007; Landers, 2003). At issue are the calcium, phosphorus, and other requirements for the VLBW baby's bone growth. Without enough of these minerals, VLBW babies are at risk for osteopenia of prematurity, decreased bone mineral content that occurs mainly because of lack of adequate calcium, and phosphorus intake. VLBW babies also require higher amounts of fat-soluble vitamins because they have not laid down adequate stores before birth.

One solution to the baby's deficiency is to supplement with human milk fortifiers (HMF) containing protein, calcium, potassium phosphate, carbohydrates, vitamins, and trace minerals. Preterm infants fed human milk with human milk fortifiers have shown improved short-term weight gain and better linear and head growth over infants not fed human milk fortifiers (Kuschel & Harding, 2004; Schanler, 2007). The latest trend in nutritional supplementation is to give the preterm baby probiotics (Alfaleh et al., 2009; Lin et al., 2008), including *Bifidobacterium bifidum* and *Lactobacillus acidophilus*, in hopes of reducing necrotizing enterocolitis morbidity and mortality. Notably, lactobacillus has been cultured from mothers' milk.

Neonatologists and nutritionists continue to try to determine and refine nutritional requirements for these compromised infants. One concern is that human milk fortifiers derive from bovine proteins and therefore may pose some risk (see Chapter 9). Human milk fortifier was found contaminated with *Bacillus cereus* in one level III NICU with a cluster of 11 NEC infections. Seven patients had received human milk fortifiers before symptom onset, and nine had received one or more types of liquid formula (Wendelboe, 2010). Human milk fortifier without iron does not appear to change the antimicrobial effect of human milk, while the addition of iron reduced the antimicrobial effect against three types of bacteria and against *Candida* (Ovali et al., 2006).

Much of the research on human milk fortifiers is funded by the pharmaceutical industry. At least one firm, Prolacta Bioscience, markets human milk fortifier made from donated (noncompensated donor) human milk. Prolacta has also signed a marketing agreement with Abbott Nutritionals, a major artificial baby milk manufacturer (Prolacta Bioscience, 2009b). See Chapter 27 for more information and practice in analyzing scientific research.

Lactoengineering

Many breastfeeding advocates propose lactoengineering for preterm infants (also discussed in Chapter 9). Lactoengineering provides increased calories, carbohydrates, and proteins through the mother's hindmilk. Proteins and calcium in human milk can be separated (Czank et al.,

2009; Kent, 2004; Kent et al., 2009; Li, 2004). Creamatocrits estimate the fat and energy content of milk (Meier, 2003; Meier et al., 2002). The hindmilk that rises to the top is skimmed off and given to the baby for increased fat intake. Mothers can learn how to do this, thereby increasing their participation in their babies' care (Griffin et al., 2000). LBW infants in Nigeria grew well through lactoengineering (Slusher et al., 2003).

Human milk is clearly the nutrition of choice to promote neurodevelopment. Although the science of lactoengineering—the engineering of human milk—holds much promise for very preterm and sick babies, ethical issues exist as well. Human milk fortifiers for infants made from noncompensated donor human milk are now patented, manufactured, and sold to NICUs (Prolacta Bioscience, 2009a; Chan et al., 2007). Moreover, there are many patents on human milk components, owned primarily by the pharmaceutical industry (McClain, 2009). These ethical concerns continue to escalate as the outcomes from human milk use and human milk components are publicized. We cannot lose sight of the mother and baby in this application of technology. Health professionals in the lactation community need to protect the breastfeeding dyad as well as the fragile newborn.

Preserving the Safety of the Mother's Milk

Good maternal hygiene will ensure the safety of the mother's milk with consideration to the more fragile state of the preterm infant. Provide the mother with verbal and simple written instructions for pumping hygiene and care of her milk. Encourage her to shower daily, wash her hands thoroughly with soap before every pumping session, and dry them with paper towels that she can throw away.

The mother should immediately rinse pump parts exposed to her milk with cold water and then wash them in hot soapy water. Pump parts should be boiled daily and the milk should be stored in sterile, hard plastic or glass containers that maintain the integrity of her milk's composition. Individual NICUs have slightly different collection and storage guidelines and usually provide the mother with the desired containers. Therefore, the mother needs to store milk from each pumping session separately and label it according to the NICU's specifications. The mother should date the milk as well as the time of day it was pumped. She can ask how the hospital wishes to receive her milk and whether it should be fresh or frozen.

The hospital may request that she freeze her milk if the baby is unable to tolerate oral feedings or if the mother is unable to deliver the milk to her baby within 24 hours after she expresses it. Placing it in a cold, insulated container helps avoid thawing during transport. Freshly expressed milk is preferred for feedings when the baby is not yet able to breastfeed directly. The composition of fresh milk is most suitable for the baby, whereas frozen milk loses a portion of its protective properties, especially vitamin C. However, frozen milk is still preferable to an artificial substitute in terms of the nutrition and protection afforded the preterm infant.

Kangaroo Care

Kangaroo care, or kangaroo mother care, is a skin-to-skin care method that has moved from the fringe into the mainstream of neonatal medicine. Infants and parents benefit from kangaroo care, a method that places the baby skin to skin with his mother in close proximity to her breasts (Bergman, 2005). It allows the opportunity for the baby to become gently familiar with a new feeding environment and explore a new feeding method. Kangaroo care can begin as soon as the preterm baby's condition permits (Wight & Morton, 2007). Stable infants may begin kangaroo care even when they are still on a ventilator (Ludington-Hoe et al., 2003). Kangaroo care may actually assist in, rather than retard, recovery from respiratory distress (Swinth et al., 2003).

Kangaroo Method

For kangaroo care the mother places her baby clothed only in a diaper skin to skin, upright and prone, between her breasts. The baby and mother are then wrapped together to maintain the baby's body temperature adequately (Figure 23.5). The mother can wear a button-down shirt and no bra for ease of kangarooing. To avoid overstimulation she can sit quietly at first, with minimal or no talking, singing, stroking, or rocking. Often during this kangarooing, the baby initially is in a quiet alert state and then settles down to sleep. An interest in maintaining eye contact increases as the baby's condition improves.

Importance of Kangaroo Care

Kangaroo care offers many advantages to both the preterm baby and parents. A Cochrane review (Moore,

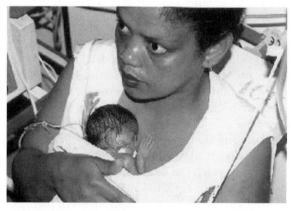

FIGURE 23.5 Kangaroo care between a mother and baby.
Source: Printed with permission of Dr. Nils Bergman.

2007) found statistically significant and positive effects of early skin-to-skin contact on breastfeeding duration. The skin-to-skin contact has a soothing effect on the baby and may contribute to the activation of central nervous system and brain function (Begum et al., 2008). The baby cries less, heart rate and respirations are more regular, and sleep periods improve. Oxygenation is better and the baby can maintain body temperature within acceptable levels (Ludington-Hoe et al., 2004). Babies who receive kangaroo care tend to gain weight faster (Suman, 2008) and leave the hospital earlier (Ruiz-Peláez et al., 2004). Kangaroo care is an affordable method of preterm care in developing countries. Survival for preterm LBW infants has been found to be significantly higher for babies receiving kangaroo care within the first 12 hours of life (Worku & Kassie, 2005).

The benefits of kangarooing are long term as well, with less crying noted at 6 months of age and a decreased rate of serious infection in the 6 months after kangaroo care (Sloan, 1994). Kangaroo care effectively decreases neonatal pain from heel sticks and promotes greater parental participation in caring for and comforting the baby (Johnston et al., 2003). Mothers feel more attached to their babies and more confident in caring for them when they use kangaroo care (Hurst, 1997). Kangarooing provides fathers the opportunity to bond with their baby as well and should be encouraged.

Kangaroo care increases the success of breastfeeding for the preterm infant. More of these babies were exclusively breastfed at the end of the Suman (2008) study (98 percent compared with 76 percent in conventional care). Time spent lying quietly by the breast—becoming familiar with the scent, sight, and sensations—gradually develops into rooting, licking, and tasting. This is a very important step in the baby's progress toward exclusive breastfeeding. As the baby becomes stronger and more alert, kangarooing leads to the baby latching onto the breast with active suckling. A small study showed greater improvement in milk production in mothers who practiced kangaroo care for about 4 hours per week than in mothers who did not practice this skin-to-skin contact (Hurst, 1997).

Transition to the Breast

NICU staff can support parents in their transition to breastfeeding by providing a conducive atmosphere and assisting them as needed. Parents can assist the baby's transition from gavage feedings to breastfeedings as well. The mother can continue to place drops of her milk on a breast pad and leave it in her baby's isolette to increase familiarity with her scent. During gavage feedings, she can hold her baby at her breast to increase the association with sucking and eating. Support and instruction from hospital staff at this critical time helps ensure a smooth transition for the baby and mother as they begin breast-feeding.

Initial Feedings

Encourage the mother to approach feedings in a relaxed and unhurried manner. Initial feedings at the breast for preterm infants involve only minimal feeding, interspersed with much resting time. Assure the mother that this is normal and expected. It is a time when she and her baby are getting to know one another, and it involves much practice at first. Ideally, the location should be quiet and private and near any needed equipment. The mother should avoid any unnecessary stimulation from bright lights, loud noises, or stroking, rocking, or talking to her baby. Too much outside stimulation can be overwhelming. Additionally, learning this new skill of feeding at the breast requires a great deal of the baby's attention. Any fussiness can be calmed through kangarooing the baby near the breast without focusing on feeding.

The mother can massage her breast before and during the feeding to encourage her baby to nurse. Some mothers use a breast pump to initiate milk flow. Holding her baby in the side-sitting (also football or clutch) or cross-cradle position enables her to see and handle her baby with optimal control. She can begin the feeding by holding her baby at the level of the breast and supporting his or her entire body. Jaw and cheek support can help increase the baby's milk intake. The mother can accomplish this by holding her breast with the Dancer hand position which supports her baby's jaw at the same time as she minimizes the weight of her breast in the baby's mouth (see Figure 14.3 in Chapter 14).

If her baby experiences gulping and choking, an adjustment in the mother's and baby's positions improves milk flow. The mother can hold her baby so the back of the throat is somewhat higher than the breast, or she can sit in a semi-reclined position. She can also express her milk before the feeding, which allows her baby to nurse with a less intense milk flow and enables the baby to "practice" sucking without being overwhelmed by milk.

Monitoring Intake and Weight

Your instruction and support during these early feedings are quite valuable to the mother, who may feel overwhelmed by this new experience. Mothers frequently worry about what to expect of their preterm baby and how to know they have enough milk. Learning how to determine when the baby is in a pattern of nutritive, or high-flow, sucks and swallows is reassuring to mothers. Mothers can also become familiar with the special devices used during the baby's transition to the breast. A tube-feeding device, for instance, may encourage more effective sucking at the breast.

The mother may need to follow early breastfeedings with supplementary feedings. For increased calories she can feed her baby the creamy portion of expressed milk that rises to the top or the hindmilk expressed after a breastfeeding. The neonatologist may recommend test weights to determine milk intake at the breast to calculate supplement needs. Electronic scales provide an accurate measurement of the preterm infant's milk intake at the breast (Meier et al., 1994, 1990). Test weights are reassuring and easy to perform (Hurst et al., 2004). You can provide mothers with encouragement about their progress with pumping and, eventually, breastfeeding.

Taking the Preterm Infant Home

When her baby is nearing hospital discharge, the mother's emotions can range from excitement and anticipation to apprehension and dread. The day she has been waiting for is finally approaching, and yet her baby still seems so fragile. Rooming-in with her baby in the hospital for several days before discharge eases this transition for the mother. It allows her to function independently, with help available when she needs it. Because nighttime care of the infant seems especially threatening to new parents, a 24-hour rooming-in is option is especially valuable.

Discharge Guidelines

Within certain parameters, preterm infants typically leave the hospital when they reach 35 weeks' gestational age. The infant must demonstrate a sucking reflex and have few respiratory problems. There must be no signs of disease or complications, and the baby must exhibit a weight gain of two-thirds to 1 ounce per day. Some hospitals discharge an infant as small as 3.5 pounds (1600 g) when the baby's condition allows it. ELBW babies (born at less than 2 pounds, 3 ounces [or 1000 g]), and babies who have serious medical complications such as respiratory, heart, or neurological problems remain hospitalized for a longer time.

Special Care at Home

Because a preterm baby requires special care at home, parents cannot treat their baby as they would a full-term baby simply because the baby has left the hospital. Preterm infants must be protected from infectious illness and other conditions that could compromise their health. The baby needs close medical supervision, particularly when medical problems are evident. Caution parents against expecting their baby to catch up very quickly developmentally. It may take as long as 2 years for a preterm baby to reach the developmental state of a full-term baby of the same age. However, the overall outlook for preterm babies is excellent, and more reach their full physical and mental potential than in the past.

Parents can explore the resources available for ongoing care, especially if their baby has developmental delays or neurological problems. Early intervention assistance programs through government, schools, and other organizations may be available (March of Dimes, 2009).

Test Weights

One of the main worries of mothers who take their preterm infant home is how to tell if direct breastfeeding provides enough milk. Kavanaugh et al. (1997, 1995) and Meier et al. (1994, 1990) recommend home use of electronic balance scales to help mothers recognize that their babies are consuming adequate milk. They contend this enables many mothers to continue breastfeeding who would have quit otherwise because their anxiety over milk transfer outweighed their desire to nurse.

Some breastfeeding supporters worry that the use of in-home test weights may imply that the mother's milk is inadequate. They see it as medicalizing breastfeeding and putting stress on the mother regarding her "performance." Although this concern has merit for a healthy, full-term baby, preterm or ill infants who may not feed effectively need close monitoring. Mothers studied reported that in-home measurement of milk intake by test weighing had been or would have been helpful (Hurst et al., 2004). Those who used scales experienced no increased stress or lower achievement of breastfeeding goals compared with mothers who did not perform test weights. Monitoring milk transfer reassures many mothers that their baby is getting enough milk.

As with any breastfeeding intervention or device, parents may consider the use of in-home scales for test weights as either a help or a hindrance. You can explain the rationale behind the test weights and empower the parents to choose what they wish to do. If the parents choose not to use in-home test weights, caution them to have frequent weight checks until their baby demonstrates a pattern of adequate weight gain.

Breastfeeding at Home

If the hospital does not provide outpatient breastfeeding follow-up, the mother should be referred to a community-based lactation consultant who can help her finalize the baby's transition to direct breastfeeding. Maintaining hospital routines for the first few days can help to ease the transition for both mother and baby. The mother needs to continue expressing her milk until her baby begins to breastfeed more frequently and more efficiently. She can then gradually decrease pumping time. If her baby required supplementation or special devices at discharge, she can discontinue these gradually as well.

Follow-up eases the mother's worries as she initiates these changes. She can weigh her baby periodically as the feeding routines change. Remind her that overt hunger cues and other infant expectations do not always apply to preterm infants. Encourage her to regard her baby's gestational age, rather than age from birth, as an indicator of what to expect. Table 23.4 provides suggestions for counseling the mother of a preterm infant.

Encouraging mothers to work toward the goal of direct breastfeeding may help them continue through the difficult time of what has been described as "triple feeding" that can overwhelm and discourage a mother. Triple feeding describes the time-consuming process of direct breastfeeding, then pumping, and then feeding the pumped milk to the baby. Anticipatory guidance about what to expect with the baby's feeding behaviors after discharge may help parents make this transition more comfortably. You can encourage the parents to watch for the "miracle day" of the baby's due date, a time when many preterm babies begin to feed effectively.

Some mothers never make the transition to direct breastfeeding. They pump for their babies in the NICU and continue to pump after discharge, feeling anxious or resistant to direct breastfeeding. The following are contributing factors to this practice (Buckley & Charles, 2006):

- Inadequate milk production
- Feelings of vulnerability and lack of confidence
- Infants' immature feeding behaviors
- Lack of commitment or desire to breastfeed before the birth
- Personal choice
- Bottle feeding more convenient
- Ability of father or other family members to participate in feedings
- Avoidance of feeling embarrassed feeding in public
- Ease of pumping and storing milk
- Parental need to quantify intake
- Lack of informational and emotional support

∽ Other Babies Not Born at Term

Preterm infants are not the only ones whose gestational age requires special care at birth. Some babies—referred to as late preterm—are born near the early range of 37 weeks. Others are born at the other extreme of 42 weeks—referred to as postterm or postmature. Both extremes call for special care of the newborn. The length of hospitalization and degree of care needed depend on the baby's condition and the number of weeks before or after term birth occurs. You can familiarize parents with the typical characteristics of these babies as well as implications for breastfeeding.

TABLE 23.4 Counseling the Mother of a Preterm Infant

Mother's Concern	Suggestions for Mother
Anxiety about taking a small baby home	• Continue close medical supervision of the baby.
Anxiety about beginning breastfeeding	• Keep realistic expectations. • Allow a transition period.
The baby tires easily at the breast	• Wake the baby frequently during breastfeeding. • Stimulate the baby to nurse. • Nurse frequently for short periods as long as the baby is suckling and swallowing. • Use a nipple shield.
Weak rooting reflex	• Provide skin-to-skin contact. • Turn the baby's head toward the breast. • Help the baby open his mouth. • Form the nipple and bring the baby to the breast.
Weak suck	• Use the Dancer hand position to increase intraoral negative pressure. • Use a nipple shield.
Intermittent sucking and resting during feedings	• Plan to allow a lengthy time for each feeding.
Nipple preference	• Express milk until letdown occurs. • Avoid artificial nipples. • Use an alternate feeding method when the mother is not present for feedings.
Difficulty interesting the baby in the breast	• Provide frequent skin contact and nuzzling. • Familiarize the baby with the smell of the mother's milk.
Difficulty positioning the baby at the breast	• Use pillows to bring the baby to breast level. • Use the side-sitting hold for positioning and the Dancer hand position under the baby's chin.
Difficulty determining whether the baby is getting enough milk	• Determine with NICU staff the number of wet diapers and stools to expect each day. • Plan a schedule of follow-up visits with the baby's primary care practitioner. • Determine the minimum feeding frequency to expect and what to do if the baby does not meet that goal. • Consider renting an electronic scale for daily weights at home. Plan with baby's practitioner what weight gain to expect. Learn from nursing staff how to determine accurate weights.

Late Preterm Infant

A late preterm infant is one born between the gestational ages of 34 weeks and 0/7 days through 36 weeks and 6/7 days. Gestational age should be rounded off to the nearest *completed* week, not to the following week. For example, an infant born on the 5th day of the 36th week (35 weeks and 5/7 days) is at a gestational age of 35 weeks, not 36 weeks (Raju, 2006). The term was changed from "near term" because of concerns that it conveyed the impression that these infants are "almost term." This misconception could result in underestimating risk, less-diligent evaluation, less monitoring, and less follow-up.

Because late preterm infants appear to be healthy and competent, they often receive the same treatment as full-term infants. They are typically cared for in the normal newborn nursery and go home with the mother at 48 to 72 hours postpartum. The baby is generally able to maintain body temperature, is at or above 2,500 g, and may appear to breastfeed well in the hospital.

Late preterm infants can have characteristics that affect their ability to breastfeed (Wight et al., 2008; Meier et al., 2007). These include cardiorespiratory instability, poor temperature control, metabolic instability, immunological and neurological immaturity, and immature oral motor development. As discussed in Chapter 22, late preterm infants comprise a large percentage of the kernicterus events in the United States (Bhutani & Johnson, 2006). They are also at higher percentage of risk than full-term babies for the following problems (Melamed et al., 2009):

- Increased risk of neonatal morbidity, including respiratory distress syndrome (4.2 compared with 0.1)
- Sepsis (0.4 compared with 0.04)
- Intraventricular hemorrhage (0.2 compared with 0.02)
- Hypoglycemia (6.8 compared with 0.4)
- Jaundice requiring phototherapy (18 compared with 2.5)

Problems After Discharge

A variety of problems can develop for late preterm infants after they leave the hospital. They may move quickly from a hyperalert state to deep sleep, give very subtle hunger cues or none at all, and have a difficult time tuning out excess stimulation. There may be poor neurological organization, with an immature rooting reflex and difficulty coordinating the suck-swallow-breathe cycle. Early delivery results in decreased albumin sites and therefore an increased risk for jaundice. This can lead to sleepiness and additional difficulty with effective milk transfer (Wight & Morton, 2007). There is a 5 to 10 percent risk of readmission to the hospital due to jaundice and/or weight loss.

A late preterm baby often has low muscle tone and finds it difficult to initiate and maintain the mother's milk production due to poor lip and cheek tone. Because of the early delivery, the baby did not accomplish full development of buccal fat pads and masseter muscles. There may be anatomical incompatibility due to the mother's nipple being too large for her baby's small mouth, making it difficult for the baby to maintain a seal on the breast. He may also be unable to attach far enough back on the breast to trigger an effective milk letdown. In addition, he tires more quickly and has difficulty drawing the nipple into his mouth, maintaining a good latch, and compressing the nipple during the sucking phase.

Breastfeeding Precautions

Parents need clear and consistent teaching about what to expect from their late preterm infant. It is important to make sure the baby nurses at least eight times in 24 hours. Many of these babies do better with shorter, more frequent feedings because they tire easily at the breast. They should go no longer than 3 hours between feedings during the day, with one longer stretch of 4 hours at night if they have achieved eight feedings in 24 hours. Mothers need to watch closely for subtle hunger cues and breastfeed as often as the baby indicates a need. Realizing that hunger cues may be subtle or lacking, parents can use gentle waking techniques and plenty of skin-to-skin contact to accomplish the appropriate number of feedings in a 24-hour period (see Figure 23.6). The parents need to count voids and stools until the baby has exhibited a pattern of robust weight gain without supplementation.

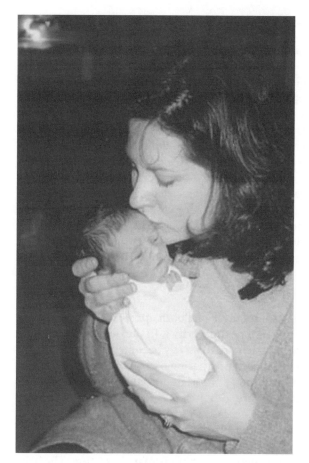

FIGURE 23.6   Mother with her late preterm infant.
Source: Printed with permission of Jan Riordan.

Physiologically, a late preterm baby is meant to be in utero sleeping and growing, not working at the breast for nourishment. Because of the baby's compromised condition, the mother cannot expect sucking alone to initiate and maintain sufficient milk production (Meier et al., 2007). The mother needs to express milk with an electric breast pump until the baby's due date arrives or until her baby is well over birth weight and milk production is well established. Pumping frequency depends on how effective her baby is at removing milk. If she pumps a minimal amount of milk after a feeding, the baby may be transferring milk well. If she pumps a significant amount of milk after a feeding, she will need to continue pumping to maintain lactation until the baby's breastfeeding ability matures and milk transfer improves. The baby's weight should be checked weekly during this time.

Some late preterm babies find it easier to transfer milk with the use of a nipple shield (Meier et al., 2000). It is important to have adequate follow-up if a nipple shield is used. Typically, however, these babies usually breastfeed well without a shield after they have grown and matured more. It often helps for mothers to realize that most late preterm babies seem to "wake up" and begin to breastfeed like term babies when they reach their due date.

Long-Term Outcomes

Researchers are reporting long-term outcomes for these infants in later life. They appear to have more school problems, including lower reading and math scores, and a greater need for special education (Chyi, 2008). Problems with visual processing and verbal skills have been observed (Baron et al., 2009), as well as a higher risk for developmental delay or disability (Morse et al., 2009). They also have higher rates of disability in prekindergarten and retention or suspension in kindergarten. Clearly, the problems associated with late preterm babies are not "transient," and the costs to society, families, and the healthcare system outweigh the convenience of elective inductions based on nebulous due dates and other nonmedical reasons (Clark et al., 2009).

Postterm Infant

A postterm infant is one born after 42 weeks' gestation. The danger of postmaturity is in the deterioration of the placenta, which progressively becomes less efficient after the normal gestation period of 37 to 42 weeks. Postterm infants may be appropriate for gestational age in body length but are often small-for-date because of the progressive decrease in placental function. Fetal oxygenation is marginal or depressed before labor, and meconium may be secreted during labor. Delivery may be through induction of labor or cesarean section. The baby has difficulty tolerating the stresses of labor and may struggle to maintain respiration, blood sugar levels, and nervous functioning. These situations generally are manageable.

The skin of some postterm infants is dry and cracked, with a texture similar to parchment paper. The skin is sagging and loose, with an absence of vernix. The baby may have profuse scalp hair as well as long fingernails and toenails. Meconium secretion produces a yellow-green staining of skin and nails.

The postterm baby may be sluggish during initial attempts at breastfeeding and may need coaxing and prodding much in the same way as a preterm baby. It is sometimes helpful to explain to the mother that even though born postterm, her baby may behave like a preterm baby initially. The strategies used to breastfeed a late preterm infant usually work well with these babies. As postterm babies put on weight, their feeding behaviors mature.

∼ Counseling a Mother Whose Baby Has Died

Perhaps the most distressing situation you will encounter professionally is caring for a mother who has lost her baby. At such a time it seems impossible to find the right words as you try to avoid painful remarks and express sensitive support. Appropriate counseling techniques, insight into the mother's emotions, and sincere empathy enable you to approach the situation comfortably, more confident in your ability to support the mother in her grief. Key components of bereavement counseling include validating the family's grief, facilitating rituals, providing mementos, and encouraging them to tell their stories (Capitulo, 2005). Although nothing can bring back their baby, sensitive and appropriate intervention can aid in healing.

Parents have specific practical needs in addition to their emotional and spiritual needs when their baby dies (Meert, 2008):

- The need for privacy
- The need for access to their child
- Opportunities to participate in their child's care
- Self-care such as a place to eat, shower, and sleep
- Physical presence of professional and personal support

What to Say to the Mother

If a grieving mother wants to talk, it is important to listen to her express her experience, without interruptions or interpretations. After listening to her relate what happened, you can let her know how sad you feel. Avoid telling her, "I know how you must feel" or "I can imagine what you are going through." You cannot begin to know what the mother is feeling unless you have experienced a similar loss. Even if you have also lost a child, this is *not* the time to talk about your own loss. Referring to your experience takes the focus off the mother's grief and minimizes it.

You can reflect back to the mother how you imagine she must feel. Appropriate statements may be "This is so heartbreaking," or, "I can't imagine the loss you feel." You can say something like, "There is nothing more painful than what you are feeling right now," or simply, "I am so sorry for your loss." Responses such as this validate her pain without taking the focus off her and her baby.

At the appropriate time you can share with the mother that other mothers who have suffered similar losses have found it helpful to talk through their feelings. This may not occur during the hospital stay and may be days or weeks later. Her grief could continue without resolution until she shares her feelings and works through them. People closest to the mother sometimes feel uncomfortable listening to her relate her birth experience and the circumstances surrounding her baby's death. She may appreciate being able to turn to you, knowing that you are concerned and interested in listening to her. Let her know you are glad to listen, assuring her that you do not want to invade her privacy.

Having an insight into the mother's feelings helps you determine how to best support her. For many mothers bonding and maternal feelings begin the day they learn they are pregnant or when they first hear their baby's heartbeat. Parents need others to acknowledge that their baby, even though born very young or stillborn, was loved before birth and was a person who meant a lot in their lives. Avoid comments such as, "At least you can have more children" or "It was for the best." Also offensive is the idea that a miscarriage or stillbirth is "nature's way" of dealing with a birth defect. The mother might rather care for an "imperfect" baby than no baby at all. The thought of replacing her deceased baby with a new one is no consolation to her right now. She is grieving for the baby she just lost. You can acknowledge her baby's importance by asking his or her name and using it during your discussion.

Grieving for Their Loss

Parental grief over the loss of a child is more intense than losing a spouse or an adult child losing a parent (Middleton et al., 1998). Parents progress through several stages of grief before their loss is resolved, typically beginning with denial and ending in acceptance of the loss. The range of emotions they experience between these two extremes appears in Figure 23.2. The time it takes parents to move from denial to acceptance varies greatly and could take as long as 3 or 4 years (Murphy, 2003). Making sense of the loss is an important predictor of grief intensity (Keesee, et al., 2008). Parents never truly "get over" the loss of a child. Their lives are irrevocably changed, and parents hold on to their relationship with their deceased child (Davies, 2004). It is never appropriate to minimize the loss of a child, even after decades have passed.

If the parents have other children, it is important they communicate openly and honestly with them about their sibling dying. Although the baby's life may be brief, consequences for survivor siblings can be life-long. Siblings born both before and after the death of an infant may be at risk and in need of psychological support. Poor family communication, unresolved parental mourning, and anxiety about their mother's health were among the issues reported by grown siblings of babies who had died. Photos and family rituals were helpful to both siblings and parents in grieving and remembering the infant. When age appropriate, clinicians should allow siblings to be active participants in the infant's brief life and death (Fanos et al., 2009).

Acceptance of the loss depends on the amount of support and understanding the parents receive from friends and family. The mother may need to talk about her baby long after most people have tired of hearing it. You may be a person she feels will be receptive, especially if you formed a bond with her. Try to key into the mother's needs and sense how often she would like to hear from you. It may be much easier for her to receive a call than to initiate a call and worry that she is bothering you. The list in Table 23.5 will help you choose your comments carefully.

Breastfeeding Concerns

A mother who has lost a child may have concerns specific to breastfeeding, especially if she and her baby were nursing. Even if she had not yet breastfed, the mother's breasts

---

TABLE 23.5 Counseling Grieving Parents

Helpful responses:

- Showing genuine concern and caring
- Listening and empathizing
- Saying you are sorry about what happened
- Allowing the mother to express her grief
- Encouraging parents to be patient with themselves
- Allowing the mother to talk about her baby
- Pointing out special qualities of the baby she lost
- Acknowledging the impact of the baby's death
- Reassuring the parents that they did everything possible for their baby
- Referring to the baby by name
- Showing your sadness and disappointment

Unhelpful responses:

- Allowing your sense of discomfort or helplessness to prevent you from reaching out to the mother
- Suggesting you know how the mother feels
- Suggesting the mother will feel better after some time
- Appearing to tell parents what they should feel or do
- Changing the subject when the baby is mentioned
- Trying to find something positive about the baby's death
- Remarking that the parents can have other children
- Suggesting that parents should be grateful for other children they have
- Suggesting that the baby's care by the parents or medical personnel was inadequate
- Avoiding use of the baby's name for fear of causing pain for the mother
- Appearing overly cheerful or casual

may fill with milk a few days after delivery and can become engorged and painful. Your anticipatory guidance will help her through this process. She can relieve the fullness without stimulating her breasts to the extent that she produces more milk, by expressing only enough to relieve discomfort. She can use the same comfort measures as for engorgement (see Chapter 16). Continuous application of cabbage leaves to the breasts promotes the milk drying up and offers the mother relief. She can replace the cabbage leaves about every 2 to 3 hours, or once they have wilted. Ibuprofen, if approved by her caregiver, and ice packs may also help relieve pain.

A mother who has been pumping to maintain milk production for a preterm or ill baby will have more difficulty ending lactation. She needs to continue pumping and decrease slowly in a weaning pattern to avoid problems associated with abrupt weaning. A mother who was nursing her baby may also need to express milk to decrease milk production gradually. Mothers who nursed or expressed milk for their babies often find comfort in knowing they gave their babies the best possible care, both nutritionally and emotionally. Many bereaved mothers donate their milk to a milk bank for a period of time. Donating milk to help save another baby's life can add to the mother's emotional healing. You can suggest this to the mother and put her in contact with the nearest milk bank, if she is interested.

Support for Parents

Healthcare providers are better able to support healing care when they are trained in perinatal loss. Caregivers can demonstrate a caring presence to parents through their words and actions by creating opportunities for the parents to meet their needs (Meert et al., 2005). Parents have a need to stay connected with their child at the time of death. They need time and privacy with their family to begin grieving for their loss. They have the right to hold or see their baby after the demise. If they elect to visit with their baby before discharge, a staff member can bring the baby to the mother's room wrapped in warm blankets. This practice is particularly helpful for parents of a stillborn infant.

Parents benefit from memories and mementos that bring them comfort in the future. Many hospitals provide memory boxes to hold mementos of the baby's birth. Pictures can help parents put their baby's death into perspective. Offering parents an opportunity to take pictures can provide them with a treasured image of their child. Some hospitals take pictures of the deceased infant for parents to keep. A staff member can cleanse, dress, and swaddle the infant for the pictures. This can be especially important to parents who choose not to see their infant at the time of death. Often, these parents have the desire to see their baby months later, when it is too late. Giving parents their infant's identification bracelet is further validation of his importance to them as a family member and another memento of their brief time with him.

Encourage parents to seek information about their options with hospital personnel and their baby's caregiver. If requested, hospital chaplains typically baptize stillborn infants. Some hospitals have nurses or other staff authorized to baptize a baby. Hospital staff can also arrange for the baby's transfer to a funeral home. Caregivers, especially the mother's midwife or labor nurse, often attend the funeral. If you have cared for the mother and baby, your attendance is appropriate and acknowledges the baby's importance. Your presence means a lot to families, even if they are not able to express their appreciation at the time.

Parents who lose a child may find comfort through altruistic acts such as organ donation, volunteer work, and charitable fund raising. Connection with others is important to their spiritual healing. Connecting with other parents who experienced a similar loss can help them and encourage them to express their feelings. Becoming involved in a support group can help them heal while they maintain connection with their baby (Meert et al., 2005). They may benefit from professional counseling, available through local clergy and social service organizations. Long after time passes parents may continue to need to talk about their loss. They benefit from the ongoing support they receive from other parents and professionals in a support group. There are many support groups for grieving parents, often affiliated with a hospital or medical center. Two such programs are Compassionate Friends (www.compassionatefriends.org) and Resolve Through Sharing (www.bereavementprograms.com).

〜 Summary

Lactation consultants are valuable members of the healthcare team caring for the high-risk infant. You are a significant advocate and resource for parents of a high-risk infant, even after discharge. You can help the mother provide her milk for her baby's care and make the transition to breastfeeding. You can support the mother as she works through her feelings related to this unexpected outcome, feelings that encompass much more than breastfeeding. Your support helps her develop realistic expectations and plan for her baby's nutrition. This may occur long before her baby is able to breastfeed directly. You can guide the mother through the initiation of pumping and handling her stored milk. Be available to her to support early breastfeeding and to guide her through the transition of bringing her baby home from the hospital. Compassion and experience help you support a mother whose baby has died. Your participation in the mother's healthcare team is critical in these special circumstances.

∼ Chapter 23—At a Glance

Applying what you learned—

Concerns of parents of a high-risk infant:

- Initiating and maintaining milk production
- A delay in breastfeeding
- Worry about the baby's survival
- Feelings of guilt, loneliness, and anxiety
- Strain on their relationship
- Desire for privacy and time alone with their baby

Counseling preterm parents in the hospital:

- Ask the baby's caregivers for explanations and clarification.
- Seek out sources of support and community resources.
- Provide gentle, warm, and loving touch.
- Express milk for their baby.
- Participate in feeding, bathing, and diapering their baby.
- Kangaroo their preterm infant.
- Encourage nonnutritive sucking on an emptied breast.

Counseling preterm parents at home:

- Read hunger cues and infant responses that show signs of overstimulation.
- Plan for frequent feedings at home with long periods of rest.
- Stimulate letdown and manage fluctuations in milk production.
- Support the baby's jaw with the Dancer hand position.
- Monitor the baby's intake and weight at home.
- Base expectations on gestational age, rather than age from birth.

Counseling late preterm parents:

- Plan for short, frequent feedings.
- Allow no longer than 3 hours between feedings during the day.
- Watch closely for subtle hunger cues.
- Use gentle waking techniques and plenty of skin-to-skin contact.
- Use a nipple shield as necessary.

Counseling parents who lose a baby:

- Help them arrange time and privacy with their baby.
- Express your concern and sorrow.
- Use reflective listening and be available.

- Key into the mother's needs and sense how often she would like to hear from you.
- Help the mother relieve fullness without stimulating more milk.
- Refer the mother to a milk bank if she wishes to donate milk.
- Refer parents to a support system and help them learn their rights and options.

∼ References

Abouelfettoh A, et al. Cup versus bottle feeding for hospitalized late preterm infants in Egypt: a quasi-experimental study. *Int Breastfeed J.* 2008;3:27.

Academy of Breastfeeding Medicine. Clinical protocol number #1: transitioning the breastfeeding/breastmilk-fed premature infant from the neonatal intensive care unit to home, 2004. www.bfmed.org. Accessed October 15, 2009.

Alfaleh K, et al. Probiotics reduce the risk of necrotizing enterocolitis in preterm infants: a meta-analysis. *Neonatology.* 2009;97:93-99.

Amaizu N, et al. Maturation of oral feeding skills in preterm infants. *Acta Paediatr.* 2008;97:61-7.

American Academy of Pediatrics (AAP). Parenting corner Q&A: premature infants. April 2007. http://www.aap.org/publiced/BR_Preemie_HealthRisks.htm. Accessed October 27, 2008.

American Academy of Pediatrics (AAP). Work Group on Breastfeeding. Breastfeeding and the use of human milk. *Pediatrics.* 2005;115(2):496-506.

Anderson G. Current knowledge about skin to skin (kangaroo) care for preterm infants. *Breastfeeding Rev.* 1993;8:364-373.

Anderson G. Skin to skin: kangaroo care in Western Europe. *Am J Nurs.* 1989;89:662-666.

Arockiasamy V, et al. Fathers' experiences in the neonatal intensive care unit: a search for control. *Pediatrics.* 2008;121:e215-e222.

Arora J, et al. Effect of oil massage on growth and neurobehavior in very low birth weight preterm neonates. *Indian Pediatr.* 2005;11:1092-1100.

Baron I, et al. Visuospatial and verbal fluency relative deficits in 'complicated' late-preterm preschool children. *Early Hum Dev.* 2009;85(12):751-754.

Begum E, et al. Cerebral oxygenation responses during kangaroo care in low birth weight infants. *BMC Pediatr.* 2008;8:51.

Bergman N. Kangaroo mother care. Overview: physiology and research of KMC; January 27, 2005. www.kangaroomothercare.com. Accessed October 28, 2009.

Bhutani V, Johnson L. Kernicterus in late preterm infants cared for as term healthy infants. *Sem Perinatol.* 2006;30:89-97.

Birch J, Newell S. Gastroesophageal reflux disease in preterm infants: current management and diagnostic dilemmas. *Arch Dis Child Fetal Neonatal Ed.* 2009;94:F379-F383.

Birnbaum R, Limperopoulos C. Nonoral feeding practices for infants in the neonatal intensive care unit. *Adv Neonatal Care.* 2009;9:180-184.

Blaymore-Bier J, et al. Breastfeeding infants who were extremely low birth weight. *Pediatrics*. 1997;100:E3.

Boekel S. Gastroesophageal reflux: the breastfeeding family's nightmare. Presentation at ILCA International Conference, Washington, DC, July 27, 2000.

Boss R, et al. Adolescent mothers in the NICU: how much do they understand? *J Perinatol*. 2010;30(4):286-290.

Brown G. NICU noise and the preterm infant. *Neonatal Netw*. 2009;28(3):165-173.

Buckley K, Charles G. Benefits and challenges of transitioning preterm infants to at-breast feedings. *Int Breastfeed J*. 2006; 1:13.

Capitulo K. Evidence for healing interventions with perinatal bereavement. *MCN Am J Matern Child Nurs*. 2005;30:389-396.

Chan G, et al. Effects of a human milk-derived human milk fortifier on the antibacterial actions of human milk. *Breastfeeding Med*. 2007;2:205-208.

Chen C, et al. The effect of breast- and bottle feeding on oxygen saturation and body temperature in preterm infants. *J Hum Lact*. 2000;16:21-27.

Chin N, Solomonik A. Inadequate: a metaphor for the lives of low-income women? *Breastfeed Med*. 2009;4:S41-S43.

Chyi L. School outcomes of late preterm infants: special needs and challenges for infants born at 32 to 36 weeks gestation. *J Pediatr*. 2008;153:25-31.

Clark S, et al. Neonatal and maternal outcomes associated with elective term delivery. *Am J Obstet Gynecol*. 2009;200: 156.e1-156.e4.

Cleveland LM. Parenting in the neonatal intensive care unit. *JOGNN*. 2008;37:666-691.

Collins C, et al. Avoidance of bottles during the establishment of breast feeds in preterm infants. *Cochrane Database Syst Rev*. 2008;CD005252.

Cregan M, et al. Initiation of lactation in women after preterm delivery. *Acta Obstet Gynaecol Scand*. 2002;81:870-877.

Czank C, et al. A method for standardizing the fat content of human milk for use in the neonatal intensive care unit. *Int Breastfeed J*. 2009;4:3.

Dall'Oglio I, et al. Breastfeeding promotion in neonatal intensive care unit: impact of a new program toward a BFHI for high-risk infants. *Acta Paediatr*. 2007;96(11):1626-1631.

Darcy A, et al. A descriptive study of noise in the neonatal intensive care unit: ambient levels and perceptions of contributing factors. *Adv Neonatal Care*. 2008;8(5 Suppl): S16-S26.

Davies R. New understandings of parental grief: literature review. *J Adv Nurs*. 2004;46:506-513.

Di Fiore J, et al. Technical limitations in detection of gastroesophageal reflux in neonates. *J Pediatr Gastroenterol Nutr*. 2009;49:177-182.

Dougherty D, Luther M. Birth to breast—a feeding care map for the NICU: helping the extremely low birth weight infant navigate the course. *Neonat Netw*. 2008;27:371-377.

Dyer K. Identifying, understanding, and working with grieving parents in the NICU, Part I: identifying and understanding loss and the grief response. *Neonat Netw*. 2005a;24:35-46.

Dyer K. Identifying, understanding, and working with grieving parents in the NICU, Part II: strategies. *Neonat Netw*. 2005b;24:27-40.

Fanos J, et al. Candles in the snow: ritual and memory for siblings of infants who died in the intensive care nursery. *J Pediatr*. 2009;154:849-853.

Gabay M. Galactagogues: medications that induce lactation. *J Hum Lact*. 2002;18:274-279.

Goines L. The importance of quiet in the home: teaching noise awareness to parents before the infant is discharged from the NICU. *Neonatal Netw*. 2008;27(3):171-176.

Gomes C, et al. Surface electromyography of facial muscles during natural and artificial feeding of infants. *J Pediatr*. 2006;82:103-109.

Gonzalez A, et al. Weight gain in preterm infants following parent-administered Vimala massage: a randomized controlled trial. *Am J Perinatol*. 2009;26:247-252.

Griffin T. Family-centered care in the NICU. *J Perinat Neonatal Nurs*. 2006;20:98-102.

Griffin T, et al. Mothers' performing creamatocrit measures in the NICU: accuracy, reactions, and cost. *JOGNN*. 2000;29: 249-257.

Groh-Wargo S, Sapsford A. Enteral nutrition support of the preterm infant in the neonatal intensive care unit. *Nutr Clin Pract*. 2009;24(3):363-376.

Hale T. *Medications and Mothers' Milk*, 14th ed. Amarillo, TX: Hale Publishing; 2010.

Hartmann P. Initiation and establishment of lactation with special reference to mothers who deliver pre-term. Presented at the Amarillo Conference on Human Lactation: Current Research and Clinical Implications: Breastmilk for Preterm Babies, Amarillo, Texas, October 21, 2004.

Henderson J, et al. Effect of preterm birth and antenatal corticosteroid treatment on lactogenesis II in women. *Pediatrics*. 2008;121:e92-e100.

Henderson J, et al. Effects of antenatal corticosteroids on urinary markers of the initiation of lactation in pregnant women. *Breastfeed Med*. 2009;4:201-206.

Ho Y, et al. The impact of massage therapy on motor outcomes in very low birth weight infants: a randomized controlled pilot study. *Pediatr Int*. Sep 15, 2009. [Epub ahead of print]

Howland L. Preterm birth: implications for family stress and coping. *Newborn Infant Nurs Rev*. 2007;7:14-19.

Hurst N. Skin to skin holding in the NICU influences maternal milk volume. *J Perinatol*. 1997;17:213-217.

Hurst N, et al. Mothers performing in-home measurement of milk intake during breastfeeding of their preterm infants: maternal reactions and feeding outcomes. *J Hum Lact*. 2004;20:178-187.

Johnson A. Engaging fathers in the NICU: taking down the barriers to the baby. *J Perinat Neonatal Nurs*. 2008;22:302-306.

Johnston C, et al. Kangaroo care is effective in diminishing pain response in preterm neonates. *Arch Pediatr Adolesc Med*. 2003;157:1084-1088.

Jones P, Carter B. Resuscitating the extremely low-birth-weight infant: humanitarianism or hubris? *AMA J Ethics Virtual Mentor*. 2008;10:665-669.

Kavanaugh K, et al. Getting enough: mothers' concerns about breastfeeding a preterm infant after discharge. *JOGNN*. 1995;24:23-32.

Kavanaugh K, et al. The rewards outweigh the efforts: breastfeeding outcomes for mothers of preterm infants. *J Hum Lact*. 1997;13:15-21.

Keesee N, et al. Predictors of grief following the death of one's child: the contribution of finding meaning. *J Clin Psychol.* 2008;64(10):1145-1163.

Kent J. Breastmilk calcium for the pre-term baby. Presented at the Amarillo Conference on Human Lactation: Current Research and Clinical Implications, Breastmilk for Pre-term Babies, Amarillo, Texas, October 22, 2004.

Kent J, et al. Why calcium in breastmilk is independent of maternal dietary calcium and vitamin D. *Breastfeed Rev*17: 5-11; 2009.

Kent J, et al. Breast volume and milk production during extended lactation in women. *Exp Physiol.* 1999;84:435-447.

Klaus M, et al. *Bonding: Building the Foundations of Secure Attachment and Independence.* New York: Perseus; 2000.

Kramer M, et al. Promotion of Breastfeeding Intervention Trial (PROBIT) Study Group. Breastfeeding and child cognitive development: new evidence from a large randomized trial. *Arch Gen Psych.* 2008;65:578-584.

Kumar A, et al. Spoon feeding results in early hospital discharge of low birth weight babies. *J Perinatol.* 2010;30(3):209-217.

Kuschel C, Harding J. Multicomponent fortified human milk for promoting growth in preterm infants. *Cochrane Database Syst Rev.* 2004;1:CD000343.

Landers S. Maximizing the benefits of human milk feeding for the preterm infant. *Pediatr Ann.* 2003;32:5.

Lang S. *Breastfeeding Special Care Babies*, 2nd ed. London: Bailliere Tindall; 2002.

Ledo A, et al. Human milk enhances antioxidant defenses against hydroxyl radical aggression in preterm infants. *Am J Clin Nutr.* 2009;89:210-215.

Li C. Variations in the composition of breastmilk and its fortification for pre-term babies. Presented at the Amarillo Conference on Human Lactation: Current Research and Clinical Implications, Breastmilk for Pre-term Babies, Amarillo, Texas, October 22, 2004.

Lin H, et al. Oral probiotics prevent necrotizing enterocolitis in very low birth weight preterm infants: a multicenter, randomized, controlled trial. *Pediatrics.* 2008;122:693-700.

Lucas A, et al. A randomized multicenter study of human milk versus formula and later development in preterm infants. *Arch Child Dis.* 1994;70:F141-F146.

Lucas A, et al. Breast milk and subsequent intelligence quotient in children born preterm. *Lancet.* 1992;339:261-264.

Lucas A, et al. Randomized outcome trial of human milk fortification and developmental outcome in preterm infants. *Am J Clin Nutr.* 1996;64(2):142-151.

Lucas A, et al. Randomised trial of early diet in preterm babies and later intelligence quotient. *BMJ.* 1998;317:1481-1487.

Ludington-Hoe S, et al. Randomized controlled trial of kangaroo care: cardiorespiratory and thermal effects on healthy preterm infants. *Neonat Netw.* 2004;23:39-48.

Ludington-Hoe S, et al. Safe criteria and procedure for kangaroo care with intubated preterm infants. *J Obstet Gynecol Neonatal Nurs.* 2003;32:579-588.

March of Dimes. www.marchofdimes.com. Accessed November 1, 2009.

Massaro A, et al. Massage with kinesthetic stimulation improves weight gain in preterm infants. *J Perinatol.* 2009;29:352-357.

McClain V. Human milk patent pending. What's wrong with patenting human milk components? October 28, 2009.

http://vwmcclain.blogspot.com. Accessed November 1, 2009.

McNeil D. The incidence and correlates of feeding problems in premature infants post neonatal intensive care. University of Calgary, Department Of Community Health Sciences. Calgary, Alberta. July 2008. http://dspace.ucalgary.ca/bitstream/1880/46809/1/McNeil_2008.pdf. Accessed October 28, 2009.

Meert K. Exploring parents' environmental needs at the time of a child's death in the pediatric intensive care unit. *Pediatr Crit Care Med.* 2008;9:623-628.

Meert K, et al. The spiritual needs of parents at the time of their child's death in the pediatric intensive care unit and during bereavement: a qualitative study. *Pediatr Crit Care Med.* 2005;6:420-427.

Meier P. Bottle and breastfeeding: effects on transcutaneous oxygen pressure and temperature in preterm infants. *Nurs Res.* 1988;37:36-41.

Meier P. Supporting lactation in mothers with very low birth weight infants. *Pediatr Ann.* 2003;32:317-325.

Meier P, et al. A new scale for in-home test-weighing for mothers of preterm and high risk infants. *J Hum Lact.* 1994;10:163-168.

Meier P, et al. Increased lactation risk for late preterm infants and mothers: evidence and management strategies to protect breastfeeding. *J Midwifery Womens Health.* 2007;52: 579-587.

Meier P, et al. Mothers' milk feedings in the neonatal intensive care unit: accuracy of the creamatocrit technique. *J Perinatol.* 2002;22:646-649.

Meier P, et al. Nipple shields for preterm infants: effect on milk transfer and duration of breastfeeding. *J Hum Lact.* 2000; 16:106-114.

Meier P, et al. The accuracy of test weighing for preterm infants. *J Pediatr Gastroenterol Nutr.* 1990;10:62-65.

Meier P, et al. The Rush Mothers' Milk Club: breastfeeding interventions for mothers with very-low-birth-weight infants. *JOGNN.* 2004;33:164-174.

Melamed N, et al. Short-term neonatal outcome in low-risk, spontaneous, singleton, late preterm deliveries. *Obstet Gynecol.* 2009;114(2 Pt 1):253-260.

Melnyk B, et al. Reducing premature infants' length of stay and improving parents' mental health outcomes with the Creating Opportunities for Parent Empowerment (COPE) neonatal intensive care unit program: a randomized, controlled trial. *Pediatrics.* 2006;118:e1414-e1427.

Melnyk BM, Feinstein NF. Reducing hospital expenditures with the COPE (Creating Opportunities for Parent Empowerment) program for parents and premature infants: an analysis of direct healthcare neonatal intensive care unit costs and savings. *Nurs Adm Q.* 2009;33:32-37.

Middleton W, et al. A longitudinal study comparing bereavement phenomena in recently bereaved spouses, adult children and parents. *Aust N Z J Psychiatry.* 1998;32:235-241.

Mitoulas L. Pumping frequency and duration and milk yields in preterm mothers. Presented at the Amarillo Conference on Human Lactation: Current Research and Clinical Implications, Breastmilk for Pre-term Babies, Amarillo, Texas, October 21, 2004.

Moore E, et al. Early skin-to-skin contact for mothers and their healthy newborn infants. *Cochrane Database Syst Rev.* 2007;(3):CD003519.

Morse S, et al. Early school-age outcomes of late preterm infants. *Pediatrics*. 2009;123:e622-e629.

Morton J. Breastfeeding the preterm infant: lessons for all. Presented at the Amarillo Conference on Human Lactation: Current Research and Clinical Implications, Breastmilk for Pre-term Babies, Amarillo, Texas, October 21, 2004.

Morton J, et al. Combining hand techniques with electric pumping increases milk production in mothers of preterm infants. *J Perinatol*. 2009;29:757-764.

Murphy S, et al. Bereaved parents' outcomes 4 to 60 months after their children's deaths by accident, suicide, or homicide: a comparative study demonstrating differences. *Death Studies*. 2003;27:39-61.

Nyqvist K. Early attainment of breastfeeding competence in very preterm infants. *Acta Paediatr*. 2008;97:776-781.

Nyqvist K, Engvall G. Parents as their infant's primary caregivers in a neonatal intensive care unit. *J Pediatr Nurs*. 2009;24:153-163.

Nyqvist K, et al. The development of preterm infants' breastfeeding behavior. *Early Hum Dev*. 1999;55:247-264.

Ovali F, et al. Effects of human milk fortifier on the antimicrobial properties of human milk. *J Perinatol*. 2006;26:761-763.

Parker K. The harried life of the working mother. Pew Research Center, October 1, 2009. www.pewsocialtrends.org. Accessed October 22, 2009.

Pinelli J, Symington A. Non-nutritive sucking for promoting physiologic stability and nutrition in preterm infants. *Cochrane Database Syst Rev*. 2005;4:CD001071.

Pohlman S. The primacy of work and fathering preterm infants: findings from an interpretive phenomenological study. *Adv Neonatal Care*. 2005;5(4):204-216.

Prolacta Bioscience. www.prolacta.com. Accessed February 15, 2010.

Prolacta Bioscience. Abbott co-promotion agreement frequently asked questions; October 4, 2009b. http://www.prolacta.com/faq_abbott.php. Accessed February 15, 2010.

Raju T. Epidemiology of late preterm (near-term) births. *Clin Perinatol*. 2006;33(4):751-763; abstract vii.

Renfrew M, et al. Breastfeeding promotion for infants in neonatal units: a systematic review. *Child Care Health Dev*. 2010;36(2):165-178.

Ruiz-Peláez J, et al. Kangaroo mother care, an example to follow from developing countries. *BMJ*. 2004;329:1179-1181.

Schanler RJ. Evaluation of the evidence to support current recommendations to meet the needs of premature infants: the role of human milk. *Am J Clin Nutr*. 2007;85:625S-628S.

Shaker C, Woida A. An evidence-based approach to nipple feeding in a level III NICU: nurse autonomy, developmental care, and teamwork. *Neonatal Netw*. 2007;26(2):77-83.

Sisk P, et al. Lactation counseling for mothers of very low birth weight infants: effect on maternal anxiety and infant intake of human milk. *Pediatrics*. 2006;117:e67-e75.

Sloan N, et al. Kangaroo mother method: randomized controlled trial of an alternative method of care for stabilised low-birthweight infants. Maternidad Isidro Ayora Study Team. *Lancet*. 1994;344(8925):782-785.

Slusher T, et al. Promoting the exclusive feeding of own mother's milk through the use of hindmilk and increased maternal milk volume for hospitalized, low birth weight infants (1800 grams) in Nigeria: a feasibility study. *J Hum Lact*. 2003;19:191-198.

Smith M. Influence of breastfeeding on cognitive outcomes at age 6–8 years: follow-up of very low birth weight infants. *Am J Epidemiol*. 2003;158:1075-1082.

Suman RP, et al. Kangaroo mother care for low birth weight infants: a randomized controlled trial. *Indian Pediatr*. 2008; 45:17-23.

Sweet L. Expressed breast milk as 'connection' and its influence on the construction of 'motherhood' for mothers of preterm infants: a qualitative study. *Int Breastfeed J*. 2008;3:30.

Swinth J, et al. Kangaroo (skin-to-skin) care with a preterm infant before, during, and after mechanical ventilation. *Neonat Netw*. 2003;22:33-38.

Thoyre SM, Carlson J. Occurrence of oxygen desaturation events during preterm infant bottle feeding near discharge. *Early Hum Dev*. 2003;72:25-36.

Vickers A, et al. Massage for promoting growth and development of preterm and/or low birth-weight infants. *Cochrane Database Syst Rev*. 2004;CD000390.

Vohr B, et al. National Institute of Child Health and Human Development (NICHD) National [*sic*] Research Network. Persistent beneficial effects of breast milk ingested in the neonatal intensive care unit on outcomes of extremely low birth weight infants at 30 months of age. *Pediatrics*. 2007; 120:e953-e959.

Vohr B, et al. National Institute of Child Health and Human Development (NICHD) Neonatal Research Network. Beneficial effects of breast milk in the neonatal intensive care unit on the developmental outcome of extremely low birth weight infants at 18 months of age. *Pediatrics*. 2006;118: e115-e123.

Weiss S, et al. Improving parent satisfaction: an intervention to increase neonatal parent-provider communication. *J Perinatol*. Oct 22, 2009. [Epub ahead of print]

Wendelboe A, et al. Cluster of necrotizing enterocolitis in a neonatal intensive care unit: New Mexico, 2007. *Am J Infect Control*. 2010;38(2):144-148.

Wheeler B. Human-milk feeding after NICU discharge. *Neonat Netw*. 2009;28:381-389.

Wheeler R, et al. Calcium and phosphorous supplementation following initial hospital discharge in 1800 gm birthweight breastfed infants. *Am J Perinatol*. 1990;7:389-390.

Wight N, et al. *Best Medicine: Human Milk in the NICU*. Amarillo, TX: Hale Publishing; 2008.

Wight N, Morton J. Human milk, breastfeeding, and the preterm infant. In: Hale T, Hartmann P. *Hale & Hartmann's Textbook of Human Lactation*. Amarillo, TX: Hale Publishing; 2007.

Wolf L, Glass R. *Feeding and Swallowing Disorders in Infancy*. San Antonio, TX: Therapy Skill Builders; 1992.

Worku B, Kassie A. Kangaroo mother care: a randomized controlled trial on effectiveness of early kangaroo other care for the low birthweight infants in Addis Ababa, Ethiopia. *J Trop Pediatr*. 2005;51:93-97.

World Health Organization/United Nations Children's Fund. Meeting on infant and young child feeding. *J Nurs Midw*. 1980;25:31-38.

Wrotniak B, et al. The relationship between birth weight and feeding maturation in preterm infants. *Acta Paediatr*. 2009; 98:286-290.

When Breastfeeding Is Interrupted

Ideally, a breastfeeding mother and her baby are together throughout lactation with no separations or interruptions in feedings. Unfortunately, in today's world this is often not possible. Total direct breastfeeding is not even desired by some mothers. Some separations of a mother and baby are temporary, whereas others are regular and long term. A separation may be for a few hours or a few days. The mother may be away on a daily basis because of returning to work or school or over a long period because of illness and hospitalization. Some of these separations may not involve missed feedings. Others require milk expression and the use of an alternative feeding method during the mother's absence. Mothers who experience such separations have special needs related to managing feedings and maintaining milk production, and will benefit from emotional support and encouragement.

～ *Key Terms*

Antibodies
Caregiver
Child care
H1N1 influenza
Hospitalization
Reverse cycle nursing
Ronald McDonald House
Short-term separation
Working mother

～ *Managing Breastfeeding Through a Separation*

Separation from her baby can create stress and anxiety for a new mother, especially when the separation is a result of illness. You can help relieve some of the mother's anxieties by accepting and supporting her decisions concerning breastfeeding. Those who combine breastfeeding with a daily or prolonged separation benefit from advice about expressing milk and maintaining milk production. You can help a mother obtain a pump and offer practical suggestions for its use. A strong sense of commitment and motivation will help her overcome any potential difficulties and pressures that may confront her. This discussion focuses on how you can help a mother whose separation from her baby affects her breastfeeding.

The Mother's Needs

Separation from her baby is challenging for a mother, especially when feedings are missed. Attitudes of family members, child care arrangements, and time management are all issues. She needs to express milk regularly to relieve fullness and to maintain milk production. Her baby must also be willing to accept nourishment by an alternative feeding method during her absence. Planning ahead allows time to work through her baby's possible rejection of the chosen feeding method.

The mother may experience conflicting emotions about the separation and about continuing to breastfeed despite obstacles. With effective use of counseling skills you can listen and respond to the mother's concerns about the cause of the separation, especially if her baby remains hospitalized. This accommodation of separation and breastfeeding can be a trying time for her family, and your support and encouragement are helpful.

Timing of the Separation

Mothers often have no control over the timing of a separation. For example, a working mother may have a limited maternity leave, or an unexpected hospitalization may be necessary for either mother or baby. Mothers who have flexibility in the timing of a separation can delay missed feedings until milk production is well established. Barring any interference, most mothers have breastfeeding well established by the time the baby is 2 months old and a mother can accommodate a separation more easily after that time. The transition is even smoother if a separation is delayed until about 6 months, when the baby is old enough to begin eating complementary foods. At that time there is less need for supplemental feedings while the mother and baby are apart. There are also many factors unrelated to breastfeeding, such as the emotional needs of the mother and baby, as well as separation anxiety, which occurs at around 9 months. The mother ideally can assess her particular situation to determine when the separation is least disruptive.

Maintaining Milk Production

A mother's milk production may diminish to some extent when she experiences a substantial separation from her baby. The key to maintaining milk production to the level the baby needs is to remove milk from the breasts to trigger further production. Many mothers who are away from their babies on a regular basis find it convenient to express milk routinely, typically at times when the baby would nurse if they were together. Some mothers prefer to express only enough milk to relieve discomfort during the separation. Thus, they allow their milk production to diminish slightly and feed their babies infant formula rather than breastmilk during their absence. The mother cannot remove milk from her breasts as effectively as the suckling of a healthy, robust baby. You can teach her how to hand express or how to access and use a breast pump.

Nourishing the Baby

When a mother is away from her baby during feeding times, she must arrange for her baby's nourishment until she returns. If she does not have sufficient breastmilk, her baby may need to be supplemented with donor milk or formula. A baby who is old enough to receive complimentary foods will not need as much breastmilk during the mother's absence. Depending on the baby's age and the length of her absence, she can arrange for her baby to be supplemented with juice, water, or solid foods.

Experimenting with feeding methods for at least 2 weeks before the separation helps the baby learn to accept nourishment by some means other than breastfeeding. Although a bottle may be convenient for the caregiver, some parents are concerned that it can cause a young baby to develop a nipple preference that could interfere with breastfeeding. Feeding the baby with a cup eliminates the possibility of nipple preference, though it may require more time for feeding. Cup feeding actually has advantages if the caregiver is willing to spend the extra time. Slowing down artificial feedings to emulate breastfeeding allows the baby to register satiety and not be as likely to overfeed.

Choice of Bottle Nipple

If the mother chooses bottle feeding during separations, the type of nipple she uses may be important (Ferrante et al., 2006). A nipple that encourages the baby's mouth to open wide may accommodate the transition from breast to bottle more easily for a very young baby. Many babies accomplish this wide gape with a nipple that has a large base. However, some babies tend to clamp down on the nipple at the narrowest part and do not take the bottle in deeply to the wide base. Mothers therefore may need to try more than one type of nipple to learn which works best for their baby. Because most women's nipples are short, a bottle with a short teat is preferable to a longer one. The key factor for many babies seems to be more the rate of flow it allows than the type of nipple (Wilson-Clay & Hoover, 2008; Kassing, 2002). Be aware that even "slow flow" nipples drip milk. See Chapter 21 for more information about selecting a nipple.

Babies supplemented with bottles have been found to be "significantly more fretful during breastfeeding" (Huang, 2009, p. 423). More mothers whose babies received bottle supplementation perceived less sufficient milk production than mothers whose babies were supplemented by cup. Cup feeding appeared to be better than bottle feeding when supplementary formula was needed for medical treatment.

Motivation to Continue Nursing

Motivation and determination are critical factors for a mother continuing to breastfeed despite a separation from her baby. Some mothers believe they must wean their babies when a separation occurs. You can assure mothers that breastfeeding is compatible with any length of separation. If weaning becomes necessary, you can encourage the mother to focus on the quality of her breastfeeding rather than the duration. If the separation has prompted the mother to compromise her initial breastfeeding goals, she can still work toward a satisfying experience if she remains flexible and positive.

If a mother's commitment to breastfeed waivers at the time a separation occurs, she might use the opportunity to wean her baby. On the other hand, some mothers who want to continue nursing may have moments of discouragement when faced with a separation. Be sensitive to messages that signal conflicted feelings: "I guess I should wean . . .", "I will have to wean . . .", or "I guess she doesn't want to nurse . . .". Draw the mother out with open-ended questions and reflective listening to help the mother clarify her situation, identify her options, and validate her choices. By assessing her motives and tailoring your assistance accordingly, you can help each mother achieve her desired outcome. Mothers who deal with separation benefit from a great deal of support and practical suggestions, whether the decision is to continue nursing or to wean.

Coping with Difficulties

A separation between mother and baby can create physical consequences related to breastfeeding as well as emotional tension and anxiety. The mother must remove milk from her breasts regularly to avoid leaking, plugged ducts, engorgement, lowered milk production, and possible mastitis. Despite being diligent in expressing her milk, she may still experience problems because hand expression or pumping does not remove milk from her breasts as efficiently as her baby does when suckling.

If the baby is hospitalized, traveling back and forth to the hospital taxes the mother's energy reserves. She may also have returned to work, school, or other responsibilities that add further to her exhaustion. Urge the mother to pay close attention to obtaining adequate rest. This is especially important if the separation is due to the mother's illness, to aid her recovery as well as build or maintain her milk production. You can encourage her to take small, quiet rest periods without the distraction of television or other media. Sometimes mothers need "permission" to rest because of the demands on their time. The mother needs to be mindful of her food intake as well. Skimping on her nutrition can affect her sense of well-being and her ability to function efficiently. Drinking something directly before or during the times she expresses helps her remember to supply herself with adequate fluids.

At times, a baby may demonstrate a strong desire to remain with the mother while at other times, the baby appears to reject her and seems more attached to the caregiver. This can be either a source of comfort to the mother or a source of jealousy and anxiety. Many mothers experience a sense of guilt about a separation, regardless of whether it is planned or unplanned and whether it is optional or unavoidable. This feeling of guilt may relate to the mother's absence from her baby or to her original goals for breastfeeding. Such guilt may motivate a mother to reconsider her options and alter her situation. You can help a mother cope with these anxieties by supporting her during the separation as well as when she and her baby reunite and resume breastfeeding.

After the Separation

If a separation results in a decline in milk production, the mother can hand express or pump to rebuild it. She may

TABLE 24.1   Counseling a Mother Who Is Separated from Her Baby

Mother's Concern	Suggestions for Mother
Overfullness or leaking	• Express milk during the absence. • Wear breast pads when away. • Nurse directly before and after the absence.
Low milk production	• Delay the separation until milk production is well-established (around 2 months). • Practice milk expression so you can express regularly during missed feedings. • Drink to thirst. • Nurse frequently when with the baby.
Feeding the baby	• Have the caregiver feed the baby the mother's milk or formula. • Use a cup to avoid bottles if nipple preference is a concern. • Practice alternate feedings before the separation to make sure the baby will accept the method.

be able to encourage nursing by feeding her milk to her baby through a tube-feeding device at the breast. Many mothers use galactogogues to boost their milk production. The baby may need supplemental feedings for a while as well until milk production increases sufficiently. Arranging for help with household chores can allow the mother time to renew her breastfeeding connection with her baby. See the suggestions in Chapter 21 for getting the baby back to the breast. In addition, Table 24.1 presents suggestions for counseling a mother who is separated from her baby.

Short-Term Separations

Most mothers will be away from their babies during a usual feeding time at some point during their breastfeeding. Such short-term absences sometimes help a woman settle into her role as mother and caretaker of a small baby. They offer a break from the routine and minutia of baby care and can help a new mother maintain a positive outlook. A brief time away can strike a compromise between stay-at-home mothering and outside interests such as schooling, part-time work, volunteer work, sports, exercise classes, or other activities. A mother may have other responsibilities that necessitate a short absence as well, such as doctors' appointments or attending functions for other family members. She may wish to simply plan an evening out with her partner, go to the hairdresser, or shop with a friend.

A mother can try to time outings to avoid missed feedings, or it may be possible for the baby to accompany her. For occasions when the baby stays home, the mother can provide expressed milk to be fed with an alternative feeding method. She can express milk in the morning and throughout the day for several days before the planned separation, storing her milk in the refrigerator or freezer. If she becomes uncomfortably full or experiences leaking while away, she can express milk for comfort and to avoid breast problems. She can use manual expression or carry a hand-held pump for that purpose. Many pumps have car adapters for use. Table 24.2 offers suggestions for helping a mother who must plan for a hospitalization.

TABLE 24.2   Preparing for Hospitalization

Points to Consider	Suggestions for Mother
Explore your options	• Learn if hospitalization is necessary. • Request a second opinion. • Learn if hospitalization can be delayed until the baby is older and milk production is established. • Learn whether early discharge is possible if home nursing care is arranged. Contact local Visiting Nurses Association for home care.
Be assertive regarding your wishes	• Discuss all concerns and wishes with your physician to avoid separation or to work toward minimizing missed feedings. • Examine hospital policies concerning rooming-in and the use of hospital breast pumps.
Become well informed	• Learn about hospital procedures and factors surrounding hospitalization. • Review informed consent as discussed in Chapter 4. • Contact local and Internet resource groups.
Keep clear, well-organized records	• Record expenses for income tax deductions for child care, travel, and breast pump rental, as these may be paid by insurance. • Record all details of your care plan and provide copies for yourself, your physician, and the hospital.
Prepare for transportation to and from the hospital	• Arrange for someone to drive you to and from the hospital.

When the Mother Is Ill

Whenever a mother contracts an infection—whether it be a cold, fever, or more serious illness—her body responds by producing antibodies in her milk that help to protect her breastfeeding baby (Hanson, 2007). Although some viruses are transmitted through her milk, in most cases the presence of antibodies to counteract them offsets any potential harm to the baby. Often, a more likely mechanism of disease transmission from the mother to her baby is through touching and close mouth and nose contact, not through her milk.

When the mother becomes ill, exposure to her baby already has occurred through contact during her most contagious period. Therefore a breastfeeding mother who develops a cold or fever does not need to worry about infecting her baby through her milk. The most effective treatment for the baby is to continue to nurse while the mother receives any necessary medication.

Educate the mother on precautions such as washing her hands with plain soap and water before nursing. If soap and water are not available, she can use an alcohol-based hand cleaner to cleanse her hands before feeding her baby. She should avoid coughing or sneezing in the baby's face and, if possible, only family members who are healthy should care for the baby. If the mother is sick and there is no one else to care for the baby, the Centers for Disease Control and Prevention (CDC, 2009b) advises wearing a face mask, if available and tolerable. Parents should cover their mouth and nose with a tissue when coughing or sneezing (CDC, 2009b). The mother also needs to rest and follow the treatment prescribed by her caregiver to return to good health quickly and not compromise her milk production.

H1N1 Influenza

The H1N1 influenza, a new strain of swine flu, created a worldwide pandemic in 2009. During an influenza pandemic, pregnant women are considered high risk based on experience with previous pandemics and with seasonal influenza. The mother's milk is an infant's primary option for immunological protection against respiratory infection. Therefore the H1N1 crisis offered unprecedented opportunities for lactation consultants to work closely with other professionals in the healthcare community to ensure infant welfare while breastfeeding. It raised awareness of the importance of breastfeeding and of the important role of lactation consultants on the mother's and baby's healthcare team.

The close interaction between the mother and her baby during feedings prompted many in the healthcare arena to consider whether this strain of flu warranted special precautions. A newborn's immature immune system, the constant close contact with the mother during breastfeeding, and multiple opportunities for exposure to droplet infection created cause for concern for the vulnerable newborn. The risk of transmission to the newborn is through droplet exposure to newborn mucosal surfaces during coughing and not through the mother's milk. At the center of debate was whether the mother could continue to breastfeed her baby, as is the case with other forms of influenza.

CDC Guidelines The CDC issued guidelines in November 2009 that apply to intrapartum and postpartum hospital settings for uncomplicated term deliveries (CDC, 2009a). In the event of a similar influenza pandemic, mothers and healthcare workers can refer to the CDC website for current guidelines. The 2009 guidelines state that during labor and delivery, a surgical mask should be placed on the infected mother and antiviral therapy begun as soon as possible. The infant should also be bathed early. After delivery the mother should be placed in a single-patient room with the baby placed in an isolette in the same room. If an isolette is not available, the baby should be placed in a bassinet at least 6 feet from the mother.

The guidelines provide a two-step process for postpartum and newborn management, with guidance for hospital discharge planning as well.

- Step 1: Assist the mother to express her milk and have a healthy caregiver feed it to the baby. When the mother simultaneously has been on antiviral medication for 48 hours, has been afebrile for 24 hours without the use of antipyretic medication, and is able to control and cover coughs and secretions, she may transition to step 2.
- Step 2: Initiate contact and direct feeding between the mother and baby. The mother should continue to wear a mask, adhere to strict hand hygiene, and continue to control and cover coughs and secretions.

After discharge the mother should continue the step 2 precautions for 7 days after symptom onset and until she has been symptom free for 24 hours. Family members should adhere to the same hygiene precautions and cough etiquette and avoid exposing the baby to any potentially ill caregivers. All caregivers of infants less than 6 months of age should be vaccinated.

Academy of Breastfeeding Medicine Guidelines The Academy of Breastfeeding Medicine (2009) recommended that breastfeeding continue even if the mother is suspected of having the H1N1 influenza virus, because the baby would most likely have been exposed to the virus before the mother's symptoms appeared. They encourage continued breastfeeding for mothers taking either of the two antiviral medications prescribed to treat or prevent the H1N1 infection. Furthermore, if breastmilk is only part of an infant's diet, it is suggested that the mother increase the amount of breastmilk the infant receives during an influenza outbreak. Precautions include careful hand washing, control of coughing to avoid droplet exposure, and antiviral therapy for the mother—ideally within 48 hours of onset of the symptoms. Use of a mask is also suggested (Lawrence & Bradley, 2009).

Hospitalization of the Mother

In most cases a mother hospitalized due to illness or injury can continue to breastfeed, provided that she is not consuming medication that could be harmful to her baby. If rooming-in is permitted, she can ask to be assigned to a floor that accommodates a young baby, such as in obstetrics. Depending on the mother's condition, she may need another adult in the room to help her care for her baby. If rooming-in is not possible, she can arrange for someone to bring her baby to the hospital during the day and stay to care for the baby and help during feedings if necessary. Another option is for someone to bring the baby to the hospital intermittently throughout the day to breastfeed.

If a mother is so ill or in such postoperative pain that she is physically unable to breastfeed, nursing staff can be instrumental in helping the mother maintain lactation. Knowledge about breastfeeding, maternal medications, pumping, and breastmilk storage will enable them to advocate for sustaining breastfeeding (Wenner, 2007). The following are suggestions for the caregiver:

- Encourage rest, good nutrition, and hydration.
- Support efforts to breastfeed and reinforce the benefits for mother and infant.
- Provide privacy as needed.
- Assist the mother with supporting any surgical area with pillows.
- Encourage the mother to take postoperative analgesia to alleviate pain.
- Promote good hand washing, limited contact with the infant's face, and continued breastfeeding as the best ways to prevent transfer of infection from mother to infant.
- Reassure the mother that medications and procedures have been investigated and breastfeeding will not harm the infant.

Failing to address a woman's lactation when she is in acute or emergency care can lead to more severe physical complications, such as mastitis or a breast abscess. If the mother is having a long surgery or is incapacitated afterward, the nursing staff should be trained to use a breast pump to remove the mother's milk (Dumphy, 2008). Interdepartmental knowledge and support of breastfeeding in areas that serve women, such as medical, surgical, and emergency departments, provide critical continuity of care.

Family members and lactation staff can advocate for preserving the mother's lactation until she is able to voice her wishes. In cases where the mother has severe mastitis or an abscess and decides to wean, she should recover from the mastitis before initiating weaning. It is important that she continue to remove milk from her breasts during the course of the mastitis (Academy of Breastfeeding Medicine, 2008; Wilson-Clay, 2008; Berens, 2004).

Continuing to nurse through a complicated medical situation may not be the best choice for every woman. If breastfeeding would compromise her medical condition or if she finds it difficult to cope, pumping or weaning may be better alternatives. On the other hand, many mothers have continued to breastfeed throughout a hospitalization. One mother underwent a breast biopsy on an outpatient basis without ever missing a feeding. Another mother underwent a mastectomy, pumping and discarding her milk during bouts of chemotherapy. She continued to breastfeed her 2-year-old on the remaining breast when the drugs cleared from her system.

Although a mother's medical condition can make nursing or caring for her baby challenging, her determination and advance planning, when elective, ease these difficulties. Mothers benefit from help in planning for the hospitalization, managing breastfeeding or pumping during the hospital stay, and returning to a regular routine after returning home.

When the Baby Is Hospitalized

Having a hospitalized baby is always stressful for parents and there are additional challenges when the baby breastfeeds. A baby may remain hospitalized for a prolonged period after birth or may return to the hospital due to complications, a contagious illness, or injury. Traveling back and forth to the hospital can be very tiring for a mother, especially if the hospitalization occurs directly after the birth, at a time when she needs to give attention to her own recovery. Frequently, the mother has other children requiring her attention and care as well.

If the baby is in a high-risk center, the mother can ask about having him transferred to a facility closer to her home after his condition has stabilized, where she can visit him more easily. Be aware that insurance companies, including public assistance (Medicaid in the United States), may not agree to a transfer of care such as this.

Most mothers want to remain with their babies throughout the hospitalization. They can inquire about rooming-in policies for mothers of sick babies. Most major hospitals have corporate-sponsored housing available, such as Ronald McDonald houses or family rooms. Newer children's hospitals have been designed with fam-

ilies in mind. A baby occasionally contracts a contagious illness requiring isolation from other babies in a special isolation room. Most often the mother is safe rooming-in with her baby, and she can request this option.

Exclusive breastfeeding was observed in 57.1 percent of infant patients readmitted to the hospital for respiratory infections in Brazil. In 35.4 percent of the cases, breastfeeding was interrupted by the introduction of infant formula during hospitalization. This was possibly due to inadequate hospital infrastructure and insufficient support from health professionals (Souza et al., 2008).

Breastfeeding is analgesic for painful bloodletting procedures, such as heel sticks (Dilli et al., 2009; Saitua et al., 2009; Shah et al., 2009; Uga et al., 2008; Osinaike et al., 2007). The mother can negotiate with caregivers to nurse her baby during these procedures. A baby who must undergo surgery benefits from the mother's presence immediately before and after the procedure. Physicians generally request that a patient consume nothing within 8 hours preceding surgery. However, human milk digests so quickly that a baby's stomach empties much more quickly, and the baby would be very hungry by the time of surgery if not permitted a later feeding.

The mother can ask her baby's caregiver how soon she can nurse before and after surgery. American Society of Anesthesiologists (1999) guidelines allow clear fluids up to 2 hours, breastfeeding up to 4 hours, and formula up to 6 hours before surgery. Lawrence (2005) suggests providing comfort measures before surgery, including a pacifier. Because pacifiers generate saliva, parents need to discuss this with the anesthesiologist. An alternative measure is for the mother to nurse the baby on a pumped breast. However, because some milk is always present, this should also be discussed with the anesthesiologist. The mother can also ask to be with her baby in the recovery room, although hospital policy may preclude this option.

If the mother needs to pump to maintain milk production, she can ask about using a hospital breast pump so she can express milk regularly during her baby's stay. If the baby cannot receive the mother's milk, pumping still is important for her to maintain milk production.

After the Hospitalization

When the mother and baby are together at home again, they will benefit from frequent contact and support. The mother may need to increase milk production if breastfeeding was interrupted during the hospitalization. If the separation was for an extended period, she may need to relactate to continue breastfeeding. Even if the mother and baby were able to nurse during the hospitalization, they may require help reestablishing their breastfeeding routine. The anxiety and worry about the situation that precipitated the hospitalization does not necessarily subside when they settle in at home. The mother may appreciate having a compassionate, concerned listener to help her talk through her emotions.

∼ Supporting Working Mothers

Many mothers face regular separations from their baby, most often due to a return to work or school. Mothers are the fastest growing segment of the U.S. workforce, and most mothers with young children work outside the home. In 2007 only about one-fourth of all married-couple families in the United States had a stay-at-home mother, as reported by the U.S. Census Bureau (2009). With only one-fourth of mothers staying at home with their babies, this means that a large percentage of mothers are employed outside the home. Combining working and breastfeeding is therefore prevalent among the mothers you see.

Twenty-six percent of working mothers in the United States return to work within 2 months of the birth of their child, and 41 percent by 3 months. Over 56 percent of mothers with children under age 6 were in the labor force in 2008 (U.S. Department of Labor, 2009). Over 39 percent of these mothers are the primary wage earners in their families, and 24 percent are co–wage earners (Center for American Progress, 2009).

In Japan 15 percent of mothers work full-time and 25 percent are employed part-time (Organization for Economic Cooperation and Development, 2008). Other industrialized nations share similar rates of maternal employment with children under the age of 6:

- United Kingdom: 59 percent
- Germany: 62.7 percent
- France: 65.9 percent
- Portugal: 68 percent
- Sweden: 80 percent (Sweden.se, 2009)

Obstacles to Working and Breastfeeding

Working outside the home negatively affects breastfeeding initiation and duration. Although mothers who work outside the home initiate breastfeeding at the same rate as mothers who stay at home, continuation rates decline sharply (Chuang et al., 2010). Mothers with a maternity leave of 6 months or less discontinue breastfeeding earlier than those who have longer than 6 months and those who delay their return to work for up to 18 months after birth. Many U.S. women receive very short paid maternity leaves. The CDC (2009b) reported the following:

- Such brief times off can affect breastfeeding initiation and duration.
- Only about one-third of women are eligible for fully paid maternity leave.
- Partially paid leave is an option for only about 1 in 5 women.
- On average, fully paid leave is 2.2 weeks long and partially paid is 1.5 weeks.

Obstacles to continued breastfeeding in the United States include an economic system that expects workers to have no domestic encumbrances, public refusal to acknowledge and accommodate breastfeeding, and a male-dominated ideological commitment to adult autonomy (Hausman, 2009). Women therefore return to work after childbirth juggling professional roles with their new family roles. Most put in a double day, fulfilling job requirements while striving to meet the nurturing needs of their child (Greenberg & Avigdor, 2009; Hochschild & Machung, 2003). Even well-educated healthcare professionals who understand and embrace the health importance of breastfeeding find it hard to continue breastfeeding their own children.

You are in a position to help mothers work through the conflicting goals of motherhood and career. Worldwide, only 10 percent of men and women favor mothers of small children working full time (Kelley et al., 2009). Supporting mothers to stay home with their child validates the importance of motherhood in a culture dominated by materialism (Palmer, 2009). Online nonprofit and grass roots organizations such as mothersandmore.org, mops.org, and momsrising.org offer support, validation, and networking for mothers.

Many mothers with the financial option embrace the idea of sequencing their family and work lives, allowing them to "have it all"—just not all at once (Weaver-Zercher, 2007). Media and Internet resources can aid mothers to advocate for their families and for flexible employment choices. However, mothers who are most vulnerable to economic discrimination and employer harassment may have low-income, non-native, or illegal immigration status and may be unaware of resources. Greater outreach and education can benefit and empower these mothers to nurture their children while achieving more economic justice.

Unaware Breastfeeding Can Continue

Counseling efforts need to focus on educating women about the feasibility of combining employment with breastfeeding. Realizing that she must return to work, a mother may expect to be unable to breastfeed her baby. Mothers who return to work full time before 6 months are less likely to be breastfeeding at the 6 month mark

(Cooklin et al., 2008). These women need practical advice as well as encouragement and support from healthcare providers, society, and the workplace to balance breast-feeding and paid employment.

Mothers who return to paid work often give up breastfeeding because of the challenges they faces. Breast-feeding is just as challenging for professional women as for those in other types of employment. One group of mothers in managerial and/or professional occupations who continued to breastfeed had difficulty because breast-feeding was "taboo" within the workplace (Gatrell, 2007). They were compelled to either quit breastfeeding or con-ceal it. Another group of mothers returning to work cited space, time, and nonsupport as affecting their ability to continue to breastfeed (Payne & James, 2008).

Of 365 female urologists in the United States sur-veyed about maternity leave, workplace policies, and breastfeeding, 70 percent took 8 weeks or less of leave. Twenty-two percent were dissatisfied with their breast-feeding duration, citing work as a factor (Lerner et al., 2010). Breastfeeding initiation rate among female physi-cians surveyed in Canada was 96.6 percent, with more than 50 percent nursing for longer than 7 months. Doc-tors who graduated in 1980 or later breastfed their babies for longer (Duke et al., 2007).

Societal and employer attitudes are pivotal in encour-aging and supporting continued breastfeeding. Part-time work, lack of lengthy separations from their babies, sup-portive work environments, and childcare options help breastfeeding to continue (Johnston & Esposito, 2007). Healthcare providers have a unique opportunity to help working mothers continue breastfeeding when they return to work (Angeletti, 2009). Common obstacles and guidance and support include:

- Maternity leave—arranging as long a leave as possible
- Milk expression—building up a store of milk
- Milk production—the importance of letdown and breast massage
- The child's needs—infant cues, reverse-cycle feeding, and breastfeeding support groups

Lack of Societal Support

The lactation consulting profession does an exemplary job of empowering women to initiate breastfeeding. How-ever, many of society's attitudes, particularly those that involve a woman's return to work or school, do not sup-port an atmosphere conducive to the mother continuing to breastfeed. This is evident in both attitude and action. It can result in women considering childbirth and breast-feeding as an interruption in their "real" life, with careers and lifestyles touted as a priority over the value of child rearing. Many times the corporate and cultural expecta-tion is to place their career or lifestyle ahead of their baby.

In Kenya, a culture supportive of breastfeeding, 94.1 percent of working mothers breastfeed and work an aver-age of 46.2 hours per week (Lakati et al., 2002). In Greece, mothers returning to work initiate breastfeeding at higher rates than their stay-at-home counterparts (Bakoula et al., 2007). Iran follows the International Labor Organiza-tion (ILO) standards for breastfeeding employed women, but only for government employees and mothers with employer-paid or self-paid insurance (Olang, 2009; ILO, 2005).

It is challenging to combine employment with long-term breastfeeding in a culture that fails to support breast-feeding. In industrialized cultures breastfeeding and working are often described as a "juggling" act, a period in women's lives when they enter motherhood, establish breastfeeding, and return to paid work. Breastfeeding needs to be considered in the context of a woman's life, including all her roles and activities (Mulford, 2008). Maternity leave of 6 weeks or less fails to provide the sup-port necessary to accommodate these various roles and activities. Pediatricians can encourage patients to take maternity leave and can advocate for extending paid post-partum leave and flexibility in working conditions.

Industrialized societal cultures seem to view employ-ment as a socially acceptable reason for mothers to wean. This leads to mothers believing that few occupations allow them to combine breastfeeding with employment. China is the world's most populated country, with great diver-sity of ethnic groups and breastfeeding rates. Despite the diversity in urban and developed areas, maternal return to paid work is universally considered as an important rea-son for quitting breastfeeding or early introduction of complementary food (Xu et al., 2009).

U.S. welfare reform requires that recipients work and in many states these work requirements apply to mothers whose children are only a few months old. Thus, lowered breastfeeding rates are an unfortunate consequence (Bent-ley, 2003; Haider, 2003). African American mothers, who have lower breastfeeding initiation rates, were more likely than white mothers to quit breastfeeding to return to work in one study (Hurley et al., 2008). Cultural support and national health policies related to employment, health, and early childhood are important for increasing the rates of employed breastfeeding women (Galtry, 2003).

Fear of Job Loss

There is ongoing concern about women illegally losing their jobs during maternity leave (ILO, 2005). The United States, Swaziland, Liberia, Lesotho, and Papua New Guinea are the only countries among 173 surveyed in 2007 that fail to guarantee paid maternity leave to new mothers (Snow & Kriskey, 2009). In an economic recession some Ameri-can women are afraid to take their maternity leave for fear of losing their job (Snow & Kriskey, 2009).

The Maternity Protection Coalition supports women's right to breastfeed and work by advocating for improved maternity protection entitlements (World Alliance for Breastfeeding Action, 2009). "The Maternity Protection Kit: A Breastfeeding Perspective" is an important resource for lactation consultants and employers (Maternity Protection Campaign, 2002). The coalition consists of the International Baby Food Action Network (IBFAN), the International Lactation Consultant Association (ILCA), the LINKAGES project, and the World Alliance for Breastfeeding Action (WABA). The maternity protection kit is designed for breastfeeding advocates interested in working toward better maternity protection laws, regulations, and workplace policies. It provides information, resources, and tools for breastfeeding educators.

Unaccommodating Work Environment

Employers play a critical role in mothers' success with breastfeeding when mothers work full time (Mills, 2009). The quality and support of the mother's workplace has the potential to increase breastfeeding rates among working women. Employer-sponsored childcare increased the likelihood of breastfeeding to 6 months after birth by 47 percent in one study. Allowing the mother to work an average of 8 of her work hours at home per week increased the probability of breastfeeding initiation by 8 percent and breastfeeding to 6 months by 16.8 percent (Jacknowitz, 2008).

A U.S. Navy study found that although most female officers with children and two-thirds of enlisted mothers initiate breastfeeding, about one-third have stopped by the time they return to duty (Uriell et al., 2009). Almost half of enlisted women and over one-third of officers indicated they were not given a comfortable, secluded location for breastfeeding or pumping, although the majority are given time to do so. Two-thirds of enlisted women and half of officers reported that they stopped breastfeeding for a work-related reason (Uriell et al., 2009).

Among a group of maternal factory workers almost 67 percent breastfed during their maternity leave for an average of 56 days (Chen et al., 2006). Only 10.6 percent of these mothers continued to breastfeed after returning to work, despite workplace lactation rooms and breast pumping breaks. The mothers continuing were mostly office workers and those aware of the company's breastfeeding-friendly policies. A 2007 Cochrane Review found no trials evaluating the effectiveness of workplace interventions in promoting breastfeeding among women returning to paid work after childbirth (Abdulwadud & Snow, 2007).

Employee awareness and education are needed among businesses and organizations offering lactation support. In one study almost 80 percent of mothers desired to continue breastfeeding after returning to work (Kosmala-Anderson & Wallace, 2006). However, 90 percent of respondents were unaware of their employers' lactation policies. Employers need to do a better job of informing their employees about their policies and services supporting breastfeeding. Women need to learn prenatally about the services, including the location of facilities for expression and policies for working flexible hours and taking pumping breaks.

Some women discover their return to work is marked by resentment from colleagues or less favorable treatment by supervisors. Negative treatment takes the form of a lower position, job loss, verbal abuse, or social isolation (ILO, 2005). The ILO correlates the importance of maternal and infant health with the right to continue nursing upon return to paid work, with clean facilities. Legislation in at least 92 countries provides for breastfeeding breaks beyond regular employee breaks (ILO, 2005). A Breastfeeding Promotion Act introduced in the United States would guarantee working mothers the right to breastfeed their children at their workplaces (U.S. Breastfeeding Committee, 2009).

Overall employer attitudes and practices toward breastfeeding mothers are discouraging (Stewart-Glenn, 2008). Many women report employment as a barrier to breastfeeding. Additionally, women who believe nursing while working causes additional work and stress are apt to not initiate it. Employers most frequently cite monetary reasons (i.e., decreased productivity) for not supporting breastfeeding.

Combining Work and Breastfeeding

When a mother combines breastfeeding with a work situation that separates her from her baby, many factors can affect her success. Women who are most likely to continue breastfeeding while working are older and more educated. It is harder for nonmanagement employees to breastfeed (Chen, 2006). However, education and position are no guarantees of smooth workplace breastfeeding, as discussed above.

Timing of the mother's return to work has an impact on the length of time she breastfeeds. Delaying a return to work to at least 3 months postpartum appears to extend breastfeeding duration (Galtry, 2003; Taveras, 2003). Breastfeeding duration is more affected for women with inflexible jobs, for nonmanagers, and for mothers with high psychosocial distress in their lives (Guendelman et al., 2009).

Mothers in the United Kingdom who were either employed part time or self-employed were more likely to breastfeed for at least 4 months than full-time working mothers (Hawkins, 2007). Likewise, the longer a mother stays home the more likely she is to breastfeed for at least 4 months. Mothers are also more likely to breastfeed for at least 4 months when their employer offers family-friendly or flexible work arrangements or they receive maternity pay and additional payments.

Family Considerations

Seeking assistance and information in the prenatal period enables a woman to explore her options for returning to work. There are many creative solutions available for incorporating motherhood and breastfeeding into her life. She may even find that her goals alter after she is home with her baby. Information and classes on breastfeeding and working offer practical advice for women who plan to combine employment and breastfeeding. They can explore options that promote their productivity while keeping them with their babies and enabling them to meet their babies' needs. Many online resources are available to help families explore factors involved in making decisions about staying home, working, and childcare options (National Association of Child Care Resource & Referral Agencies, 2009). There are also many money management websites, classes, and seminars to help parents stretch their earnings.

Options and Support at Work

Encourage the mother to explore employment options and seek input from her employer. She should become familiar with her employer's policies regarding maternity leave, her legal rights, and any issues involved with her return to work as they relate to her child's needs, including breastfeeding. The following questions relate to employment rights:

- What resources are available to her?
- How long can she stay on maternity leave? Are there any options for extending her leave?
- Can she alter, reduce, or eliminate hours at work?
- Does her employment provide flexible working options, such as job sharing, on-site child care, telecommuting from home, flex hours, or part-time hours?
- Does her work require separation from her baby, or is an alternative available that can keep her with her child?
- Can she begin a home-based business that does not require her to leave her baby?

You can provide relevant information to the mother to help her communicate her needs to her employer and coworkers. She can point out to them that breastfeeding gives the baby health benefits, thereby reducing the number of illnesses and thus lost time from her work to care for her baby. She can discuss her plans and enlist support from her employer, immediate supervisor, and coworkers. This can help her gauge the amount of support she will receive when she is ready to return to work.

The mother can check the provisions of her health insurance plan for the cost of lactation assistance or a breast pump. Descriptions of model programs and breastfeeding promotion within the insurance industry are available in "Health Plans' Innovative Programs in Breastfeeding Promotion." This monograph explores eight case studies of companies that promote breastfeeding coverage and provide benefits to their breastfeeding employees (American Association of Health Plans, 2001).

Feeding Options

You can help the mother explore feeding options for her baby. Having child care available on-site or nearby makes it possible to breastfeed on breaks throughout the day. Most mothers need information about breast pumps to express milk for missed feedings (Figure 24.1). Before she returns to work, the can begin collecting milk for later separations. Some mothers reverse their child's nursing cycle by providing most or all feedings at times when they are together, referred to as reverse-cycle nursing. Others opt for artificial baby milk for feedings during the separation and breastfeed when they are with their baby. Being a WIC recipient, having no access to breast pumps, unacceptability of pumping at work, and difficulties with nursing in public all contribute to formula supplementation (Holmes et al., 2009).

Childcare Options

When separation is necessary, the quality of substitute child care is a crucial concern for parents. Governmental

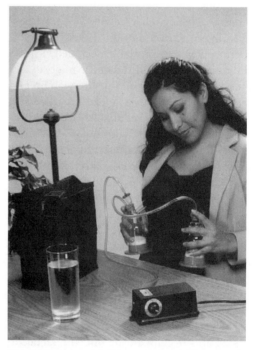

FIGURE 24.1   Mother pumping while at work.
Source: Printed with permission of Bailey Medical Engineering.

child care is provided in many countries. In Sweden, 87 percent of children aged 2 years attend day care, increasing to 97 percent for children aged 5 years (Sweden.se, 2009). The quality of child care varies widely, from "less than minimal" to "good" (National Association of Child Care Resource & Referral Agencies, 2009). In the United States a variety of arrangements is used by parents.

In 2005, 60 percent of children less than age 6 years required child care from someone other than the parents, with 22 percent cared for in daycare centers or by in-home providers (U.S. Department of Health and Human Services [USDHHS], 2009). Children who began care early in life and were in care 30 or more hours a week were at increased risk for stress-related behavioral problems. Difficulties interacting with peers or insensitive parents elevated these children's risk. Children in high-quality care centers had higher language scores and early school achievement, especially when they came from disadvantaged backgrounds. Childcare arrangements with six or more children increased the likelihood of communicable illnesses and ear infections (Bradley & Vandell, 2007).

Addressing childcare issues honestly with mothers helps them make informed choices. The American Academy of Pediatrics, the American Academy of Family Physicians (AAFP), and the National Association of Child Care Resource & Referral Agencies provide extensive childcare checklists for parents. They can all be accessed at the National Institute of Health's website (www.nlm.nih.gov). When the mother interviews childcare providers, she can address the needs of breastfeeding babies, the use of her milk, and alternative feeding methods. She can also acquaint the provider with the positive aspects of breastfeeding such as the fact that breastfed babies are less fussy, have fewer illnesses, have less diaper odor, spit up less, and their spit-up will not stain clothing. With the resurgence in breastfeeding, more childcare facilities train their staff in the correct handling of human milk and working with breastfeeding families. Some childcare centers actively advertise to breastfeeding families and use breastfeeding promotional materials as well (CDC, 2005). Both the mother and her substitute childcare provider need to feel comfortable with the arrangement. You can provide information that is useful for both of them, particularly facts related to milk storage and handling. Mothers need to be aware of the increased risk of illness for the baby if they stop breastfeeding at the same time as they begin day care.

Returning to Work

A mother who is returning to work must learn a new routine and integrate her maternal role with her workplace role. She is experiencing a degree of separation from her child, with its accompanying worries and doubts about how her child will fare. You can provide support and information to help her form solutions to the challenges associated with breastfeeding and employment. She will especially benefit from ideas to enhance her letdown and increase efficiency with her expression times.

When the time comes for the mother's return to work, several suggestions make the transition a bit smoother for both her and her baby. Scheduling her first day back to work in the middle of the workweek may allow the mother to feel less overwhelmed. If the return to work is a bit rocky, she and her baby have more time to recoup and get ready for a full workweek. Packing a bag for her baby and herself the night before work avoids a harried morning start and allows an opportunity to snuggle and feed her baby before beginning the workday. She might also explore returning to work part time initially, either in terms of days per week or hours per day.

Breastfeeding Routine

With employment and childcare arrangements made before her baby's birth, the mother can focus on initiating good breastfeeding practices and using her support systems for information and encouragement. As she settles in at home, devoting her time to enjoying her new baby and forging their relationship benefits both mother and baby.

About 2 to 3 weeks before her return to work the mother can begin the hands-on planning for her baby's needs while they are separated. As she familiarizes herself with breast pump use or manual expression, your assistance can help the mother learn these techniques and increase her self-confidence. She can begin expressing on the unused breast at the end of a feeding or express between feedings. In addition to practicing her technique, this enables her to begin storing milk for her baby.

Practicing for the Separation

In the weeks before separation the mother can begin practicing with the feeding method she has chosen. Enlisting the help of another person familiar to the baby will increase the likelihood that the baby will be receptive to being fed by someone other than the mother. That person can feed the mother's expressed milk at a comfortable temperature to encourage the baby to accept the new method of feeding. If using a bottle with an artificial nipple, warming the nipple to body temperature makes it more appealing to the baby. Occasionally, a baby will refuse any alternative method while his mother is nearby, so she may need to leave the immediate area. It is also best not to try a new feeding method when the baby is too hungry to deal with something new and unfamiliar.

As she becomes more proficient with expressing her milk and her baby is more accepting of the new feeding method, the mother can do several trial runs with the baby's substitute care provider. She can begin to gradually ease into a feeding routine that mimics her work schedule. As she finds herself in the midst of these intense changes, encourage her to keep open communication with those closest to her. Combining caring for a young baby with employment requires adjustments in other areas. Housework and errands may become less of a priority as the mother considers what must be done, what can wait, what can be streamlined for greater efficiency, and who is able to do it best.

Combining employment with caring for a young baby presents challenges, regardless of how the mother feeds her baby. Breastfeeding can temper these challenges by providing a unique way to reconnect before and after the day's work. The first feeding at the end of the workday provides special time for the mother and baby to be alone with one another. It helps the mother obtain the rest she needs and to reconnect with her baby. Breastfeeding's health benefits, in turn, reduce the working mother's stress. If the baby is kept nearby at nighttime, breastfeeding only minimally interrupts their sleep and provides the mother the opportunity for rest during nighttime hours. Some mothers reduce the need to express milk during working hours by encouraging their babies to reverse their nursing cycle so that more of their waking hours are at night.

Childcare Provider

By the time the mother returns to work, she and her substitute care provider need to have decided on the baby's feeding plan. The mother can provide a written list of instructions related to the care of her milk and her baby's special preferences. She and her care provider can review the baby's feeding method and watching for signs of hunger so the baby does not become overly hungry. She may want her baby held in the same position for feedings as for breastfeeding. Some babies will not take a bottle in the same position as breastfeeding, however, and may do better when held in a different position such as on the caregiver's lap facing outward. It is important to place the baby in charge of drawing in the bottle nipple rather than the caregiver controlling it. The mother can teach the caregiver paced feeding, described in Chapter 21, to avoid overfeeding and stress. If the feeding method is something other than a bottle, such as cup feeding, the caregiver should be trained and observed in feeding the baby with the alternate method.

The mother and care provider need to communicate closely about the amount of milk consumed at feedings and how the baby handles an artificial nipple and feedings in general. Avoiding a feeding too close to the time the mother is to arrive ensures that her baby is hungry and eager to nurse. This relieves the mother's breast fullness and facilitates their coming back together at the end of the day. If the baby seems especially hungry just before the mother's return, the caregiver can provide only a partial

feeding. If her baby is cared for outside the home, the mother may want a quiet place at the caregiver's site to breastfeed when she arrives. Some women prefer to drive home immediately to settle in with their baby. Still others prefer the baby be fed before their arrival and will pump at home. Discussing the mother's wishes helps make the transition at the end of the workday as smooth as possible.

Expressing Milk at Work

During her absence the mother will need to express milk regularly to maintain milk production and avoid engorgement, mastitis, plugged ducts, or excessive leaking. She will benefit from your support as she prepares to return to work and after she has implemented her plans. Part of this support can include information about the importance of expressing her milk. When the mother understands its importance, she is more likely to be committed to doing it. Knowing how her baby will benefit from her milk can comfort the mother when she feels discouraged. She will be reassured knowing that she is providing her baby with health and nutrition that no one can duplicate. Furthermore, breastfeeding saves money for her family by avoiding the cost of infant formula, the various feeding devices, and medical costs incurred due to more illnesses.

Pumping Routine The expressing routine the mother developed at home may change after she returns to work. She will gradually learn to blend the expressing strategy she refined at home with her new work routine. Ideally, she can work toward matching her lactation breaks to her baby's feeding needs. At a minimum she should respond to any uncomfortable fullness in her breasts.

If her baby is still quite young, the mother may find it best to express milk every 3 hours while at work. With a double breast pump, about 10 to 15 minutes pumping time is usually sufficient to stimulate milk production and remove the available milk. If she uses a single pump or hand expression, she needs about 20 minutes for the process. As her baby grows older, the time needed for pumping decreases.

Ideally the mother can express her milk in a place with privacy, a comfortable chair and room temperature, and options for passing the time while expressing her milk. She can massage her breasts and, if possible, apply moist heat to help her relax and promote letdown. Stimulating her senses in a way that reminds her of her baby also helps. She could have her baby's recorded sounds, a picture, or even an article of clothing with her. Some mothers have webcams at work that enable them to see their baby in real time.

Storing Her Milk The milk the mother expresses at work can be stored in quantities her baby will take at one feeding. Although initially this amount may be uncertain, the amount needed at a feeding becomes clearer as she and her baby settle into a routine. Her freshly expressed milk can remain at room temperature safely for up to 6 to 8 hours (CDC, 2007). Regardless of the manner in which she stores her milk, keeping it cooled on her commute home will preserve the milk safely for refrigeration when she arrives home. See Chapter 21 for more discussion of collecting and storing expressed milk.

Mother's Comfort and Adjustment

The mother may notice that her milk production fluctuates as she adjusts physically to her new routine. This change could be a byproduct of missed feedings as well as emotional swings associated with being separated from her baby. If she experiences delays in expressing her milk, her breasts can become uncomfortably full and may leak. Some mothers keep a complete change of clothes at their workplace for when leaking occurs. Prints rather than solid colors help to conceal breast fullness, leaks, or lopsidedness. The mother can also keep a jacket or sweater handy and wear breast pads to absorb leaked milk. Clothing needs to allow easy breast access for pumping at work, as well as for nursing her baby just before leaving for work and on reuniting after work.

Routine After Work Planning her time after work hours is equally as important as the mother's routine during work. Breastfeeding provides an opportunity to relax with her baby when they reunite at the end of the workday. Planning quiet time with her baby as a priority over other demands can help the mother deal with her after-work pressures. Some babies react to the separation by increasing their frequency and duration of feedings. This is helpful to both the mother's milk production and her need for rest. If it leads to reverse-cycle nursing, the mother can be encouraged to take her baby to bed with her to meet her need for rest.

Support for the Mother The benefits of support for an employed breastfeeding mother extend beyond the mother and child. Employers find that employee morale and loyalty increase, with less time lost from work for a sick baby because of the protection the baby receives from breastfeeding. Fewer days off work translate to lower healthcare costs for the company. When employers take an active interest in the families of their employees, they improve cohesiveness and productivity within the company.

Many resources are available for women who combine motherhood and working. One book mothers find helpful is *Nursing Mother, Working Mother* (Pryor & Huggins, 2007). Local breastfeeding support groups often offer evening or weekend meetings to accommodate working mothers. Interestingly, lactation consultants and breastfeeding counselors have noticed that working mothers continue to breastfeed far longer than they originally planned, some for as long as 3 or 4 years. These mothers benefit from the reassurance that extended breastfeeding is a biological norm, albeit not always a cultural one. You can recommend resources such as toddler nursing groups and books such as *Mothering Your Nursing Toddler* (Bumgarner, 2000).

⁓ Breastfeeding-Friendly Workplace

Supportive employers accommodate mothers so they can continue breastfeeding after they return to work. Many breastfeeding women return to work soon after the birth of their baby. Consequently, employers significantly influence a woman's ability to continue breastfeeding. There has been a trend in the workplace to create a more family-friendly environment for working parents. *Working Mother* magazine conducts an annual survey and compiles a list of the 100 best companies for working mothers. A survey of the best 100 companies to work for in the United States (*Working Mother,* 2009) found that 100 percent of them offered an on-site lactation/mothers' room compared to 25 percent nationally. Ninety-four percent of these companies offered lactation support services compared to only 6 percent nationally.

Employer Support for Breastfeeding

Simple measures can provide breastfeeding support in the workplace, with procedures that are practical, safe, and easy to implement economically. A wide range of occupations has implemented the components of a breastfeeding support program for the workplace as described in Table 24.3. The maternity protection kit, described above, and "The Business Case for Breastfeeding," described in the next paragraph, as well as resources from other breastfeeding proponents are the appropriate resources to support mothers' rights to breastfeed.

A program from the USDHHS (2009), "The Business Case for Breastfeeding," educates employers on supporting breastfeeding employees in the workplace. The comprehensive program emphasizes how such support contributes to the business' success and offers tools to help employers provide:

- Worksite lactation support
- Privacy for breastfeeding mothers to express milk
- Employee guidance on breastfeeding and working
- Lactation specialist and health professional resources to educate employers

Employers who support breastfeeding employees often are more positive toward breastfeeding overall (Dunn et al., 2004). Because companies operate on a profit basis, you can

TABLE 24.3   Components of a Workplace Breastfeeding Support Program

Adequate	Expanded	Comprehensive
Facilities		
A clean, private, comfortable multi-purpose space (that is not a bathroom) with an electrical outlet in order to pump milk or to breastfeed.	A breastfeeding mothers' break room (BMBR) for use only by breastfeeding women.	A breastfeeding mothers' break room (BMBR) (or rooms) close to women's worksites.
Employee provides her own breast pump.	Employer provides one multi-user electric breast pump, and employees provide their own collection kits.	Employer provides collection kits. Additional multi-user electric pumps are provided if needed.
Table and comfortable chair.	Improved aesthetics to promote relaxation.	Room large enough to accommodate several users comfortably.
Sink, soap, water, and paper towels. If these are very far, extra time is allowed for cleaning hands and equipment.	Items listed in "Adequate" column are available near the BMBR.	Items listed in "Adequate" column are available in the BMBR.
Employee supplies cold packs for storage of milk.	Employer makes available refrigerator space designated for food near BMBR.	Employer provides a small refrigerator in the BMBR for storage of human milk.
Written Company Policy		
Employer grants a 6-week unpaid maternity leave.	Employer grants a 12-week unpaid maternity leave (FMLA).	Employer offers a 6- to 14-week paid maternity leave (ILO).
Employer allows creative use of accrued vacation days, personal time, sick days, and holiday pay after childbirth.	In addition, employer allows part-time work, job sharing, individualized scheduling of work hours, compressed work week, or telecommuting.	In addition, mother can bring child to work, caregiver can bring child to workplace, or on-site day care is available.
Employer allows 2 breaks and a lunch period during an 8-hour work day for expressing milk or breastfeeding the child.	Employer allows expanded unpaid breaks during the work day for expressing milk or breastfeeding the child.	Nursing breaks are paid and are counted as working time.
Workplace Education		
Company breastfeeding support policy is communicated to all pregnant employees.	New employees, supervisors, and coworkers all receive training on the breastfeeding support policy.	Breastfeeding education is offered to the partners of employees who are expectant fathers.
Employer provides a list of community resources for breastfeeding support.	Employer contracts with skilled lactation care provider on an "as needed" basis.	Employer hires a skilled lactation care provider to coordinate a breastfeeding support program.

Source: Printed with permission of the United States Breastfeeding Committee.

educate businesses and mothers in your community about the benefits to employer support for breastfeeding employees (Texas Department of State Health Services, 2008):

- Cost savings of $3 for every $1 invested in breastfeeding support
- Less illness among breastfed children of employees
- Reduced absenteeism to care for ill children
- Lower healthcare costs (an average of $400 per baby over the first year)
- Improved employee productivity
- Higher employee morale and greater loyalty
- Improved ability to attract and retain valuable employees
- Family-friendly image in the community

Employer Breastfeeding-Friendly Program

One way employers can support breastfeeding mothers is by providing extended paid maternity leave so a mother can remain at home with her baby for as long as possible. They can incorporate breastfeeding breaks into the mother's work schedule or give mothers the option of bringing their baby to work to avoid missed feedings. They can provide information about child care or, better yet, provide child care at or near the worksite. Some companies offer prenatal and postpartum programs for parents. Employers can also accommodate mothers with appropriate physical facilities for tending to their breastfeeding needs, as well as a policy of support among coworkers.

Lactation Room

The biggest challenge to establishing facilities for breastfeeding mothers may be finding available space for pumping that is private. Progressive employers provide a lactation room for their employees with a lockable door to prevent embarrassing interruptions. A screen inside the door offers additional privacy. The climate in the lactation room should be nonstressful and soothing, perhaps enhanced by quiet music and reading material. Providing a refrigerator for the mother's milk is another gesture that shows a commitment to her efforts. It is also helpful to have a mirror so she can check to be sure her clothes are back in place before leaving the room. The room needs comfortable chairs with arm support and a table or desk on which the mother can place her breast pump, her baby's picture, a beverage, and other items she may need. Employees on maternity leave and those who are pregnant can receive information about the lactation room so they are aware their employer supports breastfeeding. This helps demonstrate the importance of the program.

A U.S. survey of companies reported 25 percent with on-site lactation/mother's rooms and 5 percent with lactation support services (Society for Human Resource Management, 2009). Figure 24.2 shows breakdown of support by company size. You can help a mother achieve breastfeeding support at work by suggesting ways to approach her employer about developing a lactation program. She can survey other employees to learn how many are pregnant, how many plan to breastfeed, and how many would use a lactation room. This helps garner support for the program ands provides concrete data to present to the employer. Likewise, she can gain support from fellow employees, another breastfeeding mother or breastfeeding advocate, the corporation's nurse, a wellness program director, or a health educator. Collaboratively, they can determine the best way to approach the employer and the necessary preparations beforehand.

Company Size	On-site Lactation/ Mother's Room	Lactation Support Services
Small (1–99 Employees)	12%	2%
Medium (100–499 Employees)	26%	3%
Large (500 or More Employees)	38%	10%

Source: Data from Society for Human Resource Management. 2009 Employee Benefits Survey Report. June 28, 2009. http://www.shrm.org/Research/SurveyFindings/Articles/Pages/2009EmployeeBenefitsSurveyReport.aspx. Accessed March 1, 2010.

FIGURE 24.2   U.S. company support for breastfeeding.

It is best to present the idea of a lactation room to the employer in a written proposal that identifies the required time, space, and environment. Suggesting more than one option often increases the likelihood of the mother and employer coming to an agreement. The mother should also be prepared to discuss alternative solutions and make compromises in her original plan. The proposal should indicate potential costs and whether the company's budget can support those costs. Indicating the cost-to-benefit ratio illustrates long-term savings to the company in healthcare costs. Attaching relevant research on the health savings of breastfeeding lends further credence to the proposal. The mother can also demonstrate to the employer that the cost of a lactation program will be less than the cost of training a new employee.

Company-sponsored lactation programs enable mothers to maintain milk production for their babies so they can continue breastfeeding to 6 months. A goal of Healthy People 2010 is to have 50 percent of mothers breastfeeding for this length of time. In a survey of 462 women in 5 companies, 97.5 initiated breastfeeding and 57.8 percent continued for at least 6 months (Ortiz et al., 2004). They expressed milk in the workplace for a mean of 6.3 months, with the average age of the baby 9.1 months when the mother stopped pumping.

Some employers place a sign-in book in the lactation room to track and report the number of employees from different departments who use the space. Employees can be encouraged to provide feedback on the conditions of the station and offer suggestions for improvement. Usually, the employees express gratitude and praise. One woman even wrote a book based on notebook journals kept by a group of women during their visits to the company's employee lactation room (Colburn-Smith & Serette, 2007).

Time to Express Milk or Breastfeed

The time allotted for mothers to express their milk needs to be valued and respected by everyone within the work environment. This employee accommodation is not comparable with a coffee break or other personal time away from the work area. It is a health practice for the mother and baby, grounded in a significant amount of research. Most mothers express their milk about twice a day and spend under an hour when they are embraced by a supportive employment environment (Slusser et al., 2004).

Employers are encouraged to allow the mother freedom to leave her workspace when she determines the need. She requires enough time to reach the room, time for unhurried milk expression, and time to return to her workspace. Allowing time for cigarette breaks seems to be standard in many companies. A break for breastfeeding—a healthy choice—certainly warrants the same accommodation!

Positive Environment

The support of management is crucial to a mother's ability to balance work with breastfeeding. Some employees may make negative comments about the mother's efforts. Ironically, male coworkers often seem to support breastfeeding employees more than other women do. A positive climate established by management encourages coworkers to support the mother in a meaningful way. Company policy needs to incorporate protection of the mother's right to pumping time and intolerance of nonsupport or sexual harassment from other employees. The policy can establish the expectation that coworkers will not question or complain about the mother's time away from work to tend to her breastfeeding needs.

Some employers have a lactation consultant on call for any concerns or special situations that arise. Employers are a significant contributor to mothers reaching their breastfeeding goals. You can be instrumental in helping employers in your community establish policies that support their breastfeeding employees. Stressing both the financial and health benefits strengthens your efforts.

Formula Company Initiatives for Working Mothers

Formula manufacturers have targeted working mothers as a hot market for their products. Abbott Labs collaborated on two marketing tools with Working Mother Media, the publisher of *Working Mother* magazine. "Business Backs Breastfeeding," initiated in 2004, was presented as a comprehensive workplace lactation program to help businesses support breastfeeding mothers upon their return to work. "As an infant nutrition company, Ross Products

has a long history of providing breastfeeding education materials to mothers and healthcare professionals" (Abbott Labs, 2007, p. 3). The program enables Abbott entry to hundreds of businesses to create brand awareness and loyalty under the guise of creating goodwill and the perception of community service.

"Workplace Lactation Programs: Good for Working Families. Good for Business" was initiated by Abbott in 2009 in conjunction with Corporate Voices for Working Families, a consortium representing 50 large corporations on public policy issues. This program is promoted as supporting low-income, hourly working mothers in pumping (Corporate Voices for Working Families, 2009). When the mother visits the Abbott site to order breastfeeding supplies, she must wade through multiple layers of formula advertising and "choices" about infant feeding. These programs undermine a woman's confidence in breastfeeding and promote the perception that infant formula is a healthy alternative to a mother's milk. "Choosing" to breastfeed after returning to work and the difficulty of pumping are emphasized. The corporate template and handouts advertise Abbott's bottle nipples.

∼ Summary

It is important to help mothers manage times when they are away from their babies and miss feedings. A mother who is ill or whose baby is ill needs practical ways to manage her milk production and the baby's feeding needs. Your support is a valuable resource to a mother throughout the stress of a hospitalization. Most separations are due to social or economic needs and may be accommodated by planning on the mother's part. You can help the mother recognize her options in providing her milk to her baby. Continued assistance after she has implemented her plans helps her find ways to fine-tune her pumping, milk storage, use of alternative feeding methods, and other changes in her breastfeeding routine. Developing or managing a corporate lactation program, or being on call for assistance, provides essential support and encouragement to working mothers as they blend breastfeeding with employment.

∼ Chapter 24—At a Glance

Applying what you learned—

Counseling a mother through a separation:

- Ensure her baby feeds from an alternative method during her absence.
- Express milk regularly to relieve fullness and maintain milk production.

- Plan the least disruptive timing for the separation, when possible.
- Avoid leaking, plugged ducts, engorgement, and mastitis.
- Get adequate rest and nutrition.

Counseling mothers about illness and hospitalization:

- Pump to maintain milk production.
- Decrease the baby's exposure by careful hand washing before contact.
- Room-in with another adult in the room to help her care for her baby.
- Have the baby brought to the hospital throughout the day to breastfeed.
- Nurse before and after surgery.

Counseling a mother who returns to work:

- Recognize conflicting goals of motherhood and career.
- Realize goals may change after the baby arrives.
- Discuss her wishes, plans, needs, and concerns with family, friends, coworkers, and employer.
- Contact the International Lactation Consultant Association for a maternity protection kit and the USDHHS for "The Business Case for Breastfeeding."
- Explore work and childcare options that protect breastfeeding.
- Breastfeed uninterruptedly and bond with baby until return to work.
- Practice for the separation with the childcare provider and feeding method.
- Plan for milk expression, enhancing letdown, collection, and storage of milk.
- Plan for relieving breast fullness and leaking.
- Plan quiet time for breastfeeding after return from work.
- Inquire about a workplace breastfeeding support program.

~ References

Abbott Labs. Business Backs Breastfeeding: a flexible workplace program for breastfeeding mothers; October 2007. Accessed February 28, 2010.

Abdulwadud O, Snow M. Interventions in the workplace to support breastfeeding for women in employment. *Cochrane Database Syst Rev.* 2007;18(3):CD006177.

Academy of Breastfeeding Medicine. ABM clinical protocol #4: mastitis review; May 2008. www.bfmed.org. Accessed October 28, 2009.

Academy of Breastfeeding Medicine. Breastfeeding and H1N1 influenza A: information for physicians; May 6, 2009. http://www.bfmed.org/Media/Files/Documents/pdf/H1N1%20and%20Breastfeeding%20-%20for%20physicians.pdf. Accessed November 3, 2009.

American Association of Health Plans. Health Plans' innovative programs in breastfeeding promotion; August 2001. www.aahp.org. Accessed November 3, 2009.

American Society of Anesthesiologists. Task Force on Preoperative Fasting. Practice guidelines for preoperative fasting and the use of pharmacologic agents to reduce the risk of pulmonary aspirations: application to healthy patients undergoing elective procedures. *Anesthesiology.* 1999;90:896-905.

Angeletti M. Breastfeeding mothers returning to work: possibilities for information, anticipatory guidance and support from US health care professionals. *J Hum Lact.* 2009;25:226-232.

Bakoula C et al. Working mothers breastfeed babies more than housewives. *Acta Paediatr.* 2007;96:510-515.

Bentley M. Breastfeeding among low income, African-American women: power, beliefs and decision making. *J Nutr.* 2003;133:305S-309S.

Berens P. Breast complications while breastfeeding. Presented at the La Leche League of Texas Area Conference, San Antonio, Texas, June 12, 2004.

Bradley R, Vandell D. Child care and the well-being of children. *Arch Pediatr Adolesc Med.* 2007;161:669-676.

Bumgarner N. *Mothering Your Nursing Toddler.* Schaumburg, IL: La Leche League International; 2000.

Center for American Progress. The Shriver report; 2009. www.awomansnation.com. Accessed November 1, 2009.

Centers for Disease Control and Prevention (CDC). CDC guide to breastfeeding interventions (Shealy K, et al.). Atlanta, GA: USDHHS, CDC; 2005. www.cdc.gov/breastfeeding/pdf/breastfeeding_interventions.pdf. Accessed November 6, 2009.

Centers for Disease Control and Prevention (CDC). Interim guidance: considerations regarding 2009 H1N1 influenza in intrapartum and postpartum hospital settings; November 10, 2009a. (Replaces earlier guidelines, Considerations regarding novel H1N1 flu virus in obstetric setting; July 6, 2009.) http://www.cdc.gov/h1n1flu/guidance/obstetric.htm. Accessed December 2, 2009.

Centers for Disease Control and Prevention (CDC). New data reveal insight into moms' complex infant feeding decisions. October 6, 2009b. www.cdc.gov/Features/Breastfeeding. Accessed November 6, 2009.

Centers for Disease Control and Prevention (CDC). Proper handling and storage of human milk. May 22, 2007. www.cdc.gov/breastfeeding/recommendations/handling_breast milk.htm. Accessed September 27, 2009.

Chen Y, et al. Effects of work-related factors on the breastfeeding behavior of working mothers in a Taiwanese semiconductor manufacturer: a cross-sectional survey. *BMC Public Health.* 2006;6:160.

Chuang C, et al. Maternal return to work and breastfeeding: a population-based cohort study. *Int J Nurs Stud.* 2010;47(4):461-474.

Colburn-Smith C, Serette A. *Milk Memo: How Real Moms Learned to Mix Business With Babies-and How You Can, Too.* New York: Penguin Books; 2007.

Cooklin A, et al. Maternal employment & breastfeeding: results from the longitudinal Study of Australian children. *Acta Paediatrica.* 2008;97(5):620-623.

Corporate Voices for Working Families. Workplace lactation: workplace lactation programs: Good for Working Families. Good for Business™; February 2009. www.corporatevoices .org/lactation. Accessed November 1, 2009.

Dilli D, et al. Interventions to reduce pain during vaccination in infancy. *J Pediatr.* 2009;154:385-390.

Duke P, et al. Physicians as mothers: breastfeeding practices of physician-mothers in Newfoundland and Labrador. *Can Fam Physician.* 2007;53:886-891.

Dumphy D. The breastfeeding surgical patient. *AORN J.* 2008; 87:759-766.

Dunn B, et al. Breastfeeding practices in Colorado businesses. *J Hum Lact.* 2004;20:170-177.

Ferrante A, et al. The importance of choosing the right feeding aids to maintain breast-feeding after interruption. *Int J Orofac Myol.* 2006;32:58-67.

Galtry J. The impact on breastfeeding of labour market policy and practice in Ireland, Sweden, and the USA. *Soc Sci Med.* 2003;57:167-177.

Gatrell C. Secrets and lies: breastfeeding and professional paid work. *Soc Sci Med.* 2007;65(2):393-404.

Greenberg C, Avigdor B. *What Happy Working Mothers Know: How New Findings in Positive Psychology Can Lead to a Healthy and Happy Work/Life Balance.* Hoboken, NJ: John Wiley & Sons; 2009.

Guendelman S, et al. Juggling work and breastfeeding: effects of maternity leave and occupational characteristics. *Pediatrics.* 2009;123:e38-e46.

Haider J. Welfare work requirements and child well-being: evidence from the effects on breast-feeding. *Demography.* 2003;40:479-497.

Hanson L. The role of breastfeeding in the defense of the infant. In Hale T, Hartmann P. *Hale & Hartmann's Textbook of Human Lactation.* Amarillo, TX: Hale Publishing; 2007.

Hausman BL. Motherhood and inequality: a commentary on Hanna Rosin's "The Case Against Breastfeeding." *J Hum Lact.* 2009;25:266-268.

Hawkins S, et al.Millennium cohort study child health group. The impact of maternal employment on breast-feeding duration in the UK Millennium Cohort Study. *Public Health Nutr.* 2007;10(9):891-896.

Hochschild A, Machung A. *The Second Shift.* New York: Penguin Group; 2003.

Holmes A, et al. A barrier to exclusive breastfeeding for WIC enrollees: limited use of exclusive breastfeeding food package for mothers. *Breastfeed Med.* 2009;4:25-30.

Huang Y, et al. Supplementation with cup-feeding as a substitute for bottle-feeding to promote breastfeeding. *Chang Gung Med J.* 2009;32(4):423-431.

Hurley K, et al. Variation in breastfeeding behaviours, perceptions, and experiences by race/ethnicity among a low-income statewide sample of Special Supplemental Nutrition Program for Women, Infants, and Children (WIC) participants in the United States. *Matern Child Nutr.* 2008;4:95-105.

International Labour Organization (ILO). Maternity at work: a review of national legislation. Findings from the ILO's Conditions of Work and Employment Database. (Öun I, Trujillo G). Geneva, Switzerland: ILO, 2005. http://www .ilo.org/public/english/protection/condtrav/pdf/wf-iogpt-05.pdf. Accessed November 1, 2009.

Jacknowitz A. The role of workplace characteristics in breastfeeding practices. *Women Health.* 2008;47:87-111.

Johnston ML, Esposito N. Barriers and facilitators for breastfeeding among working women in the United States. *JOGNN.* 2007;36:9-20.

Kassing D. Bottle-feeding as a tool to reinforce breastfeeding. *J Hum Lact.* 2002;18:56-60.

Kelley S, et al. Support for mothers' employment at home: conflict between work and family. *Int J Public Opin Res.* 2009; 21:98-110.

Kosmala-Anderson J, Wallace LM. Breastfeeding works: the role of employers in supporting women who wish to breastfeed and work in four organizations in England. *J Public Health.* 2006;28:183-191.

Lakati A, et al. Breast-feeding and the working mother in Nairobi. *Public Health Nutr.* 2002;5(6):715-718.

Lawrence RA. Lactation support when the infant will require general anesthesia: assisting the breastfeeding dyad in remaining content through the preoperative fasting period. *J Hum Lact.* 2005;21:355-357.

Lawrence RA, Bradley JS. Advice regarding breastfeeding for mothers with possible H1N1 infection. *AAP News*; 2009. http://aapnews.aappublications.org/cgi/content/full/aapnews .20091012-1v1. Accessed December 1, 2009.

Lerner L, et al. Satisfaction of women urologists with maternity leave and childbirth timing. *J Urol.* 2010;183(1):282-286.

Maternity Protection Campaign. Mulford C(ILCA) and Omer-Salim A.(IMCH). May 14, 2002. www.waba.org.my/whatwe do/womenandwork/breastfeedingandtheworkplace.htm. Accessed February 28, 2010.

Mills S. Workplace lactation programs: a critical element for breastfeeding mothers' success. *AAOHN J.* 2009;57:227-231.

Mulford C. Is breastfeeding really *invisible*, or did the health care system just choose not to notice it? *Intl Breastfeed J.* 2008;3:13.

National Association of Child Care Resource & Referral Agencies. We CAN do better: 2009 update. NACCRRA's ranking of state child care center regulation and oversight. Arlington, VA: NACCRRA; 2009. www.naccra.org. Accessed November 10, 2009.

Olang B, et al. Breastfeeding in Iran: prevalence, duration and current recommendations. *Int Breastfeed J.* 2009;4:8.

Organization for Economic Cooperation and Development. The future of the family to 2030: a scoping report. OECD International Futures Programme. December 19, 2008. www .oecd.org/dataoecd/11/34/42551944.pdf. Accessed February 28, 2010.

Ortiz J, et al. Duration of breast milk expression among working mothers enrolled in an employer-sponsored lactation program. *Pediatr Nurs.* 2004;30:111-119.

Osinaike B, et al. Effect of breastfeeding during venepuncture in neonates. *Ann Trop Paediatr*. 2007;27:201-205.

Palmer G. *The Politics of Breastfeeding: When Breasts are Bad for Business*, 3rd ed. London: Pinter & Martin; 2009.

Payne D, James L. Make or break. Mothers' experiences of returning to paid employment and breastfeeding: a New Zealand study. *Breastfeed Rev*. 2008;16:21-27.

Pryor G, Huggins K. *Nursing Mother, Working Mother*, rev ed. Boston: Harvard Common Press; 2007.

Saitua I, et al. Analgesic effect of breastfeeding when taking blood by heel-prick in newborns. *An Pediatr*. 2009;71:310-313.

Shah V, et al. Effectiveness and tolerability of pharmacologic and combined interventions for reducing injection pain during routine childhood immunizations: systematic review and meta-analyses. *Clin Ther*. 2009;31(Suppl. 2):S104-S151.

Slusser W, et al. Breast milk expression in the workplace: a look at frequency and time. *J Hum Lact*. 2004;20:164-169.

Snow K, Kriskey S. More women forced to reduce maternity leave under stress of the economy: some new mothers concerned about their families' finances as they contemplate leave. *ABC News*, June 16, 2009.

Society for Human Resource Management. 2009 Employee Benefits Survey Report. June 28, 2009. www.shrm.org/Research/SurveyFindings/Articles/Pages/2009EmployeeBenefitsSurveyReport.aspx. Accessed February 28, 2010.

Souza E, et al. Impact of hospitalization on breastfeeding practices in a pediatric hospital in Salvador, Bahia State, Brazil. *Cad Saude Publ*. 2008;24:1062-1070.

Stewart-Glenn J. Knowledge, perceptions, and attitudes of managers, coworkers, and employed breastfeeding mothers. *AAOHN J*. 2008;56:423-429.

Sweden.se. The official gateway to Sweden; 2009. www.sweden.se/eng. Accessed November 3, 2009.

Taveras E. Clinician support and psychosocial risk factors associated with breastfeeding discontinuation. *Pediatrics*. 2003;112(1 Pt 1):108-115.

Texas Department of State Health Services. Nutrition Services Section. Mother friendly worksite program. Stock #13-58; October 2008. http://www.dshs.state.tx.us/wichd/WICCatalog/PDF_Links/13-58%20Mother%20Friendly%20Worksite_lr.pdf. Accessed November 10, 2009.

Uga E, et al. Heel lance in newborn during breastfeeding: an evaluation of analgesic effect of this procedure. *Riv Ital Pediatr*. 2008;34:3.

Uriell Z, et al. Breastfeeding in the navy: estimates of rate, duration, and perceived support. *Mil Med*. 2009;174:290-296.

U.S. Breastfeeding Committee. Breastfeeding Promotion Act; November 4, 2009. www.usbreastfeeding.org/Portals/0/Virtual-BPA-Briefing-Packet-2009-11-4.pdf. Accessed November 12, 2009.

U.S. Census Bureau. America's families and living arrangements: 2007 (Kreider R, Elliott D). Current Population Reports, P20-561. Washington, DC: U.S. Census Bureau; 2009.

U.S. Department of Health and Human Services (USDHHS), Health Resources and Services Administration, Maternal and Child Health Bureau. *Child Health USA 2008–2009*. Rockville, MD: U.S. Department of Health and Human Services; 2009.

U.S. Department of Labor (USDL), News Bureau of Labor Statistics. Employment characteristics of families in 2008. USDL 09-0568, May 27, 2009. http://stats.bls.gov/news.release/archives/famee_05272009.pdf. Accessed February 28, 2010.

Weaver-Zercher V. Mother in the house. Christian Century, Feb. 6, 2007. www.bnet.com. Accessed November 2, 2009.

Wenner L. Care of the breastfeeding mother in medical-surgical areas. *Med Surg Nurs*. 2007;16:101-104.

Wilson-Clay B. Case report of methicillin-resistant *Staphylococcus aureus* (MRSA) mastitis with abscess formation in a breastfeeding woman. *J Hum Lact*. 2008;24:326-329.

Wilson-Clay B, Hoover K. *The Breastfeeding Atlas*, 4th ed. Austin, TX: Lactnews Press; 2008.

Working Mother. 2008 Best vs Rest. 2009. http://www.workingmother.com/web?service=vpage/3298. Accessed June 2, 2010.

World Alliance for Breastfeeding Action. Women, work and breastfeeding: campaigning for maternity protection at the workplace. www.waba.org.my/womenwork/campaign.html. Accessed November 4, 2009.

Xu F, Qiu L, Binns CW, Liu X. Breastfeeding in China: a review. *Int Breastfeed J*. 2009;4:6.

Long-Term Maternal and Infant Conditions

The goal of breastfeeding advocates is empowering mothers to have positive experiences nursing their babies. Some mothers require special assistance with breast-feeding. Chronic health conditions in either the mother or the infant have the potential to alter the normal course of breast-feeding. When an infant is born with a health condition or neurological disorder, the effect on family members and their relationships depends on the type and severity of the disorder. The medical expertise and emotional support available to parents are also factors. Parents can overcome many feeding challenges when they learn adaptations for achieving a fulfilling, nurturing breastfeeding relationship.

～ Key Terms

Acetone
Acquired
  immunodeficiency
  syndrome (AIDS)
Alactogenesis
Anomaly
Autoimmune disorder
Bariatric surgery
Cleft lip
Cleft palate
Cystic fibrosis
Cytomegalovirus
Diabetes
Down syndrome
Duarte variant
Endometriosis
Epinephrine
Epstein-Barr
Eustachian tube
Exocrine system
Flash heat treatment
Galactosemia
Goiter
Grommet
Hepatitis C
Herpes

Human
  immunodeficiency
  virus (HIV)
Hydrocephalus
Hypernatremic
Hypertension
Hyperthyroidism
Hypothyroidism
Infertility
Insufficient milk supply
  (IMS)
Lactogenesis
Lymphocytes
Multipara
Obesity
Obturator
Otitis media
Palatal repair
Phenylalanine
Phenylketonuria
Pierre Robin sequence
Polycystic ovary syndrome
  (PCOS)
Postpartum thyroiditis
Pretoria pasteurization
Primipara

Propylthiouracil
Raynaud's phenomenon
Rheumatoid arthritis
Scleroderma
Seroconversion
Sjögren's syndrome
Spina bifida
Submucosal cleft palate

Systemic lupus
  erythematosus
Thyroid disorder
Transplacental
Tuberculosis
Varicella zoster
Vasospasm

～ Special Maternal Health Conditions

Some maternal medical conditions can have an impact on breastfeeding. Any condition requiring medication raises the question of whether a mother can safely nurse her baby. Other disorders may affect a woman's energy or otherwise impair her ability to breastfeed. Health conditions discussed in this chapter include autoimmune disorders, infertility, obesity, bariatric surgery, diabetes, thyroid disorders, cystic fibrosis, and phenylketonuria (PKU). Several viruses that a mother may contract are addressed as well, with discussion of their safety with breastfeeding.

Autoimmune Disorders

An estimated 50 million Americans are afflicted by an autoimmune disease. Autoimmune diseases occur when the immune system misfires and attacks the cells, tissues, or organs it normally protects. All autoimmune diseases show evidence of a genetic predisposition, and they tend to cluster in families. Environmental triggers such as diet, sunlight, and a preceding infection may play a role in triggering the diseases in individuals with a genetic predisposition.

There are more than 80 autoimmune diseases, which clinicians now consider to be a group of disorders (U.S. Department of Health and Human Services [USDHHS], 2005). Some genes are specific to a certain disease, whereas others predispose to autoimmunity in general. Autoimmune diseases share many common symptoms, and often an individual has more than one disease. Some of the autoimmune diseases more familiar to the public are multiple sclerosis, Graves' disease, scleroderma, Raynaud's phenomenon, inflammatory bowel disease, ulcerative colitis, Crohn's disease, lupus, Sjögren's syndrome, and rheumatoid arthritis.

Fibromyalgia has gained recognition as a distinct clinical entity that often accompanies other autoimmune disorders. It exhibits a characteristic pattern of specific, intensely tender trigger points on the body. Chronic fatigue immune dysfunction syndrome may have an autoimmune component as well, because it is often associated with circulating antinuclear autoantibodies.

Women are three times more likely to be affected by an autoimmune disease than men (American Autoimmune Related Diseases Association, 2009). Table 25.1 presents the ratio of female-to-male occurrence in common autoimmune diseases. Women are most vulnerable during their reproductive years, and the predominance among women may reflect the involvement of female hormones in the regulation of immune response. About 75 percent of diagnosed women are in their childbearing years, making it likely that some of the women in your

TABLE 25.1 Autoimmune Diseases and the Female-to-Male Ratios of Occurrence

Disease	Female-to-Male Ratio
Hashimoto's thyroiditis	10:1
Systemic lupus erythematosus	9:1
Sjögren's syndrome	9:1
Antiphospholipid syndrome, secondary	9:1
Primary biliary cirrhosis	9:1
Autoimmune hepatitis	8:1
Graves' disease	7:1
Scleroderma	3:1
Rheumatoid arthritis	2.5:1
Antiphospholipid syndrome, primary	2:1
Autoimmune thrombocytopenic purpura	2:1
Multiple sclerosis	2:1
Myasthenia gravis	2:1

Sources: Sinaii N, et al. High rates of autoimmune and endocrine disorders, fibromyalgia, chronic fatigue syndrome, and atopic diseases among women with endometriosis: a survey anyalysis. *Hum Reprod.* 2002;17(10):2715-2724. American Autoimmune Related Diseases Association, Inc., 2009. www.aarda.org/women_and_autoimmunity.php.

care will have an autoimmune disease. Many may have an undiagnosed autoimmune disease, because those who are afflicted often exhibit symptoms for several years before they are correctly diagnosed.

Counseling Implications

What does this all mean to you as a lactation consultant? First, by understanding the nature of autoimmune disease, you may recognize symptoms such as chronic fatigue and pain as potential red flags for women in your care. You can then suggest they consult their caregiver. Proper diagnosis is one of the most difficult challenges related to autoimmune disease. You can suggest that these women learn the medical history of their immediate and extended family. They can make a list of symptoms, even those that are seemingly unrelated, dating back as far as they can recall. Finding informed caregivers who have experience with autoimmune disease is one of the most important factors in obtaining a correct diagnosis. Many individuals seek second, third, and fourth opinions over several years before they finally receive an appropriate diagnosis and treatment.

Second, you can be alert to potential symptoms that could affect these women during lactation. Although not all autoimmune diseases directly affect breastfeeding, the chronic fatigue and pain associated with many of the autoimmune diseases can affect a woman's coping abilities and mental outlook. Certain medications may relieve symptoms for some of the diseases, and you can share appropriate information about the safety of taking these and other medications while breastfeeding.

Endometriosis and Immune Disorders

Women with endometriosis have a higher incidence of autoimmune disorders than the general female population. Rates of hypothyroidism are 9.6 percent compared with 1.5 percent in the general population, and rates of allergies with fibromyalgia or chronic fatigue are 88 percent compared with 18 percent in the general population (Sinaii et al., 2002). Because 41 percent of women with endometriosis have fertility problems, you may see quite a few of these women who become pregnant through assisted reproduction and then have problems with lactation. A thorough medical history helps identify markers.

Other Implications for Breastfeeding

Sjögren's syndrome is an autoimmune disease that attacks the tear, salivary, and other secretory glands and impairs their ability to produce moisture. In most cases the autoimmune response affects the tear ducts, salivary glands, and vagina (National Institute of Neurological Disorders and Stroke, 2008). There is no evidence that it has an effect on the mammary glands. However, because the breast is a secretory organ, the possibility of a correlation bears scrutiny. Sjögren's syndrome can be a marker for other diseases, including scleroderma. Some autoimmune diseases, such as multiple sclerosis, may improve during pregnancy. Others may worsen before or after childbirth.

Some autoimmune diseases, such as thyroid diseases, increase the risk of infertility and miscarriage (Ogunyemi, 2009; Poppe et al., 2008, 2007; Negro et al., 2007). Women with lupus have about a 10 percent rate of miscarriage, and their pregnancies should be treated as high risk (Lupus Foundation of America, 2007). Lactation is associated with remission or reduction of symptoms in autoimmune diseases, including inflammatory bowel disease (Moffatt et al., 2009) and multiple sclerosis (Langer-Gould et al., 2009). Breastfeeding also lowers mothers' risks for developing rheumatoid arthritis (Oliver & Silman, 2009; Pikwer et al., 2009).

As discussed in Chapter 9, human milk has protective factors that reduce the infant's risk of autoimmune disease. These include inflammatory bowel diseases such as Crohn's disease and ulcerative colitis (Barclay et al., 2009; Thompson et al., 2000), juvenile diabetes (Quinn, 2010; Brugman et al., 2009; Ip et al., 2009, 2007; Goldfarb, 2008; Luopajärvi et al., 2008), juvenile arthritis (Hanson, 2007; Løland et al., 2007; Young et al., 2007), multiple sclerosis (Tarrats et al., 2002; Pisacane et al., 1994), and celiac disease (Tooley et al., 2009; Olsson et al., 2008; Ivarsson et al., 2002). Mexico has experienced a rise in the incidence of multiple sclerosis as breastfeeding has decreased (Tarrats et al., 2002). Because of the genetic links in autoimmune diseases, mothers are wise to breastfeed their children. Not breastfeeding increases the risks of developing any of the scores of immune diseases.

Raynaud's Phenomenon

Raynaud's phenomenon is a neurovascular condition that is believed to affect about 3 percent of the general population (USDHHS, National Institute of Arthritis and Musculoskeletal and Skin Diseases [NIAMS], 2009). The primary form (not associated with another disease) usually appears between 15 and 25 years of age and is more common in women than men. It also appears to occur more frequently in colder climates. This may be due to people with the disorder having more Raynaud's attacks in colder climates.

Pain in the extremities when exposed to cold is a marker for Raynaud's, which is a disorder of the small blood vessels in the skin. During a Raynaud's attack, restricted blood flow in the extremities causes numbness and a "pins-and-needles" sensation. Sometimes a dull pain and clumsiness occur. Skin color changes of the extremities occur in a sequence of white (blanching or pallor) to blue (cyanotic) and then to red (rubor) as blood returns to the area. Raynaud's can also affect the nose and ears. A Raynaud's attack may affect a woman's dexterity and ability to relax during a feeding. Cold is more apt to cause an attack when accompanied by physical or emotional stress. Sometimes stress alone causes vasoconstriction without exposure to cold. Given the stressors of birth and postpartum adjustment, it is not surprising that lactation consultants see many women with these symptoms.

Injuries such as frostbite or surgery can cause Raynaud's phenomenon. Regular use of machinery such as chain saws and vibrating drills can damage the small blood vessels. Other activities that may worsen the condition include frequent typing and piano playing (USDHHS NIAMS, 2009). Certain drugs and medical conditions can cause secondary Raynaud's, including some heart, blood, and migraine headache medications. The following conditions may cause secondary Raynaud's:

- Scleroderma—a thickening and hardening of the skin and other body tissues
- Systemic lupus erythematosus—a chronic inflammation of the skin and organ systems
- Rheumatoid arthritis—a chronic inflammation and swelling of tissue in the joints
- Blood flow reduction—problems that slow or stop blood flow in a vessel, such as inflammation and hardening of the arteries (arteriosclerosis)
- Nerve problems—problems that affect the nerves supplying the muscles
- Pulmonary hypertension—a condition in which pressure rises in the blood vessels of the lungs

Caffeine and nicotine increase the severity of Raynaud's due to increased blood vessel constriction. You can caution mothers that consuming caffeine or smoking may worsen their symptoms. Increasing intake of vitamin B_6 has helped some mothers. However, very high doses (600 mg) are associated with lower milk production. Vitamin B_6 passes readily into milk and too much can harm an infant's liver (Hale, 2010). Hale suggests a maximum intake of 25 mg/day of vitamin B_6. Newman and Kernerman (2009) advise that if vitamin B_6 fails to work within a week, it probably will not produce results. Calcium channel blockers, such as nifedipine, have been helpful for some mothers with Raynaud's (Hale & Berens, 2002).

Raynaud's and Nipple Soreness

As described in Chapter 16, a Raynaud-like phenomenon can cause vasospasms of the nipple. Mothers describe the pain as a stinging, tingling, burning, very painful sensation that persists after a feeding. The same triphasic color change occurs on the nipple as with the extremities in true Raynaud's (Page & McKenna, 2006; Reilly & Snyder, 2005; Anderson et al., 2004). A poor latch and/or suck may often be the cause of such a vasospasm. Many mothers find that when the latch improves, the baby no longer compresses the nipple to cause vasospasm. Sometimes, however, the baby may latch effectively but the mother still experiences this kind of pain. Women who have true Raynaud's usually are aware of it before pregnancy, though mothers may report never having symptoms before the baby's birth. Some mothers with nipple vasospasms report the pain also occurs when they are exposed to cold.

For some mothers your validation that their nipple pain has a medical cause will be a big relief. Many times their pain is dismissed by healthcare providers because they are lactating and the lactating breast is viewed as a temporary condition (Mulford, 2008). Refer the mother to her caregiver for evaluation and treatment, with current medical study references if her physician is not familiar with nipple vasospasm in the breastfeeding woman. If she is on any of the medications associated with secondary Raynaud's, her physician may be able to adjust or change them.

If you have helped a mother fix her baby's latch and she is still experiencing vasospasms, other measures may provide relief (USDHHS NIAMS, 2009):

- Seek treatment with medications, avoiding aggravating medications.
- Control stress and exercise regularly.
- Apply dry or moist heat immediately after breastfeeding.
- Wear warm socks, gloves, hat, and scarf to protect the entire body from the cold.
- Avoid putting hands in cold water.
- Remove food from the refrigerator or freezer with gloves or potholders.
- Try to avoid cuts, bruises, and other injuries to the affected areas.
- Limit activities such as keyboarding, texting, sewing, or other detail work.
- Reduce or eliminate caffeine, nicotine and other vasoconstrictors.
- Try chiropractic, acupuncture, and/or biofeedback care.
- Consult a doctor if questions or concerns develop.

Now that so many women initiate breastfeeding, healthcare providers are encountering this Raynaud's-like phenomenon more frequently and are less dismissive of it. Page and McKenna (2006) note that nipple vasospasm is severely painful and can lead to weaning if untreated.

The mother's physician may be the first one to evaluate her symptoms. Nifedipine (a beta channel blocker) treatment can be successful for these patients.

Diabetes

Diabetes mellitus is the sixth leading cause of death in the United States (about 70,000 annually). Occurrence rates are 13.7 percent among men and 11.7 percent among women aged 30 years and over (Danaei et al., 2009). The diabetes population and related healthcare costs are expected to at least double (to 44.1 million people and to $336 billion) in the next 25 years (Huang et al., 2009).

The three classifications of diabetes mellitus are insulin-dependent or type 1 diabetes, type 2 diabetes, and gestational diabetes. Gestational diabetes typically resolves after delivery. However, these women are at higher risk for converting to type 2 diabetes. Understanding how diabetes affects the body helps you counsel diabetic women appropriately. Diabetes occurs because of either insufficient insulin production or inefficient use of insulin by the body's cells. Unable to metabolize carbohydrates for energy, the body burns fat as its energy source. When the fat metabolizes, increased amounts of ketones are excreted into the urine. With the kidneys unable to keep up with the input of ketones, blood sugar level is affected. Uncontrolled blood sugar levels can cause coma and death. Diabetes results in slow wound healing and neuropathy. It is associated with other morbidities and causes of death.

Before the discovery of insulin in 1922, babies of diabetic mothers often died; the mothers often died as well. Risks are still high for diabetic mothers and their babies. The baby has twice the risk of serious injury at birth, triple the probability of cesarean delivery, and four times the rate of admission to a neonatal intensive care unit. The more poorly controlled the mother's sugar levels, the higher the risk of these outcomes (Moore, 2009).

Women who do not breastfeed and children who are not breastfed are at higher risk for developing diabetes (American Dietetic Association, 2009). Diabetic women may have difficulty conceiving, because they can experience delayed menarche, menstrual abnormalities, and premature menopause. However, diabetic women who are able to control their glycol (sugar) levels experience fertility rates close to nondiabetic women (Livshits & Seidman, 2009).

Babies of Diabetic Mothers

Babies of diabetic mothers are at risk for being large for gestational age. These babies are at high risk to be supplemented with artificial milk due to hypoglycemia (low blood sugar) at birth. Ironically, large-for-gestational-age babies are also at higher risk for developing diabetes, and it is the early exposure to bovine proteins that is believed to be the triggering allergic event (Luopajärvi et al., 2008; Holmberg et al., 2007; Tiittanen et al., 2006). Animal studies suggest that maternal transmission of autoantibodies is a critical factor in lowering the risk for developing type 1 diabetes (Washburn et al., 2007). Moreover, the factors associated with maternal type 1 diabetes, short breastfeeding duration and the baby's large birth size, predispose children to overweight during childhood (Hummel et al., 2009).

Because of the increased risk for infant susceptibility to developing diabetes, many parents do not want their baby receiving formula in the hospital. Increasingly, mothers are coping with the risk of supplementation by expressing their colostrum prenatally (Forster et al., 2009; Walker, 2009; Barlow, 2006). Starting after 37 weeks' gestation, the mother can hand express a small amount at a time and freeze it. In Forster et al.'s study, none of the mothers experienced hypoglycemia after expressing. Most of the mothers felt positive about expressing prenatally. A median of 39.6 mL of colostrum was obtained over 14 days.

Breastfeeding with Diabetes

With modern monitoring techniques, both in the hospital and at home, most diabetic women carry their babies to term and breastfeed with few complications. Diabetic women are often highly motivated to breastfeed when they are well educated about the sequelae of the disease and about the health impact of not breastfeeding. Mothers who take ownership of their health have a good working knowledge of nutrition because of their condition.

A diabetic mother needs to monitor her blood sugar levels carefully, manage her breastfeeding appropriately, and work closely with her caregivers, who may include an obstetrician, a pediatrician, and an endocrinologist. A woman's insulin needs drop dramatically after the delivery of the placenta. Therefore an insulin-dependent mother must conduct frequent blood glucose tests in the first few days postpartum to determine her requirements. Insulin levels fluctuate erratically until lactation is established and fluctuate again when weaning occurs. Careful monitoring is essential during these times.

Diabetes type can be a significant predictor of breastfeeding initiation. One study found that women with gestational diabetes both intended to and breastfed more than women with type 1 and type 2 diabetes at 2 weeks after birth (Soltani & Arden, 2009). Mothers with type 1 diabetes have been found to breastfeed less and for a shorter duration than those in the general population (Kreichauf et al., 2008). Breastfeeding duration of at least 4 weeks was associated with a reduced risk for overweight at 2 years of age in this study. Protection for the infant

appears to be dose dependent and related to exclusive breastfeeding (Ip et al., 2009, 2007; Sadauskaite-Kuehne et al., 2004).

There is evidence that lactogenesis is delayed by up to 2 to 3 days in insulin-dependent diabetics compared with nondiabetics. This phenomenon does not seem to interfere with the mother's overall lactation outcome. However, it is important to be aware of the possibility of delayed lactogenesis and counsel mothers appropriately. Breastfeeding early and regularly postpartum is especially important for diabetic mothers to assist stage II lactogenesis (Walker, 2009; Hurst, 2007). ILCA's Inside Track handout sheet on breastfeeding with diabetes, *Breastfeeding with Diabetes: Yes, You Can!,* is a helpful tool, especially for low-literacy mothers (Walker, 2006). Diet-controlled diabetic women have no breastfeeding restrictions. Insulin-dependent women may breastfeed safely while continuing insulin therapy throughout lactation.

Diabetic women are prone to yeast infections, which can affect both the mother's vaginal area and nipples. Moisture provides a breeding ground for fungus and can cause nipple soreness. Mothers can help avoid this complication by keeping the nipples dry between feedings. If sore nipples fail to respond to the usual treatment, a yeast infection may be the cause (see Chapter 16 for a discussion of thrush). The delicate balance of diet, insulin, and exercise can be disturbed by an infection, or by digestive or emotional upset. Reducing stress and removing milk regularly from her breasts helps a mother to avoid plugged ducts and mastitis. If mastitis occurs, the mother must monitor her blood sugar closely and make necessary adjustments in her treatment regimen.

Diabetic Treatment During Lactation

Diabetes treatment is highly individual. Many diabetic women feel their healthiest and have better control over their diabetes during lactation than at any other time in their lives. Some women may need to increase, rather than decrease, their dosage of insulin. Because of an altered hormone balance, diabetic women may experience improved glycemic control throughout lactation. Sugar is absorbed from the mother's system to produce the energy needed for milk production. Additionally, lactose is a component in the mother's milk, and the activity of breastfeeding expends more calories. This combination of factors often permits a higher caloric intake and lower insulin dosage.

Diabetic mothers generally require an increase in calories, carbohydrates, and protein during lactation. This varies with every woman, and precise dietary guidelines need to be part of the new regimen a mother plans with her caregiver. If her blood sugar climbs too high, the mother will release acetone and transmit it to her baby through her milk. After several days of exposure to high acetone levels, the baby can develop an enlarged liver. An increase of carbohydrates, possibly accompanied by an increased insulin dosage, controls the risk of acetone migrating into the mother's milk. If blood sugar is too low, the woman may experience diabetic shock, releasing epinephrine into her system and inhibiting letdown and milk production. Tight control of blood sugar levels helps prevent these complications.

During any interruption in breastfeeding, and especially during weaning, the mother should adjust her caloric intake and insulin dosage to compensate for the decrease in utilization of sugar for lactation. Whenever sugar is present in her urine, the mother must increase her insulin dosage gradually and reduce her caloric intake to respond to her nursing schedule. If the interruption is short-lived, a simple reduction in food intake may be sufficient, with no change in insulin dosage.

Insulin Resistance and Metabolic Syndrome

Metabolic syndrome is the term used for a cluster or group of symptoms that occur together and promote the development of coronary artery disease, stroke, and type 2 diabetes. Metabolic syndrome is estimated to affect at least a quarter of the U.S. population, and especially afflicts older adults. Symptoms of metabolic syndrome include (USDHHS, National Institutes of Health, 2009):

- High blood pressure
- High blood sugar levels
- High levels of triglycerides
- Low levels of high-density-lipoprotein ("good") cholesterol
- Too much fat around the waist

Although there is no definitive agreement on the cause of metabolic syndrome, researchers believe it may result from insulin resistance. The constant build-up of sugar in the blood sets the stage for disease later in life. Some patients with insulin resistance receive treatment with metformin and glitazones, which increase the body's sensitivity to insulin (Garruti et al., 2009; Galluzzo et al., 2008). Oral contraceptives are also effective (Radosh, 2009; Silva et al., 2006). Symptoms of insulin resistance pertinent to childbearing women include:

- High weight gain in pregnancy
- Preexisting obesity
- Gestational diabetes
- High cholesterol
- Hypertension
- Acanthosis nigricans
- Development of skin tags during pregnancy

Obesity

Obesity is rampant in both the industrialized and developing world, with more than a billion overweight adults, 300 million of whom are clinically obese. Obesity is defined as having a body mass index of 30 or greater. Body mass index is calculated from a person's weight and height. It indicates body fatness and weight categories that may lead to health problems. Obesity adds to the global burden of chronic disease and disability (World Health Organization [WHO], 2009a). It is a major risk factor for cardiovascular disease, hypertension, stroke, cancer, and type 2 diabetes.

The causes of obesity are multifaceted. As populations become more urban, diets have changed from high complex carbohydrates to a higher proportion of fats, saturated fats, and sugars. Simultaneously, work has become less physically demanding and people burn fewer calories. Automated transport, home technology, and more passive leisure interests result in less physical activity as well (WHO, 2009a).

Obesity rates in the United States have increased dramatically over the past 20 years. In 2008 only one state (Colorado) had a prevalence of obesity less than 20 percent. Obesity rates in 32 states were equal to or greater than 25 percent. Six states (Alabama, Mississippi, Oklahoma, South Carolina, Tennessee, and West Virginia) had a prevalence of obesity equal to or greater than 30 percent (Centers for Disease Control and Prevention [CDC], Division of Nutrition, Physical Activity and Obesity, 2009). Almost half the women of childbearing age in the United States are overweight (24.5 percent) or obese (23 percent). Black women are 2.25 percent more likely to be overweight than non-Hispanic white women, which seems to be related to educational and socioeconomic factors (Vahratian, 2009).

Lactation consultants have the opportunity to help break the obesity trend by empowering overweight mothers to breastfeed and thereby protect their infants against obesity. Many women seem to lose weight while breastfeeding. Exclusive breastfeeding can eliminate postpartum pregnancy weight retention by 6 months postpartum in many women, with weight gain reduced in all but the heaviest women (Baker et al., 2008).

Breastfeeding and Obesity

Obesity is a factor in delayed onset of a mother's milk (Hurst, 2007; Rasmussen, 2007a; Hilson et al., 2004). Studies show a blunted prolactin response in postpartum obese women (Rasmussen & Kjolhede, 2004). The complex interplay between insulin, progesterone, and estrogen may result in delayed onset of lactogenesis II. Furthermore, maternal obesity is associated with low breastfeeding rates and with short duration of breastfeeding (Donath & Amir, 2008; Amir & Donath, 2007), possibly because of delayed lactogenesis and the physical difficulties of positioning.

Many obese women have large breasts. A Danish study reported that women with large breasts and/or obesity found it more difficult to initiate breastfeeding than to continue to breastfeed. Difficulty was lowest for women with large breasts, higher for obese women, and highest for obese women with large breasts (Katz et al., 2009). Making adjustments for large breasts and obesity need to be addressed separately when helping a breastfeeding dyad.

A mother who is obese and/or large breasted can find it difficult to position the baby for nursing. The following practical steps can help these women breastfeed:

- Place the breast on a pillow to take the weight off the baby.
- Place a small rolled blanket or washcloth under the breast to provide lift.
- Recline and place the baby prone on top of the breast (see Chapter 14 on prone or biological nurturing).
- Nurse in a side-lying position with the breast resting on the bed.
- Support the breast with a "sling"—a commercial sling attached to the bra or one fashioned by tying the corners of a baby blanket together.

The special aids large-breasted or obese women need for positioning can make it more difficult to breastfeed discretely in public (Rasmussen, 2007a) and may discourage mothers from breastfeeding. These women also may have significant body image issues that make them reluctant to breastfeed. Breasts are an intrinsic part of a woman's self-identity and are especially sexualized in the Western culture. Distorted body image traits can increase discomfort with breastfeeding and lead to early cessation (Roth, 2006).

Your approach when helping these women needs to be nonjudgmental, with reassurance about the normalcy of breastfeeding and that breasts are designed for infant nutrition. Emotional and practical support from other breastfeeding mothers and a postpartum breastfeeding support group may help mothers more than anything to accept their body image and their breasts' biological function. *Hale & Hartmann's Textbook of Human Lactation* devotes an entire chapter to obesity and breastfeeding (Rasmussen, 2007b).

Bariatric (Weight Loss) Surgery

Bariatric surgery has risen in popularity, as obesity levels have soared in affluent cultures. The incidence of this surgery in the United States increased nearly six times, from 2.4 to 14.1 per 100,000 adults, over 10 years (Trus et al., 2005). Bariatric surgery is weight loss surgery to limit either the amount of food a person can eat or the amount of food a person can digest. Gastric bypass surgery has increased from 55 percent of all bariatric procedures in 1990 to 93 percent of such procedures in 2000 (Trus et al., 2005). Bariatric surgery carries major risks and complications, including infections, hernias, blood clots, and death. Moreover, without dramatic lifestyle, psychological, and emotional changes, many patients are at risk for regaining weight.

Eligibility guidelines for bariatric surgery are that the woman be at least 80 pounds overweight. However, bariatric surgery has become so popular that it has been performed on people weighing less. Diabetes, heart disease, and sleep apnea are reasons for performing such surgery at lower weights (USDHHS, National Institute of Diabetes and Digestive and Kidney Diseases, 2009). Adolescents are increasingly opting for bariatric surgery, with a five-fold increase in the number of adolescent bariatric procedures performed in the United States from 51 in 1997 to 282 in 2003 (Schilling et al., 2008).

Obesity lowers fertility rates. A reproductive health study found that 13.1 percent of women who had bariatric surgery were diagnosed with polycystic ovary syndrome (PCOS) (Gosman, 2009). Infertility occurred in 41.9 percent of the women who had tried to conceive. Women who were obese by age 18 were more likely to report PCOS and infertility and less likely to have ever been pregnant compared with women who became obese later in life. Future pregnancy was important to 30.3 percent of women younger than 45 years, and one-third of them planned pregnancies within 2 years of bariatric surgery. Pregnancy during a period of rapid weight loss is not recommended, and these women should use some sort of conception prevention (Kombol, 2006).

Bariatric patients have major nutritional concerns postsurgery and need to observe the nutritional advice they receive in conjunction with their surgery. Gastric bypass surgery carries a greater risk than the banding procedure in which the stomach size is decreased. Nutritional iron, vitamin A, vitamin B_{12}, vitamin K, folate, and calcium deficiencies can result in maternal complications, such as severe anemia, as well as fetal complications, such as congenital abnormalities, intrauterine growth retardation and failure to thrive (Guelinckx et al., 2009).

The limited studies on breastfed infants of bariatric mothers (Wardinsky et al., 1995; Grange & Finlay, 1994; Doyle et al., 1989) focus on the lack of vitamin B_{12} in the infant. One infant failed to thrive and the mother was anemic with milk low in fat and calorie content (Martens et al., 1990). It is important to refer these women to a nutritionist or dietitian. Be aware that some women do not adhere to the nutritional supplementation guidelines, which are advised for life. Areas of key nutritional concern in a lactating woman who underwent bariatric surgery (Stefanski, 2006) include:

- Calories
- Vitamin B$_{12}$
- Folate
- Calcium
- Water-soluble vitamins, including vitamin D and vitamin C
- Iron
- Fat-soluble vitamins
- Protein
- Fat

Stefanski (2006) recommends testing these mothers' nutritional status during pregnancy and after birth and to supplement as needed. These tests should measure complete blood count, albumin, folate, vitamin B$_{12}$, calcium, phosphorus, and 25-dehydroxy-vitamin D. The infants should also be evaluated and monitored for appropriate growth, adequacy of vitamin B$_{12}$, calcium, and folate levels throughout the breastfeeding experience. Signs of problems for the baby include fussiness, poor weight gain, lethargy, or inadequate voiding or stooling.

A handout on *Breastfeeding After Weight Loss Surgery* (Kombol, 2008), available from ILCA, will help you when working with a mother who has had bariatric surgery. Open-ended questions and thorough history taking help to identify women who have had such surgery. Some mothers may not think of gallbladder or bariatric surgery during a history, because they may believe the history focuses on surgery that affects the breast. A complete history is especially important when babies have low weight gain or failure to thrive.

The following information is important when taking a history (Kombol, 2006):

- When and what kind of surgery was performed
- Related surgeries such as plastic or breast surgery
- Complications from the procedure
- Weight pattern
- Nutritional practices and supplements taken
- Physician recommendations
- Current nutritionist/dietitian

Infertility and Insufficient Milk Supply

When you take a mother's history, be sure to ask about any previous infertility or miscarriage. Miscarriages and infertility can result from thyroid disorders, which are associated with insufficient milk supply (IMS). Many women with a history of infertility have problems with milk production. Primary IMS and infertility seem to be related, although fertile mothers also can have IMS. Additionally, some mothers who conceive by reproductive technology can have ample milk production.

Primary IMS differs from a delay in lactogenesis. Distinguishing factors of a delay in lactogenesis include cesarean delivery, hypertension, edema, hormonal birth control, diabetes, retained placenta, obesity, or a theca lutein cyst as discussed in Chapter 7. IMS also differs from secondary lactation failure, which results from external causes such as scheduling, infrequent feedings, medications, hormonal birth control, or herbs. Secondary failure may also result from conditions in the baby, such as prematurity, ineffective latch or suck, or oral anomalies such as ankyloglossia (Hurst, 2007).

When assessing a mother with IMS, pay careful attention to her breast development. Note the shape, symmetry, and vein prominence. Ask her about breast growth such as cup size changes during puberty and pregnancy. Ask about the level of breast fullness or engorgement after delivery and whether she felt her milk "coming in." Measure the space between her breasts, and palpate the breasts to determine their composition: the amount of glandular and fatty tissue and whether they are soft, flaccid, lumpy, or knotty (West & Marasco, 2008; Marasco, 2003). Hypoplasia and spacing between the breasts (intramammary spacing) greater than 1.5 inches are markers for IMS (West & Marasco, 2008; Huggins et al., 2000). Color Plates 5, 6, 7, and 8 compare normal and hypoplastic breasts.

Multiparas typically have lower serum levels of prolactin postpartum than primiparas, and their babies take in significantly more milk. Multiparas are believed to have an increased number of prolactin receptors in their mammary glands to bind with circulating prolactin, which is either reflected in or results in the lower serum levels of the hormone (Zuppa et al., 1988). This is supported by reports of other second-time mothers who produced significantly more milk (Kelley, 2003; Ingram et al., 2001).

Medications such as metoclopramide, domperidone, and metformin have helped some women with IMS. Metformin is an insulin-sensitizing agent that enhances insulin sensitivity in the liver and muscle, thus improving glycemic (sugar) control. Improved metabolic control with metformin may be associated with moderate weight loss.

Prolactin resistance, a possible explanation for alactogenesis (absence of the onset of stage II lactogenesis), may act much like insulin resistance, which suggests a possible genetic link (Zargar et al., 1997). Prolactin resistance may have caused alactogenesis in three births of a woman with normal breast development and an adequate pituitary prolactin reserve (Zargar et al., 2000). Another woman who had insufficient glandular tissue with her first child was later diagnosed with luteal phase defect and was treated with natural progesterone. She was able to exclusively breastfeed her second child, which suggests that the progesterone may have stimulated mammary gland growth (Bodley & Powers, 1999).

Polycystic Ovary Syndrome

PCOS is a common endocrine disorder in about 5 to 10 percent of women in their childbearing years. It may develop due to genetic and environmental factors, including obesity (Allahbadia & Merchant, 2008). Frequently, mothers with insufficient milk production may have either a PCOS diagnosis or symptoms consistent with the syndrome (West & Marasco, 2008; Marasco, 2003; Marasco et al., 2000).

PCOS is the leading cause of infertility in women and has multiple symptoms. It is associated with the accumulation of many incompletely developed follicles in the ovaries. The condition typically causes irregular menstrual cycles, scanty or absent menses, multiple small cysts on the ovaries (polycystic ovaries), mild to severe hirsutism (excessive hair), and infertility. Many women who have this condition develop diabetes with insulin resistance (USDHHS, Office on Women's Health, 2005). Some women with PCOS conceive spontaneously, whereas others require infertility assistance.

Weight loss is the first action suggested to women with PCOS (USDHHS, Office on Women's Health, 2005). Some women have observed an increase in their milk production while using metformin, one of the medications used to treat the condition. Very little metformin passes through to the baby, and studies of its use for 6 months postpartum suggest safety and efficacy (Glueck et al., 2007). The relationship of hormonal disorders to insufficient milk production is an area of ongoing research. Mothers who fit these profiles and are using metformin or other medications can be encouraged to join the International Registry for Lactation Research at www.ibreastfeeding.com.

Mothers with PCOS are often extremely motivated to breastfeed because of their difficulty conceiving. Breastfeeding can help heal a fragile body image battered from infertility and, often, repeated miscarriages. It is discouraging for women who struggle with infertility, achieve pregnancy through assisted reproductive technology and then struggle to achieve full milk production. Faced with yet another challenge, these mothers may quickly decide to wean and need you to validate their choice with sensitivity.

It is difficult to predict lactation outcomes for women with PCOS. Improving insulin resistance may help to increase milk production, and treating women prenatally may improve health outcomes (Creanga et al., 2008; Nestler, 2008; Essah et al., 2006) as well as milk production (Gabbay & Kelly, 2003). Some breastfeed easily and even experience an oversupply of milk, while others experience undersupply (Kelley, 2003).

Because PCOS affects far more than lactation, a mother with PCOS symptoms or IMS benefits from referral for a thorough physical and hormonal analysis. PCOS carries lifelong health risks with greater chances of developing several serious, life-threatening diseases. Women with PCOS are at higher risk for:

- Impaired glucose tolerance, with more than 50 percent of women with PCOS experiencing type 2 diabetes or prediabetes before the age of 40
- Cardiovascular disease, with a 4 to 7 times higher incidence of heart attack than women of the same age without PCOS
- High blood pressure
- High levels of low-density-lipoprotein (bad) cholesterol and low levels of high-density-lipoprotein (good) cholesterol
- Endometrial cancer

A case control study with 36 PCOS mothers tested androgen levels throughout pregnancy and the 6-month study period. Higher androgen dehydroepiandrosterone sulfate levels at gestational weeks 32 and 36 showed a weak negative association with breastfeeding in the women with PCOS. Other levels of androstenedione, testosterone, sex-hormone binding globulin, or free testosterone did not (Vanky et al., 2008). At 1-month postpartum, 75 percent of the PCOS mothers breastfed exclusively and 14 percent did not breastfeed, compared with 88 percent of the control subjects who breastfed. Rates for breastfeeding at 3 and 4 months postpartum were equal, as were problems with sore nipples and seeking lactation help.

Thyroid Disorders

Thyroid disorders in women are very common and relate to a woman's reproductive cycle. Even slight hypothyroidism (low thyroid) can increase rates of miscarriage, fetal death, and cognitive deficits in babies. Hyperthyroidism (overactive thyroid) during pregnancy is a cause for concern. Testing thyroid-stimulating hormone (TSH), triiodothyronine, and thyroxine levels before pregnancy, during pregnancy, and postpartum for mothers who complain of unusual fatigue or anxiety or who have markers for hyperthyroidism or hypothyroidism is appropriate (Rashid & Rashid, 2007). Because of hormonal fluctuations during pregnancy, pregnant women require close monitoring when they have thyroid therapy.

Hypothyroidism

Hypothyroidism results from a deficiency in thyroid secretion. Symptoms include sluggishness, low blood pressure, dry skin, obesity, and sensitivity to cold. Replacement therapy with natural or synthetic hormone preparations can eliminate these effects. When thyroid supplementation is properly managed, the mother can breastfeed with no risk to her baby's health. The supplementation she receives merely brings the mother's thyroid to a normal level. Therefore the amount of thyroid secretion the baby receives through her milk is equal to that of any other breastfeeding mother.

There is one word of caution for a mother who is severely hypothyroid and receiving unusually high dosages of thyroid supplement. The additional thyroid that passes to her baby through her milk can mask latent hypothyroidism in her baby during the course of breastfeeding. After weaning begins and the level of thyroid intake decreases, a baby with latent hypothyroidism could suffer neurological damage. Most hospitals screen for congenital hypothyroidism as a part of the newborn screening (Sahai & Marsden, 2009).

Although hypothyroidism is a marker for infertility, many women with thyroid disorders are able to conceive through assisted reproductive technologies (Poppe et al., 2008, 2007). There seems to be a link between untreated hypothyroidism and insufficient milk production. If a mother contacts you regarding low milk production and has a history of thyroid problems, you might recommend complete thyroid testing. Thyroid testing may also be in order when a mother presents with low milk production that has no identifiable cause.

Goiter

Adequate iodine intake is necessary for normal thyroid function. Insufficient iodine may lead to a goiter, which is an enlargement of the thyroid gland, resulting in a thick-looking neck or double-chin appearance. An adequate concentration of iodine in breastmilk is needed for optimal neonatal thyroid hormone stores and to prevent impaired neurological development (Azizi & Smyth, 2009). Iodine levels in human milk respond quickly to the mother increasing her intake, either by consuming iodine-rich foods or by taking supplements. The WHO recommends daily iodine intake of 250 mcg for lactating mothers (WHO, 2007b).

Hyperthyroidism

Hyperthyroidism is a condition in which the thyroid is overactive and produces too much thyroid hormone. Thyroid hormone controls many body processes, and excessive levels can affect heart rate and blood pressure. Hyperthyroidism is diagnosed through blood tests that reveal abnormally high thyroid hormone levels and low levels of TSH produced by the pituitary gland. Low TSH levels in the blood are the most reliable test of most hyperthyroidism. In rare cases the pituitary gland produces excess amounts of TSH, thereby increasing levels of both TSH and thyroid hormones in the blood. Graves' disease is a form of hyperthyroidism in which pressure occurs on the eyes from supporting muscles, resulting in a staring, wide-eyed appearance. Graves' disease is associated with pernicious anemia, vitiligo, diabetes mellitus type 1, autoimmune adrenal insufficiency, systemic sclerosis, myasthenia gravis, Sjögren's syndrome, rheumatoid arthritis, and systemic lupus erythematosus (Yeung et al., 2009).

Methimazole, a common medication for the treatment of hyperthyroidism, is considered compatible for use in breastfeeding mothers (Hale, 2010). Propylthiouracil is also used in lactating women and may be preferable because only small amounts are secreted into the milk (Hale, 2010). Encourage a mother to research her disease and to let her endocrinologist or other healthcare specialist know that continuing to breastfeed is important to her. She can share current evidence-based information to help protect her breastfeeding plans.

Scans using radioisotopes as part of the diagnostic process may require temporary weaning. The length of breastfeeding cessation is contingent on the type of radioactive agent used and the mother can ask the radiology department what kind of agent they will use. Hale's *Medications and Mothers' Milk* (2010) contains information on these agents and the length of their half-lives. The Nuclear Regulatory Commission's guidelines are available through www.ibreastfeeding.com. The mother can pump during the brief cessation and can save the milk. The radioisotopes break down in the pumped milk, just as they do in the body; she can ask to have her milk tested before use if she is concerned about its safety.

Postpartum Thyroiditis

Postpartum thyroiditis causes a mother's thyroid function to fluctuate, resulting in either transient hyperthyroidism or hypothyroidism. Postpartum thyroiditis may be an immunological flare after the immune suppression of pregnancy (Stagnaro-Green, 2004). This transient dysfunction usually resolves within a year after birth. The prevalence of postpartum thyroiditis ranges from 1.1 to 16.7 percent of all mothers, with a mean prevalence of 7.5 percent. Insulin-dependent diabetics have a threefold increase in the prevalence of postpartum thyroiditis. Approximately 25 percent of women with a history of postpartum thyroiditis develop permanent hypothyroidism within 10 years. A mother with markers for either hyperthyroidism or hypothyroidism should contact her doctor for further evaluation and care.

Cystic Fibrosis

Cystic fibrosis (CF) is an inherited disease that affects the exocrine system. In most people mucus, sweat, saliva, and digestive juices are thin and watery. The defective gene in CF makes these secretions thick and sticky causing them to clog ducts and tubes throughout the body, including the pancreas and lungs. Macronutrient content (fats, sugars, and proteins) is reported to be reduced during flare-ups of pulmonary disease (Shiffman et al., 1989), which can compromise nutritional status. Adults with CF are at increased risk for diabetes mellitus (Mackie et al., 2003). Continual monitoring of nutrition is critical for mothers with CF.

Of the 70,000 people afflicted with CF worldwide, about 30,000 are American (CFF, 2009). Advances in research and medical treatments have extended the lifespan for people with CF and many with the disease live into their 30s, 40s, and beyond. Many of these young adults marry and have children. Whereas some mothers with CF maintain a normal pregnancy with appropriate maternal and fetal weight gain, others find either their CF complicates the pregnancy or is adversely affected by the pregnancy (Edenborough et al., 2008). One study found a higher rate of miscarriage, preterm births, and perinatal deaths among mothers with CF (Kent & Farquharson, 1993).

During lactation these mothers can maintain their weight and support healthy infant growth (Michel & Mueller, 1994). Breastfeeding duration tends to be less than 3 months (Luder et al., 1990). Breastfeeding experiences among mothers in several CF centers were not always positive, suggesting a need for criteria to predict and support a successful outcome.

Although people with CF may have hypernatremia (too much salt in the blood), the breastmilk has not been shown to be hypernatremic, indicating that breastfeeding is possible (Kent & Farquharson, 1993). Milk from two mothers with CF was found to be normal. Breastfeeding women with CF must give careful attention to their nutritional requirements. The disease may compromise the mother nutritionally, and the caloric requirements of breastfeeding may further compromise her nutritional status.

Some researchers question the amount of bacterial exposure to the breastfeeding infant because people with CF are usually chronic carriers of *Staphylococcus aureus*, a potential pathogen (Welch et al., 1981). However, the infection passes to the baby not through the mother's milk but by close contact with the mother. Consequently, exposure occurs regardless of feeding method. Furthermore, lymphocytes in the mother's milk become sensitized to pathogens and provide protection to her breastfed baby.

Maternal Phenylketonuria

PKU is an inherited error of metabolism caused by a deficiency in the amino acid enzyme phenylalanine hydroxylase. When this enzyme is inactive or is inefficient, the concentration of phenylalanine in the body can build up to toxic levels. Mental retardation, organ damage, and posture abnormalities can result from this excessive phenylalanine (National Center for Biotechnology Infor-

mation, 2007). Psychological problems, including poor self-esteem, agoraphobia, and autistic-like behaviors, have been reported in PKU patients, both those who follow their prescribed special diet and those who do not. Subtle attention and performance deficits may persist (Arnold, 2009).

PKU occurs in an estimated 1 in 15,000 births. Turkey has the highest rate in the world, with 1 in 2,600 births. High occurrence is reported in the Yemenite Jewish population as well as in regions of Europe, Italy, and China (Arnold, 2009). The success of newborn screening for PKU, with resulting dietary management, has led to many babies with PKU growing to maturity and having children of their own. This has led to maternal PKU, a situation with potential dangers for a developing fetus. A woman who had PKU as an infant needs to return to a special PKU diet during her pregnancy. The phenylalanine overload in her body resulting from a regular diet can affect her fetus' growing brain. Brain damage occurs before birth, regardless of whether the baby inherits PKU. The resulting mental retardation, heart defects, and other serious congenital anomalies (e.g., orofacial clefting and bladder exstrophy) have been classified as maternal PKU syndrome (Gambol, 2007). Hanley (2008) reported on 60 women with previously undiagnosed PKU who bore a total of 119 children, virtually all of whom were profoundly damaged.

A woman may not even be aware that she had PKU as an infant. The phenylalanine overload during infancy may not have been high enough to cause the disease, although it still could be high enough to cause brain damage in her developing fetus. Because the special diet may be discontinued as early as 5 years of age, she may not remember why she was on a special diet at an early age. When a woman becomes pregnant or, better yet, when she plans to begin a family, she should ask her parents about her medical history as an infant. A woman who delays childbearing into later adulthood may find her parents passed away before she thought to ask about her early history.

Any woman planning pregnancy can request that her caregiver perform a simple test for PKU. Preconception counseling with her physician helps her plan a healthy pregnancy (ACOG, 2009). Breastfeeding is a part of the healthiest outcome possible. In one case twin sisters with PKU initiated special diets before conception and during pregnancy. Both sisters breastfed for several months and their babies maintained normal phenylalanine levels (Fox-Bacon et al., 1997).

Infectious Diseases

Some maternal infections are chronic while others are acute. Table 25.2 lists the most common diseases you may encounter, along with recommendations for breastfeeding.

TABLE 25.2 Maternal Infections and Corresponding Breastfeeding Management for Healthy Term Infants

	Infection/Disease	Microbial Agent(s)	Breastfeeding Recommendation
Bacteria	Mastitis and breast abscesses	*Staphylococcus aureus, Streptococcus* species Gram negatives: *Escherichia coli* Rarely: *Salmonella* species, *Cryptococcus*	Continue breastfeeding unless there is obvious pus, in which case pump and discard from the infected breast and continue breastfeeding with the other breast. *Mycobacteria, Candida,*
	Tuberculosis (TB)	*Mycobacterium tuberculosis*	Main route of transmission is airborne. With active TB, delay breastfeeding until mother has received 2 weeks of appropriate anti-TB therapy; provide TB prophylaxis for infant.
	Urinary tract infection	Gram negatives: *E. coli*, etc.	Continue breastfeeding.
	Bacterial infection—abdominal wall, post-cesarean section	Skin microbes	Continue breastfeeding.
	Diarrhea	*Salmonella, Shigella, E. coli, Campylobacter*	Continue breastfeeding; practice good hand hygiene.
	Other bacterial infections in which the mother's physical condition and general health are not compromised	Wide range of bacterial microbes	Continue breastfeeding.
Parasites	Malaria	*Plasmodium* species	Continue breastfeeding.
Fungi	Candidal vaginitis	*Candida*	Continue breastfeeding; practice good hand hygiene.
Viruses		Cytomegalovirus	Continue breastfeeding.
	Hepatitis	Hepatitis A virus	Continue breastfeeding; immunoglobulin prophylaxis for the infant; practice good hand hygiene.
		Hepatitis B virus (HBV)	Continue breastfeeding; routine prevention of infant HBV infection with hepatitis B immune globulin at birth; immunization with HBV vaccine.
		Hepatitis C virus	Continue breastfeeding.
	Herpes	Herpes simplex virus type 1 and type 2	Continue breastfeeding; practice good hand hygiene. If there are lesions on breasts, interrupt until lesions are healed (crusted).
	Chicken pox, shingles	Varicella	Continue breastfeeding; for perinatal varicella-zoster virus, give VZIG; for postpartum, consider VZIG.
		Enterovirus	Continue breastfeeding; practice good hand hygiene.
		HIV	Contraindicated; see text for details.
		HTLV-1, HTLV-2	Contraindicated.
		Parvovirus	Continue breastfeeding.
		West Nile virus	Continue breastfeeding.

HTLV-1, human T-cell lymphotrophic virus type 1; VZIG, varicella-zoster immune globulin.

Source: Canadian Paediatric Society. Maternal infectious diseases, antimicrobial therapy or immunizations: very few contraindications to breastfeeding. *Can J Infect Dis Med Microbiol.* 2006;17(5):270-272. Reprinted by permission of Pulsus Group, Inc.

If you encounter mothers with less common infections, timely referenced information and recommendations on infectious diseases are available from the CDC (www .cdc.gov), the American Academy of Pediatrics (AAP) (www.aap.org), the Academy of Breastfeeding Medicine (ABM) (www.bfmed.org), and the WHO (www.who.int).

Tuberculosis

Tuberculosis is a bacterial disease that usually attacks the lungs, although it can attack other body parts as well. Tuberculosis was once the leading cause of death in the United States. It occurs more often in people from countries outside the United States (CDC, 2009b). The WHO estimated 9.27 million cases of tuberculosis globally in 2007, with about 1.3 million deaths unrelated to HIV (WHO, 2009b).

A mother with active tuberculosis may breastfeed with certain precautions. When maternal disease is discovered before birth, treatment must begin immediately during pregnancy and infant prophylaxis must begin at birth (CDC, 2009a). When active maternal disease is discovered after the baby is born, all contact between the mother and baby is suspended until appropriate therapy is initiated and continued for at least 2 weeks. This contact includes breastfeeding. During the interruption in breastfeeding, the mother can express and discard her milk every 2 to 4 hours to establish and maintain milk production (Lawrence & Lawrence, 2005).

Rarely, tuberculosis can occur within the breast. Breast tuberculosis constitutes less than 0.1 percent of all known breast diseases and comprises up to 3 percent of all treatable breast lesions in developing countries (Akçay et al., 2007). Breast tuberculosis usually presents as a solitary, ill-defined, unilateral hard lump situated in the upper outer quadrant of the breast (Baharoon, 2008).

Hepatitis B

Hepatitis B is a virus that affects the liver. It has not been found to be transmitted through breastfeeding and is therefore not a reason to delay breastfeeding (CDC, 2009c). The CDC recommends that infants born to hepatitis B–infected mothers receive hepatitis B immune globulin and the first dose of hepatitis B vaccine within 12 hours of birth, with the second and third doses at normal intervals. The baby should be tested between 9 and 18 months of age to verify that the vaccine worked and the infant is not infected with hepatitis B through exposure to the mother's blood during birth. All mothers who breastfeed should take good care of their nipples to avoid cracking and bleeding.

Hepatitis C

Hepatitis C is a virus that affects the liver and is spread by contact with an infected person's blood. The risk of moth-

ers transmitting the hepatitis C virus to their infants through their milk appears to be quite low. About 5 to 6 percent transmission occurs in women who have hepatitis C RNA in their blood at the time of birth (Buescher, 2007). Up to half of infant infection appears to occur during pregnancy (Mok et al., 2005). The CDC has found no documented evidence that breastfeeding spreads the hepatitis C virus. The virus is transmitted through infected blood and not through human milk. Therefore hepatitis C virus infection is not a contraindication to breastfeed (CDC, 2009c). Buescher (2007) recommends that a mother with hepatitis C whose nipple is cracked or bleeding not breastfeed on the affected side and not use the milk from that breast until the wound has healed.

Herpes

Herpes is a viral infection that is contracted through direct contact with an active lesion or body fluid of an infected person. Herpes can pose a major health hazard to an infant, including blindness and death. There are several diseases in the herpes family, and the degree of danger varies among them. Herpes infections all share a common structure, have similar biological behavior, are transmitted by a virus, and are highly contagious. Several herpes infections manifest themselves as skin lesions that begin as small red pimples. They develop into fluid-filled blisters and then dry up and heal. Varicella-zoster (chickenpox and shingles) and the herpes simplex viruses fall into this group. During the active phase the blisters cause a burning, tingling, and itching sensation, often accompanied by fever and enlarged lymph nodes (Arduino & Porter, 2008).

Exposure to active herpes lesions can be fatal to a neonate, so all active lesions must be covered to prevent exposure. The AAP (2005) states that breastfeeding is acceptable if there are no herpetic lesions in the area or if active lesions on the breast are covered. However, if a lesion is present on the nipple the mother cannot breastfeed or feed her milk to her infant from that breast until the lesion heals. The mother can express milk to maintain production in that breast and discard the milk.

Epstein-Barr Epstein Barr is a virus that affects the central nervous system. The Epstein-Barr virus—also called infectious mononucleosis—is acquired by most people in childhood and usually affects young adults up to age 35. It is known as the "kissing disease" because it is transmitted through human saliva. Epstein-Barr virus remains a lifelong dormant infection in some cells of the body's immune system. Epstein-Barr virus infection rates between breastfed and bottle fed infants in one study were similar, suggesting breastfeeding is not a primary source for infection (Kusuhara, 1997). Huang et al. (1993) found no detectable risk factors for breastfeeding associated with primary Epstein-Barr virus. Epstein-Barr virus may trigger rheumatoid arthritis. It is also associated with nasopharyngeal carcinoma and Burkitt's lymphoma, two rare cancers (CDC, National Center for Infectious Diseases, 2006).

Varicella-Zoster The varicella-zoster virus affects the central nervous system and causes chickenpox and shingles. Chickenpox is usually contracted by children, whereas shingles is generally an adult affliction. Both zoster infections are contracted through direct contact or through droplets from the nose or mouth.

Contracting varicella during pregnancy carries risks for both the baby and the mother, including the rare occurrence of congenital varicella syndrome, which occurs when the mother has chickenpox up to 20 weeks' gestation. Congenital varicella syndrome consists of severe birth defects, including vision impairment, neurological damage, and skin and limb deformities. If the mother contracts chickenpox in the third trimester, the infant may develop herpes zoster during the first 1 or 2 years (Smith & Arvin, 2009). If the mother is infected at the time of delivery, she must be isolated from her infant until the lesions heal completely. With either of the zoster viruses, unless there are lesions on her breast the mother can feed her milk to her baby (AAP, 2005).

A baby whose mother develops chickenpox up to 7 days before delivery or up to 28 days after delivery must receive zoster immune globulin, the chickenpox vaccine. Mothers may breastfeed when their baby has a chickenpox infection or exposure. After delivery a mother who contracts chickenpox or shingles does not need to be isolated from her baby. If children at home have chickenpox and the mother does not test positive for antibodies, the newborn needs to receive the vaccine. The baby does not need to be isolated from siblings with chickenpox, regardless of having received zoster immune globulin (Heuchan & Isaacs, 2001).

Herpes Simplex Both herpes simplex viruses are contracted through close contact with an infected person who is shedding virus from the skin. The virus lies dormant in the nervous system, remaining asymptomatic until it becomes active. Common activating agents are fever, physical or emotional stress, lowered immunity as with illness or pregnancy, exposure to sunlight, and certain foods or drugs. The infection can be present in the infant without any maternal history of herpes, usually presenting with upper and lower respiratory symptoms, a hoarse cry, and fever.

Herpes simplex 1 (cold sore or fever blister) usually appears as an open sore on the mouth and nose areas. Herpes simplex 2 (genitalis) is usually transmitted through sexual contact, producing painful blisters on the skin and the moist lining of the sex organs. In addition to the other herpes simplex symptoms, herpes genitalis causes painful intercourse, urinary problems, and swelling in the groin area. Herpes simplex virus transmitted from mother to child around the time of delivery can cause potentially fatal disease in the newborn. Women who experience their first genital herpes simplex virus infection in pregnancy are at the highest risk of transmitting the virus to their newborn (Jones, 2009). Treatment in late pregnancy with oral acyclovir and valacyclovir has helped limit the recurrence, the shedding of herpes simplex virus at delivery, and the necessity for cesarean delivery. The effect of these drugs in helping prevent in utero infection is unknown. Neonates who contract the disease usually do so through direct contact with the infected tissue. Mortality and morbidity rates are extremely high for infants exposed to herpes genitalis during vaginal birth. If a woman has had active lesions within 3 weeks of delivery, she should have a cesarean section to ensure her baby's safety.

Cytomegalovirus The sixth member of the herpes family is cytomegalovirus (CMV), a virus that usually produces few, if any, symptoms and tends to reactivate intermittently without symptoms. Symptoms include fatigue, fever, swollen lymph glands, pneumonia, and liver or spleen defects. Nearly all adults are infected with CMV by the age of 50. If a mother becomes infected with CMV while pregnant, the baby can be affected, with possible hearing loss and learning disabilities.

CMV can be shed in bodily fluids of the infected person, including breastmilk. Healthy, term infants can be breastfed even when the mother is shedding the virus in her milk (Lawrence, 2006; Lawrence & Lawrence, 2005). Breastfed babies may receive passive immunity to CMV through their mothers' milk. Preterm babies are at risk for becoming ill if the mother is positive for CMV (Hamprecht et al., 2001; Omarsdottir et al., 2007; Schleiss, 2006). Degree of prematurity correlates to the risk of contracting CMV, with infants below 1,000 g birth weight and below 30 weeks gestational age at high risk of acquiring a symptomatic infection. In one study of very-low-birth-weight babies fed their mother's seropositive milk, the lower the gestational age and underlying chronic diseases were related to symptomatic infection (Capretti et al., 2009). Another study confirmed this, reporting a high maternal load and prolonged virus excretion in the milk as risk factors for transmission to very-low-birth-weight infants (Jim et al., 2009).

The greatest danger of CMV to breastfeeding infants is the possibility of seroconversion if the infant of a seronegative mother receives donor milk from a seropositive mother (Dworsky et al., 1982). Because the infant has not received transplacental antibodies, the infection could be life threatening. This is especially dangerous for preterm infants or infants who are immunologically impaired.

Pasteurization at 62°C for 8 minutes can destroy CMV in human milk. Although pasteurization destroys some of the milk's immunological properties as well, it provides donor recipients protection from CMV and is the standard for milk bank processing. See Chapter 21 for more on human milk banking.

Human T-Cell Lymphotrophic Virus Type 1

Human T-cell lymphotrophic virus type 1 (HTLV-1) is believed to be transmitted by sexual contact, blood exposure, and breastfeeding (Pimenta et al., 2008). It is linked to adult T-cell leukemia/lymphoma, a rare and aggressive T-cell lymphoma. A retrovirus, HTLV-1 infects only T cells and about 2 to 5 percent of patients infected with the HTLV-1 develop adult T-cell leukemia/lymphoma (O'Connor, 2008). The HTLV-1 virus is in the same class of virus as the HIV/AIDS virus. It is found in specific geographical areas, including Japan, the Caribbean, South and Central America, West Africa, and the southeastern United States. Freezing can eliminate the HTLV-1 infectivity of the milk (Ando et al., 2004) and enable infants to receive their mothers' milk.

Human Immunodeficiency Virus (HIV)

HIV is a retrovirus that destroys the human immune system. It can lead to acquired immune deficiency syndrome (AIDS), in which the body cannot fight off viral, bacterial, mycobacterial, and fungal pathogens. HIV is spread through sexual contact and through exposure to blood. HIV/AIDS is a major global health emergency that affects all regions of the world. It causes millions of deaths and suffering to millions more. HIV/AIDS especially affects children and mothers. The AIDS virus is the leading cause of death and disease among women between the ages of 15 and 44 (WHO, 2009c).

Global AIDS Epidemic Since the beginning of the global AIDS epidemic, almost 60 million people have been infected with HIV and 25 million people have died of HIV-related causes. Young people account for about 40 percent of all new adult (aged 15+) HIV infections worldwide. Sub-Saharan Africa is the region most affected, home to 67 percent of all people living with HIV and 91 percent of all new infections among children.

When left untreated, HIV quickly leads to infection, disease, and death. The outlook for the prevention and treatment of HIV remains grim. Continued global promiscuity and drug use sustain high infection rates. UNAIDS (2009) reports that fewer than 40 percent of young people have basic information about HIV and less than 40 percent of people living with HIV know their status. The number of new HIV infections continues to outstrip the numbers on treatment. For every two people

starting treatment, a further five become infected with the virus.

Recommendations for HIV and Breastfeeding HIV is transmitted through sexual contact, contaminated body fluids, and intravenous drug use. It is transmitted from mother to infant during pregnancy, delivery, and (it is believed) through breastfeeding. WHO (2007a) reports that HIV transmission through breastfeeding of any kind without any interventions is believed to range from 5 to 20 percent.

The 2009 revised WHO recommendations for infant feeding in the context of HIV/AIDS call for earlier initiation of antiretroviral therapy for adults and adolescents, the delivery of more patient-friendly antiretroviral drugs (ARVs), and prolonged use of ARVs to reduce the risk of mother-to-child transmission of HIV. WHO recommends that HIV-positive mothers or their infants take ARVs while breastfeeding to prevent transmission.

Increased evidence shows that ARV interventions to either the HIV-infected mother or HIV-exposed infant can significantly reduce the risk of postnatal transmission of HIV through breastfeeding. The potential of ARVs to reduce HIV transmission throughout the period of breastfeeding highlights the need to focus on how child health services communicate information about ARVs to prevent transmission through breastfeeding (WHO, 2009d). The 2009 guidelines seek to balance HIV prevention with protection from other causes of child mortality (such as not breastfeeding) and to integrate HIV interventions into maternal and child health services (Table 25.3). Humprey (2010) observes that efforts to ameliorate the effect of HIV on children may lead to stronger promotion of breastfeeding as a means to reduce the 1.4 million child deaths occurring each year due to suboptimal breastfeeding.

Unfortunately, the WHO guidelines identify donor milk as the second nutritional choice when mother's own milk is not available rather than the first choice. Donor milk from an HIV-negative mother is a healthier option than artificial infant milk. Promoting artificial milk as the preferred option seems in opposition to WHO/United Nations Children's Fund (1980) own feeding choices hierarchy: "where it is not possible for the biological mother to breastfeed, the first alternative, if available, should be the use of human breast milk from other sources."

Some researchers seek to promote relactation by healthy, non-HIV/AIDS grandmothers to breastfeed babies whose mothers are HIV/AIDS positive (Ogunlesi et al., 2008). Relactating to feed abandoned and orphaned infants, or where the mother is too sick to nurse, is reportedly an age-long tradition in most cultures, especially in African countries. Nacro et al. (2009) found that 74 percent of 300 women surveyed in Faso Burkina would

TABLE 25.3 2009 WHO Breastfeeding Recommendations for HIV-Positive Mothers

	Recommendation
Antiretroviral therapy	• Mothers known to be HIV-infected should be provided with lifelong antiretroviral therapy or antiretroviral prophylaxis interventions to reduce HIV transmission through breastfeeding.
	• If a woman received treatment during pregnancy, her child should be treated from birth until the end of the breastfeeding period.
Breastfeeding	• Mothers known to be HIV-infected (and whose infants are HIV uninfected or of unknown HIV status) are strongly urged to exclusively breastfeed for the first 6 months of life.
	• They should continue to breastfeed up to 2 years or beyond.
	• Heat-treated, expressed breastmilk may be *an interim feeding strategy* for an infant with low birth weight or other high-risk condition, when the mother is temporarily unable to breastfeed, as a means to wean, or if antiretroviral drugs are temporarily unavailable.
Weaning	• Breastfeeding should stop only when a nutritionally adequate and safe diet without breastmilk can be provided.
	• When HIV-infected mothers stop breastfeeding, they should stop gradually within 1 month.
	• Mothers or infants who have been receiving ARV prophylaxis should continue prophylaxis for 1 week after breastfeeding is fully stopped.
After weaning	
Infants < 6 mo of age	• Commercial infant formula milk if home conditions are affordable, feasible, acceptable, sustainable and safe, or expressed
	• Heat-treated breastmilk
Children > 6 mo of age	• Commercial infant formula if home conditions are affordable, feasible, acceptable, sustainable, and safe
	• Animal milk (boiled for infants under 12 months)
	• Complementary foods

Source: World Health Organization (WHO). Rapid advice: revised WHO principles and recommendations on infant feeding in the context of HIV; November, 2009d. http://www.who.int/child_adolescent_health/documents/hiv_if_principles_recommendations_11 2009.pdf. Accessed December 1, 2009. Used with permission of WHO.

accept breastfeeding by a wet nurse if they themselves were HIV/AIDS positive. A large number (69.8 percent) would be willing to be a wet nurse for the infant born to an HIV-infected woman.

Horvath et al. (2009) noted that the risk of HIV transmission from mixed feeding after 6 months may be less than the risk of severe malnutrition from stopping breastfeeding completely. In addition to exclusive breastfeeding during the first few months of life, the use of ongoing antiretroviral prophylaxis to the infant is shown to be helpful in preventing the transmission of HIV to infants from breastfeeding mothers.

An improvement in early testing—polymerase chain reaction—allows infants as young as 6 weeks old to be tested. Polymerase chain reaction is especially useful for testing infants, because only an estimated 40 percent of the infants who test antibody positive for HIV are really infected; the others are temporarily carrying their mother's antibodies (AIDS.org. 2009). In the industrialized world, where replacement feeding is considered acceptable, feasible, affordable, sustainable, and safe, the current recommendations are for HIV-positive mothers to not breastfeed (AAP, 2005).

AnotherLook, a nonprofit organization started by La Leche League International founder Marian Tompson, is dedicated to gathering information, raising critical questions, and stimulating research about breastfeeding in the context of HIV and AIDS. Their 2003 "Call to Action" (Figure 25.1) aims to ensure the best maternal and infant health outcomes. AnotherLook asserts that current research, policy, and practice that focus on reducing transmission neglect the impact of not breastfeeding on morbidity, mortality, and health.

Heat Treating Mothers' Milk and Microbicides Another alternative for an HIV-positive mother is heat treating, or home pasteurization, of her expressed milk (Buescher, 2007). This option depends on the mother's motivation, health, and ability to express her milk. WHO (2009d) affirms that heat treatment does not appear to significantly alter the nutritional composition of breastmilk and assert that breastmilk treated with this method should be nutritionally adequate to support an infant's growth and development. Therefore heat treatment of expressed milk from mothers known to be infected with HIV could be a potential approach to safely providing breastmilk to exposed infants. Further research is needed before supporting heat-treatment as a long-term solution. In the meantime, WHO suggests heat treatment as an interim strategy rather than for the full duration of breastfeeding.

There are two types of heat treatment. Pretoria pasteurization is a method in which the milk is placed into water already heated from 56°C to 62°C in an aluminum pot for about 15 minutes (Jeffery et al., 2003, 2001). The flash heat method places the container of milk into a pan

We acknowledge the possibility that HIV may be transmitted through breastfeeding and that there is an urgent need for feeding guidelines. However, there is currently no published scientific evidence showing that infants born to mothers who are HIV-positive would be healthier and/or less likely to die if they were not breastfed. In light of the above, we call for immediate action to provide:

- Clear, peer-reviewed research, with careful ongoing follow-up, which will provide sound scientific evidence of optimal infant feeding practices that lead to the lowest morbidity and mortality.
- Concise, consistent definitions of feeding methods, testing methods, HIV infection and AIDS.
- Development of research-based infant feeding policies which are feasible to implement in light of prevailing social, cultural and economic environments; which address breastfeeding (particularly exclusive breastfeeding) as a critical component of optimal infant health; and which fully consider the impact of spillover mortality/morbidity associated with infant formulas.
- Epidemic management from a public health perspective, with the focus on primary prevention, careful, unbiased surveillance, and the achievement of overall population health with the lowest rates of morbidity and mortality.
- Evidence-based practices which protect the rights of both mothers and infants including education, true informed consent, support of a mother's choice, and avoidance of coercion.
- Funding to support the above actions and those programs which improve maternal/child health in general such as prenatal and postnatal care, nutrition, basic sanitation, clean water, and education, as well as exclusive breastfeeding until clear scientific evidence supporting the abandonment of breastfeeding is available.
- Continued commitment by local and global researchers, policy makers, health workers, and funding bodies to basic scientific, medical, public health, and fiduciary principles in responding to this critical issue.

In summary, we call for answers to critical questions not currently being addressed that will foster the development of policies and practices leading to the best possible outcomes for mothers and babies in relation to breastfeeding and HIV/AIDS.

FIGURE 25.1 Infant feeding and HIV/AIDS: A call to action.
Source: Printed with permission of AnotherLook.

of water, where it is heated to a rolling boil and then removed. Both methods have shown to be effective as a means to inactivate HIV in breastmilk (Israel-Ballard et al., 2007, 2005). Heat-treated milk is observed to have safe bacterial levels up to 8 hours at room temperature (Israel-Ballard et al., 2006). Most breastmilk immunoglobulin activity survives the flash heat method, suggesting that flash-heated milk is immunologically superior to breastmilk substitutes (Chantry et al., 2009). In a third option researchers used microbicides to inactivate HIV in expressed milk (Hartmann et al., 2006). This method,

which does not require heat treatment, is capable of preserving the milk's nutritional and immune status.

Counseling HIV-Positive Mothers You can present current and evidence-based information, recommendations, and guidelines to HIV-positive women and encourage them to discuss options with their physician. Because of the impact of HIV/AIDS on breastfeeding and the financial motivation that pharmaceutical and formula manufacturers have to decrease breastfeeding, it is important that you stay current with HIV/AIDS research. The AIDS pandemic has enabled formula manufacturers to reach lucrative new markets where government enforcement of the International Code of Marketing of Breastmilk Substitutes has previously hampered their marketing efforts. Read any negative studies on human milk and breastfeeding with critical analysis, and note any competing interests. Search past the popular press articles to the original research studies behind them. Filter them through the lens of your critical thinking and research skills, as presented in Chapter 27.

∼ Special Infant Health Conditions

As a lactation consultant you will undoubtedly encounter an infant whose physical condition affects breastfeeding. Parents typically respond with shock and guilt at having a baby born with a congenital disorder or birth defect. They often progress through the classic cycle of grief, including denial, anger, rejection, and mourning for the "perfect" child. There is no set pattern or time progression for these emotions. Circumstances may also cause a mother to mourn the opportunity for a "normal" breastfeeding experience. You can be most helpful by listening and taking cues from the parents. Allow the mother to work freely through her feelings until she reaches a point of acceptance. Recognize that acceptance may not be reached during the typically brief time you work with the family.

The nutritional benefits derived from human milk are especially important to a compromised baby. Breastfeeding may help a mother accept a challenging situation, confident that she is doing everything possible to comfort and nurture her baby. The bonding facilitated by breastfeeding can lessen emotional stress and help the family through this difficult transition. At times, the infant's condition may prevent direct breastfeeding or even receiving breastmilk at all. Infant conditions presented here include PKU, galactosemia, cleft lip, cleft palate, and neurological impairment.

Phenylketonuria

PKU results from the infant lacking an enzyme needed to change phenylalanine, an amino acid in food protein, into a form the body can use. If PKU remains untreated, the body becomes overloaded with phenylalanine. Skin rashes, convulsions, mental impairment, and other problems can result. As noted above in the maternal health condition of phenylketonuria, PKU occurs in approximately 1 in 15,000 births. An infant with PKU appears healthy at birth, with diagnosis through a simple blood test that is part of standard newborn screening in most countries.

Treatment initiated promptly during the first weeks of life can avoid permanent damage. Phenylalanine intake for an infant with PKU requires strict monitoring and a diet that restricts the level of phenylalanine intake while providing a protein amount sufficient to allow appropriate growth. Continuing this diet regimen throughout the person's lifetime may help preserve normal cognitive function.

Implications for Breastfeeding

The level of phenylalanine in human milk is low (approximately 40 mg/dL) when compared with cow's milk and other artificial baby milk, which range from 73 to 159 mg/dL. The infant's diet is adjusted for phenylalanine based on weekly blood tests. After control is established, 20 ounces of human milk daily, along with a supplement of phenylalanine-free formula, meet the infant's requirements of phenylalanine. Direct breastfeeding and supplementation with a phenylalanine-free formula provide good metabolic control and improve the growth and development of PKU children with early diagnosis (Cornejo et al., 2003).

Low-phenylalanine or phenylalanine-free formula was designed to be supplemented with cow's milk or a cow's milk–based formula. Consequently, vitamin and mineral supplements may be required to augment the nutrients present in the mother's milk. If not, the addition of phenylalanine-free formula to the infant's diet could result in a decrease of nutrient absorption. Additional fluid requirements may be minimal because of the lower solute load of human milk.

Breastfeeding helps maintain the mother–infant bond and ensures adequate milk production. It may also reduce the emotional stress for parents when they learn their baby has a chronic illness. There is evidence that PKU babies who do not receive human milk initially have lower IQs and developmental outcomes than those who receive human milk (Lawrence & Lawrence, 2005; Riva et al., 1996).

Formula fed infants have exhibited lower levels of arachidonic acid than breastfed PKU babies. Researchers found a weak positive association between plasma long-chain polyunsaturated fatty acids at diagnosis, which is lower in artificially fed infants, and neurodevelopmental indices through the first year of life (Agostoni et al., 2003).

The growing trend is to add fish oil–based DHA supplements to infant and child diets (Koletzko et al., 2009; Giovannini et al., 2007; Agostoni et al., 2006). The focus of the research appears to be on mimicking the function of the fatty acids in human milk, with little acknowledgment of its biological importance. There are many constituents of human milk, and nothing can replicate mothers' milk and the nurturing of the baby at the breast.

Eighty percent of health centers surveyed encouraged a combination of breastfeeding and a protein substitute for PKU infants (Ahring et al., 2009). However, the researchers found no one dietary management strategy, with marked differences in target blood phenylalanine levels, the dosages of protein substitute dosages, daily phenylalanine allowance, and the definition of foods that could be eaten without restriction. Another survey also found disparities in measurements, calling for a more unified approach to patient care (Van Spronsen et al., 2009). A Cochrane review could not draw conclusions about the short- or long-term use of protein substitute in phenylketonuria due to the lack of adequate or analyzable trial data. They suggest that protein substitute use continue to be monitored with care (Yi & Singh, 2008).

A Brazilian study (Kanufre et al., 2007) followed 70 PKU infants, with half breastfed and half fed formula. The breastfed group was given a phenylalanine-free formula by bottle every 3 hours and breastmilk ad lib during the intervals. The phenylalanine blood levels returned to normal within a median of 8 days for the breastfed infants and within 7 days for the formula infants. Phenylalanine level results were normal 87 percent of the time for the breastfed group compared with 74.4 percent for the formula-only group. The researchers concluded that breastmilk is the appropriate source of phenylalanine in these babies and that reinforcement of the mother–baby emotional bond has a positive impact on acceptance of the disease and compliance with treatment.

Managing Breastfeeding

Physicians may interrupt breastfeeding while they stabilize phenylalanine levels and determine the infant's diet prescription. The mother can express her milk during this time to maintain production. After control is established (with the level of phenylalanine below 10 mg/dL) and the amount of phenylalanine-free formula needed has been determined, the mother's milk can be added to the infant's diet.

Some physicians may recommend an alternative that allows the mother to continue breastfeeding without interruption while control is being established, using one of two procedures. One method is to allow the infant to continue nursing and to offer a phenylalanine-free formula at each feeding, while maintaining a consistent daily intake of a prescribed volume of human milk and phenylalanine-free formula. The other method is to substitute a phenylalanine-free formula for one or two breastfeedings per day, with the mother expressing her milk at the missed feedings. A drawback to both methods is the infant's prolonged exposure to potentially toxic levels of phenylalanine. However, frequent analysis of the infant's serum can monitor this closely (Purnell, 2001; Duncan & Elder, 1997).

The standard approach for supplementing babies with PKU is to give the baby phenylalanine-free formula within 15 minutes of any supplemental food containing protein, such as human milk, thus ensuring efficient use of amino acids. Feeding the prescribed amount of phenylalanine-free formula through a tube-feeding device at the breast saves the mother time and preserves the quality of the breastfeeding bond. Although powdered formula can clog the tubing, mixing the formula with warm water and reblending it just before pouring it into the container can avoid this.

If the phenylalanine formula is given separately from the breast, absorption of nutrients in the mother's milk may be less efficient. There is a risk of the baby filling up on the mother's milk and not completing the second feeding of phenylalanine formula. Van Rijn et al. (2003) found that alternating breast and phenylalanine-free formula feedings enables babies to receive hindmilk and drink to satiety for both feedings. There was no statistically significant difference in metabolic control and growth within the first 6 months using this method of alternating feedings. This study suggests that such an approach is more convenient for parents and safe for otherwise healthy babies with PKU. Managing PKU with a combination of breastfeeding and low-phenylalanine formula provides easier maintenance of satisfactory phenylalanine blood levels. This diet helps avoid long-term neurological deficits and the adverse effects of uncontrolled maternal PKU in babies born of mothers with the disease (Purnell, 2001).

If levels of phenylalanine are high during the initial prescription phase, the baby could be breastfed once or twice a day after pumping. Although not consuming much milk, the baby stimulates milk production and receives the emotional benefits of being at the breast. After pumping, the mother can feed the phenylalanine-free formula to her baby and then breastfeed. This avoids the baby becoming frustrated from hunger. The mother can also use a tube-feeding device while the baby nurses on a breast she just pumped. If the volume of the mother's milk increases too rapidly, she can reduce feedings on a just-pumped breast or use only one breast at a feeding. If the mother's milk volume is low, she can nurse more frequently to increase milk production.

PKU diagnosis is reconfirmed between 3 and 12 months of age with a natural protein load calculated to provide a specific amount of phenylalanine for 3 days.

This is usually in the form of cow's milk or an evaporated milk formula. If the mother does not wish to interrupt breastfeeding during this time, the phenylalanine content of her milk can be measured to minimize error.

Dietary Changes

Because dietary requirements change as an infant with PKU grows, the mother can ask that the energy content of her milk be evaluated to determine if a dietary adjustment is required. Guidelines for introducing solid foods are mostly the same as for any other breastfeeding infant. High-phenylalanine foods such as eggs, meat, cheese, and milk should be avoided.

Weaning a baby with PKU from the breast requires more structure than weaning other breastfeeding babies. To maintain a healthy balance, the mother must monitor phenylalanine intake closely and replace each dropped feeding with the appropriate amount of phenylalanine-free or low-phenylalanine formula or solid foods. Weaning may need to occur earlier than usual if physicians have difficulty controlling the baby's phenylalanine levels. When considering weaning, the mother should designate a target date and estimate what her baby's weight will be to determine the requirements for phenylalanine, protein, and energy at that time. She can then consult with a nutritionist specializing in PKU to calculate the amounts of phenylalanine-free or low-phenylalanine formula and other supplements needed.

Counseling the Mother of a PKU Baby

When unique circumstances place restrictions on a mother's nursing pattern, she will need a great deal of support as well as advice on how to manage feedings and monitor her baby's intake. An infant with PKU can breastfeed safely with appropriate monitoring and special care. This requires motivation, access to daily or weekly blood checks for the baby, a support system, and a cooperative medical team. The mother may have difficulty maintaining milk production, and the additional worry about her baby may affect her letdown reflex. She also may be prone to plugged ducts or mastitis because of restricted feedings, so she should express milk whenever necessary.

Periodic test weighing is necessary to track the amount of breastmilk the baby consumes, with the amounts of phenylalanine-free formula being measured before the feeding. Daily weight checks of the baby with an electronic scale measure average intake of the mother's milk. Many medical professionals have learned more about breastfeeding PKU babies and work with mothers toward a positive outcome. The American Academy of Family Physicians (2007) supports breastfeeding of PKU infants.

Galactosemia

Galactosemia is an inherited disease in which the liver enzyme that changes galactose to glucose is absent. Galactose is a simple sugar found in lactose, referred to as milk sugar. Screening for galactosemia is one of the tests in newborn assessment. There are three types of galactosemia identified, each caused by particular gene mutations and affecting different enzymes involved in breaking down galactose:

- Type I—classic galactosemia—is the most common and most severe form of the condition. It occurs in 1 in every 30,000 to 60,000 newborns. Infants with type I galactosemia soon develop feeding difficulties, lethargy, failure to thrive, jaundice, liver damage, and bleeding. They can also develop bacterial infections and go into shock.
- Type II—galactokinase deficiency—causes fewer medical problems, but affected infants develop cataracts. Occurrence is less than 1 in every 100,000 newborns.
- Type III—galactose epimerase deficiency—can cause cataracts, delayed growth and development, intellectual disability, liver disease, and kidney problems. Symptoms range from mild to severe. Type III is very rare (U.S. National Library of Medicine, 2009).

Galactosemia requires immediate and total weaning from all milk—including human milk—as well as other foods that contain galactose (American Academy of Family Physicians, 2007). The infant is placed on a special formula that is free of galactose.

Duarte Variant

Although infants with galactosemia are generally unable to breastfeed, those with a form of classic galactosemia, known as the Duarte variant, are an exception. These infants have varying levels of enzyme activity and may be able to breastfeed. It is imperative for the parents to consult with a specialist such as a pediatric metabolic geneticist or endocrinologist for ongoing guidance. Dietary options with Duarte variant are either restricting lactose and galactose in the diet for a year or so and then gradually introducing these items and testing for the patient's response or no restrictions at all (Ficicioglu et al., 2008; Parents of Galactosemic Children, Inc., 2006). If the baby is breastfed, galactose levels need to be monitored carefully (Ganesan, 1997). Some nondairy formula may be needed; however, this is not always the case, and each infant needs to be assessed and followed individually. Elsas (2007) notes that galactose may prevent sequelae such as cataracts, ataxia, dyspraxic speech, and cognitive deficits.

Cleft Lip and Cleft Palate Defects

A cleft lip or cleft palate can affect the infant's ability to generate suction and obtain adequate nourishment. A cleft is an opening in the upper lip or palate, or both, caused when these oral structures fail to fuse during the first trimester of pregnancy. A cleft in the palate results in an opening to the nasal cavity in the roof of the mouth. Clefts can occur on one side of the mouth (unilateral) or both sides (bilateral). There can be a cleft of the lip only, a cleft of the palate only, or, most commonly, a cleft of both the lip and palate. Clefts can occur as part of other congenital anomalies, syndromes, and medical complications (March of Dimes, 2007). These require specialized medical care and often preclude breastfeeding.

Rates of occurrence for a cleft birth defect vary, depending on the type of cleft. Clefts can range from mild to very severe and are among the most common birth defect, with approximately one case of orofacial cleft in every 500 to 550 births (Tolarova, 2009a). A combination of cleft lip and cleft palate occurs more frequently in people of Asian and Native American ancestry and least frequently in African Americans.

According to the March of Dimes (2007), when isolated and unaccompanied by another birth defect the occurrence of babies born with clefts in the United States each year is about:

- 6,800 with oral–facial clefts each year
- 4,200 with cleft lip/palate
- 2,600 with isolated cleft palate

A child born with a cleft usually faces continuous treatment until adulthood, involving plastic surgery, orthodontics, management of ear fluid, and sometimes speech therapy. Each child's condition is unique, and treatment plans vary. Cleft palate treatment centers offer a comprehensive team approach to each child's needs. The child's prognosis and outcome are generally excellent, unless the cleft is a part of a more serious syndrome.

Otitis media is a common occurrence among children with cleft palates. This happens despite cleft repair and early treatment with feeding plates, called grommets or obturators, probably because of eustachian tube dysfunction. Aniansson et al. (2002) found a significant correlation during the first 18 months of life between longer duration of feeding with breastmilk and a lower incidence of otitis media.

Parents' Reactions to a Cleft

Parents' reactions to their baby's condition are affected by the type of cleft. Predictably, facial visibility of an unrepaired cleft lip, with or without a cleft palate, leads to an immediate emotional response. An isolated cleft palate is

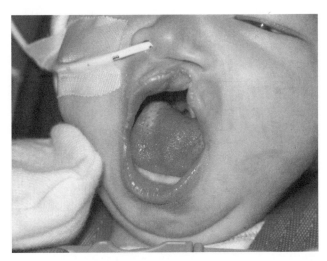

FIGURE 25.2 Infant with cleft prior to surgery.

Source: Printed with permission of Hollye Long.

visible only when the infant cries and, therefore, elicits less of an emotional response. Generally, surgery to repair a cleft lip is performed much sooner (at about 3 months of age) than that of a cleft palate (at about 1 year), although there is a growing trend to provide earlier cleft palate repair. Figure 25.2 (before surgery), Figure 25.3 (immediately after surgery), and Figure 25.4 (aged 20 months) show an infant with a unilateral cleft lip and palate who underwent early palatal and lip repair at 11 days old. The baby transitioned to direct breastfeeding by 6 weeks of age.

You can provide encouragement by commenting on how well a mother is doing in her maternal role and on her baby's positive attributes. Avoid comments that minimize the parents' concerns or deny the mother's reac-

tions. It is unrealistic to tell parents that surgery performs such miracles that afterward no one will ever know their child had a cleft. Despite tremendous surgical advances and remarkable results, traces of the cleft will exist.

Although children with cleft defects are affected by peer teasing (Hunt et al., 2007; Noor & Musa, 2007), most children and adults with repaired cleft defects do not appear to experience major psychosocial problems. Some specific consequences that occur include behavioral problems, dissatisfaction with facial appearance, depression, and anxiety (Hunt et al., 2005). Not surprisingly, the type of cleft correlates to the degree of self-concept, facial appearance satisfaction, depression, attachment, learning problems, and interpersonal relationships. A Chinese study reported lower self-esteem among patients with a cleft (Cheung et al., 2007).

In one study parents generally regarded the craniofacial team with satisfaction, while reporting they often received poor feeding advice from other caregivers who had low levels of knowledge and difficulty handling the situation (Johansson & Ringsberg, 2004). Both parents and patients report similar responses and significant satisfaction levels with the treatment provided by the cleft team in another survey (Noor & Musa, 2007). The features most important for the patients and their parents, in decreasing order of priority, were teeth, nose, lips, and speech.

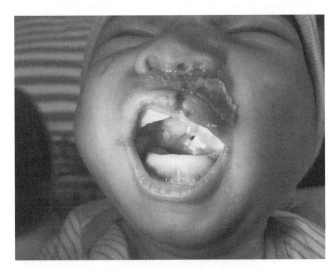

FIGURE 25.3 Infant immediately after cleft surgery.

Source: Printed with permission of Hollye Long.

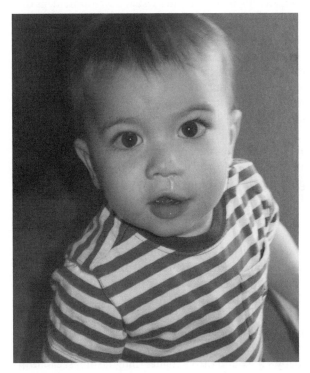

FIGURE 25.4 Infant 20 months after cleft surgery.

Source: Printed with permission of Hollye Long.

Breastfeeding Adjustments with a Cleft

Like all babies, human milk is the optimal food for babies with clefts. Babies have fewer ear infections, and any milk that leaks into the nasal cavity is less irritating than artificial formula. Breastfeeding, whether nutritive or not, aids in proper orofacial development and enhances bonding between the mother and baby. The birth order of the infant can have some effect on breastfeeding outcome. Multiparas, who typically establish milk production better initially than primiparas, may have an easier time lactating. The breastfeeding assistance a mother needs depends on the type of cleft her infant has.

Methods of feeding infants with clefts are often difficult and time consuming, especially in the early weeks. Parents may feel discouraged or apprehensive about feeding their baby and require support in overcoming their fears and dealing with obstacles. A Brazilian study found a low prevalence of breastfeeding in cleft babies, mainly due to sucking inability. Complete cleft lip and palate was the primary cause that affected sucking. The authors observed that dietary habits in babies with cleft lip and palate are more risky, with some of these babies receiving fruit juices and sugar (da Silva, 2003). A feeding protocol for cleft infants is available from the ABM (2007). The immunological properties of human milk can be particularly valuable to these children because of the higher incidence of otitis media (ABM, 2007). Additionally, breastfeeding offers these children improved speech development and aids in their visual development, as discussed in Chapter 9.

Breastfeeding with a Cleft Lip   An isolated cleft lip presents no physiological impediment to breastfeeding. The baby can usually nurse at the breast well and may be able to mold the open cleft around a breast more easily than around a small rubber nipple. In many cases the breast tissue fills the cleft to seal it off (Wilson-Clay & Hoover, 2008). The mother can place her thumb over a cleft lip while her baby nurses to improve the seal if necessary (Figure 25.5). The mother benefits greatly from support and encouragement, despite the relative ease with which she can accomplish breastfeeding.

Breastfeeding with a Cleft Palate   A cleft palate poses more of a challenge with breastfeeding than does a cleft lip. With a unilateral cleft palate the breast needs to enter the baby's mouth on the side of the cleft in such a way that the cheek on the side of the defect touches the breast. When the cleft is bilateral, the breast should enter the baby's mouth at midline. Feeding in a position that keeps the baby's nose and throat higher than the breast can minimize milk leaking into the nasal cavity. The baby can straddle the mother's body while being held upright or in a side-sitting position.

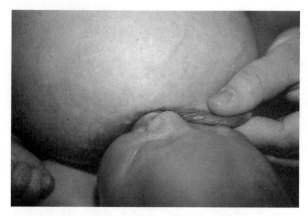

FIGURE 25.5   Using the "teacup" hold to plug cleft lip.
Source: Printed with permission of Kay Hoover and Barbara Wilson-Clay.

Some babies with a cleft palate choke often during feeding. Choking and milk leaking through the nose occur frequently in babies with cleft palates, regardless of feeding method. Although feeding can be time-consuming and frustrating in general, it often becomes easier after the first month. Breast pumping maintains milk production, makes milk readily available at the beginning of a feeding, and removes milk that remains in the breast after a feeding. Short, frequent feedings prevent the infant from tiring. Skin-to-skin contact with the mother and initiating a feeding before the baby is completely awake will help encourage feeding.

A breastfeeding begins with an infant's tongue drawing the nipple into the mouth. The tongue and palate create a vacuum to maintain hold of the breast, and the baby's gums compress the breast to promote milk flow. With a cleft palate, because of the opening between the baby's mouth and nose, the baby is unable to maintain hold of the breast and create a vacuum. Infants with a cleft lip and palate or a cleft of the soft and at least two-thirds of the hard palate have demonstrated less efficient sucking patterns than their noncleft peers (Masarei et al., 2007). They used shorter sucks, a faster rate of sucking, higher ratios of suck-swallow, and a greater proportion of intraoral positive pressure generation.

A study with bottle feeding found that babies with smaller clefts (i.e., cleft lip or minor soft palate clefts) were more likely to generate normal levels of suction and compression compared with their counterparts with larger clefts (Reid et al., 2007). Effective feeders were more likely to have smaller clefts and demonstrated higher suction pressures than babies with satisfactory or poor feeding ability. To compensate for this inability, the mother can cup her breast as she brings her baby toward her to latch and continues to hold her breast in the baby's mouth throughout the feeding.

Because having a cleft of the palate prevents creating a vacuum in the oral cavity, the baby may very likely not be able to create the suction required in breastfeeding (Wilson-Clay & Hoover, 2008). The mother can pump and feed her expressed milk to her baby to supplement feedings at the breast. Specialty feeders, such as the Pigeon Cleft Palate Nurser, the Hazelbaker Feeder, and the Medela SpecialNeeds (previously named Haberman) Feeder, are available. Familiarize yourself with such alternative feeders so you can counsel parents about their use. If parents find that spoon feeding results in excessive spillage or that tube feeding takes too long and tires the infant, you can help them find a feeding method that works for them and their baby. The parents' cleft palate team will instruct them to be very attentive to their baby's weight pattern and to monitor weight gain with weekly weight checks.

A baby with a cleft palate needs a complete breastfeeding assessment to determine the ability to transfer milk directly from the breast (after lactogenesis II has occurred). Pre- and postfeed weights are an important management tool for this population and should be used until it is determined whether the baby consistently transfers milk adequately from direct breastfeeding. Milk transfer may be easiest at the beginning of a feeding when the breast is firmer. The mother may not feel that the sucking sensation is particularly strong, especially if she has had the experience of breastfeeding other children. These babies sometimes have difficulty extracting the hindmilk from the breast. Massaging the breasts before and during the feeding increases milk flow and makes it easier for her baby to transfer milk.

A baby who is able to transfer milk from direct breastfeeding needs to go to breast on cue and with great frequency in the newborn period. The mother should aim for 8 to 12 feedings in 24 hours, initiating feedings if the baby fails to exhibit hunger cues. Counting voids and stools is an important marker for intake as well.

Breastfeeding with a Cleft Lip and Palate If the baby has both a cleft lip and palate, the techniques discussed relative to a cleft palate apply. Long-term use of a breast pump for expressing milk is likely to be even more necessary. A more extensive cleft produces the most difficulty with feedings. Many mothers pump exclusively and provide their milk through an alternative feeding method until the cleft palate is repaired. Putting her infant to breast as often as possible enhances bonding and nipple stimulation for milk production. "Comfort" nursing may also aid in jaw development.

Breastfeeding with a Submucosal Cleft Palate Because it is difficult to detect, a submucosal cleft of the soft palate can escape the newborn screening process. In this condition a layer of skin covers a cleft in the soft palate, which

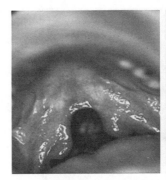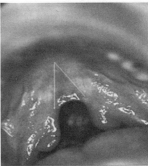

FIGURE 25.6   Submucosal cleft.
Source: Printed with permission of Dr. Marie M. Tolarova.

sometimes appears as a bluish midline discoloration (Figure 25.6). The salivary glands may be involved as well and can cause drooling. A bifid (forked) uvula, a short soft palate with muscle separation (furrow) in the midline, and a bony notch in the posterior of the hard palate are all markers for a submucosal cleft (Tolarova, 2009a).

Sometimes an occult (hidden) submucosal cleft is not discovered until the child begins speaking and hypernasal speech is noted or because of feeding difficulties or recurrent otitis media (Stal & Hicks, 1998). At times the cleft eludes diagnosis. A submucosal cleft makes it difficult for the newborn to maintain sufficient vacuum to sustain a suck. If you work with an infant with breastfeeding difficulties and you observe the above symptoms, refer the mother to her baby's physician for evaluation by a specialist such as an ear, nose, and throat specialist. A submucosal cleft can be a symptom of other more serious problems, such as velocardiofacial syndrome or chromosomal defects. Surgical repairs may be performed (Nasser et al., 2008).

Surgical Repair

Infants with a cleft lip, with or without a cleft of the palate, usually have lip repair surgery between 2 and 3 months of age. Some physicians permit infants to resume breastfeeding immediately after surgery. A mother who is not able to breastfeed during this time can express her milk and feed it to her baby through an alternative method. She could also freeze milk in preparation for the surgery. Because breastfeeding difficulties primarily involve the palate, repair of a cleft lip usually does not alter nursing ability significantly. Nonetheless, lip repair provides an important psychological lift to the parents.

Some cleft palate teams fit obturators over part of the cleft palate to assist in feeding (Figure 25.7). The baby still cannot create negative intraoral pressure, so assisted feeding is required (Karayazgan et al., 2009; Desiate & Milano, 2008). The use of nasal stents helps minimize deformities and stretches the skin for repair (see Figure 25.8). Obturators are used to position the palate for repair

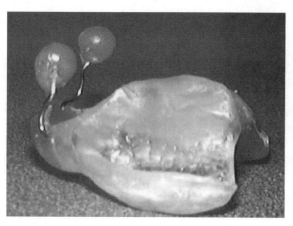

FIGURE 25.7 Obturator to bridge the gap in a cleft palate.

Source: Printed with permission of Dr. Scott Franklin.

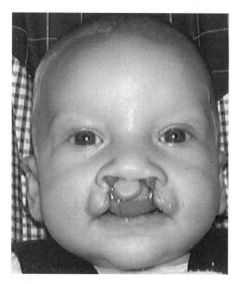

FIGURE 25.8 Nasal stent used in cleft surgery.

Source: Printed with permission of Dr. Scott Franklin.

and to prevent dental arch collapse. Although experts dispute its effectiveness for this purpose, an obturator sometimes produces psychological benefits for parents.

Some surgical teams perform lip repair during the first few weeks postpartum and early palatal repair is also becoming more frequent. Palatal growth has historically determined when the surgery may be performed. Many parents are now choosing early palatal repair and may opt for surgery soon after birth. Earlier surgery can produce a smoother transition to full breastfeeding. Although many mothers find it difficult to transition to breastfeeding, clinicians and parents should consider each baby's feeding strengths and limitations and never automatically dismiss the possibility of breastfeeding (Wolf & Glass, 1992).

You can work with the mother after lip or palate repair surgery to help her and her baby learn to breastfeed nutritively. If the baby is unable to achieve nutritive breastfeeding, any breastfeeding has value for comfort, oral development, and bonding. You can encourage the mother to continue to provide her milk to minimize her child's risk for ear and respiratory infections. Practical feeding suggestions from other mothers can offer insights into managing breastfeeding in this situation. Support groups can be helpful, and Internet resources offering parental support abound, including blogs and forums. Some cleft teams include lactation and nutritional support members.

Pierre Robin Sequence

Pierre Robin sequence is an anomaly characterized by micrognathia (a receding lower jaw) and displacement at the back of the tongue combined with a cleft palate and an absence of a gag reflex (Figure 25.9). Pierre Robin sequence, increasingly shortened to "Robin sequence," was originally thought to be a specific disease. It now refers to a grouping of clinical findings that may relate to other disorders, thus the name change from "syndrome" to "sequence" (Olasoji, 2007). This sequence may be isolated, due to uterine growth restriction of the jaw, or it may be related to over 46 different syndromes (Tolarova, 2009b). If uterine growth restriction is the cause, the jaw begins to develop after birth. If it is due to a disorder, micrognathia continues and is a marker for other problems.

An infant with Pierre Robin can suffer severe respiratory distress and have difficulty maintaining an airway, particularly during the newborn period. This can lead to difficulty thriving (Wolf & Glass, 1992) and some of these babies require endotracheal intubation and gavage feeding. Pierre Robin is associated with genetic disorders, most commonly Stickler's syndrome, a connective tissue disorder that can cause blindness. The possible severity of airway obstruction and concerns over survival usually make direct breastfeeding unlikely. Babies with Pierre Robin are an exception to the "back to sleep" rule for prevention of sudden infant death syndrome. Infants with this condition should not be put on their backs to prevent the tongue from falling back into the airway (Demetroulakos, 2007).

Pierre Robin sequence occurs in varying degrees and an infant with a very slight case may be able to breastfeed. An infant who cannot breastfeed initially can receive the mother's expressed milk. After the infant with Pierre Robin sequence gets through the crucial early stages of life and has developed sufficiently to maintain an airway without difficulty, the outcome is positive. The mother may be able to put the baby to breast at this time, depending on the caregiver's recommendations. Sometimes the baby's

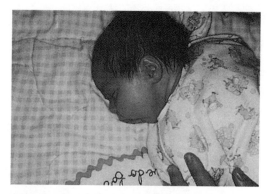

FIGURE 25.9   Infant with Pierre Robin sequence.

Source: Printed with permission of Jane Bradshaw.

position in utero is the cause of the Pierre Robin deformity. When this is the cause, jaw growth usually catches up to normal by 4 to 6 years of age.

Support for the Parents

Parents need direct information about expected difficulties in feeding and care of these babies. They need to know signs and symptoms of illness, possible complications, and information on deferring future treatment. Parents report being overwhelmed with too much information during a time of initial emotional stress. Learning how to deal with the feelings of friends and family is also a concern. It is helpful to give parents information in gradual doses during the newborn period. They may benefit from the repetition of facts as they progress through the range of emotional reactions and become more receptive to explanations and suggestions. Support is crucial and extremely valuable.

Understanding the emotions involved with cleft defects and staying current on the trends in cleft treatment help you provide reassurance and tactful, realistic information to parents. This is especially the case for those who work in community care beyond the initial newborn period. You will be most likely to encounter cleft patients if you work in a children's hospital; a pediatric clinic; Women, Infants, and Children (WIC) or other public health clinic; or in private practice. If you work in any of these practice settings, you will benefit your clients by developing your understanding, comfort, and expertise with the treatment and outcomes for these babies and children. Networking with cleft palate repair teams will increase your practice abilities as well.

Many new parents, especially those of first-born children with clefts, tend to attribute all behavior and problems of the infant to the cleft rather than realizing that much is part of the usual newborn pattern. You can help parents put the cleft into proper perspective and to view their child as normal in other respects. Encourage the mother to become an advocate for her child and to

become comfortable with questioning and understanding all aspects of her child's treatment. It is very important that you avoid evaluating or judging the mother's breastfeeding experience. The cleft palate feeding regimen can be trying, frustrating, and extremely time consuming. Help her recognize success in every effort.

Some mothers are unable emotionally or physically to continue breastfeeding for as long as they might have planned. It is important to recognize a mother's disappointment, provide support and information about weaning, and remind her how her baby benefited from the breastfeeding relationship and her milk. Additionally, support groups for parents of children with cleft palates exist in many parts of the country. They can give parents a unique, useful opportunity to relate to others who have dealt positively with the experience See Table 25.4 for counseling tips for parents about cleft lip and cleft palate and Appendix H for parent resources.

TABLE 25.4   Counseling Parents About Cleft Lip and Palate

- Lip usually molds around the breast.
- If necessary, cover the cleft with a finger to ensure good suction.
- Massage the breasts before nursing to promote milk flow.
- Hold the breast in the baby's mouth.
- With a unilateral cleft, the breast enters on the side of the defect. The baby's cheek on the side of the defect should touch the breast.
- With a bilateral cleft, the breast enters at midline. The baby's body straddles the mother.
- Use a feeding plate (obturator) to partially cover the cleft.
- Closely monitor weight gain, wet diapers, and frequency of feedings.
- Express milk after feedings and during surgical repair; feed the milk to the baby with the appropriate feeding device.
- Pump or hand express after feedings to adequately remove milk from the breast and stimulate milk production.
- Wear breast shells between feedings to stimulate milk production.
- Feed the baby in an upright position to avoid choking or milk leaking from the baby's nose.
- Push the baby's chin to his or her chest to stop choking and then resume the feeding.
- Use short, frequent feedings.
- Nurse while the baby is still sleepy.
- Use a tube-feeding device at the breast to encourage the baby to nurse.

Spina Bifida

Spina bifida, a neural tube defect present at birth, results in a gap in the bone that surrounds the baby's spinal cord. Spina bifida occurs worldwide in an average of 1 case per 1,000 births. Marked geographic variations occur, with the highest rates in Ireland and Wales. France, Norway, Hungary, Czechoslovakia, Yugoslavia, and Japan have the lowest rates. Although there is a genetic component, the preconception addition of adequate folic acid (400 mcg/day) to women's diets has reduced spina bifida rates (Foster, 2009). Surgical repair may be unnecessary if the gap is very small. When the gap is large enough to allow parts of the spinal cord to protrude, surgery may be required. Most of these infants have weakness or paralysis of the lower extremities. Surgery to repair the defect usually occurs as soon as possible—within 24 to 48 hours after birth. The infant will be in the neonatal intensive care unit after surgery, and the mother will need help expressing and transporting her milk.

The baby can go to the breast as soon as it is allowable. After the mother positions herself comfortably, a helper can carefully lift the baby and bring him to her, supporting him with pillows and making sure the mother's position avoids pressure on the baby's spinal column. Although feeding times will be brief until the baby has recovered from surgery, longer feedings can begin as the baby grows stronger. The recovery process may take several weeks, during which time the mother can pump her milk for her baby. Recognize that she may need assistance with breastfeeding after her baby arrives home.

Down Syndrome

Down syndrome, a chromosomal disorder in which the baby is born with an extra chromosome, occurs in an estimated 1 in 732 births (Sherman et al., 2007). The infant has oval eyes that slant slightly upward, a protruding tongue that seems too large, abnormally shaped ears, a wide flattened nose, and hypotonicity (low muscle tone). Other features include a short neck, white spots on the iris of the eye (called Brushfield spots), a deep transverse crease on the palm of the hand (Palmer's crease), and a short stature (Figure 25.10).

Diagnosis of Down syndrome is confirmed by a blood test to determine if extra material from chromosome 21 is present (USDHHS, National Institute of Child Health and Human Development, 2007). Because the test can take up to 2 weeks, parents may experience a long waiting period of chronic anxiety and grief.

A Down baby's growth and development, although slower than that of an uncompromised child, usually allows most of the same physical activities as with other children. Human milk's immunological factors and easy

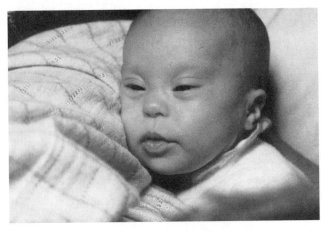

FIGURE 25.10   Infant with Down syndrome.
Source: Printed with permission of Sarah Coulter Danner.

digestibility make it especially beneficial to a Down baby, who may have incomplete heart and gastrointestinal development, respiratory infection, digestive upset, and obesity. The baby may have a lower tendency toward obesity from receiving human milk in infancy (Grummer-Strawn et al., 2004; Toschke et al., 2002).

Pisacane et al. (2003) found a 30 percent breastfeeding rate among infants with Down syndrome admitted to the neonatal unit. Reasons given by mothers for not breastfeeding include infant illness, frustration or depression, perceived milk insufficiency, and difficulty with sucking. A Dutch study found no significant difference in breastfeeding rates for children with and without Down syndrome. The adequacy of energy and nutrient intakes was similar as well (Hopman et al., 1998). Down syndrome significantly delays the age at which the baby begins receiving solid food, which can be deleterious to oral–motor development.

Most babies with Down syndrome are able to breastfeed. Cardiac complications may be present, most likely in a mild form that allows breastfeeding to take place with little difficulty. At the other extreme, however, a cardiac condition may be so severe that the activity required for breastfeeding is too stressful and may be contraindicated. In a study of 59 breastfed infants with Down syndrome, 31 had no difficulty establishing sucking, 4 were slow for less than 1 week, 8 took 1 week to establish sucking, and 16 took longer than 1 week. Severe cardiac anomaly was associated with the infant having poor sucking ability. The authors concluded that Down syndrome does not cause initial feeding problems in all infants and stated that their mothers need a lot of support (Aumonier & Cunningham, 1983). A newer study found that 66.7 percent of 225 mothers initiated breastfeeding of their Down baby, with 30 percent of them discontinuing breastfeeding at 3 to 6 months (Al-Sarheed, 2006).

Breastfeeding Management with Down Syndrome

Encourage the mother to view early breastfeedings with her Down baby as practice sessions. She and her baby can get to know one another, and the mother can learn how to hold and rouse her baby. If she needs to stimulate her baby to an alert state for nursing, the rousing techniques presented in Chapter 14 are helpful. Hypotonia will cause the baby's head, arms, and legs to be loose and floppy. Difficulty rooting and sucking because of weak reflexes, sluggishness, and becoming easily fatigued at the breast can make it difficult for the baby to remove milk sufficiently. Although extra feeding assistance and patience are needed in the early days, muscle tone will improve as the baby learns to nurse and exercises the facial muscles.

Any of the conventional breastfeeding positions work well for an infant with Down syndrome. The mother can minimize the effort required from her baby during feedings by paying careful attention to positioning and watching for signs of fatigue. With the head and body well supported, the baby can reserve energy for nursing. His head should be slightly flexed but not drooped too far forward. A position that places the baby's throat slightly higher than the mother's nipple prevents choking and gagging, especially if the mother leans back slightly to allow her nipple to tilt upward. The side-lying position seems to work well for many of these babies, with the baby supported by several pillows and the baby's head propped higher than the rest of the body. The side-sitting (also football or clutch) hold gives the mother greater ability to form and control her breast.

Pressing down on the baby's chin encourages a wide open mouth. When the baby latches, the mother can check that the bottom lip turns outward and not inward over the alveolar ridge. The typically flaccid, flat tongue initially may be unable to cup around the nipple and form a trough to carry the milk to the back of the throat. The mother can press down on the center of his tongue with her finger several times before each feeding to help her baby learn to shape the tongue appropriately. With the Dancer hand position, she can cup her baby's chin with light pressure on the cheeks from her thumb and index finger and her other three fingers supporting her breast.

To facilitate milk exchange, the mother can massage and express milk to initiate letdown before putting her baby to breast. Her goal is to nurse for at least 10 to 12 minutes on each breast every 2 to 3 hours, initiating feedings if her baby does not give cues. If her baby has difficulty sucking, she can express milk after the feeding and feed it to her baby. Because a Down baby may be passive, the mother needs to initiate feedings frequently by observing and responding to subtle signs of wakefulness, such as lip and eye movements.

Typically, an infant with Down syndrome gains weight and grows in length more slowly than the average infant, regardless of feeding method. Special growth charts for children with Down syndrome reflect this. Slow weight gain by itself is not an indication that breastfeeding is providing insufficient nourishment. If the mother expresses milk after every feeding to ensure adequate stimulation for copious milk production and if she feeds her baby the expressed hindmilk, she will probably meet her baby's nutritional needs through her milk.

Hydrocephalus

Hydrocephalus is an excessive accumulation of cerebrospinal fluid in the intracranial cavity. It results from interference in the flow or absorption of fluid through the brain and the spinal canal causing the infant's head to enlarge as fluid increases. In most cases the baby has a high-pitched cry, muscle weakness, and severe neurological defects. Breastfeeding is possible with adjustments in positioning. The infant's head needs to be slightly higher than the breast and frequent feedings will help to avoid reflux.

Neurological Impairment

Infants with neurological damage or impairment can have varying degrees of mental deficiency and learning ability. A severely brain-damaged infant is unable to maintain concentration because of an extremely poor attention span. Reflexes that were instinctive at birth are forgotten, requiring that the mother teach them to her baby. The baby also requires constant and continual reinforcement of learned abilities. Thus infants with neurological damage may require ongoing techniques and assistance to accomplish effective attachment and sucking for breastfeeding (Genna, 2008).

Babies who are born with a neurological impairment have a higher percentage of premature births and therefore may require longer hospitalization than most babies. Generally, these mothers need assistance and support to compensate for their babies' low muscle tone as well as patience while the baby learns and relearns how to suck. The mother may need to deal with separation from her baby, as well as the baby preferring bottle feeds due to sucking weakness. Depending on its severity, neurological impairment results in the infant rarely having a fully developed or strong suck and swallow reflex. Because a mature suck and swallow reflex is essential for transferring milk from the breast, breastfeeding is more challenging and feedings take more time for these infants. The degree of difficulty depends on the severity of the impairment and the mother's ability to cope with the emotional stress and practical aspects of breastfeeding.

The severity of brain damage determines the degree to which an infant is able to breastfeed. In many cases the infant's brain mechanism does not pick up the impetus to perform specific functions. Although reflexes may be present, the baby may not have the ability to coordinate them with the stimulus. Although the reflexes for rooting and sucking are satisfactory in an uncompromised infant, they may be insufficient to enable an infant with brain damage to breastfeed. Whereas the baby may respond to these reflexes in the early months, the reflexes regress from instinct to a learned ability, and the baby may continually forget how to nurse. Additionally, the baby may have difficulty swallowing, resulting in gagging and choking. Nursing the baby in an upright position and stroking downward under the chin to aid swallowing may help (Wolf & Glass, 1992).

Short, frequent feedings compensate for the difficulty a brain-damaged infant has in maintaining concentration and losing interest in nursing before transferring milk adequately. Because her infant may become very frustrated waiting for milk to release, the mother can express her milk to initiate letdown before putting her baby to breast. For a baby who is able to maintain a latch and seal, a tube-feeding device may also be useful for nourishing the baby while at the breast. Babies with neurological defects need to be followed closely to ensure adequate intake, recognizing that supplementation with the mother's expressed milk may be necessary.

Sensory Processing Disorder

Sensory integration is the process of our brain taking input from our five senses and forming a functional composite that enables us to comprehend the world around us. When sensory integration does not develop normally, problems in learning, development, or behavior may result. Previously called sensory integration disorder, the condition is now termed sensory processing disorder and describes a pattern of dysfunction in children and adults who have atypical responses to ordinary sensory stimulation (Miller et al., 2009). The Sensory Processing Disorder Foundation (2010) estimates that 1 in every 20 children experiences symptoms significant enough to affect full participation in everyday life.

A study analyzing the backgrounds of children with autistic spectrum disorder and sensory processing disorder found that the incidence of jaundice was 3 to 4 times higher in both groups than in unaffected children. Rates of breech position, cord wrap or prolapse, assisted delivery methods (particularly forceps and suction deliveries), and high birth weight were greater in both groups as well. Incidence of preterm birth was higher in the autistic spectrum disorder group but not significantly different from the sensory processing disorder group. These children also had a high frequency of absent or brief crawling phase

and high percentages of problems with ear infections, allergies, and maternal stress during pregnancy (May-Benson et al., 2009). A hyporesponsive baby, one with low registration of sensory input, may fail to suckle when put to the breast. A hyperresponsive baby, one with high registration of input, also called sensory defensive (Kranowitz, 2006), may be hypertonic, easily overstimulated, and aversive to the breast.

If you observe a baby with feeding difficulties who exhibits any or some of these behaviors, referral back to the baby's physician and a list of occupational or physical therapists who specialize in sensory integration is appropriate. Special feeding strategies may help babies at both ends of the spectrum transition to breastfeeding more effectively. A hyporesponsive infant may respond to being held upright and finger feeding as well as gentle massage to the face, mouth, and palate. Strategies for the hyperresponsive baby include deeper pressure touch, swaddling, swinging the baby gently from head-to-toe in a blanket before feeding, or self-attachment (Genna, 2008).

Sensory processing disorder is complex, and the baby will need the care of an occupational or physical therapist. If you are able to attend the baby's evaluation or therapy, you can offer valuable insights from a feeding perspective and help the mother advocate for continued breastfeeding. Many occupational and physical therapists have little experience working with breastfeeding infants. This interdisciplinary approach benefits everyone on the team, especially the mother and baby (Weiss-Salinas & Williams, 2001).

Support for Parents of Special Needs Infants

Parents of compromised infants may experience shock and grief at the birth of their "less than perfect baby." Grief can last for years, often accompanied by a sense of helplessness and loss of control (Kyle, 2008). Breastfeeding can help them form an attachment to their baby as they work through their emotions. These mothers benefit from a great deal of support and encouragement. Praise them for their efforts and remind them of all the beneficial aspects of breastfeeding for an infant with special needs. Referral to a support group can help them deal with their grief while in the company of other parents who are in the same situation and help them learn to celebrate their baby's uniqueness.

Parents of neurologically impaired infants need an extensive network of support, and you are an important member of their support team. Reinforce the mother's commitment to breastfeed, and praise her for her diligence in coping with difficulties. Encourage parents to draw on each other for strength and support, and put them in touch with special support groups for parents of challenged children. See Table 25.5 for counseling suggestions. Although neurological impairments are not

TABLE 25.5 Counseling a Mother of a Neurologically Impaired Infant

Mother's Concern	Suggestions for Mother
Baby has difficulty grasping the breast	• Position the baby close to the breast and adequately support his body. • Position the baby's lower lip outward from his gum. • Press the baby's tongue down to create a groove for the nipple. • Use the Dancer hand position to support the breast and the baby's chin.
Baby has difficulty sucking	• Feed milk by a cup, dropper, or spoon.
Baby gags or chokes during feedings	• Position the baby's head so his throat is slightly above the nipple. • Stroke downward under the chin to aid swallowing.
Baby loses interest after several minutes of nursing	• Pre-express milk to initiate letdown. • Express milk onto the nipple or into the corner of the baby's mouth. • Nurse more frequently for 5-minute periods at a time. • Use a tube-feeding device to maintain milk flow and encourage sucking.

common, lactation consultants may find that babies with impairment exhibit similar feeding problems (Moe, 1998). If you encounter a baby with an impairment, you may find it helpful to research breastfeeding in light of other conditions.

It is common for a mother to experience negative feelings at times about her compromised baby. This mother's depression can be much more severe than postpartum depression, and she will need a great deal of support. See Chapter 19 for more information on postpartum depression. You may be the only person with whom she can express her true feelings. She needs to know you are there for her and that you genuinely care. It may be difficult for you to deal with a situation like this, and you need to draw on support from those close to you. You cannot "fix" the baby. Your role is to provide lactation support.

∼ Summary

Mothers may face challenging circumstances involving their health, their baby's health, or both. Some mothers reach their breastfeeding goals despite these obstacles. Others may need to change their goals to accommodate their special situation. Your assistance will be valuable to them as they navigate their unexpected parenting journey, including any necessary accommodations in breastfeeding. You can help them see ways in which breastfeeding and/or breastmilk help meet the needs of their babies. Despite maternal health conditions, mothers can establish enriching and sound breastfeeding practices that do not compromise the health of either the mother or baby. Breastfeeding helps normalize the relationship between a mother and her compromised baby and optimizes the baby's health through human milk.

∼ Chapter 25—At a Glance

Applying what you learned—

Counseling mothers with special health needs:

- Autoimmune diseases such as chronic fatigue, Sjögren's syndrome, and Raynaud's phenomenon may affect breastfeeding.
- There is a correlation between endometriosis, infertility, and autoimmune disorders.
- Breastfeeding may reduce the risks of children developing an autoimmune disease.
- Obesity is increasing in the Western world and may affect the onset of milk production.
- Bariatric surgery for obesity carries lifelong nutritional implications.
- Women with gestational diabetes are at higher risk of converting to type 2 diabetes.
- Insulin levels in diabetic women may fluctuate erratically until lactation is established and again when weaning is initiated.
- Diabetic women are prone to yeast infections.
- Some mothers with primary IMS respond to metoclopramide or domperidone.
- Decreasing insulin resistance may help increase milk production for women with PCOS.
- Properly managed thyroid supplementation is not a risk to an infant's health.
- Thyroid hormone that passes through the mother's milk can mask latent hypothyroidism in the baby.
- Mothers with cystic fibrosis can breastfeed, with attention to special nutritional needs.

- Mothers with tuberculosis can breastfeed with certain precautions and treatment.
- Mothers are at low risk of transmitting hepatitis C to their infants through breastfeeding.
- Active herpes lesions must be covered to prevent infant exposure.
- A mother with chickenpox at delivery must be isolated from her newborn until the lesions heal; her milk can be given to her infant if there are no lesions anywhere on her breast.
- Breastfed babies may receive passive immunity to CMV through breastmilk and transplacental antibodies.
- Very-low-birth-weight preterm babies are at risk for illness from CMV-positive mothers' milk.
- Recommendations for HIV-positive women in developed countries are that they should not breastfeed if they can safely formula feed or obtain donor milk.

Counseling the mother of a compromised infant:

- For a baby with a cleft lip, breastfeeding may be easier than bottle feeding.
- Breastfeeding with a cleft palate presents breastfeeding challenges.
- Massaging the breasts before and during the feeding increases milk flow and makes it easier for the baby to transfer milk.
- Phenylalanine intake for an infant with PKU must be strictly monitored throughout breastfeeding and through structured weaning.
- Mothers can feed their PKU baby phenylalanine-free formula through a tube-feeding device at the breast.
- A baby with complete galactosemia cannot consume human milk.
- A baby with Duarte's form of galactosemia may be able to breastfeed with careful monitoring and some nondairy formula.
- In a neurologically impaired infant, rooting and sucking regress from instinct to a learned ability, requiring continual teaching and coaxing.

Breastfeeding a compromised infant:

- Put the baby to breast with great frequency in the absence of cues—at least every 2 hours—in the newborn period.
- Hold the baby upright with nose and throat higher than the breast.
- Provide skin-to-skin contact.
- Begin a feeding before the baby is completely awake.

- Nurse for brief, frequent periods to avoid tiring the baby.
- Recognize signs of fatigue, cardiac complications, hypotonia, and difficulty rooting and sucking.
- View early breastfeeding as practice sessions.
- Press down on the center of the tongue, and use the Dancer hand position to assist the baby as needed.

Counseling mothers of babies with special health needs:

- Help parents deal with emotions and stages of grief for the "perfect" child.
- Avoid comments that minimize parents' concerns or deny a mother's reactions.
- Give parents information in gradual doses during the newborn period.
- Help parents view their child as normal in other respects.
- Avoid judging mothers' breastfeeding decisions.
- Help the mother with pumping and provide follow-up care after discharge home.
- Recognize symptoms of hyporesponsive and hyperresponsive babies, teach parents coping mechanisms, and refer to specialists.

∼ References

Academy of Breastfeeding Medicine (ABM). ABM clinical protocol #17: guidelines for breastfeeding infants with cleft lip, cleft palate, or cleft lip and palate; 2007. www.bfmed.org. Accessed November 28, 2009.

Agostoni C, et al. A randomized trial of long-chain polyunsaturated fatty acid supplementation in infants with phenylketonuria. *Dev Med Child Neurol.* 2006;48:207-212.

Agostoni C, et al. Plasma long-chain polyunsaturated fatty acids and neurodevelopment through the first 12 months of life in phenylketonuria. *Dev Med Child Neurol.* 2003;45:257-261.

Ahring K, et al. Dietary management practices in phenylketonuria across European centres. *Clin Nutr.* 2009;28:231-236.

AIDS.org. PCR test now available; 2009. www.aids.org. Accessed November 28, 2009.

Akçay M, et al. Mammary tuberculosis—importance of recognition and differentiation from that of a breast malignancy: report of three cases and review of the literature. *World J Surg Oncol.* 2007;5:67.

Allahbadia GN, Merchant R. Polycystic ovary syndrome in the Indian Subcontinent. *Semin Reprod Med.* 2008;26:22-34.

Al-Sarheed M. Feeding habits of children with Down's syndrome living in Riyadh, Saudi Arabia. *J Trop Pediatr.* 2006; 52:83-86.

American Academy of Family Physicians. AAFP policy statement on breastfeeding. Breastfeeding position paper; 2007.

www.aafp.org/online/en/home/policy/policies/b/breast feedingpositionpaper.html. Accessed March 18, 2009.

American Academy of Pediatrics (AAP). Section on breast-feeding. Breastfeeding and the use of human milk. *Pediatrics.* 2005;115:496-506. http://aappolicy.aappublications.org/cgi/reprint/pediatrics;115/2/496.pdf. Accessed November 10, 2009.

American Autoimmune Related Diseases Association, Inc. Autoimmune disease in women. Autoimmunity: A major women's health issue. http://www.aarda.org/women_and_autoimmunity.php. Accessed November 15, 2009.

American College of Obstetricians and Gynecologists (ACOG). Committee on genetics. ACOG Committee Opinion #449: Maternal phenylketonuria. *Obstet Gynecol..* 2009;114(6): 1407-1408.

American Dietetic Association. Position of the American Dietetic Association: Promoting and supporting breast-feeding (James D, Lessen R). *J Am Diet Assoc.* 2009; 109(11):1926-1942.

Amir L, Donath S. A systematic review of maternal obesity and breastfeeding intention, initiation and duration. *BMC Pregnancy Childbirth.* 2007;7:9.

Anderson J, et al. Raynaud's phenomenon of the nipple: A treatable cause of painful breastfeeding. *Pediatrics.* 2004;113(4): e360-e364.

Ando Y, et al. Long-term serological outcome of infants who received frozen-thawed milk from human T-lymphotropic virus type-I positive mothers. *J Obstet Gynaecol Res.* 2004;30(6):436-438.

Aniansson G, et al. Otitis media and feeding with breast milk of children with cleft palate. *Scand J Plast Reconstr Surg Hand Surg.* 2002;36(1):9-15.

AnotherLook. Infant feeding and HIV/AIDS: A call to action; 2003. www.anotherlook.org. Accessed March 7, 2005.

Arduino PG, Porter SR. Herpes simplex virus type 1 infection: Overview on relevant clinico-pathological features. *J Oral Pathol Med.* 2008;37(2):107-121.

Arnold G. Phenylketonuria. *Medscape;* February 13, 2009. http://emedicine.medscape.com/article/947781-overview. Accessed November 12, 2009.

Aumonier M, Cunningham C. Breast feeding in infants with Down's syndrome. *Child Care Health Dev.* 1983;9(5):247-255.

Azizi F, Smyth P. Breastfeeding and maternal and infant iodine nutrition. *Clin Endocrinol.* 2009;70(5):803-809.

Baharoon S. Tuberculosis of the breast. *Ann Thorac Med.* 2008;3(3):110-114.

Baker J, et al. Breastfeeding reduces postpartum weight retention. *Am J Clin Nutr.* 2008;88(6):1543-1551.

Barclay A, et al. Systematic review: The role of breastfeeding in the development of pediatric inflammatory bowel disease. *J Pediatr.* 2009;55(3):421-426.

Barlow C. Ulcerative colitis, pregnancy, prenatal expression and breastfeeding. *Breastfeed Rev.* 2006. http://findarticles.com/p/articles/mi_6804/is_3_14/ai_n28395387/?tag=content;col1. Accessed March 18, 2010.

Bodley V, Powers D. Patient with insufficient glandular tissue experiences milk supply increase attributed to progesterone treatment for luteal phase defect. *J Hum Lact.* 1999;15(4): 339-343.

Brugman S, et al. Prolonged exclusive breastfeeding reduces autoimmune diabetes incidence and increases regulatory T-cell frequency in bio-breeding diabetes-prone rats. *Diabetes Metab Res Rev.* 2009;25(4):380-387.

Buescher S. Human milk and infectious diseases. In Hale T, Hartmabnn P. *Hale & Hartmann's Textbook of Human Lactation.* Amarillo, TX: Hale Publishing; 2007; 193-212.

Capretti M, et al. Very low birth weight infants born to cytomegalovirus-seropositive mothers fed with their mother's milk: a prospective study. *J Pediatr.* 2009;154:842-848.

Celiker M, Chawla A. Congenital B_{12} deficiency following maternal gastric bypass. *J Perinatol.* 2009;29(2):640-642.

Centers for Disease Control and Prevention (CDC), Division of Nutrition, Physical Activity and Obesity, National Center for Chronic Disease Prevention and Health Promotion. Overweight and obesity; October 26, 2009. www.cdc.gov/obesity/index.html. Accessed October 31, 2009.

Centers for Disease Control and Prevention (CDC). Fact sheet: tuberculosis and pregnancy; June 1, 2009a. www.cdc.gov/tb/publications/factsheets/specpop/pregnancy.htm. Accessed November 15, 2009.

Centers for Disease Control and Prevention (CDC). Fact sheet: tuberculosis. Trends in tuberculosis, 2008; September 17, 2009b. www.cdc.gov/tb/publications/factsheets/statistics/TBTrends.htm. Accessed November 20, 2009.

Centers for Disease Control and Prevention (CDC). Hepatitis B and C infections; October 20, 2009c. www.cdc.gov/BREASTFEEDING/disease/hepatitis.htm. Accessed November 20, 2009.

Centers for Disease Control and Prevention (CDC), National Center for Infectious Diseases. Epstein-Barr virus and infectious mononucleosis; May 16, 2006. www.cdc.gov/ncidod/diseases/ebv.htm. Accessed November 20, 2009.

Chantry C, et al. Effect of flash-heat treatment on immunoglobulins in breast milk. *J Acquir Immune Defic Syndr.* 2009; 51(3):264-267.

Cheung L, et al. Psychological profile of Chinese with cleft lip and palate deformities. *Cleft Palate Craniofac J.* 2007; 44(1):79-86.

Cornejo V, et al. Phenylketonuria diagnosed during the neonatal period and breast feeding. *Rev Med Chil.* 2003;131(11): 1280-1287.

Creanga A, et al. Use of metformin in polycystic ovary syndrome: a meta-analysis. *Obstet Gynecol.* 2008;111(4):959-968.

Cystic Fibrosis Foundation (CFF). About Cystic Fibrosis: What You Need to Know; 2009. www.cff.org. Accessed March 17, 2010.

da Silva D. G., et al. Breast-feeding and sugar intake in babies with cleft lip and palate. *Cleft Palate Craniofac J.* 2003; 40(1):84-87.

Danaei G, et al. Diabetes prevalence and diagnosis in US states: analysis of health surveys. *Population Health Metrics.* 2009; 7:16.

Demetroulakos J. Pierre Robin syndrome. U.S. National Library of Medicine. *Medline;* October 24, 2007. www.nlm.nih.gov/medlineplus/ency/article/001607.htm. Accessed November 28, 2009.

Desiate A, Milano V. Preparation of feeding obturators for newborns with cleft palate: Clinical and laboratory procedures. *Minerva Stomatol.* 2008;57(9):459-466.

Donath S, Amir L. Maternal obesity and initiation and duration of breastfeeding: data from the longitudinal study of Australian children. *Matern Child Nutr.* 2008;4(3):163-170.

Doyle J, et al. Nutritional vitamin B12 deficiency in infancy: three case reports and a review of the literature. *Pediatr Hematol Oncol.* 1989;6:161-172.

Duncan LD, Elder S. Breastfeeding the infant with PKU. *J Hum Lact.* 1997;13(3):231-235.

Dworsky M, et al. Persistence of cytomegalovirus in human milk after storage. *J Pediatr.* 1982;101:440-443.

Edenborough F, et al. European Cystic Fibrosis Society. Guidelines for the management of pregnancy in women with cystic fibrosis. *J Cyst Fibros.* 2008;(Suppl 1):S2-S32.

Elsas L. U.S. National Center for Biotechnology Information. Galactosemia; September 27, 2007. www.ncbi.nlm.nih.gov/bookshelf/br.fcgi?book=gene&part=galactosemia. Accessed November 28, 2009.

Essah P, et al. Effects of short-term and long-term metformin treatment on menstrual cyclicity in women with polycystic ovary syndrome. *Fertil Steril.* 2006;86(1):230-232.

Ficicioglu C, et al. Duarte (DG) galactosemia: a pilot study of biochemical and neurodevelopmental assessment in children detected by newborn screening. *Mol Genet Metab.* 2008;95(4):206-212.

Forster D, et al. Diabetes and antenatal milk expressing: a pilot project to inform the development of a randomised controlled trial. *Midwifery.* July 15, 2009. [Epub ahead of print]

Foster M. Spina bifida. Medscape; July 15, 2009. http://emedicine.medscape.com/article/1266529-overview. Accessed November 28, 2009.

Fox-Bacon C, et al. Maternal PKU and breastfeeding: case report of identical twin mothers. *Clin Pediatr.* 1997;36:539-542.

Gabbay M, Kelly H. Use of metformin to increase breastmilk production in women with insulin resistance: a case series. Abstract presented at the Academy of Breastfeeding Medicine Eighth International Meeting Physicians & Breastfeeding: Controversy, Challenge & Change. Chicago, Illinois, October 16-20, 2003.

Galluzzo A, et al. Insulin resistance and polycystic ovary syndrome. *Nutr Metab Cardiovasc Dis.* 2008;18(7):511-518.

Gambol PJ. Maternal phenylketonuria syndrome and case management implications. *J Pediatr Nurs.* 2007;22(2):129-138.

Ganesan R. Borderline galactosemia. *New Beginnings.* 1997;14(4):123-124.

Garruti G, et al. Adipose tissue, metabolic syndrome and polycystic ovary syndrome: from pathophysiology to treatment. *Reprod Biomed Online.* 2009;19(4):552-563. www.rbmonline.com/4DCGI/Article/Detail?38%091%09=%203884%09. Accessed March 18, 2010.

Genna CW. *Supporting Sucking Skills in Breastfeeding Infants.* Sudbury, MA: Jones and Bartlett; 2008.

Giovannini M, et al. Phenylketonuria: dietary and therapeutic challenges. *J Inherit Metab Dis.* 2007;30(2):145-152.

Glueck C, et al. Chapter 17: Polycystic ovary syndrome: pathophysiology, endocrinopathy, treatment, and lactation. In Hale T, Hartmann P. *Hale & Hartmann's Textbook of Human Lactation.* Amarillo, TX: Hale Publishing; 2007; 343-353.

Goldfarb M. Relation of time of introduction of cow milk protein to an infant and risk of type-1 diabetes mellitus. *J Proteome Res.* 2008;7(5):2165-2167.

Gosman G, et al. Reproductive health of women electing bariatric surgery. *Fertil Steril.* 2009 Oct 6 [Epub ahead of print].

Grange DK, Finlay JL. Nutritional vitamin B12 deficiency in a breastfed infant following maternal gastric bypass. *Pediatr Hematol Oncol.* 1994;11(3):311-318.

Grummer-Strawn L, et al. Does breastfeeding protect against pediatric overweight? Analysis of longitudinal data from the centers for disease control and prevention pediatric nutrition surveillance system. *Pediatrics.* 2004;113(2):e81-e86.

Guelinckx I, et al. Reproductive outcome after bariatric surgery: a critical review. *Hum Reprod Update.* 2009;15(2):189-201.

Hale T. *Medications and Mother's Milk*, 14th ed. Amarillo, TX: Hale Publishing; 2010.

Hale T, Berens P. *Clinical Therapy in Breastfeeding Patients.* Amarillo, TX: Pharmasoft; 2002.

Hamprecht K, et al. Epidemiology of transmission of cytomegalovirus from mother to preterm infant by breastfeeding. *Lancet.* 2001;357:513-518.

Hanley W. Finding the fertile woman with phenylketonuria. *Eur J Obstet Gynaecol Reprod Biol.* 2008;137(2):131-135.

Hanson L. Chapter 10: The role of breastfeeding in the defense of the infant. In Hale T, Hartmann P. *Hale & Hartmann's Textbook of Human Lactation.* Amarillo, TX: Hale Publishing; 2007; 159-192.

Hartmann S, et al. Biochemical analysis of human milk treated with sodium dodecyl sulfate, an alkyl sulfate microbicide that inactivates human immunodeficiency virus type 1. *J Hum Lact.* 2006;22(1):61-74.

Heuchan A, Isaacs D. The management of varicella-zoster virus exposure and infection in pregnancy and the newborn period. Australasian Subgroup in Paediatric Infectious Diseases of the Australasian Society for Infectious Diseases. *Med J Aust.* 2001;174(6):288-292.

Hilson J, et al. High prepregnant body mass index is associated with poor lactation outcomes among white, rural women independent of psychosocial and demographic correlates. *J Hum Lact.* 2004;20:18-29.

Holmberg H, et al. Short duration of breastfeeding as a risk factor for B-cell autoantibodies in 5 year old children from the general population. *Br J Nutr.* 2007;97:111-116.

Hopman E, et al. Eating habits of young children with Down syndrome in The Netherlands: Adequate nutrient intakes but delayed introduction of solid food. *J Am Diet Assoc.* 1998;98(7):790-794.

Horvath T, et al. Interventions for preventing late postnatal mother-to-child transmission of HIV. *Cochrane Database Syst Rev.* 2009;CD006734.

Huang E, et al. Projecting the future diabetes population size and related costs for the U.S. *Diabetes Care.* 2009;32:2225-2229.

Huang L, et al. Primary infections of Epstein-Barr virus, cytomegalovirus, and human herpesvirus-6. *Arch Dis Child.* 1993;68(3):408-411.

Huggins K, et al. Markers of lactation insufficiency: a study of 34 mothers. In: Auerbach K (ed). *Current Issues in Clinical Lactation*. Sudbury, MA: Jones and Bartlett; 2000: 25-35.

Hummel S, et al. Predictors of overweight during childhood in offspring of parents with type 1 diabetes. *Diabetes Care*. 2009;32(5):921-925.

Humphrey J. The risks of not breastfeeding. *J Acquir Immune Defic Syndr*. 2010;53(1):1-4.

Hunt O, et al. Parent reports of the psychosocial functioning of children with cleft lip and/or palate. *Cleft Palate Craniofac J*. 2007;44(3):304-311.

Hunt O, et al. The psychosocial effects of cleft lip and palate: a systematic review. *Eur J Orthod*. 2005;27(3):274-285.

Hurst N. Recognizing and treating delayed or failed lactogenesis II. *J Midwifery Womens Health*. 2007;52(6):588-594.

Ingram J, et al. Breastfeeding: it is worth trying with the second baby. *Lancet*. 2001;358(9286):986-987.

Ip S, et al. A summary of the Agency for Healthcare Research and Quality's evidence report on breastfeeding in developed countries. *Breastfeed Med*. 2009;4(Suppl 1):S17-S30.

Ip S, et al. *Breastfeeding and Maternal and Infant Health. Outcomes in Developed Countries*. Rockville, MD: Agency for Healthcare Research and Quality; 2007.

Israel-Ballard K, et al. Bacterial safety of flash-heated and unheated expressed breastmilk during storage. *J Trop Pediatr*. 2006;52(6):399-405.

Israel-Ballard K, et al. Flash-heat inactivation of HIV-1 in human milk: A potential method to reduce postnatal transmission in developing countries. *J Acquir Immune Defic Syndr*. 2007;45(3):318-323.

Israel-Ballard K, et al. Viral, nutritional, and bacterial safety of flash-heated and Pretoria-pasteurized breast milk to prevent mother-to-child transmission of HIV in resource-poor countries: A pilot study. *J Acquir Immune Defic Syndr*. 2005;40(2):175-181.

Ivarsson A, et al. Breast-feeding protects against celiac disease. *Am J Clin Nutr*. 2002;75(5):914-921.

Jeffery B, et al. Determination of the effectiveness of inactivation of human immunodeficiency virus by Pretoria pasteurization. *J Trop Pediatr*. 2001;47(6):345-349.

Jeffery B, et al. The effect of Pretoria pasteurization on bacterial contamination of hand-expressed human breastmilk. *J Trop Pediatr*. 2003;49(4):240-244.

Jim W, et al. High cytomegalovirus load and prolonged virus excretion in breast milk increase risk for viral acquisition by very low birth weight infants. *Pediatr Infect Dis J*. 2009; 28(10):891-894.

Johansson B, Ringsberg K. Parents' experiences of having a child with cleft lip and palate. *J Adv Nurs*. 2004;47(2):165-173.

Jones C. Vertical transmission of genital herpes: prevention and treatment options. *Drugs*. 2009;69(4):421-434.

Kanufre V, et al. Breastfeeding in the treatment of children with phenylketonuria. *J Pediatr*. 2007;83(5):447-452.

Karayazgan B, et al. A preoperative appliance for a newborn with cleft palate. *Cleft Palate Craniofac J*. 2009;46(1):53-57.

Katz K, et al. Danish health care providers' perception of breastfeeding difficulty experienced by women who are obese, have large breasts, or both. *J Hum Lact*. Nov 12, 2009. [Epub ahead of print].

Kelley C. PCOS and breastfeeding: breastfeeding update. San Diego County Breastfeeding Coalition 3:1,3; September 2003. www.breastfeeding.org/newsletter/v3i3/page1.html. Accessed November 20, 2009.

Kent F, Farquharson D. Cystic fibrosis in pregnancy. *CMAJ*. 1993;149(6):809-813.

Koletzko B, et al. Omega-3 LC-PUFA supply and neurological outcomes in children with phenylketonuria (PKU). *J Pediatr Gastroenterol Nutr*. 2009;48(Suppl 1):S2-S7.

Kombol P. ILCA's inside track: a resource for breastfeeding mothers. Breastfeeding after weight loss surgery. *J Hum Lact*. 2008;24(3):341-342.

Kombol P. Lactation issues and bariatric surgery. Presented at the 2006 ILCA Conference, Philadelphia, PA; 2006. www.ilca.org under study modules for fee. Accessed October 30, 2009.

Kranowitz C. *The Out-of-Sync Child: Recognizing and Coping with Sensory Integration Dysfunction*, rev. ed. New York: Perigee; 2006.

Kreichauf S, et al. Effect of breastfeeding on the risk of becoming overweight in offspring of mothers with type 1 diabetes. *Dtsch Med Wochenschr*. 2008;133(22):1173-1177.

Kusuhara K, et al. Breast milk is not a significant source for early Epstein-Barr virus or human herpesvirus 6 infection in infants: a seroepidemiologic study in 2 endemic areas of human T-cell lymphotropic virus type I in Japan. *Microbiol Immunol*. 1997;41(4):309-312.

Kyle G. Breastfeeding my baby with Down syndrome. *New Beginnings*. 2008;25(2):24-26.

Langer-Gould A, et al. Exclusive breastfeeding and the risk of postpartum relapses in women with multiple sclerosis. *Arch Neurol*. 2009;66(8):958-963.

Lawrence R. Cytomegalovirus in human breast milk: Risk to the premature infant. *Breastfeed Med*. 2006;1:99-107.

Lawrence R, Lawrence R. *Breastfeeding: A Guide for the Medical Profession*, 6th ed. St. Louis, MO: Elsevier-Mosby; 2005.

Livshits A, Seidman D. Fertility issues in women with diabetes. *Womens Health*. 2009;5(6):701-707.

Løland B, Nylander G. Human milk, immune responses and health effects. *Tidsskr Nor Laegeforen*. 2007;127(18):2395-2398.

Luder E, et al. Current recommendations for breast-feeding in cystic fibrosis centers. *Am J Dis Child*. 1990;144(10):1153-1156.

Luopajärvi K, et al. Enhanced levels of cow's milk antibodies in infancy in children who develop type 1 diabetes later in childhood. *Pediatr Diabetes*. 2008;9(5):434-441.

Lupus Foundation of America. Pregnant and healthy: moms-to-be with lupus cope with the fears and risks; 2007. www.lupus.org. Accessed November 16, 2009.

Mackie A, et al. Cystic fibrosis-related diabetes. *Diabet Med*. 2003;20(6):425-436.

Marasco L. Insufficient milk supply explored: causes, recent research, and theories. Presented at the La Leche League International 2003 Lactation Specialist Workshop, Series XVIII, Austin, Texas, March 29, 2003.

Marasco L, et al. Polycystic ovary syndrome: a connection to insufficient milk supply? *J Hum Lact*. 2000;16(2):143-148.

March of Dimes. Cleft lip and cleft palate; February 2007. www.marchofdimes.com/professionals/14332_1210.asp. Accessed November 28, 2007.

Martens W, et al. Failure of a nursing infant to thrive after the mother's gastric bypass for morbid obesity. *Pediatrics.* 1990;86(5):777-778.

Masarei A, et al. The nature of feeding in infants with unrepaired cleft lip and/or palate compared with healthy non-cleft infants. *Cleft Palate Craniofac J.* 2007;44(3):321-328.

May-Benson T, et al. Incidence of pre-, peri-, and post-natal birth and developmental problems of children with sensory processing disorder and children with autism spectrum disorder. *Front Integr Neurosci.* 3:31; 2009. Epub Nov 11, 2009.

Michel S, Mueller D. Impact of lactation on women with cystic fibrosis and their infants: A review of five cases. *J Am Diet Assoc.* 1994;94:159-165.

Miller L, et al. Perspectives on sensory processing disorder: a call for translational research. *Front Integr Neurosci.* 2009;3:22.

Moe J, et al. Breastfeeding practices of infants with Rubinstein-Taybi syndrome. *J Hum Lact.* 1998;14(4):311–315.

Moffatt D, et al. A population-based study of breastfeeding in inflammatory bowel disease: Initiation, duration, and effect on disease in the postpartum period. *Am J Gastroenterol.* 2009;104(10):2517-2523.

Mok J, et al. European Paediatric Hepatitis C Virus Network. When does mother to child transmission of hepatitis C virus occur? *Arch Dis Child Fetal Neonatal Ed.* 2005;90(2): F156-F160.

Moore T. Diabetes mellitus and pregnancy. Medscape; May 21, 2009. http://emedicine.medscape.com/article/127547-overview. Accessed November 12, 2009.

Mulford C. Is breastfeeding really *invisible*, or did the health care system just choose not to notice it? *Intl Breastfeed J.* 2008;3:13.

Nacro B, et al. Prevention of mother to child transmission of HIV in Burkina Faso: Breastfeeding and wet nursing. *J Trop Pediatr.* October 7, 2009.

Nasser M, et al. Interventions for the management of submucous cleft palate. *Cochrane Database Syst Rev.* 2008; CD006703.

National Center for Biotechnology Information. Phenylketonuria; 2007. www.ncbi.nlm.nih.gov/bookshelf/br.fcgi? book=gnd&part=phenylketonuria. Accessed November 12, 2009.

National Institute of Neurological Disorders and Stroke. Sjögren's syndrome; May 14, 2008. www.ninds.nih.gov/disorders/sjogrens/sjogrens.htm. Accessed November 16, 2009.

Negro R, et al. Euthyroid women with autoimmune disease undergoing assisted reproduction technologies: The role of autoimmunity and thyroid function. *J Endocrinol Invest.* 2007;30(1):3-8.

Nestler JE. Metformin in the treatment of infertility in polycystic ovarian syndrome: An alternative perspective. *Fertil Steril.* 2008;90(1):14-16.

Newman J, Kernerman E. Vasospasm and Raynaud's phenomenon. Rev. 2009. www.nbci.ca/index.php?view=article& catid=5%3Ainformation&id=52%3Avasospasm-and-raynauds-phenomenon&format=pdf&option=com_content&Itemid=17. Accessed November 16, 2009.

Noor S, Musa S. Assessment of patients' level of satisfaction with cleft treatment using the Cleft Evaluation Profile. *Cleft Palate Craniofac J.* 2007;44(3):292-303.

O'Connor O. Getting the facts: Adult T-cell leukemia/lymphoma (HTLV-1). Lymphoma Research Foundation; 2008. http://www.lymphoma.org/atf/cf/%7B0363CDD6-51B5-427B-BE48-E6AF871ACEC9%7D/HTLV.PDF. Accessed March 18, 2010.

Ogunlesi T, et al. Non-puerperal induced lactation: An infant feeding option in paediatric HIV/AIDS in tropical Africa. *J Child Health Care.* 2008;12(3):241-248.

Ogunyemi D. Autoimmune thyroid disease and pregnancy. Medscape; June 3, 2009. http://emedicine.medscape.com/article/261913-overview. Accessed November 30, 2009.

Olasoji H. Pierre Robin syndrome: An update. *Niger Postgrad Med J.* 2007;14(2):140-145.

Oliver J, Silman A. What epidemiology has told us about risk factors and aetiopathogenesis in rheumatic diseases. *Arthritis Res Ther.* 2009;11(3):223.

Olsson C, et al. Difference in celiac disease risk between Swedish birth cohorts suggests an opportunity for primary prevention. *Pediatrics.* 2008;122(3):528-534.

Omarsdottir S, et al. Transmission of cytomegalovirus to extremely preterm infants through breast milk. *Acta Paediatr.* 2007;96(4):492-494.

Page S, McKenna D. Vasospasm of the nipple presenting as painful lactation. *Obstet Gynecol.* 2006;108(3 Pt 2):806-808.

Parents of Galactosemic Children, Inc. What is Duarte galactosemia? 2006. www.galactosemia.org/galactosemia.asp. Accessed November 28, 2009.

Pikwer M, et al. Breastfeeding, but not use of oral contraceptives, is associated with a reduced risk of rheumatoid arthritis. *Ann Rheum Dis.* 2009;68(4):526-530.

Pimenta F, et al. Prevalence ratio of HTLV-1 in nursing mothers from the state of Paraiba, Northeastern Brazil. *J Hum Lact.* 2008;24(3):289-292.

Pisacane A, et al. Breastfeeding and multiple sclerosis. *Br J Med.* 1994;308:1411-1412.

Pisacane A, et al. Down syndrome and breastfeeding. *Acta Paediatr.* 2003;92(12):1479-1481.

Poppe K, et al. Medscape. The role of thyroid autoimmunity in fertility and pregnancy. *Nat Clin Pract Endocrinol Metab.* 2008;4(7):394-405.

Poppe K, et al. Thyroid disease and female reproduction. *Clin Endocrinol.* 2007;66(3):309-321.

Poppe K, Velkeniers B. Female infertility and the thyroid. *Best Pract Res Clin Endocrinol Metab.* 2004;18(2):153-165.

Purnell H. Phenylketonuria and maternal phenylketonuria. *Breastfeed Rev.* 2001;9(2):19-21.

Quinn M. Diabetes, diet and autonomic denervation. *Med Hypotheses.* 2010;74(2):232-234.

Radosh L. Drug treatments for polycystic ovary syndrome. *Am Fam Physician.* 2009;79:671-676.

Rashid M, Rashid M. Obstetric management of thyroid disease. *Obstet Gynecol Surv* 2007;62(10):680-688.

Rasmussen K. Association of maternal obesity before conception with poor lactational performance. *Annu Rev Nutr.* 2007a;27:103-121.

Rasmussen K. Chapter 20: Maternal obesity and the outcome of breastfeeding. In: Hale T, Hartmann P. *Hale & Hartmann's Textbook of Human Lactation.* Amarillo, TX: Hale Publishing; 2007b: 387-402.

Rasmussen K, Kjolhede C. Prepregnant overweight and obesity diminish the prolactin response to suckling in the first week postpartum. *Pediatrics.* 2004;113:e465-e471.

Reid J, et al. Sucking performance of babies with cleft conditions. *Cleft Palate Craniofac.* 2007;44(3):312-320.

Reilly A, Snyder B. Raynaud phenomenon. Review. *Am J Nurs.* 2005;105(8):56-65.

Riva E, et al. Early breastfeeding is linked to higher intelligence quotient scores in dietary treated phenylketonuric children. *Acta Paediatr.* 1996;85:56-58.

Roth M. Could body image be a barrier to breastfeeding? A review of the literature. *Leaven.* 2006;42(1):4-7.

Sadauskaite-Kuehne V, et al. Longer breastfeeding is an independent protective factor against development of type 1 diabetes mellitus in childhood. *Diabetes Metab Res Rev.* 2004;20(2):150-157.

Sahai I, Marsden D. Newborn screening. *Crit Rev Clin Lab Sci.* 2009;46(2):55-82.

Schleiss MR. Acquisition of human cytomegalovirus infection in infants via breast milk: natural immunization or cause for concern? *Rev Med Virol.* 2006;16(2):73-82.

Sensory Processing Disorder (SPD) Foundation. About SPD; March 18, 2010. www.spdfoundation.net/aboutspd.html. Accessed March 18, 2010.

Sherman S, et al. Epidemiology of Down syndrome. *Ment Retard Dev Disabil Res Rev.* 2007;13(3):221-227.

Shiffman M, et al. Breastmilk composition in women with cystic fibrosis: Report of two cases and a review of the literature. *Am J Clin Nutr.* 1989;49:612-617.

Schilling P, et al. National trends in adolescent bariatric surgical procedures and implications for surgical centers of excellence. *J Am Coll Surg.* 2008;206(1):1-12.

Silva R, et al. Polycystic ovary syndrome, metabolic syndrome, cardiovascular risk and the role of insulin sensitizing agents. *Arq Bras Endocrinol Metabol.* 2006;50(2):281-290.

Sinaii N, et al. High rates of autoimmune and endocrine disorders, fibromyalgia, chronic fatigue syndrome and atopic diseases among women with endometriosis: a survey analysis. *Hum Reprod.* 2002;17:2715-2724.

Smith C, Arvin A. Varicella in the fetus and newborn. *Semin Fetal Neonatal Med.* 2009;14(4):209-217.

Soltani H, Arden M. Factors associated with breastfeeding up to 6 months postpartum in mothers with diabetes. *JOGNN.* 2009;38(5):586-594.

Stagnaro-Green A. Postpartum thyroiditis. *Best Pract Res Clin Endocrinol Metab.* 2004;18(2):303-316.

Stal S, Hicks M. Classic and occult submucous cleft palates: a histopathologic analysis. *Cleft Palate Craniofac J.* 1998; 35(4):351-358.

Stefanski J. Breast-feeding after bariatric surgery. *Today's Dietitian.* 2006;8(1):47.

Tarrats R, et al. Varicella, ephemeral breastfeeding and eczema as risk factors for multiple sclerosis in Mexicans. *Acta Neurol Scand.* 2002;105(2):88-89.

Thompson N, et al. Early determinants of inflammatory bowel disease: use of two national longitudinal birth cohorts. *Eur J Gastroenterol Hepatol.* 2000;12(1):25-30.

Tiittanen M, et al. Finnish TRIGR Study Group. Dietary insulin as an immunogen and tolerogen. *Pediatr Allergy Immunol.* 2006;17(7):538-543.

Tolarova M. Cleft lip and palate; March 23, 2009a. Medscape. http://emedicine.medscape.com/article/995535-overview. Accessed November 28, 2009.

Tolarova M. Pierre Robin malformation; March 25, 2009b. Medscape. http://emedicine.medscape.com/article/995706-overview. Accessed November 28, 2009.

Tooley K, et al. Maternal milk, but not formula, regulates the immune response to {beta}-lactoglobulin in allergy-prone rat pups. *J Nutr.* 2009;139(11):2145-2151.

Toschke A, et al. Overweight and obesity in 6- to 14-year-old Czech children in 1991: protective effect of breast-feeding. *J Pediatr.* 2002;141(6):764-769.

Trus T, et al. National trends in utilization and outcomes of bariatric surgery. *Surg Endosc.* 2005;19(5):616-620.

U.S. Dept. Health and Human Services (USDHHS), National Institute of Arthritis and Musculoskeletal and Skin Diseases (NIAMS). Raynaud's phenomenon; April 2009. www.niams.nih.gov/Health_Info/Raynauds_Phenomenon/default.asp#2. Accessed November 15, 2009.

U.S. Dept. Health and Human Services (USDHHS), Office on Women's Health. Autoimmune Disease; January 1, 2005. http://www.womenshealth.gov/FAQ/autoimmune-diseases.cfm#1. Accessed November 15, 2009.

U.S. Dept. Health and Human Services (USDHHS), National Institute of Diabetes and Digestive and Kidney Diseases. Weight loss surgery; September 8, 2009. www.nlm.nih.gov/medlineplus/weightlosssurgery.html. Accessed November 20, 2009.

U.S. Dept. Health and Human Services (USDHHS), National Institutes of Health. Metabolic syndrome; November 19, 2009. http://www.nlm.nih.gov/medlineplus/metabolic syndrome.html. Accessed November 23, 2009.

U.S. Dept. Health and Human Services, National Institute of Child Health and Human Development. Down syndrome; February 16, 2007. www.nichd.nih.gov/health/topics/down_syndrome.cfm. Accessed November 28, 2009.

U.S. National Library of Medicine. Genetics home reference. Galactosemia; November 20, 2009. http://ghr.nlm.nih.gov/condition=galactosemia. Accessed November 28, 2009.

UNAIDS. Global facts and figures, 2009. www.unaids.org. Accessed November 27, 2009.

Vahratian A. Prevalence of overweight and obesity among women of childbearing age: Results from the 2002 National Survey of Family Growth. *Matern Child Health J.* 2009; 13(2):268-273.

Van Rijn M, et al. A different approach to breast-feeding of the infant with phenylketonuria. *Eur J Pediatr.* 2003;162(5): 323-326.

van Spronsen F, et al. PKU-what is daily practice in various centres in Europe? Data from a questionnaire by the scientific advisory committee of the European Society of Phenylketonuria and Allied Disorders. *J Inherit Metab Dis.* 2009;32(1):58-64.

Vanky E, Carlsen S. Breastfeeding in polycystic ovary syndrome. *Acta Obstet Gynaecol Scand.* 2008;87(5):531-535.

Walker M. Breastfeeding with diabetes: yes you can! *J Hum Lact.* 2006;22(3):345-346.

Walker W. *Breastfeeding Management for the Clinician: Using the Evidence,* 2nd ed. Sudbury, MA: Jones and Bartlett; 2009.

Wardinsky T, et al. Vitamin B12 deficiency associated with low breast-milk vitamin B12 concentration in an infant following maternal gastric bypass surgery. *Arch Pediatr Adolesc Med.* 1995;149:1281-1284.

Washburn L, et al. The postnatal maternal environment influences diabetes development in nonobese diabetic mice. *J Autoimmun.* 2007;28(1):19-23.

Weiss-Salinas D, Williams N. Sensory defensiveness: a theory of its effect on breastfeeding. *J Hum Lact.* 2001;17(2):145-151.

Welch M, et al. Breast-feeding by a mother with cystic fibrosis. *Pediatrics.* 1981;67:664-666.

West D, Hirsch E. *Breastfeeding after Breast and Nipple Procedures: A Guide for Healthcare Professionals.* Amarillo, TX: Hale Publishing; 2008.

West D, Marasco L. *The Breastfeeding Mother's Guide to Making More Milk.* New York: McGraw-Hill; 2008.

Wilson-Clay B, Hoover K. *The Breastfeeding Atlas,* 4th ed. Austin, TX: Lactnews Press; 2008.

Wolf L, Glass R. *Feeding and Swallowing Disorders in Infancy.* San Antonio, TX: Therapy Skill Builders; 1992.

World Health Organization (WHO). Global strategy on diet, physical activity and health. Obesity and overweight; 2009a. www.who.int/dietphysicalactivity/publications/facts/obesity/en/ Accessed November 20, 2009.

World Health Organization (WHO). HIV and infant feeding: update based on the technical consultation held on behalf of the Inter-agency Team (IATT) on Prevention of HIV Infections in Pregnant Women, Mothers and their Infants, Geneva, 25-27 October 2006. WHO; 2007a. http://whqlibdoc.who.int/publications/2007/9789241595964_eng.pdf. Accessed November 27, 2009.

World Health Organization (WHO). Prevention and control of iodine deficiency in pregnant and lactating women and in children less than 2-years-old: conclusions and recommendations of the Technical Consultation. *Public Health Nutr.* 2007b;10(12A):1606-1611.

World Health Organization (WHO). WHO report 2009. Global tuberculosis control: Epidemiology, strategy, financing. WHO; 2009b. www.who.int/tb/publications/global_report/2009/key_points/en/. Accessed November 21, 2009.

World Health Organization (WHO). Women and health. Today's evidence. Tomorrow's agenda. WHO; 2009c. http://whqlibdoc.who.int/publications/2009/9789241563857_eng.pdf. Accessed November 27, 2009.

World Health Organization (WHO). Rapid advice: revised WHO principles and recommendations on infant feeding in the context of HIV; November, 2009d. http://www.who.int/child_adolescent_health/documents/hiv_if_principles_recommendations_112009.pdf. Accessed December 1, 2009.

World Health Organization (WHO) and United Nations Children's Fund. WHO/UNICEF meeting on infant and young child feeding. *J Nurse Midwifery.* 1980;25:31-39.

Yeung J, et al. Graves' disease. *Medscape*; June 4, 2009. http://emedicine.medscape.com/article/120619-overview. Accessed November 18, 2009.

Yi S, Singh R. Protein substitute for children and adults with phenylketonuria. *Cochrane Database Syst Rev.* 2008;4: CD004731.

Young K, et al. Perinatal and early childhood risk factors associated with rheumatoid factor positivity in a healthy paediatric population. *Ann Rheum Dis.* 2007;66:179-183.

Zargar A, et al. Familial puerperal alactogenesis: Possibility of a genetically transmitted isolated prolactin deficiency. *Br J Obstet Gynaecol.* 1997;104(5):629-631.

Zargar A, et al. Puerperal alactogenesis with normal prolactin dynamics: Is prolactin resistance the cause? *Fertil Steril.* 2000;74(3):598-600.

Zuppa A, et al. Relationship between maternal parity, basal prolactin levels and neonatal breast milk intake. *Biol Neonate.* 1988;53(3):144-147.

Role of the IBCLC

Professional Considerations

A lactation consultant is an integral member of the breast-feeding mother's healthcare team, a position accompanied by tremendous responsibilities. Your professional growth will take you through a progression of stages as you acquire the role of lactation consultant. The process is similar to the acquisition of the parental role described in Chapter 19. As you navigate through this journey, you learn to appreciate the importance of formal lactation education and extensive clinical experience. This chapter explores networking with colleagues and participating in your professional association, resources that form an essential part of your support system. Safeguards for providing appropriate care to mothers and babies are discussed in terms of professional certification and standards of practice. You will learn to recognize your limitations and when you need assistance. This awareness helps you maintain a positive perspective and enables you to give the best of yourself to mothers and infants.

⌁ *Key Terms*

Care plan	Internship
Certification	Job description
Client relationship	Legal considerations
Clinical experience	Liability
Code of ethics	Networking
Curriculum vitae	Pitfalls
Documentation	Professional burnout
Follow-up	Record retention
HIPAA	Referral system
Informed consent	Role acquisition
IBCLC	Standards of practice
IBLCE	Universal precautions
ILCA	

⌁ *Acquiring the Role of Lactation Consultant*

Moving into any new role is a dynamic process, whether it involves a new career or parenthood. Acquiring the parental role describes four stages of role acquisition—the anticipatory stage, the formal stage, the informal stage, and the personal stage (Bocar & Moore, 1987). This process from novice to expert, adapted to the context of entering the lactation profession (Barger, 2009), examines the stressful and exciting journey from initial learner to confident practitioner. In many cases a novice lactation consultant has previously achieved a level of expertise in a related healthcare role such as nurse, midwife, or physician. A novice lactation consultant who embarks on acquiring the role of a confident International Board Certified Lactation Consultant (IBCLC) progresses from feeling vulnerable to criticism in a new role to attaining a new status of expert (Cusson & Strange, 2008).

Anticipatory Stage

The anticipatory stage is the beginning of your journey toward acquiring a level of expert performance. Contact with a lactation consultant who helped you with your breastfeeding may have sparked an interest to help other women. You may be a health professional seeking to expand your role with women and children. Perhaps your interest emerged from the enjoyment you experienced breastfeeding your own children. Typical of the anticipatory stage, your perception of being a lactation consultant may be somewhat idealized. You may seek the "perfect" job in a clinic or hospital setting and envision making a substantial salary doing something you love.

It is customary at this beginning stage to gather information from a variety of sources, including other lactation consultants, your professional association, the certification board, providers of lactation education, and professional journals. You will soon recognize how much there is to learn and the scope of formal training you will need. This will direct you to enroll in a lactation management course and perhaps some required college courses to fill education gaps. You will also seek sources for supervised clinical instruction to acquire the necessary clinical practice skills. As an IBCLC intern you will begin to work with a mentor as you acquire the clinical experience necessary toward becoming certified. Your internship marks the beginning of the formal stage of your role acquisition.

Formal Stage

The formal stage starts when you begin to provide direct care to mothers and babies. You rely on formalized expectations to define your role in objective, written terms. These expectations are based on the seminal documents that guide the lactation profession, all of which are available on the Internet. This is an excellent time to join local breastfeeding coalitions and your professional association, the International Lactation Consultant Association, which maintains standards of practice for lactation consultants (ILCA, 1999). The International Board of Lactation Consultant Examiners (IBLCE, 2004) monitors a code of ethics for IBCLCs that governs the IBCLC's actions. Two documents developed jointly by ILCA and IBLCE—*Clinical Competencies for IBCLC Practice* (IBLCE, 2003) and the *Scope of Practice* for IBCLCs (IBLCE, 2008)—guide interns as they acquire the necessary skills and define the activities for which lactation consultants are educated and those in which they are authorized to engage. Your place of employment will further define your role and responsibilities through a written job description tailored to that particular institution.

These documents guide you through this formal stage of becoming a lactation consultant and help you assess your acquisition of skills. As you put what you have learned into practice, you begin to break down some of your preconceived ideas and teachings. Working with increasing numbers of mothers and babies shows you there are many ways to approach situations and you begin to identify conflicting advice among the "experts" on many aspects of breastfeeding care. At the same time, you might practice rigidly and formally according to your perceived "rules" as you try to do everything right. Wanting to do everything the "right" and "best" way, you begin to choose from more than one method to determine your own practices.

At this point in your development, you may feel uncertain and uncomfortable veering from a standard care plan to form decisions based on the needs of an individual mother and baby. For example, you may have learned that bottles contribute to a baby developing a preference for an artificial nipple or that a "good" lactation consultant does not use a nipple shield. Therefore you may be reluctant to use either of these and fail to recognize circumstances when they might be appropriate.

During the formal stage of acquisition, although you are eager to work independently, you probably welcome the security of a mentor to guide you. Reactions and comments from a mentor have a great impact on you, and you will appreciate that person's moral support and affirmation as you progress toward independence. You learn how to apply your knowledge to individualize your practices for each mother and baby. You soon believe you are performing the essential plans of care adequately and your comfort level in caring for new mothers increases. You gain confidence sharing your knowledge and skills with colleagues and may welcome others observing your interactions with mothers and babies. You no longer believe that you must have all the answers and gain confidence to move on to the next stage of role acquisition, the informal stage.

Informal Stage

The informal stage is punctuated with continued growth and increasing self-confidence as you work independently with mothers and babies. You begin to modify the rigid rules and directions you had sought out and followed during the formal stage. You are increasingly comfortable considering all the different approaches to care and weighing various options as you work through problem solving.

Networking with other lactation consultants helps you mature in your role, as you continue to learn the many ways to approach various aspects of breastfeeding care. Attending professional conferences increases your knowledge and varies your exposure to many different styles and ways of practicing as a professional lactation consultant. Your interactions with mothers and other lactation consultants become more spontaneous, with less fear of imperfection. If you are not already certified by this time, you are ready to sit for the certification exam and achieve the credential of IBCLC. You then enter the personal stage, your final stage in acquiring your role as a lactation consultant.

Personal Stage

Having reached the personal stage, you continue to evolve further in your role to develop a style that reflects your personality. You are better able to understand the motives and whims of new mothers and to adjust your teaching and guidance to complement their individual preferences. You recognize that mothers are responsible for their choices, and you learn not to feel guilty about undesirable outcomes. Consequently, you are more accepting of a mother who chooses a path that you regard as less than optimal.

Although you seek other opinions, you are quick to discard them if they are incompatible with your personal approach. You look critically at research and adapt it to your practice. You are comfortable in your role as a lactation consultant and enjoy opportunities to teach others through staff training and conference presentations. This is also the stage in which you might take the lead in helping to create coalitions and in advocating for breastfeeding. You promote the IBCLC credential and may be comfortable assuming leadership roles in your professional association and other advocacy organizations.

Facilitating Role Acquisition

Aspiring lactation consultants each progress through these stages at their own pace, guided by their comfort level at each point in the process. Other lactation consultants serve as valuable mentors during the formal stage, and you might model yourself after experienced colleagues you have observed. It is through exposure to a variety of lactation practitioners that you emerge with your own unique approach. The flexibility you adopt in your approach enables you to develop personalized plans of care for mothers and babies. In the personal stage you may serve as a model to other aspiring lactation consultants. After several years practicing as a lactation consultant and recertifying, you may consider mentoring novice lactation consultants as they join the profession.

Recognizing this dynamic process of role acquisition illustrates that there are few hard-and-fast rules about working with mothers and babies. You learn to adapt theory and book knowledge to each new situation. Practices continue to change as researchers and practitioners discover and understand more about breastfeeding and human lactation. Clinicians whose practices do not change substantially throughout their career have failed to remain current with new information that surfaces continually. Remaining open to new practices and seeking out new research-based information ensure that you continue to practice optimally in meeting the needs of mothers and babies.

~ Preparing for the Profession

There are several modes of entry into the lactation consulting profession. Some individuals are licensed healthcare providers who add lactation consulting to existing work in maternal and child health, including nursing, midwifery, dietetics, and physician practice. Some have advanced degrees in related fields such as education, psychology, human development, or another area that complements lactation consulting. Others have degrees in unrelated fields and change the direction of their careers after having experienced breastfeeding and wanting to help other women. Some enter from a background as a breastfeeding support counselor and may or may not have a college degree.

New practices and recommendations appear continually, sometimes making it difficult to remain current. You need to be aware of controversies regarding new practices and to consider them with respect to basic information and solid research. You are then able to decide carefully whether newer ideas are better than older ones. Anyone who wishes to work in a helping role with breastfeeding mothers has a professional responsibility to give optimal, evidence-based care. Remaining current is essential to your growth and development as a clinician.

Lactation Education

The knowledge and skill base in the lactation field is broad and extensive. In the early years of the profession, many entrants to the field gained their knowledge through self-directed learning. As the profession has evolved, formal education in lactation management is available in programs of varying length and scope.

Beginning in 2012, the requirements for pre-certification education increases from 45 hours to 90 hours for first-time candidates; it must be completed within 5 years immediately prior to exam application. In addition, candidates who are not recognized health professionals must also complete 8 semesters of postsecondary higher education and 6 continuing education topics (see Table 26.1).

A comprehensive lactation program addresses the disciplines reflected in the certification exam blueprint,

TABLE 26.1   2012 IBLCE Non-Lactation Education Requirements for First-Time Candidates

Equivalent of 1 semester of postsecondary higher education in:
- Biology
- Human anatomy
- Human physiology
- Infant and child growth and development
- Nutrition
- Psychology or counseling or communication skills
- Introduction to research
- Sociology or cultural sensitivity or cultural anthropology

Continuing education in:
- Basic life support (e.g., CPR)
- Medical documentation
- Medical terminology
- Occupational safety, including security, for health professionals
- Professional ethics for health professionals (e.g., Code of Ethics)
- Universal safety precautions and infection control

Source: International Board of Lactation Consultant Examiners. www.iblce.org. Printed with permission.

described in Table 26.2. In addition, exam candidates must have completed postsecondary courses in anatomy and physiology; sociology, psychology, or counseling; child development; and nutrition. Courses in adult learning and counseling techniques are especially important, because you use these skills frequently when educating and supporting mothers and when educating families and professionals. Furthermore, breastfeeding programs need to address attitudes as well as knowledge (Brodribb et al., 2008). A lactation consultant needs the competence to evaluate situations and apply knowledge, skills, and attitude in both routine and nonroutine lactation management.

The trend in lactation education in many parts of the world is toward postsecondary, multidisciplinary pro-

TABLE 26.2 IBLCE Blueprint Disciplines

Disciplines

A. Anatomy

B. Physiology and Endocrinology

C. Nutrition and Biochemistry

D. Immunology and Infectious Disease

E. Pathology

F. Pharmacology and Toxicology

G. Psychology, Sociology, and Anthropology

H. Growth Parameters and Developmental Milestones

I. Interpretation of Research

J. Ethical and Legal Issues

K. Breastfeeding Equipment and Technology

L. Techniques

M. Public Health

Chronological Periods

1. Preconception

2. Prenatal

3. Labor/birth (perinatal)

4. Prematurity

5. 0–2 days

6. 3–14 days

7. 15–28 days

8. 1–3 months

9. 4–6 months

10. 7–12 months

11. Beyond 12 months

12. General principles

Source: Printed with permission of the International Board of Lactation Consultant Examiners.

grams offered at colleges and universities that combine classroom instruction with clinical experience (Howett et al., 2006). Academic accreditation for lactation programs was launched in July, 2011 by the Accreditation and Approval Committee (AARC) on Education in Human Lactation and Breastfeeding (AARC, 2011). As increasing numbers of programs emerge, wide availability of formal postsecondary education will provide an avenue for young people to prepare for the lactation consultant profession through postsecondary study just as they would other professions. Achieving consistency and quality among lactation education programs can lead toward increased availability of accredited programs to prepare future members of the profession. With sufficient numbers of accredited postsecondary programs available for aspiring lactation consultants, the profession can work toward a goal of requiring graduation from an accredited program before certification. This raises the prominence of the IBCLC credential and the lactation consultant profession even further.

Clinical Competency

Clinical education is a significant component of the lactation consultant's formal preparation for the profession. Ideally, hands-on clinical experience is incorporated throughout the student's educational program, with broad-based exposure to the numerous sites where lactation consultants work. Acquisition of clinical skills requires guidance and coaching by an experienced professional who helps the student progress from novice to competent clinician. A structured program for supervised, clinical experience provides opportunities for the student to learn and practice skills in a variety of settings. This enables the novice clinician to progress toward expertise and an understanding of patient care.

Requirements for candidates of the certification exam include extensive clinical hours. You may be able to arrange with a hospital-based lactation consultant to mentor and supervise you in providing services for mothers while you gain experience. Some hospitals have lactation clinics located within their facilities that offer extended postpartum experiences. You might also volunteer or work in a physician's office; Women, Infants, and Children agency; or other clinic.

The *Clinical Competencies for IBCLC Practice* (2010) identifies specific experiences needed to prepare for the certification exam and to work as an IBCLC. The text, *Clinical Experience in Lactation: A Blueprint for Internship* (Kutner & Barger, 2010), gives clear guidelines for finding broad-based clinical experiences. It includes worksheets and study questions that cover the essential elements in each clinical experience. Both publications ensure balance in preparing for the profession. A well-rounded lactation consultant needs clinical experience in the various settings that serve breastfeeding mothers and babies, as well as clinical experience with various infant ages. This can be acquired in community support groups, health clinics, home visits, and maternity/infant care areas in the hospital such as the neonatal intensive care unit, labor and delivery, and postpartum mother–baby units.

Certification

IBLCE develops and administers the certification examination for lactation consultants. The IBLCE examination is internationally recognized as a measure of competence in lactation consulting, administered in multiple languages and at numerous sites around the world. Since 1988 the IBLCE certification program has been continuously accredited by the National Commission for Certifying Agencies. Candidates who pass the exam are awarded the designation International Board Certified Lactation Consultant, or IBCLC.

Many professionals who work in the maternal and infant health fields incorporate their knowledge of breastfeeding into an existing practice. A pediatric nurse practitioner, physician, midwife, dietitian, or nurse may wish to become more skilled in helping breastfeeding mothers and babies. Some may decide to specialize in the care of breastfeeding mothers and infants through certification as an IBCLC.

A comprehensive course in lactation management is essential to anyone who plans to specialize in lactation. However, completion of a course alone does not provide the safeguards and standards garnered through professional certification. Although some lactation courses bestow the title "certified" to their graduates, this designation alone does not meet the standard of criterion-referenced testing and periodic recertification required by the IBCLC credential.

～ Professional Practice

Lactation consultants work in concert with primary practitioners who care for the infant and mother. You provide a level of care that facilitates continued health and wellness, particularly as it relates to breastfeeding and early parenting. As a board certified lactation consultant, you focus on helping breastfeeding women and their families achieve their breastfeeding goals.

Scope of Practice

In 2008 ILCA and IBLCE collaborated to clarify the role of the lactation consultant in a new *Scope of Practice* for IBCLCs (IBLCE, 2008), presented in Appendix B. The aim of a scope of practice is to protect the public by ensuring safe, competent, and evidence-based care. *The Scope of Practice* affirms that lactation consultants have specialized knowledge and clinical expertise in breastfeeding and human lactation and describes the activities in which lactation consultants are authorized to engage.

Lactation consultants have the duty to uphold the standards of the profession; to protect, promote, and support breastfeeding; to provide competent services for mothers and families; to report truthfully and fully to the mother's and/or infant's primary healthcare provider and to the healthcare system; to preserve client confidence; and to act with reasonable diligence.

Standards of Practice

Lactation consultants are charged with providing quality care to the public and accepting responsibility for that care. Quality and service constitute the core of a profession's responsibility to the public. Supporting that belief, ILCA developed the *Standards of Practice for Lactation Consultants* (ILCA, 1999), presented in Appendix C. Standards of practice identify "stated measures or levels of quality" that serve as models for the conduct and evaluation of practice (Association of Women's Health, Obstetric and Neonatal Nursing, 2009). You can uphold the standards of the profession by working within your scope of practice. Demonstrating clinical competence, accountability, ethical practice, and legal responsibility are core to maintaining professional standards. You can achieve this by:

- Respecting the privacy of the mother–child relationship
- Obtaining clients' written consent before providing care
- Communicating relevant information to the primary caregiver (or caregivers)
- Collaborating with and referring to other healthcare professionals as appropriate
- Learning national and international issues and trends in maternal/newborn care and women's health
- Maintaining the IBCLC credential
- Participating in self-evaluation, peer review, continuing education, and other activities to ensure quality practice
- Critically evaluating and incorporating research findings to provide evidenced-based practice
- Recognizing limitations in your knowledge or skills
- Exercising principles of optimal health, safety, and universal precautions
- Maintaining an awareness of conflict of interest in all aspects of work

- Participating in appropriate professional organizations
- Lending support to colleagues

∼ *Code of Ethics*

Members of the health profession are guided by a set of principles that outlines the commitments and obligations to self, client, colleagues, society, and the profession. These principles set forth a code of ethics that protects the health, safety, and welfare of the public by establishing and enforcing qualifications of certification and for issuing voluntary credentials to individuals who have attained those qualifications. The *Code of Ethics* for IBCLCs (IBLCE, 2004) governed and monitored by IBLCE applies to all individuals who hold the credential of IBCLC.

The *Code of Ethics* holds IBCLCs accountable for their practice and requires that they "act in a manner that safeguards the interests of individual clients, justifies public trust in her/his competence, and enhances the reputation of the profession" (IBLCE, 2004, p. 1). The full *Code of Ethics* is presented in Appendix A. Among the tenets are mandates for:

- Objectivity and respect for unique needs and values of individuals
- Nondiscrimination on the basis of race, creed, religion, gender, sexual orientation, age, and national origin
- Fulfilling commitments in good faith and free of conflict interest or personal bias, with honesty, integrity, fairness, and confidentiality
- Competent practice based on current, evidence-based information that is presented truthfully and enables clients to make informed decisions
- Responsible and professional judgment, recognizing the need to seek counsel and make appropriate referrals
- Complying with requirements for continued certification
- Reporting circumstances that violate the *Code of Ethics* or may compromise standards of practice and care of colleagues
- Refusing favors from clients that may be interpreted as seeking preferential consideration
- Submit to disciplinary action and withdraw voluntarily from professional practice if personal circumstances affect practice in a manner that could harm the client
- Comply with the *International Code of Marketing of Breastmilk Substitutes* and subsequent resolutions that pertain to health workers
- Understand, recognize, respect, and acknowledge intellectual property rights

Ethical Practice

Ethical practice intends that a lactation consultant not undermine the primary caregiver's position. It is best to try to work within the parameters of the caregiver's advice as much as possible. At the same time a moral and ethical dilemma can occur when a lactation consultant recognizes the need for a particular action and is not permitted to follow through because of caregiver or employer policies or other restrictions. When a disagreement occurs, it is important to discuss the discrepancy with the caregiver and explain the reason for your position. If a mother asks you for a referral to another physician, lactation consultant, or other caregiver, make it a practice to suggest at least three names to avoid appearing to recommend one over another.

If you work in private practice, inform the client of your fees before you initiate an assessment. You may wish to post fees in your office. If you work in private practice, when asked over the telephone what the fees will be, you can respond, "As a lactation consultant in private practice, my fees are similar to those of a medical office visit. An office or home visit is $__ and generally lasts about __ hours. You may pay by cash, credit card, or check at the end of the consultation." If you make breastfeeding equipment available as a service to mothers, you are expected to charge the standard fees for each item. Inform mothers of all fees at the beginning of the consultation to avoid misunderstandings later. Some lactation consultants post fees on their websites.

Make sure that rental equipment such as breast pumps are scrupulously cleaned and in good working condition. Pumps in rental stations should be returned to the manufacturer for servicing within 2 years. Check with the manufacturers of the pumps you are interested in carrying to find out their current requirements for a rental station. If you rent digital scales, you should invest in a calibration weight and check them before and after each rental for accuracy.

Ethical practice requires a clear understanding of biomedical ethics as well as the professional *Code of Ethics* for lactation consultants. To promote an understanding of professional ethics, IBLCE requires a minimum of 5 continuing education hours in ethics every 5 years to maintain certification. Also see Chapter 3 for a general discussion of ethics.

Examples of Ethical Situations

A variety of situations can occur that cause a lactation consultant to consider possible ethical implications of their actions. Having a framework for decision making helps you analyze and resolve such ethical dilemmas (Noel-Weiss & Walters, 2006). Much dialogue regarding ethics in lactation consultancy revolves around compliance with the *International Code of Marketing of Breastmilk Substitutes*. Other common themes are the use of alternative therapies, scope of practice, and legal aspects of practice. A few ethical dilemmas are presented here as examples (Barger, 2009). Questions appear at the end of each scenario to identify relevant issues and serve as a catalyst for considering how to respond in similar circumstances.

Ethical Situation One

A pediatrician refers Heather and her daughter Samantha to you. Samantha is 6 weeks old and is 5 ounces beyond birth weight. As you take a history and assess breastfeeding, Heather tells you that she feeds Samantha on a 3-hour schedule during the day. Samantha sleeps about 8 hours at night and breastfeeds about 6 times in a 24-hour period. You suggest that Heather feed Samantha more often and wake her at night to increase her weight and Heather's milk production. You talk with her about watching for hunger cues and trying to increase the number of feedings each day.

Heather indicates that it is important for Samantha to stay on their schedule based on what she learned in a parenting class at her church. The program discourages cue-based feedings and teaches that babies should sleep through the night by 6 to 8 weeks of age. In addition, she learned that to increase the numbers of feedings would cause Samantha's metabolism to "go into chaos." You probe a bit further and learn that for the first 4 or 5 weeks Samantha would cry for up to 40 minutes at a time. Because Heather had learned from the program that babies will not eat well if mothers feed them more frequently than every 3 hours, she left Samantha in her crib to "cry it out." She tells you, "It is important for babies to learn that the parents are in control."

You share your concerns about Samantha's weight and suggest that Heather use a supplemental feeding device at the breast. You also recommend that she express her milk between feedings to increase her milk production. Although Heather rejects both suggestions, she agrees to supplement Samantha after each feeding until her weight improves.

Consider the following issues:

- How much do you "push" to salvage breastfeeding for this mother and baby?
- What will you say to her about her parenting methods?
- What follow-up will you provide?
- What information will you provide to her physician?

Ethical Situation Two

You have started lecturing about breastfeeding in several areas of your state. A hospital in a city about 4 hours from you has invited you to present a 1-day conference. During the process of planning your presentation you learn that a major manufacturer of infant formula is one of the conference sponsors. Your code of ethics does not specifically forbid you from taking money from the formula industry. However, you feel uncomfortable agreeing to speak at the conference. As you discuss it with one of your colleagues, she tells you, "You ought to go ahead with it. It would be better that you give the presentation rather than a formula representative. At least that way you will know the attendees receive appropriate information."

Consider the following issues:

- If you speak at the conference, what underlying message does it send?
- Do the ends justify the means? You know you would give good information, but at what cost to your personal ethics?
- How can you participate in the conference without taking formula money and without forgoing compensation?

Ethical Situation Three

You are a newly certified lactation consultant working in your community hospital. On several occasions mothers have told you that their pediatrician gave them very outdated breastfeeding information. You have witnessed this same prominent physician speak sarcastically with staff who do not agree with him. Most pediatricians in your community are supportive of breastfeeding and have been receptive to learning more about appropriate breastfeeding care. You are working with a mother who has this pediatrician for her baby. How can you help her within the context of her relationship with her pediatrician?

Consider the following issues:

- Will you speak with the pediatrician and if so, what approach will you take?
- How will you correct the misinformation mothers receive?
- If the pediatrician continues to give misinformation, what actions can you take without jeopardizing your new job?

∼ Legal Considerations

Lactation consultants must practice within the laws of the geopolitical region in which they live and must respect the mother's and baby's rights to privacy and issues that are confidential in nature. To protect yourself legally, it is imperative that you obtain liability insurance before practicing as a lactation consultant if such insurance is required in your geopolitical region. If you work for a hospital or government agency and perform only those duties within that scope of practice, your employer's liability insurance should provide sufficient coverage. Privately employed lactation consultants need to secure some form of professional liability insurance. See Appendix H, Online Resources, for source information.

HIPAA Regulations

In 1996 the United States passed the Health Insurance Portability and Accountability Act (HIPAA) to provide federal protections for the privacy of patients' protected health information. The act prohibits the use or disclosure of protected health information unless authorized by the patient. HIPAA also ensures privacy and confidentiality of research participants unless they authorize the use or disclosure of their information. Furthermore, it prohibits any reuse or disclosure of the information unless required by law.

The act allows certain incidental uses and disclosures that occur as a byproduct. You can guard against violating a client's privacy through incidental disclosure by speaking quietly and avoiding use of client names when in public areas. If you e-mail or fax client reports, a confidentiality notice such as the one in Figure 26.1 ensures that your transmittal complies with HIPAA regulations. You can further protect privacy by isolating or locking file cabinets that contain client records, using a password on your computer, and destroying research identifiers at the earliest opportunity. Although suspected child neglect or

abuse does not fall within HIPAA privacy restrictions, you still have authorization and a legal duty to report such instances to appropriate public health authorities.

If practicing privately you should have a HIPAA Notice of Privacy Practices posted in your office or on your website. Also provide a copy to your clients when you make home visits. Clients should sign a form acknowledging receipt of the HIPAA information. The *Core Curriculum for Lactation Consultant Practice* (ILCA, 2007) contains detailed information for meeting HIPAA requirements, along with sample forms. See Appendix H for sources of additional software and forms.

Client Relationships

Accepting a client creates certain expectations and duties that are contractual in nature. Those duties exist regardless of whether clients pay for your services. Once that relationship is established, you have a duty to render the appropriate level of care unless the client authorizes your withdrawal. You have a duty to refer the client to another caregiver and not to abandon the client if you are unable to render appropriate care.

Establishing a Relationship

A relationship is established whenever you and the mother have contact, whether in person or over the telephone. In some cases you create a client relationship simply by the act of making an appointment. When a mother arrives by previous appointment, you are obligated to give her care or to make alternate arrangements by referring her to another competent practitioner. If you discover a problem that is beyond your competency during an assessment, you must inform the mother of your concerns. Make sure she understands she will need follow-up care, and refer her to a competent practitioner when the problem is beyond your level of competency.

Telephone Contacts

Telephone conversations can create a client relationship if you indicate acceptance or give comments in the nature of treatment. The content of the conversation determines whether it constitutes a relationship. You can avoid creating this relationship through several measures. First, when receiving a call identify yourself and obtain the name of the person who is calling. You may listen to the caller's complaints and, if the mother makes an appointment, clarify that the appointment is to evaluate whether you can accept her as a new client. If the mother makes no appointment, you can inform her of her options, such as going to the emergency room or contacting an appropriate caregiver or another lactation consultant without creating a relationship. Bear in mind that as soon as you give

---

The attached pages are my report of a recent lactation consultation. If you received this transmission in error, please respect the privacy of the people involved. Contact [your name, phone or fax number, or email address] to tell me I have sent it to the wrong recipient. Destroy the report you received by mistake.

This report contains information that falls under the privacy sections of the Health Insurance Portability and Accountability Act of 1996. When you read it, you will see personal information and details about a mother and her baby. I have obtained consent from the mother involved to transmit this report to her healthcare providers, as required by the International Board of Lactation Consultant Examiners Code of Ethics and the International Lactation Consultant Association Standards of Practice.

FIGURE 26.1   Confidentiality notice to include with fax or e-mail communication.

Source: Printed with permission of Elizabeth C. Brooks, JD, IBCLC.

comments in the nature of advice you have created a relationship with the client.

Where No Relationship Exists

Some interactions do not create a client relationship. If a physician requests that you see a patient or review the patient's record, this does not constitute a relationship. However, if the physician relies on you for lactation advice and you are aware of this, a relationship between you the patient is implied, and you want to see the patient as soon as possible. If you work in a hospital, generally no relationship exists between you and mothers after discharge. However, this rule does not apply if the mother contacts you through a hospital telephone contact.

Duration of a Relationship

Whenever you have an established relationship with a client, you are legally required to continue care until the need for your services no longer exists, until the mother withdraws from your care, or until you withdraw in a manner that does not constitute "abandonment" of the mother. If you choose to withdraw from the relationship, you must give the mother appropriate notice of your intentions, either by talking with her or by sending a written notice. In the letter you should state the mother's status, any need for follow-up care, and your intention to withdraw by a definite stated date that allows the mother time to seek alternative care. You must indicate that until the stated date you are available for emergencies. In addition, you must state that the mother's physician can obtain a copy of all records with written permission of the mother. Be aware that a client's failure to pay does not justify your withdrawal without giving her sufficient opportunity to obtain alternative care. After notifying the mother of your intent, you must refer her to a competent replacement or to a specialist if her problem is outside a lactation consultant's competence.

You can avoid the potential of abandonment by performing services when needed. When a physician asks you to evaluate a patient, you can tell the patient verbally, "I have been contacted by Dr. _____ to evaluate you and your baby." Also, write this in the patient's chart. When you terminate the relationship, tell the patient and write in the chart, "I am signing off this case and will no longer follow this patient. However, I will remain available if I am notified that additional consultations or assistance are required."

Substituting your services with those of another lactation consultant does not constitute abandonment. To avoid problems you can notify the replacement of case details, both verbally and in writing, after securing permission from the mother. If a client fails to keep a follow-up appointment or to follow your advice, there are safeguards to ensure that the client understands the nature of the condition and the risks of failing to seek medical attention. Provide her with an opportunity to visit you for counseling or care. Although you share all this verbally with the client, you also need to follow it up in writing.

Informed Consent

It is important that you obtain informed consent before providing care to mothers. Although informed consent may not be a legal requirement in some places of residence, you are wise to discuss specific topics with mothers so they are fully informed. You want to discuss the nature of the mother's problem, the proposed treatment, and reasonable alternative treatments. Inform the mother of the chance of success with the proposed treatment as well as any inherent risks. Make sure she understands the consequences of failing to undergo treatment. You can explore alternative treatments and risks with colleagues to learn what they explain to their clients. Consult current medical literature as well to document frequency and severity of risks so you can include this in your consent form.

Standard consent forms ordinarily do not provide sufficient information about disclosures made to the patient or client to establish that consent was adequately informed. Lactation consultants in a busy practice can ensure adequate legal protection by preparing an information sheet for the courses of treatment. Both you and the mother should sign the form, attesting to the fact that the mother acknowledges receipt of the information. Retain one copy for your files and give another copy to the mother. Generally, competent adults are capable of giving valid consent for infants. Therefore the mother's signed consent covers both her care and that of her infant. In addition to consent forms for treatment, you may want to include permission for photographs to use for educational purposes. You can also attach photographs to the mother's chart; for example to document the status of her breasts and nipples before and after treatment.

Record Retention

Client records provide a history of the mother's and infant's health that are helpful to other care providers. Your geopolitical region defines how long you must retain records. Records help comply with statutes and other regulations in your geopolitical region, obtain third-party payment by substantiating fees, and defend against professional negligence suits. In addition, patient records (with identifiers removed) are a great source of research projects and are useful when preparing teaching presentations.

If you work in a physician's office, the state's medical practice act or licensing statutes may dictate the type of information to be included in a patient's record. In the

United States these typically include a written record of patient history, examination results, and test results. To remain accredited, a hospital's records must contain identification data, patient medical history, reports of relevant physical examinations, diagnostic and therapeutic orders, evidence of appropriate informed consent, clinical observations, reports of procedures and tests, and conclusions at the termination of hospitalization or evaluation of treatment. You should keep a record of telephone calls, written correspondence, and appointment calendars. These demonstrate that you followed up on a mother's care or responded to a complaint in a timely fashion. They also demonstrate dates of appointments or the mother's failure to keep an appointment.

Avoiding Liability

Becoming familiar with your local laws regulating the practice of medicine will help you avoid placing yourself at risk for liability. Familiarize yourself with protocols in your practice setting and always perform within your scope of practice. The *Core Curriculum for Lactation Consultant Practice* (ILCA, 2007) contains important reading on the topic of liability. Ensure that you are protected continuously by professional liability insurance and that you build positive relationships with patients and respect their autonomy to safeguard against lawsuits. Avoid guaranteeing results or creating unrealistic expectations, and empower parents to make informed decisions rather than relying on you to direct their actions.

Recognize when a case may be beyond your level of competence or when you may not have time to handle it. Document everything you do as well as what you choose not to do and why. Avoid making negative notations in a mother's record that could be seen later, keeping in mind that a mother can request to see her records at any time. Organize your workspace and keep necessary paperwork accessible to make it convenient for documenting what you do. Keep a copy of everything you document. If you are in private practice, you may want to consider incorporating your practice to limit your personal liability. Consulting a business attorney before you open your practice is a worthwhile investment.

〜 Developing Resources

You are not alone in your efforts to promote, protect, and support breastfeeding. The field of lactation consulting has grown tremendously since the creation of ILCA and IBLCE in 1985. By 2010 there were over 19,000 lactation consultants certified as IBCLCs worldwide. Opportunities abound for networking with others for advice on a particular issue. It is important to make sure you know experienced lactation consultants with whom you can

network. With the growth of the lactation consulting profession, there are increasing numbers of knowledgeable and skilled professionals to serve as a mentor until you feel competent and confident in your abilities. Even after becoming a qualified IBCLC, you will continue to benefit from mentoring and networking with other experienced clinicians.

Continuing Education

Becoming a member of ILCA brings you in contact with thousands of lactation professionals worldwide and provides access to a wealth of resources. Membership includes subscriptions to the *Journal of Human Lactation* and the association's online newsletter. These periodicals share new research and practical tips, case studies, and innovative approaches. Appendix H lists other professional newsletters and journals.

Professional conferences provide valuable networking opportunities for lactation professionals and other breastfeeding advocates, and ILCA members receive a discount on registration to the annual ILCA conference. ILCA national affiliates and chapters offer a variety of continuing education opportunities, and ILCA offers online study modules on numerous topics. Online networking opportunities are available through ILCA discussion boards. *Lactnet*, a professional listserv, shares breastfeeding information and the opportunity to ask questions of a large number of colleagues at one time.

Professional Referral Sources

Throughout your career in the lactation profession, you may encounter an unusual breastfeeding situation, a medical question, or another circumstance that you cannot address adequately with your existing information. Establishing professional resources helps you deliver complete and correct information in your services and support to aid women in breastfeeding. Developing contacts with people in areas that enhance your consulting enables you to establish an advisory relationship so that you may call on them when questions arise. Hospitals, physicians, dietitians, pharmacies, medical libraries, service organizations, and colleges are all valuable resources.

Cultivating contacts in related fields will help you provide mothers in your care access to the information and services they need. Keep a list of referral resources such as physical therapists, occupational therapists, speech and language therapists, clinicians who will clip a frenulum, craniosacral therapists, acupuncturists, chiropractors, herbalists, and other specialists. In addition to establishing personal resources, you can develop a reference library with current breastfeeding texts and periodicals. You might also keep a lending library or an updated list of books and other materials that may be of interest to parents.

~ *Promoting Your Services*

Learning how many lactation consultants already work in local hospitals, physicians' offices, and clinics helps you determine the market for employment in your community. If you plan to begin a private practice, determine how many other private practice lactation consultants are located within comfortable driving distance for parents in your community. After you have settled on the best potential settings for employment, decide which services you can offer to fill the needs of your target market. Establishing baseline data on breastfeeding statistics helps you demonstrate a need for your services. Record the number of mothers who initiate breastfeeding and the length of time they continue. Identify current policies, practices, and attitudes. Determine breastfeeding resources that are currently available for parents and caregivers and develop a plan to fill the gap.

Referrals

Maintaining a referral system is integral to the quality of your assistance to breastfeeding women. Women who receive breastfeeding education and support prenatally are more likely to achieve their goals. Therefore if you work in a hospital setting, you can ensure that mothers who give birth in your hospital receive this exposure before they deliver. Because lactation consultants in private practice depend on referrals for their entire practice, it is especially important that parents and others in the community know how to access those services. This includes hospitals, birthing centers, physicians, midwives, childbirth educators, breastfeeding support groups, community groups, pharmacies, providers of breastfeeding accessories, and others who encounter expectant or new mothers. Check out websites that provide lists of local lactation consultants for parents and ask that you be included. Chapter 2 presents referral suggestions specific to individual practice settings.

Community Awareness

You need your community to be aware of your services irrespective of your work setting. You can obtain free community exposure in a variety of ways. Consider providing outreach programs to educate the public about breastfeeding. Presenting breastfeeding information to high school classes as part of their health curriculum enables you to reach adolescents (see Chapter 28). Newspapers often print articles about members of the community who have recently achieved special honors.

Participating in health fairs, trade shows, and charities further advertises your services. World Breastfeeding Week and IBCLC Day are ideal times to sponsor a breastfeeding program in your community and highlight the services available from a lactation consultant. A local radio or television station may be willing to conduct an interview as well.

Offering to speak in the community helps you develop a reputation as an authority on breastfeeding. Educating childbirth instructors and other health professionals in your area opens doors for later referrals and relationships. Consider offering professional discounts or in-kind services to groups such as your local breastfeeding coalition, ILCA affiliate, or support group. Something as simple as bringing refreshments or breastfeeding literature when you visit other healthcare professionals may make an impression that brings you to their mind later.

You can develop an attractive logo for your private practice that identifies you easily to prospective clients and referral sources. Use the logo on your e-mail, brochures, business cards, letterhead, postcards, and other materials that promote your services. Consider developing a website advertising your services. Website design ranges from free, simple, do-it-yourself sites to customized, detailed sites that offer clients the ability to shop and pay online. If you sell breast pumps and other accessories, a Web presence is especially effective for reaching most of today's mothers, who are accustomed to using the Internet for purchases. Custom Web design can be very expensive, so you may benefit from comparing costs and features for your needs. You should ask the Web designer for the cost of ongoing maintenance, as well as the initial design. Many lactation consultants have embraced social networking with a presence on networks such as Facebook, MySpace, LinkedIn, and Twitter.

You can produce promotional items such as pens, note pads, magnets, and buttons that advertise your services. A consistent, professional look to all printed material speaks well for you. A professional appearance and demeanor also have a great impact on the impressions you make. If you have been wearing scrubs or a uniform in a hospital or clinic environment and are beginning private practice or speaking publicly, invest in a small professional wardrobe. Many lactation consultants speak at conferences and have found professional clothing that does not wrinkle and is travel friendly a worthwhile investment.

Résumé or Curriculum Vitae

A well-written résumé or curriculum vitae (referred to as a CV) helps you make a professional impression to a potential employer. Employment agencies and computer software programs can help you develop this document. You can begin by taking a personal inventory of your background, work experience, and strengths. There are distinct differences between a résumé and a CV. Your choice depends on what you have learned about the facility and which format you feel will pique their interest. The purpose of both documents is to highlight your talents. Include a cover letter that states the kind of position you are seeking and why you are applying to the particular facility. Follow up with a telephone call a short time later to request an interview. Many large organizations require that candidates apply for the position online and upload their résumés.

Résumé

A résumé is a brief, one- to two-page, promotional piece that identifies a specific job or interest. Personal data to include are name, address, telephone number, fax number, and e-mail address. Begin with a brief statement of your objective or career goal and any skills and abilities that may be useful in the position you are seeking. This may include such things as the number of years you have worked as a lactation consultant, knowledge of foreign languages, public speaking abilities, artistic talents, and computer capabilities. Follow this with a history of your education, employment, formal education, and other professional training. List dates of graduation, degrees or certificates received, major and minor subjects, and any scholarships or honors. You can organize your work history either by job or by function.

Work History by Job   List each job separately, even if you held more than one position at the same facility. List dates of employment, name and address of the employer, nature of the business, the position that you held, specific job duties, any special assignments or use of special equipment, your scope of responsibility (e.g., how many people you supervised, the degree of supervision you received), and noteworthy accomplishments (backed by concrete facts and figures).

Work History by Function   List functions, fields of specialization, and types of work you performed related to your present employment objectives. Describe briefly the work you have done in each of these fields, without breaking it down by jobs. You could also list volunteer activities related to your present objectives, such as breastfeeding counseling.

References   It is imperative that you represent your experience and skills honestly. Four or five references are usually appropriate, from among former employers or mentors who have worked with you in clinical or internship settings and have seen your skills and mother–baby interaction firsthand. Many people, to keep the résumé short, state "References provided upon request" and take

the reference sheet with them to give to the prospective employer at the face-to-face interview.

Curriculum Vitae

A CV is an extensive, scholarly piece that reflects all your professional activity. It begins with your name, address, telephone number, fax number, and e-mail address. List your educational background, professional practice, academic appointments, memberships to professional associations, and any publications or articles you have written. Indicate outside professional interests and related community and consultant activities as well as professional presentations and licensure. If your CV has several pages, you can prepare a one-page abbreviated version with a note at the bottom indicating that the complete CV is available on request. Conference planners often request a CV from potential speakers.

Job Description or Proposal

Approaching a potential employer with a formal job proposal strengthens your potential for employment. A prospective employer may be receptive if you request a position on a trial basis for a period of 6 months, perhaps working as a freelance, independent contractor. During that time you can train staff, establish breastfeeding protocols, and collect data to justify the continuation of your position. Below is a list of possible elements to include in a job description or a proposal for a position as a lactation consultant. Items are categorized in terms of the type of activity and expertise required. Because not all items apply to a particular position, determine the facility's specific needs to personalize your proposal based on their needs. Try to identify the appropriate person to receive the proposal, which is often the person in charge of maternity services.

Cover Letter or Introductory Remarks

You can begin the proposal with rationale for establishing a lactation consultant position. Give a brief description of your role on the mother's and infant's healthcare team, and describe how you see yourself functioning in the facility. Describe the benefits of having a lactation consultant on staff, including the cost-to-benefit aspect of your services for the facility.

Objectives

Demonstrate that the establishment of a lactation consultant position enhances the facility's reputation in the community as a provider of health care to mothers and babies. Point out that the increased number of mothers who choose to deliver there because of the facility's reputation will fund your position. Cite that with a lactation consultant on staff the facility will:

- Provide a positive breastfeeding experience for both the mother and baby
- Promote bonding between the mother and her baby
- Promote healthier babies and mothers
- Provide consistent breastfeeding teaching and support
- Increase the incidence of mothers choosing to breastfeed
- Increase the incidence of mothers continuing to breastfeed at 6 months
- Decrease the incidence of unresolved breastfeeding problems
- Reduce the incidence of readmission to the hospital or ill-child visits

Teaching Services

Indicate the educational programs you can provide to both parents and staff:

- Teach prenatal infant feeding classes
- Teach in-hospital breastfeeding classes
- Teach postpartum classes
- Provide inservice education for staff
- Assist with orientation of staff
- Maintain a resource center for patient and staff materials
- Conduct bedside teaching of staff through a mentorship or preceptor program

Services to Mothers and Infants

Identify the services you can offer to mothers:

- Individual consultation during the hospital stay, which may include:
  - Conducting daily rounds with breastfeeding mothers
  - Giving anticipatory guidance to mothers
  - Performing a breastfeeding assessment
  - Revisiting mothers who are experiencing problems
  - Developing a plan of care with the mother
  - Providing problem-solving advice and support
  - Documenting teaching and progress on patient charts
- Coordinate or provide home follow-up through telephone calls, written correspondence, or personal visits
- Provide a 24-hour hotline where mothers can call and have their questions answered immediately, or a 24-hour warm line where mothers leave a message on an answering machine or voice mail and the call is returned later

- Refer mothers to a support group and other community resources
- Coordinate counseling and support of mothers who wish to provide their milk for a high-risk infant
- Coordinate dispensing of breastfeeding devices
- Provide an outpatient lactation clinic for weighing infants and discussing problems

Working with Staff

Indicate the manner in which you will work with staff:

- Initiate case conferences and confer with staff on patient needs
- Serve as a resource for staff, physicians, and support group counselors
- Consult with the mother's and baby's primary care providers
- Discuss appropriate referrals with primary care providers
- Provide on-call service for consultations with staff
- Participate as a team member with staff and physicians to provide comprehensive care
- Coordinate or participate in a breastfeeding committee

Writing, Reviewing, and Revising Printed Materials

A lactation consultant needs the writing and editing skills necessary for developing and revising printed materials and protocols. Indicate the materials you can provide:

- Standards of care that support breastfeeding
- Breastfeeding policies
- Breastfeeding care plans
- A charting system for documentation, teaching, and progress notes
- Patient literature
- Monthly breastfeeding newsletter for staff
- Statistics to assess the effectiveness of your services

Professional Requirements

Learn the preferences in the facility regarding credentials and experience required for a lactation consultant to practice there. Some facilities may require a degree in another area of health care (e.g., nursing). Be sure to include any education and experience that complements the position you are seeking. This serves the purpose of a conventional résumé by identifying skills and abilities that make you attractive for the position you are seeking. Stress the importance of hiring a board-certified lactation consultant as opposed to someone without the IBCLC credential. Your list may include:

- IBCLC-certified through the IBLCE
- Member of ILCA
- Graduate from a lactation management course (name the course)
- Graduate from a school of nursing or other facility (name the school)
- Current licensure in the state in a related field
- College degree(s)
- Skills, knowledge, and attitude to promote breastfeeding
- Communication skills for interactions with patients, families, and colleagues
- Knowledge of cultural, psychological, psychosocial, nutritional, and pharmacological aspects of breastfeeding
- Understanding of current breastfeeding practices and research findings
- Participation in continuing education through seminars, workshops, networking, and relevant professional journals
- Support for the facility's philosophy and policies

Fee for Services

Profit is the bottom line in any business and it is no different in healthcare. Previous sections of the job proposal identify how your services will enhance the facility's delivery of care. This section demonstrates how the facility can cover the cost of your services and perhaps even generate new revenue. One way to do this is to indicate areas in which the facility can charge a fee for your services. For example, some insurance companies reimburse for lactation services and you can check the status of the insurance carriers for women in your community and in the facility. Fee-for-service offerings may include:

- In-hospital assistance
- Prenatal classes
- Home or outpatient follow-up (including telephone counseling with an unlimited 24-hour hotline, an office visit, or a home visit)
- Outpatient consultation services

Equipment and Other Resources

The facility will want to anticipate any additional expenses your position requires. Therefore in your proposal indicate the initial investment required in terms of equipment and other resources. The list may include:

- Office space
- Desk and chair
- File cabinets

- Computer and printer
- Telephone and fax machine or online fax service
- Answering machine or voice mail
- Internet access
- Beeper
- Comfortable cushioned armchair or sofa
- Electric breast pumps and other breastfeeding devices
- Infant scale
- Secretarial support
- Funds for reference books and continuing education

∿ Educating the Healthcare Team

The lactation consultant's role extends beyond helping mothers and babies. Lactation consultants are pivotal in helping other members of the healthcare team remain current with knowledge and clinical skills in breastfeeding care. An important goal for lactation professionals is to achieve a continuum of supportive breastfeeding care for mothers and babies. For mothers to receive the best possible advice and support, the providers on their healthcare team must be knowledgeable in lactation and have the necessary skills to facilitate learning. When health practitioners find it necessary to refer routine situations to a lactation consultant for assistance, the mothers, infants, and staff can lose valuable time. The longer a mother has a problem, the longer it takes to resolve it. By empowering physicians, nurses, and other caregivers to provide necessary assistance and support, you can help minimize the problems that mothers may experience.

Gaps in Knowledge and Skills

As discussed in Chapter 2, a knowledge deficit regarding breastfeeding exists in all areas of health care (Szucs et al., 2009; Nakar et al., 2007; Hellings & Howe, 2004; Cantril et al., 2004; Taveras et al., 2004a; Beal et al., 2003; Power et al., 2003). There appears to be a gap between knowledge and self-efficacy as well. An Iraqi study found that although primary healthcare physicians had good basic knowledge about the process of breastfeeding they were deficient in problem solving (Al-Zwaini et al., 2008). The need to address these gaps in knowledge and self-efficacy extends to nursing students as well (Spatz, 2005; Spatz & Sternberg, 2005). Additionally, an Australian study demonstrated that although midwives recognized the importance of immediate skin-to-skin contact for newborn infants, few understood its significance for facilitating correct attachment and effective suckling (Cantril et al., 2004). Another study cited statistically low knowledge among childcare teachers and directors on ways to adequately store breastmilk and formula (Clark et al., 2008).

Formal education in most nursing and medical schools fails to provide adequate knowledge and skills in breastfeeding management and support. A 2007 study found that breastfeeding information in nursing textbooks is at times inaccurate and inconsistent (Phillipp et al., 2007). Statistics show that health professionals who care for mothers and babies need more effective training in supporting breastfeeding (Clifford & McIntyre, 2008; Shah et al., 2005). One study revealed that obstetrical providers were least confident in resolving problems with milk production, whereas pediatric providers were least confident in resolving problems with breast and nipple pain (Taveras et al., 2004b). Mothers need a strong continuum of knowledgeable support throughout their healthcare team.

Clinicians report having limited time during preventive visits to address breastfeeding problems as a barrier to promoting breastfeeding (Taveras et al., 2004b). It may be more likely, however, that gaps in knowledge and skills affect the comfort level of healthcare professionals in promoting and supporting breastfeeding. According to a study in Puerto Rico, although physicians and residents recognized the benefits of breastfeeding, most did not encourage exclusive breastfeeding (Leavitt et al., 2009). Formal education can help eliminate such barriers to breastfeeding promotion and support (Caldeira et al., 2007). General practitioner registrars (resident medical students) in Australia acknowledged that gender and personal experience with breastfeeding influenced their attitudes, perceived knowledge, and confidence with breastfeeding issues (Brodribb et al., 2007). Such an approach fails to provide evidence-based assistance and support.

Teaching Breastfeeding Care

Knowledge gaps may account for the sparse breastfeeding-friendly practices in many developed countries. These trends have influenced health professionals in Greece to advocate feeding practices that fail to promote exclusive breastfeeding (Pechlivani et al., 2008). Studies support the value of education in establishing supportive practices. Labarere et al. (2005) suggest that brief training programs for practicing physicians contribute to improving breastfeeding outcomes. Law et al. (2007) reports that increasing midwives' knowledge of breastfeeding support in the immediate postpartum period may be a cost-effective way of improving the ability of mothers to begin and continue to breastfeed successfully.

Swanson and Power (2005) contend that nurses and midwives have a crucial role in communicating positive views on breastfeeding to new mothers. Clinical experience is a significant component in improving knowledge among members of the mother's healthcare team (Anderson & Geden, 1991). Programs that teach correct breast-

feeding management and effective communication and counseling techniques can facilitate improved knowledge and skills among nursing staff. Training hospital nursery staff in breastfeeding guidance is a potential, cost-effective intervention even in settings with relatively high breastfeeding rates (Shinwell et al., 2006). Practical problems in accessing training make it difficult for health professionals to stay up-to-date with new evidence (Tennant et al., 2006). Even baby-friendly hospitals find it challenging to remain current. A follow-up assessment in Brazil found that only 82 percent of the 167 baby-friendly hospitals continued to meet all 10 steps. Regular staff training was recommended (de Araújo & Schmitz, 2007).

A U.K. study reported that caregivers who have longer experience with breastfeeding support were more competent and that those already competent were most likely to want more updating (Wallace & Kosmala-Anderson, 2007). Lactation consultants are challenged with generating more enthusiasm among caregivers who most need the knowledge and skills to support breastfeeding families. In one study where learners reportedly had poor knowledge of evidence-based policy, there was a stated preference for training with a practical component (Wallace & Kosmala-Anderson, 2007). Busy clinicians may be receptive to practical, clinical instruction that helps them improve their skills and confidence. Spatz and Sternberg (2005) describe an education plan that enables nursing students to influence breastfeeding practices and culture by carrying out community-based breastfeeding advocacy projects. The approach includes a needs assessment, a list of community resources, and development of a project to promote breastfeeding.

An interactive course increases health practitioners' knowledge of breastfeeding practice (Kronborg et al., 2008). A study in Sri Lanka assessed the effectiveness and feasibility of staff training and supportive supervision on the job. The proportion of mothers who breastfed their infants exclusively for 6 months improved from 19 to 70 percent after the intervention (Agampodi & Agampodi, 2008). Offering group inservice programs and individual clinical mentoring helps achieve consistent care for mothers and babies. In hospital practice, if a staff member asks for help in assisting a mother and baby, the lactation consultant can use the opportunity to teach the staff member while assisting the mother (see Figure 26.2). Inservice programs can be planned to meet the needs of both new and experienced staff. You might consider holding occasional seminars with more involved information in addition to short breastfeeding updates at unit meetings or on bulletin boards. You can also participate in the orientation of new staff members (Stokamer, 1993).

The American Academy of Pediatrics (2009) published a breastfeeding curriculum to help residents develop confidence and skills in breastfeeding care. The program is designed to help residency program directors

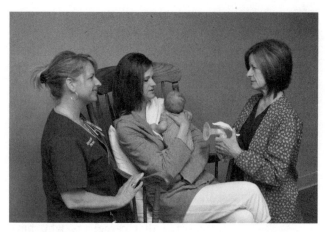

FIGURE 26.2   Staff nurse observes as the IBCLC works with a mother and baby.

Source: Printed with permission of Anna Swisher.

and faculty incorporate breastfeeding education into existing curricula. It can be applied to pediatrics, family medicine, preventive medicine, internal medicine, and obstetric/gynecologic residency programs. In testing the curriculum the AAP recognized that residents need to learn about breastfeeding in a supportive environment. This led to a landmark decision by the AAP to endorse the Ten Steps to Successful Breastfeeding, with exception to the ban on pacifiers because of the association of their possible role in reducing sudden infant death syndrome. In their letter of endorsement, AAP President David Tayloe stated, "the endorsement of these Ten Steps is integral to improving the overall care that mothers and babies receive in maternity facilities in the United States and is particularly helpful to our national effort to promote breastfeeding" (Tayloe, 2009, p. 1).

Creating Enthusiasm Among Staff

Staff education can be both formal and informal. You could launch a breastfeeding initiative with a motivational program for the staff, perhaps in conjunction with World Breastfeeding Week. A workshop or conference energizes people and generates enthusiasm for learning more about breastfeeding. A breastfeeding bulletin board with monthly updates can include highlights of particular staff members who have done something noteworthy related to breastfeeding. Post breastfeeding messages where people are likely to read them, such as in the locker room or on the back of the stall door in the restroom. When staff attends a breastfeeding program, you can show your appreciation with a badge that identifies them to mothers as someone who can help them with their breastfeeding questions.

You can begin a class with a needs assessment or a quiz to whet their appetites. Let them know that the purpose is to receive their input to design a program to meet

their needs. Because disgruntled members may need to voice negative feelings or raise contentious issues, it is important that time be planned for questions and comments. Many times these people can become your most supportive allies when they know you have heard them and respect their feelings and concerns.

A receptive learning climate enhances your effectiveness in teaching other staff members about breastfeeding care. Providing opportunities to role play situations in a classroom setting helps relieve anxiety and makes the anticipated situation less awkward when confronted with it in practice. Chapter 4 discusses the use of humor as a communication tool. In many ways humor is simply allowing your humanness to shine through by a willingness to make mistakes in front of colleagues. You are a role model to them and it is instructive for them to see that in the real world we all make mistakes and recover from them. Humor is graphic and creates mental images that help the learner remember better and longer. Modeling the use of humor by weaving it into your teaching shows staff how they can use humor as a communication tool with mothers.

∾ Maturing Through Experience

At times, lactation consulting may present discouraging experiences. Inevitably, something will occur that you cannot correct or prevent. At such a time it is helpful to talk with an understanding colleague to express your frustrations or doubts. The following sections describe some circumstances that may occur during your career.

Lack of Compliance

You will invariably encounter mothers who do not follow through on your advice and experience what you consider to be negative results. Some of these outcomes may occur because of what you consider inappropriate or ill-advised action by the mother. A mother may wean unexpectedly or earlier than you would consider optimal. Another may supplement with formula or introduce solid foods at an early age. It is discouraging when a mother fails to follow your advice. It is equally frustrating to see breastfeeding deteriorate because a mother has chosen not to follow suggestions and advice that were best for her baby. Keep in mind that what a mother does with your advice is her responsibility, as are the consequences of her actions. As long as you have given the appropriate support and information, you have fulfilled your obligation to the mother. You must then step back and respect her choice.

Medical Complications

It is discouraging for both you and the mother when a highly motivated and determined mother is unable to breastfeed for medical reasons. You may tend to view it as failure on your part. Other times, more tragic events may leave you feeling helpless, such as a baby dying or a mother having had radical breast surgery that prevents breastfeeding. These events can affect you deeply when you have cultivated a caring relationship with the mother. You may find it difficult to remove yourself emotionally from the situation and may need to work through the grief process just as the mother does.

External Interference

Some discouraging situations involve people other than the mother in your care. Perhaps her partner is unsupportive and resents your involvement. A member of the medical community may be unsupportive of your efforts or may consistently give incorrect breastfeeding information. While these situations can make it difficult to provide necessary help and advice to a mother, they offer opportunities as well. You can educate the partner or caregiver and try to determine the cause of the misinformation or lack of support. You can be open and frank with the mother about her partner's feelings and arrange follow-up contacts at times when the partner is not at home. You can give literature to the mother to share with her caregiver and encourage her to also share the positive aspects of her breastfeeding. You can suggest she seek another caregiver's opinion if she seems receptive.

Pitfalls in Counseling

Every mother is unique, with her own personality and personal limitations. Approaching each mother with a focus on her individual needs ensures that you help her reach her goals. Our own personality and communication styles can sometimes interfere with the manner in which we approach and help mothers. Examining your own personal style and consciously working to mitigate any weaknesses helps you overcome potential roadblocks in your communication with mothers.

Not Accepting Your Limitations

Because mothers and members of her healthcare team consider lactation consultants as experts, it is difficult to admit when we don't know something. Acknowledge when you do not have all the answers and need to get help from outside sources. Realize that your influence on a mother's behavior is limited and that your role is to encourage her to determine her own solutions. Recognize when a mother needs referral to another caregiver, and do not attempt to handle a situation that is beyond your expertise.

Getting Overly Involved

Mothers can sometimes become overly dependent on a caregiver's assistance to the point that they fail to recognize and utilize their own resources. If a mother seems to rely on you too much, encourage her to take charge of her own decisions. Build her confidence, and offer her information with minimal guidance. When problems are serious and outside the realm of breastfeeding, encourage her to contact her physician, mental health professional, religious advisor, or other sources of advice and support. You are not the mother's professional guidance counselor and she needs to understand that your services are restricted to breastfeeding and related topics.

If you are a licensed counselor or psychologist who has been counseling a mother in breastfeeding and the nature of the contact changes, you need to renegotiate your relationship formally. Furthermore, it is not a good practice to counsel family members or close friends. Because of the emotional ties, you may have very strong emotions about the choices the parents make. If breastfeeding goes well, the mother may become overly dependent on you and fail to mature in her mothering experience as quickly as she otherwise might. If breastfeeding does not go well she may blame you regardless of the reason, thus harming your personal relationship. It is usually wise to refer family members or friends to another lactation consultant and maintain your role as a loving family member or friend.

Discussing Your Breastfeeding

Mothers often ask their lactation consultant about her personal breastfeeding experience. If a mother asks how long you breastfed, it is important to maintain a professional relationship with her. It is doubtful that she really wants to know about your breastfeeding experience. More likely, she has a question about her own breastfeeding. Capitalizing on your counseling skills helps you determine the real purpose of the question. You might say, for example, "You're wondering how long to breastfeed your baby." Discussing aspects of your life diminishes the mother's experience and it is important that you keep the discussion focused on her. At times, it may be appropriate to give a short answer and immediately return the focus to her, without elaborating on your personal experience.

Making Value Judgments

It may be challenging to remain objective and avoid conveying value judgments to mothers. Remember that your role with mothers is to empower them as informed consumers. You are responsible for giving correct and appropriate information and advice. What the mother does with that advice is her choice and her responsibility. Encourage mothers to make decisions that fit into their lifestyle, and then support their choices. Always leave mothers with a graceful exit if they are not comfortable with your suggestions. Clearly state, "Only you know what you and your family can deal with at this time"—and mean it!

Interrupting

One of the greatest challenges in communication is allowing the other person to talk uninterrupted and not interjecting your own thoughts. Becoming an effective listener involves the use of counseling skills to draw out the mother and engage her in conversation. Resist the urge to interrupt with comments before the mother finishes her train of thought. Avoid attempts to change the subject until the mother has explored it sufficiently. This pitfall is common in many social and professional interactions. Avoiding it often requires practice and careful attention to your communication skills.

Overwhelming the Mother

Avoid falling into the trap of overwhelming mothers with too much advice and information. Remember to restrict the amount of information you give to a mother at any one time. As a rule, offer only three suggestions at a time. As in the art world, less is more! You can always follow up a contact with a telephone call or e-mail to determine if your plan worked. Clearly explain to the mother that there are more options and if this suggestion does not work, she can call you for more help.

Being Too Solution Oriented

There is always the risk of focusing too much on solutions at the expense of other factors in a mother's life that need to be explored. This risk is common in helping roles within the health profession, and especially true in a hospital where staff time is limited. You can avoid overlooking important factors by listening carefully for feelings and concerns the mother expresses. Gather impressions from what she is *not* saying through observing her body language. Allow the mother time to define her situation and work toward solutions. The entire consultation should follow the mother's and baby's pace, not yours. Engage in problem solving only after you have gathered sufficient information and impressions.

Failing to Follow Up

Routine follow-up with clients indicates whether your advice has been helpful. It is an essential final component of every interaction. Always follow through to learn if the mother's situation has improved and to offer support. Make sure mothers know who they may contact when they need help or feel discouraged. If you will be away for an extended period of time, arrange for someone to receive your calls so mothers receive help when they need it. Follow-up may involve referring the mother to community resources when it is apparent that you cannot resolve her problem while she is in your care. Make it a practice to consider a consultation unfinished until appropriate follow-up is arranged.

∽ Avoiding Professional Burnout

Working in a caring profession such as the medical field carries a risk of emotiobnal stress and burnout. Stress, emotional exhaustion, and burnout are widespread in many industrialized countries (Gustafsson et al., 2008) and within the medical profession specifically (Saleh et al., 2009; Viviers et al., 2008; Soler et al., 2008). When multiple stresses are not managed and controlled they can lead to professional burnout, anxiety, and depression (Holt & Ladwa, 2008). Burnout may occur any time that you become overly involved in your work. Although almost everyone feels burned out to some degree at times, idealists who have high standards and believe they must do all the work themselves tend to burn out more quickly in their efforts to achieve perfection. This need for perfection can lead to lack of enthusiasm, a low tolerance level, and a loss of creativity and openness to change.

Signs of Emotional Burnout

A host of studies throughout the world associate an increased risk of burnout with the inability to cope with emotional exhaustion, low work satisfaction, and depersonalization (Devereux et al., 2009; Kania et al., 2009; Orzechowska et al., 2008; Onder & Basim, 2008; Orbáiz et al., 2008; Escribà-Agüir et al., 2008; Lourel & Gueguen, 2007). When burnout occurs, you may distance yourself from a mother, and it is only by releasing your feelings and tension that you can return to the mother and give compassionate care. Case conferences, similar to those used by social workers, can help lactation consultants learn and grow. Sharing concerns with colleagues helps you recognize when you are too emotionally or unprofessionally involved with a client. Signs of emotional burnout include:

- Tunnel vision
- Loss of coping skills
- Lack of focus and concentration
- Inability to manage time
- Irrational behavior; a feeling of being on an "emotional roller coaster"
- Irritation
- Avoiding obligations and other avoidance behaviors
- Feeling that life is out of control
- Physical pain or weakness
- Physiological reactions such as weakness, fatigue, insomnia, listlessness, depression, or anxiety attack

Job Satisfaction

To progress past emotional burnout, you first need to recognize that the problem you are experiencing is with your job and not with you. Chronic work stress and unfavorable work conditions are associated with burnout and job dissatisfaction (Bellingrath et al., 2009; Kanai-Pak et al., 2008; Viviers et al., 2008). Factors in your life outside your job can affect your satisfaction at work as well. Emotional burnout is a response to unrelieved stress that occurs when you fail to achieve a balance. Challenges of a changing society, increased work-related stress, and decreasing social security contribute to emotional stress (Hillert, 2008; Price, 2008).

Job dissatisfaction can result from an imbalance between the effort you expend and the rewards you receive in your job. Low social support from colleagues and superiors contributes to job stress (Lavoie-Tremblay et al., 2008; Sakata et al., 2008). Perceptions of reciprocity in relationships with supervisors and peers have particular influence on the level of burnout (Prins et al., 2008). Receiving cooperation and validation from colleagues increases a sense of satisfaction in our work life. High levels of empowerment and the ability to influence our work situation reduce work-related stress and lower levels of burnout (Hochwälder, 2008; Wadensten et al., 2008). Additionally, having had higher prior levels of empowerment can be associated with greater burnout (Hochwälder, 2008). Novice lactation consultants who had high levels of empowerment in a related healthcare role may find it challenging as they move forward in acquiring expertise in their new role.

A study in Sweden found high job demands to be a significant predictor of symptoms of emotional exhaustion. Downsizing and lack of support from superiors and fellow workers and low decision authority also contributed (Magnusson Hanson et al., 2008). Job demands and lack of resources lead to constant psychological overtaxing, exhaustion, and cynicism. This emotional burnout and stress can cause high levels of absenteeism, low morale, mental fatigue, and exhaustion (Braithwaite, 2008).

High achievers who are full of enthusiasm and high expectations may fear not achieving self-imposed goals, resulting in disappointment and frustration. Failure to live up to our ideals increases the risk of burnout (Gustafsson et al., 2008; Daloz et al., 2007). Conflict between personal values and the values of the employer can also result in a feeling of powerlessness to change something we consider important. This can be magnified when combined with moral distress from knowing an ethically appropriate action and being unable to take that course (Beumer, 2008; Silén, 2008). This can be taxing for lactation consultants whose employers violate the International Code by accepting gratuities from formula manufacturers and distributing formula discharge bags.

Job satisfaction and emotional health can significantly influence the quality of care that health professionals provide (Bakker et al., 2008; Glass & Rose, 2008;

Kanai-Pak et al., 2008; Wadensten et al., 2008; Daloz et al., 2007; Tabolli et al., 2006). Furthermore, time constraints and staff shortages contribute to stress and can impact on the quality of patient care (Holt & Ladwa, 2008; Mohale & Mulaudzi, 2008; Moola et al., 2008; Shimizutani et al., 2008; Viviers et al., 2008). Developing better time management skills often improves circumstances at work. An overwhelming workload may result from lack of planning, prioritizing, or delegation skills. Measures to control these aspects of your job can prevent burnout and lead to increased job satisfaction and quality of care.

Predictability at work is an important component of job control (Väänänen et al., 2008). Higher levels of job satisfaction are associated with positive coping strategies and a self-confident, optimistic approach (Golbasi et al., 2008). Self-efficacy has been shown to be protective for psychological well-being (Schwerdtfeger et al., 2008). Age, resources, meaningful work and impact are other significant predictors of job satisfaction. Being involved in developing work goals and making important changes can decrease work stress and help to lower the risk of burnout (Li et al., 2008). Opportunities to self-schedule or job share are potential approaches to increase job satisfaction, especially among the younger generation (Wilson et al., 2008). Mentoring has also been identified as a good tool for supporting the quality of job performance (Holt & Ladwa, 2008). Individual and group counseling can help reduce emotional exhaustion (Rø et al., 2008). Receiving support and encouragement from peers and being recognized for good performance increase job satisfaction and reduce the risk of burnout (Holt & Ladwa, 2008).

Delegating responsibilities helps you put your valuable time and energy into the most important functions. Training others on the staff to take calls and answer basic breastfeeding questions gives ownership to others and enables everyone to focus on priorities. Furthermore, empowering others to provide the first levels of care to breastfeeding mothers helps minimize the types of problems that cause stress. If you are in private practice, develop a referral list of two or three colleagues whose abilities you respect and ask one of them to take your referrals when you feel overwhelmed. You can record a message on your voicemail or answering machine letting callers know you are unavailable and refer them to your colleague.

Balancing Work and Home

The nurturing nature of the lactation profession impels many caregivers to provide constant access to mothers whenever a concern or problem arises. Lactation professionals and others who care for breastfeeding mothers are often available to clients 24 hours a day. We are in danger of emotional exhaustion and professional burnout any time we fail to achieve a balance between professional responsibilities and personal needs (Miedema et al., 2009; Saleh et al., 2009; Lourel & Mabire, 2008; Soler et al., 2008).

It is often difficult for us to admit to our limitations and recognize that trying to be everything for everyone is unrealistic and impractical. When you attempt to do too many things, you cannot give your best to what is most important. Establishing personal boundaries and prioritizing the demands on your time help you achieve balance and reduce stress. You cannot give the best of yourself when you feel stressed and stretched to the limit. Learn to limit the commitments you place on your time and to say no when others ask more of you than you can give. Screen your telephone calls when you feel unprepared to answer the telephone, and respond to messages at a more conducive time.

Recapturing personal time to enjoy family, friends, and favorite activities helps you overcome burnout. Take the time to cultivate and nurture relationships with the important people in your life, remembering that you also need time for the *most* important person in your life— you! Plan special time to relax, pamper yourself, and enjoy activities that your busy schedule has not allowed. Use visualization and slow, deep breathing to relax and reclaim your strength and perspective. Physical exercise or a massage can also help rejuvenate you. Your ability to maintain perspective and find humor in situations is especially important during times of stress. People with a sense of humor are healthier, happier people!

Renewing Enthusiasm

Learn how to recognize situations that make you feel uncomfortable and work through them by discussing them with a colleague. Networking at conferences and affiliated meetings is a perfect opportunity for getting rejuvenated in the lactation field. Spending time with others in similar situations and learning new techniques can breathe new life into a job that is wearing you down. You can expand your learning further by reading journals and technical books, and by increasing networking through serving on committees and becoming active in your professional association.

If lack of cooperation and support from others creates work stress, you may need to use a new approach or find other avenues for garnering their support. If you enjoy community outreach, you could speak to clinics, high school health classes, and local organizations. If you enjoy writing, you could write an online blog, newsletter, or column on breastfeeding for your local newspaper. You may also enjoy writing a column for a breastfeeding or parenting website. If you enjoy teaching, you can teach lay counselors in the community or mentor new lactation consultant interns. You can work at the local, state, national, or global level in breastfeeding promotion efforts. When you redefine your goals and relate them to your actions in this manner, you will be on your way toward developing a satisfying new role for yourself.

～ Summary

The lactation consultant, an integral member of the mother's healthcare team, must continually grow and thrive in the profession. Appropriate education and clinical experience prepares you to enter the profession. Understanding the stages of acquiring your new role helps you anticipate each new challenge. Availing yourself of the networking and support from colleagues and your professional association enhances your effectiveness with mothers and babies. Becoming certified and adhering to the profession's standards of practice and ethics ensures that you provide appropriate care to mothers and babies. Recognizing your limitations and seeking assistance when appropriate enable you to give your best effort to mothers. As you mature in your professional role, balancing your professional and personal life helps you avoid burnout and maintain enthusiasm for lactation counseling.

～ Chapter 26—At a Glance

Applying what you learned—

Your growth as a lactation professional:

- Recognize your progression through the stages of role acquisition.
- Complete a lactation management course.
- Acquire clinical experience with a mentor, using the profession's clinical competencies.
- Become IBCLC certified.
- Obtain liability insurance.
- Follow the profession's code of ethics and standards of practice.
- Network with other lactation professionals to mature in your own role.
- Attend conferences and read professional journals to learn new clinical practice and research.
- Join your professional association and use its resources.

Your role with mothers:

- Recognize what constitutes a client relationship and provide appropriate care.

- Obtain informed consent and retain records appropriately.
- Build positive relationships with the mothers in your care.
- Avoid guaranteeing results or creating unrealistic expectations for mothers.
- Empower parents to make their own decisions, and accept their choices.
- Work within the parameters of other caregivers' advice as much as possible.

Establishing yourself in the profession:

- Develop resources and contacts in areas that enhance your consulting.
- Determine the market for lactation consultants in your community.
- Provide prenatal breastfeeding education and support.
- Market your services through a website, social networking, brochures, business cards, health fairs, and other community events.
- Offer to speak in the community to build recognition as an authority.
- Develop a résumé or curriculum vitae and a job proposal based on the needs of the facility where you wish to work.
- Teach breastfeeding care to all members of the healthcare team to provide consistency.
- Launch a breastfeeding initiative with a motivational program for the staff.
- Use creativity and humor to create a receptive learning climate.
- Learn how to deal with misinformation and lack of support.
- Achieve a balance between professional responsibilities and personal needs.
- Recognize signs of emotional burnout and learn how to minimize it.
- Find new challenges and goals to renew your enthusiasm.
- Accept your limitations and avoid becoming overly involved, discussing your own breastfeeding, making value judgments, interrupting, or overwhelming mothers.
- Use counseling skills to avoid being too solution oriented.
- Provide follow-up to mothers.

∼ References

Accreditation and Approval Review Committee (AARC) on Education in Human Lactation and Breastfeeding. Morrisville, NC: www.aarclactation.org. Accessed May 24, 2011.

Agampodi SB, Agampodi TC. Effect of low cost public health staff training on exclusive breastfeeding. *Indian J Pediatr*. 2008;75(11):1115-1119.

Al-Zwaini EJ, et al. Knowledge of Iraqi primary health care physicians about breastfeeding. *East Medit Health J*. 2008; 14(2):381-388.

American Academy of Pediatrics (AAP). Breastfeeding residency curriculum. http://www.aap.org/breastfeeding/curriculum. Accessed October 29, 2009.

Anderson E, Geden E. Nurses' knowledge of breastfeeding. *JOGNN*. 1991;1;20:58-63.

Association of Women's Health, Obstetric and Neonatal Nursing. *Standards for Professional Nursing Practice in the Care of Women and Newborns*, 7th ed. Washington, DC: AWHONN; 2009.

Bakker AB, et al. How job demands, resources, and burnout predict objective performance: a constructive replication. *Anxiety Stress Coping*. 2008;21(3)::309-324.

Barger J. Certified Lactation Specialist Course. Wheaton, IL: Lactation Education Consultants; 2009.

Beal A, et al. Breastfeeding advice given to African American and white women by physicians and WIC counselors. *Public Health Rep*. 2003;118(4):368-376.

Bellingrath S, et al. Chronic work stress and exhaustion is associated with higher allostatic load in female school teachers. *Stress*. 2009;12(1):37-48.

Beumer CM. Innovative solutions: the effect of a workshop on reducing the experience of moral distress in an intensive care unit setting. *Dimens Crit Care Nurs*. 2008;27(6):263-267.

Bocar D, Moore K. *Acquiring the Parental Role. Lactation Consultant Series #16*. New York: Avery Publishing Group; 1987.

Braithwaite M. Nurse burnout and stress in the NICU. *Adv Neonatal Care*. 2008;8(6):343-347.

Brodribb W, et al. Breastfeeding and Australian GP registrars: their knowledge and attitudes. *J Hum Lact*. 2008;24:422-430.

Brodribb WE, et al. Gender and personal breastfeeding experience of rural GP registrars in Australia: A qualitative study of their effect on breastfeeding attitudes and knowledge. *Rural Remote Health*. 2007;7(3):737.

Caldeira AP, et al. Knowledge and practices in breastfeeding promotion by family health teams in Montes Claros, Brazil. *Cad Saude Publ*. 2007;23(8):1965-1970.

Cantril R, et al. Midwives' knowledge of newborn feeding ability and reported practice managing the first breastfeed. *Breastfeed Rev*. 2004;12(1):25-33.

Clark A, et al. Assessing the knowledge, attitudes, behaviors and training needs related to infant feeding, specifically breastfeeding, of child care providers. *Matern Child Health J*. 2008;12(1):128-35.

Clifford J, McIntyre E. Who supports breastfeeding? *Breastfeed Rev*. 2008;16(2):9-19.

Cusson RM, Strange SN. Neonatal nurse practitioner role transition: the process of reattaining expert status. *J Perinat Neonatal Nurs.* 2008;22(4):329-337.

Daloz L, et al. Feeling of non-acknowledgment at work, disappointment and burnout, an exploratory study [in French]. *Sante Ment Que.* 2007;32(2):83-96.

de Araújo M, Schmitz B. Reassessment of baby-friendly hospitals in Brazil. *J Hum Lact.* 2007;23(3):246-252.

Devereux JM, et al. Social support and coping as mediators or moderators of the impact of work stressors on burnout in intellectual disability support staff. *Res Dev Disabil.* 2009; 30(2):367-377.

Escribà-Agüir V, et al. Effect of psychosocial work environment and job satisfaction on burnout syndrome among specialist physicians [in Spanish]. *Gac Sanit.* 2008;22(4):300-308.

Glass N, Rose J. Enhancing emotional well-being through self-care: the experiences of community health nurses in Australia. *Holist Nurs Pract.* 2008;22(6):336-347.

Golbasi Z, et al. Relationships between coping strategies, individual characteristics and job satisfaction in a sample of hospital nurses: cross-sectional questionnaire survey. *Int J Nurs Stud.* 2008;45(12):1800-1806.

Gustafsson G, et al. Meanings of becoming and being burnout: phenomenological-hermeneutic interpretation of female healthcare personnel's narratives. *Scand J Caring Sci.* 2008;22(4):520-528.

Hellings P, Howe C. Breastfeeding knowledge and practice of pediatric nurse practitioners. *J Pediatr Health Care.* 2004; 18(1):8-14.

Hillert A. Burnout—a new disease [in German]? *Versicherungsmedizin.* 2008;60(4):163-169.

Hochwälder J. A longitudinal study of the relationship between empowerment and burnout among registered and assistant nurses. *Work.* 2008;30(4):343-352.

Holt VP, Ladwa R. Mentoring. A quality assurance tool for dentists. Part 1: The need for mentoring in dental practice. *Prim Dent Care.* 2008;15(4):141-146.

Howett M, et al. Designing a university-based lactation course. *J Hum Lact.* 2006;22(1):104-107.

International Board of Lactation Consultant Examiners (IBLCE). *Clinical Competencies for IBCLC Practice.* Falls Church, VA: IBLCE; 2011.

International Board of Lactation Consultant Examiners (IBLCE). *Scope of Practice for International Board Certified Lactation Consultants.* Falls Church, VA: IBLCE; 2008. http://www.iblce.org/upload/downloads/ScopeOfPractice-March2008.pdf. Accessed March 8, 2010.

International Board of Lactation Consultant Examiners (IBLCE). *The Code of Ethics: International Board Certified Lactation Consultants.* Falls Church, VA: IBLCE; 2004.

International Lactation Consultant Association (ILCA). *Standards of Practice for Lactation Consultants,* 2nd ed. Raleigh, NC: ILCA; 1999.

International Lactation Consultant Association (ILCA) (Mannel R, et al., eds.). *Core Curriculum for Lactation Consultant Practice,* 2nd ed. Sudbury, MA: Jones and Bartlett; 2007.

Kanai-Pak M, et al. Poor work environments and nurse inexperience are associated with burnout, job dissatisfaction and quality deficits in Japanese hospitals. *J Clin Nurs.* 2008;17(24):3324-3329.

Kania ML, et al. Personal and environmental characteristics predicting burnout among certified athletic trainers at National Collegiate Athletic Association institutions. *J Athl Train.* 2009;44(1):58-66.

Kronborg H, et al. Health visitors and breastfeeding support: influence of knowledge and self-efficacy. *Eur J Public Health.* 2008;18(3):283-288.

Kutner L, Barger J. *Clinical Experience in Lactation: A Blueprint for Internship,* 3rd ed. Wheaton, IL: Lactation Education Consultants; 2010.

Labarere J, et al. Efficacy of breastfeeding support provided by trained clinicians during an early, routine, preventive visit: a prospective, randomized, open trial of 226 mother-infant pairs. *Pediatrics.* 2005;115(2):e139-e146.

Lavoie-Tremblay M, et al. Creating a healthy workplace for new-generation nurses. *J Nurs Scholarsh.* 2008;40(3):290-297.

Law SM, et al. Breastfeeding best start study: training midwives in a "hands off" positioning and attachment intervention. *Matern Child Nutr.* 2007;3:194-205.

Leavitt G, et al. Knowledge about breastfeeding among a group of primary care physicians and residents in Puerto Rico. *J Community Health.* 2009;34:1-5.

Li IC, et al. The relationship between work empowerment and work stress perceived by nurses at long-term care facilities in Taipei city. *J Clin Nurs.* 2008;17(22):3050-3058.

Lourel M, Gueguen N. A meta-analysis of job burnout using the MBI scale [in French]. *Encephale.* 2007;33(6):947-953.

Lourel M, Mabire C. The effort-reward imbalance and negative spill-over between professional and personal life among dairy farmers: effects on job burnout [in French]. *Sante Publique.* 2008;20(Suppl 3):S89-S98.

Magnusson Hanson LL, et al. Demand, control and social climate as predictors of emotional exhaustion symptoms in working Swedish men and women. *Scand J Public Health.* 2008;36(7):737-743.

Miedema B, et al. Crossing boundaries: family physicians' struggles to protect their private lives. *Can Fam Physician.* 2009; 55(3):286-287.

Mohale MP, Mulaudzi FM. Experiences of nurses working in a rural primary health-care setting in Mopani district, Limpopo Province. *Curationis.* 2008;31(2):60-66.

Moola S, et al. Critical care nurses' perceptions of stress and stress-related situations in the workplace. *Curationis.* 2008;31(2):77-86.

Nakar S, et al. Attitudes and knowledge on breastfeeding among paediatricians, family physicians, and gynaecologists in Israel. *Acta Paediatr.* 2007;96(11):1712-1713.

Noel-Weiss J, Walters G. Ethics and lactation consultants: developing knowledge, skills, and tools. *J Hum Lact.* 2006; 22(2):203-212.

Onder C, Basim N. Examination of developmental models of occupational burnout using burnout profiles of nurses. *J Adv Nurs.* 2008;64(5):514-523.

Orbáiz VR, et al. Burnout syndrome epidemiology [in Spanish]. *Rev Enferm.* 2008;31(7-8):29-38.

Orzechowska A, et al. The burnout syndrome among doctors and nurses [in Polish]. *Pol Merkur Lekarski.* 2008;25(150): 507-509.

Pechlivani F, et al. Infant feeding and professional advice in the first half of the 20th century in Greece. *Breastfeed Rev.* 2008;16(3):23-28.

Phillipp BL, et al. Breastfeeding information in nursing textbooks needs improvement. *J Hum Lact.* 2007;23(4):345-349.

Power M, et al. The effort to increase breast-feeding. Do obstetricians, in the forefront, need help? *J Reprod Med.* 2003; 48(2):72-78.

Price B. Strategies to help nurses cope with change in the healthcare setting. *Nurs Stand.* 2008;22(48):50-56.

Prins JT, et al. The relationship between reciprocity and burnout in Dutch medical residents. *Med Educ.* 2008;42(7):721-728.

Rø KE, et al. Counselling for burnout in Norwegian doctors: one year cohort study. *BMJ.* 2008;11:337.

Sakata Y, et al. Effort-reward imbalance and depression in Japanese medical residents. *J Occup Health.* 2008;50(6): 498-504.

Saleh KJ, et al. Recognizing and preventing burnout among orthopaedic leaders. *Clin Orthop Relat Res.* 2009;467(2): 558-565.

Schwerdtfeger A, et al. Self-efficacy as a health-protective resource in teachers? A biopsychological approach. *Health Psychol.* 2008;27(3):358-368.

Shah S, et al. Breastfeeding knowledge among health workers in rural South Africa. *J Trop Pediatr.* 2005;51(1):33-38.

Shimizutani M, et al. Relationship of nurse burnout with personality characteristics and coping behaviors. *Ind Health.* 2008;46(4):326-335.

Shinwell ES, et al. The effect of training nursery staff in breastfeeding guidance on the duration of breastfeeding in healthy term infants. *Breastfeed Med.* 2006;1(4):247-252.

Silén M, et al. Workplace distress and ethical dilemmas in neuroscience nursing. *J Neurosci Nurs.* 2008;40(4):222-231.

Soler J, et al. Burnout in European family doctors: the EGPRN study. *Fam Pract.* 2008;25(4):245-265.

Spatz D. The breastfeeding case study: a model for educating nursing students. *J Nurs Educ.* 2005;44(9):432-434.

Spatz D, Sternberg A. Advocacy for breastfeeding: making a difference one community at a time. *J Hum Lact.* 2005; 21(2):186-190.

Stokamer C. In-service breastfeeding program development: needs assessment and planning. *J Hum Lact.* 1993;9:253-256.

Swanson V, Power KG. Initiation and continuation of breast-feeding: theory of planned behaviour. *J Adv Nurs.* 2005; 50(3):272-282.

Szucs KA, et al. Breastfeeding knowledge, attitudes, and practices among providers in a medical home. *Breastfeed Med.* 2009;4(1):31-42.

Tabolli S, et al. Job satisfaction, burnout and stress amongst nursing staff: a survey in two hospitals in Rome [in Italian]. *G Ital Med Lav Ergon.* 2006;28(Suppl 1):49-52.

Taveras E, et al. Mothers' and clinicians' perspectives on breastfeeding counseling during routine preventive visits. *Pediatrics.* 2004a;113:e405-e411.

Taveras EM, et al. Opinions and practices of clinicians associated with continuation of exclusive breastfeeding. *Pediatrics.* 2004b;113(4):e283-e290.

Tayloe D. American Academy of Pediatrics. Letter to WHO and UNICEF on AAP endorsement to the WHO/UNICEF Ten Steps to Successful Breastfeeding; August 25, 2009. http://www.aap.org/breastfeeding/files/pdf/Ten-Stepswosig.pdf. Accessed October 29, 2009.

Tennant R, et al. Barriers to breastfeeding: a qualitative study of the views of health professionals and lay counsellors. *Community Pract.* 2006;79(5):152-156.

Väänänen A, et al. Lack of predictability at work and risk of acute myocardial infarction: an 18-year prospective study of industrial employees. *Am J Public Health.* 2008;98(12): 2264-2271.

Viviers S, et al. Burnout, psychological distress, and overwork: the case of Quebec's ophthalmologists. *Can J Ophthalmol.* 2008;43(5):535-546.

Wadensten B, et al. A cross-cultural comparison of nurses' ethical concerns. *Nurs Ethics.* 2008;15(6):745-760.

Wallace LM, Kosmala-Anderson J. Training needs survey of midwives, health visitors and voluntary-sector breastfeeding support staff in England. *Matern Child Nutr.* 2007; 3(1):25-39.

Wilson B, et al. Job satisfaction among a multigenerational nursing workforce. *J Nurs Manag.* 2008;16(6):716-723.

World Health Organization. *International Code of Marketing of Breast-milk Substitutes.* Geneva, Switzerland: World Health Organization; 1981.

Critical Reading and Review of Research

There are three kinds of lies: lies, damn lies, and statistics.

—Attributed to Benjamin Disraeli by Mark Twain

By studying this and other texts, you learn a lot of state-of-the-art information and many techniques to use in your practice as a lactation consultant. The ability to critically read and interpret scientific literature is a necessary skill to keep your practice current. This chapter provides background information on the processes of science used in scientific journal articles. A "how-to" section on the structure and critical reading of scientific articles is aimed at readers who have little previous experience. Two mock articles with commentary provide an opportunity to practice the techniques presented to prepare you for reviewing a real article. You can savor the satisfaction of knowing you are offering families the most carefully considered, evidence-based practice they can receive from a thoughtful lactation professional.

～ Key Terms

Abstract
Anchors
Assumptions
Average
Bell curve
Bias
Blinded
Case studies
Case-control study
Chi-square
Cohen's kappa

Cohort
Confidence intervals
Confounding variables
Control group
Convenience
Correlation
Cronbach's alpha
Cross-sectional study
Dependent variable
Descriptive study
Distribution and range

Electronic publishing (Epub)
Evidence-based practice
Fabrication
Falsification
Experiment
Generalize
Homogeneity
Human subjects review
Hypothesis
Independent variable
Instruments
Internal validity
Likert scale
Mean
Meta-analysis
Nonprobability
Normal distribution
Odds ratio
Open access
Operationalize
Outcome
Output variables
Oximeter
Peer review
Plagiarism
Population

Probability
Prospective study
P value
Qualitative study
Random assignment
Randomized clinical trials
Regression
Relationship
Reliability
Research reports
Retrospective study
Review articles
Sample
Slope
Speculation
Spurious
Statistically significant
Subjects
Theory
Tools
True assumptions
t test
Validity
Variables
Variation

⌒ Online Journals

Access to scientific journals and research articles is dramatically easier than in previous decades thanks to the Internet. Every major journal has a website. Articles are available online either with free access, membership, or an individual fee. Many times, articles appear online before the print journal. When this is the case, you will see a notation such as "Epub 2009 June 20" (Epub stands for "electronic publication"). For example: Xu X, Dailey AB, Freeman NC, Curbow BA, Talbott EO. The effects of birthweight and breastfeeding on asthma among children aged 1–5 years. *J Paediatr Child Health*. 2009 Oct 19. [Epub ahead of print] PubMed PMID: 19845842. The information "PubMed PMID: 19845842" in the citation above is the identifying number for the article where it appears in PubMed, the database for the National Library of Medicine. This powerful database has a sophisticated search engine to list thousands of scholarly journal articles on virtually any topic.

The Directory of Open Access Journals service covers free, full text, quality-controlled scientific and scholarly journals. Its goal is to cover all subjects and languages. Accessible online journals, subject specific pre- and e-print archives and collections of learning objects are a valuable supplement to published scientific books, journals, and databases (Directory of Open Access Journals, 2009). *International Breastfeeding Journal* (2009) is an example of an open access journal. It covers all aspects of breastfeeding, from original research to case studies to editorials.

⌒ Types of Articles in Scientific Journals

Scientific journals contain many types of articles. Commonly, the first prose to appear is an editorial, and some journals print more than one. Editorials are very interesting and important to read. The editor is a prominent person in the field whose knowledge is broad and whose perspective on how the field is changing is often insightful. It is important to recognize that editorials are not studies and do not report on a particular study. Therefore they cannot be subjected to the kind of critical analysis this chapter addresses. However, editorials do offer reasoned opinions from someone who is usually an expert in the field on which they are writing. The editorial may either be a guest editorial, or the piece may be written by the editor or member of the editorial staff at the journal.

Case Studies

Case studies are a type of article published by many biomedical journals. They report on one or more cases of a problem, diagnosis, or treatment. A case study often appears because there is interest in a particular topic; however, because the diagnosis is unusual or treatment risky, it is unlikely that any experiments take place. An example of this in lactation literature is a case study of mothers who need to use a medication not often prescribed during breastfeeding. Typically, the physician who treated the mother describes her medical history and circumstances leading to the medication's use. A description and discussion of the outcomes for the mother and baby follow. Such a case study has a sample of one mother and one baby. The absence of comparison subjects or comparison treatment prevents critical analysis. It is still important information to retain, however, because it may be the only information available on the use of a particular drug during lactation. The information may help guide an especially difficult decision in clinical practice. However, because of its limited nature, a case study cannot form the basis for generalizing to most breastfeeding mothers and babies.

Meta-Analyses

Meta-analysis is a technique that combines the data and results of several studies to improve the strength of the conclusions. Although meta-analyses are important studies, the analysis approach discussed in this chapter does not apply to them. If you read a meta-analysis, you may want some help from a researcher or statistician before you implement the recommendations made in the study. Scientific journals still publish a lot of debate questioning the validity of the criteria for a good meta-analysis. Because this type of study relies heavily on statistical assumptions, clinicians often need help in judging their quality. Often, such articles contain the words "meta-analysis" in their titles or abstracts, so you should be able to identify them fairly easily.

Review Articles

Review articles are written by one or more experts in the field who summarize and often critique the best and worst studies published on a topic. They differ from a meta-analysis in that they do not combine the data and results as a meta-analysis does. The opinions of the experts clearly play a role in the selection and the critical analysis of the articles to review. Little or no original data appear in a review article. Therefore this chapter does not cover critical reading of this type of article.

If you wish to learn about an area of clinical research that is new to you, reading a review article can be very productive. You can discover some of the most recent information, some of the important scientists in the field, and some of the current controversies. Most of these articles contain the word "review" in the title or abstract. If you want to find a review article, you can use the word "review" in your database search or in your request to the librarian. The Cochrane Collaboration publishes Cochrane reviews in *The Cochrane Library* four times a year. Each issue contains all existing reviews, plus new and updated reviews. Cochrane reviews explore "the evidence for and against the effectiveness and appropriateness of treatments (medications, surgery, education, etc.) in specific circumstances" (Cochrane Collaboration, 2009).

Clinical Practice

Clinical practice articles often appear in journals for applied sciences such as nursing, dietetics, physical therapy, and medicine. Authors with experience in a particular diagnosis, problem, deficit, or preventive technique write these articles to share their accumulated wisdom with other clinicians. The *Journal of Human Lactation*, for example, usually has several of these articles in each issue, offering valuable insights from one lactation consultant to another.

Because such articles do not study a problem scientifically, there are usually no presentations of data in graphs, tables, or figures. There also are no hypotheses or research questions. There may be some summary information about how, for example, mothers who followed protocol X coped with problem Y. However, there is no comparison group or an attempt to show that protocol X is better than some other protocol. Although these articles are helpful, there is no substantive test of the authors' ideas. Therefore they do not constitute the same quality of evidence for changing care practices as research does.

Research

Research articles put a long-held belief or new idea to a scientific test. Researchers subject themselves and their work to the processes of scientific investigation and to the scrutiny of their peers. They take the risk that their colleagues may find their work wanting. Therefore, as lactation consultants, we must approach the work of our colleagues respectfully. Each article deserves careful attention, both for the growth of our human understanding about lactation and for the benefit of the families in our care. Research articles follow the basic structure described in the following sections.

∼ *Structure of a Scientific Article*

Most scientific articles follow a format that provides a maximum amount of information in a limited amount of journal space. You learn to appreciate well-written journal articles that condense information effectively. You come away knowing exactly what the researchers did and why. They have explained what they wish they had done differently and what they can justifiably conclude from their work. With practice, you derive a clear sense of whether or not you agree with their conclusions, and you can give clear reasons for your decisions. The growth of the science of lactation depends on this clear communication and on feedback to researchers.

Identifying Information

At the very top of many scientific journals, especially the European ones, is information identifying the journal using its standard abbreviated name. For example, *Acta Paediatr* is the abbreviation for the journal *Acta Paediatrica*, a Scandinavian journal. Although the format for the name, volume number, pages, and year of publication varies from one journal to another, the format used by *Acta Paediatrica* illustrates the commonalities. All this information is very handy to have at the top of the first page of the article. Those journals that do not put it at the top usually put it at the end of the abstract or somewhere else on the first page.

An example is *Acta Paediatr.* 91(3):267-274; 2009:

- *Acta Paediatr* is the journal's abbreviation.
- 91 is the volume of the journal. Most journals publish one volume every year; however, some publish two volumes per year.
- 267–274 are the pages where the article is located. Most journals paginate continuously for 1 year. Volume 91 begins with page 1. If the first issue for that year ends at page 112, then the second issue begins at page 113, and so on. This continuous pagination is the reason many journals do not include the issue number in the identifying information; it is not necessary. However, some do include it, usually right after the volume. In the example, (3) is the volume number. Many journals publish an issue monthly. Some, like the *Journal of Human Lactation*, publish quarterly. Others, like *Lancet*, publish weekly. When you look up an article or request one from a library, it is important to copy the numbers from the reference list carefully.
- 2009 is the year of publication. In some journals the year appears directly after the name of the journal.

Title of the Article

A well-chosen title tells you a lot about an article. In some journals the title explains the main finding and may be two sentences long. This helps busy readers choose which articles are highest priorities for their reading.

Authors

As you read research regularly, you begin to recognize the research interests of particular lactation scientists who publish several articles on aspects of a limited scope of problems. Many times, you can acquire a good reference list on a single topic just by knowing a few researchers' names and noting the references in their articles. If you do not have a library where you can perform a computer search and do not have Internet access, you can build your own library of articles by authors' names. This will help when you are preparing a presentation or documenting the need for a practice change.

Abstract

Most journals ask authors to write a brief summary of (1) the reason they performed the study, (2) a description of the main subjects and methods, (3) the findings, and (4) the conclusion. This is the abstract. The abstract is often the best guide for deciding whether the article is worth reading. Although it may not answer all your questions about the study, it does indicate what the authors thought was most important about their study. Abstracts vary in length and format and from one journal to another. Each journal sets its own requirements.

Introduction

The authors usually spend a few paragraphs explaining why they chose to study the problem cited in the article. Many studies receive funding from a particular source. The authors need to justify their acceptance of funding from the source, and that kind of justification is often contained in the introduction. You may also find clues to why the authors made certain decisions, such as why they only studied infants younger than 6 weeks old or collected data only during a particular season.

Review of the Literature

The purpose of this section of the article is to explain the issues surrounding the problem studied and review past research. Many funding sources will not support a study on a question that has received a great deal of past research. Therefore the researcher must either identify an aspect of the problem that was not covered or demonstrate that past research has not clarified an important point. The literature review narrows down the subject of interest. It cites previous studies and their findings and shows how the current study is different or better. Authors sometimes also explain weaknesses of past studies that their current study will correct.

In some journals (the *New England Journal of Medicine*, for example), the review of the literature is combined with the introduction. There may not even be a heading to identify this first part of the article. Nearly all articles contain a discussion of the research problem and of past studies before they begin to explain the current research. Literature reviews could be very long, and journals usually want them to be limited to the most relevant studies. If you read such a review and do not find a study cited there that you know is available, space considerations could be the reason.

Methods

The goal of the methods section is to tell the reader how the scientists operationalized the hypotheses and questions they studied. This section often begins with a description of subject recruitment. A member of the research team may have recruited subjects with certain criteria in mind (such as a previous preterm birth or giving birth to twins). Alternatively, subjects may have volunteered to be part of the study after hearing about it through a childbirth class or a newspaper advertisement. Sometimes the study relied on charts or other records and the subjects were unaware of the study. Usually, journals require the authors to state whether the study obtained approval from a human subjects review group and that the subjects gave informed consent.

Instruments

The methods section describes the tools (instruments) used to measure the outcome under study. The instrument may be a written questionnaire or survey, an electronic balance scale, a chemical test, biopsy, or ultrasound. The authors often explain the methods in much detail, including the way in which different measurement instruments led to the results. For example, a milk sample collected early in a feeding will probably not have the same proportion of hindmilk as a sample from a breast that was drained more fully. One study takes early samples of milk and finds low vitamin A levels. The other study takes a sample after a complete feeding and finds higher vitamin A content. The difference might be due to the greater fat content in the complete feeding sample because vitamin A is fat soluble.

Definition of Terms

The methods section defines the terms used in the study. When the authors include "breastfeeding dyads," they need to define what they mean by breastfeeding. Was it exclusive breastfeeding or partial breastfeeding? Did they ask mothers about the amount of supplemental formula the baby consumed, or did they actually measure it?

Statistical Methods

Statistical methods usually appear in the methods section. The authors define what methods they used and why they chose those particular ones. They may explain that they applied more than one statistical test to the data to strengthen the conclusions. This can be the least familiar part of the article to read. However, if you keep track of statistical terminology, you can develop a list of tests that you can look up in a text.

Results

The most important study results often appear in graphs, tables, or charts. The title of the table or graph explains its topic. A key below the table explains the statistical significance of the results. Another helpful use of tables is to summarize information about the subjects. Tables often compare the experimental group with the control group on relevant characteristics.

Most authors phrase their results very carefully. Because their article has been through peer review, they usually cannot claim findings that are not fairly well supported by the work they present. However, reading only the results or the abstract of a study can limit the reader's understanding of both the general problem and this particular study's approach to it. Many clinicians are tempted to read just the results because it seems like so much work to wade through the methods. Making the effort to understand the methods, though, may prevent clinicians from inappropriately adopting a recommended change in practice that does not really fit their clinical practice. The results of a study, in other words, need to be considered in the context of the rest of the article so the findings can be judged based on the specifics of that study.

Discussion

The discussion is the easiest part of the article to read. The authors explain their reason for conducting the study, review more of the relevant literature, sum up their most important results, and suggest applications and further research. They also explain any weaknesses or problems with the project. Some of these explanations are in response to the comments of peer reviewers. These can be very helpful to a reader who is too unfamiliar with a particular area of research to think of alternative methods or interpretations. Although the earlier parts of the article are standard and prescribed by the journal itself, the discussion shows more of the authors' thinking and creativity. By the time a study is complete and ready for publication, the researchers have raised many questions in their minds, which they often explore in the discussion.

References, Literature, and Bibliography

In this final section you find the articles that the authors cite in their review of the literature. It includes any article cited in their methods section if they used a method described in a separate article. Many journals also permit the listing of additional articles related to the main topic.

～ Critical Reading of a Scientific Article

This discussion of critical reading suggests an order in which to read the parts of an article. For beginners, it might be helpful to use this standard approach with the first several articles you read. Using this method helps you compare in a defined way the strengths and weaknesses of a study. This improves your ability to determine why studies differ in their findings and clarify why you find a particular study unsatisfying. As you acquire more experience, you can create your own approach.

The process of critical reading does not lend itself to a "recipe" format. If it did, you and another reader would come to the same conclusions every time. By reading critically, your opinion will differ from other readers. If you reread an article at a later time, you may assess its strengths and weaknesses differently from the first time you read it. This is where the fun lies in critical reading: in the challenge of the puzzles the science investigates.

Some readers are frustrated when they cannot clearly label a given study as "good" or "bad," and they either reject it entirely or apply every finding. Most studies are a mixture of well-done science and things that merit improvement. Honest investigators admit this in the discussion section. These imperfections reveal the nature of science. Science is a process, not a body of facts written in a textbook. The evidence for or against "truth" accumulates over time, as the result of many imperfect studies. Clinicians who want to find the best science to use in their practice realize they must keep reading because there is no final story. The process of following the development of our human understanding of a particular problem is fascinating and exciting once you are familiar with the tools scientists use to share their work with one another.

After the following discussion of critical reading, two mock articles are presented. Using the format described you will answer each question for yourself as you progress through each article. You will get more out of this process if you actually try to be critical at each stage rather than just reading the answers the text provides (of which you should also be critical!). Finally, you will review some general themes of critical reading. They are not the final words on the subject, as your own experiences are valuable too. Expect to grow as a reader and as a clinician from your continuing efforts to consider the science of lactation carefully. The following sections describe the steps to critical reading.

Step 1: Look at the Title

A well-written title indicates the subject of the article. From reading the title, determine what you expect the article to present. Sometimes, a title may lead your thinking along one track and the article turns out actually to be about a different facet than you were expecting. When you are aware of what you had expected, you can adjust more readily to what the authors really meant.

Be aware that bias can be reflected in the wording of the title. A recent analysis found that "formula is rarely named in publication titles or abstracts as an exposure increasing health risk. In 30 percent of cases, titles imply misleadingly that breastfeeding raises health risk. Initiatives to increase breastfeeding have described the importance of accurate language and well-informed health professional support. If widespread, this skew in communication of research findings may reduce health professionals' knowledge and support for breastfeeding" (Smith et al., 2009, p. 350).

What Do You Know About the Topic?

Consider what you already know about the subject. Try to be specific in terms of what you know from other studies, textbooks, lectures, and experience. Do you know, for example, that sore nipples usually decrease by day 5 to 10 postpartum? Do you know that in the Hispanic community, support for breastfeeding from the mother's mother may be more important than support from the baby's father? Have sources taught you that processing at high temperatures decreases immunoglobulins?

Taking time to review what you know helps you recognize discrepancies between your knowledge and what the authors claim later in the article. There may be legitimate reasons for those discrepancies. The scientists may have learned something new, for instance. Your reading will be more critical if you identify your own knowledge before you begin. Usually, this does not take very long. You may have chosen to read the article because of its importance for a problem that already interests you and that you have encountered several times in practice. What you already know about it will be easy to recall. With new subject matter, your knowledge is limited, so that review does not take very long either!

How Would You Have Studied the Topic?

Consider how you would have studied the topic. If you are new to reading research, you may not have many ideas. Nevertheless, try this step anyway. If the topic is breastfeeding twins, where would you have gone to find subjects? Would you want any specific age of twins? Would gender of the babies be relevant? If a mother had other children, would that affect the findings? If the twins were born before 35 weeks, could that complicate the causes of problems you are studying? Do you need to find twins who were exclusively breastfed?

For the question you are asking, is it possible to do an experiment, or can you simply observe mothers and babies who have made their own choices? Will it be easy to come up with 20 or more twin sets that meet the criteria, or is the problem so unusual that the number of subjects will be small? Does the problem occur in one ethnic or cultural group more than in other groups? If so, do you want to do a comparative study or focus more on just one group? The more questions you ask yourself about how you would have done the study, the more readily you grasp the significance of the choices the researchers made.

What Will You Expect to Find?

What should result from your brief review is a short list of aspects you expect to find in the study. For example, you may expect the study to include both first-time breastfeeders and experienced ones. On the other hand, you may expect it to include only preterm infants weighing over 2,500 grams. If the result turns out to be different from your expectations, you will be very interested in the reasons. This may lead you to uncover a deficiency in the study.

Step 2: Read the Authors' Names

Noting author names is helpful, especially if you have read a previous work by the author or authors and found the work to contain a problem. You should determine whether the authors corrected the problem in this study. If the authors studied a related problem previously in a way you thought was valuable, it will alert you to any changes in their methods or focus. If you have never read work by these authors, noting their names gives you a reference point for future reading.

Step 3: Read the Abstract

Reading the abstract is the first point at which you confirm whether your assumptions about the study are correct. The abstract should briefly tell you the main characteristics of the subjects and methods. If a study's colicky babies are older than 6 months of age and you wanted information for 6-week-old infants, you may stop reading and look for a different article. If the abstract proclaims an article to be about treating engorgement but does not mention the use of cabbage leaves, you want to read the introduction and literature review to determine the reason for the omission.

The article may report a finding that contradicts what you know about the subject. Do not let this cause you to stop reading. Reading the abstract alerts you to the importance of specific aspects of the study that may justify the unexpected findings. The abstract may give you your first hint of the results the investigators believe warrant their recommendations. Knowing the direction in which they want to apply their findings prepares you to read for specific inclusions or exclusions in their work. For example, they may state in the abstract that they believe all new mothers should receive a DVD on positioning or Internet resource list to take home with them. You may want to determine whether they included any low-income women in their study (who may not have a DVD player at home or access to the Internet). They may suggest that all new mothers need a visit from a lactation consultant before discharge. You may question whether they measured the lactation knowledge of the nursing staff or whether they included any mothers who had nursed previous babies.

Reading the abstract heightens your awareness of what the scientists believe is most important about their study. The abstract does not include much rationale for decisions made by the investigators. You must read the entire study for that. However, questioning while you read the abstract helps you get more out of the article itself.

Step 4: Study the Tables and Graphs

Make a quick overview of the tables and graphs to determine how many there are, their titles, and whether they are understandable. The most helpful tables have a title that tells the main idea, a source of the data (e.g., from a survey or from patient charts), and clear labels on each column and row, including the units of measurement (i.e., mL, kg, sec, and so on). Some provide percentages of the total that each subgroup represents as well as statistical test results.

For each table or graph ask yourself why the authors chose to put this particular information in a summary form. Often, it is to save space, because there is not enough space in many journals for the authors to present their "raw" data (the actual numbers they collected or measured). They therefore summarize quantitative information in tables, graphs, and charts. Tables are often the simplest way to capture a large amount of quantitative information in concise form. A table or graph may highlight an unusual aspect of their sample, method, or results. If a treatment produced a dramatic improvement in the patients' problems, for example, a graph may show that most clearly.

Take special note of graphs or tables that display results you consider minor while ignoring results that seem to be more important. You may become aware of a bias in such a presentation. Also, ask yourself if the table agrees with the text. This seems very basic. However, sometimes the text portrays one picture and the table another. If you cannot explain this in a plausible way, it may be a flaw in the article or an editorial error. Evaluate

tables first by their clarity of presentation. Then, as you read the article, make sure the table agrees with the text.

Pay particular attention to whether the number of subjects reported in the tables is the same as described in the text. The number of subjects who gave consent to participate initially is often greater than the number who participated in any particular aspect of the study. For example, the authors may have explained their study to several childbirth preparation classes and obtained consent from 50 couples to observe the first breastfeed. What could happen to reduce that number? The researchers might have been out of town when two of the couples delivered. Perhaps two mothers were so tired after delivery that they refused to allow the researcher to observe them. Maybe three mothers decided not to breastfeed. This reduces the sample size to 43 couples. Therefore if you read that 50 couples granted consent and then see that the total number of observations was 43, you might need to reread the part of the article that describes what happened to the other 7 couples. As long as the tables and text agree and there is an explanation of any apparent discrepancies, you can use the information in the tables to decide if your clients or patients are similar to the ones studied. You can also decide whether the tables and figures support the findings and reasoning claimed by the researchers.

Graphs should have clear titles and labels, designed to portray the data accurately. You need to look carefully at the scale of the graph. In the graph in Figure 27.1 the scale goes from 0 to 20, so the height of the curved lines looks lower and less impressive than the height of the curves in the graph in Figure 27.2, in which the scale goes from 0 to 7. Either scale could be appropriate depending on the definition of the pain scale. However, the graphs create different reactions in the viewer. Because the slope or angle of the lines in Figure 27.2 is steeper than that of Figure 27.1, it appears that the change in pain was different from that shown in Figure 27.2. Actually, both are the same.

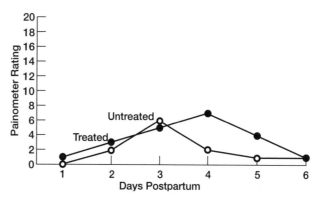

FIGURE 27.1 Changes in nipple soreness on scale of 0 to 20.

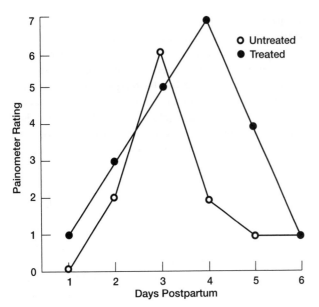

FIGURE 27.2   Changes in nipple soreness on scale of 0 to 7.

Therefore, although graphs can be very helpful, they can also be misleading and require careful scrutiny.

Second, suppose this study was one in which each woman was her own control, randomly assigned to treat one nipple and not the other. Suppose further that the authors claim that the treated nipple was in pain for less total time than the untreated nipple. Although you might agree with that conclusion, you might wonder if it was a fair test. Perhaps some of the babies sucked more vigorously on the untreated nipple, causing it to be more painful than the treated nipple on day 1. This example is probably not what the authors would publish because it represents only one subject. You can see that the details of a graph can both clarify and confuse your understanding.

There are many additional kinds of tables, graphs, and charts. Their purposes range from summarizing basic information to clarifying complex patterns found in the data. When you read the results to decide whether the evidence supports the findings, you want to look closely at these graphics. Critical analysis includes judging their clarity and consistency with the rest of the article.

Step 5: Read the Results

Read the results to get firmly in your mind what the authors claim to find. You need to understand their claims to read about their methods effectively. Pay particular attention to the subjects in the study and the relationships between variables. The first time you read the results section, determine whether the results are what the authors expected based on their theories and hypotheses.

Before you read the article any further, get the results clear in your mind and whether those results were predicted or not.

Subjects

This section of the article tells you what their final sample was. Identify the subjects who actually ended up in the study. Perhaps the researchers intended an equal portion of first-time breastfeeding mothers and experienced breastfeeding mothers. You then need to decide whether the sample was appropriate for the question they asked and whether the results are justified based on the kind of subjects they acquired. Most researchers try very hard to anticipate a certain number of study dropouts. However, they are sometimes unlucky (or plan poorly), and more subjects drop out from one group than from the other. Consider whether their results could have been different if their original plan had worked. Dropouts can affect the results. Some leave the study because their problem resolves quickly and they no longer need the treatment. Some leave because there are side effects of the treatment they cannot tolerate. Others drop out because the research process is a burden. Some families move before the study is completed.

Consider the implications of each reason for dropping out of the study. If the dropouts had remained in the study, might the findings have been different? Suppose a study of women who returned to employment at 6 weeks postpartum was trying to determine what factors made it likely that they would continue breastfeeding to 12 weeks. One factor to study might be employer support. The researchers might enroll women in the hospital who were planning to return to work at 6 weeks and continue nursing until at least 12 weeks. If a few women drop out because they expect lack of support from their employer, the remaining subjects would disproportionately include more mothers who expect support from their employers. It would then be likely that both those who continued and those who stopped expected support. This might lead the researchers to conclude that there was no difference between the two groups in terms of support. In reality, a higher proportion of those who expected no support simply left the study. The dropouts caused the study to suffer from homogeneity with respect to employer support, preventing detection of a difference in the "employer" factor.

Relationships

The investigators usually tell you that their study found a relationship between two or more variables. For example, they may have found a relationship between giving discharge packs containing formula to new mothers and early discontinuation of breastfeeding. The discharge packs are the independent variable and the duration of breastfeeding is the dependent variable. Think about all the logical steps needed to substantiate that finding.

Data Should Be Consistent with the Claims In the discharge pack example, one result could be that more of the mothers who received discharge packs needed to stop breastfeeding earlier than did the mothers who did not receive packs. The number of mothers who stopped compared with those who continued must be significantly different in a statistical sense—statistically significant. It also needs to be convincingly different to you. Similarly, "early" weaning must be meaningfully different from "late" weaning.

There Must Be No Other Equal or Better Explanation In the discharge pack example, determine whether the data can rule out other possible competing explanations. Did more mothers in the discharge pack group have sore nipples? Was there a higher proportion of preterm infants? Were there more mothers who only intended to breastfeed for 6 weeks or less? Ruling out these possible explanations makes it more likely that the discharge pack itself is the cause of the early weaning.

A Plausible Mechanism Must Link the Two Variables In the discharge pack example, the mechanism for this causation might be that a discharge pack is a subtle signal to the mother that her healthcare professionals do not really believe she can make sufficient milk for her baby. Because she then doubts the adequacy of her milk production, she weans early.

Step 6: Read the Methods (or Subjects and Methods)

The topics covered in this section are the most important to your critical reading because they determine whether the authors can justify their conclusions. The design of the study, the definitions of terms, the tools for measurement, and the statistical tests all contribute to your evaluation and are covered in the next section.

Design of the Study

There are several shorthand ways of describing the design of the study to a scientific audience. When you recognize these basic study designs, you can understand aspects of subject selection, data gathering, and comparisons that are drawn. You also know the kinds of conclusions warranted by the study's design.

Retrospective Study A retrospective study uses two comparison groups. The case subjects have the problem under examination, and the control subjects do not. Designing a study by designating case subjects first results in a design based on output variables. Output variables describe the subjects after follow-up or treatment. For example, the case subjects might be babies readmitted to the hospital with weight loss in excess of that expected during the first week of life. The control subjects would be babies without such weight loss, possibly found by a search of the charts in a pediatric practice. The purpose of such a comparison might be to determine whether there were any differences in the number of feedings or stools in the first 4 days of life or differences in the highest bilirubin level achieved that could be associated with the need for readmission. Such a retrospective study is a case-control study.

When the methods section declares that the design is retrospective, you expect to read a description of the groups chosen for comparison. You then want to decide whether the groups were appropriate. Retrospective studies greatly depend on records kept before researchers conducted the study. If a retrospective study concluded that babies who had stooled only once during their first 24 hours were at higher risk of readmission, you want to know whether the record keeping of stools passed was accurate. In a retrospective study the use of existing records may be all that is possible. The evidence gained from such a study may not be as strong as when the record keeping is more deliberate and planned.

Prospective Study In a prospective study subjects are sampled based on input variables that are believed to influence the outcomes. A prospective study might be one in which the authors held staff education classes and designed new record-keeping tools before data collection began. From the starting date forward in time, the staff would be asked to keep careful count of the number—and perhaps color and size—of the stools on a certain cohort of babies designated as infants born from January 1 to June 30, 2009. If the number of stools related to the risk of readmission for weight loss, there would be greater confidence in this prospective study than in the retrospective one. The researchers ensured the accuracy of data collection before the study. Another term for prospective studies is cohort studies.

Cross-Sectional Study A cross-sectional study relies on record keeping or memory, much as a retrospective study does. However, researchers do not begin by identifying an affected group. Rather, they gather data from everyone at the same time. In a study about stooling and readmission rates in a cross-sectional design, for example, researchers might collect data at the time of all infants' 2-month visits. After gathering data researchers identify the affected group (readmitted infants, in this example). Researchers compare the information about their stools, feedings, and bilirubin levels with the same information for the unaffected group. Cross-sectional studies are adequate for suggesting causative factors and relevant variables. The possibility that the data collection was too dependent on recall or missed too many possible subjects on the collection day or days limits confidence in their findings.

Descriptive Study A descriptive study lists many relevant variables of a defined sample rather than compare two groups. A family practice office might want to know the characteristics of its childbearing families before designing a preconception class. The study might describe how many families in the previous year had borne a first child, how many had a second child, how many breastfed and for how long, and so on. Even though researchers gathered the information from one particular sample, they might publish their findings so that other family practices with similar types of families might benefit from the information. Descriptive studies require a thorough and careful description of the sample. Readers can then understand the degrees of similarity and difference between their own groups of families and the one studied.

Qualitative Study Another type of descriptive study is the qualitative study. In this type of study researchers observe subjects and events in a natural setting rather than establishing a control. These researchers are often looking for the meaning of an event or practice to the person experiencing it. Variables in a qualitative study usually are not measured in numbers, and differences between variables are not expressed numerically. Qualitative variables are often words that the researcher believes change together, that is, category labels. For example, as "ethnic heritage" changes, so does the "critical support person."

Qualitative research emphasizes getting a sense of the whole or comprehending the emergent properties of an experience instead of breaking down a phenomenon or experience into parts. Qualitative studies in breastfeeding, for instance, have described the feelings of women who breastfed a child for several years, as well as the empowerment of low-income women through breastfeeding. When you are evaluating such studies, you can use the more general ideas in this chapter. Because qualitative work by itself does not claim that practice should change in a particular way, qualitative research critique is discussed separately later in this chapter.

Experiments and Trials In research about breastfeeding it is less common to find studies designed as experiments. Problems that involve humans are difficult to conduct as experiments. However, researchers might study comparisons of equipment or differences between animals experimentally. The best information about a problem that involves humans comes from studies called randomized clinical trials. They are similar to experiments. These trials attempt to avoid bias in the compar-

isons they draw. If the trial is blind as well, then knowledge of which treatment the patient received remains secret until analysis of the data begins. In that way the patient's or lactation consultant's assessment of the effectiveness of treatment is not influenced by knowing to which treatment group the patient belonged. Treatment groups are as similar as possible at the beginning of the study, with great effort to identify any differences that exist. Furthermore, the groups are treated the same in all ways except for the treatment itself.

Suppose there was a new drug to eliminate mastitis caused by *Staphylococcus aureus*. To conduct a blinded study, researchers disguise the new and old drugs, perhaps by using identical capsules, and administer them in the same manner. In that way no one could tell one from another. Only a system of codes detects the difference for later analysis. Both groups are otherwise healthy, first-time breastfeeders of babies 2 to 6 months old. Therefore the groups are as similar as possible. The mastitis is diagnosed and its severity graded by strict criteria and by the same two clinicians for all subjects. Recommendations for other aspects of treatment (pain relief, treatment of baby, and so on) are the same for all subjects. In a tightly controlled study like this, differences in cure rates between the two drugs are more likely to be attributable to the drugs than in a case-control or other less controlled study.

There are several reasons why more studies are not blinded, randomized trials. First, ethical concerns preclude random assignment of people to potentially poorer treatments. Second, it is difficult to control many of the variables about people that result in comparison groups of humans who are different in many ways. Third, very large numbers of subjects are required when a trial attempts to study prevention of problems. Fourth, precision in measuring "soft" outcomes—such as quality of mother–child attachment—is lower. Funding and recognition for researchers tend to be greater when their study outcomes are "harder" and more quantifiable. Your critical analysis of clinical trials involves judgments about the researchers having adequately identified and controlled important variables.

Definitions

You should identify the important terms used in the article. These are the key concepts of the study. They may include breastfeeding, supplementation, multipara, infant, pain, treatment, exercise, and so on. In this section of the article the authors should define these terms clearly enough that you know who or what was included and excluded.

If the authors studied only multiparas, were they women with previous breastfeeding experience, or did the authors assume they had previously breastfed without specifically asking them? If they identified experienced breastfeeders, does it matter to the study's conclusions whether the previous experience was positive or negative? Is the age of the multiparas important? Is their experience coping with other stressful situations or child-rearing problems significant?

Not all multiparous women are the same. You should keep in mind what the results were and consider how the definition of multipara in the study might affect the results. All the possible differences in multiparas are variables. Critically reading the definitions includes being able to state how a different or clearer definition could change the results or the interpretation of the results.

Tools (Instruments)

Scales for weighing babies, survey questions, diet diaries, and pain ratings are examples of tools. Some tools may be intimidating if you are not familiar with them. You may not be able to analyze the tool completely if it is new to you. Still, you want to read the study because you may encounter similar tools in later reading. In addition, you should have some basic idea of how a defined term was measured to decide its applicability to your situation.

In the better studies the tools have undergone testing. Good tools should measure the dependent variable consistently. The reliability of the measurement from one time to the next may be part of the reason the investigators chose to use this tool. Authors may assume some familiarity with the type of tool without explaining the general type in much detail. For example, they expect healthcare professionals to know what a Likert scale is and how a pulse oximeter is used. Although they do not describe their Likert scale in detail, they should tell how it is different from others (whether it is a 5-point or a 7-point scale, for example). They should also tell whether the placement of the pulse oximeter was on a finger or toe. Any details about the tool itself or its use should be described clearly, so that you do not have serious questions about whether the quirks of their method are more responsible for their results than the explanation for the results that they expound.

It is not necessary that the authors publish the entire tool in the article. Its length, developmental status, or potential profitability may prevent its publication. Examples or short versions of a survey's questions may help you decide whether the tone or complexity of the questions could have influenced the way subjects answered them. If you have serious concerns about the quality of the questions, you can often write to the authors through the journal and request more information. Even if you agree with a study's conclusions, you may not want to use the study in a formal presentation until you have learned more about the tool so you can adequately answer your audience's questions.

Operationalizing

When you put together the definitions and the tools, you should understand how the researchers operationalized their concepts. Suppose they are studying the change in pain after the application of a treatment. They should tell you how they define pain. It is often the subject's verbal or written report of her pain. Alternatively, the definition might involve videotaping subjects before and after the treatment and watching for changes in facial expression.

A different tool measures each definition of pain. The tool for verbal reports might be a 10-point scale in which the anchors (words used at specific points on the scale to describe what that number means) are "1 = no pain" and "10 = the worst pain you can imagine." You can then understand that the researchers operationalized the concept "pain" by asking the subject herself to place a mark on the scale that best represented her pain before the treatment and again at a specified time afterward.

The critical reading of this operationalization involves both its clarity and your judgment about its validity. The validity of a pain measure is often supported by expert review or by comparing the current pain tool with an older one and finding that the two agree. Although pain is very difficult to measure due to its subjectivity, what is important is the person's determination of the amount of pain and whether that determination changes.

A scale that reflects the changes is the operationalization of the pain. The construction of measurement scales is the subject of many research articles. You may want to investigate previously tested tools if you decide to design a scale yourself. Below are several common methodological concerns in lactation research.

Methodological Concerns in Lactation Research

- Test weighing is not uniform. At present, this is usually resolved by careful instruction of the people who weigh the babies and by the use of electronic digital scales that are highly calibrated.
- It is difficult to equate the volume of expressed milk to the volume produced. Such volumes can be quite different unless good quality pumps are used, pumping duration is adequate, milk lets down, and the study accounts for time of day.
- Observing and measuring the breastfeeding process disturbs the natural process.
- It is difficult to obtain a representative milk sample. Milk composition varies by length of time postpartum, time of day, proportion of breast drained, and gestation of the infant.
- Changing method of feeding is a one-direction change. With rare exceptions, mothers do not usually switch from formula to breastfeeding. If a mother

changes feeding methods, it is usually a change from human to artificial. Therefore when studies encompass babies who have been fed for any length of time, some in the group usually have breastfed at some point and then bottle fed. None has fed in the reverse order. This can make it difficult to interpret growth differences. To improve growth, mothers may try to switch to formula, but they cannot switch to breastfeeding. Most researchers believe that there are ways to overcome this built-in direction, but that may complicate interpretation.

- Studies of environmental contaminants often use human milk because it is easier to obtain than blood or other body tissue and because milk fats promote the accumulation of some chemicals in milk. However, the media may misunderstand the use of milk, implying that finding a pollutant in milk automatically means that feeding human milk is harmful.

- Studies of effects of breastfeeding on women's bone mineralization have sometimes been misunderstood because the time it takes to recover bone mass that was mobilized during lactation has been longer than the length of the study.

When you have read and thought about the methods, think back to the results. Do the study design, definitions, tools, and operationalizations allow for the conclusions the scientists made? How could they have done the study differently to make you believe that the conclusions were more justified? What additional information about the methods would help you evaluate the findings even more thoroughly?

Statistics

A brief description of the main statistical approach used to evaluate the data is usually found within the methods section of the article. For lactation consultants this section may be the most difficult to decipher because the language is so specialized. As you have learned, a lot of meaningful critical analysis can occur, even without judging the statistical techniques used. To some extent you must rely on the peer-review process to catch any major problems in the statistics. The more you read breastfeeding research, the more you become familiar with some of the common approaches used in certain research designs. The examples presented in the following sections help you understand some of these more common statistical ideas and tests.

Statistical Theory Statistical theory is based on probability, a mathematical discipline that focuses on trying to precisely answer finely tuned questions about uncertain events. Statistical theory uses probability to answer real questions based on real data (Dean & Illowsky, 2009). For

example, if one is wondering whether the Euro coin is biased (i.e., tends to land heads more often than tails or vice versa) you might flip the coin, say, 100 times and record how often heads results from those 100 flips. Statistics would then allow you to take the observed number of heads (the data) and see if there is convincing evidence of a bias. For example, if you observe only 37 heads in the 100 flips, a pattern that would happen less than 1 percent of the time if you were flipping a fair coin, you would conclude that the coin has some bias. Sample size (the number of data points) is important. If there is an interesting trend (for example, if low-birth-weight babies tend to have lower IQ scores later in life), the larger the sample, the more likely we would see this pattern in the data in a way that convinces us of the reality of what was observed.

Study Frequency When you study the frequency of breastfeeding by mothers and their babies at 10 days of age in your city, you are studying a sample of the whole population of 10-day-old breastfed babies and their mothers (in the world, and maybe throughout human history). If your goal in studying the frequency in this sample was to publish in a textbook that the "normal" or "usual" or "average" frequency for all human babies at 10 days was x, then you would be trying to make a statement about the population by studying a sample of it. If your sample is large (500 subjects or more) there is far less chance of an error in your estimate of x than if your sample is only 20 subjects.

Good studies aim for the largest sample size they can reasonably get. The statistical analysis tells the power of that sample size. Power relies on more than sample size. However, sample size is what researchers have the most control over, so they try to maximize it. For most purposes researchers want a power of 0.80 (80 percent) or higher. If the power of a test is low, then the reason for failing to find a significant difference between two groups could be that the sample selected was too small for that difference to show up, not that there is no real difference. A power of 80 percent means that the data have an 80 percent probability of correctly rejecting the null hypothesis.

Statistical Tests Statistical tests are valid only when applied correctly. To be valid, each test assumes certain things about the data. If those assumptions are not true, the test should not be used. Sometimes in the methods section there is a brief statement about why a certain test was used and whether or not a particular assumption was met. There are few hard-and-fast rules in statistical analysis. Statisticians disagree, just as lactation consultants do, about which should be the first solution to try.

Discussions about assumptions often speak to potential readers who are researchers and statisticians who might disagree with the choice of statistical test. One such discussion sometimes centers on whether or not the assumption of a normal distribution of the data is true. A normal distribution describes much of the infinite data we could collect about the natural world. A normal distribution, plotted on a graph, looks like a bell curve. Look, for example, at the graph entitled "How much milk the 1-month-old infant takes at a single episode at breast" (see Figure 27.3).

The left end of the graph shows a few babies who take very tiny amounts, perhaps when nursing is very frequent and short. The right end shows a few babies who take a very large amount. Assuming that most babies take in about 120 mL, the center of the graph (the large hill or bell) represents what the bulk of babies do. Between the center and each extreme is a gradual slope.

Now, instead, suppose the data on milk intake actually comes from a distribution that looks like the graph in Figure 27.4. Here, the bulk (greatest number of values) of the data is at one extreme, not in the middle. The left side rises quickly with a long slope off to the right. Perhaps this is a group of preterm infants at 1 month of age whose intake tends to be less than that of full-term infants. A statistical test that was attempting to predict what happens

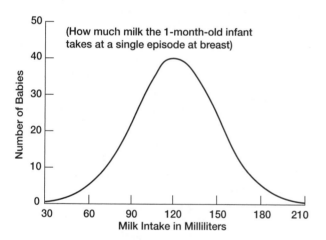

FIGURE 27.3   Centered bell curve.

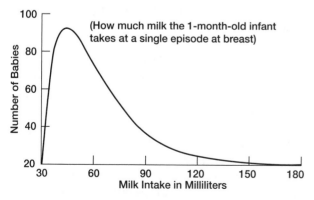

FIGURE 27.4   Unbalanced bell curve.

in the bulk of this distribution by expecting it to be a normal distribution would be way off. The middle in this distribution is far to the left of where it would be with normal distribution of the data. The data in Figure 27.4 require a statistical test designed for this particular distribution. It is very important that researchers and statisticians carefully choose which tests to use and that they look at all the underlying assumptions, including distribution of the data.

Statistical Significance Statistical significance, or lack of significance, is determined by applying a statistical test to a fact about the data (a result) and calculating the probability of obtaining that result (or more extreme result). The probability is reported as a *P* value. Most researchers want *P* values that are 0.05 or lower. The *P* value measures the risk of rejecting a true null hypothesis. Researchers want the chance of falsely stating that there is a real difference between two groups to be 5 percent or less.

Confidence intervals (CIs) provide information about the statistical significance of a result. CIs are the range within which a population's true value is expected to be found. Usually, a 95 percent CI is reported. This describes the other possible results that are close to the one that actually came from the data and that are likely to contain the true population value. So, if the mean (average) of the weight gain from the study's sample was 200 g and the 95 percent CI was 185 to 215 g, then it is likely that the population's true weight gain is somewhere between 185 and 215 g.

Large CIs (from 50 to 350 g, for this example) do not tell you very much. Nearly every weight gain falls somewhere in that interval, so you cannot tell the difference between a usual one and a more extreme one. Large CIs often arise when the sample size is small. Furthermore, if you are trying to compare, for example, the weight gains in two different groups and you expect them to be different, you do not want their CIs to overlap. So, if the mean for group A (breastfed) is 200 g (95 percent CI, 185 to 215 g) and the mean for group B (formula fed) is 220 g (95 percent CI, 205 to 235 g), the intervals share the values 205 to 215 g. These shared values mean that the real average weight gain could be the same for both groups. These CIs would not allow you to claim you had found a statistically significant difference between the two groups. (See "odds ratio" below for another example of the use of a CI.)

Common Statistical Tests and Terms This section on common statistical tests and terms can help you understand some of the tests you are most likely to encounter.

Chi-Square. There are several slightly different versions of the chi-square test. It is typically used to determine whether the proportions in two groups are significantly different. You may want to determine, for example, if the proportion of experienced breastfeeders who have mastitis is the same as the proportion of first-time breastfeeders who have mastitis. Large chi-square values usually lead to low, statistically significant *P* values.

Cohen's Kappa. Cohen's kappa is calculated when two observers rate the same event on a scale and the researcher wants to show that the two raters are in close agreement. Values at 0.7 or higher are considered good.

Cronbach's Alpha. A Cronbach's alpha test is often reported when the researcher is trying to give evidence of the reliability of an instrument. Values can range from 0.0 to 1.0. The closer they are to 1.0, the better the reliability.

Odds Ratio. Odds ratio is not a statistical test; rather, it is a way to summarize the relative proportion of illness in two different groups. For example, you may want to compare the proportion of breastfed babies who get otitis media with the proportion of artificially fed babies who do, under certain similar conditions. If you found that 2 of 10 breastfed babies developed otitis media and 4 of 10 formula fed babies did, the ratio of those odds is 0.2/0.4 = 0.5. The odds of the breastfed baby getting an ear infection were one-half the odds of the baby who failed to receive human milk's protection.

The only way an odds ratio could equal 1 is if the odds for both groups are the same. CIs for odds ratios might be written like this: "0.5 (95% CI, 0.35–0.60)." This means that the best estimate of the odds ratio could be anywhere from 0.35 to 0.60. Significant CIs for the odds ratio should not contain "1" (0.90–1.05, for example) because that would mean the odds ratio could be 1. This is another way of saying that the odds for the breastfed baby were the same as the odds for the artificially fed baby. In studies comparing breastfed infants, bottle fed infants, and differing risks, we would expect to find that the breastfed babies had less risk.

Regression. Regression is a technique used to try to understand the relationship between variables. Simple regression relates one predictor variable (or independent variable) to one outcome variable (or dependent variable). Multiple regression relates several variables to one outcome variable. Logistic regression relates one or more variables to a dichotomous outcome (two-possibility) variable. This addresses a question such as, "Do maternal satisfaction, infant weight gain, and family support with the first breastfed child relate to the decision to breastfeed or not breastfeed [dichotomous outcome] the next child?" Regression methods usually try to estimate how much change there is in the outcome variable for a one-unit change in the predictor variable. For example, "How much change occurs in infant crying time for each additional half-hour of being carried in a baby sling?"

t Test. Use of a *t* test is to decide between two contradictory hypotheses about the mean of a sample. For example, you may want to know if the average weight gain of breastfed infants in hospital A is the same as the average weight gain for all breastfed babies in the United States (where the national average is often considered a "norm" or "true" population value). A slightly different *t* test could be used to compare the average gain of babies in hospital A with that of babies in hospital B.

Step 7: Read the Introduction and Literature Review

You can now read the introduction and literature review to understand some of the decisions the researchers made in light of the results they found and the methods they used. You can ask yourself whether the authors' justification for doing the study seems adequate to you. Most articles start out by stating that some expert bodies recognize the superiority of breastfeeding. They may then say that although breastfeeding by all mothers is preferable, there is such-and-such a problem that prevents near-universal breastfeeding. They might claim their study is going to address that problem, shed light on it, and help move humankind toward more breastfeeding.

Often, the authors explain and reference the theory underlying their approach to the problem and the hypothesis they want to test. Somewhere in this line of reasoning is the explicit or implicit statement of why the authors chose this particular problem to study.

The literature review is used to show how their study is different from what has been done before and how their study is an improvement. If they have done a good job of this reasoning, they convince you that (1) the problem is significant, (2) no one has adequately addressed it before, and (3) their approach is superior. You can use your experience and your reading of other articles and books to decide whether they have convinced you of this. The questions to ask yourself are discussed in the following section.

Questions to Guide Your Reading

- Do you believe this is a significant problem? Have they explained why? If you were a professional who is interested but not very experienced in lactation, would their explanation be convincing?
- Are the summaries of the articles they cite to explain their study accurate? If you know the studies they cite, did they do a good job of stating the conclusions?
- If you know any of the studies, do you believe they are appropriate ones to use? For example, if the new study you are reading is about colic-like symptoms in fully breastfed babies but the cited studies included

partially breastfed babies, what parts can legitimately be compared and what parts have to be different? Suppose the new study wants to use removal of dairy products from the mother's diet as a treatment. That could be a clear change in an exclusively breastfed baby's diet. But in a baby who is also receiving some cow's milk formula, a comparable change in diet would need to include removal of the formula. On the other hand, the older study may have found that first-born infants suffered more colic-like symptoms and the new study might want to examine birth order. That aspect of both studies is more similar than exposure to cow's milk because birth order does not directly relate to cow's milk or maternal diet. If you do not know any of the studies cited, you will not be as able to judge their appropriateness. You will grow in your ability to do this as you read more.

- Did they omit any studies that you would have included? Do you know about previous research (even if you do not know the exact title or authors' names) that also addresses this problem but that the authors left out? If it is an area of research with several previous studies, lack of space may be the cause. However, it may happen by design if the authors do not want to mention contrary studies, especially if those studies rejected what the authors wish to convey. Leaving out relevant studies may also result from an inadequate literature search. However, usually peer reviewers demand that prospective authors read and include the most important articles. Leaving out relevant studies may not be too damaging to readers who know the background information well. It can portray a misleading picture of the state of knowledge to those unfamiliar with the background information.

- Are the methods that were used in previous studies explained fully enough that you can judge whether the authors' use or rejection of them in the new study is appropriate? For example, in a study of infection rates in children who attend day care versus those who do not attend day care, the literature review may describe the use of "written parental diaries" as the method. The authors may tell you that they propose to use the same method as previous studies, having parents record weekly whether the child had fever, sore throat, medical visits, and so on. Suppose they find that children in day care have no different infection rates than stay-at-home children, although previous studies have found a difference. The authors may have failed to mention that in the older study parents recorded symptoms on a daily basis and received biweekly calls and cards to remind them to do so. That may explain why the older study found differences in rates while the new study does not. You

are looking for ways in which the current study is different from and similar to the older studies cited in the literature review. The authors should be clear about those aspects that are relevant to the current study.

Step 8: Read the Discussion

There usually is a link between the literature review and the discussion. The authors may explain the link in the beginning of the discussion section. You should ask yourself whether the intentions the researchers declared based on their review of the current state of knowledge carried through to the methods and results. Ask if they did something different from the earlier cited studies and, if so, whether it was an improvement.

In the discussion the researchers may summarize their results in a less formal way. They may offer an interpretation of the results that puts their findings into the context of other studies conducted on the same problem. You should consider whether their findings are as important as the authors claim and whether the state of knowledge about the problem is now more complete or clearer.

Speculation

The authors may stretch the interpretation of their findings into a more speculative understanding of some aspect of the problem. An example of this is a study that found that peanut butter and jelly sandwiches correlated with higher milk production. Suppose the authors had found evidence in the literature review that a chemical in peanuts could cause an appetite increase in lab animals. They put these two ideas together to suggest that the reason peanut butter and jelly sandwiches are associated with higher milk production is that the sandwiches stimulated appetite in breastfeeding mothers who eat them. Their study did not really look at either the chemistry of peanuts or the overall calorie intake of mothers. Nevertheless, they speculate that such a causal mechanism exists.

It is your job, as a critical reader, to judge how plausible, realistic, and rational that link is. You do not know if the link is correct, but you need to think about whether it could be real and whether further suggestions by the authors along this line of reasoning are worth considering.

Suggestions for Further Research

Often, the next step the researchers take is to suggest further research. Some suggestions are to test the speculations they made. Other suggestions are to fill in the gaps in the understanding of the problem that remain in spite of the knowledge gained from their study.

Flaws or Weaknesses

The authors may acknowledge in the discussion some of the flaws or weaknesses you detected in reading the article. You can decide whether your assessment of the flaws (and their impact on the confidence you have in the results) is the same as that of the authors. If you believe the problems are more serious than the authors acknowledge, you want to read their justification as generously as you can. On the other hand, if the authors fail to note a flaw you have uncovered, you should try to understand why. This may be just another opportunity to reinforce your critique, but it could be that the goal or methods as explained further in the discussion are different from your original understanding of them.

Step 9: Read the Results Again

When you first read the results section, you were trying to understand what the authors claimed to have found. This time, read to decide whether you believe those claims were justified. You probably formed some judgments about this already, having read the methods and discussion. The following suggestions lead you to look even more closely at the logic of the relationships between variables that the authors claim to have found. Recall the three steps discussed previously:

1. Data need to be consistent with the claims.
2. There must be no other equal or better explanation.
3. A plausible mechanism must link the two variables.

Data Consistent with Claims

Are the data consistent with the claims? Consider again the example of the study testing the effect of discharge packs on the duration of breastfeeding. If the study had 100 subjects (50 in the pack group and 50 in the nonpack group) and if 15 in the pack group weaned "early" but only 5 did in the nonpack group, is that a convincing difference to you? This difference would be statistically significant at $P = 0.05$. That is, there is only a 1 in 20 chance that a difference of 15 versus 5 (or a more extreme difference) occurred by chance. Therefore, statistically speaking, it is probable that the difference between the numbers of early weaners in the two groups is a real difference and not a chance occurrence. However, you could ask whether that difference is clinically important. Do 10 more "late" weaners out of 50 achieve enough additional health and relationship benefits to warrant discontinuing discharge packs?

This question is not just about statistics but also about values. Many healthcare providers probably consider this valid and important evidence against discharge packs. Skeptics, however, might say, "Well, if discharge packs are so bad, then how did 35 of 50 mothers go on to wean late in spite of them?" Considering answers to such questions helps you think about the study and formulate responses you could use if you presented this study to skeptics.

Another Possible Explanation for the Relationship

Is there another possible explanation for the claimed relationship between variables? To continue looking at the logical steps, think about another way of presenting the numbers. Instead of defining "early" and "late" and comparing the proportions in each group, suppose the average number of weeks of breastfeeding was computed in the pack group versus the nonpack group.

You need to take a close look at whatever numbers the authors present. Usually, you find that they have chosen appropriate ways to measure and summarize their data. Nevertheless, you may find that you have questions about their numbers that make you reluctant to agree with their conclusions.

Averages and Distribution Range If the study found that those who received packs breastfed for 18 weeks and those who did not breastfed for 20 weeks, would you believe this was an important difference? This could be a statistically significant difference between the groups, depending on the group sizes and the degree of variation in the averages. Whenever an average (mean) is reported, you may want to know the distribution and range of each group's length of breastfeeding. An average can be misleading if one subject (or a small number) has an extremely short or extremely long duration. Figure 27.5 demonstrates the number of different ways a group could breastfeed for an average of 18 weeks.

Group 1 had many people who actually breastfed for 18 weeks and four people who breastfeed for a shorter or longer amount of time. In this kind of distribution the average gives a good representation of the typical behavior in the group. The range is 25 – 11 = 14 weeks. Group 2 had only one person who breastfed the "average" length of time and two people whose duration was very different from the average (outliers), 2 and 50. The range in these data is 48 (50 – 2 = 48). The range in group 1 was smaller.

You might legitimately question whether the extremes in group 2 had much in common with the average. Specifically, you might wonder whether the 2-week person had a difficult problem, such as a baby with ankyloglossia and a severe cardiac defect, so that she would have breastfed only 2 weeks regardless of whether she received a discharge pack. After asking yourself that question, you should look in the results section to determine whether the authors describe the mothers' reasons for weaning. If that information is absent or not collected, the

Group 1	Group 2	Group 3
25 weeks	50 weeks	29 weeks
20 weeks	19 weeks	27 weeks
18 weeks	18 weeks	26 weeks
18 weeks	17 weeks	25 weeks
18 weeks	16 weeks	24 weeks
18 weeks	16 weeks	23 weeks
18 weeks	15 weeks	22 weeks
18 weeks	14 weeks	2 weeks
16 weeks	13 weeks	1 week
11 weeks	2 weeks	1 week
180 weeks	180 weeks	180 weeks

FIGURE 27.5 Ten subjects who breastfed an average of 18 weeks.

authors cannot claim that discharge packs alone made a difference in the groups.

Looking closely at the numbers to determine if they are consistent with the claims may suggest a possible alternative explanation for the study's findings. At least a few mothers may have had an extremely difficult problem that would have led to short breastfeeding, regardless of whether or not they received a pack. Excluding these mothers' durations from the calculation of duration might change the study's results. Of course, you cannot know that the results would change. Nevertheless, if the authors' data make you suspicious, you might ultimately be less willing to accept and apply their findings.

Another example of looking closely at the "average" is the other extreme in group 2. Suppose the mother who breastfed for 50 weeks was in the discharge pack group. You might ask, "If discharge packs are so bad, how did this woman manage to continue to breastfeed for so long?" Several possible explanations exist, and you might wonder whether the authors asked what the mothers did with the packs. Did they use them? If yes, how old was the baby? Did they discard the pack? If you read some of the real studies of discharge packs, you will find that the authors rarely ask this question. Instead, there is an assumption that mere receipt of a pack probably encourages formula use. Although this may be true, the results would be stronger with data collected on actual use of the packs as well as formula use in the nonpack group.

Hidden Differences Between Groups In group 3 no one breastfed to 18 weeks, and there is quite a clear separation into two subgroups, one who nursed for 2 weeks or less and the other who nursed for at least 22 weeks. Such a split might make you think about the possibility of a major

difference within the group. Perhaps, for example, the two subgroups received substantially different amounts of support. The subgroup who breastfed longer may have had three or more support people, whereas the subgroup who breastfed less may have had two or fewer support people. So, although this entire group breastfed for an average of 18 weeks, that average does not well represent the real story about the group. By trying to explain the duration of breastfeeding using an average, the authors may have missed an alternative explanation for their findings related to differences in support.

Many studies try to avoid potential alternative explanations for their findings by avoiding major hidden differences between groups (like the difference in support cited earlier) through random assignment of subjects to groups. The idea is that if mothers are assigned by chance to receive a discharge pack, differences other than receipt of a pack between groups are approximately the same in both groups. Differences that could confuse the explanation of findings are called confounding variables. In randomized assignment to groups, there is approximately the same number of multiparas, people with good support, people with inverted nipples, and so on in both groups. Therefore all the reasons they could have stopped breastfeeding early is the same in both groups except for receipt of a discharge pack. Random assignment, then, allows researchers to conclude that the reason the women stopped breastfeeding must be the single relevant difference between the groups—receipt of a discharge pack.

The best studies go even further and check whether random assignment worked. In such studies the authors report whether the groups were different at baseline in some important ways. As their colleague, you need to consider whether they checked on the right things. For example, if you believe lack of support is important in early weaning, did the scientists check their groups to be sure that, say, the average number of support people reported by mothers in the pack and nonpack groups was not statistically different? This checking for the differences and similarities achieved by random assignment is reported in the methods or results section. It is not possible to check for all differences. However, it is important to check for a few major ones, and it is up to you to decide whether the researchers omitted anything critical. If they did, you may be less likely to use the findings of the study.

Most articles related to the practice of helping women with breastfeeding do not have randomized groups. Rather they use a convenience (nonprobability) sample. Therefore, for a study about discharge packs, the sample might be the first 100 breastfeeding mothers after the starting date (in which mothers 1 to 50 do not get packs and 51 to 100 receive packs). Checking the basic similarity of groups is even more important in convenience samples than in randomized ones.

Plausible Mechanism for Relationship

Is there a plausible mechanism for the claimed relationship between variables? This may be the most difficult of the logical steps for which to find clear evidence in the article. Sometimes authors address the reason lanolin seems to help heal sore nipples, for example, in the literature review or in the discussion section. They usually do not address this in the results section unless they have studied the possible mechanism along with the relationship between variables.

For example, along with testing whether lanolin led to faster healing, they may have taken microscopic photos of cell changes in nipple skin to see if the differences in cell changes might explain healing differences. In many studies researchers hypothesize the mechanism itself and do not study it directly. This is especially true when the variables are not physiological but rather psychological or sociological.

Demonstrating a plausible mechanism for how peer support enables longer durations of breastfeeding than professional support does is not straightforward. Yet many mechanisms for important relationships between variables related to breastfeeding are in the "not straight-forward" category. Instead of dismissing research because of an inability to demonstrate mechanisms convincingly, most scientists and clinicians instead require plausibility and thoughtful consideration of mechanisms. In your critical reading you want to consider whether a mechanism is discussed and whether you judge that mechanism to be reasonable. If there is very little consideration of how and why the variables are related as the study found them to be, you may be less likely to accept the study's findings.

Spurious Relationships Sometimes there is little discussion of mechanism because the mechanism is obvious. The greatest danger in the lack of a plausible mechanism is the acceptance of a relationship that is actually spurious. Spurious relationships between variables are those that look statistically significant but have resulted from a correlation with no underlying meaning.

Suppose that lactation consultant Lila Cecilia found that of her last 500 clients, the ones whose babies' home nurseries were painted lavender had a statistically significantly longer duration of breastfeeding than those whose nurseries were any other color. Suppose, further, that Lila had determined that no alternative explanations adequately fit her data. She really did not know why the color of the nursery mattered but she claimed that breastfed babies should have their nurseries painted lavender.

Many readers might guess Lila had failed to study hard enough to find the explanation. Most readers would not rush out and tell their clients to repaint their nurseries. They would not be convinced because there is no plausible relationship between nursery color and breastfeeding duration. The numeric relationship Lila found was probably spurious.

Any time a study finds a relationship for which the authors present no plausible mechanism, it could be spurious. This most often happens when researchers just happen to notice some correlation in their data that was not the main relationship they were studying. In doing a variety of manipulations of the data, sometimes a relationship surfaces that is statistically significant. Although the authors may mention this "finding" in their article, it is not good science to claim it as a major result. Instead, they can consider the mechanisms and recommend further research.

Scientific Research Misconduct Be aware that misconduct occurs in the world of academic research. In a meta-analysis of surveys on research misconduct, it was found that about 2 percent of scientists admitted to having fabricated, falsified, or modified data or results at least once. A third of them admitted to other questionable research practices as well. Misconduct was reported more frequently by medical and pharmacological researchers than by others (Fanelli, 2009). Fanelli describes fabrication as the invention of data or cases, falsification as the willful distortion of data or results, and plagiarism as the copying of ideas, data, or words without attribution.

Misconduct was exposed recently regarding research findings of Dr. Ranjit Chandra. Chandra's work on allergies in infants and children was cited in journals and textbooks (including previous editions of this text) for years. In the late 1980s Nestlé launched an infant formula, Nestlé Good Start, that the company claimed could reduce infants' risk of developing allergies. Chandra reported findings to justify the claims. Much of his work has since come under intense scrutiny for academic fraud. One of his studies was discredited and retracted by the periodical that initially published it, the *British Medical Journal*. A CBC national documentary reported that much of Dr. Chandra's research may have been fraudulently produced (Infant Feeding Action Coalition, 2006). This illustrates the potential for corruption in industry-funded research where lack of controls and accountability exist.

It can be challenging to detect when errors or misconduct occur. A study found that peer reviewers for journals seem to prefer studies with positive findings. When asked to rate two bogus manuscripts, most trained peer reviewers strongly preferred the paper with positive findings. Five errors were placed in both papers using the same mistakes in the same places within the manuscript. Errors were overlooked more often in the positive paper than in the equivocal one (Raloff, 2009).

∼ *Practicing Critical Reading Skills*

Now you are ready to practice using the ideas and the steps for critical reading presented earlier. Using steps 1 through 9 read the following two mock articles in the suggested order. You should consider the questions presented in each section. You may find it helpful to make notes to yourself as you go through the process so you can compare your ideas with those presented in the commentary that follows each mock article.

Before you read the commentary, return to the beginning of Critical Reading of a Scientific Article and apply the process to the article. Consider each part separately and in the order suggested, and make notes to yourself about the strengths and flaws you find. Then compare your ideas with those that follow. You probably have some ideas not mentioned here. As long as you can justify them logically or by reference to other studies, your commentary is valuable.

First Practice Article

Sore Nipple Treatments: Gooeypaste Works Best

I.M. Wright

Journal of Supposed Things, Vol. 21, pp. 5–10, 2009.

Abstract

Sore nipples are one of the obstacles many women need to overcome to continue breastfeeding. Thirty women began using Gooeypaste, warm water compresses, or lanolin when their nipples became sore. After 3 days Gooeypaste provided more pain relief than the other treatments as measured on the Pain Relief Self-Rating. Gooeypaste should become the standard treatment for breastfeeding-related nipple soreness.

Introduction

Breastfeeding is acknowledged by healthcare professionals worldwide as the best way to feed infants.[2–4] However, women who intend to breastfeed for many weeks or months are sometimes stopped by the development of nipple soreness, which makes breastfeeding intolerable.[4,5] No single measure or combination of measures has been found to reliably reduce pain and increase healing. Although prevention is surely the best policy, the need for treatment is evident. This study was designed to investigate the effectiveness of a new product against two standard treatments.

Review of the Literature

Pain with breastfeeding has been shown to be an important reason for early weaning in several studies[1,4,5] and may include pain due to engorgement or candidiasis as well as sore nipples. Positioning is important to the prevention of soreness. Sometimes, comfortable positioning is not achieved with the first few feedings, and, by then, enough nipple damage is done that pain results. In addition, nipple pain may occur later in breastfeeding when the baby tries to interact with the world while nursing or when solid foods begin. Cando[6] found that warm water compresses applied for 15 minutes after every feeding relieved pain better than two other measures. In a study by Workhard,[7] lanolin felt soothing to mothers with nipple soreness.

Relief from pain has been measured in many different ways. In keeping with the Ouchless[8] theory of pain perception, tools that measure the patient's perception of pain were reviewed for possible use. The Painometer, a self-rated, five-question scale, was believed to be the most convenient for a busy, new mother to use. The scale has been used before in postoperative patients and was found to correlate with the use of medication. In addition to the questions about degree of pain, there are three questions about coping with the pain.

In Helpful Hospital's Mother-Baby Unit, obstetricians prescribed lanolin for routine use by breastfeeding mothers. Some nurses encouraged mothers to use warm water, but mothers' actual use of these products and the relief provided by them had never been evaluated. When the new product, Gooeypaste, developed by Phunny Pharmaceuticals, became available, the staff decided it was time to conduct a study.

(Continued)

Subjects and Methods

Table 27.1 describes the subjects of the study. Subjects were recruited from the Mother–Baby Unit on the day of their postpartum stay when they first began to develop sore nipples. Except for mothers who had undergone cesarean births, most were discharged by 24 to 48 hours. When a nurse identified a mother with soreness who agreed to participate in the study, an envelope was pulled from the enrollment drawer. The envelopes were in random order (10 envelopes each for warm water, lanolin, and Gooeypaste), and each contained instructions for the mother and nurse on which treatment was to be used. Each also contained three copies of the Painometer that the mother was to complete at 24, 48, and 72 hours after she first started using her assigned treatment.

While the subjects were hospitalized, nurses reminded them to complete the scale. The nurses collected them and stored them anonymously with codes that identified the treatment used and whether this was the 24-, 48-, or 72-hour scale. For subjects who went home before all scales were completed (this included almost all subjects), nurses called mothers to remind them to complete the scales and return them in the envelopes provided. If the mother seemed especially unlikely to return her scales, nurses asked mothers the scale's questions over the telephone and recorded them. Results were analyzed by odds ratios for the odds of experiencing less pain by day 3. In addition, the mother's responses on the questions about coping were analyzed by comparing means.

TABLE 27.1   The Subjects of the Study.

	Gooey-paste	Warm Water	Lanolin
Maternal age (mean)	22.3 yrs	25.3 yrs	24.2 yrs
Breastfed previous baby	8	5	4*
Female infants	5	7	3
Infant birthweight (mean)	3500 g	3405 g	3200 g
Number of infants who had alternative feedings prior to starting the study	1	2	3

*No statistically significant differences between groups, p = 0.15.

Results

Thirty new mothers agreed to participate in the study. Of these, 28 went home before they completed all the scales. All mothers were called at the appropriate follow-up times for reminders. As a result, all 30 had completed scales for all three measurement times.

For 15 mothers, pain worsened from 24 to 48 hours after the first treatment. Three of those were using Gooeypaste, five using warm water, and seven using lanolin. Pain remained the same for two mothers from each group. It improved for five mothers using Gooeypaste, three using warm water, and one using lanolin. By 72 hours eight mothers using Gooeypaste noted improvement, whereas six using warm water and four using lanolin reported improvement in pain.

The odds ratio for decreased pain at 72 hours comparing Gooeypaste to lanolin was 1.3. The odds ratio comparing Gooeypaste to warm water was 2.0. Both were statistically significant at $P = 0.05$.

The average score for optimism was higher in the Gooeypaste group than in the other treatment groups (see Table 27.2). Although that trend was nonsignificant, optimism remains an important part of pain relief.

TABLE 27.2   Pain Score.

	Mean Pain Score at Each Time*		
	24 hours	48 hours	72 hours
Gooeypaste	7	8	5
Warm water	6	8	6
Lanolin	7	9	7

*Mean for the 10 mothers using that method.

Discussion

Although this is a small study, Gooeypaste appears to be an important measure to consider for the treatment of sore nipples. Further studies with larger groups of patients are needed to confirm these findings. Because the Gooeypaste mothers were also more optimistic, they will probably go on to breastfeed in greater numbers to meet their personal goals. The nursing staff at Helpful Hospital is currently working with the obstetric staff to include Gooeypaste as an alternative treatment for sore nipples in breastfeeding mothers.

References

1. Healthy World Alliance. Breastfeeding best for babies. *HWA.* 56:123-125; 2008.
2. Bet U, Wynn R. Nutrition experts endorse breastfeeding. *Nutrition Group Reports.* 25:2-5; 2008.
3. Up G. Support for breastfeeding grows. *Child Health Studie.s* 50:3-9; 2007.
4. Rocks M. A study of engorgement. *Human Nurturing.* 23:21-28; 2006.
5. Complete D. Weaning from breast. *Feeding Babies Journal.* 11:335-339; 2009.
6. Cando Y. Providing relief for breastfeeding problems. *HA.* 58:130-140; 2009.
7. Workhard S. The many uses of lanolin. *Journal of the Natural Products Industry.* 12:22-26; 2007.
8. Ouchless T. A theory of pain: The patient knows. *Human Nurturing.* 1:70-80; 1998.

Note: The author wishes to express gratitude to Phunny Pharmaceuticals for the provision of Gooeypaste, lanolin, and copies of the Painometer.

Discussion of First Practice Article

Title Your considerations of this article can begin by asking yourself what you believe the article is about just from reading the title. Because this article focuses on treatment, information about the cause of the soreness is certainly important. Did the author look at causes? Will the results vary depending on the cause? Sore nipples due to continued pacifier use and resultant tongue movements are expected to take longer to resolve than the initial tenderness of getting started breastfeeding. Therefore if the author did not ensure that the causes were the same in the comparison groups, the results might differ for that reason alone, no matter what the treatment was.

Also, consider what you already know. Because early soreness is often due to poor positioning, did the author measure attempts at correct positioning? Other studies demonstrate that much nipple soreness diminishes with time. However, no treatments to date have reduced that time dramatically. A control group that does not use any treatment might be important to determine the baseline pain experience to judge whether any of the treatments is better than just the passage of time.

Does the title suggest surprises? What is Gooeypaste? It must be a new product and so may be available only to researchers. In addition to measuring pain, will the study attempt to document wound healing as some research has done?

If you had designed a study on nipple soreness, would you have limited the ages of the babies? Would you have limited the previous experience of the mothers? Both of these factors might influence the expected duration and ability to cope with the pain. If the groups have underlying differences in such variables, the expectation that their pain experience would be the same is not justifiable.

Authors' Names This author is not one you have read before (since he or she is fictitious!). You would ordinarily want to keep this name in mind for future reading.

Abstract Which of the aspects of the study that you thought about from looking at the title does the abstract clarify? For one, the abstract does not clarify much about the mothers' experience or the babies' ages. Because the abstract recommends Gooeypaste, you would expect to find a strong relationship (documented later in the results) between its use and pain relief.

Tables and Graphs Table 27.1 tells more about the subjects. You may have many questions after you look at this table. The average maternal age is not the same in the groups, and the author reports no tests to check whether the differences are statistically significant. The author,

and you, may decide that there is no clinically significant difference; that is, that age differences like these are not likely to contribute in important ways to how the mothers respond to treatment.

You are probably more concerned about the differences between the treatment groups in the numbers who have breastfed previously. The Gooeypaste group has twice as many mothers who previously breastfed as does the lanolin group. Although the statistical test showed the groups to be not statistically significantly different, that may be because each treatment group has only 10 subjects, a small sample. Before you apply the results of this study to your practice, you might want to see a study in which the experienced breastfeeders are represented equally (or closer to equally) in each treatment group.

A further consideration, not clear from this table and seldom considered in the literature, is whether those previous breastfeeding experiences were favorable. Many women, when asked if they breastfed a previous child, say "yes" even if they only breastfed for 1 week and that week was full of problems. The level of confidence and the interpretation of pain for such women are likely to be different from that of an experienced breastfeeder who met her goals and overcame problems.

The number of female infants looks different in each group as well. However, unless you know of research that links gender of the infant to pain perception or treatment effectiveness, it probably does not matter. Do you believe that infant birth weight could be an important difference between treatment groups? None of these groups has an average that makes us think about preterm babies. However, if you reread the abstract, there is no statement that all babies were full term. Therefore it is possible that any of the groups could have a preterm baby in it.

We might be especially concerned that the lanolin group had more preterm babies than the other two groups. Preterm babies may take longer to learn effective sucking and, thereby, affect their mother's pain perception. We do not know for sure (1) that there are preterm babies in the lanolin group or (2) that preterm babies necessarily correlate with differences in healing sore nipples. Nevertheless, we do know that many preterm babies are more difficult to nurse in the first few days. Therefore we wonder whether there might be a hidden difference between the treatment groups, such as prematurity, for example. The difference could alter the explanation for the reported faster pain relief in the Gooeypaste group. Such an unanswered question may be serious enough that we may not want to apply this study's findings without more information.

The author also reports the number of infants who received alternative feedings before starting the study. The table does not clarify whether the feedings were by bottle or cup, so we hope that information is in the text. Statistical tests are absent, so you must consider the possibility that the differences are important clinically. How might bottle feeding or cup feeding affect the mothers' pain perception? Notice that the table does not tell how many times each of the babies who received an alternative feeding were fed that way. It only tells how many babies (out of 10 in each group) were fed by some other method.

Now take your critical reading of this table another step further. By now, you may have collected doubts about the underlying similarity of the lanolin group and the Gooeypaste group. That is, you may be concerned that (1) the number of mothers who previously breastfed differs; (2) there may be more small, possibly preterm, babies in the lanolin group; and (3) there are more babies who had alternative feedings in that group as well. Before reading the text of the article, you have begun to suspect that the groups may have started differently, both before they developed sore nipples and before they used treatments. These differences are potentially associated with sore nipples (unlike gender of the infants, which, although different between groups, is probably not related to pain). It is possible that these differences could be an alternative explanation for the different pain perceptions between the groups rather than the different treatments. Keep these doubts in mind as you read the next table and the remainder of the text.

Table 27.2 reports average pain scores for each group. Does this seem to you to be the most meaningful way to analyze the data? Could the author instead have shown a table of improvement versus no improvement? Do we know enough about the Painometer to know what a "7" means? There was no discussion of how many points were on the scale, or what the descriptive anchors were at each end. We would also expect a table like this to report whether the pain score averages are different for each treatment group.

Looking at the numbers—without a statistical analysis—would you anticipate a clinically important difference to be demonstrated for Gooeypaste? That is, is there a big difference between Gooeypaste and the other treatments? With experience, you will come to answer that question for yourself, even without statistics, and then can compare your impression to what the statistical tests demonstrate. In fact, there does not seem to be a very remarkable difference between the groups at any of the times. If the mothers are rating their pain on a scale of 1 to 10 and they are reporting, on average, pain of 5, 6, or 7 at 72 hours after their pain started, they are probably still having an important amount of pain that might affect their overall breastfeeding experience.

A more difficult judgment to make is whether averaging the pain levels makes any sense. Often, when using scales like this that require people to mark specific defined

anchor points, it is difficult to know what an intermediate point represents. It is important to look at the instructions the author gave to the subjects about completing the scale. It could be that they were encouraged to mark a place anywhere along the line. In that event the author would also need to explain how a quantity was assigned to a mark that fell between two points, such as between 3 and 4. Instead of averaging, some studies might try to sum the amount of time each woman spent at each pain level and compare the sums between groups.

One other aspect of the study is evident from this table. In thinking about designing a sore nipple study after reading the title, the need for a no-treatment group was identified. Yet, no such group appears to have been used for comparison. You might also wonder why the pain scores do not appear in a table because that was the focus of the study. You can reasonably expect the author to explain this omission in the text.

Results What does the author claim? First, the author claims that the Gooeypaste group was 2.7 times as likely to experience decreased pain at 72 hours as the lanolin group and 6 times as likely as the water group. This finding was statistically significant. Second, the author claims that the optimism level of the Gooeypaste group was higher than that of the other groups, but statistical significance was not attained.

Independent variables in this study include Gooeypaste, lanolin, and water. Dependent variables include nipple soreness and optimism. Potential confounding variables are the cause of pain, experience of the mothers, quality of positioning, and age of the babies. Applying the three logical steps to this article:

1. The statistical significance of the odds ratios means the data on pain is consistent with the first claim. The claim about optimism is less clear.

2. From the results section, are you reassured that the author ruled out other possible explanations? Probably not, because the author did not show in the results that the three groups were similar in their potential confounding variables. As you read the rest of the article, you will be interested to determine whether the subjects had enough in common that the only important difference between them was the treatment they were using.

3. Does the author suggest a plausible mechanism for how the treatment affects pain? Not to this point in the article, though that is often reserved for either the review of the literature or the discussion. The kinds of mechanisms you might be expecting to read later in the article are topical anesthesia, faster wound healing, anti-inflammatory effects, or others.

Subjects We do not know whether the mothers were first-time or experienced breastfeeders because the author did not report this. The proportion of these mothers in each treatment group could be significant if more experienced mothers persisted simply because they had been through similar pain before or had a higher level of confidence, or both. We do not know age and education level of the mothers or their intended breastfeeding duration, factors related to general commitment to breastfeeding.

Cesarean birth may differ from vaginal birth in several ways: (1) general rate of recovery from birth, (2) difficulty of birth, (3) more professional breastfeeding help for mothers who have undergone cesarean birth due to longer stays, and (4) possibly later milk induction.

We do not know how many times each mother breastfed before pain developed. Nor do we know how often she breastfed afterward. These factors might affect pain intensity and duration and, therefore, the likelihood of relief. The effectiveness of feeding by the baby might also tell something about the quality of latch. There is no mention of routine help with and observations of positioning.

Nurse or physician preferences for the older treatments do not seem to have prevailed, and neither were they accounted for in the design. If nurses who favored warm water encouraged its use before group assignment, for example, the mothers might have continued with that as well as with their other assigned treatment.

The Painometer was not administered at a baseline time. This means it is possible the Gooeypaste mothers actually started the study with a lower pain level than the other groups, so their level of pain might indeed be lower at 72 hours for that reason alone. Because we know little about the scale, we do not know if it tries to measure absolute levels of pain ("the worst pain I've ever felt" to "the least pain I've ever felt") or if it just measures changes in pain perception over time.

Methods The design of this study followed the outline of a clinical trial with randomly assigned treatments. However, it is not a good example of a clinical trial because of its failure to control for several variables. Thus the design of a study alone is not sufficient to guarantee the quality of the resulting evidence.

Telephoning mothers was a good way to increase compliance with the scale. However, investigators should separately have analyzed the scales for which the nurses asked the questions from the mailed ones to be certain there was no tendency to answer differently when speaking directly to a nurse. Compliance with the treatment plan was not reported as validated in any way. Often, if patients do not affirm that they have indeed followed the treatment plan a certain amount of the time, it is not considered an adequate test of the treatment and the data are discarded. Assuming that they followed the plan could lead to invalid conclusions.

What do you think of the operationalization of the variables? The independent variables were not thoroughly described. As has been addressed, the ingredients in Gooeypaste were not discussed to help us understand its pharmacological action. It would also be helpful to have an explanation of the way mothers were instructed to use the warm water and vitamin E. Did they use these after every feeding or four times a day? Before the lanolin was applied, were they instructed to air dry their nipples? Was the Gooeypaste to be removed before the next feeding or allowed to soak in? (If its ingredients had been explained, we might have this answered.)

In some studies the difference between the effectiveness of treatments turns out to be related to the ease of using the treatment rather than any specific action of the treatment itself. As already discussed, the lack of detail about the Painometer makes it difficult to judge what the measurements mean in Table 27.2. However, operationalization of "pain" and "optimism" via such a scale is an accepted way to measure these dependent variables.

The confounding variables are not defined sufficiently or even acknowledged. Even though random assignment was used, it is a small sample. The researcher should have checked on whether some basic variables occurred in similar proportions in all the groups. In addition to the experience of the mothers and the quality of positioning already discussed, several more potential influences on treatment effect could confuse the interpretation of the data. Were any of the mothers experiencing problems establishing milk production, either because of the pain or for some other reason? If so, they might be inclined to feed more often, possibly necessitating more uses of a treatment. Conversely, they might have been so discouraged that they used the treatment less often.

Some readers of this study might ask why there is such a seemingly common problem with early sore nipples in this hospital. (It would have helped if the author had defined the percentage of all mothers that the 30 subjects represent.) Could it be that the nurses have very different skills in helping breastfeeding mothers and that poor positioning is not detected early? Or, contrary to the author's intent, could it be that many of the mothers had only the initial nipple tenderness that improves without actual treatment beyond attention to positioning? Perhaps a hospital postpartum unit would be a good place to test Gooeypaste.

When analyzing a study, it is important to step back from its original premises and ask these basic questions. However, it is often difficult to answer them. Instead, we usually have to accept some of the assumptions and choices the author made and then build a critique based on that. Even when the initial conditions of the study are not ideal, the results can still have value.

Literature Review Nipple pain is a widely acknowledged problem for breastfeeding mothers. There is no great need to establish this from the literature, although there are articles the author could have cited. Types or causes of pain may not all respond to the same treatment. It is therefore important that the literature review be related to the type of pain in the proposed subjects. In this study it is not likely that candidiasis is a common cause of pain so early postpartum, so it is unclear why the author mentioned it. Superficial treatment is not likely to relieve engorgement, so its inclusion seems inappropriate.

The article by Cando was the only reference for warm water treatment. It is likely that the author intended to follow the protocol for its use described therein. However, there are no details about frequency of use, fabric used for application, temperature of the compresses, or air-drying afterward. These omissions make it more difficult to judge whether it was a more complex or time-consuming regimen to follow than that for Gooeypaste or lanolin.

Similarly, there is no description of the protocol for lanolin use. Although the author reports that mothers found lanolin to be soothing, there is no finding presented about its effect on healing or continuation of breastfeeding. Apparently, the main reason that lanolin was compared was that some of the obstetricians favored it.

For both studies, it would be helpful to know whether the subjects studied were similar to those in the current study. Further, did pain relief correlate with longer duration of breastfeeding or more satisfaction with breastfeeding? Many studies do not report longer outcomes such as duration or satisfaction. However, as lactation science matures, it will be important to include these as dependent variables because they are the more important goals.

Readers may not be familiar with the Ouchless theory of pain cited by the authors. They need more description before they can judge its applicability to postpartum nipple soreness. Even if we agree that patient perception of pain is very important, there are other aspects of the pain that are also important—its severity, its duration, its association with an obvious wound, and its meaning to the mother. If the theory suggests that some other aspects of the mother's perception are important to the ultimate resolution of the pain, the author should have measured those aspects as potential confounding variables.

Discussion Readers cannot judge how adequately the author used the literature reviewed (see Methods, earlier), so the link to the discussion is missing. In addition, the author does not introduce any further literature in this section and has not delved into the problem of sore nipples to try to understand the causes. Instead, the scope of the study has been limited to treatment. This is not necessarily bad. It does mean that the implications for practice are more difficult to derive because we cannot generalize to any causes of sore nipples except those that occurred in the study. Because we do not learn what those are, the best we can do is apply the findings to patients whose soreness develops during their hospital stay. Had the author sought to define the causes of the subjects' pain, the discussion might have speculated about why Gooeypaste was especially helpful to these mothers.

In light of the finding that optimism scores were not statistically significantly different between the treatment groups, is the following statement justified: "Because the Gooeypaste mothers were also more optimistic . . . ."? No, it is not. The lack of significance means that Gooeypaste could appear higher on the optimism scale simply by chance. Watch carefully for such claims. If you had not read the results, the discussion might mislead you. The suggestion that optimism may lead to longer nursing is reasonable. However, it would have provided even better evidence for Gooeypaste's effectiveness if the researcher had also studied the proportion of mothers in each group who breastfed until at least 3 months, for example, or who met their goals. The author does admit the need to replicate these findings in a larger sample, and that is an important admission.

Results Revisited The data do seem consistent with the claim that soreness decreases faster for those women who use Gooeypaste. Nevertheless, the control of confounding variables (alternative explanations) was unknown. Remember that when they started treatment there was no assurance that the groups were similar and no information about variables such as breastfeeding experience, adequacy of positioning, or many others. The author depended heavily on the random assignment of this small sample but did not check on its effectiveness. Therefore something else may explain why Gooeypaste seemed to work so well. There is also no plausible mechanism discussed.

The data on optimism are not consistent with the claim that Gooeypaste mothers are more optimistic because of the lack of statistical significance. What are the implications for your practice? You would not begin using Gooeypaste immediately in your postpartum clients. You might design a better randomized trial in your work setting and write up a research report. You might investigate Gooeypaste further by contacting the manufacturer for ingredients, mechanism of action, and any studies they conducted. When you find this number of flaws in a study and when they are so basic, you should not adopt the practice change recommended by the author without considerable further investigation.

References Because these references are fictitious, it is difficult to determine whether important ones were included or not. One of these references is older, from 1998, but that is not necessarily negative (Amir, 2006). In scientific literature you frequently see seminal or classic works that have broken new ground. Just a few examples in the lactation field include research like Niles Newton's work on the science of lactation in the 1940s (Newton & Newton, 1948), Jelliffe's traditional society work in the 1950s (Jelliffe, 1956), and Mavis Gunther's studies on nipple pain and general lactation in the 1940s (Gunther, 1945). Newer examples of seminal or groundbreaking research include Donna Geddes (neé Ramsay) and colleagues' ultrasound imaging of the lactating breast and infant sucking (Ramsay et al., 2005) and Paula Meier and colleagues' work with preterm infants (Meier et al., 2000). You may see these references over and over again in lactation research literature.

The most important deficiency in our fictitious study is the lack of a reference for the Painometer. See also the "Note" following the reference list. It tells you that a manufacturer of Gooeypaste partially funded the study. Although that is not necessarily an indication of bias, you should think about that possibility. Notes about sources of funding are not always present in articles, but it is important to pay attention when they are. Moreover, whenever you read research that casts a negative slant on human milk or a positive slant on artificial feeding, note the researchers' names. An Internet search easily reveals any commercial affiliations they may have that would potentially create bias. Researchers should always declare any competing interests, but they don't always do so (Fanelli, 2009).

Comments You may have uncovered other questionable aspects of this sore nipple study that make you uncomfortable in applying its findings. Critical reading can lead to many questions. This study would probably never have made it to publication in its present form because of the deficiencies identified. It illustrates questions that took the process of critical reading in whatever direction occurred to you. You undoubtedly found still more criticism within the commentary.

Rigorous peer review of this article would, no doubt, have required that the author provide a citation for the Painometer, additional data about the pain scores and other ways of comparing them, a change in the wording about the claim that Gooeypaste was related to higher optimism, and more information about the potential confounding variables. That is the purpose of peer review—to present to readers a good-quality article without fundamental flaws so that what remains is valuable information (though not perfect), and so that the judgments required of readers are about more subtle or more arguable dimensions of the study.

Second Practice Article

Nursing Strikes—Identifying Patterns
by Emma Halter and Makit Gogh
Journal of Intermittent Phenomena. 13:44-47; 2010.

Abstract

A questionnaire was distributed to over 700 breastfeeding mothers in two suburban pediatric practices. Of this group, 200 reported having had experience with their babies refusing to nurse. There was a great deal of variation in reasons for refusing—in measures tried, in other life events, and in mothers' feelings. Stress and biting may be two types of events that precipitate refusals. Teaching mothers about possible nursing refusals in prenatal classes may help them realize they can overcome such discouraging events.

Introduction

Breastfeeding mothers often report[1,2] that their babies display a sudden lack of interest in breastfeeding that persists long enough to cause concern about hunger and dehydration. The mothers also experience engorgement. These "nursing strikes" can be the reason for the introduction of formula, and weaning may follow soon after. For mothers who intended to continue breastfeeding longer, such unplanned weaning is emotionally difficult. Pediatric experts agree that continuing breastfeeding for 6 months to 1 year is best for infant health.[3] Some scientists found that mothers believe that nursing strikes are related to the return of their menses[2] or to starting oral contraceptives.[4] There has been little attempt to study this phenomenon. As a first step we collected data on breastfeeding couplets in two private pediatric practices and looked for patterns. The study was approved by the Review Board of Busy Hospital, and subjects gave written, informed consent.

(Continued)

Subjects and Methods

Participants were mothers of currently breastfeeding infants who were recruited by lactation consultants, nurses, and nurse practitioners in two large, suburban group pediatric practices. From March 1, 2009 to May 31, 2009 all nursing mothers whose babies had appointments for any reason were invited to complete a questionnaire while they waited to see their providers. Those who needed help with child care to complete the survey received that help.

The questionnaire (Figure 27.6) was developed by the authors after reviewing the books for mothers and professionals that suggest causes and remedies. It was designed to be concise so that mothers could finish it while they waited for their appointments (about 10 minutes to complete). Descriptive statistics were calculated for most responses. Correlations were determined for demographic characteristics and responses.

Your help with this questionnaire is greatly appreciated. We are trying to understand why some babies occasionally stop breastfeeding for a few feeds. Please answer as fully as you can, and feel free to add any comments you would like.

1. Are you currently breastfeeding? ___ Yes ___ No
2. How old is your breastfed baby? _____
   How old are you? _____
3. Is this your first breastfed baby? ___ Yes ___ No
   A. If yes, do you have other children? ___ Yes ___ No
      If yes, how many? ___
   B. If no, how many other children have you breastfed? ___
4. With your currently breastfeeding baby, if you have had any of the following problems at *any* time, please check:
   ___ Difficulty latching on
   ___ Sore nipples
   ___ Teething
   ___ Engorgement
   ___ Breast infection
   ___ Plugged milk ducts
   ___ Baby refused to breastfeed
   ___ Baby had a cold or stuffy nose that interfered with feeding
   ___ Biting
5. Since your baby was born, have you resumed your menstrual periods? ___ Yes ___ No
   A. If yes, how old was your baby when the first period started? _____
6. Please check any of the following birth control methods you have used since this baby was born and the age of the baby when you started using it:

Method	Age of baby when started use
___ Condoms (male or female)	_____
___ Natural family planning	_____
___ Lactational amenorrhea	_____
___ Depo-Provera shots	_____
___ Birth control pills	_____
___ Intrauterine device (IUD)	_____
___ Tubal ligation	_____

7. Has your baby ever stopped breastfeeding for at least 24 hours? ___ Yes ___ No

   If no, you have finished this questionnaire. Thank you very much.

   If yes, how old was your baby at the time? _____

   If yes, please check all of the following that you feel apply to your situation, or write a brief description of why you think the baby stopped nursing:

Breastfeeding stopped for at least 24 hours because:
   ___ Mother needed a medicine and was advised to temporarily stop nursing.
   ___ Mother and baby were separated by a trip, a storm, or other unexpected event.
   ___ Baby had surgery.
   ___ Baby was too ill to breastfeed.
   ___ Baby was jaundiced.
   ___ Mother had sore nipples that needed rest.
   ___ Baby was teething.
   ___ Mother returned to work.
   ___ Baby had bitten mother and stopped nursing soon after.
   ___ Baby refused to nurse but would take other food.
   ___ Unknown. The reason for stopping was never clear.
   ___ Other: Please describe why you think your baby stopped nursing:

8. If your baby had stopped nursing for at least 24 hours, please check all of the following that describe your feelings during the time your baby did not breastfeed:
   ___ Concerned breastfeeding was finished for good.
   ___ Worried about hunger or dehydration.
   ___ Concerned about breasts becoming engorged.
   ___ Relieved to have a short break.
   ___ Confused about what was happening.
   ___ Confused about the cause of the refusal to nurse.
   ___ Thought baby might be sick.
   ___ Other. Please describe:

9. If your baby had stopped nursing for at least 24 hours, please check all of the following actions you tried to help resume feeding:
   ___ Just kept trying to nurse in the usual ways.
   ___ Just gave my baby time to feel better.
   ___ Called the lactation consultant, physician's office, or breastfeeding counselor (e.g., La Leche League).
   ___ Talked to a family member or friend.
   ___ Nursed my baby when he/she was very sleepy.
   ___ Increased the amount of skin-to-skin contact we had.
   ___ Took a bath with my baby.
   ___ Used a sling or pack.
   ___ Tried to reduce the stress in my life.
   ___ Other. Please describe:

Thank you so much for your help. If you would like to learn the results of this study, please let us know at your next appointment.

FIGURE 27.6   Appendix A: Questionnaire for nursing strikes.

(Continued)

Results

During the 3-month period, the combined practices had 1,032 breastfeeding couplet visits. Because some couplets had multiple appointments, 955 different couplets were offered a questionnaire. Of those, 780 agreed to complete the survey. For various reasons only 600 questionnaires were actually complete enough to use. Of these, 400 had never had the problem of the baby refusing to nurse for 24 hours. Of the 200 refusers, 30 had stopped nursing at a few days old because of jaundice in the infant. Another 70 mothers identified medication, surgery, illness, separation, and maternal sore nipples (see Table 27.3). Teething was the cause 30 mothers indicated.

These causes, although stressful and needing remedies, were not the most perplexing. The nursing strikes of interest were those that 70 mothers marked as unknown reason, other reason, or preference for another food. Of course, because these mothers were nursing at the time of the appointment, they had overcome the strike. Many of the events that occurred near a nursing strike also occurred in couplets that never experienced a strike. The two strongest correlations were an increase in family stress and biting (see Table 27.4). However, together these included only 15 percent of couplets who experienced nursing strikes.

TABLE 27.3 Reasons for Stopping Nursing as Determined by Mothers.

Newborn jaundice	30
Medication	10
Surgery	12
Illness of baby	20
Maternal sore nipples	15
Separation of mother and baby	13
Teething	30
	130

TABLE 27.4 Correlations Between Unexplained Nursing Strikes and Recent Events for Breastfeeding Dyads.

Event	Number of Dyads	*r* (Correlation)
Resuming menses within 1 week of strike (<3 mo old)	5	0.21
Resuming menses	3	0.15
Starting birth control within same month	2	0.09
Increase in family stress	15	0.55
Biting	16	0.59

Discussion

Mothers need lactation professionals who are aware of the potential for nursing strikes and who can encourage them to not give up. That is probably the most important message of this study. Short periods of refusal to nurse are common. Determining a cause is very difficult. Based on this survey we suggest educating mothers in prenatal classes about possible refusals. Cautioning them against responding strongly to biting and emphasizing the importance of stress management may be the most specific strategies that emerge from these data (see Table 27.5). There is no evidence herein that resuming menses or starting the birth control pill, as suggested by others, is causal.

TABLE 27.5 Remedies Used by Mothers to Overcome Nursing Strikes.

Remedy	% of Mothers Who Used It
Time and patience	83
Calling lactation professional	80
Nursing during sleep	50
Skin-to-skin soothing	55
Bathing together	30
Sling or pack	34
Trying to reduce stress	42

References

1. Complete D. Weaning from breast. *Feeding Babies Journal*. 14:120-125; 2008.
2. Empp A. Common concerns of breastfeeding mothers in a food assistance program. *Nutrition Group Reports*. 55:37-41; 2009.
3. Healthy World Alliance. Breastfeeding best for babies. *HA*. 56:123-125; 2008.
4. Wilgot E. Postpartum menstrual cycles. *Annals of Families*. 33:293-255; 2000.

Discussion of Second Practice Article

Title How will the authors define "nursing strike"? Although experienced breastfeeding mothers may speak of this phenomenon as though everyone agrees on it, a clear definition is necessary to determine clearly associated variables. What do you believe should be included and excluded? You might expect to see refusal to nurse by the baby for a certain length of time (more than one feeding) and for no obvious reason. Would it be reasonable to allow certain probable causes and disallow others?

When attempting to explore a previously understudied phenomenon like this, there are many possible choices for the definition, none of which is right or wrong. Rather, clarity is the most important criterion for judging the choices—so that investigators, subjects, and readers all agree on which breast refusals constitute nursing strikes.

What "patterns" do you consider based on the title? Do the authors intend to see whether babies at a particular age are more likely to go on strike? Will they study whether increased bottle use or separation (common when babies start day care) often precede strikes? For mothers who have breastfed other children, is it likely that prior instances of strikes in the older child correlate with more strikes in the current nursing baby? Many patterns are possible, and you can compare the patterns you would like to see investigated to what the researchers chose.

What study design does the title suggest? Is this a trial to determine whether certain events cause or specific treatments cure nursing strikes? Do you know of other studies of this phenomenon that have gained enough basic information to conduct such a trial? For this exercise the topic of nursing strikes was chosen because there is not much literature on it. Therefore a descriptive study of some sort is more likely at this point in the development of knowledge.

If the authors intended to conduct a qualitative study, what kind of data might they collect? They might ask mothers to tape record the feelings they remember having and the effect on their confidence when the baby went on strike. Alternatively, they might try to include mothers from many different cultures and compare the ways the mothers describe the experience of nursing strikes. If they do a quantitative study, they might try to find patterns by using correlation between variables as an outcome measure.

Authors' Names Again, because this is a mock article, you will not find these authors' names in any database. However, for an actual article, if you wanted to know whether the authors had published on this topic previously, you could search an online database such as PubMed (www.pubmed.org) or EBSCO (ebscohost.com) by author name. That would be a worthwhile effort if you need the most complete information available.

Abstract The fact that 200 mothers claim experience with breast refusal might be surprising. This should start you thinking about the definition again. The definition may indicate that many more mothers have had strikes than your experience suggests. Alternatively, it could be that this problem is much more widespread than anyone realizes simply because no one has sought to study its prevalence before.

The source of subjects was two pediatric suburban practices. Will the authors provide more demographic data on maternal income, education, race, ethnic heritage, and type of insurance? If the sample population is primarily white, married, and middle class, will the results apply to mothers in other groups? The authors used a questionnaire, which requires literacy. Did they determine whether any subjects had trouble reading English? Did they provide the questions in another language? Did the nature of the tool exclude mothers with visual disabilities or language barriers? Why did they single out biting and stress as events to mention in the abstract? Were these especially strong findings, or the only findings that mothers can modify? What is their reasoning for suggesting that prenatal education might help?

Table 27.3: Reasons for Stopping Nursing as Determined by Mothers Note first that only 130 of the 900 mentioned in the abstract appear in this table. You will want to read why in the text. Are there reasons for nursing strikes that you had thought of that are not in this list? The investigators should explain their reasons for these choices. Note that no descriptive statistics, such as percentages, or any tests of significance appear in this table.

Table 27.4: Correlations Why the focus on "unexplained" strikes, and how was that defined? Why do the events listed in this table differ from the "reasons" given in Table 27.3? Although the correlation statistic r is presented, no statistical significance is reported. None of the correlations is high ($r = 0.7$ or above) in many definitions. Do moderate correlations like 0.55 and 0.59 represent the most powerful of the possible variables associated with strikes? Has something been left out of the study inadvertently? The text of the article should address all these questions. The explanations may be too complex to include as footnotes to the table.

Table 27.5: Remedies Did all the mothers who completed this survey successfully overcome nursing strikes? If so, they do not represent all the mothers who have experienced strikes, because weaning occurs after strikes in some unknown proportion of cases. How would limiting the data collection to mothers who have successfully overcome strikes limit the applicability of the findings? Are there other remedies the authors should have included?

Results First, note that the mothers targeted by the researchers were breastfeeding at the time of the appointment. Apparently, mothers who had stopped breastfeeding after a strike were not included. Regarding the claims, the strongest correlations between variables included in the questionnaire were the correlation between strike and biting and between strike and stress. The descriptive data appear to support the claim, but there is no report of statistical tests. In terms of ruling out alternative explanations:

1. Do the investigators offer any analysis of whether mothers who did not agree to participate were similar to or different from the mothers who participated? (This problem is similar to the "dropout" problem discussed in the Critical Reading section under "Results.") Some of these mothers may be unable to read English. Without knowing more about the non-participants, it is difficult to know how to apply (generalize) the results.

2. Is the list of preceding events such as medication, surgery, and jaundice in Table 27.3 sufficiently explanatory to exclude them from the study of nursing strikes? They are potential confounding variables if the essence of a nursing strike is that there is no "obvious" explanation. This is where definitions and the purpose of the investigation need to be very clear to interpret the data properly.

3. Are there plausible mechanisms suggested or investigated for the relationships the authors found? Typically, the results section does not discuss the mechanism unless it was the focus of the study. In a descriptive study it is important to think about how the relationships might work for the results to be taken seriously. Even if no strong evidence is available for a mechanism, if it does not violate known principles of physiology or human behavior, it is plausible. Both biting and stress could plausibly relate to a nursing strike in a baby. As you read more of the article, you should be able to determine whether you believe the authors' explanations.

Methods What is the design of this study? It is descriptive and cross-sectional. It takes a snapshot of the couplets in one area on a limited-time basis and contacts them only once, so it looks at a cross-section of the population. It is also correlational; the researchers used a structured instrument to measure variables and then sought statistically significant relationships.

Was the definition of nursing strike clear and appropriate? From the questionnaire itself, rather than from the article, you can determine that the definition was "stopped nursing for at least 24 hours." Knowledgeable professionals could disagree with this definition. Some

might prefer a different time period or different wording. What is crucial is that the authors and mothers mean the same thing when they use this definition.

If there were a big discrepancy in understanding, the internal validity of the study would be in jeopardy. Because this is such a new area of research, the investigators could have done some work before this big study to be more certain about the meaning of this definition. They could have conducted a pilot study and talked in more depth with women about their experiences with nursing strikes. They might have suggested different definitions until the mothers and researchers agreed that they were identifying the same phenomenon. They also could have asked lactation and child development experts for their opinions on the definition.

If you were to use this study to try to convince childbirth educators or pediatricians to address nursing strikes, it is very important that you discuss nursing strike as defined in this article and that you not extend the findings to some other looser or stricter definition. The choices listed in the questionnaire are not defined for mothers but most are probably reasonably clear. If you can think of multiple, significantly different interpretations for any of the phrases, you may have identified a less valuable part of the data.

Questionnaire Look at the questionnaire itself. There are entire courses on how to design questionnaires to obtain unbiased information. You could ask many questions about the quality of this one. Even if reasonable people would disagree, it is important to think about some aspects of it. Here are just a few ideas about specific questions:

1. Item 1 does not ask whether the mother is breastfeeding exclusively or partially. With a baby younger than 6 months of age, the nursing strike could have been the cause of a switch to partial breastfeeding. The investigators cannot determine such a switch from this question.

2. Questions such as item 3 about previous breastfeeding experience often fail to ask whether the experience overall was positive or negative.

3. In item 4 it is not clear what information or relationship the investigators were seeking. It might have been useful to ask the age at which the mother experienced the problem to determine whether it was close in time to the strike. It should probably have an "other" category in case the mother wants to list problems she has had. Among ones that might bear some relationship to nursing strikes are those in which the baby has had some frustration in getting enough milk. These may include delayed lactogenesis, delayed or overactive milk ejection, nipples that needed reshaping, or bottle feeding that led to poor breast sucking.

4. In item 6 some of the contraceptive methods listed may not be familiar to all mothers, but those who had used them would probably recognize them.

5. Item 7 does not allow for multiple instances of nursing strikes. As a result some mothers may list multiple causes, intending them to refer to separate events. Often, researchers ask mothers to reflect the most recent occurrence in their answer.

6. In item 8 the age of the baby greatly influences the mother's concern about a nursing strike. With babies who are taking solid foods and other liquids, a 24-hour nursing strike may not be alarming. Therefore it might be important to discuss the correlations separately for different age groups.

Subjects could be characterized by age, the number of children they have, the number of children they breastfed, return of menses, use of contraception, and problems experienced. Other variables that might influence their nursing strike experience and interpretation, such as ethnic group or planned duration of breastfeeding, are not included. This often happens in descriptive studies. You will have to decide whether the information is useful to you even with some deficiencies.

Introduction and Literature Review Because there is little research on this topic, the review is somewhat limited. Some authors seek what they believe is related research from other topics that cover the hypotheses they wish to highlight. For example, if they related nursing strikes to stress in the mother, they might study other research on mother–infant stress responses. These authors chose to look for patterns in a large number of couplets without a specific hypothesis. If you knew of articles they failed to include, you might judge their effort to be incomplete.

Discussion If this is a representative cross-section of breastfeeding mothers, the authors' statement that nursing strikes are common is probably true. However, we are not sure just what group this sample represents, and we know that it does not represent mothers who weaned after a nursing strike. Therefore it can only be a piece of the puzzle. On the other hand, if nursing strikes are very common and most nursing mothers handle them smoothly, then it would be very important to understand how they coped to help those who wean as a result.

The suggestion to educate mothers about nursing strikes is difficult to argue with, although doing it in the usual childbirth class may not be the best time. Similarly, although education about biting and stress are appropriate, we cannot expect them to resolve the problems of nursing strikes based on this study alone. Furthermore,

although the authors claim to have found no evidence that resuming menses or starting birth control pills caused strikes, this does not constitute the best evidence. We would believe that a prospective study that queried mothers about strikes beginning shortly after birth and carefully recorded other possibly relevant variables on a regular basis would more likely detect a relationship.

Results Revisited Depending on how convinced you are that this sample resembles your patients, you may want to initiate research yourself. At the very least you could include questions about nursing strikes in more of your routine follow-up calls. This study, like many descriptive studies, raises more questions than it answers. To review, the moderate correlation of stress and biting with strikes (although the statistical significance is unknown) is consistent with the claim that these are two of the more common preceding events. The biggest failure of this study is its inability to rule out alternative explanations because of study design, poorly characterized sample, and inadequate definitions. Although the authors discuss implications for practice, there could be a lot of disagreement on clinical implications because of the degree of uncertainty about so many possible confounders.

References This appears to be a relevant list. Even though the mothers in reference 2 may be a different sample than the ones in this study, the authors use that reference only to suggest what others have noted, which is appropriate.

～ Summary

The process of critique presented in this chapter is structured around the parts of a scientific article because that is how most clinicians use it. However, the more general themes of the process of critical reading, as outlined in the following list, are not determined solely through the article's sections. As a clinician who wants to decide whether to apply the results of a study to your work, you want to determine the following:

1. What did the authors choose to include and exclude in their literature review, in their subjects, in the survey questions, and in the comparisons they made in data analysis? Did they adequately explain and justify their choices? Did their choices make the sample patients or study situation so different from your practice that you cannot justifiably use the results?

2. What else could the authors have done? Why did they not do that? Could they have included more mothers? Could they have studied them for a longer period? Could there have been a more diverse ethnic base? Could they have included a control group?

3. For every limitation of the study identified by answering questions 1 and 2, what might have been the impact on the study's findings? For example, if you believe the authors should have included more low-income women, how might that have affected the finding that intending to breastfeed more than 12 weeks is the best predictor of continuing to breastfeed at least 6 weeks? You may be reasoning that the low-income women in your practice must return to work by 6 weeks. Therefore very few mothers even plan to breastfeed past 6 weeks, and some other predictor variable would tell you more about what enables them to continue to 6 weeks. When critically reading your scientific colleagues' work, it is not enough to say what they should have done differently. You need to justify your critique by stating how that might have changed the study's results.

Critically reading a scientific article is a skill that grows with experience and strengthens your practice as a lactation consultant. Learning how to read and analyze scientific articles opens many doors for your continued learning. Self-direction and self-education are hallmarks of the professional lactation consultant. You are well along on the road of lifelong education. As you mature in your practice, keep your eyes open for opportunities to research and publish studies. Your opportunities may range from case studies to large prospective studies on breastfeeding families. You could have a big impact on the understanding of lactation!

∾ Chapter 27—At a Glance

Facts you learned—

- Editorials, although insightful, are not studies or critically reviewed.
- Scientific research is not without problems and fraud. Read critically and question, question, question!
- Case studies report on instances of a problem, diagnosis, or treatment; they cannot be used to generalize.
- Meta-analyses combine data from several studies to test conclusions.
- Reviews are written by experts who analyze the best and worst studies, with little or no original data.
- Clinical practice articles are reports of applications in real life.
- The Internet has fueled a growing trend for open access (free use) journals and articles.
- Research reports put a long-held belief or new idea to a scientific test.

- Titles explain main findings and may be two sentences long.
- Authors tend to publish profusely in a specific, narrow discipline.
- Many studies are funded by and some even published by the pharmaceutical industry.
- Abstracts are brief summaries that explain a study.
- Introductions contain the purpose, parameters, and restraints of the study.
- Literature reviews explain previous research.
- Methods describe how researchers operationalized the hypothesis, how subjects were recruited, tools used to measure outcomes, surveys, scales, tests, definition of terms, and statistical methods.
- Results are often displayed in graphs, tables, and charts; they are peer reviewed for accuracy.
- Discussion reviews study reasons and other relevant literature, summarize results, and suggest applications and further research.
- References and the bibliography list all citations referred to in the article.
- Study design may be retrospective, case-control, prospective, cross-sectional, survey, descriptive, qualitative, experiment, or trial.
- Tools (instruments) measure dependent variable consistently.
- Statistical theory is based on probability.
- Study frequency is based on samples of populations.
- Statistical tests include distributions, centered and unbalanced bell curves, CIs, chi-square, Cohen's kappa, Cronbach's alpha, regression, and t tests.
- Odds ratio is a summary of relative proportion in two different groups.

Applying what you learned—

- Look at the title of the article and consider what you know about the topic, how you would have studied it, and what you expect to find.
- Read the authors' names and the abstract.
- Identify terms and key concepts.
- Study the tables and graphs, and read the results.
- Read the methods to determine whether the authors can justify their conclusions.
- Read the introduction and literature review and consider significance, accuracy, appropriateness of studies, omissions, and thoroughness of explanations.
- Read the discussion and watch for speculation, suggestions for further research, and flaws or weaknesses.

- Read the results again to check that data are consistent with claims and that there is no other equal or better explanation.
- Watch for spurious relationships.
- Determine what the researchers chose to include and exclude and why.
- Research any article or scientist about which/whom you have questions. Ties to industry may or may not be disclosed in the publication (although they should be).

〜 *References*

Amir L. International Breastfeeding Journal: introducing a new journal. *Int Breastfeeding J.* 2006;1:1. www.international breastfeedingjournal.com/content/1/1/1. Accessed October 3, 2009.

Cochrane Collaboration. www.cochrane.org. Accessed October 4, 2009.

Dean S, Illowsky B. *Collaborative Statistics.* Houston: Rice University Connexions Project; 2009. http://cnx.org/content/col10522/1.36. Accessed October 4, 2009.

Directory of Open Access Journals. www.doaj.org. Accessed October 4, 2009.

Fanelli D. How many scientists fabricate and falsify research? A systematic review and meta-analysis of survey data. *PLoS ONE.* 2009;4(5):e5738.

Gunther M. Sore nipples: causes and prevention. *Lancet.* 1945;2:590-593.

Infant Feeding Action Coalition Canada (INFACT). Nestlé scientist's false claims exposed. February 7, 2006. www.infactcanada.ca/Chandra_Feb72006.htm. Accessed October 5, 2009.

International Breastfeeding Journal. www.internationalbreast feedingjournal.com; 2009. Accessed October 4, 2009.

Jelliffe D. Breast feeding in technically developing regions (with especial reference to West Bengal). *Courier.* 1956;6(4):191-195.

Meier P, et al. Nipple shields for preterm infants: effect on milk transfer and duration of breastfeeding. *J Hum Lact.* 2000;16(2):106-114; quiz 129-131.

Newton M, Newton N. The let-down reflex in human lactation. *J Pediatr.* 1948;33(6):698-704.

Raloff J. Journal bias: novelty preferred (which can be bad). *Science News.* September 11, 2009. www.sciencenews.org/view/generic/id/47297/title/Journal_bias_Novelty_preferred_%28which_can_be_bad%29. Accessed October 5, 2009.

Ramsay D, et al. Anatomy of the lactating human breast redefined with ultrasound imaging. *J Anat.* 2005;206:525-534.

Smith J, et al. Health professional knowledge of breastfeeding: are the health risks of infant formula feeding accurately conveyed by the titles and abstracts of journal articles? *J Hum Lact.* 2009;25(3):350-358.

28

Breastfeeding Promotion and Change

Excellence can be attained if you
Care more than others think is wise,
Risk more than others think is safe,
Dream more than others think is practical,
And expect more than others think is possible.

—Anonymous

Promoting breastfeeding presents unique challenges in societies where artificial feeding is perceived as the norm. Undertaking the challenge of breastfeeding promotion requires strong, confident leadership. You need to understand other points of view and work for everyone's mutual benefit in order to win colleague and administration support. This approach enables you to build a strong team that can arrive at creative solutions. Being an effective change agent requires skills in assertiveness and persuasion and an appreciation for the importance of giving recognition and praise. Understanding why others resist change helps resolve conflicts and identifies common goals, so that you can move on to define problems, goals, and strategies.

Capitalizing on various personality styles contributes to productive group dynamics. Major international initiatives support your promotion efforts as you seek to remove obstacles toward achieving breastfeeding-friendly practices. Chapter 1 presents an historical perspective on infant feeding and highlights major initiatives to support, protect, and promote breastfeeding. This final chapter focuses on ways you can provide leadership in breastfeeding promotion and facilitate change that continues to empower women to breastfeed.

～ *Key Terms*

Ad Council
Assertiveness
Baby-Friendly Hospital
  Initiative
Breastfeeding Awareness
  Campaign
Breastfeeding committee
Breastfeeding promotion
Change agent
Conflict resolution
Difficult people
Formula manufacturer
  advertising
Global Strategy for Infant
  and Young Child
  Feeding
International Baby Food
  Action Network
  (IBFAN)
Infant Feeding Action
  Coalition Canada
  (INFACT)

International Code of
  Marketing of
  Breastmilk Substitutes
Joint Commission Media
  Watch
National Alliance for
  Breastfeeding Advocacy
  (NABA)
Paradigm
Personality types
Persuasion
Resistance to change
Seven Habits of Highly
  Effective People
Team building
Ten Steps to Successful
  Breastfeeding
World Alliance for
  Breastfeeding Action
  (WABA)
World Health Assembly
  (WHA)

∿ *Strong Leadership*

It is not surprising that people prefer to work with people they like. Human nature draws us to people who are cheerful, generous, and considerate of others. People who possess these qualities find it easier to generate cooperation from those around them. Others may need to make a concerted effort to present themselves in a manner that achieves the same results.

Part of being an effective leader is instilling confidence in others. People respond well to a leader who is self-confident, assertive, and forthright. The key to being influential is to focus on solutions, priorities, and action. An effective problem solver looks for problem areas and then focuses on solutions. After establishing goals, be aware of the priorities that helps you achieve them and be willing to take risks to put your ideas into action. Be approachable, listen attentively, and guard against snap judgments. All these attributes build a strong team and garner support for your breastfeeding and other healthcare initiatives.

Effective Behavior

The approach that Stephen Covey (2004) presents in his book, *The 7 Habits of Highly Effective People*, provides a helpful structure for examining ways to promote breastfeeding. Covey states that an effective person is proactive, establishes goals, sets priorities, and is genuinely open to others' ideas. The effective person works toward mutual benefits for both sides of an issue, promotes unity, and actively seeks self-renewal, both physically and mentally. The practices described in the next section will contribute to your success in facilitating real change in breastfeeding promotion.

Choose to Be Effective

Stephen Covey asserts that behavior is a function of our decisions and not our conditions. Although it is human nature to react immediately to events, there is always a gap between a stimulus and our response to that stimulus. The key to our effectiveness is how we use that gap. A spontaneous response is usually impulsive and based on feelings aroused by particular conditions. Such an impetuous reaction lacks forethought and may not lead to responsible action.

A proactive person recognizes that we each have the ability to choose our responses. It is not what happens to us but our response to what happens to us that determines the outcome. We can take the initiative to create circumstances and make things happen by first reflecting on our options and thinking through possible actions. Our responses may not always produce the desired results. Nonetheless, when we make mistakes, it is important to acknowledge them, learn, and go on. Making mistakes is part of being a leader and a problem solver—it simply means we are trying! Baseball players know they have countless strikeouts for every home run they hit. Leadership is a learning process, strengthened as much by every failure as by every success. Eleanor Roosevelt stated that no one can make us feel inferior without our consent. Responding to mistakes with purposeful insight is a sign of strength.

In bolstering your effectiveness as a leader, consider how you respond to questionable practices or unsupportive coworkers. A reactive response might be to defend what you are trying to accomplish by arguing your position and backing up your argument with research articles and other documentation. In a proactive response you might first try to learn the reasons for resistance to or disinterest in your proposal. Understanding what has led to a situation is an important first step to exploring appropriate solutions and garnering support.

Start with a Blueprint

An effective planner thinks first and then acts. Imagine if an architect were to begin building a new structure without first having created a blueprint. Likewise, where would a traveler be without first mapping out a route? Planning begins with visualizing the process of getting to where you want to be. Knowing what you want the result to be dictates how you plan to arrive there. Mapping it out on paper with specific goals, and visualizing it in your mind, help you solidify a workable plan. The next step is to determine how to accomplish the goals you set so that you arrive at your desired result. Leadership and vision must always precede any action. As a lactation consultant, you are in an ideal position to provide leadership and vision to others in improving breastfeeding promotion and practices.

Creating a personal mission statement further guides your actions. You can begin with the blueprints for breastfeeding promotion provided by the Ten Steps to Successful Breastfeeding (World Health Organization, 1989) and the Global Strategy for Infant and Young Child Feeding (World Health Organization, 2003). These seminal documents help focus your efforts and guide the development of appropriate breastfeeding policies and protocols. They will help you identify current practices that can stay in place as well as other areas that need improvement. Your end goal is healthy mothers and babies. Keeping this result in mind will help you determine how to get there.

Focus on What Is Important

Be mindful to not allow seemingly urgent matters to get in the way of important issues that need your attention.

People often become so overly involved in what they perceive to be *urgent* that what is *important* receives little or no attention. Devoting your time to what is important is a product of careful time management and usually requires that you learn to say "no" to others and "yes" to yourself. An effective person practices self-management, makes decisions, and then acts on them. You can learn to distinguish between what is urgent and what is important by recognizing they often are not the same. Focusing on what is important helps prevent your efforts from being diverted to distractions, crises, or obstacles. It enables you to prioritize important changes, develop a timeline, and stay committed to your goals.

As you establish priorities and a timeline, it is important to designate tasks to a particular time and person. There are a variety of ways to organize and execute goals and tasks around priorities, ranging from notes and checklists to calendars (both print and electronic), appointment books, and daily planners. Effective leaders are comfortable delegating tasks to others and trusting others to come through for them. You may need to settle for things being done differently from you would have done them—and perhaps done not as well. Nonetheless, relinquishing control to others and nurturing their growth are essential to developing a strong team. Such trust brings out the best in people and leads to enthusiastic and productive teamwork. The only way to build a strong team is to bring out the best in the other team members.

If your goal is to establish a strong continuum of care for breastfeeding mothers and babies, teaching other members of your staff how to assist mothers enables you to delegate this responsibility to others. The harsh reality is that time is at a premium in health care, especially in hospitals and health clinics where staffing is low. Nonetheless, supportive breastfeeding practices need not tax an already busy day for maternity staff or caregivers with other responsibilities. You cannot expect cooperation and compliance until you ensure that others are equipped to carry through appropriately. Therefore, identify the essential elements breastfeeding mothers need to learn and teach other staff how to help mothers in those areas. Focusing on the essential areas and practicing effective time management will help you achieve your goals.

Work Toward Mutual Benefit

Initiating change and planning promotion efforts require strong teamwork. Recognize that your success cannot be achieved at the expense of others. All parties need to feel good about the outcome. An essential goal, therefore, is to create mutual benefits for both sides of an issue. If two opposing sides are unable to compromise, creative thinking will help you consider whether an acceptable third alternative exists. Help each side understand that the result may not be just "your way" or "my way," but a better way. An effective team works together to determine acceptable results and identify new options to achieve those results.

A well-managed team ensures that all members of the team operate on an even playing field. Establishing the expectation that everyone leaves their credentials, personalities and personal agendas at the door helps to achieve this. An effective leader identifies the key issues and concerns and keeps everyone focused on topics rather than on personalities or job titles. In planning and decision making, you want to include those who are receptive to the change as well as those who you anticipate will resist. List the needs and concerns of people on both sides of an issue, and work toward everyone's mutual benefit. If there appear to be losers on a particular issue, look for ways that both parties can benefit so there are only winners.

Understand Other Points of View

Attempting to see an issue from another person's point of view enhances communication and garners support. In everyday communication, people do not generally listen with the intent to understand. We tend to focus on our own needs and fail to recognize that the way we view a problem often *is* the problem. Effective listening requires patience, openness, and a true desire to understand. When you are genuinely open to other people's ideas, they are more likely to be open to yours. Make it a practice to listen until you are able to explain the other person's point of view as well as they can. Furthermore, be open to allowing others' arguments and points of view to influence your thinking. The better you understand, the more you can appreciate others' views. Reflective listening helps you listen with intent and openness, paving the way to mutually developed, creative solutions.

To successfully motivate other people to change, it is important that you understand their reasons for resistance. Recognize that changes you propose may conflict with the way things "have always been done." Attempt to understand specific concerns and worries and to see an issue the way others see it. One effective method for doing this is to role play the discussion of an issue with another colleague, placing yourself in the role of the resistor. Such an exercise helps you see the concerns more clearly so you can determine counterarguments.

Listen attentively and with an open mind to others' arguments and concerns. Although it can be instinctive to assign negative motives to those with whom you disagree, it helps to remember that most healthcare professionals enter the healthcare field because they care deeply about helping others. Everyone's end goal in breastfeeding is to meet the needs of mothers and babies. There are simply differences of opinion on what that constitutes and how to get there. Remain open to flexibility and compromise as you and your team work through the differences to achieve consensus on how to move forward.

Build a Strong Team

Another Covey principle is that the whole is greater than the sum of its parts. An effective team builds on each person's strengths and compensates for weaknesses as it works toward achieving unity. An effective leader helps team members learn to sidestep negative energy and resist taking criticism personally. Communicating back and forth until the team reaches a solution that is mutually comfortable fosters trust and cooperation. As members increasingly feel ownership of a problem, they become more engaged and ultimately part of the solution. Remaining open to new alternatives and compromises helps you facilitate team members taking ownership of the proposed changes.

An effective team-building climate is one in which it is safe and comfortable for everyone to air disagreements and concerns. Differences in point of view can provide valuable resources, insights, and perceptions. A variety of opinions and approaches adds to your knowledge and understanding. Two people can disagree and both can be right—they just interpret differently. Validating everyone's perspective helps the team achieve its goals.

Take Care of Yourself

Covey says that to be an effective person you need to be healthy, both physically and mentally. This means paying attention to exercise, nutrition, and stress. Additionally, using your value system to guide what you say and do helps to keep you focused in a positive direction. Getting and staying in touch with your inner self helps you draw on your innate enthusiasm and energy. Continue to learn and share information with the staff, helping them stay focused on the vision and bringing out the best in each of them. Cultivate relationships, especially with people you perceive as adversaries, while keeping the team on track and working cooperatively.

∿ Increasing Self-Confidence

Self-confidence is an essential factor in actively facilitating change. How you perceive yourself and your abilities has a tremendous influence on how you project yourself to others. Additionally, "your attitude will determine your altitude." In other words, how successful you view yourself to be often determines your level of success. If you focus on your faults rather than on your strengths, you may prevent yourself from soaring to great heights.

The principles outlined in this section help you maintain perspective and increase your ability to take action in a self-assured manner (Browder, 1994). Much of your attitude involves the vocabulary you use in self-talk. If you continually expect to fail, you probably will fail! Replace any negative thoughts such as, "I hope I don't . . .," with positive self-talk such as, "I will. . . ." Tell yourself how confident you are. Rather than saying, "I wish I were . . ." or "I should be . . . ," tell yourself, "I am. . . ." Table 28.1 contains powerful statements to replace those that convey less affirmative messages. Positive and negative thinking are both learned habits. You can recondition your mind to think positively by replacing negative thoughts with positive ones. Approach every situation with the belief that you will succeed. Focus on the best way to do the job right, and visualize yourself doing it!

Effective leaders do not allow fear of failure to undermine their self-confidence. If you want good things to happen, you have to make them happen; sometimes that requires taking a risk. If you make mistakes along the way, congratulate yourself for taking a risk. Learn to view your mistakes as lessons, not failures, and to regard a mistake as just another way of doing things. When you make a mistake—and you will—acknowledge it and regard it as a learning experience. Making mistakes is proof that you are trying! Trust in your ability to learn, and help others trust in their ability to learn from their mistakes as well. This is especially important when your efforts to change practices require others to learn new skills. Coping with failure builds strength and wisdom. Help others recognize that every defeat is another step toward success.

TABLE 28.1 Powerful Language

Don't Say	Do Say
I have to . . .	I'll be glad to . . .
I'm no good at . . .	I'm getting better . . .
I failed . . .	Here's what I learned . . .
I'm going under . . .	I'm bouncing back . . .
This drives me crazy . . .	I can find a better way . . .
I can't do anything about it . . .	It's my responsibility to change . . .
We should have it ready by . . .	We will have it ready by . . .
Generally speaking, I tend to think . . .	I believe . . .
Do you have any questions?	What questions do you have?
It's not my fault. I couldn't help it.	I'm sorry. It was my responsibility.

The concept of "emotional intelligence" describes factors that come into play when people with high IQs fail while people with average IQs succeed. Emotional intelligence includes such attributes as self-awareness, impulse control, persistence, zeal, self-motivation, empathy, and social deftness (Goleman et al., 2002; Goleman, 1997). These qualities can help you succeed in your goals, earning breastfeeding support and optimized health outcomes for mothers and babies.

~ Increasing Assertiveness

Caregivers who serve breastfeeding women are predominantly female, as are most nurses. Lactation consultants practicing in a hospital setting typically are perceived in much the same way as nurses, a profession that has historically had little power in the hierarchical, male-dominated healthcare industry (Manojlovich, 2007). Additionally, women often are concerned that others may perceive their assertiveness negatively and interpret it as aggressive behavior. Employee response to such powerlessness can lead to passive-aggressive behavior, frustration, and burnout.

Embracing assertive behavior as a strong asset helps you become comfortable with your assertiveness when presenting your ideas to others. An important first step is to analyze assertive behavior in others. Identify what it is about others that you admire, observing what they say and how they say it, and deciding which approaches and traits you want to emulate.

Next, analyze your behavior and the ways you respond in situations that call for assertiveness. Do others listen when you have something important to say? Are you able to convince others to comply with your wishes? Analyze times when you were assertive and times when you were not. Think back on times when you were perceived to come across as aggressive. Consider the language you used in each situation, including nonverbal messages you conveyed. You might even record your behavior; documenting how you behaved in various situations, what worked, and what you could have done differently to be more effective.

The next step is to practice assertiveness in your interactions with family, friends, coworkers, neighbors, and store clerks. Visualize yourself being assertive, and role play situations with others. When you feel confident that you can approach an issue with assertiveness, undertake an easy challenge first—one you feel certain will succeed. If the results are not what you had planned, examine why it did not go the way you wanted and reflect on what you can do differently. Keep a positive attitude, and adjust your approach with the next challenge. The important thing is that you not allow one setback to discourage you from continuing to work toward more assertive behavior.

~ Becoming a Change Agent

Healthcare professionals are in an ideal position to plan and implement changes to benefit mothers and babies. Recognizing the need for change is the first step in the process of planned change (Ellis, 1992). A need for change is exemplified, for example, in the way in which U.S. culture perceives infant feeding. Examining breastfeeding in a cultural context involves both the mother's culture within her family and support system and the cultural expectations and beliefs within her birth environment. Because most U.S. infants are born in hospitals, this requires attention to the culture and traditions within the hospital as it relates to infant feeding (Mulford, 2008, 1995).

Cultural beliefs evolve from the way in which members of that culture perceive their world. Figure 28.1 illustrates how two people can look at the same image and perceive it very differently. One person readily sees an aristocratic young woman with a stylish hat. Another sees a haggard old woman with a large nose, wearing a scarf. Neither perception is right or wrong; each person simply sees one image more readily than the other. In other words, one image stands out more clearly than the other and is recognized more easily. However, another more

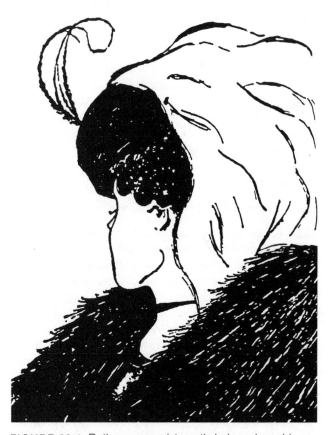

FIGURE 28.1 Both a young aristocratic lady and an old woman can be seen in this illustration.

subtle image also is present and can be perceived with greater effort.

Understanding this duality in perception sheds light on the challenge inherent in breastfeeding promotion. There are two very different perceptions of infant feeding throughout the world. In much of the Western world baby bottles are readily associated with infant feeding with bottle feeding the norm and expectation of the general population. To meet the challenge of increasing breastfeeding rates and acceptance, society therefore needs to change how it *perceives* infant feeding. In your efforts to promote breastfeeding, you need to recognize this perception of bottle feeding for infants. You cannot persuade others to change their perceptions and beliefs. Change must happen from the inside out and at a pace that is comfortable for those who are undergoing the change. Understanding *why* others may be resistant helps you in your efforts to facilitate meaningful change.

Anticipating Resistance to Change

Unfortunately, not everyone will share your enthusiasm for making dramatic changes in breastfeeding policies and practices. You will undoubtedly meet with some degree of resistance in your efforts to institute changes. As common as change is, people do not always receive it well. A change in routine can be very unsettling, creating tension and stress. Unless a change is handled effectively, the changed practice risks being undermined or sabotaged. The change could result in employee turnover, political battles, and a drain on money and time. There are substantial financial issues at stake in U.S. hospitals, most of which receive "free" formula from manufacturers in return for serving as the manufacturers' unpaid marketing arm to consumers (Walker, 2007a, 2007b; Merewood & Philipp, 2000). Recognizing that resistance is a natural part of the change process helps you capitalize on it and use it as a tool.

Seven Stages of Resistance to Change

There is a descending scale of resistance to change, with the most resistant person arguing that there is no problem and thus no change needed. People who are most likely to embrace change acknowledge a problem exists and enthusiastically help to bring about the desired outcome. The stages of resistance presented here are adapted from educational materials developed by SARAR International and published by World Neighbors in Action (Anand, 2005). Some possible arguments against breastfeeding promotion appear with each stage. With some minor adaptations from the original version, the seven stages are as follows:

1. There is no problem. I know human milk is good for babies, but artificial baby milk is perfectly safe. Formula has fed babies for decades. Furthermore, women have a right to choose how they want to feed their babies and they shouldn't be made to feel guilty if they choose to bottle feed.

2. I recognize there is a problem, but it's not my responsibility. I accept that breastfeeding is superior to artificial feeding. But I can't get involved. I don't have the time. Someone else will do it.

3. I accept there is a problem, but I doubt anyone's ability to change it. We have a problem with infant feeding, but the formula companies are too strong and influential and our society does not see a problem. Society will never embrace a breastfeeding culture.

4. I accept there is a problem, but I'm afraid to get involved. We have a problem, but I'm afraid to try to do anything about it. If I make too many waves, I might lose my job. I'm afraid of what others will think of me. I'm afraid of the time commitment.

5. We believe we can do something about it, and I will begin to look for solutions. We have a problem with infant feeding. I want to empower women and help improve infant health. I will get involved, but I'm still unsure it will make a difference.

6. We know we can do it and obstacles will not stop us. I know I can make a difference. Working together we can change things. Let's get started!

7. We did it! Now we want to share our results with others. We finally have policies and procedures that promote breastfeeding, and our staff is following the guidelines. We have returned control to mothers and babies and are empowering women to reach their breastfeeding goals.

It is likely that several of these stages of resistance are represented among the various members of a group. A group goal is to foster a climate in which each person advances to stage 5, where the focus is on group effort rather than a single person taking responsibility. When individuals reach this stage, they are on their way to achieving the desired goal of empowerment.

Every member of the group needs to respect the process of change their colleagues undertake. Each person enters the process at varying stages in their acceptance of the anticipated change. Thus, members need time and patience to progress at their own rate and cannot be expected to jump forward several stages at once. Members enter the process at varying stages along the continuum and progress at a pace corresponding to their level of comfort.

Many times, the greatest resister becomes one of the staunchest advocates when given the opportunity to progress through the necessary stages that lead to understanding and embracing the change. Some individuals may seem to slide backward during the period of change, depending on specific issues or information that surface. Furthermore, the group needs to accept that some people never change their opinions or beliefs. Patience and flexibility are cornerstones to establishing consensus for moving forward with positive change.

Resistance to the Ten Steps to Successful Breastfeeding

As discussed earlier, the Ten Steps to Successful Breastfeeding can serve as your guide to instituting changes in breastfeeding policies and practices. By anticipating the reasons people may resist these guidelines, you can select an approach to help resolve issues before they become obstacles. Table 28.2 identifies the types of responses that may occur relative to each of the steps for breastfeeding promotion.

Reasons for Resistance to Change

The previous section described the stages of resistance people experience when confronted with the prospect of change. Understanding the possible source for resisting the *idea* of change, in other words, an individual's motives, helps you determine your most effective approach.

Loss of Control

How people greet a change depends on the degree to which they feel they are in control of it. Some people who resist a change in routine may worry about losing their feeling of self-efficacy or power. Just as loss of control can lead to resistance, ownership typically leads to commitment. It is important at every step in the process to recognize that change is exciting when it is done *by* us and is threatening when it is done *to* us. Increasing each person's involvement and participation and empowering them with legitimate choices promote ownership of the change.

Uncertainty

Some people may have a sense of uncertainty about where a proposed change will lead. They may, for example, worry about how it could alter their daily routines and career plans. You can help to allay doubts and fears by openly sharing what is happening with everyone involved. Avoid springing decisions on others without sufficient groundwork or preparation. Furthermore, dividing a big change into several small steps over an extended period allows others the opportunity to settle into one part of a change before experiencing the next step. People who have no time to prepare mentally can feel threatened by a change, and their natural reaction is to resist. Making sure everyone understands what will take place and when to expect more information helps to minimize uncertainty.

Difference

Things are different whenever change occurs, and some people simply want things to remain the same. With

---

TABLE 28.2 Responses to Arguments Against the Ten Steps to Successful Breastfeeding

Step 1	*Have a written breastfeeding policy that is routinely communicated to all healthcare staff.*
Stage of Resistance	**Argument**
There is no problem	We've had a policy for years. It's working well enough.
	We've been functioning well enough without one.
It's not my responsibility	I have too much to do already.
	I wouldn't know where to even begin writing a policy.
No one can do it	Even if we had a policy, no one would follow it.
	Mothers aren't motivated enough to breastfeed, so why bother.
I can't get involved	There are too many on the staff opposed to it.
	I wouldn't be able to get support from the supervisor or manager.
Let's begin	I can explore policies in other hospitals.
	I can contact ILCA to locate resources.
We can do it	Let's bring people together from all departments to work on it.
	Let's survey our patients to learn how satisfied they are.
We did it!	**We accomplished our goal!**

(Continued)

TABLE 28.2 Responses to Arguments Against the Ten Steps to Successful Breastfeeding (*Continued*)

Step 2	*Train all healthcare staff in skills necessary to implement this policy.*
Stage of Resistance	**Argument**
There is no problem	We have IBCLCs, so we don't need to train the rest of the staff.
	Our nurses know what they need to know about breastfeeding.
It's not my responsibility	I don't have time to train everyone.
	I wouldn't know where to even begin with training.
No one can do it	The staff would never agree to 18 hours of training.
	We don't have enough money or time to train the entire staff.
I can't get involved	Staff would resent my suggesting that they need the training.
	I wouldn't be able to get support from the supervisor/manager.
Let's begin	I can explore how other hospitals do their training.
	I will take an extensive course in lactation.
We can do it	Let's survey staff to find out what they know about breastfeeding.
	Let's form a committee with people from several departments.
We did it!	**We accomplished our goal!**

Step 3	*Inform all pregnant women about the benefits and management of breastfeeding.*
Stage of Resistance	**Argument**
There is no problem	We give help and advice to mothers when they are in the hospital.
	Teaching breastfeeding will create guilt in those who don't.
It's not my responsibility	Mothers learn what they need to know in their childbirth classes.
	It's the mother's responsibility to read and seek information.
No one can do it	We realize we need to, but we don't have the resources.
	If women want to bottle feed, it's our responsibility to help them.
I can't get involved	I don't have time to do prenatal teaching with everything else.
	I wouldn't be able to get support from the supervisor/manager.
Let's begin	I can explore breastfeeding initiation rates in other hospitals.
	I can make a questionnaire to screen mothers with difficulties.
We can do it	Let's survey our patients to find out how satisfied they are.
	Let's explore what we can improve in the labor and delivery department.
We did it!	**We accomplished our goal!**

TABLE 28.2 Responses to Arguments Against the Ten Steps to Successful Breastfeeding (*Continued*)

Step 4	*Help mothers initiate breastfeeding within a half-hour of birth.*
Stage of Resistance	**Argument**
There is no problem	We start breastfeeding as soon as the mother gets to her room. Most babies are too sleepy to breastfeed right away.
It's not my responsibility	If she breastfeeds after delivery, relatives will have to wait to see the baby. Babies get too cold in the delivery room.
No one can do it	The labor and delivery staff would never support such a policy. There are too many procedures that need to be done at that time.
I can't get involved	The staff is getting tired of all my suggestions about breastfeeding. I'm not very good at persuading people.
Let's begin	I can find someone in labor and delivery who will be receptive to change. I can teach the staff about the importance of early initiation of breastfeeding.
We can do it	Let's try it on a short-term trial basis and then evaluate it. We can find ways to keep babies warm.
We did it!	**We accomplished our goal!**
Step 5	*Show mothers how to breastfeed and how to maintain lactation, even if they should be separated from their infants.*
Stage of Resistance	**Argument**
There is no problem	Breastfeeding is a natural instinct; we don't need to teach it. There are plenty of support groups who will help them.
It's not my responsibility	If the baby is in the NICU, those nurses are responsible for it. I can't possibly see every breastfeeding mother.
No one can do it	We don't have enough staff to spend the time required for this. A lot of our staff don't believe in pushing breastfeeding.
I can't get involved	I wouldn't get support from my supervisor for the time it will take. Staff won't spend so much time with breastfeeding mothers.
Let's begin	I can encourage staff to accompany me on rounds. I can propose telephone follow-up for breastfeeding mothers.
We can do it	Let's survey our patients about what would have helped them. Let's explore a program to mentor staff in breastfeeding.
We did it!	**We accomplished our goal!**

(Continued)

TABLE 28.2 Responses to Arguments Against the Ten Steps to Successful Breastfeeding (*Continued*)

Step 6	*Give newborn infants no food or drink other than breastmilk, unless* medically *indicated.*
Stage of Resistance	**Argument**
There is no problem	We never do anything unless it is medically indicated. I am legally responsible to see that the baby is not dehydrated.
It's not my responsibility	I can't influence physician policies. Purchase of formula is an administrative decision, not mine.
No one can do it	Administration will never agree to begin purchasing formula. Formula companies will withdraw other funding if we make this change.
I can't get involved	I would not be able to get support from the supervisor/manager. What about jaundice? This could be dangerous.
Let's begin	I can explore how other hospitals have begun purchasing formula. I can teach staff the importance of exclusive breastfeeding.
We can do it	Let's review reasons we have been giving formula and water. Let's invite some mothers in to discuss how they managed.
We did it!	**We accomplished our goal!**
Step 7	*Practice rooming-in—allow mothers and infants to remain together—24 hours a day.*
Stage of Resistance	**Argument**
There is no problem	We have better security if babies are kept in the nursery. Babies could choke if they stay in the mother's room.
It's not my responsibility	Mothers are tired after laboring and delivering. That is an administrative decision.
No one can do it	If babies stay with their mothers, nursery staff will lose their jobs. Mothers do not want to keep their babies in the room.
I can't get involved	I will never get support from administration. The pediatricians will not examine babies in the mothers' rooms.
Let's begin	I can explore rooming-in policies at other hospitals. I can teach staff the importance of keeping babies with mothers.
We can do it	Let's invite pediatricians to meet with the breastfeeding committee. Let's record how much time babies spend away from their mothers.
We did it!	**We accomplished our goal!**

TABLE 28.2 Responses to Arguments Against the Ten Steps to Successful Breastfeeding (*Continued*)

Step 8	*Encourage breastfeeding on demand.*
Stage of Resistance	**Argument**
There is no problem	It is more efficient having scheduled feeding times. Babies need to get on a schedule as early as possible.
It's not my responsibility	I can do it with the mothers I see, but I can't see all of them. The babies must be fed at least two times on every shift.
No one can do it	Staff routines would be disrupted too much. It would be too hard to monitor babies for hypoglycemia without a schedule.
I can't get involved	Staff routines would be disrupted too much. This would be much too confusing.
Let's begin	I can teach staff the importance of the mother and baby setting the pace. I can help staff learn to recognize and teach feeding cues.
We can do it	Let's keep statistics to see if schedules make a difference. Let's try it for 6 months to see how it works.
We did it!	**We accomplished our goal!**

Step 9	*Give no artificial teats or pacifiers (also called dummies or soothers) to breastfeeding infants.*
Stage of Resistance	**Argument**
There is no problem	We have to test to see if the baby can suck and swallow. Babies have strong sucking needs and need pacifiers to keep calm.
It's not my responsibility	If parents want them, it is not my position to discourage it. Everyone uses pacifiers, so what's the big deal?
No one can do it	I'm the only one in the hospital who considers this to be a problem. Pacifiers are a part of our culture, just like baby bottles.
I can't get involved	The staff will think it takes too long to feed with a cup or spoon. There is nothing to document the use of cups for feeding babies.
Let's begin	I can teach staff about sucking preference and confusion. I can teach the staff how to cup feed a baby.
We can do it	Let's review why we give formula and water. Let's teach mothers to put the baby to breast rather than give a pacifier.
We did it!	**We accomplished our goal!**

(Continued)

TABLE 28.2 Responses to Arguments Against the Ten Steps to Successful Breastfeeding (*Continued*)

Step 10	Foster the establishment of breastfeeding support groups and refer mothers to them on discharge from the hospital or clinic.
Stage of Resistance	**Argument**
There is no problem	We have the information at the desk if the patient requests it. Women in those groups make mothers feel guilty if they wean early.
It's not my responsibility	It is the mother's responsibility to seek help. The physician will refer her if there is a problem.
No one can do it	We don't have enough resources to start a support group here. The counselors do not always give sound advice and information.
I can't get involved	If I do this, I'll have to do it on my own time. I don't have time to keep updating the referral list.
Let's begin	I can visit community support groups and foster a strong link. I can offer to train mother-to-mother support counselors.
We can do it	Let's give a name and telephone number to breastfeeding mothers. Let's explore an outpatient clinic and/or support group.
We did it!	**We accomplished our goal!**

Source: Reprinted by permission of Judith Lauwers.

change, people will be obligated to question familiar routines and habits. They must actively think about behavior they had taken for granted, needing to "reprogram" their daily routines. You can help others find their comfort level by minimizing the number of changes and leaving as many habits and routines unchanged as possible. Conducting an inventory of your practices will help you identify what you are doing right and what needs to be adjusted.

Loss of Face

Some people may believe that a proposed change implies that the old ways were wrong. They may fear looking foolish because of past actions and may feel embarrassed and self-conscious. People with deeply personal reasons for resisting breastfeeding promotion need help putting past actions into perspective. Help others appreciate that their past actions were based on what was considered appropriate at the time. As new research and new knowledge about breastfeeding become available, practices evolve and change. Praise others for their accomplishments under the old conditions, and thank them for their willingness to change to meet present needs. Help them understand that you, too, have changed your practices, and encourage them to view the change positively.

Competence

Understandably, the prospect of change often causes concern about future competence. It is natural for people to worry about their ability to be effective after the change. New ways often demand an entirely new set of competencies and they may wonder, "Can I do it?" or "How will I do it?" Some may be forced to start over again with a new way of doing things. Equipping everyone with the necessary knowledge and skills for doing their jobs under the new rules is critical to the success of your new practices. You can ensure that others feel competent by providing sufficient training, giving positive reinforcement, and providing ample opportunity for them to practice new skills without judgment. A formal mentorship program or other method of supervised training allows people to observe and practice in a nonthreatening setting.

Disruption

It is important to acknowledge that a proposed change can be disruptive to some of the people involved. For example, it may interrupt plans or projects that others believe are as worthy as the one you propose. Meeting a deadline or attending a meeting may intrude on people's personal time. The time commitment required could interfere with days they are not scheduled to work and with planned family activities. Staff members may be concerned that instituting the change requires more energy, time, and mental preoccupation. They may be required to go "above and beyond" their usual efforts. Be sure to validate these concerns and to give support and recognition for this extra effort. Introduce changes with flexibility, and be sensitive to the effect the process has on those who must implement the change and operate in a new way.

Past Grievances

The goal of leaving personalities and positions at the door is for everyone to enter the process on even footing and with an open mind. In reality, however, this rarely happens. Understandably, unresolved grievances from the past can surface as you approach others with your proposed change. Perhaps one person sought your support for a previous activity and was not satisfied with your response or your seeming lack of support. Undercurrents of professional jealousy or other resentments may obstruct your efforts at achieving unity within the group. Perhaps your predecessor alienated staff with an offensive approach and your motives are questioned. Addressing past issues that could color attitudes and responses to your proposed change clears the air so everyone can focus on the present issues.

Real Threat

When your change is in place, it most likely will alter people's routines. The traditional way of doing things is replaced with new routines and a new set of expectations that challenges people to modify their practices. The process that took place may transform relationships with colleagues as well. Despite your efforts at collaboration and unity, instituting the change may have created winners and losers, resulting in people losing status or power.

For example, if a proposed change would institute 24-hour rooming-in as a standard in your facility, babies would no longer remain in a central nursery. A particular nurse may have worked in the central nursery for the past 20 years because her greatest enjoyment is taking care of "her" babies. If babies spend the majority of their time in the mothers' rooms, this nurse's daily routine will change dramatically. She may adapt or may dislike the change enough to resign.

Everyone needs a chance to let go of the past and needs a supportive climate in which to do so. Be sensitive to the loss of routines, comforts, traditions, and relationships. Avoid any pretense or false promises and accept that a perceived threat sometimes is real and that a person may find the change too difficult or too disruptive.

Conflict Resolution

Introducing change results in a certain degree of conflict. While on the surface it may seem helpful to try to avoid conflict or pretend that it does not exist, this attitude can actually lead to further conflict (Dana, 2000; Mayer, 2000). Embracing conflict as a natural part of the change process enables you to manage it more rationally and productively. Bringing conflicts out in the open allows honest, frank, and positive relationships to develop among group members. Conflict can actually be very constructive; it makes people revved up and more receptive to finding creative solutions. Conflict helps us realize and validate our values, and it is through conflict that people learn to understand others and recognize the value of working together.

Inevitably, further conflicts will surface as the process of change continues. It is better to address such issues as they arise, no matter how minor they may seem. You want to foster an environment in which honesty prevails and where neither side keeps an "account" of grievances against the other. Recognize that people work to satisfy their own personal needs, often a need for money, power, or identity. People generally want others to accept them as they are and to like and appreciate them. Consequently, to resolve conflict, you must meet the other person's needs as well as your own.

Be Sensitive to Others

Sensitivity to another person's circumstances is important in all communication. Avoid confronting conflict in a public setting or in the presence of others who are uninvolved. Keep in mind that you are attempting to change behaviors, not people. To establish and maintain solid relationships, you need to remain focused on the solution rather than on individual problems. Find ways group members can join together to work through conflicts that stand in the way of reaching your goals. Because conflict involves both issues and feelings, you must get emotions out of the way before you can solve problems. When emotions surface, reflecting them back through active listening recognizes and validates them. It is only then that you can move on to address problems and work toward solutions.

Identify Common Goals

In addressing a conflict, it may help first to determine basic goals that you share with the other person. Establishing common ground can help set the stage for debating respective strategies for moving forward. One common objective is empowering mothers and babies to achieve their goals. With that as a starting point, you can begin to discuss strategies to accomplish it. After establishing what you have in common, you need to figure out how to meet on common ground with other related issues.

Finding outcomes with mutual benefit sets a tone of cooperation and problem solving and puts both of you on the same side, instead of remaining adversaries.

Coping with Difficult People

Invariably, you will have at least one person on your team whom others regard as difficult. You have tried everything in your arsenal to work with this person cooperatively. You have validated feelings and acknowledged concerns, and yet you continually meet with resistance. A change in approach may achieve more positive results. Recognize that you cannot change the other person. Moreover, you cannot directly change the way that person responds to you. What you can change is the way you relate to that person. Finding a more effective way to communicate and present yourself can indirectly influence how the other person will respond.

Approaching a Difficult Person

- Be positive. Give recognition and praise for accomplishments, and avoid placing blame.
- Prepare for interactions by writing down exactly what you plan to say. In addition to helping you prepare, this helps release any underlying negativism before an actual confrontation.
- Use appropriate body language. Face the person squarely, sit or stand erect, and lean forward to demonstrate a desire to interact and communicate in a meaningful way.
- Give your undivided attention and respond both verbally ("I see . . . , I'm with you") and nonverbally (nodding, smiling, and maintaining eye contact).
- Avoid distractions when speaking. Do not focus on what you anticipate the other person will say. Focus on your goal, and keep an even pace.
- Recycle the other person's message to make sure you understood it correctly. After you have sent the message, pause for a response before continuing to speak.

The Aggressor   Some difficult people are aggressive to the point of being hostile. Having a strong sense of what others should do and how they should do it, they can be abrasive, abrupt, intimidating, and relentless. Their goal is to prove that you are wrong and they are right. You need to stay as dispassionate as possible with such a person. An angry person cannot stay overtly angry for long if you remain calm. Listen attentively, look them directly in the eye, and be ready to interrupt them. On the other hand, if they interrupt you, hold your ground and say, "You interrupted me, let me finish." It is important not to allow an aggressor to take control with negative energy.

The Saboteur   You may find yourself dealing with someone who sabotages your efforts from behind the scenes. This person does not engage in direct confrontation yet can be as divisive as one who confronts you openly. Never ignore a sniper! You need to expose their undermining efforts either privately or in a group setting. Otherwise, they will continue to breed discontent at every turn.

One type of sabotage that can occur in a hospital setting may come in the form of opposition or threats from formula manufacturers (Walker, 2007b, Merewood & Philipp, 2000). One formula company ceased printing a hospital's mother–baby care booklet because breastfeeding rates were getting too high to justify their "free" printing. One manufacturer labels its water bottles with the words "do not use for breastmilk storage." This enables them to promote brand awareness while at the same time creating negative imagery about breastfeeding.

The Wet Blanket   A wet blanket can infect others by dampening enthusiasm and undermining positive thinking. This person argues, "It won't work" or "It's no use" and refuses to buy into what the group is trying to accomplish. One way to challenge such a person is to ask them for ideas on positive, realistic ways to solve problems. Take their complaints seriously and ask, "What's the worst possible scenario?" Put the matter back in their hands and engage them in considering solutions. Capitalize on the strength they bring to the group for identifying things that can go wrong with implementation of any policy or procedure. Engaging their talents in this way gives them value and enables them to contribute to the process.

The Expert   Be aware of people who consider themselves experts. Although their demeanor may seem pompous and arrogant, they are usually very productive and talented. Avoid trying to assert yourself as the expert and instead show that you respect their opinion and ask them to explain their point further. Allowing them to be the expert may help you accomplish your goal. Be prepared and accurate in your interactions with these people. If their opinion is at odds with your recommendations, make sure what you recommend is evidence based and has peer-reviewed research to support it. You can ask politely for the same evidence for their recommendations as well.

Divisiveness in a Meeting   Attention to meeting dynamics can help neutralize the efforts of a difficult person. When you are confronted by a difficult person in a meeting, try to get involvement from others in the group. Obtain their input and support before the meeting. During the meeting you might ask for their reactions, for example, "How would you . . .", "What do you think of . . .", "How many would agree?" Even where you sit in a meeting can help to reduce divisiveness. If you expect conflict with a particular person, arrange to sit directly next to them and avoid placing yourself directly across from the person, as this heightens the potential for conflict. It is more difficult to spar with someone who is sitting immediately next to you.

Food is a great neutralizer in meetings and sales organizations have used "free" food to capture attendance for years (Stolberg & Gerth, 2000). The social dynamics of passing through a line, handing a plate of cookies to someone, or commenting on food increases goodwill. It is socially acceptable to finish chewing and swallowing and then take a drink of water before answering. Therefore, the mechanics of eating enables you to pause for time to think and reduces impatience for those waiting for a response.

Using Humor as a Tool for Change

Humor is an invaluable tool for facilitating change and diffusing resistance. Humor makes it possible for us to survive in "the system." It leads toward a greater awareness of the strengths and weaknesses in the present system, new ways to respond and express creativity, and the survival and productivity of valuable human resources (Jackson, 1985). The comic relief of humor injected into a situation often presents a new perspective and leads to compromise. A leader who maintains a good sense of humor inspires tremendous loyalty and enthusiasm (Yerkes, 2001). Humor leads to the creation of a positive climate and fosters an energized work environment. Learn how to maintain humor in your quest for change and to infuse humor in others.

∽ Beginning the Process of Change

The first step to creating change is to believe that you can do it! Margaret Mead taught us, "Don't ever say one person can't change the world. It is the only thing that ever has." A confident attitude and systematic preparation increase the ability to garner support for the anticipated change. Gathering supporting research, evaluating current practices, and defining the problems leads to developing an action plan for implement the change.

Art of Persuasion

Attitude and communication style affect the ability to overcome the challenge of persuading others to embrace a new change. Benjamin Franklin said, "The aim of persuasion is not to confront other people, but to appreciate their points of view and try to move them generally in your direction." Franklin used the acronym TALKING to describe his success at persuasion, with each letter standing for one of seven keys to successful persuasion (Humes, 1992):

- Timing—It's not good enough to have the right message. You must also choose the right moment.
- Appreciation—If you want someone else to accommodate a request, you should learn to appreciate the other person's problems and concerns.
- Listening—Learn to listen well enough to find out what you need and how best to sell it to the other person. Feed back their own words, using their words to sell the point.
- Knowledge—Learn where the other person is coming from and how to get them where you want to go.
- Integrity—Never misrepresent your fundamental beliefs or motives.
- Need—The three most persuasive words in the English language are "I need you." When you must ask people for something, the best way to convince them is to show them they are uniquely qualified to give it to you.
- Giving—Learn the value of giving. If you insist on everything, you may wind up with nothing.

Doing Your Homework

Your effectiveness in initiating change depends on how well you prepare before you approach others with your ideas. For example, if you want to work toward your facility becoming baby friendly, first consider which policies and procedures need to be changed. Before you approach anyone with your ideas, collect as much supporting data as possible for each change you have in mind. Such preparation before approaching others will be central to your success.

Gather Data

An essential first step in initiating change is to gather supporting research, and lots of it! Accumulate information needed to support your proposed change, including current policies and practices and the consequences of the way you are operating. Document breastfeeding initiation rates, as well as continuation rates at 2 weeks, 3 months, and 6 months. Learn how your rates compare with other hospitals in your community. Survey mothers about the breastfeeding support they receive in your hospital to learn what was good or bad and what could be improved.

Record all the data you collect and incorporate it into your goals for change. For example, if 65 percent of mothers in your hospital initiate breastfeeding, you may set a goal that in 12 months the initiation rate will be 70 percent. The following year the goal can be a rate of 75 percent, and so on. You can do the same for increasing breastfeeding duration and other improvements in breastfeeding care.

Comparing your facility's findings with national, state, provincial, or local statistics is also instructive. For example, in 2003, the percentage of mothers who initiated breastfeeding ranged from 51.2 percent in Louisiana to 90.3 percent in Alaska. This range of initiation rates illustrates that the community's needs are very different in Louisiana than in Alaska (Suellentrop et al., 2006). Therefore, your strategies and goals need to reflect where you reside.

Evaluate Your Facility

After gathering your data and research, you can next assess which of your present policies and practices are research based and in line with current recommendations. Where you determine a need for change, prepare detailed rationale for the change. Write down anticipated arguments, along with your possible responses to each one. Identify alternative approaches and methods in case you experience obstacles. This careful evaluation is an essential step in the process of change. It will prepare you for responding to those who present obstacles and arguments. The best defense is a strong offense, shored by evidence-based research. After a change has been proposed and discussed, write down any unanticipated arguments that surfaced and note any adjustments needed in your approach.

Model for Planned Change

An important part of your process will be developing a systematic plan for structuring the change. Most planning begins with defining a problem and goal, determining the change agent, and then designing a well-defined plan of action. In your plan for your facility to become baby friendly, you can examine other hospitals that have achieved official Baby-friendly Hospital designation. Resources such as Women, Infants, and Children (WIC), Loving Support, and Wellstart are other models that can be adapted to fit your hospital's needs.

Define the Problem

For every change you wish to institute, define the problem that makes that change necessary. Rather than stating a problem globally in terms of lack of support for breastfeeding, define each specific problem area where changes need to occur. For example, you may cite low initiation rates, high rates of engorgement, or large numbers of babies who have difficulty with latch. Determine the

change agents, in other words, the people who will be the most effective leaders in proposing and instituting the particular change. Identify those people and positions the change will affect, and involve representatives from all affected areas in the process so that everyone has ownership in the change.

Define Goals and Strategies

Determine whether you hope to change behavior, attitudes, values, procedures, policies, or perhaps the entire structure. You can then identify specific objectives—short term, intermediate and long term—and develop a timeline for planning and implementing the change. A goal of increasing the incidence of breastfeeding, for example, may have a short-term objective of increasing the rate to 58 percent, an intermediate objective of 68 percent, and a long-term objective of 75 percent. Reflect all these objectives in the timeline.

With objectives established, you are ready to develop an action plan and strategies. Try to anticipate all the issues involved in each individual objective. Be sure to address the education required for empowering the staff to implement the change, as well as how the change will be communicated. Consider which procedures and policies need to be altered and how the changes will affect people's levels of authority or power.

Implement the Change

After you have defined the problems, goals, and strategies, you are ready to implement the change. As you do so, be sure to monitor everyone's responses to learn if any unanticipated problems arise. If problems occur, resolve them immediately so you can maintain a high level of commitment among the staff. Evaluate both the positive and negative outcomes. Too often, this step of evaluation receives little attention. Failing to evaluate the outcomes associated with the change could jeopardize long-term success. When the change has become ingrained procedurally, you can take the final step of linking it to the overall organizational structure and standardizing it.

Planning a Breastfeeding Committee

Your chances of success will be greater when change occurs through some form of concerted group effort. A breastfeeding committee or task force can serve this purpose. If you do not already have a breastfeeding committee in your facility, you may want to consider establishing one. You can approach the person in charge of maternity services to discuss how breastfeeding is going in your facility. In a hospital, for example, this may be the nurse manager or nursing director. In a low-key manner you can ask, "Have you noticed that our breastfeeding initiation rate is 20 percent lower than in the hospital across town?" This or another issue you wish to explore can spark an interest that could be pursued casually over lunch or at another convenient time. This discussion marks the beginning of your committee and the beginning of your initiative for change!

Members of the Team

The constitution of a committee influences its success, and you will want to put careful thought into the makeup of the members on a committee. You want the committee to be large enough that if a couple of members are absent, the meeting can still go on as planned. Each person's level of support for breastfeeding is important as well. Group dynamics will benefit from including people whom you have identified as allies, those you expect will resist, and those who seem to be neutral. Having such diversity in the group and getting buy-in from potential resistors helps avoid sabotage or a perception that the cards are stacked in favor of one group over another. Many times, the greatest resistors become some of the most avid supporters after they understand the issues involved.

A quality improvement representative is a valuable member of a breastfeeding committee. All U.S. hospitals accredited by the Joint Commission are required to have a process in place for quality improvement. This motivates hospitals to identify problem areas and make improvements. Because quality improvement efforts aim to increase customer satisfaction, their mission mirrors that of breastfeeding advocates in focusing efforts on what is best for the baby and mother (Cadwell, 1997).

Attempt to have the group represent all areas the change will affect. In a hospital, areas affected may include obstetrics, labor and delivery, postpartum, neonatal intensive care, and pediatrics. Consider other areas and people who have contact with breastfeeding mothers and babies as well. These may include technicians, housekeeping personnel, and management as well as community professionals in home care, pharmacy, and speech pathology. Bringing together representatives of all these groups to form an interdisciplinary team enables all those affected by the change to participate equally in the process. Changes in breastfeeding practices and policies are ideally suited to a quality improvement approach.

Types of Personalities

The personalities of the specific people on a committee are important to group dynamics. Every personality type contributes positive traits to a group. The variety of personal attributes and diversity with which people approach issues demonstrates the value of including the entire range of personalities in a group process. Capitalizing on the best of each style contributes to the group's dynamics and productivity.

Kahler (2008) identified six basic personality types prevalent among North Americans (Table 28.3): feelers (reactors), thinkers (workaholics), funsters (rebels), believers (persisters), dreamers (dreamers), and doers (promoters). Feelers form the largest group, about 30 percent of the population. They are compassionate and react quickly to the feelings of others. Feelers respond to assurances that you are happy to have them on your team. Thinkers comprise 25 percent of the population. They are logical and organized and want you to get to the point and just tell them the facts. Funsters (rebels), another 20 percent of the population, are creative, spontaneous, and playful. They enjoy stimulating contact with other people and dislike rigid schedules. Believers (persisters) are conscientious, observant, and dedicated. Representing 10 percent of the population, their strong beliefs make it difficult for them to accept criticism from others. It helps to let them know how much you value their character and accomplishments. Dreamers, another 10 percent of the population, are imaginative and like solitude and quiet surroundings. You may need to take the initiative with them and give them personal space. Doers (promoters) form the final 5 percent of the population. They are persuasive, charming, action oriented, and are firm and direct. It is easy to see that each of these personalities will contribute positively to group dynamics.

Another method of comparing personality types divides them into five categories: synthesist, idealist, pragmatist, analyst, and realist (Bramson, 1992). Although synthesists are often labeled as troublemakers because they seek conflict, they also provide debate and creativity to the group process. Idealists are good at articulating goals and providing a broad view of issues. However, because of their extremely high standards, idealists can suffer deep disappointments. Pragmatists are resourceful, adaptable and sensitive to what appeals to others, and willing to experiment and to settle for small gains. Nonetheless, they also look for immediate results and find it difficult to focus on long-range plans. Analysts are methodical, accurate, thorough, and persistent. They rationalize, are stubborn and strong-minded, and look for one best way to do something. Realists are confident, practical, and good at delegating. They focus on both facts and opinions, provide drive and momentum, and are interested in concrete results. Because realists are forthright and dogmatic, they sometimes seem domineering. Nevertheless, others can count on them to get the job done and to rarely be wrong. It is easy to see the strengths each of these personalities offer to the group.

Dynamics of a Team Meeting

After committee members are in place, the group can begin to meet regularly. The fact that not all members of the team share a common purpose should not prevent

TABLE 28.3 Six Personality Types

Personality Type	Percent of N.A. Population	Characteristics
Feelers (Reactors)	30%	• Compassionate, sensitive, warm • Nurturing and giving; create harmony • React quickly to feelings of others • Will respond to assurances that you are happy to have them on your team
Thinkers (Workaholics)	25%	• Logical, responsible, organized • Take in facts, ideas, and synthesize • Will want you to get to the point and just tell them the facts
Funsters (Rebels)	20%	• Creative, spontaneous, and playful • Enjoy stimulating contact with other people • Humorous, able to enjoy the present • Dislike rigid schedules
Believers (Persisters)	10%	• Conscientious, observant, and dedicated • Strong beliefs make it difficult to accept criticism from others • Ability to express opinions, beliefs, judgments • Let them know how much you value their character and accomplishments
Dreamers (Dreamers)	10%	• Imaginative, reflective, calm • Like solitude and quiet surroundings • Able to see big picture • Work well with things and directions • May need to take the initiative with them and give them personal space
Doers (Promoters)	5%	• Persuasive, charming, adaptable • Action oriented • Experience world by doing • Ability to be firm and direct

Source: "Six Personality Types" from *The Process Therapy Model: The Six Personality Types with Adaptations* by Taibi Kahler, PhD. Copyright © 2008 Taibi Kahler Associates, Inc. All rights reserved. Reprinted by permission of Kahler Communications, Inc.

them from cooperating to reach group goals. The ultimate group goal is to find creative solutions that are mutually beneficial. A smoothly functioning team requires empathy and a willingness to encourage the best from others. Members of the group can be asked to identify specific problems and then determine how and where to start making changes.

As a group leader withholding your own agenda until the group has processed the issues helps you learn their needs. In the process, your agenda may take a different shape if you are open to hear what others say. Knowing when to keep quiet, sit back, and let the discussion flow helps you avoid the trap of beginning with a rigid pre-planned agenda. After you have stated your position or proposal, stop and let others respond. For group members to take ownership of a change, they each need to be a part of designing it. It is important that you learn as much as possible about the needs of each member before proposing solutions.

Take It Slow and Easy

It is important that you not try to change everything all at once. Many routines and practices can probably remain in place. First recognize the strengths of the organization by identifying what is right with the present system. Underscore with members of the group all the positive policies and practices that already provide good care to mothers and babies.

After you target areas where improvements are needed make sure everyone has realistic expectations for how the changes will occur. Recognize that major change cannot occur quickly and that it could take as long as 10 years for your facility to reach its full potential in protecting, supporting, and promoting breastfeeding.

As you prioritize the changes, consider the anticipated level of difficulty in convincing others to support each change. Starting with a change likely to garner the most support gives you a greater chance of success. For example, it may be much easier in a hospital setting to begin regular breastfeeding rounds than to eliminate mothers being given discharge bags from a formula company. Changes that are least disruptive to routines or least controversial are likely to meet with greater acceptance. Move slowly to issues perceived as more complicated or potentially problematic. At the same time, recognize that the change that seems easiest to you may not be the one that others favor.

Establishing a record of accomplishment with several of the easier changes prepares you for going on to the more challenging ones. Leave the toughest hurdles until you have several of the less controversial and less difficult changes in place. The success of instituting the earlier changes instills a greater level of confidence for moving on to the others. Additionally, after some of the changes are in practice, people may be better able to see the larger picture and be more willing to support the tougher changes.

Give Recognition and Praise

Everyone likes to be recognized for doing something correctly. This is especially true when they believe they have gone out of their way to provide good care. People respond favorably to positive feedback and expressions of gratitude. Sharing the praise with others gives well-earned recognition as well. Make sure others know the progress they made. For example, "Did you hear how much Mrs. Robinson appreciated Sheryl's help in getting her baby to latch?"

Creative incentives and rewards can encourage everyone's participation and compliance. You might award a button or pin for completing a breastfeeding module or attending an inservice program, a pizza party when a breastfeeding course is completed, or a designated breastfeeding counselor of the month. If you work for a large hospital, you could ask for a presence on the facility's website to publicize your services and the hospital's commitment to breastfeeding, and to post breastfeeding information. You can post a bulletin board with lactation updates, new policies, committee reports, summaries of professional research, and articles from newspapers, the Internet and professional journals. You could also publish a newsletter to send to physician offices. Such efforts can create cooperation and goodwill among those who care for breastfeeding women and their babies.

Ultimately, people have very basic needs they want to meet through their work. Although priorities may vary, most people share many of the same desires. They want work that is interesting and challenging. They want appreciation expressed for their efforts. They want to be involved in and important to the overall scheme. They want job security and reasonable pay. They want opportunities for career growth and advancement. Helping them meet these needs reaps the support and cooperation necessary for meeting your own needs.

∼ Turning the Tide in Breastfeeding Promotion

Breastfeeding promotion takes place at personal, institutional, political, and global levels. There is a great deal of support for breastfeeding promotion among the international healthcare community, governments, and organizations committed to protecting the health of infants and young children. Breastfeeding promotion initiatives recommend restrictions on inappropriate marketing of infant formula, citing the health risks inherent in aggressive promotion.

To understand the challenges inherent in breastfeeding promotion, the obstacles need to be clear. Examining the motives and actions of the infant formula industry provides a clear picture of the obstacles in breastfeeding promotion. The use of infant formula is an instantly recognizable obstacle to breastfeeding promotion efforts. Other less overt barriers can present challenges as well. Recognizing these challenges helps you develop strategies to capitalize on your promotion efforts.

Approaches to Promoting Breastfeeding

Opportunities for breastfeeding promotion present themselves in many spheres of influence affecting mothers' infant feeding decisions. Promotion strategies can target family, friends, health professionals, peer counselors, employers, and the communities in which mothers live (Bridges, 2007). Hospitals, physician practices, and employers are in the business of satisfying customer needs. In this regard breastfeeding promotion is no different from the marketing of any other health practice that improves the consumer's well-being. An institution adds value to its services by adopting a consumer-focused marketing strategy. Parents and infants are the consumers whose needs must be met. Breastfeeding-friendly practices provide a framework within which they can achieve their goals.

Breastfeeding promotion is a form of social marketing, and effective marketing strategies increase awareness of breastfeeding's importance. Marketing involves promotions used by businesses to convert people's needs and wants into profitable company opportunities (Kotler & Keller, 2008). Social marketing became popular when marketers applied the same principles used to sell products to "selling" ideas, attitudes, and behaviors. Social marketing seeks to influence social behavior and benefit the target audience and society as a whole (Weinreich, 2006). Although breastfeeding promotion initiatives use initiation and duration rates as markers for success, the ultimate goal is to return breastfeeding to a natural activity and to normalize it within the cultures of mothers and families.

Breastfeeding Promotion to Mothers

Breastfeeding promotion involves motivation, training, and coordination of the efforts of many people. Its success depends on the quality of education and support offered to mothers. In fact, educational programs are the single most effective intervention on initiation and short-term duration of breastfeeding (Guise et al., 2003). Educating mothers and families about breastfeeding within a context of risks and benefits helps inform mothers and promotes their commitment to exercise their right to breastfeed (Knaak, 2006). Including fathers in education programs has been shown to increase exclusive breastfeeding as well (Susin & Giugliani, 2008).

A woman's attitude toward child care and parenting is pivotal in her infant feeding decision. As discussed in Chapter 3, knowledge, social influence, and exposure to breastfeeding are significant in forming these attitudes. Normalizing breastfeeding during adolescence and young adulthood helps women develop favorable attitudes toward breastfeeding their children. Furthermore, understanding women's attitudes toward pregnancy and breastfeeding can lead to new strategies for promoting and maintaining breastfeeding (Sandes et al., 2007). More research is needed regarding factors that influence breastfeeding decisions, including maternity care practices, interactions with healthcare professionals, and workplace support (Scanlon et al., 2007).

Reach Mothers at Multiple Levels Breastfeeding promotion messages targeted at mothers need to reach them on multiple levels. A comprehensive approach places breastfeeding promotion and advocacy within the context of women's lives, in all aspects of their private and public lives (Mulford, 2008). Promotion strategies need to consider the composition of a mother's personal network beyond her socioeconomic or demographic characteristics (Fonseca-Becker & Valente, 2006). Generational traits and peer influence can strongly influence personal decisions, including the choice of infant feeding. Lactation consultants and other breastfeeding advocates can find this discouraging when a family member chooses not to breastfeed despite their support and encouragement.

The importance and benefits of breastfeeding are being incorporated into the curriculum of elementary school classes and high school home economics classes in the Philippines (Tubeza, 2009). School personnel are also mobilized in communicating health messages related to infant and young child feeding to students, teachers, and parents. Adolescents raised in an environment where breastfeeding rates are low may never have seen a baby nursing. Exposing them to visual representations of nursing mothers and introducing the topic to them in age-appropriate messages will reach them at a time when their own sexuality is emerging. Offering to teach classes at local schools provides an important community service and enables you to answer questions for young children and adolescents that may form the basis for later infant feeding decisions. Figure 28.2 provides a sample teaching outline for a high school class.

Opening discussion
- What have you heard about breastfeeding? (address misconceptions and concerns)
- Were you breastfed?
- Have you seen anyone breastfeed?
- Do you plan to breastfeed your children?

Paradigms of infant feeding
- Show illustrations that depict two possible interpretations (see Figure 28.1); relate to infant feeding practices
- Show images of animals nursing their young; relate to the normalcy of humans nursing

Changes in infant feeding practices
- Technological revolution and infant formula manufacturing
- World War II and women remaining in the workforce
- Return to breastfeeding as prevailing infant feeding method

Why we need to return to breastfeeding
- Health importance to babies, mother, family, society
- How breastmilk protects the baby and mother

Show video that:
- Depicts women breastfeeding
- Shows how breastfeeding works
- Puts breastfeeding into the context of lifestyle

Closing discussion
- Reactions to video and seeing women breastfeeding
- Discuss how class may have altered previous answer

FIGURE 28.2 High school class on breastfeeding.

Promotion efforts need to reflect particular circumstances in women's lives. Factors associated with early cessation of exclusive breastfeeding include being an adolescent mother, having fewer than six prenatal visits, use of a pacifier within the first month, and difficulty with latch. Developing promotion strategies to address these barriers helps to increase exclusive breastfeeding (Santo et al., 2007). Breastfeeding promotion among working women needs to be geared toward the mother, her social network, and the entire community (Johnston & Esposito, 2007) as well as mother–infant attachment and maternal sensitivity (Yoon & Park, 2008). Activities to promote exclusive breastfeeding should be intensified for adolescent mothers and for those whose prenatal care was less than ideal. These activities should reinforce the ill effects of pacifiers and should also include appropriate instruction for these mothers in correct breastfeeding technique. Promotion efforts need to address trends among women living within resource-poor settings as well (Sibeko et al., 2005).

Address Cultural Factors Cultural norms can influence the types of marketing strategies to which families respond favorably. Promotion strategies need to reflect an understanding of a woman's cultural heritage, including recognizing deep-rooted cultural beliefs that prohibit exclusive breastfeeding. Conventions and expectations from family members in one Zambian community were significant barriers in preventing the message of exclusive breastfeeding from being translated into practice (Fjeld et al., 2008). Similar barriers exist among Hispanics and other cultures as well. Understanding the heritage, cultural traditions, and acculturation of these women enhances their breastfeeding experience and promotes optimal breastfeeding practices (Hernandez, 2006). Black women have lower rates of breastfeeding than white and Mexican-American women. Promotion efforts targeted specifically at this group helps to increase breastfeeding rates among the black population.

Address Health Factors Over the past decade breastfeeding promotion changed from a positive message of breastfeeding's benefits to a risk-based message of the unfavorable consequences of *not* breastfeeding. Although this shift may appear subtle to some, it represents a deliberate marketing shift that underscores the health imperative of breastfeeding for mothers and babies. Risk-based messages encourage social and institutional change and may encourage others in the mother's life to value breastfeeding. On a cautionary note, however, we need to ensure that such risk-based messages don't cause us to fail to recognize and respond to mothers' perceived barriers (Heinig, 2009). Perceived barriers can be strong motivators in making decisions; thus, dispelling any misperceptions is an important first step in promotion efforts.

Women's social and economic status needs to be improved to provide choice for all women regardless of race or class. Only when breastfeeding represents a true choice for all women will it truly be fair to women (McCarter Spaulding, 2008). Breastfeeding promotion is especially critical among populations at high risk. Lack of awareness among mothers and lack of support from health workers and communities are largely to blame for only 39 percent of infants in developing countries being exclusively breastfed (UNICEF, 2005). Interventions to promote exclusive breastfeeding could potentially prevent 13 percent of all deaths of children younger than 5 years old in developing countries and are the single most important preventive intervention against child mortality (Jones et al., 2003). Cost savings in the United States alone could amount to $13 billion per year (Bartick & Reinold, 2010). Promotion of breastfeeding among Native American women was part of a type 2 diabetes prevention intervention (Murphy & Wilson, 2008).

Growth charts by the WHO constitute normal infant growth and development. This is in contrast to past practice, which treated breastfeeding as the optimal, rather than the normal, way to feed babies. One researcher suggests that a "breast is best" message actually may be coun-

terproductive in promoting breastfeeding as the norm (Berry & Gribble, 2008). Idealization of breastfeeding may inadvertently reinforce a perception that formula feeding is the standard way of feeding babies. Strategies and messages that normalize breastfeeding abandon the "breast is best" message in favor of messages that promote breastfeeding as a biological norm.

Breastfeeding Promotion Within the Healthcare Profession

Changes are occurring in health care around the globe. In the United States, for example, the length of stay after birth has altered dramatically in the past decade in response to new trends in health insurance. These changes affect everyone working in the healthcare field. Insufficient staffing, lack of continuity, ineffective guidelines, and lack of commitment interfere with implementing breastfeeding-friendly practices (Bulhosa et al., 2007). Promotion of breastfeeding must fit into the context of these aspects of the healthcare system.

Most women make their infant feeding decision before delivery, yet little promotion of breastfeeding occurs in most prenatal practice settings (Dusdieker et al., 2006). Breastfeeding promotion should also be incorporated into pediatric outpatient settings with specially trained pediatric staff (Böse-O'Reilly et al., 2008). Increasing women's breastfeeding empowerment and efficacy in clinical settings is an effective promotional strategy (Kang et al., 2008). Interactive interventions are effective during pregnancy and combining prenatal and postnatal interventions has a larger effect on increasing breastfeeding duration than either pre- or postnatal interventions alone (Hannula et al., 2008). Combining these interventions with peer support or peer counseling further increases short-term breastfeeding rates (Chung et al., 2008a). Effective hospital interventions include hands-off teaching, support, and encouragement. After hospital discharge, home visits, telephone support, and peer support are effective.

Breastfeeding promotion and support within health care needs to be patient centered and multidimensional. Especially important among adolescent mothers, promotion efforts need to be developmentally appropriate as well (Feldman-Winter, 2007). Culturally and linguistically sensitive breastfeeding promotion and postpartum support services are also needed (Sutton et al., 2007). The development of supportive breastfeeding policies can formalize an institution's support. See the examples of breastfeeding-friendly policies for hospitals (Figure 28.3), pediatric practice (Figure 28.4), obstetric practice (Figure 28.5), home health practice (Figure 28.6), and a pediatric unit (Figure 28.7). Mothers whose care is coordinated by a healthcare team from these types of breastfeeding-friendly practices

1. All pregnant women and new mothers will be informed of the nutritional and health benefits and basic management of breastfeeding.

2. Staff will presume the mother is breastfeeding unless the mother informs the staff otherwise.

3. Mothers will be helped to initiate breastfeeding within an hour of birth unless maternal or neonatal complications intervene.

4. All nursing mothers will be given instructions on hand expression of milk. If they should be separated from their infants, nursing mothers will be given specific instructions on breastfeeding and how to maintain lactation (pumping). Mothers who have not begun breastfeeding within 8 to 12 hours of birth will begin milk expression.

5. Breastfeeding newborns will be given no food or drink other than human milk unless medically indicated and a specific order is written by the physician. A list of medical indications for using human milk substitutes is provided.

6. Breastfeeding babies will be given pacifiers only at the direction of the mother. The risks and benefits of using artificial nipples (pacifiers, bottles) will be explained to the mother.

7. Infants who need supplementation will be tube fed at the breast or cup fed unless medically contraindicated.

8. Rooming-in will be encouraged; babies are to be kept with their mothers 24 hours a day. Mothers will be taught how to cosleep with their infants safely.

9. Mothers will be taught to watch for infant feeding cues, and will breastfeed their babies on demand rather than on a predetermined schedule. Mothers will be encouraged to breastfeed their babies a minimum of 8 times in 24 hours.

10. Mothers will be given information about breastfeeding support groups and lactation consultants prior to discharge from the hospital.

11. Each healthcare professional who cares for mothers and infants at this facility is expected to maintain the skills and knowledge necessary for implementation of this policy.

FIGURE 28.3 Baby-Friendly hospital breastfeeding policy.

Source: Printed with permission of Marsha Walker, RN, IBCLC.

1. Develop or implement a current breastfeeding protocol for use in your practice that is communicated to all staff. Provide copies to those who cover for you.

2. Arrange for all staff to attend inservices that teach the skills necessary to implement the protocol.

3. Inform all pregnant women about the benefits and management of breastfeeding. Give written, noncommercial prenatal information on breastfeeding, refer parents to breastfeeding classes, and encourage fathers to attend.

4. Help mothers initiate and maintain breastfeeding during hospital rounds. Perform newborn exam in the mother's room, showing her how well-designed her baby is for breastfeeding.

5. If mother and baby are separated due to illness, prematurity, and so on, confirm that an electric breast pump is available for expressing milk, and that milk is expressed at least 8 times in 24 hours. A prescription may be written for human milk, if necessary, to cover the cost of renting an electric breast pump.

6. Avoid the use of sterile water, glucose water, or formula for breastfeeding newborn infants, unless medically indicated. Adequate amounts of milk are present at delivery in the form of colostrum.

7. Encourage mothers to room-in 24 hours a day in the hospital. This protects the baby from disease in the nursery, provides opportunities for unrestricted contact and feeding, and encourages mothers to become aware of their baby's needs and rhythms.

8. Advise mothers to feed their infants on cue, 8 to 12 times each 24 hours. Teach behavioral feeding cues to avoid underfeeding or overhunger, with resulting infant behavioral disorganization.

9. Avoid the use of artificial nipples and pacifiers in newborn breastfeeding infants. This approach decreases the incidence of nipple preference and its sequelae.

10. Have available on staff a nurse practitioner or lactation consultant whose responsibility can include prenatal teaching, hospital rounds, call-in times, and visits for breastfeeding questions or problems. Or refer such situations to a lactation consultant in the community. Refer mothers to breastfeeding support groups for mother-to-mother support.

FIGURE 28.4 Ten steps to a Baby-Friendly pediatric practice.

Source: Printed with permission of Marsha Walker, RN, IBCLC.

receive optimal support and care in their breastfeeding efforts.

Hospital Promotion Efforts Hospitals and maternity centers offer many opportunities for promoting breastfeeding to families and caregivers. Globally, hospital practices vary considerably in their promotion and support of breastfeeding. Despite global promotion efforts, many mothers receive marginal or no in-hospital breastfeeding care. Conflicting advice, misconceptions, and inconsistencies between theory and practice affect the course of breastfeeding for mothers. Maternity nurses may acknowledge, for example, that sucking promotes milk production, yet they may advise formula supplements if a mother appears not to have enough milk. Mothers need consistent technical assistance from caregivers who empower them to reach their goals and follow the health guidelines of exclusive breastfeeding for at least 6 months.

Hospital policies and practices have a role and responsibility in the promotion and duration of breastfeeding (Manganaro et al., 2009). Promotion strategies need to remove barriers during labor, delivery, recovery, and postpartum (Komara et al., 2007). Removing promotional materials that detract from breastfeeding is

1. Create and implement a breastfeeding promotion and support policy for use in your practice that is communicated to all staff. Provide copies to those who cover for you.
2. Arrange for all staff to attend inservices that teach the skills necessary to implement the protocol.
3. Inform all pregnant women about the benefits and management of breastfeeding. Give written, noncommercial information on breastfeeding. Recommend that parents attend prenatal breastfeeding classes that include fathers. Refer parents to childbirth education classes.
4. Help mothers initiate breastfeeding within 1/2 hour of birth. Place and leave the infant on the mother's chest to promote the prefeeding sequences of behavior that leads to proper latch, suck, and organization of breastfeedings.
5. If mother and baby are separated due to illness, prematurity, and so on, confirm that an electric breast pump is available for expressing milk; that milk is expressed at least 8 times in 24 hours; that no nipple soreness, engorgement, or breast problems arise from the use of the pump.
6. Avoid the use of sterile water, glucose water, or formula for breastfeeding newborn infants, unless medically indicated. Adequate amounts of milk are present at delivery in the form of colostrum.
7. Encourage mothers to room-in 24 hours a day in the hospital. This protects the baby from disease in the nursery, provides opportunities for unrestricted contact and feeding, and encourages mothers to become aware of their baby's needs and rhythms.
8. Advise mothers to feed their infants on cue, 8 to 12 times each 24 hours. Teach behavioral feeding cues to avoid underfeeding or overhunger, with resulting infant behavioral disorganization.
9. Avoid the use of artificial nipples and pacifiers in newborn breastfeeding infants. This approach decreases the incidence of nipple preference and its sequelae.
10. Have available on staff a nurse practitioner or lactation consultant whose responsibility can include prenatal teaching, hospital rounds, call-in times, and visits for breastfeeding questions or problems. Or refer such situations to a lactation consultant in the community. Refer mothers to breastfeeding support groups for mother-to-mother support.

FIGURE 28.5 Ten steps to a Baby-Friendly obstetric practice.

Source: Printed with permission of Marsha Walker, RN, IBCLC.

1. Create a written breastfeeding policy that is research based, and provide copies of the policy to all home health staff. Include the WHO/UNICEF Code for Marketing Breastmilk Substitutes in the policy.
2. Train all healthcare staff in the Maternal–Child Services using the WHO/UNICEF 18 Hour Course. Update staff as new or revised research-based information becomes available. New staff will be given the 18-hour course beginning during orientation and completed within 1 year.
3. Inform all pregnant women about the benefits and management of breastfeeding; weave breastfeeding information into every visit. Provide written information that complies with the WHO Code. Refer all pregnant women to the prenatal breastfeeding classes within the community.
4. Inform all pregnant women of the importance of initiating breastfeeding within the first hour of life.
5. If postpartum mothers are separated from their babies, be sure they have proper equipment for milk expression and provide instruction as needed. Teach hand expression to all breastfeeding mothers. Assess breastfeeding during each home visit.
6. Give the child (ages newborn to about 6 months) no food or drink other than human milk unless *medically* indicated. Instruct mothers (prenatal and postpartum) about the risks of artificial baby milks. A list of acceptable medical reasons for human milk substitutes is included in the breastfeeding policy.
7. Encourage a "rooming-in" home environment. Explain the importance of close mother–infant contact 24 hours a day by the use of a sling, bathing together, sleeping together and so on.
8. Teach mothers the importance of their babies' cues. Explain the importance of baby-led feedings, rather than placing limitations and times on feeds. Advise mothers that 8 to 12 or more feeds in 24 hours is normal and expected.
9. Give no artificial teats or pacifiers to breastfeeding infants. Discourage their use, and instead direct the mother to breastfeed for suckling satisfaction. Explain the negative consequences of such devices.
10. Foster the establishment of breastfeeding support groups within the community, and refer mothers to them at any time.

FIGURE 28.6 Ten steps to a Baby-Friendly home health practice.

Source: Printed with permission of Debbie Shinskie.

another important strategy. Pens, pads of paper, coffee mugs, pamphlets, and other items that display names and logos of formula manufacturers undermine breastfeeding promotion efforts and send subliminal messages to staff and patients.

Implementation of breastfeeding-friendly practices is multifaceted and complicated. Global strategies such as the Baby-Friendly Hospital Initiative (BFHI) (WHO &

UNICEF, 2009) and the Global Strategy for Infant and Young Child Feeding, discussed later in this chapter, provide guidelines to assist your efforts to make changes in your facility. They help you develop hospital policies to promote breastfeeding that are practical and action oriented. Gaining staff compliance requires time, persistence, and adequate staff education. Achieving exclusive breastfeeding may be challenging in birthing facilities that

1. Have a written breastfeeding policy, and train healthcare staff caring for breastfeeding infants in skills necessary to implement thepolicy.
2. When the sick infant is admitted, ascertain the mother's wishes about infant feeding, and assist mothers to establish and managelactation as necessary.
3. Provide parents with written and verbal information about the benefits of breastfeeding and human milk.
4. Facilitate unrestricted breastfeeding and frequent human milk expression by mothers who wish to provide milk for their children, regardless of age.
5. Give breastfed children other food or drink only when age appropriate or medically indicated.
6. When medically indicated, use only those alternative feeding methods most conducive to successful breastfeeding, and restrict the use of any oral device associated with breastfeeding problems.
7. Provide facilities that allow parents and infants to remain together 24 hours a day, that encourage skin-to-skin contact as appropriate, and that avoid modeling the use of artificial feeding.
8. Administer medications and schedule all procedures so as to cause the least possible disturbance of the breastfeeding relationship.
9. Maintain a human milk bank that meets appropriate standards.
10. Provide information about community breastfeeding support groups to parents at the time of the infant's discharge from the hospital or clinic.
11. Maintain appropriate monitoring and data collection procedures to permit quality assurance and ongoing research.

FIGURE 28.7 Eleven steps to optimal breastfeeding in the pediatric unit.

Source: Printed by permission of Maureen Minchin.

deal with complex cases (Moore et al., 2007). The information in this text helps you develop educational programs to empower your staff and bring them along on the road to a breastfeeding-friendly facility. Many hospitals reach a level of breastfeeding promotion and support to qualify for official Baby-Friendly status.

Caregiver Promotion The American Academy of Pediatrics (AAP) calls for pediatricians to support breastfeeding enthusiastically. Health professionals are fundamental in breastfeeding promotion activities. Breastfeeding-friendly health care requires a genuine commitment of all health professionals who work with mothers and babies. Despite a universal recognition of the health imperative of breastfeeding, many physicians fail to support breastfeeding mothers (Taveras et al., 2004). One study showed that 48 percent of practicing pediatricians failed to recommend breastfeeding to their patients and reported few interventions to assist breastfeeding women. Neverthe-

less, these same physicians overwhelmingly reported favorable attitudes toward breastfeeding promotion (Michelman et al., 1990).

Mothers suffer from the gap that exists between physicians reporting favorable attitudes and yet demonstrating actions that fail to support mothers and fail to reflect research-based practice. One study suggests that it is a providers' culture and attitudes, not their knowledge, that most influence their efforts in breastfeeding promotion and support (Szucs et al., 2009). New strategies that focus on the attitudes and culture of physicians may help to enhance their promotion and support of breastfeeding (Barclay, 2008).

Promotion efforts need to address the relationships developed between caregivers and mothers as well. Low-income, black non-Hispanic women in a Philadelphia study expressed distrust and anxiety about the ways they were treated by nurses and physicians. Healthcare professionals need to develop trusting relationships and continuity of care as well as clear, consistent breastfeeding education and support (Cricco-Lizza, 2006).

Physicians need to be aware of the influence they exert on patients. When they distribute infant formula or vouchers to parents, they place themselves in the position of advertising and promoting a product. Such promotion contributes to the failure of women in their practice to breastfeed their infants (Donnelly et al., 2000; Howard et al., 1993). Physicians who support breastfeeding can be encouraged to educate their peers and raise their awareness of mothers' needs related to breastfeeding. UNICEF developed a pledge for physicians to sign attesting to their commitment to protect, promote, and support breastfeeding, presented in Figure 28.8 (Grant, 1994). Signing such a pledge demonstrates physicians' desire to support breastfeeding women in their practices.

Mothers benefit from breastfeeding encouragement and guidance that supports their feelings of being capable and empowered and is tailored to their individual needs. In addition to physicians, other members of the mother's healthcare team contribute to this support. There is a positive correlation between the services of lactation consultants and breastfeeding duration (Thurman & Allen, 2008). Mothers benefit from the technical assistance of a trained lactation consultant within the context of a relationship built on encouragement, guidance, and support (Memmott & Bonuck, 2006).

Breastfeeding promotion, support, and education by volunteer peer counselors improve breastfeeding duration rates in low socioeconomic populations (Smith, 2007). See Chapter 2 for further discussion of the role of peer counselors. Pediatric nurses have also been shown to have an important role in supporting breastfeeding mothers so they are able to continue breastfeeding (Hunt, 2006). These caregivers, in addition to maternity nurses,

Recognizing that breastfeeding plays a uniquely important role in the healthy development of infants and young children;

that no substitute can provide the complex balance of nutrients, antibodies and growth factors that make human milk the perfect food for infants;

that women have the right to make infant feeding decisions based on complete and accurate information;

that my role as a physician is one of influence, authority and trust;

that current marketing practices—including the free and low-cost distribution of human milk substitute supplies to hospitals and other parts of the healthcare system—compete against and discourage breastfeeding;

that my Government, at the 1994 World Health Assembly, affirmed that the marketing and promotion of human milk substitutes should not be conducted anywhere in the healthcare system; and

that the promotion of health and the prevention of disease are my duties and the mandates of responsible healthcare providers everywhere;

I hereby pledge to do my part to protect, promote, and support breastfeeding and to work to end the free and low-cost distribution of human milk substitutes to our healthcare systems.

Signature _____

FIGURE 28.8 Physician's pledge to protect, promote, and support breastfeeding.

midwives, and dietitians, form a team with potential for strong breastfeeding promotion.

Role of Education in Promotion Efforts The absence of formal training in breastfeeding accounts for much of the lack of tangible caregiver support. There is an urgent need to educate medical professionals as well as future medical professionals. Breastfeeding education has a significant effect on increasing initiation rates (Dyson et al, 2005). Learning about breastfeeding early in their medical training, and being surrounded by a culture in which breastfeeding is the norm, enhance caregivers' promotion efforts (Feldman-Winter et al., 2008).

Pediatricians, obstetricians, and family practice physicians need formal instruction in breastfeeding during their residency programs, with a focus on three main areas. First, the program must provide information regarding medical rationale, techniques, and problem solving. Second, it needs to address expectations, beliefs, and an acceptance of data that demonstrate the health benefits of breastfeeding. Finally, the program needs to build physicians' confidence that they can provide effective counseling and support to breastfeeding women (American Academy of Family Physicians, 2007; Saenz, 2000; Freed, 1993).

Caregivers should be exposed to breastfeeding education from the beginning of their training. The approach to caregiver education should be multidisciplinary, including both didactic instruction and clinical mentorship with knowledgeable role models. It should facilitate personal reflection and critical engagement with sociopolitical issues as well, thus allowing for collective understanding and change (Dykes, 2006). The training of healthcare providers through the BFHI is an effective, low-cost strategy for raising awareness, providing consistent information, and ensuring the appropriate breastfeeding support to mothers (Caldeira et al., 2008). The Baby-friendly model from WHO and UNICEF (2009) forms a framework for academic education, with additional elements aimed at the specific professionals (Giusti et al., 2006). Breastfeeding information in pediatric textbooks needs updating and expansion as well (Philipp et al., 2004). Course material on breastfeeding also needs to be added to the curricula of nursing schools and other centers for the training of health professionals.

Community Breastfeeding Promotion

Breastfeeding promotion goes far beyond the health community as well. Education and promotional strategies need to be targeted at both the general public and health workers in maternity units (Chung et al., 2008b). Lobbying by lactation activists can be an effective way to change public policy (Wilson-Clay et al., 2005). Promotion of breastfeeding at the government level increases the incidence and duration of breastfeeding (Merewood & Heinig, 2004; Mitra et al., 2003).

Successful government campaigns share several characteristics. They have a long-term plan for sustaining the program and sound administrative and financial management. Staff and funds are devoted exclusively to the promotion program to identify key obstacles and strategies for overcoming them. A mass media program conveys appropriate messages and materials to the target audience.

Communities need well-defined policies and strategies, financial resources, and strong political will to deliver effective promotional efforts at the community level (Bhandari et al., 2008). A social and cultural change of the whole community toward breastfeeding increases breastfeeding rates (Mordini et al., 2009). Women's current beliefs and practices are strongly influenced by traditions within their culture and community. Therefore a strategy for promoting early and exclusive breastfeeding needs to incorporate traditional beliefs and practices into modern messages on breastfeeding.

Efforts to create a breastfeeding-friendly community can begin with developing local criteria with political and social leaders in the community who are committed to the essence of the initiative. Criteria can include appropriate breastfeeding support and training to local health workers, including where and how to refer mothers for additional care. In addition, support can be established in the community to assist mothers in making appropriate choices and succeeding with them. A community-wide, mother-to-mother support system and removal of practices, distributors, shops and services that violate the *International Code of Marketing of Breastmilk Substitutes* (World Health Organization, 1981)—referred to as the Code—further this community effort.

Many regard breastfeeding as an important women's, human rights, and feminist issue. On the surface, feminism and breastfeeding may appear incompatible because breastfeeding is associated with traditional roles for women. However, breastfeeding is a holistic act that is intimately connected to all domains of life—sexuality, eating, emotion, appearance, sleeping, and parental relationships (Van Esterick, 1994). Breastfeeding confirms a woman's power to provide nutrition and nurture for her baby and challenges views of the breast as primarily a sexual object (Palmer, 2009; Stuart-Macadam & Dettwyler, 1995). Women's groups are encouraged to commit resources and time to breastfeeding promotion. Artists can portray the beauty and power of breastfeeding through paintings, photographs, poems, and plays. The media can present breastfeeding as a natural part of our culture, or can perpetuate bottle feeding as equal (Frerichs et al., 2006).

Richard Reid (1993), then Director of Public Affairs for UNICEF, urged a global return to breastfeeding as an urgent moral, health, social, and economic imperative. Coordinated community efforts to return breastfeeding to its rightful place as the cultural norm empower women to nurture their babies in the manner that nature intended.

Long-Term Strategies for Community Promotion

- Ensure that maternity centers practice all of the Ten Steps to Successful Breastfeeding.
- Take action to implement fully all articles of the International Code of Marketing of Breastmilk Substitutes and its subsequent World Health Assembly (WHA) resolutions.
- Enact and enforce legislation to protect the breastfeeding rights of working women.
- Educate communities to value women's contributions to the health of their children and thus the health of the community and the world.
- Encourage institutions to ease the tasks of motherhood with convenient antenatal care, respect from caregivers, good obstetrical services, and patient-focused delivery procedures.
- Provide women with counseling and clinical services for breastfeeding and birth spacing.

- Enlist community, health, religious, and political leaders to promote the primary healthcare principles of preventive health education and empowerment of mothers.

Global Breastfeeding Initiatives

As introduced in Chapter 1, several international initiatives guide breastfeeding promotion efforts throughout the world. Spearheaded by the WHO, the WHA, and UNICEF, these initiatives provide a beacon for breastfeeding advocates at all levels of promotion. UNICEF and the WHO have provided healthcare professionals and administrators with very clear guidelines for the establishment of policies and procedures that promote, protect, and support breastfeeding.

The International Code of Marketing of Breastmilk Substitutes, the BFHI, and the Global Strategy for Infant and Young Child Feeding continue to guide the development of breastfeeding promotion strategies. Hospitals, clinics, and physician offices throughout the world are incorporating these global guidelines into their policies and practices. With collaborative efforts of everyone in the healthcare system, the 21st century can turn the tide of infant health and ensure optimal growth of young children.

International Code of Marketing of Breastmilk Substitutes

The *International Code of Marketing of Breastmilk Substitutes* was adopted in 1981 by the WHA to promote safe and adequate nutrition for infants. The aim of the International Code is to contribute to the provision of safe and adequate nutrition for infants by protecting and promoting breastfeeding and by ensuring the proper use of breastmilk substitutes on the basis of adequate information and through appropriate marketing and distribution. One of the main principles of the International Code is that healthcare facilities should not be used for the purpose of promoting breastmilk substitutes, feeding bottles, or teats. Subsequent WHA resolutions have clarified the International Code and closed loopholes.

Elements of the International Code To uphold the International Code, healthcare facilities should not accept free or low-cost supplies of breastmilk substitutes. Breastmilk substitutes should be purchased in the same way as other foods and medicines and for at least wholesale price. There should be no promotional materials for breastmilk substitutes in the facility, and pregnant women should not receive materials that promote artificial feeding. Feeding with breastmilk substitutes should be demonstrated only by health workers and only to pregnant women, mothers, or family members who need to use them.

Breastmilk substitutes should be kept out of sight of pregnant women and mothers, and they should receive no sample gift packs with breastmilk substitutes or related supplies. Health workers and their families should accept no financial or material inducements to promote products within the scope of the International Code. Manufacturers and distributors of products within the scope of the International Code should disclose any contributions made to health workers such as fellowships, study tours, research grants, or conferences.

Unfortunately, most health workers are unaware of the International Code. Furthermore, even in countries where the International Code was made into law, many breach the law despite being aware of it (Salasibew et al., 2008). In most hospitals representatives from infant formula companies distribute free samples, gifts, and sponsorships to health staff. This occurs freely where hospital authorities have no practical rules and regulations in place to implement the International Code in their institutions. Research shows that pregnant women, mothers of infants less than 6 months old, and health workers continue to receive free products that violate the International Code (Taylor, 1998).

International Code Compliance Monitoring and education are needed to better promote the elements of the International Code, identify violations, and restrict access to families with inappropriate formula marketing messages. Legislation must be accompanied by effective information, training, and monitoring systems to ensure that healthcare providers and manufacturers comply with evidence-based practice and the International Code (Aguayo et al., 2003). Low breastfeeding rates are a challenge to the International Code, as evidenced in a Glasgow study in which primary care staff stated a need for information about breastmilk substitutes due to the high level of bottle feeding there (McInnes et al., 2007).

You can protect breastfeeding by urging colleagues and facilities to adhere to the International Code and develop an awareness of instances in which a facility violates it. Remove posters, videos, and leaflets that advertise products marketed or otherwise represented to be suitable as substitutes for human milk. Make sure instruction on the use of infant formula targets only mothers who have chosen not to breastfeed. Remove videos on artificial feeding from the hospital's television channel, for instance, and loan them individually to mothers who need the instruction.

Baby-Friendly Hospital Initiative

Goals of the BFHI are to transform hospitals and maternity facilities through implementation of the Ten Steps to Successful Breastfeeding and to end the practice of distribution of free and low-cost supplies of breastmilk substitutes to maternity wards and hospitals. Baby-friendly practices increase the likelihood that babies will be breast-fed exclusively for the first 6 months and then given appropriate complementary foods while breastfeeding continues for 2 years or beyond. The basis of the initiative is a self-appraisal process that evaluates current policies and practices and development of action plans to make necessary changes.

The BFHI and Global Strategy serve as the standard for measuring adherence to each of the Ten Steps for Successful Breastfeeding and the International Code of Marketing of Breastmilk Substitutes. Guidelines for the initiative were updated and expanded in 2009 and provide an insightful resource for developing breastfeeding promotion strategies for numerous settings. Achieving and sustaining practices necessary to protect, promote, and support optimal infant and young child feeding requires a comprehensive, multisector, multilevel effort. Guidance is available for creating baby-friendly practices in hospitals, clinics, pediatric services, physician offices, complimentary feeding, care of HIV positive mothers, and community services (WHO & UNICEF, 2009).

Hospitals with comprehensive breastfeeding policies are likely to have better breastfeeding support services and better breastfeeding outcomes (Rosenberg et al., 2008a). An inadequate or absent national program for the promotion of breastfeeding negatively influences breastfeeding practices (Zareai et al., 2007). Only 1 percent of women in a Taiwan study reported experiencing all 10-step practices during their childbirth and postpartum stay (Chien et al., 2006). An Australian study found a range of variables that appeared to negatively influence breastfeeding practices. Among them were a comparatively inadequate national promotion program and fewer adherences to the BFHI (Zareai et al., 2007). One study suggests that implementing BFHI policy could be more straightforward in smaller facilities and those with stable workforces (Moore et al., 2007).

Baby-friendly facilities are responsible for monitoring their practices and maintaining BFHI standards. After a period of time, usually 3 years, a reassessment is needed with use of the self-assessment tool or a reassessment tool. In reassessment of certified Baby-friendly Hospitals in Brazil, only 82 percent continued to meet all 10 steps (Moura de Araújo & Soares Schmitz, 2007). Likewise, exclusive breastfeeding rates declined in Baby-friendly Hospitals in the Czech Republic from 92.9 percent in 2000 to 90.3 percent in 2006 (Mydlilova et al., 2009). Achieving Baby-Friendly designation is not sufficient; facilities must make it a priority to maintain the high standards set forth in the initiative to continue to provide optimal breastfeeding care to mothers and babies.

Becoming a Baby-friendly Hospital If you are early on the road to Baby-Friendly Hospital designation, you can begin with interviewing key informants in both public and private health sectors. Review any standards of practice, curricula, studies, surveys, policies, laws, training courses, professional services, nongovernmental organizations, BFHI resources, and government agencies. Using the BFHI self-appraisal tool for your country, make a preliminary assessment of whether your facility is fully implementing the Ten Steps, adheres to the International Code, and meets the global criteria to protect, promote, and support optimal infant and young child feeding.

The hospital administrator will need to become familiar with the BFHI process and determine where responsibility lies within the hospital structure. Some hospitals appoint a committee with representatives from prenatal care, labor and delivery, postpartum wards, and neonatal intensive care. The administrator will then work with key hospital staff to fill in the self-appraisal tool using the global criteria.

You will need to collect statistics on related infant feeding and integrate the data into your maternity record-keeping system. After providing the required staff training and meeting most of the global criteria, you can request an external assessment by the national BFHI coordination group. If you fail to achieve Baby-friendly designation, you will be awarded a Certificate of Commitment and encouraged to make necessary changes before reassessment. If your self-assessment reveals you are unable to meet the global criteria, you can request a Certificate of Commitment, establish a plan for raising your standards, and prepare for the external assessment.

In 2010, Baby-Friendly USA, the national authority for BFHI in the United States, launched a new 4-D Pathway to Baby-Friendly Designation. The four pathways are:

- Discovery: register, obtain administrative support, and complete self-appraisal
- Development: develop policies, training materials, and data collection plan
- Dissemination: train staff and collect data
- Designation: implement quality improvement plan, undergo on-site assessment, and achieve official designation

Global Strategy for Infant and Young Child Feeding

Breastfeeding promotion is a centerpiece of the Global Strategy for Infant and Young Child Feeding. Endorsed by the WHA and UNICEF, the Global Strategy aims to reduce the global consequences of childhood undernutrition, specifically diarrheal disease, measles, malaria, and lower respiratory infection. The Global Strategy should be effective in further increasing optimal breastfeeding practices.

The strategy reasserts exclusive breastfeeding for the first 6 months of life and breastfeeding with appropriate complementary foods for up to 2 years and beyond. Among its tenets it calls for supporting working women, culture-specific nutrition counseling, skilled support to parents and caregivers, and appropriate response to global emergencies. Specific strategies within the healthcare system include skilled counseling, implementation of the BFHI, routine nutrition intervention, and guidance in appropriate complementary feeding.

The Global Strategy urges that hospital routines and procedures remain fully supportive of the successful initiation and establishment of breastfeeding through implementation of the BFHI, monitoring and reassessing BFHI-designated facilities, and expanding the BFHI to include clinics, health centers, and pediatric hospitals. It also urges adapting the BFHI to the feeding of infants and young affected by HIV/AIDS and ensuring that those responsible for emergency preparedness are well trained to support appropriate feeding practices consistent with BFHI's universal principles.

Lactation professionals can be instrumental in advancing the goals of the Global Strategy by developing breastfeeding protocols, challenging traditional procedures, and removing barriers that erode the mother's confidence in her ability to breastfeed. You have enormous potential to facilitate consistent care by instituting care plans for managing breastfeeding problems and conducting staff inservice education.

National Breastfeeding Awareness Campaign

A National Breastfeeding Awareness Campaign was launched in June 2004 by the Office of Women's Health in the U.S. Department of Health and Human Services, the first of its kind since 1911. The goal of the campaign was to encourage exclusive breastfeeding for 6 months and increase breastfeeding rates to 75 percent (Merewood & Heinig, 2004). The campaign, "Babies were born to be breastfed," was run by the Ad Council, a private, nonprofit organization. Public service announcements targeted the general market as well as the African American community, because rates of breastfeeding are lowest among this population. Previous Ad Council campaigns include "Rosie the Riveter," "Smokey Bear," "Crash Test Dummies," and "This is your brain on drugs."

Infant formula industry executives objected to describing the risks of not breastfeeding rather than the benefits of breastfeeding. Their lobbying efforts delayed the campaign launch by several months. Nevertheless, protests from the medical community, breastfeeding advocates, and AAP members—particularly the AAP Section on Breastfeeding Executive Committee—put the campaign back on track, although the ads were watered down with significant content removed. Despite this, the continued launch of the campaign represented a major step forward for breastfeeding advocacy in the United

States. The campaign serves as a model to the international community for promotion in other countries.

One Million Campaign

A web-based One Million Campaign was launched in 2009 as part of a global Breastfeeding Initiative for Child Survival. It was formed in partnership with the North American Aerospace Defense Command (NORAD) and the "Global Proposal for Coordinated Action of IBFAN and WABA: Protecting, Promoting and Supporting Breastfeeding through Human Rights and Gender Equality" in partnership with the Swedish International Devolvement Agency. The objective is to build public opinion to support women and mothers to breastfeed.

Infant Formula Industry

The infant formula industry is eager to ostensibly promote breastfeeding. Breastfeeding mothers are typically very health conscious. When they wean their babies from the breast, they are more likely to wean to an infant formula rather than immediately to cow's milk. Their babies are likely to receive formula until an older age than babies who received formula from birth and are more likely to receive "toddler formulas" or "add-on formulas." Mothers who begin feeding formula from birth are more likely to wean their babies to cow's milk at an earlier age.

As with any industry, individual formula manufacturers are in fierce competition with each other for customers. Because the company that looks best wins more breastfeeding mothers, they give lip service that breastfeeding is "best" and promote their product under the guise of promoting breastfeeding. They tell the public what they know they want to hear and couch it in language that appeals to them. That is simply good advertising.

Pharmaceutical Company Practices

An eye-opening and educational resource, www.nofree lunch.org, urges healthcare practitioners to provide high-quality care based on unbiased evidence rather than on biased pharmaceutical promotions. Studying the pharmaceutical industry's actions provides insight into the actions of the infant formula industry. This is to be expected because most formula manufacturers are owned by pharmaceutical companies. They promote their products in an effort to influence prescribing. They exert significant influence on provider behavior through samples, gifts, and food. They provide promotional materials and presentations that are often biased and uninformative (No Free Lunch, 2009). Failure to demand disclosure of potential conflicts of interest often reinforces the lack of disclosure by third-party messengers. Tactics aimed at shaping important decisions on health care continue to flourish.

Breastfeeding advocates see this ploy frequently, as formula companies offer "medical education" seminars and lectures for continuing nursing and medical education credits. One recent "medical lecture" featured a physician extolling the virtues of the addition of the long-chain polyunsaturated fatty acids DHA and AA to the manufacturer's infant formulas. Yet, what the audience may not have learned was that Mead Johnson was forced by the Canadian Health Department to remove its claims about DHA and AA improving IQ and vision from its Canadian advertising. They probably did not learn that these acids are made from algae and soil fungus (Agennix, 2009; E. Sterken, Director, Infant Feeding Action Coalition Canada, personal e-mail correspondence, April 27, 2004). Such marketing seminars occur routinely under the guise of continuing education.

One study investigated the issue of pharmaceutical companies invoking peer-reviewed studies to support their claims and add credence to their advertising. Of 125 citations claimed, most were from randomized clinical trials. In 45 claims the reference did not support the promotional statement, most frequently because the slogan recommended the drug in a patient group other than the one assessed in the study (Villanueva et al., 2003).

In 2002 drug companies and physicians fought a government plan to restrict gifts and other rewards that pharmaceutical manufacturers give physicians and insurers to encourage the prescribing of particular drugs. The U.S. Department of Health and Human Services observed that many gifts and gratuities have the appearance of illegal kickbacks. Drug makers admit they routinely make payments to insurance plans to market their products and reward doctors and pharmacists (Pear, 2002).

A prime example of name identification, referred to as "branding" in marketing, is the Ross logo and teddy bear trademark prominently displayed on the AAP's breastfeeding book, *New Mother's Guide to Breastfeeding.* AAP members have voiced increasing concern about the influence that corporations have on the academy (Petersen, 2002) and have urged the academy to develop a policy to ensure that commercial logos never again appear on its books and other educational materials. Some believe that pharmaceutical companies—which include formula companies—spend more on marketing, advertising, and administrative budgets than on research and development efforts (Families USA, 2002).

Influencing Healthcare Decisions

Infant formula manufacturers worldwide advertise their infant foods in medical journals and to the lay public. Hospitals receive infant formula for their nurseries at no charge, a practice that originated in the 1930s and has been criticized by health experts ever since. Hospitals receive no other product routinely without being charged

(Walker, 2007b; Merewood & Philipp, 2000). They should be required to pay for infant formula just as they do all other supplies. Any gifts given to hospitals should be legitimate, in the form of documentable research or teaching grants. Gifts should not go through the hospital's purchasing agent.

Manufacturers do not stop at giving free formula to hospital nurseries. Aggressive marketing campaigns target physicians and hospital maternity units. Hospitals and healthcare practitioners receive free equipment, architectural planning, calendars, office supplies, and other giveaways. Funding is provided for airline tickets to conferences, medical fellowships, scholarships, educational grants, and other rewards that are common to the industry, such as tickets to sporting events, dinners, and fishing trips.

Ties between formula manufacturers and associations such as the AAP and the American Medical Association run deep (Petersen, 2002; Stolberg & Gerth, 2000). In 1996 Nestlé sued the AAP, Ross Laboratories, and Mead Johnson's parent company, Bristol-Myers Squib, claiming a conspiracy to restrict trade. The suit stated that the AAP accepted millions from these manufacturers, including funds to help pay for the AAP's headquarters. In 2001 Ross was one of the top three corporate sponsors of the AAP's $65 million operating budget, contributing $500,000 or more (Petersen, 2002).

Many healthcare providers are naive about the practices of the infant formula industry. One study sought to determine how problematic experienced physicians and residents viewed common pharmaceutical marketing activities. Although activities permitted under their guidelines troubled some respondents, the views reported by others violated the guidelines (Brett et al., 2003). The entire May 2003 issue of the *British Medical Journal*, "No More Free Lunches," focused on the issue of pharmaceutical industry marketing. It discussed marketing tactics and how those tactics influence the behavior of healthcare providers.

Healthcare professionals need to recognize that accepting a "gift" implies an obligation on the receiver's part to look favorably at the giver. It causes the receiver to feel obligated to treat that person well and, ultimately, to promote their product. Editors of the *British Medical Journal* called for an end to the acceptance of "free" lunches.

The U.S. Senate continues efforts for transparency about drug company funding and financial ties between the pharmaceutical industry and medical professionals. Senator Chuck Grassley (2009) asserts that such transparency builds public confidence in research and the practice of medicine. Senator Grassley and Senator Herb Kohl introduced the Physician Payments Sunshine Act, which requires annual public reporting by drug, device, and bio-logical manufacturers of payments made to physicians nationwide.

Lactation consultants are urged to refuse funding from formula companies and others who violate the International Code (ILCA, 2007). There is no such thing as a free lunch, and someone eventually pays. For parents it is higher costs on the retail market and increased medical bills. For infants it is a higher incidence of illness, chronic disease, and death. For the public it is higher taxes and overall healthcare costs. Physicians can be instrumental in developing alternatives that take into account the best interests of patients and hospitals (Revai & Huston, 2009).

Influencing Parents

Pharmaceutical company marketing efforts increasingly target potential patients. Drug companies sponsor patient groups, and a "third-party" marketing strategy uses an apparently independent spokesperson to create higher credibility with a company's target audience (Burton & Rowell, 2003). Similar tactics are used by formula manufacturers, with company representatives presenting themselves as experts in infant nutrition. They educate parents through videos and literature (Moynihan, 2003; Young, 1990), send discount coupons and cases of free formula to their homes (Howard et al., 1994), and send them home from the hospital with free samples of formula (Donnelly et al., 2000). Studies show that the distribution of formula company–sponsored gift bags (with or without formula) undermines breastfeeding and negatively impacts exclusivity and duration (Rosenberg et al., 2008b; Donnelly et al., 2007).

Aggressive marketing exerts tremendous influence on the general public. Mass media influences the decision of women to breastfeed their newborn children. Infant formula manufacturers recognize that infant feeding decisions tend to be based on feelings and intuition rather than knowledge (Hausman, 2008). Studies report that when the frequency of hand (bottle) feeding advertisements increased, the percentage change in breastfeeding rates reported the next year generally tended to decrease (Brown & Peuchaud, 2008; Foss & Southwell, 2006). After adopting a law to regulate artificial feeding, the country of Georgia in southwest Asia experienced a sharp increase in breastfeeding rates, Baby-friendly designation at 14 maternity centers, and a decrease in the advertisement of artificial feeding products (Nemsadze, 2004).

International Code Violations

When you encounter violations of the International Code, take action to make others aware. Ask hospital administrators to reject anything that does not comply with the

International Code. Discuss violations with colleagues, and take steps to change practices that do not comply. Refuse gifts or samples of formula and prevent others from giving them to mothers, if you have the power to do so. Be aware that sponsorship of a conference by formula companies often may not be clear, and ask before agreeing to participate in the program. Because formula companies own subsidiaries that sell other products, if asked to speak or participate in a conference, find out if the sponsor or organizer has an affiliation with the pharmaceutical or infant formula industry. The International Code is in place to promote, protect, and support breastfeeding, and your compliance helps protect the interests of breastfeeding mothers and babies.

Although Japan ratified the International Code in 1994, most hospitals in Japan continue to receive free supplies of infant formula and distribute discharge packs to new mothers provided by infant formula companies. Physicians argue that although breastmilk is good, recommending that mothers breastfeed their infants places undue pressure on the mothers. They further assert that although breastmilk is good, it is appropriate for infants to receive formula routinely (Mizuno et al., 2006). Although 80 percent of pediatricians believe their hospitals should comply with the International Code, only 39 percent of obstetricians agree.

A Philippine government 1986 Milk Code, which included a ban on baby milk advertising, took effect in 2006. The Pharmaceutical and Health Care Association of the Philippines challenged its legality in court, and in October 2007 the Philippine Supreme Court lifted the ban (Associated Foreign Press, 2007). The ruling upholds the Department of Health's authority to regulate advertising of all products covered by the International Code on the Marketing of Breastmilk Substitutes. UNICEF (2007) perceives the Supreme Court ruling as a significant victory for infant, young child, and maternal health in the Philippines because it strengthens regulation of advertising and marketing practices.

The challenge to stem the irresponsible marketing of artificial baby milk parallels the lengthy efforts to reduce cigarette smoking. The fight against the tobacco industry took more than 40 years, and countering uncontrolled formula advertising will not be accomplished quickly. Members of the lactation consulting profession joined in one voice can exert tremendous pressure. Report violations of the International Code and deceptive advertising and trade practices to the U.S. Food and Drug Administration or the equivalent governmental agency in your country. Enlist the risk management executives in your organization and educate them about the organization's liability in giving away formula to patients. Concerns about formula contamination scandals have prompted several hospital systems in the United States to discontinue distributing formula bags (banthebags.org, 2010).

The Joint Commission requirement that hospitals log all formula lot numbers in case of recall has helped make this a corporate risk management decision, removing it from the local maternity unit's decision.

Action groups such as the National Alliance for Breastfeeding Advocacy, Media Watch, Infant Feeding Action Coalition, International Baby Food Action Network, and World Alliance for Breastfeeding Action (WABA) can help hold companies accountable. Your involvement with local ILCA affiliates and local breastfeeding support groups can energize and motivate you to continue to help mothers and babies realize their birthright to breastfeed and be breastfed and to work toward producing healthier families and a healthier world.

~ Summary

Demonstrating effective leadership as a lactation consultant and helping others embrace change can help return breastfeeding to the cultural norm and ensure every child's basic human right to be breastfed. Breastfeeding-friendly health care extends beyond the baby to creating an environment that is mother friendly and family friendly. Breastfeeding is an endangered practice that needs an entire culture to support and nurture it back to its full, potent strength. Major international initiatives are in place to guide and support your efforts toward promoting optimal nutrition for infants and young children.

Achieving an environment supportive of breastfeeding may seem daunting. Yet the benefits are immense. If you give more than is asked of you, you will reap great rewards. What an exhilarating feeling to be part of such a positive health-affirming effort! To get where you want to go, you need a clear vision of your overall goal. UNICEF and WHO have provided the vision with their Ten Steps to Successful Breastfeeding and Baby-friendly Hospital Initiative. The aim of the initiative is to make healthcare providers the "prime movers in recreating a world environment that supports, protects, and promotes the practice of breastfeeding—a world environment that is friendly to babies and their mothers" (Kyenkya-Isabirye, 1992).

The success of the breastfeeding promotion depends on countless small changes enacted one person at a time, hospital by hospital, and country by country. The pharmaceutical industry will continue to use its money and political power to obscure the basic truth that human milk is for human babies and cows' milk is for baby calves. Surmounting these hurdles requires the combined efforts of lactation professionals, physicians, nurses, and all other members of the healthcare profession and breastfeeding support community, as well as the most important people involved—mothers and babies!

∽ *Chapter 28—At a Glance*

Applying what you learned—

- Increase your success as a leader by choosing to be effective, making a blueprint, staying focused, working toward mutual benefit, and building a strong team.

- Use positive self-talk, and view mistakes as lessons learned.

- Increase your assertiveness by practicing assertive behavior.

- Plan and implement change, and anticipate resistance.

- Recognize reasons for resistance, and resolve conflicts.

- Gather data, and evaluate your facility.

- Define problems, goals, and strategies.

- Form a breastfeeding committee with members from areas affected by the change and different personality types.

- Pursue changes slowly, and give recognition and praise.

- Be aware of marketing practices of the infant formula industry, and refuse funding from them.

- Learn the provisions of the International Code of Marketing of Breastmilk Substitutes, follow them, and report violations.

- Promote the Baby-friendly Hospital Initiative.

- Learn components of the Global Strategy for Infant and Young Child Feeding.

- Work as an active agent for change to promote optimal nutrition for infants and young children.

∽ *References*

Agennix, Inc. www.agennix.com. Accessed December 1, 2009.

Aguayo VM, et al. Monitoring compliance with the International Code of Marketing of Breastmilk Substitutes in West Africa: multisite cross sectional survey in Togo and Burkina Faso. *BMJ*. 2003;326(7381):127.

American Academy of Family Physicians. AAFP policy statement on breastfeeding. Breastfeeding Position Paper. Leawood, KS: American Academy of Family Physicians; 2007.

Anand RK. Transforming health colleagues into breastfeeding advocates. WABA Activity Sheet No. 3. Penang, Malaysia: World Alliance for Breastfeeding Action; February 7, 2005.

Associated Foreign Press. Philippine court lifts baby milk ad ban; October 9, 2007. http://afp.google.com/article/ALeqM5jb8KMbJB9budpgTnyEq-MTpKrdLw. Accessed October 20, 2009.

Ban the Bags. Hospitals should market health, and nothing else. Bag-Free Hospitals and Birth Centers. www.banthebags.org. Accessed April 4, 2010.

Barclay L. Pediatrician promotion of breast-feeding among their patients has declined. *Arch Pediatr Adolesc Med*. 2008;162:1142-1149.

Bartick M, Reinhold A. The burden of suboptimal breastfeeding in the United States: a pediatric cost analysis. *Pediatrics*. Apr 5, 2010; DOI: 10.1542/peds.2009-1616. http://pediatrics.aappublications.org/cgi/reprint/peds.2009-1616v1. Accessed May 5, 2010.

Berry NJ, Gribble KD. Breast is no longer best: promoting normal infant feeding. *Matern Child Nutr*. 2008;4(1):74-79.

Bhandari N, et al. Mainstreaming nutrition into maternal and child health programmes: scaling up of exclusive breastfeeding. *Matern Child Nutr*. 2008;4 (1):5-23.

Bicalho-Mancini P, Velasquez-Melendez G. Exclusive breastfeeding at the point of discharge of high-risk newborns at a neonatal intensive care unit and the factors associated with this practice. *J Pediatr (Rio J)*. 2004;80(3):241-248.

Böse-O'Reilly S, et al. Promotion of breast feeding in paediatric outpatient settings [in German]. *Gesundheitswesen*. 2008; 70(Suppl 1):S34-S36.

Bramson R. *Coping with Difficult Bosses*. New York: Fireside Publishing; 1992.

Brett A, et al. Are gifts from pharmaceutical companies ethically problematic? A survey of physicians. *Arch Intern Med*. 2003;163(18):2213-2218.

Bridges N. Ethical responsibilities of the Australian media in the representations of infant feeding. *Breastfeed Rev*. 2007; 15(1):17-21.

Browder S. Super-confidence and how to get it. *New Woman Magazine*; July 1994.

Brown JD, Peuchaud SR. Media and breastfeeding: friend or foe? *Int Breastfeeding J*. 2008;3:15.

Bulhosa MS, et al. Promotion of breastfeeding by the nursing staff of a children-friendly hospital [in Portuguese]. *Rev Gaucha Enferm*. 2007;28(1):89-97.

Burton B, Rowell A. Education and debate: Unhealthy spin. *BMJ*. 2003;326:1205-1207.

Cadwell K. Using the quality improvement process to affect breastfeeding protocols in United States hospitals. *J Hum Lact*. 1997;13:5-9.

Caldeira AP, et al. Educational intervention on breastfeeding promotion to the Family Health Program team [in Portuguese]. *Rev Saude Publ*. 2008;42(6):1027-1033.

Chien LY, et al. The number of Baby-Friendly hospital practices experienced by mothers is positively associated with breastfeeding: a questionnaire survey. *Int J Nurs Stud*. 2006; 44(7):1138-1146.

Chung M, et al. Interventions in primary care to promote breastfeeding: an evidence review for the U.S. Preventive Services Task Force. *Ann Intern Med*. 2008a;149(8):565-582.

Chung W, et al. Breast-feeding in South Korea: factors influencing its initiation and duration. *Public Health Nutr*. 2008b;11(3):225-229.

Covey S. *The 7 Habits of Highly Effective People*, 15th Anniversary ed. New York: Free Press; 2004.

Cricco-Lizza R. Black non-Hispanic mothers' perceptions about the promotion of infant-feeding methods by nurses and physicians. *JOGNN*. 2006;35(2):173-1780.

Dana D. *Conflict Resolution*. New York: McGraw-Hill; 2000.

Donnelly A, et al. Commercial hospital discharge packs for breastfeeding women. *Cochrane Database Syst Rev.* 2000;2:CD002075.

Donnelly A, et al. Commercial hospital discharge packs for breastfeeding women. *Cochrane Database Syst Rev.* 2007; 18(2).

Dusdieker LB, et al. Prenatal office practices regarding infant feeding choices. *Clin Pediatr.* 2006;45(9):841-845.

Dykes F. The education of health practitioners supporting breastfeeding women: Time for critical reflection. *Matern Child Nutr.* 2006;2(4):204-216.

Dyson L et al. Interventions for promoting the initiation of breastfeeding. *Cochrane Database Syst Rev.* 2005;2: CD001688. DOI: 10.1002/14651858.CD001688.pub2.

Ellis DJ. Supporting breastfeeding: how to implement agency change. Clinical Issues in Perinatal and Women's Health Nursing. *NAACOG.* 1992;3(4):560-564.

Families USA. *Profiting from Pain: Where Prescription Drug Dollars Go.* Washington, DC: Families USA; 2002.

Feldman-Winter L, Shaikh U. Optimizing breastfeeding promotion and support in adolescent mothers. *J Hum Lact.* 2007;23(4):362-7.

Feldman-Winter LB, et al. Pediatricians and the promotion and support of breastfeeding. *Arch Pediatr Adolesc Med.* 2008;162(12):1142-1149.

Fjeld E, et al. No sister, the breast alone is not enough for my baby: A qualitative assessment of potentials and barriers in the promotion of exclusive breastfeeding in southern Zambia. *Int Breastfeed J.* 2008;5;3(1):26.

Fonseca-Becker F, Valente TW. Promoting breastfeeding in Bolivia: do social networks add to the predictive value of traditional socioeconomic characteristics? *J Health Popul Nutr.* 2006;24(1):71-80.

Foss KA, Southwell BG. Infant feeding and the media: the relationship between Parents' Magazine content and breastfeeding, 1972-2000. *Int Breastfeed J.* 2006;30:10.

Freed GL. Breast-feeding: time to teach what we preach. *JAMA.* 1993;269(2):243-245.

Frerichs L et al. Framing breastfeeding and formula-feeding messages in popular U.S. magazines. *Women Health.* 44(1):95-118; 2006.

Giusti A, et al. How Italian midwives contribute to breastfeeding promotion: a national experience of "cascade" training [in Italian]. *Ig Sanita Pubbl.* 2006;62(1):53-67.

Goleman D. *Emotional Intelligence.* New York: Bantam; 1997.

Goleman D, et al. *Primal Leadership: Realizing the Power of Emotional Intelligence.* Boston, MA: Harvard Business School Press; 2002.

Grant JP. Physician's pledge to protect, promote and support breastfeeding. New York: UNICEF; 1994.

Grassley C. Grassley continues effort for transparency about drug company money; November 18, 2009. http://grassley.senate.gov/news/Article.cfm?customel_data-PageID_1502=24170. Accessed December 4, 2009.

Guise JM, et al. The effectiveness of primary care-based interventions to promote breastfeeding: systematic evidence review and meta-analysis for the US Preventive Services Task Force. *Ann Fam Med.* 2003;1(2):70-78.

Hannula L, et al. A systematic review of professional support interventions for breastfeeding. *J Clin Nurs.* 2008;17(9):1132-1143.

Hausman BL. Women's liberation and the rhetoric of "choice" in infant feeding debates. *Int Breastfeed J.* 2008;3(1):10.

Heinig MJ. Are there risks to using risk-based messages to promote breastfeeding? *J Hum Lact.* 2009;25(1):7-8.

Hernandez IF. Promoting exclusive breastfeeding for Hispanic women. *MCN Am J Matern Child Nurs.* 2006;31(5):318-324.

Howard C, et al. Antenatal formula advertising: another potential threat to breast-feeding. *Pediatrics.* 1994;94:102-104.

Howard F, et al. The physician as advertiser: the unintentional discouragement of breastfeeding. *Obstet Gynecol.* 1993;81:1048-1051.

Humes JC. Life lessons from Ben Franklin. *Bottom Line/Personal*; June 15, 1992.

Hunt F. Breast feeding and society. *Paediatr Nurs.* 2006; 18(8):24-6.

International Lactation Consultant Association (Mannel R, et al., eds.). *Core Curriculum for Lactation Consultant Practice,* 2nd ed. Boston: Jones and Bartlett; 2007.

Jackson M. The comedy of management. In: Simms L, et al., eds *The Professional Practice of Nursing Administration.* New York: Wiley; 1985:339-351.

Johnston ML, Esposito N. Barriers and facilitators for breastfeeding among working women in the United States. *JOGNN.* 2007;36(1):9-20.

Jones G, et al. How many child deaths can we prevent this year? *Lancet.* 2003;362:65-71.

Kahler T. *The Process Therapy Model: The Six Personality Types with Adaptations.* Little Rock, AR: Taibi Kahler Associates, Inc.; 2008.

Kang JS, et al. Effects of a breastfeeding empowerment programme on Korean breastfeeding mothers: a quasi-experimental study. *Int J Nurs Stud.* 2008;45(1):14-23.

Knaak SJ. The problem with breastfeeding discourse. *Can J Public Health.* 2006;97:412-414.

Komara C, et al. Intervening to promote early initiation of breastfeeding in the LDR. *MCN Am J Matern Child Nurs.* 2007;32(2):117-121.

Kotler P, Keller K. *Marketing Management,* 13th ed. Englewood Cliffs, NJ: Prentice Hall; 2008.

Kyenkya-Isabirye M. UNICEF launches the Baby-Friendly Hospital Initiative. *MCN.* 1992;17(4):177-179.

Manganaro R, et al. Effects of hospital policies and practices on initiation and duration of breastfeeding. *Child Care Health Dev.* 2009;35(1):106-111.

Manojlovich M. Power and empowerment in nursing: looking backward to inform the future. *Online J Issues Nursing.* 2007; 12(1):1. www.nursingworld.org/MainMenuCategories/ ANAMarketplace/ANAPeriodicals/OJIN/TableofContents/ Volume122007/No1Jan07/LookingBackwardtoInformthe Future.aspx. Accessed December 1, 2009.

Mayer B. *The Dynamics of Conflict Resolution: A Practitioner's Guide.* San Francisco: Jossey-Bass; 2000.

McCarter Spaulding D. Is breastfeeding fair? Tensions in feminist perspectives on breastfeeding and the family. *J Hum Lact.* 2008;24(2):206-212.

McInnes RJ, et al. Who's keeping the code? Compliance with the international code for the marketing of breast-milk substitutes in Greater Glasgow. *Public Health Nutr.* 2007; 10(7):719-725.

Memmott MM, Bonuck KA. Mother's reactions to a skills-based breastfeeding promotion intervention. *Matern Child Nutr.* 2006;2(1):40-50.

Merewood A, Heinig J. Efforts to promote breastfeeding in the United States: development of a national breastfeeding awareness campaign. *J Hum Lact.* 2004;20(2):140-145.

Merewood A, Philipp B. Becoming baby-friendly: Overcoming the issue of accepting free formula. *J Hum Lact.* 2000; 16(4):279-282.

Michelman DF, et al. Pediatricians and breastfeeding promotion: attitudes, beliefs and practices. *Am J Health Promot.* 1990;4:181-186.

Mitra A, et al. Evaluation of a comprehensive loving support program among state Women, Infants, and Children (WIC) program breast-feeding coordinators. *South Med J.* 2003;96(2):168-171.

Mizuno K, et al. Differences in perception of the WHO International Code of Marketing of Breast Milk Substitutes between pediatricians and obstetricians in Japan. *Int Breastfeed J.* 2006;1:12.

Moore T, et al. Implementing Baby Friendly Hospital Initiative policy: the case of New Zealand public hospitals. *Int Breastfeed J.* 2007;2:8.

Mordini B, et al. Correlations between welfare initiatives and breastfeeding rates: a 10-year follow-up study. *Acta Paediatr.* 2009;98(1):80-85.

Moura de Araújo Mde F, Soares Schmitz Bde A. Reassessment of Baby-Friendly Hospitals in Brazil. *J Hum Lact.* 2007;23(3):246-252.

Moynihan R. Who pays for the pizza? Redefining the relationships between doctors and drug companies. 1: Entanglement. *BMJ.* 2003;326(7400):1189-1192.

Mulford C. Is breastfeeding really invisible, or did the health care system just choose not to notice it? *Int Breastfeed J.* 2008;3:13.

Mulford C. Swimming upstream: breastfeeding care in a non-breastfeeding culture. *JOGNN.* 1995;24(5):464-474.

Murphy S, Wilson C. Breastfeeding promotion: a rational and achievable target for a type 2 diabetes prevention intervention in Native American communities. *J Hum Lact.* 2008;24(2):193-198.

Mydlilova A, et al. Breastfeeding rates in Baby-Friendly and non-Baby-Friendly Hospitals in the Czech Republic from 2000 to 2006. *J Hum Lact.* 2009;25:73-78.

Nemsadze K. Report from the country of Georgia: Protecting and promoting breastfeeding through regulation of artificial-feeding marketing practices. *J Perinat Educ.* 2004; 13(1):23-28.

No Free Lunch. www.nofreelunch.org. Accessed December 1, 2009.

Palmer G. *The Politics of Breastfeeding: When Breasts are Bad for Business,* 3rd ed. London: Pinter & Martin, Ltd.; 2009.

Pear R. Drug makers battle plan to curb rewards for doctors. *NY Times* Late Edition—Final, Section A, Page 1, Column 6; December 26, 2002.

Petersen M. Pediatric book on breast-feeding stirs controversy. *NY Times* Late Edition—Final, Section C, Page 1, Column 3; September 18, 2002.

Philipp B, et al. Breastfeeding information in pediatric textbooks needs improvement. *J Hum Lact.* 2004;20(2):206-210.

Reid R. The baby-friendly hospital initiative: a global movement for humankind. *Int Child Health.* 1993;4(1):41-47.

Revai K, Huston R. Hospital distribution of formula discharge bags: opinions of Texas pediatricians. *Breastfeed Med.* 2009;4(3):157-160.

Rosenberg KD, et al. Impact of hospital policies on breastfeeding outcomes. *Breastfeed Med.* 2008a;3(2):110-116.

Rosenberg KD, et al. Marketing infant formula through hospitals: the impact of commercial hospital discharge packs on breastfeeding. *Am J Public Health.* 2008b;98(2):290-295.

Saenz R. A lactation management rotation for family medicine residents. *J Hum Lact.* 2000;16(4):342-345.

Salasibew M, et al. Awareness and reported violations of the WHO International Code and Pakistan's national breastfeeding legislation: a descriptive cross-sectional survey. *Int Breastfeed J.* 2008;3:24.

Sandes AR, et al. Breastfeeding: prevalence and determinant factors [in Portuguese]. *Acta Med Port.* 2007;20(3):193-200.

Santo LC, et al. Factors associated with low incidence of exclusive breastfeeding for the first 6 months. *Birth.* 2007; 34(3):212-219.

Scanlon KS, et al. Breastfeeding Trends and Updated National Health Objectives for Exclusive Breastfeeding—United States, Birth Years 2000-2004. Centers for Disease Control and Prevention. *MMWR.* 2007;56(30):760-763.

Sibeko L, et al. Beliefs, attitudes, and practices of breastfeeding mothers from a periurban community in South Africa. *J Hum Lact.* 2005;21(1):31-38.

Smith S. An analysis of Australia's changing context: the breastfeeding mother, motivation and free community-based education. *Breastfeed Rev.* 2007;15(2):21-25.

Stolberg S, Gerth J. High-tech stealth being used to sway doctor prescriptions. *NY Times;* November 16, 2000.

Stuart-Macadam P, Dettwyler K, eds. *Breastfeeding: Biocultural Perspectives.* New York: Aldine de Gruyter; 1995.

Suellentrop K, et al. Monitoring progress toward achieving Maternal and Infant Healthy People 2010 objectives—19 states, Pregnancy Risk Assessment Monitoring System (PRAMS), 2000-2003. *MMWR Surveill Summ.* 2006; 55(9):1-11.

Susin LR, Giugliani ER. Inclusion of fathers in an intervention to promote breastfeeding: Impact on breastfeeding rates. *J Hum Lact.* 2008;24(4):386-392.

Sutton J, et al. Barriers to breastfeeding in a Vietnamese community: a qualitative exploration. *Can J Diet Pract Res.* 2007;68(4):195-200.

Szucs KA, et al. Breastfeeding knowledge, attitudes, and practices among providers in a medical home. *Breastfeed Med.* 2009;4(1):31-42.

Taveras E, et al. Opinions and practices of clinicians associated with continuation of exclusive breastfeeding. *Pediatrics.* 2004;113(4):e283-e290.

Taylor A. Violations of the International Code of Marketing of Breast Milk Substitutes: prevalence in four countries. *BMJ.* 1998;316(7138):1117-1122.

Thurman SE, Allen PJ. Integrating lactation consultants into primary health care services: are lactation consultants affecting breastfeeding success? *Pediatr Nurs.* 2008;34(5): 419-425.

Tubeza P. Schools to teach breastfeeding's benefit. *Philippine Daily Inquirer*; February 16, 2009. http://newsinfo.inquirer.net/inquirerheadlines/nation/view/20090216-189569/Schools-to-teach-breastfeedings-benefit. Accessed December 4, 2009.

UNICEF. 15 Years after Innocenti Declaration, breastfeeding saving six million lives annually. Geneva/Florence; November 22, 2005. www.unicef.org/media/media_30011.html. Accessed May 12, 2009.

UNICEF. UNICEF lauds Supreme Court for lifting ban on Philippine Milk Code implementing rules. Manila, October 10, 2007. www.unicef.org/philippines/news/index.html. Accessed February 8, 2009.

Van Esterick P. Breastfeeding and feminism. *Int J Gynecol Obstet*. 1994;(Suppl 1):S41-S54.

Villanueva P, et al. Accuracy of pharmaceutical advertisements in medical journals. *Lancet*. 2003;361(9351):27-32.

Walker M. International breastfeeding initiatives and their relevance to the current state of breastfeeding in the United States. *J Midwifery Womens Health*. 2007a;52(6):549-555.

Walker M. *Still Selling Out Mothers and Babies: Marketing of Breast Milk Substitutes in the USA*. Weston, MA: NABA REAL; 2007b.

Weinreich N. What is social marketing? 2006. www.social-marketing.com. Accessed December 1, 2009.

Wilson-Clay B, et al. Learning to lobby for pro-breastfeeding legislation: the story of a Texas bill to create a breastfeeding-friendly physician designation. *J Hum Lact*. 2005; 21(2):191-198.

World Health Organization (WHO). *Protecting, Promoting, and Supporting Breastfeeding: A Joint WHO/UNICEF Statement*. Geneva, Switzerland: WHO; 1989.

World Health Organization (WHO). *Global Strategy for Infant and Young Child Feeding*. Geneva, Switzerland: WHO; 2003.

World Health Organization (WHO). *The International Code of Marketing of Breastmilk Substitutes*. Geneva, Switzerland: WHO; 1981. http://www.who.int/nutrition/publications/code_english.pdf. Accessed March 27, 2009.

World Health Organization (WHO) and UNICEF. Baby-Friendly Hospital Initiative: Revised, updated and expanded for integrated care. WHO Document Production Services, Geneva, Switzerland; 2009. www.who.int/nutrition/publications/infantfeeding/9789241594967_s1.pdf. Accessed May 12, 2009.

Yerkes L. *Fun Works: Creating Places Where People Love to Work*. San Francisco: Berrett-Koehler; 2001.

Yoon J, Park Y. Effects of a breast feeding promotion program for working women [in Korean]. *J Korean Acad Nurs*. 2008;38(6):843-852.

Young D. Breastfeeding: can it compete in the marketplace? *Birth*. 1990;17:119-120.

Zareai M, et al. Creating a breastfeeding culture: a comparison of breastfeeding practises in Australia and Iran. *Breastfeed Rev*. 2007;15(2):15-20.

Glossary

abscess   Localized collection of pus that forms from an infection that has no opening for drainage.

acculturation   Integration into a new culture.

acinus   Any small saclike structure, as one found in a gland. Also called alveolus.

acrocyanosis   Bluish tinge of the hands and feet.

acrodermatitis enteropathica   A rare long-term disease of infants. Symptoms are blisters on the skin and mucous membranes, hair loss, diarrhea, and failure-to-thrive.

active immunity   See immunity, active.

active listening   A counseling skill that involves paraphrasing a message and reflecting it back to the sender.

acute bilirubin encephalopathy (ABE)   Neurological damage caused by acute excessive bilirubin, suggested as a replacement for the term kernicterus.

adhesion   Tissue layers that adhere, or stick, to one another.

adipose tissue   Tissue made of fat cells arranged in lobes.

afterpains   Menstrual-like pains that occur in the first few days after birth as the uterus contracts to return to normal size.

alactogenesis   Absence of the onset of stage II lactogenesis.

allergen   A foreign substance that can cause an allergic response in the body.

alpha-lactalbumin   Protein in the whey portion of human milk that assists with synthesis of lactose. Bactericide against *Streptococcus pneumoniae*.

alternate massage   Technique in which the mother compresses the breast when the baby pauses during a feeding. Used to encourage suckling and increase milk production. Also called breast compression.

alveolar ridge   The bony ridge of the jaw that contains the tooth sockets.

alveoli   Tiny glands in the breast that produce milk.

amenorrhea   The absence of the monthly flow of blood and discharge of mucous tissues from the uterus through the vagina (menstruation).

amino acids   The basic building blocks that make up proteins in the body. They are the end products of protein digestion.

amylase   An enzyme that aids the breakdown of starch in digestion.

analgesia   Absence of the normal sensation of pain.

anchor   A word or phrase used at the numerical endpoints of a written scale to describe the extremes of feeling or thought measured by the scale.

anemia   A decrease in red cells in the blood, in hemoglobin, or in total volume, reducing the blood's ability to carry oxygen. Anemia occurs in about half of all pregnancies.

anesthesia   Partial or complete loss of sensation with or without memory loss as a result of disease, injury, or administration of an anesthetic agent, usually by injection or inhalation.

ankyloglossia   Tight lingual frenulum; defect of the mouth in which the membrane under the tongue is too short, limiting movement of the tongue.

anomaly   Change from what is regarded as normal; inherited problem with growth of a structure.

anovulatory   Failure of the ovaries to produce, mature, or release eggs.

anoxia   Lack of oxygen.

antibody   A protein substance that is developed in response to and interacts specifically with an antigen to form the basis of immunity.

anticipatory guidance   A form of counseling that provides encouragement, help, and guidance to prevent or minimize problems.

anticipatory stage   The first of four stages in role acquisition. The time in which one collects information and begins learning about the new role.

antigen   A substance foreign to the body, often a protein.

antimicrobial   Preventing or destroying the development of microorganisms.

apnea   Failure to breathe.

approach behavior   Signals the baby sends to indicate a willingness to interact, such as tongue extension, bringing the hand to the mouth, or rooting.

areola   The dark, circular area surrounding the nipple.

artificial baby milk   See human milk substitute.

artificial feeding   Feeding an infant anything other than human milk.

assessment   An evaluation of a patient that includes physical examination and medical history.

assimilate   (1) The process of incorporating nutrition into living tissue. (2) Becoming incorporated into a culture other than one's own.

assisted reproductive technology (ART)   Reproductive technology used to achieve pregnancy by artificial or partially artificial means, primarily in infertility treatments.

assumption   In statistics, a condition that must be true of the data for the statistical test to be used accurately.

asymmetry   Disparity in size or shape.

atopic dermatitis   Allergic tendency (possibly inherited) to rash or inflammation of the skin.

atresia   Absence of a normal body opening.

atrophy   Loss of size of a part of the body because of disease or other influences; a natural occurrence in the final stage of lactation (involution).

attachment parenting   A form of parenting that creates strong, healthy emotional bonds between children and their parents by nurturing a child's need for trust, empathy, and affection, providing a lifelong foundation for healthy, enduring relationships.

attending   A counseling skill that involves listening and observing in a noninterfering manner.

attentive listening   A counseling skill in which the listener actively focuses on the words that are heard.

augmentation, breast   Surgical procedure performed to increase the size of the breast. It can interfere with milk production.

autocrine control   Local control within a gland. In the case of the breast, the control agent is a secretory product from one type of cell that influences the activity of the same type of cell. This suggests that milk that is left in the breast acts to inhibit the production of more milk.

autonomic nerves   Nerves that have the ability to function independently without outside influence.

average   The sum of the values (in the group being averaged) divided by the number of members of the group.

avoidance behavior   Signals the baby sends to indicate an unwillingness to interact, such as frowning, wrinkling his brow, squinting, closing his eyes, or clenching his fists.

axilla   Pyramid-shaped space forming the underside of the shoulder between the upper part of the arm and the side of the chest. Also called the armpit.

∼ B

baby blues   The mild depression some women feel for several weeks after birth, frequently appearing around the third day postpartum. The mother may have bouts of tearfulness and sadness mingled with happiness and excitement. It is more common in women having their first baby.

baby friendly   Maternity care that protects, promotes, and supports breastfeeding.

Baby-Friendly Hospital Initiative (BFHI)   Health initiative of the World Health Organization and UNICEF launched in 1991 to protect, promote, and support breastfeeding.

baby-led weaning   Weaning initiated by the baby, according to the baby's own timetable.

baby training   Popular term for feeding and putting infants to sleep at specific times, including feeding on a clock schedule; emphasizes making infants go to sleep on their own without sleep "props" such as breastfeeding, rocking, bottles, or pacifiers.

bactericidal   Having the ability to destroy bacteria.

bacteriostatic   Capable of restraining the development of bacteria.

Ballard Scale   A gestational assessment tool that evaluates the tone of the infant's total body, wrist, biceps muscle, knee joint, shoulder girdle, and pelvic girdle.

bariatric surgery   Weight loss surgery to limit either the amount of food a person can eat, or the amount of food a person can digest.

basal   Referring to the fundamental or basic, as in the lowest body temperature or lowest prolactin level.

baseline   The starting value or values before a treatment or test is applied.

Bauer's response   Reflex in which pressure on the soles of the feet elicits spontaneous crawling efforts and extension of the baby's head.

bell curve   The shape of the normal distribution on a graph, resembling the shape of a bell.

bias   In sampling, bias refers to the tendency of a sample to misrepresent the whole population because some of the sample did not answer the questions. In statistics, unbiased estimators of the true value are usually desired because biased ones tend to consistently overestimate or underestimate the true value.

bifidus factor   A carbohydrate present in human milk that has anti-infective properties.

bifurcated   Splitting into two branches or parts.

bili-light   Fluorescent light used to treat jaundice.

bilirubin   A byproduct of the breakdown of the hemoglobin portion of red blood cells.

bioavailability   The amount of a nutrient, drug, or other substance that is active in the tissues.

biological nurturing   An approach to positioning for breastfeeding that allows gravity and primitive neonatal reflexes to stimulate nursing.

bisphenol A (BPA)   An organic compound with two phenol functional groups thought to be hazardous to health.

blind   A characteristic of a study in which the treatment is kept secret from the person receiving it and, often, from those giving the treatment as well.

blood incompatibility jaundice   A condition resulting from blood incompatibility between a mother and her baby that appears within the first 24 hours of life.

body language   Nonverbal messages sent by body position and gesture.

body mass index (BMI)   A measure of the body that takes into account a person's weight and height to gauge total body fat in adults.

bolus   A round mass of food or liquid ready to be swallowed; a dose of a substance given intravenously.

bonding   Interaction between parents and infant to form a unique lasting relationship.

bradycardia   An abnormal condition in which the heart contracts steadily but at a rate below normal.

breast compression   See alternate massage.

breast infection   See mastitis.

breast massage   Manual massage of the breast used to facilitate letdown and expression of milk.

breast shell   A plastic cup worn over the nipple during pregnancy and between feedings to increase nipple protractility and protect sore nipples.

breastfeeding-associated jaundice   Neonatal jaundice caused by mismanagement of breastfeeding. Also called lack-of-breastfeeding jaundice.

breastfeeding counselor   A lay counselor who assists breastfeeding mothers at a peer level.

breastfeeding diary   Daily log of the baby's feedings, wet diapers, and stools.

breastmilk jaundice   See late-onset jaundice.

breastmilk substitute   See human milk substitute.

buccal pad   A fat pad over the main muscle of the cheek. It is very evident in infants and is also called a sucking pad. It is not fully developed in preterm infants.

building hope   A counseling skill used to encourage the mother by offering hope for improvement.

burnout   A condition of becoming bored, discouraged, or frustrated.

~ C

Candida albicans   A tiny, common yeastlike fungus normally found in the mouth, digestive tract, vagina, and on the skin of healthy persons.

candidiasis   A yeastlike fungal infection, commonly afflicting the vagina that produces a thick vaginal discharge; can be transmitted to the baby at birth and result in candidiasis in his

mouth and digestive tract, which appears as white patches or ulcers. May also occur on the mother's nipples.

capillaries   Tiny blood vessels in the system that link the arteries and the veins.

caput succedaneum   A collection of fluid between the scalp and skull of a newborn. It is usually formed during labor as a result of the pressure of the cervix on the infant's head. The swelling begins to recede soon after birth.

case   A person who has the problem under study.

case-control study   Research in which cases (people who have the disease or problem of interest) are identified first, and then controls (people who are similar to cases but do not have the problem) are identified.

case study   An article in a journal describing one (or a few) instances of a diagnosis, problem, or situation that arose in practice.

casein   Component of the proteins in milk.

categorical data   Data that can be classified but not quantified, such as survey responses "very satisfied," "satisfied," "unsatisfied," "very unsatisfied."

catheter   A tubular medical device for insertion into canals, vessels, passageways, or body cavities usually to permit injection or withdrawal of fluids or to keep a passage open. Usually used during labor to drain the bladder when the mother has received anesthesia.

Centers for Disease Control and Prevention (CDC)   An agency of the U.S. Public Health Service established in 1973 to protect the public health of the nation by providing leadership and direction in the prevention and control of diseases and other preventable health conditions and to respond to public health emergencies.

cephalhematoma   Swelling caused by the pooling of blood under the scalp. It may begin to form in the scalp of a baby during labor and may slowly become larger in the first few days after birth. It may be a result of trauma, often from forceps or vacuum extraction.

certification   Process that attests to having met certain standards of the profession.

chiropractic care   Care that emphasizes diagnosis, treatment, and prevention of mechanical disorders of the musculoskeletal system, especially the spine, under the hypothesis that these disorders affect general health via the nervous system.

chi-square   A statistical term that can describe a distribution of data; can be the name for a test of categorical data.

C-hold   Technique in which the mother cups her free hand to form the letter "C," with her thumb on top and her fingers curved below the breast, well behind the areola; used to help support the breast with positioning and attachment.

cholecystokinin (CCK)   A gastrointestinal hormone that enhances digestion, sedation, and a feeling of satiation and well-being. It is released in both the infant and mother during suckling.

clarifying   A counseling skill used to make a point clear.

clavicle   The collarbone. It is a long, curved horizontal bone just above the first rib, forming the front portion of the shoulder.

cleft lip   A birth defect consisting of one or more clefts (splits) of the upper lip. This results from the failure of the upper jaw and nasal areas to fuse in the embryo.

cleft palate   A birth defect in which there is a hole in the middle of the roof of the mouth (palate). The cleft may be complete, going through both the hard and soft palates into the nasal area, or it may go only partly through. It is often linked to a cleft in the upper lip.

clinical instructor   Skilled practitioner who supervises students in a clinical setting to allow practical experience with patients. See also mentor.

clinical practice   The day-to-day work of healthcare professionals rather than the kind of care that might be given in an experimental setting.

clustered feedings   Period of almost constant wakefulness and suckling at some time of the day, generally the early evening. Also referred to as bunched feedings.

clutch hold   See side-sitting hold.

cognitive learning   The process of learning that includes perception and judgment.

Cohen's kappa   A statistical test, designed by J. Cohen (1960), to measure concordance for dichotomous data. Experts differ, but kappa values of .7 or higher are considered evidence of excellent agreement.

cohort   A group studied together because of some characteristic or experience they have in common.

cohort study   A type of research that examines the effect or effects of belonging to a particular group on some result or outcome of interest.

colic   Extreme fussiness in the baby that is characterized by a piercing cry, severe abdominal discomfort, and inability to be comforted.

colostrum   Breastmilk secreted during pregnancy, after childbirth, and before the onset of secretion of mature milk.

combined spinal-epidural anesthesia   A regional anaesthetic technique that combines the benefits of both spinal anaesthesia and epidural anaesthesia and analgesia. The spinal component gives a rapid onset of a predictable block. The indwelling epidural catheter gives the ability to provide long-lasting analgesia and to titrate the dose given to the desired effect.

community outreach   Reaching the community through programs and services.

complementary feeding   New foods added to the growing breastfed infant's diet to meet the energy and nutrient needs that are not met by human milk alone. Introduction of solid foods. In some cases this term is interpreted as "topping off" the breastfed infant with liquids other than human milk, but that is technically referred to as supplementing.

complete protein   See protein, complete.

complex carbohydrates   Carbohydrates that contain important vitamins and minerals. Complex carbohydrates take longer to digest than simple carbohydrates and do not stimulate a craving for more food. Foods in this category include vegetables, fruits, whole-grain cereals, rice, breads, and crackers.

compliance   In health care, the act of a patient following the plan of care or treatment prescribed.

confidence interval (CI)   A statistical term that states the range within which a population's true value is expected to be found.

confounding variable   A characteristic or attribute of the people in the study or their experiences that could confuse the interpretation of the study's results.

congenital   Present at birth, such as a congenital defect.

conjugation   The process by which the liver converts bilirubin into a form that can be broken down and pass into the intestine.

consent   Permission to perform a procedure.

contraception   A technique or device for preventing pregnancy.

contraindicate   To give indication against the advisability of, as in "In very few instances is breastfeeding contraindicated."

control   (1) The group in the study to whom the treatment was not given (in an experiment) or who do not have the problem of interest (in a case-control study). (2) The amount or type of regulation of study conditions the researchers can exercise.

convenience   Refers to a type of sample selected by the researcher that is not random or carefully defined but rather readily accessible.

Coombs' test   Test that measures the presence of antibodies to red blood cells in the blood.

Cooper's ligaments   Ligaments that run vertically through the breast and attach the deep layer of subcutaneous tissue to the dermis of the skin.

cord blood   Blood that remains in the umbilical cord at birth.

correlated   Shown, by a specific statistical test, to be associated.

cosleeping   Practice in which the infant sleeps with the parents.

cradle hold   The traditional sitting position whereby the mother sits with her baby's body across her abdomen. She places his head in the crook of her arm and supports his body with her hand.

craniosacral therapist   Specialist who very subtly and gently manipulates the skull, spine, and sacrum to help with minor aches and pains through to severe and persistent health problems.

creamatocrit   Percentage of cream, used to estimate the fat and energy content of human milk.

Cronbach's alpha   A special test applied to determine whether the items on a scale or tool are internally consistent, or that they measure the same concept in a similar way.

cross-cradle hold   The same holding technique as the dominant hand hold but used for the less dominant hand as well. See dominant hand hold.

cross-sectional study   Research that examines a question at one point in time (such as surveys of a neighborhood all collected within the same week).

culture   The environment that surrounds us and influences our beliefs and attitudes.

cup feeding   Alternate feeding method in which the baby is fed with a cup.

cyanosis   Bluish coloring of the skin or mucous membranes due to low oxygen levels.

cytokines   A unique family of growth factors secreted primarily from leukocytes. Cytokines stimulate humoral and cellular immune responses, as well as the activation of phagocytic cells.

～ D

Dancer hand position   Position that begins in the C-hold position. The mother then brings her hand forward so that her breast is supported with only three fingers. She bends the index finger slightly so that it gently holds the baby's cheek on one side, with the thumb holding the other cheek. This helps the baby's tongue form correctly for suckling and provides stability to help the baby stay latched. Originated by Sarah Danner and Ed Cerutti.

dehydration   Large loss of water from the body tissues.

demographics   Variables that describe basic characteristics of the subjects such as age, gender, place of residence, income, education, and ethnicity.

dependent variable   The aspect or characteristic of the subjects, or of their experience, that the researcher is trying to understand or explain. In a study of the effect of calories on weight gain, weight gain is the dependent variable.

dermis   The layer of skin just below the outer layer (epidermis). It contains blood and lymph vessels, nerves and nerve endings, glands, and hair follicles.

descriptive study   Usually, a study that begins to explore a phenomenon by describing it in detail rather than trying to control any aspects of it.

detoxify   Speed up the removal of harmful substances from the body.

diabetes   A variable disorder of carbohydrate metabolism resulting from inadequate secretion or utilization of insulin.

dichotomous outcome   A result or answer that has only two possibilities such as "Yes, No" or "True, False."

discharge planner   Hospital staff person evaluates a patient to determine readiness for discharge and gives the patient instructions until the first follow-up visit.

disorganized suck   Temporary sucking difficulty due to illness, prematurity, drugs given to the infant or mother, a delay in the first breastfeeding at birth, a neuromotor dysfunction, variations in oral anatomy or nipple preference due to the introduction of an artificial nipple.

distribution   A description of the way the values of a variable (independent or dependent) range; how many values are small, medium, and large. Often, this is shown graphically.

dominant hand hold   Position in which the mother holds her baby with her dominant hand to nurse. She holds the baby's head in her hand and supports his body with her forearm. She can nurse on the nearest breast and then move her arm with the baby across her body to the opposite breast.

donor milk   Human milk that is expressed and donated to a human milk bank to be given to another baby.

dopamine   A hormone made in the adrenal gland that acts as a prolactin inhibitor.

doula   An experienced woman who helps other women immediately before, during, and/or after delivery.

Down syndrome   A form of congenital mental retardation caused by an extra chromosome; also called trisomy 21.

drip milk   Milk that leaks from a breast without direct stimulation.

duct system (ductwork)   A system of ducts and ductules through which milk flows from the point of production out to the nipple pores.

ductule   Small duct in the mammary gland that drains milk from the alveoli into larger ducts that terminate in the nipple.

dyad   Two individuals who form one unit, each dependent on the other, such as a mother and baby.

dysfunction   Inability to function normally.

dysfunctional suck   Sucking anomaly that requires a referral to a physical, occupational or speech therapist with specialization in infant disorders.

～ E

eclampsia   Coma and convulsive seizures occurring in a woman between her 20th week of pregnancy and the end of the first week postpartum.

eczema   Swelling of the outer layer of skin that may be itchy, red, have small blisters, and weep.

edema   A local or generalized condition in which body tissues contain excessive amounts of fluid.

Edinburgh postnatal depression scale   Scale for rating the degree of postnatal depression.

ELBW   Extremely low-birth-weight infant, born weighing under 2 lb, 3 oz (1,000 g).

emergency weaning   Weaning abruptly, with no preparation or forethought.

empathetic listening   A counseling technique in which the counselor listens with the intent to understand emotionally and intellectually.

empowerment   The act of promoting or influencing self-actualization.

endocrine   Pertaining to a gland that secretes directly into the bloodstream.

engorgement   Swelling or congestion of body tissues; overfullness of the breast.

enteral   Within or by way of the intestines.

environmental contaminant   Impurity in human milk that results from contamination of the environment by such chemicals as DDT, PBB, and PCB that then enter the food chain and are consumed by the mother.

enzyme   A protein that speeds up or causes chemical reactions in living matter.

epidermis   The outer layers of the skin. It is made up of an outer, dead portion and a deeper, living portion. Epidermal cells gradually move outward to the skin surface, changing as they go, until they become flakes.

epidural anesthesia   Anesthesia produced by injection of an anesthetic into the epidural space of the spinal cord.

epiglottis   The cartilage-like structure that overhangs the trachea like a lid. It prevents food from entering the trachea by closing during swallowing.

episiotomy   A surgical incision made to enlarge the vaginal opening during childbirth.

epithelium   The covering of the organs of the body.

erythema toxicum   Pink to red macular (raised) area in newborns with a center that is yellow or white. It has no apparent significance and requires no treatment.

estrogen   The hormone that stimulates growth of the reproductive organs, including alveoli and ducts in the breasts.

ethics   The discipline dealing with what is good and bad and with moral duty and obligation; a set of moral principles or values.

eustachian tube   Tube lined with mucous membrane that joins the nose–throat cavity (nasopharynx) and the inner ear (tympanic cavity).

evaluating   A counseling technique used to examine the quality of a counseling contact.

evert   Protrude outward.

exclusive breastfeeding   Breastfeeding in which the baby receives no drinks or foods other than human milk, not even water; is given no pacifiers or artificial nipples; has no limits placed on frequency or length of a breastfeeding; and receives at least 8 to 12 breastfeedings in 24 hours, including night feedings.

excoriated   Surface of the skin that is scraped or chafed.

exocrine   Pertaining to a gland whose secretion reaches an epithelial surface either directly or through a duct.

exogenous   Derived from outside the body.

experiment   A type of research in which the scientist selects a sample and applies some treatment or performs some action on part of the sample in order to measure the differences between treated and untreated parts.

extrauterine   Occurring or located outside the uterus.

～ F

facilitating   A counseling technique used to direct a conversation in such a way that encourages the other speaker to provide information and define the situation.

failure-to-thrive (FTT)   Condition in which an infant's weight is seriously compromised. Signs are failure to regain birth weight by 3 weeks of age, weight loss of greater than 10 percent of birth weight by 2 weeks of age, deceleration of growth from a previously established pattern of weight gain, and evidence of malnutrition on examination, such as minimal subcutaneous fat or wasted buttocks.

fat-soluble vitamins   Vitamins A, D, E, and K.

fat stores   Layers of fat laid down during pregnancy that provide a reserve to help nourish the breastfeeding baby.

feedback inhibitor of lactation (FIL)   A human whey protein that enables the mammary gland to regulate its milk production; it acts to inhibit milk synthesis when milk is left in the breast.

feeding cues   See hunger cues.

fibrocystic breast   A common type of benign breast condition that causes lumpiness in the breast.

finger feeding   An alternate feeding method in which the baby sucks on the mother's or examiner's finger. A 5-, 6-, or 8-French oral gastric tube that leads to the liquid is placed along the fat pad of the finger, extending a few centimeters beyond the tip of the finger. The fat pad of the finger with the tube on it is placed into the baby's mouth far enough to elicit suckling. See also tube feeding.

fistula An abnormal passage from an internal organ to the body surface or between two internal organs.

flange To extend outward, to flare, as in the baby's lips being flanged when attached at the breast; a portion of a breast pump that is placed against the breast to form suction.

flash heat treatment Milk treatment method in which a container of milk, placed into a pan of water, is heated to a rolling boil and then removed

flatulence Excessive gas in the stomach and abdomen causing pain in the abdomen or intestines.

flexion A state of being bent or curved.

flora Normal bacteria and other microbes.

focusing A counseling skill that is used to concentrate on a point that should be explored.

follow up Provide further contact or resources.

fontanel A space between the bones of an infant's skull covered by tough membranes.

football hold See side-sitting hold.

forceps Instruments used to help a difficult childbirth, to quickly deliver a baby with breathing problems, or to shorten normal labor. The blades of the forceps are put into the vagina one at a time and applied to opposite sides of the baby's head, with the baby's head held firmly between the blades.

foremilk The lower-fat milk that is present at the beginning of a breastfeeding.

formal stage The second of four stages in role acquisition. A time in which the role is viewed more personally.

frenulum A fold of skin or mucous membrane that is attached to a part of the body and checks or controls its motion, as in the fold under the tongue.

frenum A fold of skin that anchors the upper lip to the top gum.

∼ G

galactocele A cyst that is caused by the closing or blockage of a milk duct. It contains a thick, creamy milklike substance that may be discharged from the nipple when the cyst is compressed.

galactogogue Food or drink that is believed to increase milk production.

galactopoiesis Stage III lactogenesis, which marks the establishment and maintenance of mature milk.

galactorrhea Secretion and release of milk unrelated to childbirth or breastfeeding; excessive or inappropriate milk production; also called spontaneous lactation.

galactose A simple sugar produced by the breakdown of lactose (milk sugar).

galactosemia An inherited disease of inability to process galactose, caused by lack of an enzyme.

gastroenteritis Inflammation of the stomach and intestines.

gastroesophageal reflux (GER) A backflow of acidic contents of the stomach into the esophagus that produces burning pain. It is often the result of failure of the lower esophageal sphincter to close.

gastrostomy Gavage feeding in which a tube is placed through the skin directly into the stomach.

gavage feeding A method for feeding an infant in which a tube is passed through the nose, mouth, or skin into the stomach.

generalize To extend the results of a study not just to the people studied but also to a larger group who are more or less similar to them.

genetically modified food Foods derived from genetically modified organisms.

gestation The time period from conception to birth.

gestational age The age of a fetus or a newborn, usually stated in weeks dating from the first day of the mother's last menstrual period.

gestational ovarian theca lutein cyst A cyst that develops in the ovary during gestation. During a woman's menstrual cycle, a mound of yellow tissue (corpus luteum) forms in the wall of the ovary where an egg has just been released. Its purpose is to release hormones to help prepare the body for pregnancy. If the egg is not impregnated, it shrinks and is shed during menstruation.

ghrelin A peptide hormone called the "hunger hormone."

glucuronic acid An agent that conjugates bilirubin in the liver.

glycan A polysaccharide or oligosaccharide.

goiter Enlargement of the thyroid gland, resulting in a thick-looking neck or double-chin appearance.

grommet See obturator.

grooming Gently stroking an infant's body during a feeding. This increases a mother's prolactin level.

growth spurt A period of sudden growth when the baby nurses more frequently than usual.

guiding method A counseling method that provides emotional support and encourages the sharing of feelings and concerns.

∼ H

H1N1 influenza A strain of swine flu responsible for a 2009 flu pandemic.

half-life The time needed for a drug's level in the bloodstream to go down to one-half of its beginning level.

hand expression Removal of milk from the breast by manual manipulation.

health consumerism An informed person who is a responsible decision maker concerning health care.

hematocrit A measure of the number of red cells found in the blood, stated as a percentage of the total blood volume.

hemoglobin The portion of the red blood cell that transports oxygen to all parts of the body.

high-risk infant An infant born at risk due to a particular medical condition or social situation.

hindmilk The high-fat milk resulting from the letdown reflex, which forces milk from the alveoli and washes the fat from the walls of the ducts.

Hirschsprung's disease A condition in which a part of the infant's intestines lacks proper nerve innervation and the stool is not passed easily beyond that point. These infants frequently have large, bloated abdomens from the collection of stool and gas.

HIV See human immunodeficiency virus.

HMBANA Human Milk Banking Association of North America, a multidisciplinary group of healthcare providers that sets the standards and guidelines for donor milk banking in Canada, Mexico, and the United States.

Hoffman technique A technique used to train the nipple to become graspable by manually stretching the tissue surrounding the nipple.

Holder pasteurization Heat treating at either 56ºC or 62.5ºC.

home visit A form of consultation in which the counselor or practitioner visits the mother in her home.

homogeneity Sameness. In studies that hope that two groups are different in important ways, finding sameness between them invalidates the results.

human immunodeficiency virus (HIV) Virus that slowly weakens the body's immune system, thus allowing viruses, bacteria, parasites, and fungi that usually don't cause problems to cause illness and death.

human milk Milk secreted in the human breast.

human milk bank A service established for the purpose of collecting, screening, processing, and distributing donated human milk to meet the specific medical needs of individuals for whom it is prescribed.

human milk fortifier (HMF) Nutrients added to expressed human milk to enhance the growth and nutrient balances of VLBW infants and ELBW infants.

human milk substitute Any food being marketed or otherwise represented as a partial or total replacement for human milk. Also called artificial baby milk.

human subjects review group Groups of people in research institutions and healthcare agencies who study a research proposal to be sure it does not violate people's rights or jeopardize their safety.

humoral Immunity against invaders, as with bacteria and foreign tissue. Humoral immunity is the result of the development and continuing presence of circulating antibodies that are produced by the body's defense system.

hunger cues A progression of signs that indicate a desire to feed. The baby will begin to wriggle his body, and his closed eyes will exhibit rapid eye movement (REM). He will then make mouthing movements. He will pass one or both of his hands over his head and will bring his hand to his mouth.

hydration The water balance within the body.

hyperalimentation The administration of nutrients by intravenous feeding, especially to patients who cannot ingest food through the alimentary tract, such as preterm infants.

hyperbilirubinemia A yellow coloring of the tissues, membranes, and secretions due to the presence of bile pigments in the blood; a symptom in the body. Also referred to as jaundice.

hypercapnia High carbon dioxide levels.

hyperemesis Excess vomiting that can result in weight loss and fluid and electrolyte imbalance.

hypernatremia Overconcentration of sodium in the blood, caused by an excess loss of water and electrolytes resulting from diarrhea, excessive sweating, or inadequate water intake.

hyperprolactinemia Elevated prolactin levels.

hypertension A common disorder often without external symptoms, marked by high blood pressure persistently exceeding 140/90.

hypertonia Abnormally high tension or tone, especially of the muscles.

hypocalcemia Too little calcium in the blood.

hypopituitarism See Sheehan's syndrome.

hypoplasia Incomplete or under developed organ or tissue, usually the result of a decrease in the number of cells.

hypothalamus The portion of the brain forming the floor and part of the side wall of the third ventricle. It triggers the release of hormones.

hypothesis An expected relationship between two variables expressed before a study and around which the study is designed.

hypothyroidism A condition caused by a deficiency of thyroid secretions causing low metabolism.

hypotonia Abnormally low tension or tone, especially of the muscles.

hypoxemia An abnormal lack of oxygen in the blood in the arteries.

hypoxia   Too little oxygen in the cells, characterized by rapid heartbeat, high blood pressure, contraction of blood vessels, dizziness, and mental confusion.

∼ I

iatrogenic   Induced inadvertently by a physician or surgeon or by medical treatment or diagnostic procedures.

IBCLC   International Board Certified Lactation Consultant.

IBFAT   Infant Breastfeeding Assessment Tool, which assesses the infant's behavior during a breastfeeding.

ICD-9   International Classification of Diseases.

identifying strengths   A counseling skill that helps the mother focus on positive qualities.

ignoring   The lowest level of listening.

immunity   The quality of being protected from disease organisms and other foreign bodies.

immunity, active   Long-term immunity that protects the body from new infection; gained from the production of antibodies.

immunity, passive   Immunity from antibodies carried through the placenta to the fetus or through breastmilk.

immunization   Any injection of weakened bacteria given to protect against or to reduce the effects of related infectious diseases; vaccination.

immunoglobulin   Group of five distinct antibodies in the serum and external secretions of the body that provide immunity. Immunoglobulins include IgA, IgD, IgE, IgG, and IgM.

immunological   Providing immunity to disease by stimulating antigens.

incomplete protein   See protein, incomplete.

independent variable   The aspect of the subjects or their experience that the researcher suspects may explain or predict the result or outcome. In a study of the effect of calories on weight gain, calories are the independent variable.

induce lactation   Initiate breastfeeding in a woman who has not given birth, as with an adoptive mother. Milk production is prompted by frequent nursing and other measures rather than by the delivery of the placenta.

induction   A method of artificially or prematurely stimulating labor in a woman.

inert   A chemically inactive substance.

influencing   A counseling technique used to produce positive action in the mother through the use of special skills.

informal stage   The third of four stages in role acquisition. A time of modifying, blending, and individualizing one's role.

informed consent   Consent to medical care based on sufficient education and information.

informing   A counseling technique used to educate the mother by offering her explanations to increase her understanding of situations and suggestions.

innervation   The distribution or supply of nerve fibers or nerve impulses to a part of the body.

Innocenti Declaration   Declaration to promote, protect and support breastfeeding, produced and adopted by WHO/UNICEF policymakers at the Spedale degli Innocenti, Florence, Italy in 1990.

insensible   Small amount; not perceptible.

instruments   Also called tools. Can be a variety of things used to measure such as questionnaires, photographs, tape measures, stopwatches, and so on.

intercostal   Situated or extending between the ribs.

internal validity   The assurance that extraneous variables are not responsible for the observed results.

International Board Certified Lactation Consultant (IBCLC)   A health care professional who specializes in the clinical management of breastfeeding and is certified by the International Board of Lactation Consultant Examiners.

International Board of Lactation Consultant Examiners (IBLCE)   A nonprofit corporation established in 1985 to develop and administer certification for lactation consultants.

International Code of Marketing of Breastmilk Substitutes   A set of resolutions developed in 1979 by WHO and UNICEF that regulate the marketing and distribution of any fluid intended to replace human milk, devices used to feed such fluids, and the role of healthcare workers who advise on infant feeding.

International Lactation Consultant Association (ILCA)   A global association founded in 1985 for health professionals who specialize in promoting, protecting, and supporting breastfeeding. The professional association for lactation consultants.

internship   In the field of lactation, a program for acquiring clinical practice hours toward becoming a certified lactation consultant (IBCLC).

interpreting   A counseling skill making use of an analysis of what the mother is saying.

intraductal papilloma   Benign tumor within a duct. It is often associated with a spontaneous bloody discharge from one breast.

intramuscular (IM)   Referring to the inside of a muscle, as of an injection into a muscle to administer medicine.

intrauterine   Within the uterus.

intrauterine growth rate   Normal rate of fetal weight gain; used to describe growth rate for premature infants.

intrauterine growth retardation (IUGR)   Abnormal process in which the development and maturation of the fetus is delayed by genetic factors, maternal disease, or fetal malnutrition caused by placental insufficiency.

intravenous (IV)   Referring to the inside of a vein, as of a tube inserted into a vein to provide nutrients or medication directly into the bloodstream.

intubation   Passing a tube into a body opening, as putting a breathing tube through the mouth or nose or into the trachea to provide an airway for anesthetic gas or oxygen.

inverted syringe   Device for everting the mother's nipple. The tapered end of a syringe is cut off and the plunger direction is reversed to provide a smooth surface next to the breast. The mother places the smooth end of the syringe over her nipple and pulls gently on the plunger.

involution   A normal process marked by decreasing size of an organ, as in involution of the uterus after birth.

isolette   Specialized, clear-covered infant crib that allows the infant to maintain appropriate body temperature and receive appropriate treatment; allows for continuous observation of the infant by healthcare providers; stablelet.

∼ J

jaundice   See hyperbilirubinemia.

Joint Commission   An independent, not-for-profit organization that evaluates and accredits more than 18,000 healthcare organizations in the United States, including hospitals, healthcare networks, managed care organizations, and healthcare organizations that provide home care, long-term care, behavioral health care, laboratory, and ambulatory care services, to improve the quality of health care for the public by providing accreditation and related services that support performance improvement in healthcare organizations.

∼ K

kangaroo care   Technique in which the baby is held skin to skin upright and prone between his mother's breasts, wearing only a diaper. He and his mother are then wrapped together to maintain his temperature appropriately.

kangaroo transport   Transporting neonates from their birth facility to the tertiary care center with the baby held skin to skin on the parent's or doctor's chest instead of in an incubator.

kappa   See Cohen's kappa.

kcal   The amount of heat needed to raise the temperature of 1 kg of water 17°C.

Kegel exercises   Exercises to tighten muscles surrounding the vagina, urethra, and rectum.

keratin   The tough surface layer of dead skin developed in response to pressure.

kernicterus   Brain damage caused by excessive bilirubin.

∼ L

lactase   An enzyme that increases the rate of the conversion of milk sugar (lactose) to glucose and galactose, carbohydrates needed by the body for energy.

lactation   Breastfeeding; secretion of human milk.

lactation consultant   A health professional who is board certified (IBCLC) in lactation.

lactational amenorrhea method (LAM)   Method of contraception that must meet three conditions: the mother's menses has not yet returned, the baby is breastfed around the clock without other foods in the diet, and the baby is younger than 6 months.

lactiferous   Mammary, as in lactiferous duct.

lactiferous duct   Tube that collects milk from the ductules and carries it to the nipple.

Lactobacillus bifidus   Organism in the intestinal tract of breastfed infants that discourages the colonization of bacteria.

lactocyte   Epithelial cells.

lactoengineering   Process of fortifying human milk to meet the needs of very and extremely low-birth-weight infants, through separating the fat and giving the fatty portion to the infant.

lactoferrin   An iron-binding protein that increases absorption of iron.

lactogenesis   The phase during which milk production and secretion are established. Lactogenesis occurs in three stages. Stage I is the initiation of milk synthesis, and stage II marks copious milk production. Stage III, also called galactopoiesis, refers to the establishment of a mature milk supply.

lactose   Milk sugar, the type of sugar present in human milk.

lactose intolerance   A disorder resulting in the inability to digest milk sugar (lactose) because of an enzyme (lactase) deficiency.

larynx   Part of the air passage connecting the throat with the windpipe (trachea) leading toward the lungs. The infant's larynx rises and is closed off by the epiglottis during swallowing.

LATCH method   Acronym for system to assess the infant's ability to latch onto the breast and evaluate audible swallowing as a determinant of milk intake: Latch, Audible swallow, Type of nipple, Comfort, and Hold.

late-onset jaundice   A rare type of neonatal jaundice caused by an unknown factor in the mother's milk; this condition appears between the fourth and seventh day of life. Also called breastmilk jaundice.

late preterm   Born between the gestational ages of 34 weeks and 0/7 days through 36 weeks and 6/7 days (formerly called near term).

lay counselor   Counselor who helps others on a peer level.

LBW   Low birth weight. Baby born weighing less than 5 1b, 8 oz (2,500 g).

leading method   A counseling method that entails directing a conversation to help identify options and resources, as well as to aid in developing a plan of action.

leaking   The involuntary release of human milk that usually occurs in the un-nursed breast while the baby is feeding from the other breast, the seepage of milk from a very full breast, or the expulsion of milk from the breast due to the milk letting down.

leaky gut syndrome   A condition in which the intestinal lining becomes inflamed and then thin and porous. Proteins that are incompletely digested may cross from the intestines into the bloodstream.

learning climate   The prevailing influence or set of conditions characterizing the setting in which learning takes place.

leptin   A peptide hormone in human milk that plays a key role in regulating energy intake and energy expenditure, including appetite and metabolism.

lesion   An abnormal change in structure of an organ or part due to injury or disease.

letdown   Milk ejection from the breast triggered by nipple stimulation or as a conditioned reflex.

leukocytes   Cells present in human milk that fight infection.

LGA   Large for gestational age, determined by size and weight at birth in the top 10 percent of the growth rate appropriate for gestational age.

Likert scale   A type of commonly used attitude measure that asks respondents to "strongly agree" or "strongly disagree."

lingual   Pertaining to the tongue, as in lingual frenulum.

lipase   A digestive system enzyme that increases the breakdown of fats (lipids).

lobule   A small lobe, a cluster of 10 to 100 alveoli.

local food   A collaborative effort to build more locally based, self-reliant food economies.

lochia   Discharge that is composed of blood, mucus, and tissue caused by the gradual renewal of reproductive structures after childbirth. Its color transforms from red to pink and then to white in about 2 to 4 weeks.

logistic regression   A statistical technique for studying relationships between variables that can be used when the dependent (outcome) variable is dichotomous (only two possibilities).

lymph   A thin, clear, slightly yellow fluid present in the lymphatic system. It is about 95 percent water with a few red blood cells and variable numbers of white blood cells.

lymph nodes   Small, rounded masses that function as filters in the lymph vessels to trap bacteria and cast-off cell parts. Each is a potential dam to arrest the spread of infection. They may swell and be painful when functioning in this way.

lymphatic system   Complex network of capillaries, thin vessels, valves, ducts, nodes, and organs. The lymphatic system absorbs the excess blood fluids from the tissue spaces and eventually returns them to the heart.

lymphocyte   A lymph cell or white blood cell.

lysozyme   An enzyme with antiseptic actions that destroys some foreign organisms.

～ M

macrophage   Any large cell that can surround and digest foreign substances in the body.

macrosomia   Large size at birth, associated with increased risk of diabetes and cardiovascular disease in later life and an increased risk of some cancers.

macular   Of, relating to, or characterized by a spot or spots; raised.

malignant   Medical term used to describe a severe and progressively worsening disease, most familiar as a description of cancer.

malnutrition   Inadequate nutrition due to improper diet, regardless of the number of calories consumed.

mammary organ   Exocrine gland that functions and develops independently to extract materials from the blood and convert them into milk.

mammary ridge   The line extending from the armpit to the inner thigh of the fetus, sometimes the site of an extra nipple. Also called milk line.

mammogenesis   Stage during which the breast develops to a functioning state.

mammoplasty   Breast reduction; see reduction, breast.

manual expression   See hand expression.

masseter muscle   The muscle that closes the mouth and is the principal muscle in chewing.

mastitis   An inflammation of the breast, usually resulting from a plugged duct left untreated or from a cracked nipple. Also referred to as a breast infection.

mature milk   Composition of human milk after seven to ten days postpartum.

MBA   Mother Baby Assessment, which evaluates the progress of a mother and baby as they learn to breastfeed by observing signaling, positioning, fixing, milk transfer, and ending.

mean   The average of an array of numbers.

meconium   The first stool of a newborn, greenish black to dark brown with a tarry consistency.

mentor   Experienced person who provides expertise to less experienced individuals to help them advance their careers, enhance their education, and build their networks; term used in lactation for helping students acquire clinical skills. See also clinical instructor.

meta-analysis   A method of putting together the results of many studies and reanalyzing them as if they had all been parts of one big study.

metabolic   Referring to metabolism, the sum of all chemical processes that take place in the body as they relate to the movement of nutrients in the blood after digestion.

methicillin-resistant *Staphylococcus aureus* **(MRSA)** Any strain of *Staphylococcus aureus* bacteria that is resistant to a large group of antibiotics, which include the penicillins and the cephalosporins.

mg/dL   Milligrams per deciliter.

milk bank   See human milk bank.

milk bleb   A blocked nipple pore; milk blister.

milk blister   A blocked nipple pore; milk bleb.

milk-ejection reflex   A normal reflex in a nursing mother, caused by stimulation of the nipple and resulting in the release of milk from the breast.

milk/plasma ratio   The quantity of a given drug or its metabolite in human milk in relation to its quantity in the maternal plasma or blood.

milk supply   The quantity of milk that a woman is currently producing, usually compared with the baby's requirements for milk.

milk synthesis   The process of making a compound (human milk) by joining together several elements.

minimal breastfeeding   Breastfeeding between one and three times a day, with complementary or supplementary feedings providing the remaining nourishment. Typical scenario for gradual weaning.

mixed message   A communication or impression that is indistinct or confused.

molding   Asymmetrical appearance of the baby's head after birth due to the overlapping of skull bones.

Montgomery glands   Small raised areas around the nipple that enlarge during pregnancy and lactation and secrete a fluid that lubricates the nipple.

morbidity   An illness or an abnormal condition or quality. The number of ill persons or diseases in a population.

Moro reflex   A normal reflex in a young infant caused by a sudden loud noise. It results in drawing up of the legs, an embracing position of the arms, and usually a short cry.

mortality   The number of deaths in a population.

mother-led weaning   Weaning initiated by the mother without cues from the baby.

motility   Power of motion, spontaneous motion.

mucin   A glycoprotein found in mucus; it is present in human milk, saliva, bile, salivary glands, skin, connective tissues, tendon, and cartilage.

multipara   Woman who has given live birth to more than one child.

myelin   A fatty substance found in the coverings of various nerve fibers. The fat gives the normally gray fibers a white, creamy color.

myoepithelial cells   Smooth muscle layers that enclose the alveoli and ducts of the breast.

⁓ N

narcotic analgesia   A medication that acts on the central nervous system to reduce or eliminate pain.

nasogastric   Gavage feeding with a tube passing through the nose into the stomach.

nasopharynx   Part of the throat behind the nose and reaching from the back of the nasal opening to the soft palate.

necrotizing enterocolitis (NEC)   Inflammation of the intestines and especially of the human ileum that results in tissue death.

need feeding   Feeding the baby whenever he indicates a need, in response to feeding cues. Sometimes referred to as demand or cue feeding.

neonate   The newborn infant up to 6 weeks of age.

networking   Communicating among people with common interests or needs.

neuromotor dysfunction   Impaired or abnormal functioning of the brain and motor function.

neurotransmitter   Chemical released from a nerve terminal that changes or results in the sending of nerve signals across spaces separating nerve fibers.

NICU   Neonatal intensive care unit.

nipple   The protruding part of the breast that extends and becomes firmer on stimulation.

nipple, common   A nipple that protrudes slightly when at rest and becomes erect when stimulated.

nipple, cracked   A nipple that has a crack or fissure lengthwise or crosswise along it.

nipple, flat   A nipple with a very short shank that does not become erect in response to stimulation.

nipple, inverted   A nipple that remains retracted, both when at rest and on stimulation.

nipple, inverted appearing   A nipple that appears inverted but becomes erect when stimulated.

nipple pores   Openings on the end of the nipple through which milk flows.

nipple preference   A preference by the baby for an artificial nipple over the breast, resulting from sucking alternately on the breast and an artificial nipple, which require two completely different mechanisms.

nipple, retracted   A nipple that appears graspable but retracts on stimulation.

nipple shield   An artificial nipple used over the mother's own nipple during nursing.

nonnutritive sucking   Alternate bursts of sucking and resting.

nonprobability   Refers to a type of sampling other than random. Convenience sampling is nonprobability.

normal distribution   The dispersal of data that comes from measuring many natural phenomena. It is a common assumption in statistical tests.

normal fullness   Increased amounts of blood and lymph necessary for milk production that cause the breasts to become fuller, heavier, and slightly tender; not to be confused with engorgement.

nosocomial   Hospital-acquired, as in a nosocomial infection.

nucleotides   Compounds derived from nucleic acid and secreted by mammary epithelial cells. They play key roles in function and growth of the gastrointestinal and immune systems.

nursing strike   Nursing abstinence; a baby's refusal to breastfeed.

nutritive sucking   An organized continuous sequence of long drawing sucks that produces a regular flow of milk.

≈ O

obesity   A body mass index (BMI) of 30 or greater.

obestatin   A peptide hormone in human milk that increases appetite.

obturator   A feeding plate placed over a cleft palate to aid in feeding the baby. Grommet.

odds ratio   A descriptive measure of the association between two variables. Because it is composed of the odds of one group in the numerator and the odds of another group in the denominator, if the odds are greater in the numerator, the odds ratio is greater than one.

oligosaccharide   A carbohydrate present in human milk that discourages the growth of pathogens in the intestinal tract.

online help   Topic-oriented, procedural or reference information delivered through computer software.

open-ended question   A form of question used in counseling that cannot be answered by "yes" or "no"; questions beginning with who, what, when, where, why, how, how much, and how often.

operationalize   The process of defining the concepts to be studied in terms of measurable variables and relationships, including choosing instruments or tools.

orbicularis oris muscle   Circular muscle surrounding the mouth that closes the lips.

orogastric   Gavage feeding with a tube passing through the mouth to the stomach.

osteopenia   Condition where the bone lacks sufficient minerals, usually because the number of bone cells dying exceeds the number of new ones being made by the body.

osteoporosis   A loss of normal bone density, marked by thinning of bone tissue and the growth of small holes in the bone.

otitis media   Swelling or infection of the middle ear, a common disease of childhood that is less frequent in breastfed babies.

outcome   In the context of research, outcome is usually the same as the dependent variable. More broadly, outcomes are the results of any treatment or action, whether or not that treatment is part of a research study.

outliers   Unusually small or large values for one of the variables being measured. Outliers can distort an average. Researchers often try to offer explanations for why a few values are so different from most others.

output variable   Like an outcome variable, this data element is a result or effect. In some studies the sample is selected based on an "effect" of interest such as jaundice. Babies would be studied only if they are jaundiced, or jaundice would be the output variable that divides babies into two comparison groups.

outreach counseling   To reach out to mothers, contacting them on a regular basis to offer support and anticipatory guidance to circumvent problems.

oximeter   A small clip-on instrument that noninvasively estimates the oxygen saturation of a person's blood.

oxytocin   The hormone that stimulates the smooth muscles to contract, specifically those surrounding the alveoli in the breast (causing the release of milk) and those in the uterus (causing uterine contractions); a synthetic form is Pitocin.

≈ P

paced feeding   Bottle feeding method that allows the baby to suck, swallow, and breathe as he would during breastfeeding.

paladai   Cup-feeding device used to feed babies in India that is gaining recognition in the Western world.

palatal   Referring to the palate.

palate, hard   The hard portion of the roof of the mouth.

palate, soft   The soft portion of the roof of the mouth.

palliative care   Care that lessens or relieves pain or other uncomfortable symptoms but does not provide a cure.

Palmar grasp   A reflex that curls the fingers when the palm of the hand is tickled.

paradigm shift   A change from one way of thinking to another.

parenchyma   Functional parts of an organ. In the breast, it includes alveoli and lactiferous ducts.

parenteral   Nongastrointestinal, intravenous.

passive immunity   See immunity, passive.

passive listening   A type of listening such as attending.

pathogen   Any microorganism able to cause a disease.

pathologic   That which is caused by disease.

pathological jaundice   Jaundice that results from such conditions as infections in the blood or liver, diseases of the liver, obstructions in the gastrointestinal system, and interference with the binding of the bilirubin in the bloodstream.

patient-controlled epidural anesthesia (PCEA)   A programmed infusion pump that delivers boluses of anesthetic solution on demand from the patient.

peer review   A process conducted by scientific journals in which an article submitted for publication must be read and approved by several scientists with relevant knowledge. They are peers of the authors, and they can suggest improvements or reject the article.

peptide   A molecule chain of two or more amino acids.

perception   A mental image or awareness; a judgment on or inference from what one has observed.

perineum   An area of tissue that marks externally the approximate boundary of the pelvic outlet and gives passage to the urogenital ducts and rectum; also the area between the anus and the posterior part of the external genitalia, especially in the female.

periosteum   A fiberlike covering of the bones. It has the nerves and blood vessels that supply the bones.

peripheral   Referring to the outside surface or surrounding area of an organ or other structure.

peristalsis   The wavelike, rhythmic contraction of smooth muscle.

persistent organic pollutants   Organic compounds that are resistant to environmental degradation through chemical, biological, and photolytic processes.

personal stage   The final of four stages in role acquisition. The time in which one's style evolves to be consistent with one's personality.

phagocyte   A cell that can engulf particles such as bacteria, other microorganisms, aged red blood cells, and foreign matter.

pharynx   The throat; passage for the breathing and digestive tracts.

phenylalanine   An amino acid present in food protein that can accumulate to dangerous levels in a baby with phenylketonuria.

phenylketonuria (PKU)   A hereditary disease that, if not treated early, can cause brain damage or severe mental retardation in the baby.

phototherapy   Use of a bili-light to treat infantile jaundice.

phthalates   Estrogen-mimicking compounds found in various plastics that infants can be exposed to by artificial feeding.

physiological jaundice   A common type of neonatal jaundice resulting from the normal breakdown of red blood cells and the delay in removing their byproducts from the bloodstream; it appears by the third day of life.

phytoestrogen   Estrogen present in a plant, as in the phytoestrogen in cabbage (used to treat engorgement).

Pierre Robin sequence   A condition of the newborn that consists of an unusually small jaw combined with a cleft palate, downward displacement of the tongue, and absence of a gag reflex.

PIF   See prolactin inhibitory factor.

pilot study   A small trial run of a study conducted before the main study to test processes or instruments planned for use in the main study so that problems can be worked out.

Pincer grasp   Use of the thumb and forefinger to pick up objects, usually occurring at about 8 to 9 months of age.

pinch test   A test for inverted nipples, performed by gently compressing the nipple between the thumb and forefinger and observing the amount of protrusion that results.

Pitocin   A synthetic form of oxytocin.

pituitary   A small, rounded body at the base of the brain that secretes hormones. The anterior pituitary secretes prolactin; the posterior pituitary secretes oxytocin.

placenta   The spongy structure that grows on the wall of the uterus during pregnancy and by which the baby is nourished.

plugged duct   Blockage in a milk duct caused by accumulated milk or cast-off cells.

pneumothorax   Collection of air or gas in the chest causing the lung to collapse.

polycystic ovarian syndrome   A variable disorder marked by amenorrhea, excessive hair, obesity, infertility, and ovarian enlargement; usually initiated by an elevated level of luteinizing hormone, androgen, or estrogen that results in an abnormal cycle of gonadotropin release by the pituitary gland. Also called polycystic ovarian disease, polycystic ovarian syndrome, polycystic ovary disease, and Stein-Leventhal syndrome.

polysaccharides Class of carbohydrates, such as starch and cellulose, consisting of a number of monosaccharides joined by glycosidic bonds.

pooled milk Donor human milk that is pooled and heat treated to ensure the absence of HIV, hepatitis, and other viruses and bacteria.

population The whole group of people who have some characteristic(s) under study of which the sample actually studied is just a part.

postpartum The 6-week period after childbirth.

postpartum depression A mild to moderate depression that lasts from 1 to 6 weeks postpartum. It is characterized by mood changes, sleep disturbances, and fatigue. The mother feels unable to cope with life and may have unexplained physical symptoms such as abdominal pains or headache. She may feel no attachment to the baby and worries that something is not "right." The mother may entertain occasional thoughts of suicide.

postpartum psychosis Postpartum depression that can lead to a loss of control, rational thought, and social functioning. The mother may experience overwhelming confusion and hallucinations. She may attempt to harm herself or her child.

postterm Born after 42 weeks' gestation.

posture feeding Feeding position in which the baby is positioned above the breast and has better control over milk flow. The mother lies flat on her back with her baby lying tummy to tummy on top of her. Also called prone position feeding.

power A mathematical term that represents the degree of likelihood that a given sample size and test will find a difference between comparison groups when there really is a difference.

ppm Parts per million.

praising Counseling skills used to give emotional support and encouragement to mothers.

prebiotics Nondigestible food ingredients that stimulate the growth or activity of bacteria in the digestive system that are beneficial to the health of the body.

preceptor See mentor and clinical instructor.

probiotics Dietary supplements of live microorganisms thought to be beneficial to the health of the body; lactic acid bacteria and bifidobacteria are the most common types of microbes used as probiotics but also certain yeasts and bacilli are available.

predictor variable Independent variable; the characteristic that is believed to influence the result.

premature infant See preterm infant.

prepared childbirth Conscious cooperative birth in which the woman is aware of and able to cooperate with her body.

pretending A type of listening in which the listener gives a noncommittal response, trying to be polite and really not giving any attention to the speaker.

preterm infant Infant born before 37 weeks' gestation; premature.

Pretoria pasteurization Pasteurization method in which the container of milk is placed into water already heated from 56°C to 62°C in an aluminum pot for about 15 minutes.

prevalence Frequency of disease in the population.

primipara A woman who has completed one pregnancy.

probability A probability sample is one selected by random sampling.

problem solving A counseling technique that follows a step-by-step process to arrive at a solution to a problem.

progesterone The hormone responsible for the development of the placenta and mammary glands.

projectile vomiting See vomiting, projectile.

prolactin The hormone that stimulates breast development and formation of milk during pregnancy and lactation.

prolactin inhibitory factor (PIF) A factor produced in and released from the hypothalamus that prohibits the release of prolactin.

prolactinoma A pituitary tumor that secretes prolactin.

prone Referring to the position of the body when lying face downward.

prospective study A study in which events to be studied have not yet happened, so data can be collected as the events happen rather than from old records or memory.

prostaglandin One of several strong hormonelike fatty acids that act in small amounts on certain organs.

protein, complete A protein that contains all the essential amino acids.

protein, incomplete A protein that does not contain all the essential amino acids and must be combined with a complementary protein to become complete.

protractility The ability of the nipple to be drawn out.

pustule A small blister that usually is filled with pus.

_P_ value The observed significance level of a statistical test; it measures how strong the evidence is against the hypothesis that there is no relationship.

pyloric stenosis A condition in which the outflow valve of the stomach will not open satisfactorily to permit the contents of the stomach to pass through. It is most common in firstborn white male infants and is characterized by projectile vomiting.

∾ Q

qualitative study   A study in which the measurement of variables is less important than a description of phenomena or experiences. Statistical analysis is not typically used and changes in practice are not often recommended, except at a conceptual level. Often, such studies lead to further studies.

∾ R

random assignment   The process of fairly designating participants in a study to be in a treatment or control group. The fairness is achieved by a process that cannot be influenced by the scientists or participants, such as a coin flip or use of a special random number chart.

randomized clinical trial   An experiment or experiment-like type of research in which the scientist controls many aspects of the study. Subjects are randomly assigned to their groups. Potential confounders are measured and analysis is planned before data collection.

range   The number that results from subtracting the lowest from the highest value in the data.

Raynaud's phenomenon   Sporadic attacks of interruptions in blood flow to the extremities (fingers, toes, ears, and nose), resulting in tingling, numbness, burning, and pain. Nipple vasospasms can mimic Raynaud's.

RDI   Reference Daily Intake.

reassuring   A counseling skill used to restore confidence through pointing out the normalcy of a situation.

rebirthing   Simulating the birth experience. The baby is placed on the mother's abdomen in a bath of warm water and allowed to find the breast on his own; remedial cobathing.

recall   Bring to mind or think of again.

reduction, breast   Surgical procedure to decrease the size of the breast. It can interfere with milk production. Mammoplasty.

reflective listening   See active listening.

relactation   Resumption of lactation beyond the immediate postpartum period.

reliability   The property possessed by good-quality measurement tools that ensures they measure a concept or characteristic the same way each time.

remedial cobathing   See rebirthing.

renal solute load   Amount of solutes (i.e., glucose, amino acids, potassium, sodium, and chloride) handled by the kidneys.

replicate   To repeat a study that has already been done. Often, the study is conducted on a different sample of people or in a different setting.

resection   Removal of part of an organ or structure by surgery.

respiratory distress syndrome   A condition present, usually at birth, that is characterized by delayed onset of respiration and low Apgar score; caused by the lungs not being fully developed.

respiratory syncytial virus (RSV)   Multistrain virus that causes severe respiratory disease, including bronchitis and pneumonia, in infants and children.

retention   A preservation of the aftereffects of experience and learning that makes recall or recognition possible.

retrospective study   A study in which the result of interest is identified in a group of subjects and then the past experiences of those subjects are examined to see what might have led to the result.

reverse cycle nursing   A nursing pattern in which a mother who has regular separations from her baby provides most or all of her baby's feedings at the breast at times when she and the baby are together.

reverse pressure softening   Breast massage method to help soften the areola to help the baby latch on effectively.

review   In research, a type of study published in a journal that usually does not present any new results but rather summarizes several previous studies.

rickets   Condition caused by lack of vitamin D, calcium, and phosphorus; marked by abnormal bone growth.

rooming-in   Mother and baby sharing the same hospital room, beginning as soon as possible after birth.

rooting reflex   The natural instinct of the newborn to turn his head toward the stimulation when touched on the cheek.

rotavirus   Class of viruses that cause diarrheal illness and lead to hospitalization.

∾ S

sample   The group of people or subjects who are selected to participate in a study. The sample is only part of the whole population of subjects who could be studied.

searching response   Bobbing and bouncing behavior demonstrated by the newborn at the breast.

sebaceous   Fatty, oily, or greasy, usually referring to the oil-secreting glands of the skin or to their secretions.

secretory   Having the function of secretion.

secretory IgA   One of the most common antibodies, found in all secretions of the body. IgA combines with protein in the mucosa and defends body surfaces against invading microorganisms.

selective listening   Form of listening in which the listener hears only certain parts of what is said.

self-efficacy   One's belief in the ability to perform well.

self-image   One's conception of oneself or of one's role.

sensory input   A message, perception, or awareness the mind receives while processing information.

sepsis   Infection.

seroconversion   The process by which serum shows the presence of a factor that previously had been absent, or vice versa.

seronegative   Serum that does not demonstrate the presence of a factor for which tests were conducted; tested negative.

seropositive   Serum that demonstrates the presence of a factor for which tests were conducted; tested positive.

serum   The clear yellowish fluid that remains from blood plasma after clotting factors have been removed by clot formation.

SGA   Small for gestational age, determined by size and weight at birth in the bottom 10 percent of the growth rate appropriate for gestational age. Infant whose growth was retarded and who was delivered before 37 weeks (premature) or after 42 weeks (postmature).

Sheehan's syndrome   A condition occurring after giving birth in which the pituitary gland is damaged. It is caused by a lessening of blood circulation after hemorrhaging of the womb. Also called hypopituitarism.

sibling   A brother or sister.

side sitting hold   A breastfeeding position in which the mother places the baby along her side with his feet toward her back; also known as the football or clutch hold.

simple carbohydrate   The simplest sugars that can cause a sudden rise in blood sugar level after ingestion, followed by a rapid drop and a craving for more food. When consumed in the absence of nutritional foods, simple carbohydrate foods may cause fatigue, dizziness, nervousness, or headache.

sling   An apparatus worn by an adult to carry and comfort a baby.

slope   The slope of a line on a graph as defined by its angle relative to the horizontal axis or by making a ratio of the units of rise over the units of run.

smooth muscle   The type of muscle that provides the erectile tissue in the nipple and areola.

social toxicant   Mood-changing toxicant such as tobacco, coffee, tea, alcohol, marijuana, and other social drugs.

soporific   Sleep-inducing agent, e.g., warm milk.

sphincter   A circular band of muscle fibers that narrows a passage or closes a natural opening in the body.

spina bifida   A neural tube defect present at birth that results in a gap in the bone that surrounds the spinal cord.

spinal anesthesia   A form of regional anesthesia involving injection of a local anesthetic into the cerebrospinal fluid (CSF), generally through a fine needle, usually 3.5 inches (9 cm) long.

spitting up   Baby expelling a small amount of milk from the mouth during or after feedings; common in most babies.

spontaneous lactation   See galactorrhea.

spurious   The relationship between two variables when statistical significance is found, but the significance is actually caused by a third variable that is hidden or unclear.

standards of practice   Stated measures or levels of quality that serve as models for the conduct and evaluation of practice.

stasis   A slowing or stoppage of the normal flow of a bodily fluid or semifluid.

statistical theory   The mathematical ideas about probability and infinite cases that underlie the applied tests commonly used by researchers.

statistically significant   Description of an outcome that did not happen by chance; there is some underlying relationship that caused the event.

subclinical mastitis (SCM)   Asymptomatic inflammation of mammary tissue.

subcutaneous   Under the skin.

sublingual   Under the tongue.

suck   The oral motor activity used by the baby to extract milk from the breast.

suck reorganization   Technique in which the examiner places the index finger in the baby's mouth pad side up and places slight pressure on the midline of the tongue, pulling the finger out slowly to encourage the baby to suck it back in.

suck training   Technique in which the therapist places the index finger in the baby's mouth and stimulates certain portions of the baby's oral anatomy to train him to suck.

sucking pad   See buccal pad.

suckle   The act of feeding at the breast.

summarizing   A counseling skill that entails making a summary of the important points in a conversation.

supernumerary nipple   Extra nipple, other than the one normally found on each breast, which may be present along the milk lines.

supine   Lying flat on the back.

supplementary feeding   Foods other than human milk fed to the infant in place of or after a breastfeeding. Some refer to this as "topping off" the breastfed infant with liquids other than human milk.

supply and demand   The process by which the baby increases the mother's milk production to meet his needs.

suppressor peptides   Inhibiting peptides in human milk that bring about the cessation of milk secretion during milk stasis and engorgement.

sustainable farming   Farming that integrates three main goals: environmental stewardship, farm profitability, and prosperous farming communities.

swaddle   Wrapping the baby, confining his arms and legs to inhibit the startle reflex and provide a feeling of warmth and security.

switch nursing   Frequently altering between breasts during a feeding.

syringe feeding   An alternate feeding method in which a syringe is placed into the corner or middle of the baby's mouth. Depressing the syringe releases milk into the baby's mouth.

systemic   Of or relating to the whole body rather than to a single area or part of the body.

∽ T

tail of Spence   Breast tissue that extends into the axilla.

tandem nursing   A mother nursing more than one child of different ages.

teachable moment   A time of optimal attention and capacity for learning.

tertiary   Third in order of use; belonging to the third level of sophistication of development, as in a specialized, highly technical tertiary-level healthcare facility.

thrush   See candidiasis.

tonic neck reflex   A normal infant reflex present until 3 or 4 months of age; also referred to as the "fencer position." When the baby lies on his back, he extends the arm and leg on the side of his body opposite to the direction his head is turned. This prevents him from rolling over until adequate neurological and motor development occurs.

tool   In research, used interchangeably with instrument.

trachea   A nearly cylindrical tube in the neck by which air passes to and from the lungs; windpipe.

transcutaneous bilimeter   Device that indicates bilirubin levels in the blood by measuring intensity of skin coloration.

transient nipple soreness   Nipple soreness in the first week postpartum that is temporary.

transitional milk   Milk that is present at stage II lactogenesis, around the second or third day postpartum. Blood flow within the breast increases, and copious milk secretion begins. The milk that is between colostrum and mature milk.

transplacental   Across or through the placenta.

transplantation   Removal and reattachment.

trimester   A period of 3 months, particularly used when referring to pregnancy.

trough (for mother's milk)   Channel through which the mother's milk travels formed in the center of the infant's tongue during suckling.

trough level   The lowest blood or milk level achieved by a drug during its dosing period.

true   In statistics, "true" value is used to refer to a population value. For example, if we knew the weight of every human baby born in the last 100 years, we could say, "The true value of the mean of the population is 3020.57 grams." Because we do not know the true value of the mean, we try to estimate it using research and statistics.

***t*-test**   A statistical test used on data that can be averaged, like height. It determines whether two means are significantly different from one another.

tubal ligation   One of several sterilization processes in which the fallopian tubes are blocked to prevent conception from occurring.

tube feeding   An alternate feeding method in which tubing that leads to liquid is placed against the mother's breast with a few centimeters extending beyond the end of the nipple. The baby suckles at the breast and the tip of the tube simultaneously. The flow of supplement from the container encourages him to continue suckling. See also finger feeding.

turgor   Normal strength and tension of the skin caused by outward pressure of the cells and the fluid that surrounds them.

∽ U

unconjugated   In jaundice, bilirubin that is not bound to albumin and circulates freely in the bloodstream; it can migrate toward tissues with high fat content, including the brain and nervous system.

United Nations Children's Emergency Fund (UNICEF)   An agency of the United Nations, established in 1946 and charged with protecting the lives and health of children.

universal precautions   Guidelines observed in health care that help control the transmission of infection.

urethra   The canal for discharge of urine, located in women between the vagina and the clitoris.

U.S. Department of Agriculture (USDA)   The government agency that oversees the Special Supplemental Food Program for Women, Infants, and Children, referred to as WIC.

uvula   Small cone-shaped process suspended in the mouth from the middle of the back edge of the soft palate.

∽ V

vaccine   Weakened or dead microorganisms given to a person to produce antibodies against the virus.

vacuum extraction   Vaginal delivery of the infant assisted by the use of a machine that applies suction to the infant's head.

validity   A property of research methods that conveys how well they capture or measure the phenomenon or concept under study.

vancomycin-resistant enterococcus (VRE)   Group of bacterial species of the genus *Enterococcus* that is resistant to the antibiotic vancomycin.

vancomycin-resistant *Staphylococcus aureus* (VRSA)   Strain of *Staphylococcus aureus* that has become resistant to the glycopeptide antibiotic vancomycin.

variable   A characteristic or effect of either the hypothesized "causes" or "outcomes" under study. If feeding is a partial cause of jaundice, the number and amount of feedings are variables, and the possible bilirubin levels are also variables.

variation   In statistics, it is expected that most phenomena are not exactly the same when measured over time or when measured in different individuals. The variation in the number of times each day that a breastfed baby wants to nurse and the variation in the number of feedings between different babies on the same day are both examples.

vasospasm   Sharp and often persistent contraction of a blood vessel reducing blood flow. Observed in breastfeeding mothers as nipple vasospasm. See Raynaud's phenomenon.

ventral   On the abdomen; draped on the hand.

vernix   The creamy protective coating on the newborn.

vertical transmission   The transfer of a disease, condition, or trait from a mother to her child, either in the genes or at the time of birth, as in the spread of an infection through human milk or through the placenta.

virus   A tiny organism that can grow only in the cells of another organism.

VLBW   Very low birth weight. Infant born weighing less than 3 lb, 5 oz (1,500 g).

voice tone   Pitch level, rate of speech, and volume when speaking.

vomiting   Expelling the contents of the stomach with force.

vomiting, projectile   Violent expulsion of the contents of the stomach with force enough to send it over a foot.

～ W

warm line   A telephone line that is answered by a machine or voice mail, asking the mother to leave a message for a return call.

water-soluble vitamins   Vitamin C and the B vitamins.

weaning   Discontinuation of breastfeeding by substituting other nourishment.

wet nursing   Breastfeeding an infant other than one's own.

whey   Clear fluid when milk stands, when curds are removed.

WIC   Special Supplemental Food Program for Women, Infants, and Children that helps pregnant women in the United States choose nutritious foods to have healthier babies and provides services to breastfeeding mothers, infants, and children up to 5 years of age.

witch's milk   Milk sometimes secreted by the newborn infant's breasts that disappears shortly after birth.

World Health Organization (WHO)   An agency of the United Nations charged with planning and coordinating global healthcare and assisting member nations to combat disease and train healthcare workers.

～ Y

yeast infection   See candidiasis.

A

Code of Ethics for International Board Certified Lactation Consultants

∼ Preamble

It is in the best interests of the profession of lactation consultants and the public it serves that there be a Code of Ethics to provide guidance to lactation consultants in their professional practice and conduct. These ethical principles guide the profession and outline commitments and obligations of the lactation consultant to self, client, colleague, society, and the profession.

The purpose of the International Board of Lactation Consultant Examiners (IBLCE) is to assist in the protection of the health, safety, and welfare of the public by establishing and enforcing qualifications of certification and for issuing voluntary credentials to individuals who have attained those qualifications. The IBLCE has adopted this Code to apply to all individuals who hold the credential of International Board Certified Lactation Consultant (IBCLC).

∼ Principles of Ethical Practice

The International Board Certified Lactation Consultant shall act in a manner that safeguards the interests of individual clients, justifies public trust in her/his competence, and enhances the reputation of the profession. The International Board Certified Lactation Consultant is personally accountable for her/his practice and, in the exercise of professional accountability, must

1. Provide professional services with objectivity and with respect for the unique needs and values of individuals.
2. Avoid discrimination against other individuals on the basis of race, creed, religion, gender, sexual orientation, age, and national origin.
3. Fulfill professional commitments in good faith.
4. Conduct herself/himself with honesty, integrity, and fairness.

5. Remain free of conflict of interest while fulfilling the objectives and maintaining the integrity of the lactation consultant profession.
6. Maintain confidentiality.
7. Base her/his practice on scientific principles, current research, and information.
8. Take responsibility and accept accountability for personal competence in practice.
9. Recognize and exercise professional judgment within the limits of her/his qualifications. This principle includes seeking counsel and making referrals to appropriate providers.
10. Inform the public and colleagues of her/his services by using factual information. An International Board Certified Lactation Consultant will not advertise in a false or misleading manner.
11. Provide sufficient information to enable clients to make informed decisions.
12. Provide information about appropriate products in a manner that is neither false nor misleading
13. Permit use of her/his name for the purpose of certifying that lactation consultant services have been rendered only if she/he provided those services.
14. Present professional qualifications and credentials accurately, using IBCLC only when certification is current and authorized by the IBLCE, and complying with all requirements when seeking initial or continued certification from the IBLCE. The lactation consultant is subject to disciplinary action for aiding another person in violating any IBLCE requirements or aiding another person in representing himself/herself as an IBCLC when she/he is not.
15. Report to an appropriate person or authority when it appears that the health or safety of colleagues is at risk, as such circumstances may compromise standards of practice and care.

16. Refuse any gift, favor, or hospitality from patients or clients currently in her/his care that might be interpreted as seeking to exert influence to obtain preferential consideration.

17. Disclose any financial or other conflicts of interest in relevant organizations providing goods or services. Ensure that professional judgment is not influenced by any commercial considerations.

18. Present substantiated information and interpret controversial information without personal bias, recognizing that legitimate differences of opinion exist.

19. Withdraw voluntarily from professional practice if the lactation consultant has engaged in any substance abuse that could affect her/his practice, has been adjudged by a court to be mentally incompetent, or has an emotional or mental disability that affects her/his practice in a manner that could harm the client.

20. Obtain maternal consent to photograph, audiotape, or videotape a mother and/or her infant(s) for educational or professional purposes.

21. Submit to disciplinary action under the following circumstance: If convicted of a crime under the laws of the practitioner's country that is a felony or a misdemeanor, an essential element of which is dishonesty, and that is related to the practice of lactation consulting; if disciplined by a state, province, or other local government and at least one of the grounds for the discipline is the same or substantially equivalent to these principles; if committed an act of misfeasance or malfeasance that is directly related to the practice of the profession as determined by a court of competent jurisdiction, a licensing board, or an agency of a governmental body; or if violated a Principle set forth in the Code of Ethics for International Board Certified Lactation Consultants that was in force at the time of the violation.

22. Accept the obligation to protect society and the profession by upholding the Code of Ethics for International Board Certified Lactation Consultants and by reporting alleged violations of the Code through the defined review process of the IBLCE.

23. Require and obtain consent to share clinical concerns and information with the physician or other primary healthcare provider before initiating a consultation.

24. IBCLCs must adhere to those provisions of the International Code of Marketing of Breastmilk Substitutes and subsequent resolutions that pertain to health workers.

25. Understand, recognize, respect, and acknowledge intellectual property rights, including but not limited to copyrights (which apply to written material, photographs, slides, illustrations, etc.), trademarks, service marks, and patents.

Source: Printed with permission of the International Board of Lactation Consultant Examiners.

Scope of Practice for International Board Certified Lactation Consultants (IBCLCs)

International Board Certified Lactation Consultants (IBCLCs) have demonstrated specialized knowledge and clinical expertise in breastfeeding and human lactation and are certified by the International Board of Lactation Consultant Examiners (IBLCE).

This Scope of Practice encompasses the activities for which IBCLCs are educated and in which they are authorized to engage. The aim of this Scope of Practice is to protect the public by ensuring that all IBCLCs provide safe, competent and evidence-based care. As this is an international credential, this Scope of Practice is applicable in any country or setting where IBCLCs practice.

IBCLCs have the duty to uphold the standards of the IBCLC profession by

- Working within the framework defined by the IBLCE Code of Ethics, the Clinical Competencies for IBCLC Practice, and the International Lactation Consultant Association (ILCA) Standards of Practice for IBCLCs
- Integrating knowledge and evidence when providing care for breastfeeding families from the disciplines defined in the IBLCE Exam Blueprint
- Working within the legal framework of the respective geopolitical regions or settings
- Maintaining knowledge and skills through regular continuing education Scope of Practice for IBCLCs

IBCLCs have the duty to protect, promote, and support breastfeeding by

- Educating women, families, health professionals, and the community about breastfeeding and human lactation
- Facilitating the development of policies that protect, promote, and support breastfeeding

- Acting as an advocate for breastfeeding as the child-feeding norm
- Providing holistic, evidence-based breastfeeding support and care, from preconception to weaning, for women and their families
- Using principles of adult education when teaching clients, healthcare providers, and others in the community
- Complying with the International Code of Marketing of Breastmilk Substitutes and subsequent relevant World Health Assembly resolutions

IBCLCs have the duty to provide competent services for mothers and families by

- Performing comprehensive maternal, child, and feeding assessments related to lactation
- Developing and implementing an individualized feeding plan in consultation with the mother
- Providing evidence-based information regarding a mother's use, during lactation, of medications (over-the-counter and prescription), alcohol, tobacco and street drugs, and their potential impact on milk production and child safety
- Providing evidence-based information regarding complementary therapies during lactation and their impact on a mother's milk production and the effect on her child
- Integrating cultural, psychosocial, and nutritional aspects of breastfeeding
- Providing support and encouragement to enable mothers to successfully meet their breastfeeding goals
- Using effective counseling skills when interacting with clients and other healthcare providers

- Using the principles of family-centered care while maintaining a collaborative, supportive relationship with clients

IBCLCs have the duty to report truthfully and fully to the mother and/or infant's primary healthcare provider and to the healthcare system by

- Recording all relevant information concerning care provided and, where appropriate, retaining records for the time specified by the local jurisdiction

IBCLCs have the duty to preserve client confidence by

- Respecting the privacy, dignity, and confidentiality of mothers and families

IBCLCs have the duty to act with reasonable diligence by

- Assisting families with decisions regarding the feeding of children by providing information that is evidence-based and free of conflict of interest

- Providing follow-up services as required
- Making necessary referrals to other healthcare providers and community support resources when necessary
- Functioning and contributing as a member of the healthcare team to deliver coordinated services to women and families
- Working collaboratively and interdependently with other members of the healthcare team
- Reporting to IBLCE if they have been found guilty of any offense under the criminal code of their country or jurisdiction in which they work or is sanctioned by another profession
- Reporting to IBLCE any other IBCLC who is functioning outside this Scope of Practice

Adopted March 8, 2008.

Source: Printed with permission of the International Board of Lactation Consultant Examiners.

C

Standards of Practice for International Board Certified Lactation Consultants

∾ Preface

This is the third edition of *Standards of Practice for International Board Certified Lactation Consultants* (IBCLCs) published by the International Lactation Consultant Association (ILCA). All individuals practicing as a currently certified IBCLC should adhere to ILCA's *Standards of Practice* and the International Board of Lactation Consultant Examiners (IBLCE) *Code of Ethics for International Board Certified Lactation Consultants* in all interactions with clients, families, and other healthcare professionals. ILCA recognizes the certification conferred by the IBLCE as the worldwide professional credential for lactation consultants.

Quality practice and service are the core responsibilities of a profession to the public. Standards of practice are stated measures or levels of quality that are models for the conduct and evaluation of practice. Standards of practice

- Promote consistency by encouraging a common systematic approach
- Are sufficiently specific in content to guide daily practice
- Provide a recommended framework for the development of policies and protocols, educational programs, and quality improvement efforts
- Are intended for use in diverse practice settings and cultural contexts

∾ Standard 1. Professional Responsibilities

The IBCLC has a responsibility to maintain professional conduct and to practice in an ethical manner, accountable for professional actions and legal responsibilities.

1.1 Adhere to these ILCA *Standards of Practice* and the IBLCE *Code of Ethics*

1.2 Practice within the scope of the *International Code of Marketing of Breastmilk Substitutes* and all subsequent World Health Association resolutions

1.3 Maintain an awareness of conflict of interest in all aspects of work, especially when profiting from the rental or sale of breastfeeding equipment and services

1.4 Act as an advocate for breastfeeding women, infants, and children

1.5 Assist the mother in maintaining a breastfeeding relationship with her child

1.6 Maintain and expand knowledge and skills for lactation consultant practice by participating in continuing education

1.7 Undertake periodic and systematic evaluation of one's clinical practice

1.8 Support and promote well-designed research in human lactation and breastfeeding, and base clinical practice, whenever possible, on such research

∾ Standard 2. Legal Considerations

The IBCLC is obligated to practice within the laws of the geopolitical region and setting in which she/he works. The IBCLC must practice with consideration for rights of privacy and with respect for matters of a confidential nature.

2.1 Work within the policies and procedures of the institution where employed or, if self-employed, have identifiable policies and procedures to follow

2.2 Clearly state applicable fees before providing care

2.3 Obtain informed consent from all clients before

- Assessing or intervening
- Reporting relevant information to other health care professional(s)
- Taking photographs for any purpose
- Seeking publication of information associated with the consultation

2.4 Protect client confidentiality at all times

2.5 Maintain records according to legal and ethical practices within the work setting

⌁ Standard 3. Clinical Practice

The clinical practice of the IBCLC focuses on providing clinical lactation care and management. This is best accomplished by promoting optimal health, through collaboration and problem solving with the client and other members of the healthcare team. The role of the IBCLC includes

- Assessment, planning, intervention, and evaluation of care in a variety of situations
- Anticipatory guidance and prevention of problems
- Complete, accurate, and timely documentation of care
- Communication and collaboration with other health care professionals

3.1 Assessment

3.1.1 Obtain and document an appropriate history of the breastfeeding mother and child

3.1.2 Systematically collect objective and subjective information

3.1.3 Discuss with the mother and document as appropriate all assessment information

3.2 Plan

3.2.1 Analyze assessment information to identify issues and/or problems

3.2.2 Develop a plan of care based on identified issues

3.2.3 Arrange for follow-up evaluation where indicated

3.3 Implementation

3.3.1 Implement the plan of care in a manner appropriate to the situation and acceptable to the mother

3.3.2 Utilize translators as needed

3.3.3 Exercise principles of optimal health, safety, and universal precautions

3.3.4 Provide appropriate oral and written instructions and/or demonstration of interventions, procedures and techniques

3.3.5 Facilitate referral to other healthcare professionals, community services, and support groups as needed

3.3.6 Use equipment appropriately:
- Refrain from unnecessary or excessive use
- Ensure cleanliness and good operating condition
- Discuss the risks and benefits of recommended equipment including financial considerations
- Demonstrate the correct use and care of equipment
- Evaluate safety and effectiveness of use

3.3.7 Document and communicate to healthcare providers as appropriate:
- Assessment information
- Suggested interventions
- Instructions provided
- Evaluations of outcomes
- Modifications of the plan of care
- Follow-up strategies

3.4 Evaluation

3.4.1 Evaluate outcomes of planned interventions

3.4.2 Modify the care plan based on the evaluation of outcomes

⌁ Standard 4. Breastfeeding Education and Counseling

Breastfeeding education and counseling are integral parts of the care provided by the IBCLC.

4.1 Educate parents and families to encourage informed decision making about infant and child feeding

4.2 Use a pragmatic problem-solving approach, sensitive to the learner's culture, questions, and concerns

4.3 Provide anticipatory guidance (teaching) to
- Promote optimal breastfeeding practices
- Minimize the potential for breastfeeding problems or complications

4.4 Provide positive feedback and emotional support for continued breastfeeding, especially in difficult or complicated circumstances

4.5 Share current evidence-based information and clinical skills in collaboration with other healthcare providers

Approved by the Board of Directors, October 2005.
Source: Copyright © 2005 International Lactation Consultant Association (ILCA). Reprinted by permission.

D

Clinical Competencies for IBCLC Practice*

Much of the clinical practice of the International Board Certified Lactation Consultant (IBCLC) consists of systematic problem solving in collaboration with breastfeeding mothers and other members of the healthcare team. This checklist includes most of the clinical/practical skills that an entry level IBCLC needs to be satisfactorily proficient to provide safe and effective care for breastfeeding mothers and babies. The list is designed to encompass common breastfeeding situations and the challenges that are encountered most frequently by lactation consultants. Clinical instructors may use this checklist as an appropriate guide in providing individualized education. A list of possible sites for obtaining clinical/practical experience appears at the end of the list of competencies.

Students are encouraged to become familiar with other documents that address the role of the IBCLC. The knowledge, skills, and attitude inherent in the role of an IBCLC are summarized in a list of 16 "Competency Statements" contained in the *International Board of Lactation Consultant Examiners Candidate Information Guide*. A more detailed description of the role is provided in the *Standards of Practice for IBCLC Lactation Consultants* published by the International Lactation Consultant Association (ILCA). Optimal breastfeeding care is clearly presented in 24 management strategies with rationales and references in *Evidence-Based Guidelines for Breastfeeding Management During the First Fourteen Days*, also published by ILCA.

∼ Communication and Counseling Skills

In all interactions with mothers, families, healthcare professionals, and peers, the student will demonstrate effective communication skills to maintain collaborative and supportive relationships.

The student will:

- Identify factors that might affect communication (i.e., age, cultural/language differences, deafness, blindness, mental ability, etc.)

- Demonstrate appropriate body language (i.e., position in relation to the other person, comfortable eye contact, appropriate tone of voice for the setting, etc.)
- Demonstrate knowledge of and sensitivity to cultural differences
- Elicit information using effective counseling techniques (i.e., asking open-ended questions, summarizing the discussion, and providing emotional support)
- Make appropriate referrals to other health care professionals and community resources

The student will provide individualized breastfeeding care with an emphasis on the mother's ability to make informed decisions.

The student will:

- Assess the mother's psychological state and provide information appropriate to her situation
- Include those family members or friends the mother identifies as significant to the mother
- Obtain the mother's permission for providing care to her or her baby
- Ascertain the mother's knowledge about and goals for breastfeeding
- Use adult education principles to provide instruction to the mother that will meet her needs
- Select appropriate written information and other teaching aides

∼ History Taking and Assessment Skills

The student will be able to:

- Obtain a pertinent history
- Perform a breast evaluation related to lactation
- Develop a breastfeeding risk assessment
- Assess and evaluate the infant relative to his or her ability to breastfeed
- Assess effective milk transfer

* For updated Clinical Competencies for IBCLC Practice, please visit http://www.iblce.org/upload/downloads/ClinicalCompetencies.pdf.

Documentation and Communication Skills with Health Professionals

The student will:

- Communicate effectively with other members of the healthcare team, using written documents appropriate to the geopolitical region, facility, and culture in which the student is being trained, such as consent forms, care plans, charting forms/clinical notes, pathways/care maps, and feeding assessment forms
- Use appropriate resources for research to provide information to the healthcare team on conditions, modalities, and medications that affect breastfeeding and lactation
- Write referrals and follow-up documentation/letters to referring and/or primary healthcare providers that illustrate the student's ability to identify:
- Communicate about the mother's concerns or problems, planned interventions, evaluation of outcomes, and follow-up
- Address situations in which immediate verbal communication with the healthcare provider is necessary, such as serious illness in the infant, child, or mother
- Report instances of child abuse or neglect to specific agencies as mandated or appropriate

Skills for First Two Hours After Birth

The student will:

- Identify events that occurred during the labor and birth process that may negatively impact breastfeeding
- Identify and discourage practices that may interfere with breastfeeding
- Promote continuous skin-to-skin contact of the term newborn and mother through the first feeding
- Assist the mother and family to identify newborn feeding cues
- Help the mother and infant to find a comfortable position for latching-on/attachment during the initial feeding after birth
- Identify correct latch-on (attachment)
- Reinforce to mother and family the importance of
  - Keeping the mother and baby together
  - Feeding the baby on cue—but at least eight times in each 24-hour period

Postpartum Skills

Before discharge from care, the student will observe a feeding and effectively instruct the mother about:

- Assessment of adequate milk intake by the baby
- Normal infant sucking patterns
- How milk is produced and supply maintained, including discussion of growth/appetite spurts
- Normal newborn behavior, including why, when, and how to wake a sleepy newborn
- Avoidance of early use of a pacifier and bottle nipple
- Importance of exclusive breastmilk feeds and possible consequences of mixed feedings with cow's milk or soy milk
- Prevention and treatment of sore nipples
- Prevention and treatment of engorgement
- SIDS prevention behaviors
- Family planning methods and their relationship to breastfeeding
- Education regarding drugs (such as nicotine, alcohol, caffeine, and illicit drugs) and folk remedies (such as herbal teas)
- Plans for follow-up care for breastfeeding questions and infant's medical and mother's postpartum examinations
- Community resources for assistance with breastfeeding

Problem-Solving Skills

The student will be able to:

- Identify problems
- Assess contributing factors and etiology
- Develop an appropriate breastfeeding plan of care in concert with the mother
- Assist the mother to implement the plan
- Evaluate effectiveness of the plan

Skills for Maternal Breastfeeding Challenges

The student will be able to assist mothers with the following challenges:

- Cesarean birth

- Flat/inverted nipples
- Yeast infections of breast, nipple, areola, and milk ducts
- Continuation of breastfeeding when mother is separated from her baby
- Milk expression techniques
- Maintaining milk production
- Collection, storage, and transportation of milk
- Cultural beliefs that are not evidence-based and may interfere with breastfeeding, (i.e., discarding colostrum, rigidly scheduled feedings, necessity of formula after every breastfeeding, etc.)
- Medical conditions that impact breastfeeding
- Adolescent mother
  - Strategies for returning to school
  - Maintaining milk production
- Nipple pain and damage
- Engorgement
- Plugged duct or blocked nipple pore
- Mastitis
- Breast surgery/trauma
- Overproduction of milk
- Postpartum psychological issues, including transient sadness ("baby blues") and postpartum depression
  - Appropriate referrals
  - Medications compatible with breastfeeding
- Insufficient milk supply, differentiating between perceived and real
- Weaning issues
  - Safe formula preparation and feeding techniques
  - Care of breasts

⌇ Skills for Infant Breastfeeding Challenges

The student will be able to assist mothers who have infants with the following challenges:

- Traumatic birth
- 35–38 weeks' gestation
- Small for gestational age (SGA) or large for gestational age (LGA)
- Multiples/plural births
- Preterm birth, including the benefits of kangaroo care
- High risk for hypoglycemia
- Sleepy infant

- Excessive weight loss, slow/poor weight gain
- Hyperbilirubinemia (jaundice)
- Ankyloglossia (short frenulum)
- Yeast infection
- Colic/fussiness
- Gastric reflux
- Lactose overload
- Food intolerances
- Neurodevelopmental problems
- Teething and biting
- Nursing strike/early baby-led weaning
- Toddler nursing
- Nursing through pregnancy
- Tandem nursing

⌇ Management Skills

The student will demonstrate the ability to:

- Perform a comprehensive breastfeeding assessment
- Assess milk transfer with
  - AC/PC weights, using an electronic digital scale
  - Use of balance scale for daily weights
- Calculate an infant's caloric and volume requirements
- Increase milk production

⌇ Skills for Use of Technology and Devices

The student will have up-to-date knowledge about breastfeeding-related equipment and demonstrate appropriate use and understanding of potential disadvantages or risks of the following:

- A device to evert nipples
- Nipple creams/ointments
- Breast shells
- Breast pumps
- Alternative feeding techniques
  - Tube feeding at the breast
  - Cup feeding
  - Spoon feeding
  - Eyedropper feeding
  - Finger feeding
  - Bottles and artificial nipples
- Nipple shields

- Pacifiers
- Infant scales
- Use of herbal supplements for mother and/or infant

∾ *Skills for Breastfeeding Challenges Encountered Infrequently*

The following issues are encountered relatively infrequently and may not be seen during the student's training. The entry-level lactation consultant is not expected to be proficient in these situations. The student will need to use basic skills to assist the mother and infant while seeking guidance from a more experienced IBCLC.

Infant:

- Infant with tonic bite/ineffective/dysfunctional suck
- Cranial-facial abnormalities, such as micrognathia (receding lower jaw) and cleft lip and/or palate
- Down syndrome
- Cardiac problems
- Chronic medical conditions, such as cystic fibrosis, PKU, etc.

Mother:

- Induced lactation and relactation
- Coping with the death of an infant
- Chronic medical conditions, such as MS, lupus, seizures, etc.
- Disabilities that may limit mother's ability to handle the baby easily, such as rheumatoid arthritis, carpal tunnel syndrome, cerebral palsy, etc.
- HIV/AIDS: understanding of current recommendations based on the mother's access to safe replacement feeding

∾ *Skills for Meeting Professional Responsibilities*

The student will demonstrate the following professional responsibilities:

- Conduct herself or himself in a professional manner, by complying with the IBLCE Code of Ethics for International Board Certified Lactation Consultants and the ILCA Standards of Practice; and by adhering to the International Code of Marketing of Breastmilk Substitutes and its subsequent World Health Assembly resolutions
- Practice within the laws of the setting in which she or he works, showing respect for confidentiality and privacy
- Use current research findings to provide a strong evidence base for clinical practice, and obtain continuing education to enhance skills and obtain/maintain IBCLC certification
- Advocate for breastfeeding families, mothers, infants, and children in the workplace, community, and within the healthcare system
- Use breastfeeding equipment appropriately and provide information about risks as well as benefits of products, maintaining an awareness of conflict of interest if profiting from the rental or sale of breastfeeding equipment

∾ *Sites for Acquisition of Skills*

The student may acquire clinical/practical skills in the following settings:

- Private practice IBCLC office
- Private practice obstetric, pediatric, family practice, or midwifery office
- Public health department; Women, Infants, and Children (WIC) program (in the United States)
- Hospital
- Lactation services
- Birthing center
- Postpartum unit
- Mother-Baby unit
- Level II and level III nurseries: special care nursery, neonatal intensive care nursery
- Pediatric unit
- Home health services
- Outpatient follow-up breastfeeding clinics
- Breastfeeding hotlines and warm lines
- Prenatal and postpartum breastfeeding classes
- Home births (if legally permitted)
- Volunteer community support group meetings

Source: Printed with permission of the International Board of Lactation Consultant Examiners.

Baby Feeding Requirements

Pounds	Ounces	Required Milk	Pounds	Ounces	Required Milk	Pounds	Ounces	Required Milk
5	0	13.3	7	6	19.7	9	12	26.0
5	1	13.5	7	7	19.8	9	13	26.2
5	2	13.7	7	8	20.0	9	14	26.3
5	3	13.8	7	9	20.2	9	15	26.5
5	4	14.0	7	10	20.3			
5	5	14.2	7	11	20.5	10	0	26.7
5	6	14.3	7	12	20.7	10	1	26.8
5	7	14.5	7	13	20.8	10	2	27.0
5	8	14.7	7	14	21.0	10	3	27.2
5	9	14.8	7	15	21.2	10	4	27.3
5	10	15.0				10	5	27.5
5	11	15.2	8	0	21.3	10	6	27.7
5	12	15.3	8	1	21.5	10	7	27.8
5	13	15.5	8	2	21.7	10	8	28.0
5	14	15.7	8	3	21.8	10	9	28.2
5	15	15.8	8	4	22.0	10	10	28.3
			8	5	22.2	10	11	28.5
6	0	16.0	8	6	22.3	10	12	28.7
6	1	16.2	8	7	22.5	10	13	28.8
6	2	16.3	8	8	22.7	10	14	29.0
6	3	16.5	8	9	22.8	10	15	29.2
6	4	16.7	8	10	23.0			
6	5	16.8	8	11	23.2	11	0	29.3
6	6	17.0	8	12	23.3	11	1	29.5
6	7	17.2	8	13	23.5	11	2	29.7
6	8	17.3	8	14	23.7	11	3	29.8
6	9	17.5	8	15	23.8	11	4	30.0
6	10	17.7				11	5	30.2
6	11	17.8	9	0	24.0	11	6	30.3
6	12	18.0	9	1	24.2	11	7	30.5
6	13	18.2	9	2	24.3	11	8	30.7
6	14	18.3	9	3	24.5	11	9	30.8
6	15	18.5	9	4	24.7	11	10	31.0
			9	5	24.8	11	11	31.2
7	0	18.7	9	6	25.0	11	12	31.3
7	1	18.8	9	7	25.2	11	13	31.5
7	2	19.0	9	8	25.3	11	14	31.7
7	3	19.2	9	9	25.5	11	15	31.8
7	4	19.3	9	10	25.7			
7	5	19.5	9	11	25.8	12	0	32.0

Source: Copied with permission © 1990 Kittie Frantz. Available in laminated pocket form at www.geddesproduction.com or as an app for iPhone as Breast Milk Calculator.

F

WHO Weight Charts

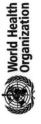

Weight-for-age GIRLS

Birth to 2 years (percentiles)

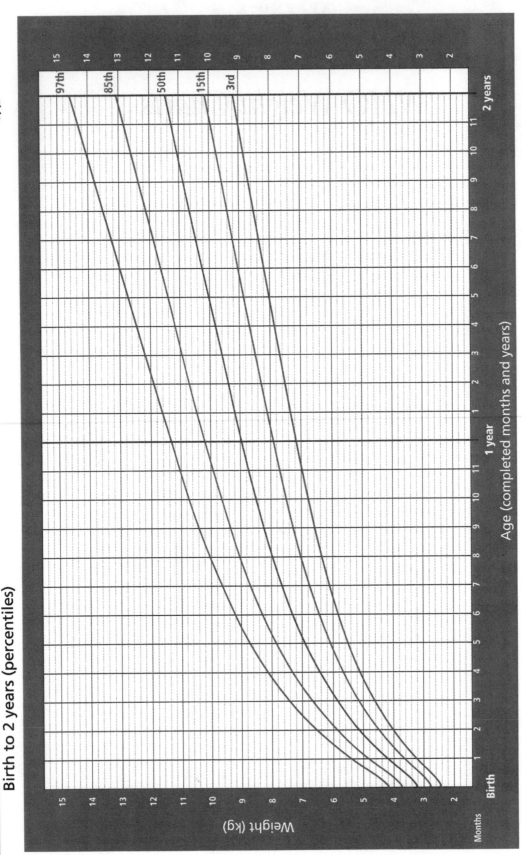

Source: WHO Child Growth Standards, Chart Catalogue, 2008 Girls Percentiles and 2008 Boys Percentiles; Weight-for-age girls, Birth to 2 years (percentiles); Weight-for-age boys, Birth to 2 years (percentiles), www.who.int. Reprinted by permission of the World Health Organization.

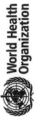

Weight-for-age BOYS
Birth to 2 years (percentiles)

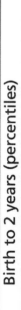

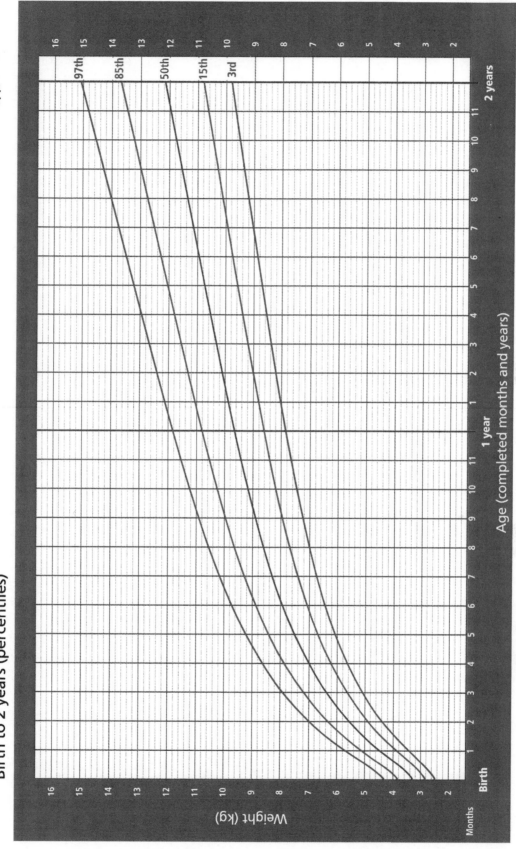

WHO Child Growth Standards

Source: *WHO Child Growth Standards, Chart Catalogue, 2008 Girls Percentiles and 2008 Boys Percentiles; Weight-for-age girls, Birth to 2 years (percentiles); Weight-for-age boys, Birth to 2 years (percentiles)*, www.who.int. Reprinted by permission of the World Health Organization.

Spanish Breastfeeding Glossary

～ General Spanish Terms

alcohol	alcohol
allergy	alergia
at least	por lo menos
aunt, uncle	tía, tío
cigarette	cigarillo
cousin	primo, prima
do not use	no usar
doctor	doctor
each day	cada día
enough	suficiente
family	familia
father	padre
good afternoon	buenas tardes
good evening	buenas noches
good morning	buenos días
grandmother	abuela
grandfather	abuelo
healthy	saludable
help you	ayudarla
hospital	hospital
how long	cuánto tiempo
how many	cuántos
how many times	cuántas veces
how much	cuánto
how often	cada cuando
husband	esposo
it's important	es importante
it's necessary	es necesario
medication	medicina
mother	mama, madre
mother-in-law	suegra
nurse (person)	enfermera
nutritionist	nutricionista
parents	padres
please	por favor
problem	problema
sister, brother	hermana, hermano
sister-in-law	cuñada
thank you	gracias
the more	cuanto más
upset	alterado
usually	usualmente
you're welcome	de nada

～ Terms Related to the Baby

baby	bebé
baby (your)	su bebé
baby blues	tristeza posparto
bonding	el apego, la bondad
bottle	biberón
bottle-fed	alimentado con biberón
burp your baby	eructe su bebé
cleft lip	labio leporino
cleft palate	paladar hendido
crying	llanto
cuddle	acurrucar abrazar
diaper rash	irritación de la piel causada por el pañal
dirty diaper	pañal(es) sucio(s) (con evacuación)
failure to thrive	retraso en el crecimiento
feeding	toma, alimentación, mamada
food allergy	alergia a las comidas
formula	fórmula
frenulum	frenillo
gain weight	aumento de peso; (ganar) peso
infant	infante
jaundice	ictericia
newborn	recién nacido
pacifier	chupete, chupón
premature	prematuro
return to work	regresar al trabajo
sleep	dormir
sling	cargador tipo hamaca
spit up	regugita
stool	evacuación
toddler	bebé mayorcito
twins	gémelos
weigh your baby	pesar el bebé
weight gain	aumento de peso
wet diapers	pañales mojados

～ Terms Related to Breastfeeding

areola	areola
breast	el pecho; el seno
breastfeeding	amamantar, dar el pecho
breastmilk	leche materna
colostrum (first milk)	calostro (la primera leche)
cue feeding	seguir la señal del bebé
dropper	gotero
flat nipples	pezones planos
good latch-on	bien prendido; buen agarre
hold (to)	tomar en brazos
hormones	hormonas
inverted nipples	pezones invertidos
lactation consultant	consultora en lactancia
latch on (to)	agarrar
leaking	se sale la leche
letdown	reflejo de eyección de la leche
lump in breast	masa en el pecho
meconium	meconio, popó negro y espeso
milk expression	extracción de la leche
night feedings	tomas nocturnas
nipple	pezón
nurse (to)	amamantar; mamar
nursing	mamada
plugged duct	conducto obstruido
pump breasts	succionar los pechos
relactation	relactancia
rooting	señales de búsqueda
sore nipples	pezones adoloridos
spoon, teaspoon	cuchara; cucharadita
sucking bursts	ráfagas de succión
suckle (to)	dar el pecho; amamantar mamar
suckling	niño lactante, que toma pecho
swallow (to)	tragar
swallow(s)	trago(s)
thrush	cándida; infección de hongo
wean	destetar
weaned	destetado
weaning	destete

～ Helpful Phrases

4 or more	cuatro o mas
5 to 6	cinco a seis
8 to 12 times	ocho a doce veces
attachment to the breast	prenderse al pecho
breast engorgement	congestión mamaria pechos hinchados
breast infection	infección mamaria; infección del pecho
breast massage	masaje del pecho
breast pads	protectores absorbentes para el pecho; pañalitos para el pecho

breast pump	sacaleches
breast shells	conchas plásticas; duras para pezones
close contact	contacto cercano
cluster feeding	período de mamadas frecuentes
cradle position	acunar, posición para tomar al niño en brazos
cross cradle position	utilizar la mano para sostener al bebé y acomodarlo al pecho opuesto
exclusive breastfeeding	dar el pecho exclusivamente
feed your baby	déle pecho a su bebé
football hold	posición lateral debajo del brazo (sandía)
growth spurts	períodos de crecimiento acelerado
hand expression	sacar la leche usando presión manual
nipple shield	protectores flexibles para el pezón; pezonera
repositioning baby	reposicionar mejor el bebe al pecho
skin to skin	tener el bebé con sólo el pañal en contra de su piel; de piel a piel
supplemental feeding	alimentación suplementaria

～ Questions and Instructions

How may I help you?	¿Cómo puedo ayudarla?
In a day, how many times do you breastfeed?	¿En un día, cuántas veces le da pecho a su bebé?
Describe a normal 24 hour day.	Descríbame un día de 24 horas.
How often does your baby nurse?	¿Cuán a menudo toma el pecho su bebé?
Can you hear your baby swallowing?	¿Puede oír los tragos de su bebé?
Does your breast feel softer after feeding?	¿Se ablanda el pecho después de una mamada?
How many wet diapers each day?	¿Cuántos pañales mojados cada día?
How many soiled diapers each day?	¿Cuántos pañales con evacuación cada día?
What color are the soiled diapers?	¿De qué color son las evacuaciones?
How much does your baby weigh?	¿Cuánto pesa su bebé ahora?
How much did your baby weigh at birth?	¿Cuánto pesó su bebé cuando nació?
Breastfeed at least 8 times each day.	Déle pecho por lo menos ocho (8) veces al día.

Do you feel pain when you breastfeed?	¿Siente dolor cuando da pecho?	If necessary, feed your baby by spoon or dropper.	Si es necesario, alimente a su bebé por cuchara o gotero.
Where?	¿Dónde?	If you think you need to give your baby formula call a lactation consultant first.	Si piensa que necesita darle fórmula a su bebé primero llameuna consejera de lactancia.
When?	¿Cuándo?		
At the beginning or during the whole feed?	¿Al comienzo o durante toda la toma?		

Source: International Lactation Consultant Association. Printed with permission.

Professional Resources

∾ Lactation Consultant Organizations

International Lactation Consultant Association (ILCA): The International Lactation Consultant Association (ILCA) is the professional association representing the IBCLC (International Board Certified Lactation Consultant) worldwide. ILCA's mission is to advance the profession through leadership, advocacy, professional development, and research. ILCA sponsors international and regional conferences to provide education and networking for members and others interested in the lactation field. ILCA also publishes the *Journal of Human Lactation*, policy and practice statements, and independent study modules. A wide variety of resource materials and professional networking is available through the association website.

ILCA; 2501 Aerial Center Pkwy, Suite 103; Morrisville, NC 27560 USA; Phone: 919-861-5577, 888-ILCA-IS-U (in U.S.); Fax: 919-459-2075; E-mail: ilca@ilca.org; www.ilca.org

International Board of Lactation Consultant Examiners (IBLCE): The International Board of Lactation Consultant Examiners develops and administers the international certification examination for lactation consultants. The IBLCE examination is the premier, internationally recognized measure of competence in lactation consulting. Founded in 1985, the IBLCE has certified more than 18,000 IBCLCs in multiple languages and at numerous sites around the world. IBLCE is accredited by the U.S. National Commission for Health Certifying Agencies.

IBLCE in The Americas and Israel; 6402 Arlington Boulevard, Suite 350; Falls Church, VA 22042 USA; Phone: 703-560-7330; Fax: 703-560-7332; E-mail: iblce@iblce.org; www.iblce.org.

IBLCE Australia: Asia Pacific, Southern Africa, Ireland, and Great Britain; P.O. Box 1533; Oxenford QLD 4210, Australia; Phone: 161 7 5529 8811; Fax: 161 7 5529 8922; E-mail: RD@iblce.edu.au; www.iblce .edu.au.

IBLCE Europe: Europe, Middle East, and North Africa; Steinfeldgasse 11; 2511 Pfaffstaetten, Austria; Phone: 143 2252 206595 ; Fax: 143 2252 206487; E-mail: office@iblce-europe.org; www.iblce-europe.org.

Accreditation and Approval Review Committee (AARC) on Education in Human Lactation and Breastfeeding: The Accreditation and Approval Review Committee on Education in Human Lactation and Breastfeeding is jointly sponsored by ILCA and IBLCE. AARC reviews and evaluates courses to determine the degree to which they meet Standards and Guidelines for educational programs. AARC then makes a recommendation to the Commission on Accreditation of Allied Health Education Programs (CAAHEP), which is a voluntary, specialized accreditation agency representing a broad range of health care disciplines.

AARC; 2501 Aerial Center Pkwy, Suite 103; Morrisville, NC 27560 USA; Phone: 919-861-5577; Fax: 919-459-2075; E-mail: info@aarclactation.org; www. aarclactation.org

∾ Medical and Lactation-Related Organizations

Academy of Breastfeeding Medicine; 140 Huguenot Street, 3rd floor, New Rochelle, NY 10801, USA; Phone: 914-740-2115, 800-990-4ABM (U.S.); Fax: 609-799-7032; E-mail: ABM@bfmed.org; www .bfmed.org.

American Academy of Family Physicians (AAFP); P.O. Box 11210, Shawnee Mission, KS 66207-1210, USA; Phone: 800-274-2237; 913-906-6000; E-mail: fp@aafp .org; www.aafp.org.

American Academy of Pediatrics (AAP); 141 Northwest Point Boulevard, Elk Grove Village, IL 60007-1098, USA; Phone: 800-433-9016; 847-434-4000; Fax: 847-434-8000; E-mail: kidsdocs@aap.org; www.aap.org.

American College of Nurse-Midwives (ACNM); 8403 Colesville Road, Suite 1550, Silver Spring, MD 20910-6374, USA; Phone: 240-485-1800; Fax: 240-485-1818; www.acnm.org.

American College of Obstetricians and Gynecologists (ACOG); 409 12th Street, P.O. Box 96920, Washington, DC 20090-6920, USA; Phone: 202-638-5577; Fax: 202-484-5107; E-mail: resources@acog.org; www.acog.org.

American Dietetic Association (ADA); 120 South Riverside Plaza, Suite 2000, Chicago, IL 60606-6995, USA; Phone: 312-899-0040, 800-877-1600 (in U.S.); Fax: 312-899-1979; E-mail: cdr@eatright.org; www.eatright.org.

American Heart Association; 7272 Greenville Avenue, Dallas, TX 75231-4596, USA; Phone: 214-373-6300, 800-242-8721 (in U.S.); TTY: 800-654-5984; Fax: 214-706-2221; www.americanheart.org.

American Medical Association (AMA); 515 North State Street, Chicago, IL 60610, USA; Phone: 312-464-5262, 800-621-8335 (in U.S.); Fax: 312-464-4184; www.ama-assn.org.

American Public Health Association (APHA); Clearinghouse on Infant Feeding and Maternal Nutrition; 800 I Street, NW, Washington, DC 20001, USA; Phone: 202-777-2742; Fax: 202-777-2534; E-mail: comments@apha.org; www.apha.org.

AnotherLook; P.O. Box 383, Evanston, IL 60204, USA; Phone: 847-869-1278; E-mail: MT@anotherlook.org; www.anotherlook.org.

Association of Women's Health, Obstetric and Neonatal Nurses (AWHONN); 2000 L Street, NW, Suite 740, Washington, DC 20036, USA; Phone: 202-261-2400, 800-673-8499 (in U.S.), 800-245-0231 (in Canada); Fax: 202-728-0575; E-mail: customerservice@awhonn.org; www.awhonn.org.

Australian Breastfeeding Association; P.O. Box 4000, Glen Iris, Victoria 3146, Australia; Phone: +61 3 98850855; Fax: +61 3 98850866; E-mail: info@breastfeeding.asn.au; www.breastfeeding.asn.au.

Baby Friendly USA; 327 Quaker Meeting House Road, East Sandwich, MA 02537, USA; Phone: 508-888-8092; Fax: 508-888-8050; E-mail: info@babyfriendlyusa.org; www.babyfriendlyusa.org.

Centers for Disease Control and Prevention; Breastfeeding Web page; www.cdc.gov/breastfeeding.

Coalition for Improving Maternity Services; 1500 Sunday Drive, Suite 102, Raleigh, NC 27607, USA; Phone: 919-863-9482; Fax: 919-787-4916; E-mail: info@motherfriendly.org; www.motherfriendly.org.

Department of Health and Human Services; Office on Women's Health; 200 Independence Avenue, SW, Room 730B, Washington, DC 20201, USA; Phone: 202-690-7650, 800-994-9662 (U.S.); Fax: 202-205-2631; www.4woman.gov/owh.

Doulas of North America; P.O. Box 626, Jasper, IN 47547, USA; Phone: 888-788-DONA; Fax: 812-634-1491; E-mail: Doula@DONA.org; www.DONA.org.

Human Milk Banking Association of North America, Inc. (HMBANA); 1500 Sunday Drive, Suite 102, Raleigh, NC 27607, USA; Phone: 919-861-4530; E-mail: info@hmbana.org; www.hmbana.org.

Infant Feeding Action Coalition; INFACT Canada; 6 Trinity Square, Toronto, Ontario M5G 1B1, Canada; Phone: 416-595-9819; Fax: 416-591-9355; E-mail: info@infactcanada.ca; www.infactcanada.ca.

Institute for Reproductive Health; Georgetown University Medical Center; 4301 Connecticut Avenue, NW, Suite 310, Washington, DC 20008, USA; Phone: 202-687-1392; Fax: 202-537-7450; E-mail: irhinfo@georgetown.edu; www.irh.org.

International Baby Food Action Network (IBFAN); P.O. Box 19, 10700 Penang, Malaysia; Phone +60-4-8905799; Fax: +60-4-8907291; E-mail: ibfanpg@tm.net.my; www.ibfan.org.

International Childbirth Education Association (ICEA); 1500 Sunday Drive, Suite 102, Raleigh, NC 27607, USA; Phone: 919-863-9487, 800-624-4934; Fax: 919-787-4916; E-mail: info@icea.org; www.icea.org.

International Labour Office; 4, Route des Morillons, CH-1211 Geneva 22, Switzerland; Phone: +41-22-799-6111; Fax: +41-22-798-8685; E-mail: ilo@ilo.org; www.ilo.org.

International Society for Research in Human Milk and Lactation; Meriter Hospital Perinatal Center; 202 S. Park Street, Madison, WI 53715, USA; Phone: 608-262-6561; Fax: 608-267-6377; E-mail: frgreer@facstaff.wisc.edu; www.isrhml.org.

La Leche League International, Inc.; P.O. Box 4079, 1400 N. Meacham Road, Schaumburg, IL 60173-4048, USA; Phone: 800-525-3243, 847-519-7730, 800-525-3243; Fax: 847-519-0035; E-mail: lllhq@llli.org; www.lalecheleague.org.

March of Dimes; 1275 Mamaroneck Avenue, White Plains, NY 10605, USA; Phone: 914-997-4488; www.marchofdimes.com.

National Alliance for Breastfeeding Advocacy (NABA); 254 Conant Road, Weston, MA 02493-1756, USA; Phone: 781-893-3553; Fax: 781-893-8608; E-mail: Marsha@naba-breastfeeding.org; www.naba-breastfeeding.org.

National Association of Neonatal Nurses; 4700 W. Lake Avenue, Glenview, IL 60025-1485, USA; Phone: 847-375-3660, 800-451-3795; Fax: 888-477-6266, International Fax: 732-380-3640; E-mail: info@nann.org; www.nann.org.

National Association of WIC Directors (NAWD); 2001 S. Street, NW, Suite 580, Washington, DC 20009, USA;

Phone: 202-232-5492; Fax: 202-387-5281; E-mail: info@nwica.org; www.nwica.org.

National Healthy Mothers, Healthy Babies; 2000 N. Beauregard Street, 6th floor, Alexandria, VA 22311, USA; Phone: 703-837-4792; Fax: 703-684-5968; info@hmhb.org; www.hmhb.org.

National Perinatal Association; 2000 North Beauregard Street, 6th floor, Alexandria, VA 22311, USA; Phone: 888-971-3295; Fax: 703-684-5968; E-mail: npa@nationalperinatal.org; www.nationalperinatal.org.

Sudden Infant Death Syndrome (SIDS); Mother-Baby Behavioral Sleep Laboratory, University of Notre Dame; Department of Anthropology, Notre Dame, IN 46556, USA; E-mail: James.J.Mckenna.25@nd.edu; www.nd.edu/~jmckenn1/lab.

Support for the Breastfeeding Employee, National Maternal and Child Health Clearinghouse, Health Resources and Services Administration; Parklawn Building, 5600 Fishers Lane, Rockville, MD 20857, USA; Phone: 888-275-4772; www.hrsa.gov.

The Joint Commission; One Renaissance Blvd., Oakbrook Terriace, IL 60181, USA; Phone: 630-792-5889; Fax: 630-792-5599; E-mail: customerservice@jointcommission.org; www.jcaho.org.

UNICEF; 3 United Nations Plaza, New York, NY 10017, USA; Phone: 212-888-7465; Fax: 212-303-7911; E-mail: information@unicef.org; www.unicef.org/programme/breastfeeding.

UNICEF Canada; Canada Square, 2200 Yonge Street, Suite 1100, Toronto, Ontario M4S 2C6, Canada; Phone: 416-482-4444, 800-567-4483; Fax: 416-482-8035; E-mail: secretary@unicef.ca; www.unicef.ca.

United States Breastfeeding Committee (USBC); 2025 M Street, NW, Suite 800, Washington, DC 20036-3309, USA; Phone: 202-367-1132; Fax: 202-367-2132; E-mail: info@usbreastfeeding.org; www.usbreastfeeding.org.

U.S. Committee for UNICEF; 125 Maiden Lane, New York, NY 10038, USA; Phone: 800-486-4233; E-mail: information@unicefusa.org; www.unicefusa.org.

Wellstart, International; P.O. Box 602, Blue Jay, CA 92317, USA; E-mail: info@wellstart.org; www.wellstart.org.

WIC Supplemental Food Programs Division, Food and Nutrition Service, U.S. Department of Agriculture; 3101 Park Center Drive, Alexandria, VA 22302, USA; Phone: 703-305-2746; Fax: 703-305-2196; E-mail; wichq-web@fns.usda.gov; www.fns.usda.gov/wic.

World Alliance for Breastfeeding Action (WABA); P.O. Box 1200, 10850, Penang, Malaysia; Phone: 604-6584-816; Fax: 604-6572-655; E-mail: waba@waba.org.my; www.waba.org.my.

World Health Organization (WHO); Avenue Appia 20, 1211 Geneva 27, Switzerland; Phone: 22-791-2111; Fax: 22-791-3111; E-mail: info@who.int; www.who.int.

～ Domestic Violence and Abuse Organizations

Adult Survivors of Child Abuse; P.O. Box 14477, San Francisco, CA 94114-0038, USA; Phone: 415-928-4576; E-mail: info@ascasupport.org; www.ascasupport.org.

National Domestic Violence Hotline; Phone: 800-799-SAFE (7233), TTY for the deaf: 1-800-787-3224; E-mail: ndvh@ndvh.org; www.ndvh.org.

Parents Anonymous, Inc.; 675 W. Foothill Blvd., Suite 220, Claremont, CA 91711-3416, USA; Phone: 909-621-6184; Fax: 909-625-6304; E-mail: Parentsanonymous@parentsanonymous.org; www.parentsanonymous.org.

～ Cleft Lip and Cleft Palate Organizations

American Academy of Otolaryngology-Head and Neck Surgery (AAO-HNS); One Prince Street, Alexandria, VA 22314, USA; Phone: 703-836-4444, TTY: 703-519-1585; Fax: 703-683-5100; E-mail: webmaster@entnet.org; www.entnet.org.

American Cleft Palate-Craniofacial Association (ACPA); 104 S. Estes Drive, Suite 204, Chapel Hill, NC 27514, USA; Phone: 919-933-9044. 800-24-CLEFT; Fax: 919-933-9604; E-mail: cleftline@aol.com; www.cleftline.org.

American Society of Human Genetics; 9650 Rockville Pike, Bethesda, MD 20814-3889, USA; Phone: 301-571-1825; Fax: 301-530-7079; www.faseb.org/genetics.

American Speech-Language-Hearing Association (ASHA); 10801 Rockville Pike, Rockville, MD 20852, USA; Phone: 301-897-5700, 800-638-8255, TTY: 301-897-0157; Fax: 301-571-0457; E-mail: actioncenter@asha.org; www.asha.org.

Children's Craniofacial Association (CCA); P.O. Box 280297, Dallas, TX 75228, USA; Phone: 972-994-9902, 800-535-3643; Fax: 972-240-7607; www.ccakids.com.

FACES—National Craniofacial Association; P.O. Box 11082, Chattanooga, TN 37401, USA; Phone: 423-266-1632, 800-3FACES3; Fax: 423-267-3124; E-mail: faces@mindspring.com; www.faces-cranio.org.

National Foundation for Facial Reconstruction; 317 East 34th St. #901, New York, NY 10016, USA; Phone: 212-263-6656; Fax: 212-263-7534; E-mail: nffr@earthlink.net; www.nffr.org.

National Institute of Child Health and Human Development; Building 31, Room 2A32, 31 Center Drive MSC

2425, Bethesda, MD 20892-2425, USA; Phone: 301-496-5133, 800-370-2943; Fax: 301-496-7102; E-mail: NICHDClearinghouse@ mail.nih.gov; www.nichd.nih.gov.

National Institute of Dental and Craniofacial Research; Building 45, Room 4AS-19, 45 Center Drive MSC 6401, Bethesda, MD 20892-6401, USA; Phone: 301-496-4261; Fax: 301-496-9988; E-mail: nidrinfo@ od31.nidr. nih.gov; www.nidcr.nih.gov.

National Organization for Rare Disorders (NORD); P.O. Box 8923, New Fairfield, CT 06812, USA; Phone: 203-746-6518, 800-999-NORD, TTY: 203-746-6927; Fax: 203-746-6481; E-mail: orphan@rarediseases.org; www.rarediseases.org.

Velo-Cardio-Facial Syndrome Educational Foundation, Inc.; P.O. Box 874, Milltown, NJ 08850, USA; Phone: 866-VCFSEFS, 800-823-7335; Fax: 732-238-8803; E-mail: info@vcfsef.org; www.vcfsef.org.

∼ Journals and Newsletters

Acta Paediatrica, Editorial Office, Building Z6:04, Karolinska Hospital, SE-171 76, Stockholm, Sweden. www.wiley.com/bw/journal.asp?ref=0803-5253&site=1.

American Journal of Obstetrics and Gynecology, C.V. Mosby Co., 11830 Westline Industrial Dr., St. Louis, MO 63141, USA. www. ajog.org.

Birth: Issues in Perinatal Care and Education, Blackwell Publishing Ltd. www.ovid.com/site.

Breastfeeding Abstracts, La Leche League International, P.O. Box 4079, Schaumburg, IL 60173-4048, USA. www.lli.org.

Breastfeeding Medicine. Journal of the Academy of Breastfeeding Medicine. www.liebertpub.com/products/product.aspx?pid=173.

Breastfeeding News. Primary Health Care Research & Information Service. www.phcris.org.au.

Breastfeeding Review, Australian Breastfeeding Association. www.breastfeeding.asn.au.

British Medical Journal, BMJ Publishing Group, PO Box 299, London WC1H 9TD, United Kingdom. www.bmj.com.

International Breastfeeding Journal. www.internationalbreastfeedingjournal.com.

Journal of Human Lactation, International Lactation Consultant Association. Sage Publications, 2455 Teller Road, Thousand Oaks, CA 91320, USA. 800-818-7243. www.sagepub.com.

Journal of Obstetric, Gynecologic, and Neonatal Nursing, Suite 200, 600 Maryland Ave., SW, Washington, DC 20024, USA. http://jognn.awhonn.org.

Journal of Pediatrics, C.V. Mosby,II 830 Westline Industrial Dr., St. Louis, MO 63141, USA. www.us.elsevierhealth.com.

Journal of the American Dietetic Association, 430 N. Michigan Ave., Chicago, IL 60611, USA. www.eatright.org.

Journal of the American Medical Association, 535 N. Dearborn St., Chicago, IL 60610, USA. www.jama.ama-assn.org.

New England Journal of Medicine, 10 Shattuck St., Boston, MA 02115, USA. www.nejm.org.

Obstetrical and Gynecological Survey, Williams and Wilkins, 428 East Preston St., Baltimore, MD 21202, USA. www.obgynsurvey.com.

Pediatrics, P.O. Box 1034, Evanston, IL 60204, USA. www.pediatrics.com.

Science, American Association for the Advancement of Science, 1515 Massachusetts Ave., NW, Washington, DC 20005, USA. www.scienceonline.org.

The Harvard Medical School Health Letter, Department of Continuing Education of Harvard Medical School, 79 Garden St., Cambridge, MA 02138, USA. www.health.harvard.edu.

The Lancet, North American Editor: Little, Brown and Co., 34 Beacon St., Boston, MA 02106, USA. www.thelancet.com.

∼ Online Resources

www.aap.org. Health Professionals Resource Guide with links to websites and publications.

www.breastfeeding.com. Video clips on benefits, working, premies, pumpng hunger cues, latching, and cup feeding.

www.breastfeedinonline.com.

www.ezzo.info. Website detailing concerns about baby training books and programs.

www.healthyarkansas.com/breastfeeding/training.html. Video clip of Anita Baker, "Giving you the best that I've got, baby."

www.healthypeople.gov. Healthy People U. S. national health objectives.

www.ilca.org. PowerPoint presentations, links to many professional resources.

www.pumpstation.com/frmvideos-1.cfm. Video clips on feeding cues, latch, and finishing the feeding.

www.seaburychicago.com. Professional liability insurance, Marsh Affinity Group Services.

www.womenshealth.gov. U.S. Dept. Health & Human Services, Office on Women's Health.

∽ Online Networking

www.ilca.org. Discussion forum.

Listserv@library.ummed.edu. Lactnet e-mail listserv.

http://neonatal.ttuhsc.edu/lact. Breastfeeding and medications forum.

∽ CD-ROMs

Breastfeeding and Human Lactation, Riordan and Wambach; CD-ROM of breastfeeding images with 4th ed, 2010. www.ibreastfeeding.com.

Breastfeeding Answers Made Simple. Amarillo, TX: Hale Publishing; 2010.

HIPAA and the IBCLC. Elizabeth Brooks; CD-ROM of privacy documents for LCs; E-mail: ecbrks@yahoo.com.

The Breastfeeding Atlas, 4th ed. Hoover and Wilson Clay; 2008. CD-ROM of breastfeeding images from 3rd edition and video clips available at: www.lactnews.com.

∽ Books, Media, and Other Products

Resources are available from many of the organizations listed in this appendix. In addition, the following businesses offer a variety of resources. There may be other product sources available. A search on the Internet will help you find everything that is available.

Cascade Health Care; 1826 NW 18th Avenue, Portland, OR 97209, USA; Phone: 503-595-1720; Fax: 503-595-1726; E-mail: info@1cascade.com; www.1cascade.com.

Childbirth Graphics, Division of WRS Group, Inc.; P.O. Box 21207, Waco, TX 76702-1207, USA; Phone: 800-299-3366, ext. 287; Fax: 888-977-7653; E-mail: sales@wrsgroup.com; www.wrsgroup.com.

Hale Publishing; 1712 N. Forest St., Amarillo, TX 79106, USA; Phone: 806-376-9900; Phone: 800-378-1317; Fax: 806-376-9901; E-Mail: books@hale-publishing.com; www.ibreastfeeding.com.

Injoy Birth Videos, Inc.; 1435 Yarmouth Ave. Suite 102, Boulder, CO 80304, USA; Phone: 303-447-2082; E-mail: custserv@injoyvideos.com; www.injoyvideos.com.

Noodle Soup; 4614 Prospect Ave #328, Cleveland, OH 44103, USA; Phone: 800-795-9295; www.noodlesoup.com.

Index

RJ
216
.L35
20

DATE DUE

GAYLORD   PRINTED IN U.S.A.

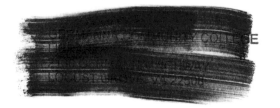